Surgical Techniques of the Shoulder, Elbow, and Knee in Sports Medicine

SECOND EDITION

Surgical Techniques of the Shoulder, Elbow, and Knee in Sports Medicine

Edited by

Brian J. Cole, MD, MBA

Professor, Department of Orthopaedics
Department of Anatomy and Cell Biology
Section Head, Cartilage Restoration Center
Rush University Medical Center
Chicago, Illinois

Jon K. Sekiya, MD

Larry S. Matthews Collegiate Professor of
Orthopaedic Surgery
Associate Professor
MedSport—University of Michigan
Ann Arbor, Michigan

Associate Editors

Geoffrey S. Van Thiel, MD, MBA

Clinical Instructor
Rush University Medical Center
Chicago, Illinois
Rockford Orthopedic Associates
Rockford, Illinois

Jack G. Skendzel, MD

Sports Medicine Fellow
The Steadman Philippon Research Institute
Vail, Colorado

SAUNDERS

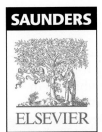

ELSEVIER

ELSEVIER
SAUNDERS

1600 John F. Kennedy Blvd.
Ste 1800
Philadelphia, PA 19103-2899

SURGICAL TECHNIQUES OF THE SHOULDER,
ELBOW, AND KNEE IN SPORTS MEDICINE

ISBN: 978-1-4557-2356-0

Library of Congress Cataloging-in-Publication Data

Surgical techniques of the shoulder, elbow, and knee in sports medicine / edited by Brian J. Cole, Jon K. Sekiya; associate editors, Geoffrey S. Van Thiel, Jack G. Skendzel.—2nd ed.
    p. ; cm.
  Includes bibliographical references and index.
  ISBN 978-1-4557-2356-0 (hardcover)
  I. Cole, Brian J.   II. Sekiya, Jon K.
  [DNLM: 1. Arthroscopy. 2. Elbow—surgery. 3. Knee—surgery. 4. Shoulder—surgery.
5. Sports Medicine—methods.   WE 304]
  RC932
  617.4′720597—dc23

                                                              2013008299

Printed in China

Last digit is the print number: 9 8 7 6 5 4 3 2 1

Senior Content Strategist: Don Scholz
Senior Content Development Specialist: Ann Ruzycka Anderson
Publishing Services Manager: Patricia Tannian
Project Manager: Carrie Stetz
Design Direction: Louis Forgione

Contents

PART 3 THE KNEE

General Principles

Surgical Techniques of the Meniscus

Surgical Techniques of the Articular Cartilage

Surgical Techniques of the Anterior Cruciate Ligament

Surgical Techniques of the Posterior Cruciate Ligament and Posterolateral Corner

Other Surgical Techniques of the Knee

VIDEO CONTENTS

Videos are available at the *Surgical Techniques of the Shoulder, Elbow, and Knee in Sports Medicine* collection online at www.expertconsult.com.

Contributors

Sami Abdulmassih, MD
Visiting Associate, Division of Sports Medicine, Department of Orthopedic Surgery and Rehabilitation, University of Iowa Hospitals and Clinics, Iowa City, Iowa

Julie E. Adams, MD
Assistant Professor of Orthopaedic Surgery, University of Minnesota, Minneapolis, Minnesota

Christopher S. Ahmad, MD
Assistant Professor of Orthopaedic Surgery, Center for Shoulder, Elbow and Sports Medicine, Columbia University, New York, New York

Answorth A. Allen, MD
Associate Professor, Weill Medical College of Cornell University, Associate Attending Physician, Hospital for Special Surgery, New York, New York

Laith Al-Shihabi, MD
Resident, Department of Orthopaedic Surgery, Rush University Medical Center, Chicago, Illinois

David W. Altchek, MD
Hospital for Special Surgery, Chief, Sports Medicine and Shoulder Service, Professor of Orthopaedic Surgery, Weill Cornell Medical College, New York, New York

Annunziato Amendola, MD
Professor, Orthopaedics and Rehabilitation, University of Iowa; Director, University of Iowa Sports Medicine Center, University of Iowa Hospitals and Clinics, Iowa City, Iowa

Kyle Anderson, MD
Director, Sports Medicine and Shoulder Fellowship, Department of Orthopaedic Surgery, William Beaumont Hospital; Team Physician, Detroit Lions, Detroit, Michigan

Wade Andrews, MD
Orthopaedic Surgeon, OSS Health, York, Pennsylvania

Paulo H. Araujo, MD
Research Fellow, Department of Orthopaedic Surgery, University of Pittsburgh, Pittsburgh, Pennsylvania; Centro de Ortopedia e Traumatologia de Brasília, Sao Paulo, Brazil

Frederick M. Azar, MD
Professor and Residency Program Director, Sports Medicine Fellowship Director, Campbell Clinic, University of Tennessee, Memphis, Tennessee

Bernard R. Bach Jr, MD
The Claude N. Lambert–Susan Thomson Endowed Professor of Orthopedic Surgery, and Director, Division of Sports Medicine and Sports Medicine Fellowship, Rush University Medical Center; Team Physician, Chicago White Sox and Chicago Bulls, Chicago, Illinois

Champ L. Baker Jr, MD
Clinical Assistant Professor, Department of Orthopaedic Surgery, Tulane University School of Medicine, New Orleans, Louisiana; Clinical Assistant Professor, Department of Orthopaedics, Medical College of Georgia, Augusta; Staff Physician, The Hughston Clinic, Columbus, Georgia

Champ L. Baker III, MD
Resident, Department of Orthopaedic Surgery, University of Pittsburgh Medical Center, Pittsburgh, Pennsylvania

Asheesh Bedi, MD
Assistant Professor, Harold and Helen W. Gehring Early Career Professor in Orthopaedic Surgery, MedSport, Department of Orthopaedic Surgery, University of Michigan, Ann Arbor, Michigan

Knut Beitzel, MD
Department of Trauma and Orthopaedic Surgery, Trauma Center Murnau, Murnau, Germany

Patrick M. Birmingham, MD
Assistant Professor, Department of Orthopaedic Surgery, Medical College of Wisconsin, Milwaukee, Wisconsin; Orthopaedic Surgeon, Northwestern Orthopaedic Institute at NorthShore University Health System, Chicago, Illinois

Debdut Biswas, MD
Department of Orthopaedic Surgery, Rush University Medical Center, Chicago, Illinois

Andrew J. Blackman, MD
Resident, Department of Orthopaedic Surgery, Washington University, St. Louis, Missouri

Matthew T. Boes, MD
Raleigh Orthopaedic Clinic, Raleigh, North Carolina

Pascal Boileau, MD
Consultant Orthopaedic Surgeon, St. James's Hospital, Dublin, Ireland

Davide Edoardo Bonasia, MD
Orthopaedic Clinic of the University of Turin, CTO Hospital, Turin, Italy

Craig R. Bottoni, MD
Chief of Surgery, Aspertar Sports Medicine Hospital, Doha, Qatar

Jay Boughanem, MD
Harvard Shoulder Service, Department of Orthopaedic Surgery, Brigham and Women's Hospital, Boston, Massachusetts

Mark K. Bowen, MD
Associate Professor of Clinical Orthopaedic Surgery, Northwestern University Medical School; Active Attending Physician, Northwestern Memorial Hospital, Chicago, Illinois

Karl F. Bowman Jr, MD
Fellow, Sports Medicine, UPMC Center for Sports Medicine, Pittsburgh, Pennsylvania

Michael B. Boyd, DO
Attending Physician, Department of Orthopaedic Surgery, St. Mary's Hospital and Deaconess Hospital, Evansville, Indiana

James P. Bradley, MD
Clinical Associate Professor of Orthopaedic Surgery, University of Pittsburgh Medical Center; Orthopaedic Surgeon, University of Pittsburgh Medical Center Shadyside and St. Margaret Hospitals; Head Orthopaedic Surgeon, Pittsburgh Steelers, Pittsburgh, Pennsylvania

William D. Bugbee, MD
Associate Professor, Department of Orthopaedic Surgery, University of California, San Diego; Attending Physician, Lower Extremity Reconstruction and Cartilage Restoration, Division of Orthopaedic Surgery, Scripps Clinic, La Jolla, California

Stephen S. Burkhart, MD
Fellowship Director, The San Antonio Orthopaedic Group, San Antonio, Texas

Joseph P. Burns, MD
Southern California Orthopedic Institute, Sports & Shoulder Team, Van Nuys, California

Charles A. Bush-Joseph, MD
Associate Professor, Department of Orthopaedic Surgery, Rush University Medical Center, Chicago, Illinois

Thomas R. Carter, MD
Emeritus Head of Orthopedic Surgery, and Consultant, Orthopedic Surgery, Arizona State University, Tempe, Arizona

Simone Cerciello, MD
Orthopaedic Surgeon and Professor, Molise University, Campobasso, Italy

Jaskarndip Chahal, MD
University Health Network and Women's College Hospital, University of Toronto, Toronto, Canada

Peter N. Chalmers, MD
Orthopaedic Surgery Resident, Department of Orthopaedic Surgery, Rush University Medical Center, Chicago, Illinois

Salma Chaudhury, MD, PhD
Orthopaedic Resident, Nuffield Department of Orthopaedics, Rheumatology and Musculoskeletal Sciences, University of Oxford, Oxford, United Kingdom

Neal C. Chen, MD
Resident, Department of Orthopedic Surgery, Harvard Combined Orthopedic Residency, Boston, Massachusetts

Emilie Cheung, MD
Assistant Professor, Shoulder and Elbow Surgery, Department of Orthopedic Surgery, Stanford University Medical Center, Redwood City, California

Robert M. Coale, MD
Orthopaedic Surgeon, Ortho West; Medical Director, Sports Medicine, Southwest General Health Center, Middleburg Heights, Ohio

Mark S. Cohen, MD
Director, Section of Hand and Elbow Surgery, Department of Orthopaedic Surgery, Rush University Medical Center, Chicago, Illinois

Steven B. Cohen, MD
Assistant Professor, Department of Orthopaedic Surgery, Thomas Jefferson University; Orthopaedic Surgeon, Rothman Institute; Assistant Team Physician, Philadelphia Phillies, Philadelphia, Pennsylvania

Brian J. Cole, MD, MBA
Professor, Departments of Orthopedics and Anatomy and Cell Biology, Section of Sports Medicine; Section Head, Cartilage Restoration Center, Rush University Medical Center, Chicago, Illinois

CPT Jay B. Cook, MD, MC, USA
Resident, Department of Orthopaedics, Tripler Army
Medical Center, Honolulu, Hawaii

Andrew J. Cosgarea, MD
Associate Professor and Director of Sports Medicine and
Shoulder Surgery, Department of Orthopaedic Surgery,
Johns Hopkins University, Baltimore, Maryland

D. Jeff Covell, MPH
Research Assistant, Cognitive Neuroscience Laboratory,
University of Kentucky College of Medicine, Lexington,
Kentucky

Matthew Craig, BS
Georgetown University School of Medicine, Washington,
DC

R. Alexander Creighton, MD
Assistant Professor of Orthopaedics, University of North
Carolina at Chapel Hill and University of North
Carolina Hospitals, Chapel Hill, North Carolina

Thomas DeBerardino, MD
Associate Professor, Department of Orthopaedic Surgery,
University of Connecticut Health Center, Farmington,
Connecticut

Scott J. Deering, MD
Fellow, Department of Orthopaedic Sports Medicine,
University of Kentucky, Lexington, Kentucky

David Dejour, MD
Orthopaedic Surgeon, Lyon-Ortho-Clinic, Lyon, France

Patrick J. Denard, MD
Clinical Instructor, Department of Orthopaedics &
Rehabilitation, Oregon Health & Science University,
Portland, Oregon; Shoulder Surgeon, Southern Oregon
Orthopedics, Medford, Oregon

Aman Dhawan, MD
Assistant Clinical Professor of Orthopaedic Surgery,
Department of Orthopaedic Surgery, UMDNJ-Robert
Wood Johnson Medical School, New Brunswick, New
Jersey

Aad A.M. Dhollander, MD, PhD
Department of Orthopaedic Surgery, Ghent University
Hospital, Ghent, Belgium

David R. Diduch, MD
Professor, University of Virginia Head Orthopaedic Team
Physician; Director, Sports Medicine Fellowship Program,
Charlottesville, Virginia

Joshua S. Dines, MD
Sports Medicine and Shoulder Service, The Hospital for
Special Surgery, Great Neck, New York

Christopher C. Dodson, MD
Rothman Institute, Department of Sports Medicine;
Assistant Professor of Orthopaedic Surgery, Thomas
Jefferson Medical College, Philadelphia, Pennsylvania

Kevin M. Doulens, MD
Clinical Fellow, Sports Medicine, Orthopaedics and
Rehabilitation, Vanderbilt University Medical Center,
Nashville, Tennessee

Alex Dukas, MD
Resident Physician, New England Musculoskeletal
Institute, Department of Orthopaedics, University of
Connecticut Health Center, Farmington, Connecticut

Neal S. ElAttrache, MD
Sports Medicine Surgeon, Kerlan-Jobe Orthopaedic
Clinic, Los Angeles, California

Gregory C. Fanelli, MD
Fanelli Sports Injury Clinic, Geisinger Medical Center,
Danville, Pennsylvania

Jack Farr II, MD
Associate Clinical Professor of Orthopaedic Surgery,
Indiana University School of Medicine; Orthopaedic
Surgeon, St. Francis Hospital and Health Centers and
Indiana Orthopaedic Hospital, Indianapolis, Indiana

Diego Fernandez, MD
Professor of Orthopaedic Surgery, Department of
Orthopaedic Surgery, University of Bern and Lindenhof
Hospital, Bern, Switzerland

John J. Fernandez, MD
Assistant Professor, Department of Orthopaedics, Rush
University Medical Center, Chicago, Illinois

Paolo Ferrua, MD
Orthopaedic Surgeon, G. Pini Orthopaedic Institute,
Milan, Italy

Larry D. Field, MD
Clinical Instructor, Orthopaedic Surgery, University of
Mississippi School of Medicine; Co-Director, Upper
Extremity Service, Mississippi Sports Medicine and
Orthopaedic Center, Jackson, Mississippi

David C. Flanigan, MD
Assistant Professor of Orthopedics, Team Physician, The
Ohio State University Athletic Department, The Ohio
State University, Columbus, Ohio

Brian Forsythe, MD
Orthopedic Surgeon, Sports Medicine Specialist, Midwest
Orthopedics, Rush University Medical Center, Chicago,
Illinois

Tyler Fox, MD
Harvard Shoulder Service, Department of Orthopaedic
Surgery, Brigham and Women's Hospital, Boston,
Massachusetts

Jonathan M. Frank, MD
Resident Physician, Department of Orthopaedics, Rush
University Medical Center, Chicago, Illinois

Rachel M. Frank, MD
Department of Orthopaedic Surgery, Rush University
Medical Center, Chicago, Illinois

Heather Freeman, PT, DHS
Shelbourne Knee Center, Indianapolis, Indiana

Freddie H. Fu, MD, DSc(Hon), DPs(Hon)
Chairman, Orthopaedic Surgery, University of Pittsburgh
Medical Center, Pittsburgh, Pennsylvania

John P. Fulkerson, MD
Clinical Professor of Orthopedic Surgery, University of
Connecticut School of Medicine, Farmington,
Connecticut

Andrew Gelven, DO
Atlanta Sports Medicine & Orthopaedic Center, Atlanta,
Georgia

Scott Gillogly, MD
Medical Staff, Department of Orthopaedic Surgery,
St. Joseph's Hospital, Atlanta, Georgia

M. Mustafa Gomberawalla, MD
Orthopaedic Surgery Resident, Department of
Orthopaedic Surgery, University of Michigan, Ann Arbor,
Michigan

Andreas H. Gomoll, MD
Instructor of Orthopaedic Surgery, Harvard Medical
School; Cartilage Repair Center, Department of
Orthopaedic Surgery, Brigham and Women's Hospital,
Boston, Massachusetts

Simon Görtz, MD
Resident Physician, Department of Orthopaedic Surgery,
University of California–San Diego, San Diego,
California

James Hammond, DO, ATC
Clinical Instructor, Bone and Joint/Sports Medicine
Institute, Department of Orthopaedics, Shoulder/Elbow/
Sports Surgeon, Naval Medical Center Portsmouth,
Portsmouth, Virginia

Michael G. Hannon, MD
Chief Resident, Department of Orthopaedic Surgery,
NYU Hospital for Joint Diseases, New York, New York

Shane Hanzlik, MD
Chief Resident, Department of Orthopedics, Case
Western Reserve University, Cleveland, Ohio

Christopher D. Harner, MD
Professor, Department of Orthopaedic Surgery, University
of Pittsburgh; Medical Director, Department of
Orthopaedic Surgery, University of Pittsburgh Medical
Center, Center for Sports Medicine, Pittsburgh,
Pennsylvania

Marc S. Haro, MD
University of Virginia, Department of Orthopaedic
Surgery, Charlottesville, Virginia

Wendell Heard, MD
Assistant Professor of Orthopaedic Surgery, Department
of Orthopaedic Surgery, Section of Sports Medicine,
Tulane University School of Medicine, New Orleans,
Louisiana

Laurence D. Higgins, MD
Chief, Harvard Shoulder Service and Sports Medicine,
Brigham and Women's Hospital, Department of
Orthopaedic Surgery, Boston, Massachusetts

Stephen M. Howell, MD
Professor, Department of Mechanical Engineering,
University of California–Davis, Sacramento, California

Nicholas D. Iagulli, MD
Mississippi Sports Medicine and Orthopaedic Center,
Jackson, Mississippi

Mary Lloyd Ireland, MD
President/Director, Kentucky Sports Medicine Clinic,
Lexington, Kentucky

Warren R. Kadrmas, MD
Fellow, Sports Medicine and Shoulder Service, Hospital
for Special Surgery, New York, New York; Staff
Orthopaedic Surgeon, Wilford Hall Medical Center,
Lackland Air Force Base, Texas

Christopher C. Kaeding, MD
Professor of Orthopaedics and Director of Sports
Medicine, Department of Orthopaedic Surgery; Head
Team Physician, Department of Athletics, The Ohio State
University, Columbus, Ohio

Richard Kang, MD
Resident, Orthopedic Surgery, Rush University Medical
Center, Chicago, Illinois

Anjan P. Kaushik, MD
University of Virginia Department of Orthopaedic
Surgery, Charlottesville, Virginia

Michael W. Kessler, MD, MPH
Assistant Professor, Department of Orthopaedic Surgery, Associate Residency Program Director, Georgetown University Hospital, Washington, DC

W. Ben Kibler, MD
Medical Director, Shoulder Center of Kentucky, Lexington, Kentucky

Matthew A. Kippe, MD
Department of Orthopedic Surgery, Hawthorn Medical Associates, North Dartmouth, Massachusetts

Pradeep Kodali, MD
Resident Physician, Department of Orthopaedic Surgery, McGraw Medical Center-Northwestern University, Chicago, Illinois

Nate Kopydlowski, BA
University of Michigan Medical School, Ann Arbor, Michigan

Marc Korn, BA
Department of Orthopaedics, Wayne State University, Detroit, Michigan

John E. Kuhn, MD
Associate Professor and Chief of Shoulder Surgery, Division of Sports Medicine, Department of Orthopaedics and Rehabilitation, Vanderbilt University Medical Center, Nashville, Tennessee

Laurent Lafosse, MD
Chairman, Alps Surgery Institute, Clinique Generale d'Annecy, Annecy, France

Robert F. LaPrade, MD, PhD
Chief Medical Research Officer, Steadman Philippon Research Institute, The Steadman Clinic, Vail, Colorado

Christian Lattermann, MD
Assistant Professor for Orthopaedics and Sports Medicine, and Director, Center for Cartilage Repair and Restoration, Department of Orthopaedic Surgery, University of Kentucky, Lexington, Kentucky

Keith Lawhorn, MD
Orthopaedic Surgeon, Commonwealth Orthopaedics and Rehabilitation, Fairfax, Virginia

Lance LeClere, MD, LCDR MC USN
Assistant Professor, Uniformed Services University of Health Sciences, Division of Sports Medicine and Shoulder Surgery, Naval Medical Center San Diego, San Diego, California

James H. Lubowitz, MD
Director, Taos Orthopaedic Institute, Taos Orthopaedic Institute Research Foundation, Taos Orthopaedic Institute Sports Medicine Fellowship Training Program, Taos, New Mexico

Jamie L. Lynch, MD
Northeast Orthopaedics & Sports Medicine, San Antonio, Texas

Nathan Mall, MD
Director, St. Louis Center for Cartilage Restoration and Repair Regeneration Orthopedics, St. Louis, Missouri

Fabrizio Margheritini, MD
University of Rome-Foro Italico-IUSM, Department of Health Science, Unit of Orthopedics and Sports Traumatology, Rome, Italy

Pier Paolo Mariani, MD
University of Rome-Foro Italico-IUSM, Department of Health Science, Unit of Orthopedics and Sports Traumatology, Rome, Italy

Augustus D. Mazzocca, MD
Assistant Professor, Orthopaedic Surgery, University of Connecticut, Farmington, Connecticut

Eric McCarty, MD
Associate Professor and Chief of Sports Medicine and Shoulder Surgery, Department of Orthopaedic Surgery, University of Colorado Health Science Center; Attending Physician, Boulder Community Hospital, Boulder, Colorado

L. Pearce McCarty III, MD
Sports and Orthopaedic Specialists, Minneapolis, Minnesota

Mark McConkey, MD
Orthopaedic Surgeon, Iowa City, Iowa

John E. McDonald, MD
Texas Orthopedics, Sports, and Rehabilitation, Austin, Texas

LCDR Lucas S. McDonald, MD, MPH, MC, USN
Department of Orthopaedic Surgery, Naval Medical Center San Diego, San Diego, California

John McMullen, MS, ATC
Director Orthopedic Service, Shoulder Center of Kentucky, Lexington, Kentucky

Emmanuel N. Menga, MD
Resident, Department of Orthopaedic Surgery, Johns Hopkins University, Baltimore, Maryland

Kellie K. Middleton, MD, MPH
Resident, Department of Orthopaedic Surgery, University of Pittsburgh Medical Center, Pittsburgh, Pennsylvania

Mark D. Miller, MD
S. Ward Casscells Professor of Orthopaedic Surgery, University of Virginia, Charlottesville, Virginia

Kai Mithoefer, MD
Department of Orthopedics and Sports Medicine, Harvard Vanguard Medical Associates, Harvard Medical School, Boston, Massachusetts

Craig D. Morgan, MD
Clinical Professor, University of Pennsylvania; Associate Clinical Professor, Thomas Jefferson University, Philadelphia, Pennsylvania; Orthopaedic Surgeon, Morgan Kalman Clinic, Wilmington, Delaware

Gregory P. Nicholson, MD
Associate Professor, Orthopaedic Surgery, Rush University Medical Center, Chicago, Illinois

Gordon Nuber, MD
Professor of Clinical Orthopaedics, Northwestern University, Chicago, Illinois

Michael O'Brien, MD
Tulane School of Medicine, Department of Orthopaedics, Tulane Institute of Sports Medicine, New Orleans, Louisiana

Kieran O'Shea, FRCSI
Consultant Orthopaedic Surgeon, St. James's Hospital, Dublin, Ireland

Michael J. Pagnani, MD
Director, Nashville Knee and Shoulder Center; Head Team Physician, Nashville Predators Hockey Club, Nashville, Tennessee

Michael Pensak, MD
Resident, Department of Orthopaedic Surgery, University of Connecticut Health Center, Farmington, Connecticut

Matthew T. Provencher, MD
Chief, Sports Medicine and Surgery, Associate Professor of Surgery, Massachusetts General Hospital and Harvard Medical School, Boston, Massachusetts

R. David Rabalais, MD
Sports Medicine and Shoulder Surgery Fellow, Department of Orthopaedic Surgery, University of Colorado Health Science Center and Boulder Community Hospital, Boulder, Colorado

Richard Rainey, MD
Fellow, Department of Orthopaedics, University of Tennessee-Campbell Clinic, Germantown, Tennessee

Andrew Riff, MD
Resident, Department of Orthopaedics, Rush University Medical Center, Chicago, Illinois

Eric Rightmire, MD
Attending Physician, Orthopedic Surgery, Jordan Hospital, Plymouth, Massachusetts; Orthopedic Surgeon, Plymouth Bay Orthopedic Associates, Duxbury, Massachusetts

David Ring, MD, PhD
Assistant Professor, Orthopaedic Surgery, Harvard Medical School; Medical Director and Director of Research, Orthopaedic Hand and Upper Extremity Service, Massachusetts General Hospital, Boston, Massachusetts

Scott A. Rodeo, MD
Associate Professor of Orthopaedic Surgery, Weill Medical College of Cornell University; Associate Attending Physician, Sports Medicine and Shoulder Service, Hospital for Special Surgery; Associate Team Physician, New York Giants, New York, New York

William G. Rodkey, DVM (Dipl), ACVS
Director, Basic Science Research, Steadman Hawkins Research Foundation, Vail, Colorado

Anthony A. Romeo, MD
Associate Professor, Department of Orthopaedics, Rush Medical College and Rush-Presbyterian-St. Luke's Medical Center, Chicago, Illinois

Marc R. Safran, MD
Professor of Orthopaedic Surgery, Associate Director of Sports Medicine, and Fellowship Director, Department of Orthopaedic Surgery, Stanford University, Stanford, California

Paulo R.F. Saggin, MD
Orthopaedic Surgeon, Instituto de Ortopedia e Traumatologia (IOT), Passo Fundo, Brazil

Dipit Sahu, MS
Consultant Orthopaedic Surgeon, Department of Orthopaedics, Sahu Hospital and Research Center, Agra, India

Michael J. Salata, MD
Assistant Professor, Division of Sports Medicine, Department of Orthopaedic Surgery; Director, Joint Preservation and Cartilage Restoration Center, University Hospitals Case Medical Center, Cleveland, Ohio

Rodrigo Salim, MD
Research Fellow, Sports Medicine, UPMC Center for
Sports Medicine, Pittsburgh, Pennsylvania

Felix H. Savoie III, MD
Professor of Clinical Orthopaedics, Department of
Orthopaedics, Section of Orthopaedic Surgery; Chief,
Section of Sports Medicine, Tulane University School of
Medicine, New Orleans, Louisiana

Aaron Sciascia, MS, ATC
Coordinator, Shoulder Center of Kentucky, Lexington,
Kentucky

Jon K. Sekiya, MD
Associate Professor, Department of Orthopaedic Surgery,
University of Michigan, Ann Arbor, Michigan

K. Donald Shelbourne, MD
Orthopaedic Surgeon, Shelbourne Knee Center,
Indianapolis, Indiana

Seth L. Sherman, MD
Assistant Professor, Department of Orthopedic Surgery,
Division of Sports Medicine, University of Missouri,
Columbia, Missouri

Lewis L. Shi, MD
Assistant Professor of Orthopaedic Surgery, Department
of Orthopaedic Surgery and Rehabilitation Medicine,
University of Chicago Medical Center, Chicago, Illinois

Keerat Singh, MD
Resident, Department of Orthopaedic Surgery and
Rehabilitation, Vanderbilt University School of Medicine,
Memphis, Tennessee

Jack G. Skendzel, MD
Sports Medicine Fellow, The Steadman Philippon
Research Institute, Vail, Colorado

Adam M. Smith, MD
Kentucky Sports Medicine, Lexington, Kentucky

Matthew V. Smith, MD
Washington University Department of Orthopaedics, St.
Louis, Missouri

Patrick A. Smith, MD
Clinical Practice at the Columbia Orthopaedic Group,
LLP, Columbia, Missouri; Director of Sports Medicine,
University of Missouri Head Team Physician, University
of Missouri, Columbia, Missouri

Stephen J. Snyder, MD
Director, Shoulder Arthroscopy Service, Southern
California Orthopedic Institute, Van Nuys, California

John W. Sperling, MD, MBA
Associate Professor, Department of Orthopedic Surgery,
Mayo Clinic College of Medicine; Consultant,
Department of Orthopedic Surgery, Mayo Clinic,
Rochester, Minnesota

Umasuthan Srikumaran, MD
Assistant Professor, Department of Orthopaedic Surgery,
Johns Hopkins School of Medicine, Baltimore, Maryland

Scott P. Steinmann, MD
Associate Professor, Department of Orthopedic Surgery,
Mayo Clinic College of Medicine; Consultant in
Shoulder, Elbow, and Hand Surgery, Department of
Orthopedic Surgery, Saint Mary's Hospital, Rochester,
Minnesota

Zachary Stender, MD
Resident, Department of Orthopaedics, New England
Musculoskeletal Institute, University of Connecticut,
Farmington, Connecticut

Eric J. Strauss, MD
Assistant Professor, Division of Sports Medicine,
Department of Orthopaedic Surgery, NYU Hospital for
Joint Diseases, New York, New York

Justin P. Strickland, MD
Resident, Department of Orthopedic Surgery, Mayo
Clinic Graduate School of Medicine, Rochester,
Minnesota

Kenneth G. Swan Jr, MD
Sports Medicine and Shoulder Surgery Fellow,
Department of Orthopaedic Surgery, University of
Colorado Health Science Center and Boulder Community
Hospital, Boulder, Colorado

Thomas Tampere, MD
Resident, Department of Orthopaedic Surgery, Ghent
University Hospital, Ghent, Belgium

Gof Tantisricharoenkun, MD, CDR
Research Fellow, Department of Orthopaedic Surgery,
University of Pittsburgh, Pittsburgh, Pennsylvania;
Orthopaedic Surgeon, Department of Orthopaedic
Surgery, Royal Thai Navy, Somdejprapinklao Hospital,
Bangkok, Thailand

Sam G. Tejwani, MD
Southern California Permanente Medical Group, Kaiser
Permanente Hospital, Department of Orthopaedic
Surgery, Division of Sports Medicine, Fontana, California

James A. Thiel, DO
Orthopaedic Surgeon, WellSpan Orthopedics, Gettysburg,
Pennsylvania

Lt Col John M. Tokish, MD, MC, USAF
Orthopedic Residency Program Director, Tripler Army
Medical Center, Honolulu, Hawaii

Jeffrey D. Tompson, MS
Clinical Research Assistant, Harvard Shoulder Service,
Massachusetts General Hospital, Boston, Massachusetts

Jeffrey M. Tuman, MD
University of Virginia, Department of Orthopaedic
Surgery, Charlottsville, Virginia

Max Tyorkin, MD
Associate Attending Physician, Orthopaedic Surgery, Beth
Israel Medical Center and Lenox Hill Hospital, New
York, New York

Tim Uhl, PhD, ATC, PT
Associate Professor of Athletic Training, Co-Director of
Musculoskeletal Laboratory, University of Kentucky,
Lexington, Kentucky

Geoffrey S. Van Thiel, MD, MBA
Clinical Instructor, Rush University Medical Center,
Chicago, Illinois; Rockford Orthopedic Associates,
Rockford, Illinois

Peter C.M. Verdonk, MD, PhD
Professor of Orthopaedic Surgery, Department of
Orthopaedic Surgery, Monica Hospitals Antwerp,
Antwerp, Belgium

René Verdonk, MD
Emeritus Professor of Orthopaedic Surgery, Department
of Orthopaedic Surgery, Ghent University Hospital,
Ghent, Belgium

Nikhil N. Verma, MD
Attending Orthopaedic Surgeon, Department of
Orthopaedic Surgery, Rush University, Chicago, Illinois

Michael Walsh, MD
Orthopaedic Surgery Resident, Department of
Orthopaedic Surgery, University of Michigan, Ann Arbor,
Michigan

Robert Waltz, MD
Department of Orthopaedic Surgery, Naval Medical
Center San Diego, San Diego, California

Bryan A. Warme, MD
HSS Sports and Shoulder Fellow, Iowa State University
Sports Medicine, McFarland Clinic, Ames, Iowa

Jon J.P. Warner, MD
Professor of Orthopaedics, Department of Orthopaedics,
Harvard Medical School; Chief, Harvard Shoulder
Service, Department of Orthopaedics, Massachusetts
General Hospital, Boston, Massachusetts

Alexander E. Weber, MD
Orthopaedic Surgery Resident, Department of
Orthopaedic Surgery, University of Michigan, Ann Arbor,
Michigan

Robin V. West, MD
Assistant Professor, Department of Orthopaedics,
University of Pittsburgh, Pittsburgh, Pennsylvania

Lucas R. Wymore, MD
Chief Resident, Department of Orthopedic Surgery,
University of North Carolina, Chapel Hill, North
Carolina

Robert W. Wysocki, MD
Orthopaedic Surgery Resident, Department of
Orthopaedic Surgery, Rush University and Rush
University Medical Center, Chicago, Illinois

Adam B. Yanke, MD
Orthopedic Surgeon, Chicago, Illinois

Preface

We are excited to present the second edition of *Surgical Techniques of the Shoulder, Elbow, and Knee in Sports Medicine*. As educators, our most formidable challenge is to teach proper decision making and the techniques required to succeed in the operating room setting. As students, we are continuously pressured to compress the learning experience outside the operating room into efficient and digestible bits of information. We all recognize the importance of having access to accurate, timely, and concise tools to supplement our knowledge base. The emergence of digital content has positively influenced our access to up-to-date information. Simply "reading" about surgical procedures seems somewhat at odds with "doing" a series of steps that require dexterity and skill. More important, the act of physical repetition is what seems to propel us along the typically steep learning curve, especially when it involves the arthroscope.

The second edition of *Surgical Techniques of the Shoulder, Elbow, and Knee in Sports Medicine* was developed with these principles in mind. The principal objective of this textbook was to maximize its value by being thorough in the breadth of open and arthroscopic procedures covered, yet remaining concise in specific content. Authors have uniformly adhered to a template that we believe will optimize an efficient learning experience that is visually consistent, simple, and descriptive. To this end, each chapter is crafted with a brief introduction, a thumbnail of only the most relevant preoperative and postoperative considerations, a thorough and visually supported step-by-step explicit description of the procedure, and a table with the most up-to-date results related to that specific procedure. Simply stated, it is exactly what you need to know before entering the operating room.

It is nearly impossible to cover every joint in a single-volume textbook. While the term "sports medicine" has broad-reaching connotations, the vast majority of the conditions faced by the orthopedic surgeon who practices sports medicine and arthroscopy involve the shoulder, elbow, and knee. Thus, *Surgical Techniques of the Shoulder, Elbow, and Knee in Sports Medicine* intentionally limits the number of joints to those most commonly seen and treated, but covers them comprehensively without exception. This edition is bigger and better, with more chapters and newer, updated information. Most important, the content is provided by authors who have largely developed and popularized the procedures discussed.

Part 1, "The Shoulder," covers the general technical aspects of shoulder arthroscopy, including patient positioning, portal placement, rehabilitation of the shoulder, and specific steps required to pass sutures and tie knots. Because so many different techniques are performed to address the same pathology, we include 16 chapters describing surgical techniques for shoulder instability, including arthroscopic and open management of bone lesions of the glenoid and humeral head. Similarly, the management of rotator cuff pathology is addressed by no less than six chapters, including single-row, double-row, and mini-open techniques, and the role of tendon transfers. Finally, this section is complemented by chapters that address the treatment of the most common entities, including SLAP tears and instability, scapulothoracic disorders, and glenohumeral arthritis. Part 1 is a stand-alone compendium of the treatment of virtually every clinical problem seen by the shoulder surgeon.

Part 2, "The Elbow," is also comprehensive in that it includes the requisite steps required to perform elbow arthroscopy, such as patient positioning, portal placement, and a review of normal arthroscopic anatomy. In addition to providing excellent chapters on the most common conditions that are treated arthroscopically (e.g., osteochondritis dissecans, stiffness, synovitis, impingement, arthritis, and lateral epicondylitis), this part also contains an entire section on the most important open elbow procedures. Surgeons who treat athletes with ulnar and lateral collateral ligament disruption, elbow stiffness, instability of the elbow, biceps tendon tears, and epicondylitis will recognize that the section on open procedures of the elbow is thorough and completely up-to-date with surgical principles and techniques.

Part 3, "The Knee," is another virtual compendium that includes the complete management of any knee-related pathology. For example, management of meniscus-related issues has led to the development of multiple techniques to excise, repair, and replace the meniscal-deficient knee. Twelve chapters thoroughly review all these techniques. Articular cartilage, the subject of stand-alone textbooks, is completely covered with the management of virtually every problem that involves cartilage short of arthroplasty. Eight chapters address every cartilage repair procedure in addition to realignment osteotomy. One of the most exciting sections is the management of the anterior and posterior cruciate ligaments. This section includes single- and double-bundle as well as inlay techniques written by the surgeons who have popularized these procedures. Finally, management of the multi-ligament-injured knee, arthrofibrosis, and patellofemoral joint completes a text that leaves the reader with little need to turn to any other resource.

Surgical Techniques of the Shoulder, Elbow, and Knee in Sports Medicine is the product of almost 3 years of hard work by its contributors. These authors are frequently asked to further the education of others, yet never seem to wane in their enthusiasm and completeness. It is an honor to work with the contributors of this textbook, and the readers will appreciate the highly edited and consistent style that completely eliminates the noise of unnecessary information.

We would like to also thank our families, who once again have created an environment where a labor of love can result in something invaluable for our students and, more importantly, for our patients. Specifically, Dr.

Cole would like to thank Emily, Ethan, Adam, and Ava for their willingness to occasionally forego a late-night story so Daddy can stay awake to edit these chapters. Dr. Sekiya would like to thank his parents, Fred and Pat Sekiya, and wife, Jennie, for their never-ending support and understanding, and their sons, Kimo and Koa. We would like to thank our co-editors for helping complete the final details of this task, Dr. Geoffrey S. Van Thiel and Dr. Jack G. Skendzel. Finally, we would thank the many people at Elsevier, including Don Scholz, Ann Ruzycka Anderson, and Carrie Stetz, for governing the entire process until the book was released. So, read the text and prepare to challenge your mentors. *Surgical Techniques of the Shoulder, Elbow, and Knee in Sports Medicine* will allow you to do just that.

Brian J. Cole, MD, MBA
Jon K. Sekiya, MD

The Shoulder

Patient Positioning, Portal Placement, Normal Arthroscopic Anatomy, and Diagnostic Arthroscopy

Peter N. Chalmers and Seth L. Sherman

Chapter Synopsis
- Diagnostic arthroscopy, while difficult to master, provides the surgeon with an important tool to evaluate the shoulder joint.
- Potential benefits are numerous, and complications infrequent.

Important Points
- Beach chair and lateral decubitus positioning have advantages and disadvantages; the practitioner should be familiar with both.
- Proper portal placement is critical.
- Understanding of normal anatomy allows recognition of pathology.

Pearls
- The beach chair position offers the greatest versatility and access.
- Separate portal sites allow superior triangulation.
- Familiarity with accessory portals can speed certain procedures.
- The glenohumeral joint may be palpated, manipulated, and repositioned.
- The practitioner should know anatomic variants.

Pitfalls
- Landmarks and portal placement sites should be marked before insufflation.
- Threaded cannulas are used whenever possible.
- Vertical orientation of the glenoid should be maintained.
- It is important to always visualize the subacromial space.

Shoulder arthroscopy has become an invaluable diagnostic and therapeutic tool for the sports medicine surgeon. Through innovative thinking and technical advancement, we continue to refine our ability to recognize and treat shoulder disorders with use of minimally invasive techniques. Shoulder arthroscopy has been shown to be both safe and effective when compared with open surgery. In a series of more than 14,000 procedures, the overall complication rate of shoulder arthroscopy was 0.56%.[1] Arthroscopic surgery offers the potential benefits of reduced operative time, decreased postoperative pain, decreased surgical scarring, improved cosmesis, and the ability to perform outpatient surgery. In addition, complications related to the subscapularis inherent to the deltopectoral approach can be avoided. Shoulder arthroscopy has demonstrated equivalent or superior outcomes to open procedures for a variety of shoulder conditions.[2-4]

Enhanced visualization of both the intraarticular and subacromial space and the ability to perform a dynamic intraoperative examination improves the accuracy of diagnostic shoulder arthroscopy. With advances in surgical techniques and instrumentation, the indications for arthroscopy treatment have also broadened to include rotator cuff pathology, labral and capsular injuries, and diseases of the articular cartilage.

PATIENT POSITIONING

Shoulder arthroscopy may be performed with use of either general endotracheal anesthesia or regional anesthesia. Benefits of regional anesthesia with a long-acting local anesthetic such as bupivacaine include enhanced postoperative pain control and improved operating room efficiency, as the block can be administered in the preoperative holding area. The surgeon may opt for a combination of the two for procedures in which muscular relaxation is critical, such as for capsular release in adhesive capsulitis. Hypotensive anesthesia will assist the surgeon by reducing bleeding that may limit arthroscopic visualization. However, care must be taken by the anesthesiologist to maintain a safe and consistent mean arterial pressure, particularly for patients with medical comorbidities, and for those placed in the beach chair position. Insufflation with dilute (1:300,000) epinephrine in the arthroscopic fluid may also improve hemostasis. In either the beach chair or the lateral decubitus position, compression boots may be placed on bilateral lower extremities for the duration of the procedure to help prevent deep venous thrombosis.

The patient may be positioned in the beach chair or the lateral decubitus position for shoulder arthroscopy. Both positions have been shown to be safe and reliable for a wide variety of shoulder arthroscopic procedures. Although surgeon preference for one position over the other may vary based on training and experience, some of the major advantages and disadvantages of each position are as follows.

Advantages of the beach chair position include ease of positioning, easier conversion to open procedures if necessary, avoidance of traction-related complications, potential for decreased intraoperative bleeding as a result of reduced venous pressure, and the ability to dynamically reposition the arm during the procedure. The last benefit is best realized by use of a pneumatic articulated arm holder for the duration of the procedure. We prefer the beach chair position for diagnostic arthroscopy, subacromial decompression, acromioclavicular (AC) joint procedures, rotator cuff repair, biceps procedures, capsular release, intraarticular debridement, and loose body removal. Advantages of the lateral decubitus position include the use of traction with the potential for improved intraarticular distraction and visualization, and the avoidance of cerebral hypoperfusion. Whereas patient positioning, dynamic shoulder evaluation, and conversion to open procedures are more cumbersome in the lateral decubitus position, they are certainly possible and should not be thought of as a reason to choose one position over the other. We prefer the lateral decubitus position for shoulder instability surgery, including labral repair (particularly for posterior labral or extensive 180- to 270-degree labral tears) and capsular plication and capsular shift procedures.

For the beach chair position, the patient is positioned supine and the back of the bed is elevated to 60 degrees (Fig. 1-1). The patient is positioned such that the medial border of the scapula is just lateral to the lateral aspect of the bed. A rolled towel placed just medial to the scapula may improve operative positioning. For the lateral decubitus position, the patient is supported with either a vacuum beanbag or a combination of bolsters, kidney rests, chest strap, foam headrest, and axillary

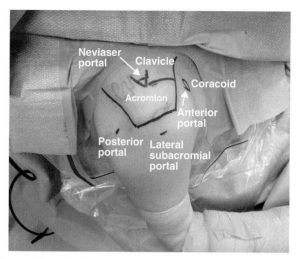

Figure 1-1. Patient in beach chair position with an articulated arm holder in place with landmarks and portals identified.

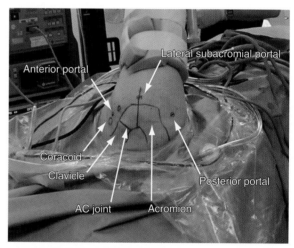

Figure 1-2. Patient in lateral decubitus position with traction in place with landmarks and portals identified. *AC,* Acromioclavicular.

roll (Fig. 1-2). Visualization may be more anatomic if the patient is tilted 20 to 30 degrees posteriorly to bring the face of the glenoid parallel to the floor. Care should be taken to protect and pad superficial bony landmarks of the lower extremities. Ten pounds of traction is typically adequate. The lowest amount of weight (maximum 15 pounds) and shortest time of traction (maximum 2 hours) necessary to perform the procedure are recommended. In addition to axial traction, joint distention may be augmented by the addition of secondary traction close to the axilla and perpendicular to the joint. Caution should be exercised with dual traction setups to avoid distal hypoxemia. Alternatively, a sterile rolled towel placed deep into the axilla may provide improved joint distention without the need for a dual traction setup. For access to the subacromial space, smaller degrees of flexion and abduction can provide inferior distraction of the humeral head and an improved subacromial view.

After induction of anesthesia but before sterile preparation and draping, an examination with the patient under anesthesia (EUA) should be performed. Both the operative and nonoperative limb should be examined, if possible. Degrees of abduction, forward elevation, and internal and external rotation in adduction and abduction, respectively, should be documented. Restrictions in motion may be observed in patients with adhesive capsulitis, glenohumeral arthritis, or frank shoulder dislocation. In patients with a history of instability, an examination for shoulder laxity should be performed via load and shift testing. After application of a force to center the humerus on the glenoid, the humerus is translated in both an anterior and a posterior direction while 90 degrees of abduction are maintained. Translation is graded as 0 for no translation, 1+ for trace translation, 2+ for translation to the edge of the glenoid, and 3+ for translation over the edge of the glenoid. Laxity to an inferiorly directed humeral force in adduction is documented as 0 for no humeral movement, 1+ for 1 cm of inferior humeral movement, 2+ for 2 cm of humeral movement, and so on.[2] If external humeral rotation dampens the inferior translation, the rotator interval may need to be addressed in addition to other sources of pathologic shoulder laxity.

After EUA the shoulder is prepared and draped in a sterile fashion. For the beach chair position, a sterile drape is placed over the arm holder for sterile intraoperative readjustment. For the lateral decubitus position, the arm is wrapped with Coban (3M, St Paul, Minnesota) for sterile arm traction up to but not including the wrist to avoid superficial radial nerve compression. Indelible ink is used to mark the anterior and posterior borders of the clavicle, borders of the acromion, and scapular spine. The AC joint and the coracoid process are identified and marked (see Figs. 1-1 and 1-2).

PORTAL PLACEMENT

Proper portal placement is essential for both surgical visualization during diagnostic arthroscopy and access of instruments used for the treatment of shoulder pathology. Improper portal placement can make even the simplest arthroscopic task seem near impossible. Planned portal sites should be marked before insufflation of the joint, to avoid obscuring palpable landmarks. The skin and subcutaneous tissue of portal sites should be infiltrated with 0.25% bupivacaine with epinephrine before incision.

Posterior Portal

In either the beach chair or lateral decubitus position, shoulder arthroscopy begins with the establishment of a posterior viewing portal. In the beach chair position this portal is classically located in the "soft spot" 2 cm medial and 2 cm inferior to the posterolateral corner of the acromion. In the lateral decubitus position the posterior portal may be positioned further laterally, just off the posterolateral corner of the acromion. An easy way to identify the posterior portal in the lateral decubitus position is to place the tip of the second finger on the coracoid process, the tip of the index finger in the soft space just posterior to the AC joint, and the tip of the thumb posteriorly over the presumed portal location. The portal lies in the sulcus between the humeral head and the glenoid. Regardless of shoulder position, an 18-gauge spinal needle is placed through the skin and into the glenohumeral joint, aiming toward the coracoid process. The joint is then insufflated with 30 to 50 mL of saline, with attention paid to ease of injection. The syringe is then briefly removed to visualize fluid egress, also confirming an intraarticular position. The spinal needle is then briskly removed and an 8-mm skin incision is made in its place through the skin and subcutaneous tissue with an 11 blade scalpel. A blunt obturator is then placed through the incision, aiming toward the coracoid process in the same trajectory as the spinal needle. Prior joint insufflation assists with shoulder distention, decreasing the risk of iatrogenic damage to the articular surface during portal placement. With the beach chair position, an assistant may provide gentle glenohumeral distraction by abducting the shoulder under the axilla while maintaining the elbow in an adducted position. Although the posterior portal theoretically takes advantage of the neurovascular plane between the teres minor muscle (axillary nerve) and the infraspinatus muscle (suprascapular nerve), it commonly pierces the belly of the infraspinatus muscle. Dangers to posterior portal placement include the axillary nerve, which lies 3 cm inferior to the placement site, and the suprascapular nerve, which lies 2 cm medial to the placement site.

Anterior Portals

The anterior portal is best placed with an "outside-in" technique, through use of a spinal needle placed under direct arthroscopic visualization (Fig. 1-3). The position of the anterior portal may vary based on the goals of the procedure. For anterior instability, placement of the portal just above the subscapularis is desirable. The portal may be placed more centrally within the rotator interval for routine diagnostic arthroscopy (Fig. 1-4). Superficially, this portal is located just lateral to the coracoid process. It travels between the deltoid muscle (axillary nerve) and the pectoralis major (lateral and medial pectoral nerves). In the deeper layer the anterior portal travels in the interval between the supraspinatus (suprascapular nerve) and the subscapularis (upper and lower subscapular nerves). The portal is also inferior to the long head of the biceps tendon (LHBT) and just

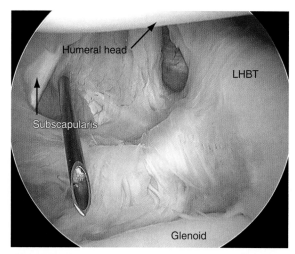

Figure 1-3. Spinal needle localization of the anterior portal in the lateral decubitus position. *LHBT,* Long head of the biceps tendon.

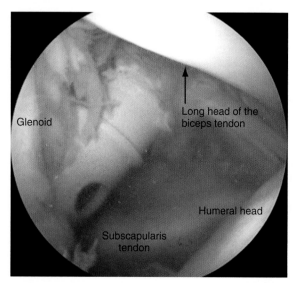

Figure 1-4. Cannula in anterior portal visualizing rotator interval, subscapularis, and biceps tendon in the beach chair position.

lateral to the middle glenohumeral ligament (MGHL). Safety of the anterior portal is ensured by making the portal under direct visualization, incising only the skin and subcutaneous tissue with the scalpel, and remaining lateral to the coracoid process, protected from critical neurovascular structures.

In addition to the standard anterior portal, an anterosuperior portal may be used for several shoulder procedures (e.g., Bankart repair, superior labral anterior-posterior [SLAP] repair, visualization during posterior labral repair). An "outside-in" approach is also used for portal placement. The spinal needle is placed through the skin, just inferior to the anterior border of the AC joint. The needle should enter the joint adjacent to the LHBT, just anterior to the leading edge of the supraspinatus. A switching stick and dilator system may be used

to assist in cannula placement for either the anterior or anterosuperior portal. Threaded cannulas may be inserted to prevent cannula back-out under the pressure of the insufflation fluid. Cannula insertion also prevents extravasation of irrigation fluid into the periarticular soft tissues and minimizes possible trauma associated with instrument insertion.

The lateral portal is useful for diagnostic and therapeutic arthroscopy of the subacromial space. This portal is established under direct arthroscopic visualization, viewing from a posterior portal. A spinal needle is placed approximately two to three fingerbreadths inferior to the lateral border of the acromion, in line with the posterior border of the AC joint. Once the location of the spinal needle has been confirmed, incision of the skin and subcutaneous tissue is followed by insertion of a blunt trocar through the deltoid and into the subacromial space. There is no internervous plane for this portal, as it transverses the deltoid muscle (axillary nerve). Care is taken not to place the portal too inferiorly (>5 cm) along the lateral aspect of the shoulder, which would place the axillary nerve at risk. This portal is useful for subacromial decompression, for rotator cuff repair, and as an adjunct or viewing portal during AC joint procedures.

Accessory Portals

Whereas diagnostic arthroscopy may require only a single anterior and posterior portal, other procedures may require a variety of portals. Accessory portals that transverse the rotator cuff musculature should be percutaneously placed, if possible, with avoidance of use of large cannulas through an otherwise intact rotator cuff tendon. An example of a useful percutaneous accessory portal is the "port of Wilmington" portal. This portal can be used for anchor placement during SLAP repair and is located 1 cm lateral and 1 cm anterior to the posterolateral corner of the acromion (see Figs. 1-1 and 1-2).[5] This portal does not have a classical neurovascular plane but pierces the deltoid and traverses through the muscle or musculotendinous junction of the rotator cuff. Other noteworthy accessory portals include a trans-subscapularis portal (useful for percutaneous anchor placement during Bankart repair), a 5/7 o'clock portal (also useful for either suture passage or anchor placement during instability surgery), and accessory lateral, anterolateral, or posterolateral percutaneous portals (useful during rotator cuff repair). The superior portal of Neviaser may also be useful for SLAP repair, rotator cuff repair, or suprascapular nerve decompression.[6] This portal is placed within the soft spot created by the clavicle anteriorly, the scapular spine posteriorly, and the acromion laterally. A spinal needle is aimed 30 to 45 degrees with respect to the skin in the coronal plane and 10 degrees posteriorly in the sagittal plane.

TABLE 1-1. Portals for Shoulder Arthroscopy

Portal Location	Insertion Site	Example of Uses
Posterior	About 2 cm medial to and inferior to the posterolateral corner of the acromion, aiming toward the tip of the coracoid process	Diagnostic arthroscopy
Anterior	Slightly lateral to the midpoint of a line drawn between the coracoid and the anterolateral corner of the acromion	Diagnostic arthroscopy, biceps tenotomy
Anterosuperior	At the leading edge of the supraspinatus tendon	Anterior instability repairs, capsulorraphy
Anteroinferior	Just superior to the subscapularis tendon	Anterior instability repairs, capsulorraphy
Lateral	Two to three fingerbreadths lateral to the lateral acromion in line with the posterior edge of the AC joint	SLAP repair, biceps tenodesis, rotator cuff repairs
Superior portal of Neviaser	Within the soft spot bordered by the acromial arch, scapular spine, and clavicle, with the needle aimed 0-45 degrees with respect to the skin in the coronal plane and 10 degrees posteriorly in the sagittal plane	SLAP repair, rotator cuff repair, suprascapular nerve decompression
Subacromial	Same insertion site as posterior portal, aiming toward anterolateral acromial edge	Acromioplasty, bursectomy, rotator cuff repairs
"Port of Wilmington"	About 1 cm lateral and 1 cm anterior to the posterolateral corner of the acromion	SLAP repair, rotator cuff repair
5/7 o'clock	Inferior edge of the subscapularis	Anteroinferior instability repairs, capsulorraphy

AC, Acromioclavicular; *SLAP,* superior labral anterior-posterior.

As is true for the standard portals, thorough knowledge of shoulder anatomy is paramount for safe and effective accessory portal placement. A brief summary of standard and accessory portals is found in Table 1-1.

DIAGNOSTIC ARTHROSCOPY AND NORMAL ARTHROSCOPIC ANATOMY

Diagnostic shoulder arthroscopy should include a reproducible and systematic evaluation of the intraarticular and subacromial space (Table 1-2). Full evaluation includes not only static visualization but also the use of palpation, tissue manipulation, and dynamic changes in glenohumeral positioning. Normal and abnormal structures should be documented through intraoperative image capture. In general, the entirety of the joint can be well visualized with a 30-degree arthroscope, but occasionally a 70-degree arthroscope is required for a complete view of the anterior and inferior recesses, respectively.

Diagnostic arthroscopy begins with the arthroscope in the posterior portal and a probe in the anterior portal (Fig. 1-5). Initial evaluation should focus on the major anterior structures that comprise and/or form the borders of the rotator interval. These include the capsular components of the rotator interval, the

subscapularis, and the biceps tendon (see Figs. 1-3 and 1-4). The superior glenohumeral ligament (SGHL) and MGHL should be visualized and probed. These ligaments act as checkreins to translation of the humeral head on the glenoid, with each ligament functioning maximally at a different glenohumeral position. The SGHL is generally visible within the superior portion of the rotator interval, traveling with the LHBT. Its superior aspect originates at the supraglenoid tubercle at the anterior aspect of the LHBT. The SGHL tightens in adduction to resist inferior translation of the humeral head. The MGHL originates from the supraglenoid tubercle and the superior labrum and traverses the rotator interval, continuing over the subscapularis tendon.[7] The MGHL resists anterior humeral excursion between 0 and 45 degrees of abduction. Considerable anatomic variation exists within the MGHL, which may exist as a well-defined structure, may resemble a cord, and may not exist at all. The Buford complex, a not uncommon MGHL variation, exists when the MGHL inserts directly onto the LHBT, leaving an area of anterior glenoid without labrum (Fig. 1-6).[8] In patients with significant anterior or inferior capsular laxity, these capsular structures may be attenuated or torn. Alternatively, patients with adhesive capsulitis will have significant scarring of the SGHL and MGHL that may involve the entire rotator interval. In these patients there may also be diffuse synovitis. These pathologic entities

TABLE 1-2. Diagnostic Arthroscopy

Arthroscopic Step	Anatomy Visualized	Pathology Visualized
Insert arthroscope posteriorly to view rotator interval	LHBT, SGHL, MGHL, subscapularis tendon	Synovitis, SLAP lesions, labral tears, ligamentous ruptures
Visualize the anterior joint inferior to the rotator interval	Subscapularis tendon	Subscapularis tears, biceps pulley lesions
Manipulate LHBT into joint, evaluate biceps anchor	Bicipital groove portion of LHBT, superior labrum, LHBT anchor	Tendonitis, fraying, tendon tears, SLAP tears
Advance arthroscope and rotate inferiorly	Subscapularis, MGHL, AIGHL, labrum, capsule	Bankart lesions, ALPSA lesions, ligamentous tears, labral tears
Turn arthroscope inferiorly and posteriorly	AIGHL, PIGHL, posterior recess	Foreign bodies, posterior capsulolabroligamentous tears
Place arthroscope in anterior portal	Posterior labrum, capsule	Reverse Bankart lesions, internal impingement
Turn arthroscope to view glenohumeral joint surfaces	Articular cartilage of humeral head, glenoid	Osteochondral lesions, cartilage defects
Turn arthroscope superiorly to view the rotator cuff	Supraspinatus and infraspinatus tendons	Fraying, synovitis, tendonitis, articular-sided partial cuff tears
Place arthroscope in subacromial space	Inferior acromion, subacromial bursa, rotator cuff, coracoid acromial ligament	Bursitis, subacromial impingement signs, bursal-sided rotator cuff tears

AIGHL, Anterior inferior glenohumeral ligament; *ALPSA,* anterior labral periosteal sleeve avulsion; *LHBT,* long head of the biceps tendon; *MGHL,* middle glenohumeral ligament; *PIGHL,* posterior inferior glenohumeral ligament; *SGHL,* superior glenohumeral ligament.

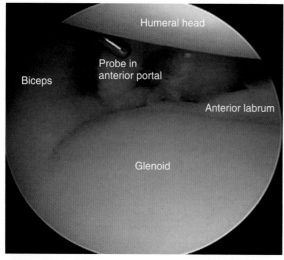

Figure 1-5. The anterior labrum, as viewed from the posterior portal with the patient in the lateral decubitus position.

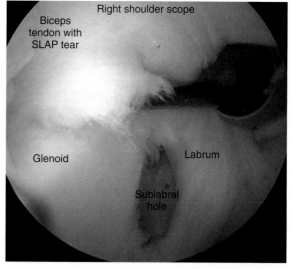

Figure 1-6. A sublabral hole, part of the spectrum of normal anterior labral variants and an aspect of the Buford complex in which the middle glenohumeral ligament inserts directly onto the anterior labrum and not the glenoid. *SLAP,* Superior labral anterior-posterior.

may cause difficulty with initial visualization and access into the glenohumeral joint.

The examination may then turn to the subscapularis tendon (see Figs. 1-3 and 1-4). The upper rolled border of the subscapularis is a well-defined anatomic landmark, defining the inferior border of the rotator interval. The subscapularis should be visualized as it inserts into the lesser tuberosity of the humerus. Forward flexion and internal rotation of the arm may assist in visualization of this insertion. A probe should be used to palpate the subscapularis, and dynamic internal and external rotation of the arm can aid in assessment of tendon integrity. In the event of a subscapularis tear, the long head of the biceps may sublux out of the bicipital groove and course inferiorly, becoming adherent to or lying just posterior to the subscapularis. A 70-degree scope may be useful for both visualization and arthroscopic fixation of subscapularis tears.

The LHBT is the next structure that should be visualized and probed. Through placement of the probe

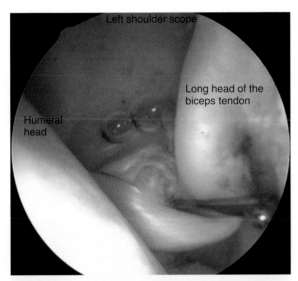

Figure 1-7. Technique for pulling the biceps tendon intraarticularly to evaluate the portion that normally lies in the intraarticular groove.

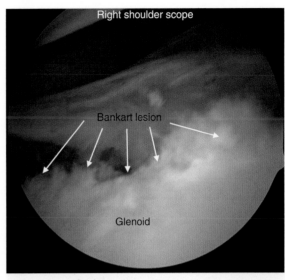

Figure 1-9. A Bankart lesion of the anteroinferior labrum and anteroinferior glenohumeral ligament.

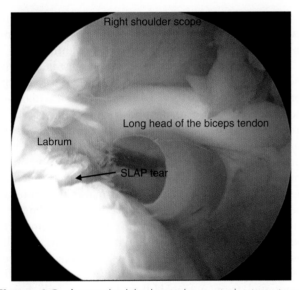

Figure 1-8. A superior labral anterior posterior tear, type II. *SLAP,* Superior labral anterior-posterior.

superior to the tendon, a portion of the biceps that lies within the bicipital groove may be pulled into the joint for inspection (Fig. 1-7). Both the upper and lower surfaces of the tendon should be visualized, looking for inflammation and/or tearing. The "lipstick lesion" of the biceps is a useful sign of bicipital tendonitis. The biceps should also be inspected at its proximal anchor site to rule out a SLAP tear (Fig. 1-8). Complete evaluation of the labral attachment of the LHBT may be performed by moving the arm from adduction and neutral rotation to 90 degrees of abduction and 90 degrees of external rotation. A tear that becomes evident with this maneuver is referred to as a *peelback lesion.*

Attention is then turned to the anteroinferior capsulolabral complex. This consists of the anterior labrum and the anterior and inferior capsular structures. The glenoid labrum deepens the glenoid fossa, enhances glenohumeral stability, and serves as the attachment site for the glenohumeral ligaments. Up to 20% of patients may have an anatomic anterior sulcus indenting the labrum, which can be differentiated from a pathologic labral lesion by smooth edges without evidence of fraying.[9] In cases of anterior instability, the anterior labrum may be torn, as in a Bankart lesion (Fig. 1-9), or may appear absent, as in an anterior labral periosteal sleeve avulsions (ALPSA).[6] In the latter case, the labrum has retracted medially and scarred to the anterior glenoid neck.

The inferior glenohumeral ligament (IGHL) complex is the next structure visualized on arthroscopic examination. Inferior capsular structures are very important to glenohumeral stability. If the inferior capsular structures are injured in isolation or in conjunction with labral tears, the arthroscopist may appreciate an increase in shoulder laxity and a positive "drive-through" sign on arthroscopic examination.[10] The IGHL is divided into the anterior (AIGHL) and posterior (PIGHL) segments These inferior ligaments resemble a hammock, tightening with shoulder abduction. The AIGHL originates between the 2- and 4-o'clock positions on the right shoulder and resists anterior humeral translation at 90 degrees of abduction and external rotation. This is the position of "apprehension" in patients with recurrent anterior instability.[7] The PIGHL originates from the 7- to 9-o'clock position on a right-sided glenoid and resists posterior humeral translation in an abducted shoulder.[11] In addition to a thorough examination of their origin at the glenoid labrum, site, the glenohumeral ligaments should be evaluated at their humeral insertion sites for rare avulsion injuries (humeral avulsion of the glenohumeral ligaments [HAGL] and reverse

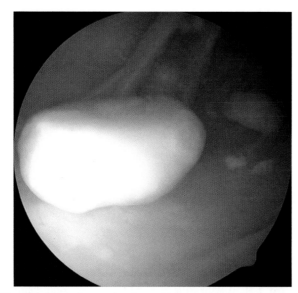

Figure 1-10. Loose bodies within the axillary pouch.

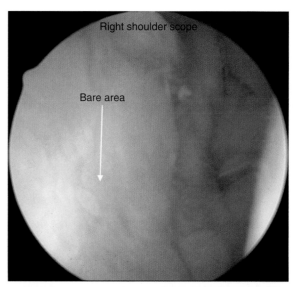

Figure 1-12. Bare area of the glenoid as viewed from the posterior portal with the patient in the beach chair position.

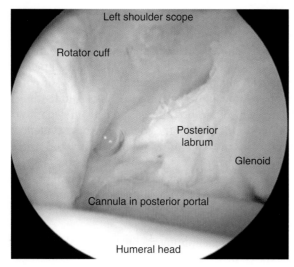

Figure 1-11. The posterior labral structures as viewed from anterior portal with the patient in the beach chair position.

humeral avulsion of the glenohumeral ligaments (RHAGL) lesions.[12] Inspection of the inferior pouch and posteroinferior recess should also include a search for loose bodies, as this is a common location for them to hide (Fig. 1-10).

After examination of the anterior and inferior capsulolabral structures, arthroscopic evaluation turns to the posterior labrum. A gross overview of the posterior labrum can be obtained by looking from the posterior portal, completing the circumferential tour of the glenoid soft tissue attachments. In cases with high suspicion for posterior labral injury, the arthroscope should be switched to an anterior or anterosuperior portal for more thorough evaluation and probing of the posterior labral and capsular structures (Fig. 1-11). In throwing athletes or football linemen, among others, a range of

posterior pathology may be appreciated, including reverse Bankart lesions, RHAGL lesions, Bennett lesions, or evidence of posteroinferior capsular tightness.

Remaining intraarticular evaluation must include the chondral surfaces of the glenoid and humerus, and the rotator cuff. Examination of the articular cartilage of the humeral head and glenoid includes the use of a probe, feeling the cartilage surfaces for evidence of softening, fissuring, or fragmentation. Internal and external rotation will aid the arthroscopist in visualization of the entirety of the humeral head. Of importance, the glenoid has a physiologic "bare area" that marks the center of the glenoid (Fig. 1-12). This reproducible landmark is an invaluable reference point for the measurement of glenoid bone loss in patients with recurrent shoulder instability. The humeral head has a similar bare area posterosuperiorly. This physiologic area must be differentiated from a true Hill-Sachs lesion, which is a pathologic osteochondral defect seen as a sequela of anterior shoulder dislocation.

The undersurface of the supraspinatus and infraspinatus can be fully evaluated from within the glenohumeral joint. The tendon insertion should be evaluated for fraying, partial or full thickness tearing, or calcification. Abduction and internal and external rotation of the humerus provide a complete view of the articular-sided tendon insertions (Fig. 1-13).

Once the glenohumeral joint has been fully evaluated, the arthroscope is moved to the subacromial space. The arm may be repositioned by changing the abduction angle (in the lateral decubitus position) or by providing inferior distraction (beach chair position) to increase the subacromial space. The trocar is withdrawn from the posterior portal so that the tip remains within the skin but superficial to the deltoid. The trocar is advanced to

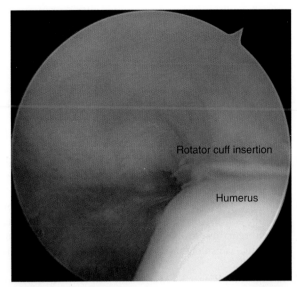

Figure 1-13. Intraarticular view of the rotator cuff insertion.

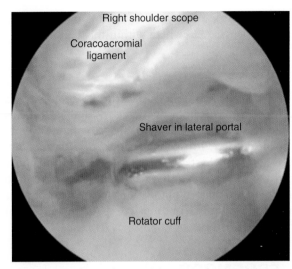

Figure 1-15. The subacromial space after partial bursectomy with the shaver in the lateral portal.

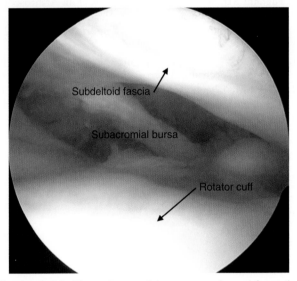

Figure 1-14. The subacromial space as viewed from the posterior portal.

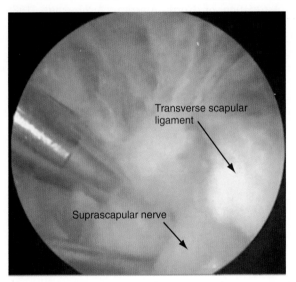

Figure 1-16. The suprascapular nerve at the suprascapular notch.

palpate the junction of the posterior acromion and the deltoid muscle. The trocar is then introduced through the deltoid and directed toward the anterolateral edge of the acromion. Once the anterolateral edge of the acromion has been reached with the obturator, sweeping motions are used to brush tissue off the undersurface of the acromion, freeing up a space for the arthroscope. The subacromial space should be visualized as a "room with a view" (Fig. 1-14). A spinal needle is used to establish a lateral working portal. If necessary, a mechanized shaver or radiofrequency device may be used to perform a thorough bursectomy for improved visualization (Fig. 1-15).

Within the subacromial space, the coracoacromial (CA) ligament insertion on the undersurface of the acromion (see Fig. 1-15) is examined. Fraying or thickening

of this ligament is indicative of subacromial impingement. Releasing or excising the CA ligament may reveal an acromial bone spur at the anterolateral corner of the acromion. Dynamic evaluation in abduction and external and internal rotation may assist in recognition of pathologic impingement or rotator cuff tear. After bursectomy has been performed, the bursal side of the rotator cuff insertion can be clearly visualized. The tendons are inspected for partial or full-thickness tears. Careful dissection medially may expose the AC joint anteriorly and the spine of the scapula posteriorly. Advanced arthroscopic evaluation includes identification and evaluation of the subdeltoid space and identification of the bicipital groove, pectoralis major insertion, and suprascapular nerve at both the suprascapular (Fig. 1-16) and spinoglenoid notches. However, these techniques are beyond the scope of this chapter and are discussed elsewhere within this text.

CONCLUSION

Shoulder arthroscopy provides the surgeon with an invaluable tool for both the diagnosis and treatment of shoulder joint and subacromial space pathology. Potential benefits of arthroscopy are numerous, and complications are rare. Systematic and reproducible diagnostic arthroscopic examination is a critical tool for the shoulder surgeon to master. Innovations in surgical technique and instrumentation continue to expand the indications for shoulder arthroscopy.

REFERENCES

1. Complications in arthroscopy: the knee and other joints. Committee on Complications of the Arthroscopy Association of North America. *Arthroscopy*. 1986;2: 253-258.
2. Cole BJ, L'Insalata J, Irrgang J, et al. Comparison of arthroscopic and open anterior shoulder stabilization. A two to six-year follow-up study. *J Bone Joint Surg Am*. 2000;82:1108-1114.
3. Davis AD, Kakar S, Moros C, et al. Arthroscopic versus open acromioplasty: a meta-analysis. *Am J Sports Med*. 2010;38:613-618.
4. Nho SJ, Shindle MK, Sherman SL, et al. Systematic review of arthroscopic rotator cuff repair and mini-open rotator cuff repair. *J Bone Joint Surg Am*. 2007;89(Suppl 3): 127-136.
5. Morgan CD, Burkhart SS, Palmeri M, et al. Type II SLAP lesions: three subtypes and their relationships to superior instability and rotator cuff tears. *Arthroscopy*. 1998;14: 553-565.
6. Neviaser TJ. Arthroscopy of the shoulder. *Orthop Clin North Am*. 1987;18:361-372.
7. Turkel SJ, Panio MW, Marshall JL, et al. Stabilizing mechanisms preventing anterior dislocation of the glenohumeral joint. *J Bone Joint Surg Am*. 1981;63:1208-1217.
8. Williams MM, Snyder SJ, Buford Jr D. The Buford complex—the "cord-like" middle glenohumeral ligament and absent anterosuperior labrum complex: a normal anatomic capsulolabral variant. *Arthroscopy*. 1994;10: 241-247.
9. Levine WN, Rieger K, McCluskey 3rd GM. Arthroscopic treatment of anterior shoulder instability. *Instr Course Lect*. 2005;54:87-96.
10. Pagnani MJ, Warren RF, Altchek DW, et al. Arthroscopic shoulder stabilization using transglenoid sutures. A four-year minimum followup. *Am J Sports Med*. 1996;24: 459-467.
11. Jobe CM. Posterior superior glenoid impingement: expanded spectrum. *Arthroscopy*. 1995;11:530-536.
12. Wolf EM, Cheng JC, Dickson K. Humeral avulsion of glenohumeral ligaments as a cause of anterior shoulder instability. *Arthroscopy*. 1995;11:600-607.

Chapter 2

Rehabilitation of the Athlete's Shoulder

W. Ben Kibler, Aaron Sciascia, John McMullen, and Tim Uhl

Chapter Synopsis

- The throwing motion is accomplished through use of the kinetic chain. Rehabilitation of shoulder injuries should involve evaluation for and restoration of all kinetic chain deficits that may hinder kinetic chain function. Rehabilitation programs focused on eliminating kinetic chain deficits and soreness should follow a proximal-to-distal pattern in which lower extremity impairments are addressed in addition to the upper extremity impairments. A logical progression focusing on flexibility, strength, proprioception, and endurance with kinetic chain influence is recommended.

Important Points

- The orthopedic surgeon has specific roles in rehabilitation that will result in optimal restoration of function in the athlete with a shoulder injury.
- Proper kinetic chain function is imperative to efficient and effective overhead throwing.
- Inefficient mechanics or physical impairments may hinder an athlete's ability to perform at optimal levels.
- Shoulder injuries are frequently associated with alterations in other parts of the kinetic chain.
- Compromised tissue or weakness or tightness of lower and upper extremity structures should be addressed as part of the total rehabilitation effort.
- Use of a kinetic chain–focused approach will aid clinicians in addressing all factors that can deleteriously affect the multisegmented throwing motion.

Clinical and Surgical Pearls

- Address soft tissue inflexibilities of upper and lower extremities.

- Facilitate scapular retraction and depression with thoracic extension.
- Encourage scapular retraction to control scapular protraction.
- Maximum rotator cuff strength is achieved only from a stabilized scapular base.
- Closed chain exercise for the glenohumeral joint should be implemented before open chain exercise.
- Work in multiple planes of motion.

Clinical and Surgical Pitfalls

- Postural abnormalities can negatively affect kinetic chain function. These should be addressed initially in rehabilitation.
- Core stability, focusing on both local and global muscles, is critical to the success of kinetic chain–focused rehabilitation.
- Inflexibilities such as pectoralis minor tightness and glenohumeral internal rotation deficit need to be assessed and treated.
- The serratus anterior is a multifunctional muscle that is imperative to the stability and mobility of the scapula. Focusing on it solely as a protractor can lead to poor rehabilitation outcomes.
- The lower trapezius is a key muscle in stabilizing the abducted arm.
- Muscle endurance should not be overlooked. High-repetition, low-load exercise will help develop muscle endurance but should be attempted after kinetic chain deficits have been corrected.

Advances in understanding the pathology and appropriate implementation of treatment for shoulder joint injuries have resulted in greater success in defining and restoring the anatomic lesions associated with shoulder dysfunction. Similarly, advances in understanding and implementation of rehabilitation principles for the shoulder have resulted in greater success in restoring the physiologic and biomechanical alterations associated with shoulder dysfunction.

Rehabilitation programs for the shoulder should focus on restoration of functional ability rather than solely on resolution of symptoms. The orthopedic surgeon and the physical therapist must identify and treat all of the structures that are limiting this functional return. Rehabilitation of the shoulder can be both difficult and complex. Multiple joints are involved, and shoulder pain or the pathology that is causing it may actually be the result of distant body biomechanical and physiologic alterations.

This chapter discusses the roles of the orthopedic surgeon in shoulder rehabilitation, presents the basic science in physiology and biomechanics as the basis for shoulder rehabilitation, and offers guidelines and clinical practices that implement the rehabilitation protocols.

THE ORTHOPEDIC SURGEON'S ROLES IN REHABILITATION

The orthopedic surgeon plays several roles in shoulder rehabilitation. The first is to understand the basic principles of the kinetic chain. The biomechanical model for striking and throwing sports is an open-ended kinetic chain of segments that work in a proximal-to-distal sequence.[1,2] The proximal segment contributions are key components of the sequential activation of body segments that is necessary to accomplish any athletic activity. The kinetic chain harmonizes the interdependent segments to produce a desired result at the distal segment. The goal of the kinetic chain activation sequence is to impart maximum velocity or force through the distal segment (the hand) to the ball, racquet, or other implement. The shoulder does not function in isolation but as a link in the kinetic chain activity that optimizes shoulder function. Alterations in any of the kinetic chain links can affect the shoulder, and alterations in the shoulder can affect the other kinetic chain links. The ultimate velocity of the distal segment is highly dependent on the velocity of the proximal segments. The proximal segments accelerate the entire chain and sequentially transfer force and energy to the next distal segment.[2-5] Because of their large relative mass, the proximal segments are responsible for most of the force and kinetic energy that are generated in

the kinetic chain.[1] As a result, lower extremity force production is more highly correlated with ball velocity than is upper extremity force production.[6]

This interaction creates two implications for shoulder rehabilitation. First, the evaluation and identification process preceding shoulder treatment and rehabilitation should include more than just local shoulder structures. The evaluation process should result in a complete and accurate diagnosis of all of the altered structures throughout the kinetic chain. Second, optimum restoration of shoulder function requires that all the kinetic chain segment interactions are reestablished to meet the individual's needs that existed before injury.

The second role of the orthopedic surgeon is to establish the complete and accurate diagnosis of the anatomic, biomechanical, and physiologic alterations that may be present in shoulder injury and dysfunction. This may seem obvious but is sometimes difficult to implement unless the entire kinetic chain is screened for alterations. Nonetheless, the actual shoulder injury is the primary factor that determines treatment and rehabilitation. This may involve tendon injury or tear, instability, or joint internal derangement, whose overt clinical symptoms can be evaluated by standard diagnostic methods. However, both nonovert local and distant alterations are frequently associated with shoulder clinical symptoms and dysfunction.

The most common local alterations are decreased shoulder internal rotation,[7] which creates altered glenohumeral translations,[7,8] altered strength or strength balance,[7] and alterations in scapular motion and position (scapular dyskinesis).[7,9-11] Inappropriate scapular motion can disrupt the normal smooth coupling of scapulohumeral movement in voluntary activation and is present in most patients with shoulder impingement. Distant alterations include lumbar muscle inflexibility and muscle weakness,[12] as well as hip and knee inflexibility.[13] Because these alterations are common findings in shoulder injury, they need to be assessed through a screening process in the clinical evaluation. This requires a clinical evaluation approach known as "victims and culprits," in which the site of symptoms is the "victim," but the "culprits" may include alterations at other sites.

The clinical evaluation should include screening tests for hip and trunk posture and functional strength. Our screening examination includes standing posture evaluation of legs and lumbar, thoracic, and cervical spine; bilateral hip range-of-motion assessment; trunk flexibility assessment; and a one-leg stability series (Fig. 2-1), which assesses control of the trunk over the leg. Any observed abnormalities should be further evaluated in more detail.

Scapular evaluation is performed from behind the patient. It should assess resting position, and the examiner should note any asymmetries with respect to bony

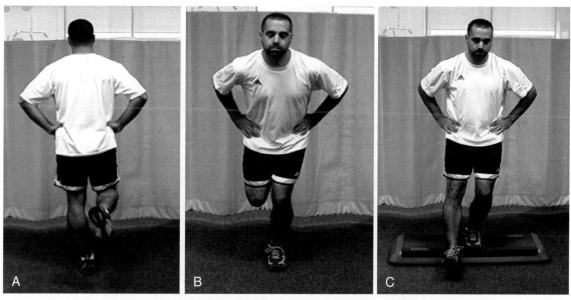

Figure 2-1. The single-leg stability series used to assess dynamic hip strength.

landmarks of the inferior angle, medial, and superior border. Dynamic motion screening involves evaluation of the same asymmetries of scapular control with weighted arm abduction and forward flexion, in both ascent and descent.[14,15] Observation of any of the three types ("yes" indicates that asymmetry is seen, "no" indicates that asymmetry is not seen) correlates highly with actual biomechanical alteration and can be reliably used as a marker of scapular dyskinesis that needs to be addressed in rehabilitation.[16]

The third role of the orthopedic surgeon is to determine the timing of entry into and exit from the rehabilitation program. In many cases, entry into rehabilitation should be started before surgery to address deficits of flexibility and strength both locally and at distant portions of the kinetic chain. In many cases, rehabilitation interventions focused on addressing the correct culprits may prevent the need for surgical intervention Postoperative entry into rehabilitation may be quite early, while the shoulder is still protected. Kinetic chain rehabilitation of the legs, trunk, and scapula may be started early, and closed-chain range of motion may be started in safe ranges determined at the time of surgery. Exit from rehabilitation should be based not only on healing of the anatomic lesion, but on normalization of physiology and biomechanics to allow functional return to the demands of the sport or activity. This requires frequent functional assessment as rehabilitation proceeds. Key functional components include range of motion, balanced strength, intact kinetic chain, and functional activities.

The fourth role is to be familiar with the phases of the rehabilitation program, the content and goals of each stage, and the criteria for progression between stages. Rehabilitation may be divided into three phases (acute, recovery, and functional) based on anatomic injury, anatomic healing, functional capabilities, and functional tasks (Fig. 2-2).

The fifth role is to guide the pace of the rehabilitation protocol. In the early stages this will be determined by the anatomic diagnosis and integrity of the anatomic repair. In later stages, it will be determined by the progressive acquisition of components of normal kinetic chain function, normal flexibility, normal strength, and sport- or activity-specific functions. This requires periodic reassessment of the patient and frequent precise communication with the physical therapist or athletic trainer. Rehabilitation should be viewed as a flow of exercises that will vary according to stages of healing and reestablishment of key points of muscle and joint function. This flow is indicated in the rehabilitation flow sheet based on categories of rehabilitation exercises (Table 2-1). In most cases it is not appropriate to abdicate the responsibility or involvement in rehabilitation by marking "evaluate and treat" on a physical therapy prescription. Even though the orthopedic surgeon does not actually provide the details of the exercises, the surgeon must be an integral part of the team that provides the rehabilitation protocol. Several guidelines can be followed to guide the flow and make sure kinetic chain principles are followed.

The sixth and most important role is communication, because the physician is ultimately responsible for the care of the patient. Establishing an open line of communication with the other members of the rehabilitation team is critical. This may be done in several ways, including written notes, prearranged protocols, sheets with specific guidelines, or direct electronic or phone

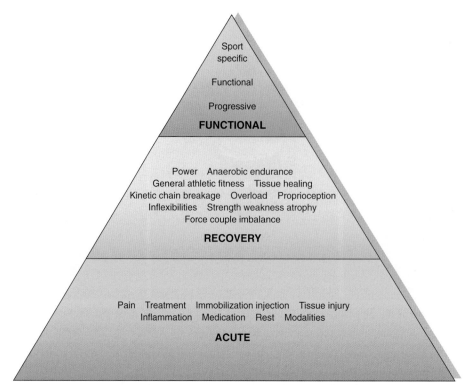

Figure 2-2. Functional progression pyramid.

communications. In an ideal situation the physician has an established working relationship with the physical therapist or athletic trainer. However, in practice this may not be the case; therefore the physician must make it clear to the patient that any questions from the rehabilitating clinician should be directed back to the referring physician. During subsequent follow-up visits, the physician should share primary concerns and precautions in the referring prescription. The notation "continue therapy" does not provide adequate communication or direction to yield optimal outcome for the patient.

GUIDELINE 1: PROXIMAL SEGMENT CONTROL

Optimum shoulder and arm function in both normal athletic activity and rehabilitation is dependent on activation of the proximal segments of the kinetic chain: the legs, pelvis, and spine. If these segments are altered in posture, flexibility, or strength, these alterations should be corrected in the early stages of rehabilitation. If and when these segments are normal, they should be used to initiate scapular and arm activation. Early in rehabilitation, the inhibited scapular muscles or the injured or inhibited shoulder muscles require a large degree of facilitation, so the role of proximal segments is increased. These exercises may be started in the early stage of rehabilitation, even in the preoperative stage, because they do not rely on shoulder motion or loading.

Practice

Specific exercises include step up–step down with trunk extension, front and side lunges, one-leg and two-leg squats, and hip flexions and extensions with trunk rotations (Fig. 2-3). These may be done on a stable surface and may progress to unstable surfaces for added difficulty and proprioceptive input.

GUIDELINE 2: SCAPULAR REHABILITATION

Scapular motion in retraction, protraction, and elevation is multiplanar. Optimal scapular motion maintains rotator cuff length/tension ratios, thereby improving force production and reducing rotator cuff energy requirements during arm motion. Scapular muscle activation precedes rotator cuff activation in the throwing or striking sequence.[17]

Loss of scapular control, or scapular dyskinesis, is noted early in shoulder injury and is very frequently associated with shoulder injury. This is possibly caused by inhibition of coupled muscle activation to elevate, depress, retract, and protract the scapula and subsequent substitute patterns of muscle activation.[18] The lower trapezius and serratus anterior appear to be most inhibited, and the upper trapezius most commonly becomes overactivated. This creates the most common manifestation of scapular dyskinesis, lack of effective retraction with a tendency toward protraction.

TABLE 2-1. Rehabilitation Flow Sheet

| | Weeks (Estimate) | | | | | | | | | |
| | Acute | | | Recovery | | | | Functional | | |
Stages (Estimate)	1	2	3	4	5	6	7	8	9	10
Proximal Segment Control										
Step up, step down	X	X	X							
Lunges	X	X	X							
Squats	X	X	X	X			X	X		
Hip extension, trunk rotation	X	X	X	X	X	X	X	X		
Scapular Rehabilitation										
Pectoralis minor–upper trapezius stretch	X*	X*	X	X						
Posterior joint mobilization	X*	X*	X	X	X					
Hip and trunk extension with scapular retraction	X	X	X	X	X					
Diagonal rotation with scapular retraction	X	X	X	X	X	X	X			
Pinches	X	X								
Scapular clock	X*	X*	X	X	X					
Low row	X*	X*	X							
Lawnmower			X	X	X	X	X	X		
Shoulder dumps			X	X	X	X	X	X		
Punches			X	X	X	X	X	X	X	
Table pushup		X	X	X						
Normal pushup plus					X	X	X	X		
Glenohumeral Rehabilitation										
Weight shifts		X*	X*	X						
Inferior glide	X*	X*	X	X	X					
Wall washes				X*	X	X	X			
Rotation diagonal					X	X	X	X	X	
Isolated rotator cuff						X	X			
Plyometrics										
Lower extremity				X	X	X	X	X	X	
Medicine ball						X	X	X	X	X
Rotation diagonals						X	X	X	X	X
Ball drops						X	X	X	X	X

*May be performed if indicated by tissue healing.
Adapted from Kibler WB, McMullen J, Uhl TL. Shoulder rehabilitation strategies, guidelines, and practice. *Oper Tech Sports Med.* 2000;8:258-267.

Practice

Hip and trunk extension patterns are used to initiate and facilitate scapular retraction. Scapular retraction exercises can be started in the preoperative or early healing stages of rehabilitation because they do not require shoulder or arm movement. Adjustments in arm position and arm load can occur as shoulder healing proceeds, and scapular control exercises should be continued throughout the intermediate

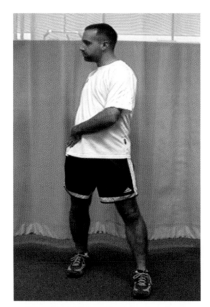

Figure 2-3. Hip extension with trunk rotation.

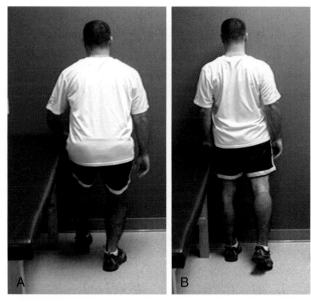

Figure 2-5. Low row exercise for serratus anterior and lower trapezius strengthening.

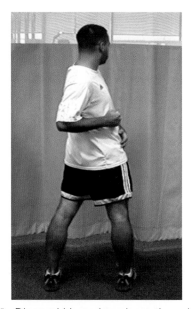

Figure 2-4. Diagonal hip and trunk rotation with scapular retraction.

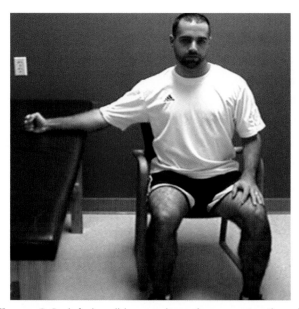

Figure 2-6. Inferior glide exercise using cocontraction of shoulder stabilizers.

recovery and sport-specific functional phases of rehabilitation.

Early-stage exercises to regain scapular retraction control include ipsilateral and contralateral hip and trunk extension with scapular retraction, diagonal hip and trunk rotation with scapular retraction (Fig. 2-4), and isometric scapular pinches.[19] These all can be done even with the arm in a sling. When arm motion and shoulder loads are safe to perform, an extremely effective set of exercises for initiation of scapular retraction and depression is the scapular stability series, including the "low row" (Fig. 2-5), inferior glide (Fig. 2-6), and

lawnmower (Fig. 2-7), which includes trunk extension, scapular retraction, and shoulder extension with the arm close to the side.[20] These may be started in isometric fashion and progressed to isotonic, concentric, and eccentric work with rubber tubing. A scapular exercise that may be done in the acute phase, when the healing tissue can tolerate mobility, is the scapular clock. This involves elevation-depression and retraction-protraction exercises with the hand on a wall or a movable object. Exercises for the recovery and functional phases include shoulder "dumps," a trunk rotation–scapula retraction–shoulder extension exercise, and punches with dumbbells

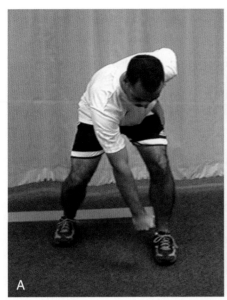
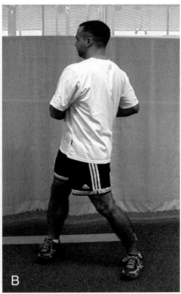

Figure 2-7. Lawnmower exercise.

or tubing, which load the serratus anterior and posterior shoulder musculature. Pushups with a plus, or full protraction, are also an advanced scapular exercise. They may be done initially on a table and then advanced to normal style.

These exercises require muscular flexibility and joint mobility. The upper trapezius and pectoralis minor are common sites of myofascial tightness, and shoulder internal rotation is frequently decreased. The anterior and superior muscle inflexibility creates a tendency for upward and forward tilt, and posterior tightness creates a "wind-up" situation of pulling the scapula forward in follow-through. Manual stretching, massage techniques, and joint mobilizations must be used to normalize these alterations.[21]

GUIDELINE 3: GLENOHUMERAL REHABILITATION

Dynamic glenohumeral stability can be improved by eliminating joint mobility deficits, thereby decreasing abnormal joint translations in the midrange of shoulder motion, by positioning and moving the glenoid socket in a "ball on a sea lion's nose" relation to the moving humerus so that concavity and compression of the joint are maintained by active rotator cuff contraction.

In this stability role, as well as in its role in humeral head depression, the rotator cuff is essentially operating as a "compressor cuff." Rotator cuff activation is coupled with and follows scapular muscle activation so that the rotator cuff muscles work from a stabilized and optimally positioned base, are physiologically activated, and are mechanically placed in an optimal length-tension arrangement to create appropriate joint stiffness.[22-24]

Joint range of motion, muscle flexibility, and adequate tissue healing are necessary so that the glenohumeral rehabilitation program will generate minimal substitute patterns. Proximal segment and scapular control are necessary for glenohumeral motion and facilitation. These controls are accomplished in the acute and recovery stages. Glenohumeral emphasis in rehabilitation of "shoulder problems" such as impingement, tendinitis, or mild instability is toward the end of the rehabilitation stages, rather than the beginning.

Integrating the rotator cuff muscles within the kinetic chain can be accomplished by "closing the chain." Activities performed with the hand in contact with a firm surface simultaneously activates the rotator cuff, scapular, and axial-humeral musculature to stabilize the humerus in the glenoid. The amount of load is proportional to the muscular activation[25,26]; therefore the rehabilitation program can be progressed by simply increasing the weight-bearing load. In addition, closed chain exercises reduce shear forces across the joint[25] as long as the humerus is kept in the scapular plane when loads are applied.

Practice

Closed chain exercise practices may be started in early rehabilitation stages with the hand in a relatively fixed position, below shoulder level on a table. Weight shifts on a table or balance board are safe when this position is used. When the arm may be raised toward shoulder height, scapular clock exercises are effective axial loading rotator cuff exercises. These exercises progress by placement of the hand on an unstable surface, such as a ball, or by use of "wall washes," in which an axial load is applied through the moving hand. An advanced axial loading exercise that transforms into open chain activity is the internal and external rotation diagonal, with the shoulder moving through 90 degrees of abduction and using rubber tubing resistance. Isolated rotator cuff exercises may be used if any local deficit is still present. Internal and external rotation strengthening should be done at the functional position of 90 degrees of abduction for most overhead athletes.

GUIDELINE 4: PLYOMETRIC EXERCISES

Power is required for shoulder function in throwing or striking. Plyometric training, through activation or stretching and shortening responses in muscles, is the most effective method of power development. Because power is generated in the entire kinetic chain, plyometric training should be done in every segment. Plyometrics can be instituted in uninjured areas early in rehabilitation but must be deferred to later stages in injured areas because of the large range of required motions and large forces developed.

Practice

Lunges, vertical jumps, and depth jumps are some methods of lower extremity plyometrics. Trunk and upper extremity plyometrics include rotation diagonals, medicine ball rotations and pushes, and ball drops.

GUIDELINES FOR PROGRESSION

Because this type of rehabilitation program focuses on functional return of kinetic chain patterns, there is less emphasis on specific stages, pathways, or specific isolated exercises and more emphasis on flow and overlap in the acquisition of functional control of the various segments. The program must be flexible enough to be applied over a wide range of the individual aptitudes. New exercises are instituted when the segment function is appropriate.

Normal pelvis control over the planted leg is a prerequisite for proximal segment control. Scapula retraction should be well established before humeral elevation strengthening activities are emphasized, as this allows coupled shoulder motion and coupled rotator cuff muscle activation. Normal glenohumeral rotation is required to decrease joint translation and motion and should be reestablished before glenohumeral strengthening is begun. If the patient shows substitute activities or is not progressing, the rehabilitation program should be modified to address underlying deficits, usually in the proximal kinetic chain, which may be limiting the progression.

GUIDELINES FOR RETURN TO PLAY

Return to play is proceeded by demonstrating proper functional activities with normal biomechanical patterns. The loads or repetitions should approximate 85% of normal demands before return to full functional activities. In overhead athletes the functional phase should be an incremental integration of functional activities. Return to play should be the natural progression of this phase. The ability to function at high levels often proceeds anatomic healing, as illustrated in a healing rotator cuff tendon.[27] The rehabilitation of the athlete is not completed when the athlete return to play, as persistent monitoring during the initial season of performance is still necessary and is primarily the responsibility of the rehabilitation specialists who is with the athlete on a more regular basis than the physician.

SUMMARY

This framework for rehabilitation is consistent with the proximal-to-distal kinetic chain biomechanical model and applies current concepts of motor control and closed chain exercises. This framework approaches the final goal—glenohumeral motion and function—through facilitation by scapular control, and scapular control through facilitation of hip and trunk activation. The orthopedic surgeon plays key roles in establishing the optimal anatomic basis for rehabilitation, overseeing the pace of the rehabilitation protocols, determining the progression between phases, and delineating the return-to-play criteria.

REFERENCES

1. Kibler WB. Biomechanical analysis of the shoulder during tennis activities. *Clin Sports Med*. 1995;14:79-86.
2. Putnam CA. Sequential motions of body segments in striking and throwing skills: Descriptions and explanations. *J Biomech*. 1993;26(Suppl 1):125-135.
3. Elliott BC, Marshall R, Noffal G. Contributions of upper limb segment rotations during the power serve in tennis. *J Appl Biomech*. 1995;11:443-447.
4. Fleisig G, Barrentine SW, Escamilla RF, et al. Biomechanics of overhand throwing with implications for injuries. *Sports Med*. 1996;21(6):421-437.
5. Hirashima M, Kadota H, Sakurai S, et al. Sequential muscle activity and its functional role in the upper extremity and trunk during overarm throwing. *J Sports Sci*. 2002;20:301-310.
6. Kraemer WJ, Triplett NT, Fry AC. An in-depth sports medicine profile of women college tennis players. *J Sports Rehabil*. 1995;4:79-88.
7. Burkhart SS, Morgan CD, Kibler WB. The disabled throwing shoulder: Spectrum of pathology Part I: Pathoanatomy and biomechanics. *Arthroscopy*. 2003;19(4): 404-420.

8. Harryman II DT, Sidles JA, Clark JM, et al. Translation of the humeral head on the glenoid with passive glenohumeral motion. *J Bone Joint Surg Am*. 1990;72(9): 1334-1343.

9. Kibler WB. The role of the scapula in athletic function. *Am J Sports Med*. 1998;26:325-337.

10. Laudner KG, Myers JB, Pasquale MR, et al. Scapular dysfunction in throwers with pathologic internal impingement. *J Orthop Sports Phys Ther*. 2006;36(7): 485-494.

11. Myers JB, Laudner KG, Pasquale MR, et al. Glenohumeral range of motion deficits and posterior shoulder tightness in throwers with pathologic internal impingement. *Am J Sports Med*. 2006;34:385-391.

12. Vad VB, Bhat AL, Basrai D, et al. Low back pain in professional golfers: the role of associated hip and low back range-of-motion deficits. *Am J Sports Med*. 2004;32(2): 494-497.

13. Robb AJ, Fleisig GS, Wilk KE, et al. Passive ranges of motion of the hips and their relationship with pitching biomechanics and ball velocity in professional baseball pitchers. *Am J Sports Med*. 2010;38(12):2487-2493.

14. McClure PW, Tate AR, Kareha S, et al. A clinical method for identifying scapular dyskinesis: Part 1: Reliability. *J Athl Train*. 2009;44(2):160-164.

15. Tate AR, McClure PW, Kareha S, et al. A clinical method for identifying scapular dyskinesis: Part 2: Validity. *J Athl Train*. 2009;44(2):165-173.

16. Uhl TL, Kibler WB, Gecewich B, et al. Evaluation of clinical assessment methods for scapular dyskinesis. *Arthroscopy*. 2009;25(11):1240-1248.

17. Kibler WB, Chandler TJ, Shapiro R, et al. Muscle activation in coupled scapulohumeral motions in the high performance tennis serve. *Br J Sports Med*. 2007;41: 745-749.

18. Kibler WB, Sciascia AD. Current concepts: Scapular dyskinesis. *Br J Sports Med*. 2010;44(5):300-305.

19. Kibler WB, McMullen J, Uhl TL. Shoulder rehabilitation strategies, guidelines, and practice. *Oper Tech Sports Med*. 2000;8(4):258-267.

20. Kibler WB, Sciascia AD, Uhl TL, et al. Electromyographic analysis of specific exercises for scapular control in early phases of shoulder rehabilitation. *Am J Sports Med*. 2008;36(9):1789-1798.

21. Borstad JD, Ludewig PM. Comparison of three stretches for the pectoralis minor muscle. *J Shoulder Elbow Surg*. 2006;15(3):324-330.

22. Kibler WB, Sciascia AD, Dome DC. Evaluation of apparent and absolute supraspinatus strength in patients with shoulder injury using the scapular retraction test. *Am J Sports Med*. 2006;34(10):1643-1647.

23. Smith J, Kotajarvi BR, Padgett DJ, et al. Effect of scapular protraction and retraction on isometric shoulder elevation strength. *Arch Phys Med Rehabil*. 2002;83:367-370.

24. Tate AR, McClure P, Kareha S, et al. Effect of the scapula reposition test on shoulder impingement symptoms and elevation strength in overhead athletes. *J Orthop Sports Phys Ther*. 2008;38(1):4-11.

25. Dillman CJ, Murray TA, Hinterneister RA. Biomechanical differences of open and closed chain exercises with respect to the shoulder. *J Sports Rehabil*. 1994;3:228-238.

26. Uhl TL, Carver TJ, Mattacola CG, et al. Shoulder musculature activation during upper extremity weight-bearing exercise. *J Orthop Sports Phys Ther*. 2003;33(3): 109-117.

27. Charousset C, Grimberg J, Duranthon LD, et al. The time for functional recovery after arthroscopic rotator cuff repair: Correlation with tendon healing controlled by computed tomography arthrography. *Arthroscopy*. 2008;24(1):25-33.

Chapter 3

Knot-Tying and Suture-Passing Techniques

Adam M. Smith, Scott J. Deering, and Mary Lloyd Ireland

Chapter Synopsis

- This chapter reviews basic principles and techniques of arthroscopic suture passage and knot tying. The authors also review basics types of instrumentation and different types of arthroscopic knots.

Important Points

- A firm understanding of available technology including different anchor types and available instrumentation is essential for a smooth arthroscopic case.
- Confidence with multiple suture-passing devices makes a case go more smoothly.
- Learn at least one sliding and one nonsliding knot.
- Practice, practice, practice your knot-tying skills.

Clinical and Surgical Pearls and Pitfalls

Suture Passing

- Create accessory portals under direct vision using a spinal needle to assess angle of entry to be able to successfully pass suture through tissue.
- An attempt should be made to place the portal in an adequate position to allow for a reasonable amount of swelling. For example, placement of the lateral portal too close to the lateral aspect of the acromion may lead to difficulty performing adequate acromioplasty and bursectomy.
- Maximize visualization before starting the reparative procedure. Remove obstructing bursa or soft tissue.
- Perform a complete survey of the joint and periarticular structures before beginning the repair. Focusing on only the known pathology may lead to missed diagnoses.
- Make a plan. Make sure all potential equipment and devices are available before the case.
- Work quickly on secondary procedures such as acromioplasty to minimize unnecessary soft tissue extravasation.

- Obtain adequate hemostasis. Failure to do so may ultimately lead to longer operative times with difficulty visualizing the structures. The anesthesia team should maintain blood pressure less than 100 mm Hg systolic to maximize visualization of work in the subacromial space via the arthroscopy.
- Prevent tangling of sutures when multiple anchors are used. We recommend that sutures from each anchor be placed in different portals to prevent entanglement. Other options include keeping the sutures "outside" of a cannula interposed between the cannula and soft tissue, or using a small stab incision to serve as a suture repository while other suture limbs are being passed.
- Different repairs require different suture passers. Gaining comfort with multiple suture-passing techniques allows for better tissue fixation and a quicker operative procedure.

Suture Tying

- A clear cannula in the working portal allows visualization and prevents soft tissue from interfering with the knot as it slides to the tissue.
- Only one set of suture should be retrieved into the working portal used for tying the knot.
- Use the portal that is best directed over the anchor to allow better suture sliding. Be sure to check that the suture slides easily before attempting to tie a sliding knot.
- If the suture does not slide, a nonsliding knot with reversed half hitches is necessary for maximum fixation to be obtained.
- Before the knot is tied, a knot pusher may be passed down the post suture to untwist the suture.[1]
- For nonsliding knots, we tie at least six half hitches, alternating the post and reversing the throws with each (underhand and overhand).

Continued

- Advanced arthroscopists may choose to forego the use of a cannula. If this method is chosen, we recommend that a ring forceps be placed around both suture limbs inside the working space and retrieved together to avoid soft tissue interposition.

- Select the suture limb that will function as the "post" that allows for best tissue approximation and compression. In a mattress suture configuration, the post can be either limb. In the simple suture configuration, pick the post away from articular cartilage. This suture limb is usually on the tissue side, allowing for maximal compression of the tissue against bone and also directing the knot away from the joint, thus avoiding articular injury from the resultant knot.[1]

- Place a clamp to the end of the suture post limb before tying a knot. This prevents the knot pusher from sliding off the post and provides resistance as the knot is tightened.

- Visualize the knot as it slides to the tissue to ensure that the tissue is compressed to the desired location.

- Maintain tension on the post limb as the knot is seated to avoid loosening.

- "Past pointing" is a technique by which the knot pusher is used to tension the knot by switching the tension to the loop limb and pushing past the knot with the post limb of suture (see Fig. 3-7). This technique allows the knot to fully seat, which increases the knot security provided by the knot's internal friction.

- After an initial sliding knot is tied, reversed half hitches on alternating posts should be thrown and seated with the knot pusher, using past pointing to prevent the knot from coming loose or backing out.

- Be patient. Allow extra time on all arthroscopic cases in the beginning.

- Practice your knot-tying skills. The time to practice is before the case when you are not under pressure. When practicing, use bigger string or rope to view the knot configuration. Dry and wet laboratories are extremely helpful and should be used for training when possible.

- Management of suture requires careful attention. You must practice and visualize your knot tying. Make it as easy and automatic as tying your shoes.

 Video

- Video 3-1: Shoulder arthroscopic knot-tying

Arthroscopic surgical techniques have advanced as technology and surgical expertise have expanded. Less invasive soft tissue repair, such as rotator cuff or labral repairs, must focus on an anatomic approach that relies on strong fixation of the tissue to either bone or other soft tissue via a surgeon-tied knot. Suture passage and knot tying remain technically challenging exercises that can frustrate any surgeon regardless of experience level. Revisit your memories of learning to tie your shoes as a child. Arthroscopic knot tying must be practiced and must become as easy as tying your shoes. This chapter reviews the basics of soft tissue suture passage and arthroscopic knot tying via standard arthroscopic instrumentation.

INSTRUMENTATION

Unlike open surgery in which the surgeon has direct access to the tissue being repaired, arthroscopic surgery requires different techniques to tie effective knots that can resist displacement and allow for healing. Arthroscopic knot-tying methods have advanced through the years along with advances in implants and instrumentation. This section focuses on the essential "tools of the trade" to make an arthroscopic procedure go more smoothly.

Suture Anchors

The advent of the suture anchor has dramatically expanded the options for tissue repair. Numerous suture anchor designs are available; anchors come in multiple sizes, allowing maximum fixation strength of tissue to bone.[2] Anchors may be made of metal, absorbable material, or plastic and should allow for sutures to slide easily through the eyelet. The anchor, when inserted into the bone, allows suture to be passed through soft tissue and affixed to the desired anatomic location in a predictable fashion. Multiple sutures may be preloaded into the anchor, allowing for multiple points of soft tissue fixation and decreased load on each suture knot.[3] Although the choice of the best anchor for each surgical procedure is beyond the scope of this chapter, a basic understanding of anchor types is advised.

Cannulas

Arthroscopic cannulas allow for suture passage through tissues, avoiding incorporation of unwanted soft tissue in the repair constructs.[4] Sutures and instruments that are not passed through a cannula can be trapped in soft tissues, causing significant difficulty in knot tying, which may result in increased operative times, less secure fixation, and generalized frustration for the surgeon. Cannulas also allow the surgeon to keep sutures organized, prevent suture entanglement, provide easy access to the joint, and facilitate visualization. The ideal cannula size to allow for passage of typical arthroscopic instruments is 8.5 to 10 mm. Cannulas are important tools that play an integral part in the surgical plan.

Arthroscopic Instruments

After insertion of the anchor, specialized instruments will be necessary to assist with management of sutures to facilitate a secure repair.[4] Suture retrievers are the workhorse of any arthroscopic procedure (Fig. 3-1). These devices can be locking or ratcheting, and function to grasp the suture. Some devices will securely hold the suture, whereas others secure the suture but allow it to slide in the jaws (suture retrieval forceps, or "loopie"). Suture retrieval forceps can facilitate removal of suture from the joint by allowing it to slide as it is extracted. This prevents the suture limb from sliding through the anchor unintentionally. Another option for suture management is the crochet hook instrument.[4] This device allows the surgeon to place the suture at various places within the joint for retrieval and passage. Some crochet hooks have a modification that allows for sutures to be pushed with the tip in addition to being pulled with the hook ("push-me, pull-me").

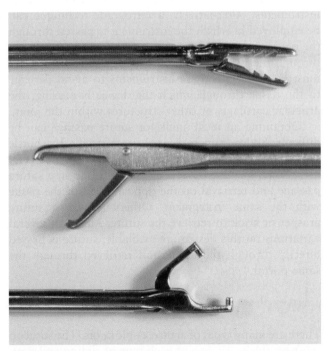

Figure 3-1. Several devices are necessary for an efficient arthroscopic repair. Suture grasping and retrieving devices are available from many manufacturers. Tissue graspers allow for positioning to allow easier passage of suture. Pictured from top to bottom: serrated grasper, tissue grasper, and suture or ring retriever.

Tissue graspers are also important for management during a repair. These devices function to grasp the tissue and apply traction. However, the grasper should not perforate or damage the tissue. This allows the surgeon to manipulate the tissue and both determine the appropriate location and tension of the torn tissue and place the tissue in positions that are amenable to suture passage. Graspers may also lock, allowing the surgeon to work with the tissue in a hands-free manner.

The arthroscopic knot pusher is another critical device used to tension knots and ensure that tissues are tightly apposed. Knot pushers come in various configurations and should be chosen based primarily on surgeon preference.[4,5] Once all knots are completed, there are also a variety of manufacturer-specific cutting devices. Some of these devices are preferentially made to cut the many different high-tensile sutures, including FiberWire (Arthrex, Naples, FL) and Ultrabraid (Smith & Nephew, Andover, MA). However, more generally, there are cutting tools that can be placed into the joint, and then the suture is loaded; other devices allow the surgeon to load the suture external to the joint and follow the suture limbs down before cutting at the knot.

SUTURE PASSAGE

Proper suture passage allows for precise placement of sutures to maximize secure tissue fixation and to minimize iatrogenic tissue injury. Various techniques have been developed to facilitate the passage of suture through soft tissue. Although a comprehensive review of suture-passing devices is not feasible, it is important for any arthroscopic surgeon to be comfortable with multiple suture-passing techniques. This allows the surgeon to accommodate intraoperative challenges and decrease operative times, as one technique is not always the easiest for any given pathology. Confidence and familiarity with these devices is necessary for an efficient arthroscopic repair.

The ability to manage the soft tissues in a gentle manner is important for avoidance of iatrogenic injury.[6] However, without fail, the key to arthroscopic and minimally invasive surgery is visualization. In our experience and observation, the failure to perform an adequate bursectomy before beginning an all-arthroscopic rotator cuff repair is the most common reason for conversion to an open procedure.[7] Convenience, cost-effectiveness, and tissue quality are deciding factors in use of any suture-passing device.

Suture Relay

Suture relay has been the workhorse of arthroscopists from its inception. Cannulated large-bore needle devices are passed through the soft tissue that is in need of repair (Fig. 3-2). These devices come in numerous shapes

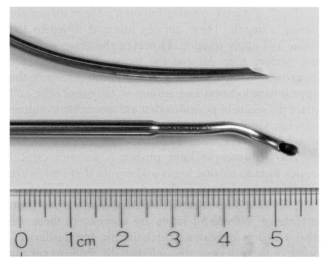

Figure 3-2. Suture lassos are the workhorse of arthroscopic shoulder surgery. Cannulated needles usually come prepackaged and have various bends and angles that assist with suture passage in otherwise difficult locations.

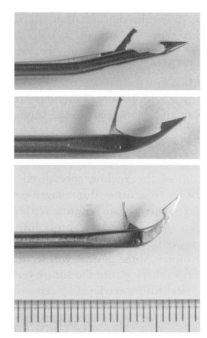

Figure 3-3. Tissue-penetrating devices are extremely valuable and can be used in antegrade or retrograde fashion to pass suture. Various angles are available to facilitate suture passage. Penetrators with a higher angle require a larger-bore cannula.

and twists to facilitate placement of the suture at the point of maximum fixation. Before the arthroscopic procedure, practice with new devices and use what works best in your hands. Suture relay devices are particularly useful for difficult-to-reach or more delicate tissues such as the labrum.

With these devices the sharp cannulated needle is passed through the tissue; a suture lasso is deployed through the needle into the joint and retrieved with the desired suture to be passed through an accessory working portal. Care should be taken to avoid tangling the suture that is to be passed with the remaining sutures. An easy technique to avoid this is to grasp the lasso and the suture in one pass, retrieving them through the same working portal. Currently we recommend the use of clear plastic cannulas when available to pass sutures to avoid soft tissue interposition in the suture.

The suture end, usually from an anchor, is then passed through the lasso. Only 10 cm or so of suture should be passed, to minimize kinking of the suture or lasso when the lasso is retrieved. The lasso is then pulled through the original portal, allowing retrieval of the desired suture. The process is repeated as necessary until all sutures have been placed.

Tissue Penetrators

Tissue-penetrating devices such as the Birdbeak (Arthrex, Naples, FL) are useful in larger spaces with more robust tissue (Fig. 3-3). These devices have sharp, pointed ends and are used to grasp or pass suture directly through the tissue. These instruments allow for precise placement of sutures through tissues and are usually passed

in an antegrade fashion to hand off the suture to other instruments. Alternatively, a retrograde technique can be employed in which the instrument is passed through the tissue and used to grasp a suture, pulling the suture through the tissue on removal of the instrument. Care must be used with these instruments to avoid damage to the tissue through which the device is passing, the articular cartilage, or other structures within the joint.

Obtaining an ideal angle for suture passage can be difficult. Suture punch devices use a needle to shuttle suture through tissue when the device is deployed (Fig. 3-4). Some of these devices allow for a one-step suture passage and retrieval on the opposite side of the tissue with the same instrument. Others require a suture grasper or hook to retrieve the suture. Although several variations on this design are available, suture is passed directly through the tissue and retrieved through the same portal.

KNOT TYPES

There are many types of arthroscopic knots. The surgeon must be able to tie one of each type of sliding and non-sliding knots. A basic review of terminology is crucial to understand the techniques described for these knots (Box 3-1). Although there are benefits to each knot type, we recommend understanding how to perform a non-sliding and at least one sliding knot.[3,8-10]

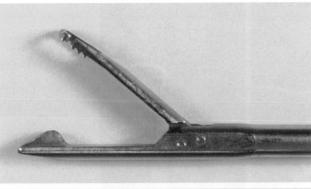

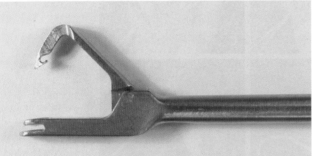

Figure 3-4. One-step suture passers were designed to minimize the number of steps involved in suture passing. In general, a suture is loaded into the end of the device and passed through the tissue. In the ideal situation, the suture is grasped by the same instrument used to pass the suture; however, this can be difficult, and we recommend performing the grasping and retrieving steps through a different portal to avoid pulling the suture out of the tissue. These devices are larger than suture relay or tissue penetrators and can be difficult to use in confined spaces. *Top:* Scorpion (Arthrex, Naples, FL). *Bottom,* Caspari Suture Punch (Arthrotek, Warsaw, IN).

BOX 3-1 Knot-Tying Terminology

Post: Suture limb around which a loop is made, used to pull knot to tissue

Loop: Suture limb used to make a loop around the post

Half-hitch knot: Single loop around the post

Knot pusher: Mechanical device used to slide a knot or loop down the post limb

---

Nonsliding Knots

Nonsliding knots consist of a series of half hitches in which the loop limb is tied around the post. The post and loop limbs can be alternated, and the direction of throws of the suture can also be varied to increase knot security.[10] Each throw of the knot must be guided to the tissue completely to ensure that a tight knot is produced. Examples of nonsliding knots are the Revo knot and alternating half hitches. Nonsliding knots must be used when the suture material does not slide freely through

the suture anchor and tissue being repaired. These can be used for any situation in which an arthroscopic knot is tied.

Sliding Knots

Sliding knots consist of a looped suture end that is passed around a shortened post limb. When the post is pulled or the knot is pushed, the knot slides down the post to the tissue. Sliding knots can be further subdivided into locking and nonlocking configurations. Nonlocking configurations do not have internal resistance to knot slippage other than friction between the suture limbs. When these knots are tied, tension must be maintained on the post limb until half hitches are thrown to provide knot security. Examples of nonlocking sliding knots include the Duncan loop and the overhand loop.

Sliding, locking knots have an internal locking mechanism that provides increased loop security while they are tied. These locking knots function by having a wrapping limb that distorts the post limb when tensioned, increasing the internal interference and preventing knot slippage. This locking mechanism is known as the *one-way ratchet effect* or the *self-locking effect*.[11] Locking knots can be further categorized as proximal, middle, or distal locking, depending on the location of the wrapping limb relative to the surgeon. Proximal-locking knots deform closer to the surgeon, whereas distal-locking knots deform closer to the tissue. Nicky's knot is an example of a proximal-locking knot; the Samsung Medical Center (SMC) (Fig. 3-5) and Tennessee slider are examples of middle-locking knots; and the Weston (Fig. 3-6) and Roeder knots are examples of distal-locking knots.[11] Proximal-locking knots can be locked more easily when tension in the knot loop is high; however, distal-locking knots tend to have less enlargement of the suture loop when the locking mechanism is deployed, so each knot has its own advantages and disadvantages.

SELECTED LITERATURE REVIEW

Much has been written on the technique and optimization of arthroscopic knot tying. Burkhart and co-workers did an elegant study in which they evaluated the configuration of sliding knots that would have adequate strength for rotator cuff repair.[3] They found that reversing posts while tying half hitches to secure sliding knots greatly increased the load to failure of the knot. Another recommendation was the use of double-loaded anchors to decrease the amount of stress to which any one knot was subjected by increasing the number of individual knots per repair. The recommendation that they provided was that to withstand maximal muscle

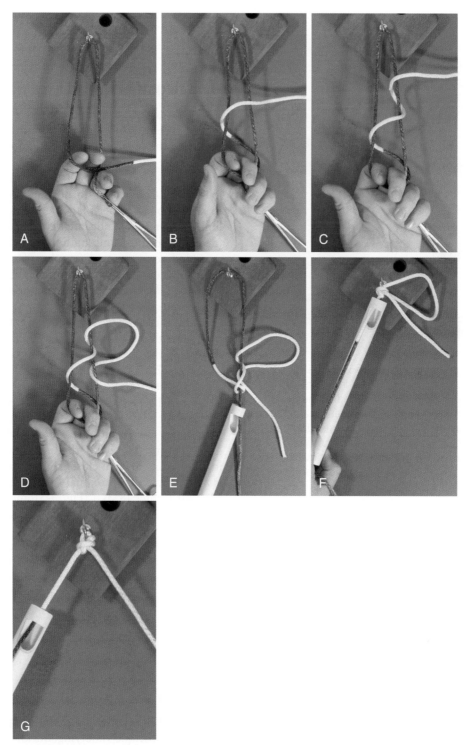

Figure 3-5. Samsung Medical Center sliding-locking knot. The post limb is colored dark blue to allow for better visualization. **A,** The loop strand is passed over the post. **B,** The loop limb is then passed under and over both suture limbs. **C,** The loop limb is then passed under and back over the post limb. **D,** The loop limb is then passed under the post just distal to the first throw. **E,** As tension is pulled on the post, a "locking loop" is formed and should be maintained, usually with the index finger. **F,** The post limb is tensioned with a knot pusher, causing the knot to slide distally. Care should be taken to avoid tightening the locking loop until the knot has adequately tensioned the tissue. **G,** While the post limb is tensioned with the knot pusher, the loop strand is then tensioned, tightening the locking loop and effectively securing the knot. This is usually followed with at least two alternating (over and under) half-hitch knots.

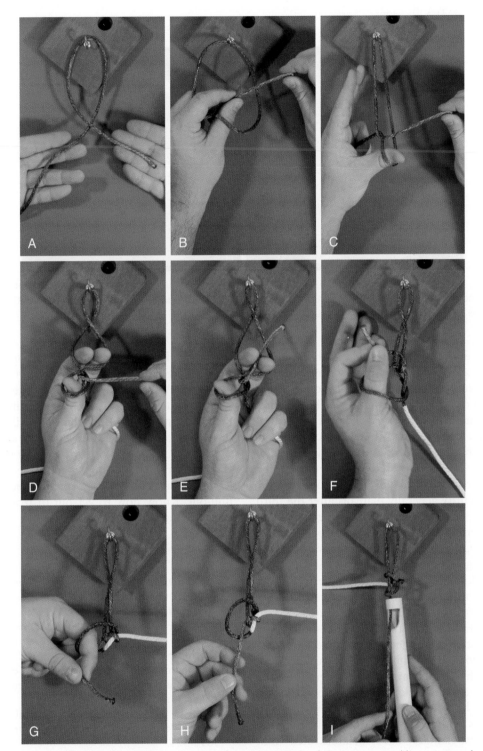

Figure 3-6. Weston knot. **A,** The post limb is placed over the loop limb of the suture, making an open loop. **B,** The index finger of the left hand passes over the open loop, and the post limb is grasped with the index finger and thumb. The post limb is then passed under and through the open loop, and the end of the suture is grasped with the right hand. **C,** The left thumb is then used to tension the suture loop while the post limb is tensioned by the right hand. **D,** The left index and second fingers are then passed under both limbs of the open loop, over the far strand and back under the near strand. Tension should be maintained on the post during this maneuver. **E,** The post strand is then passed with the right hand to between the left index and second fingers. **F,** The left index and second finger are pulled down through the open loop, allowing the post limb to be grasped by the left thumb and index finger. **G,** The post limb is then passed with the left index and thumb through the space occupied by the thumb. **H,** In this figure the post limb is not yet ready to be tensioned. The knot should be dressed by flipping the remaining open loop and gently tensioning the post so that it will slide. Tensioning of the loop strand at this stage will lock the knot and thus should be avoided. **I,** The post limb is then tensioned with a knot pusher, sliding the knot to tension the soft tissue. After adequate soft tissue tension has occurred; the loop limb is tensioned, locking the knot. This is typically followed by three alternating half hitches, while alternating the post on at least one throw.

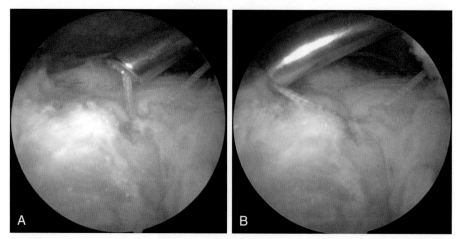

Figure 3-7. Past pointing. This technique is used to ensure that the knot is adequately tensioned. After the knot has been pushed to the tissue, **A,** the loop limb is tensioned and **B,** the knot pusher is pushed past the knot, allowing the knot to flatten and fully seat, maximizing knot security.

contraction in the rotator cuff crescent, anchors should be placed 1 cm apart with two sutures per anchor to allow for adequate healing of the torn tendon.[3]

Another area of debate is the number of half hitches necessary to secure an arthroscopic sliding knot. A biomechanical study demonstrated that self-locking knots still require half hitches to resist failure in the setting of a dynamic cyclic load.[12] The study also demonstrated that most knots require three half hitches to secure the knot and that security generally plateaus after the third half hitch (Fig. 3-7). We recommend tying three half hitches with alternating posts after a self-locking knot to prevent knot failure and increase security.

The ultimate goal in tying an arthroscopic knot is to achieve a secure knot that stabilizes the tissue and allows for healing in a tension-free environment. The gold standard to which arthroscopic knots have been compared is the open knot. Multiple studies have demonstrated that arthroscopic knots, when tied correctly, resist slippage and elongation, similar to open knots.[13,14] Arthroscopic sliding knots have also been demonstrated to be as secure as square knots tied open when the sliding knots are backed up with three half hitches with alternating posts and throw directions.[13] In addition to sliding knots, studies have demonstrated that arthroscopic square knots have equivalent strength to open square knots in resistance of elongation and ultimate failure in the setting of a cyclic load.[14]

SUMMARY

Techniques for knot tying and suture passage continue to evolve with the field of arthroscopy. Surgeons who perform arthroscopic techniques for tissue repair need to be comfortable with methods for passing suture through tissue and tying arthroscopic knots. A surgeon should have the ability to throw nonsliding and sliding knots. The best course of action is to practice knot tying before surgery and suture passage in a laboratory, if available. Arthroscopic suture passage and knot tying allow for durable repair of soft tissue injuries in a minimally invasive fashion. Techniques will continue to be developed as the burgeoning field of arthroscopy continues to develop. As with any case, be prepared for any situation in the operating room. Have a plan for problematic situations—loose knot, tangled suture, anchor pull-out. Know how to get out of trouble, and reduce your frustration level.

REFERENCES

1. Mair SD. *Aspects of Arthroscopic Knot Tying, Technique Tips AAOS/ASES Arthroscopic Management of Rotator Cuff Disease and Instability.* Chicago: Illinois; 2010.
2. Barber FA, Herbert MA, Hapa O, et al. Biomechanical analysis of pullout strengths of rotator cuff and glenoid anchors: 2011 update. *Arthroscopy.* 2011;27:895-905.
3. Burkhart SS, Wirth MA, Simonick M, et al. Loop security as a determinant of tissue fixation security. *Arthroscopy.* 1998;14:773-776.
4. Nottage WM, Lieurance RK. Current concepts: arthroscopic knot tying techniques. *Arthroscopy.* 1999;15:515-521.
5. Milia MJ, Peindl RD, Connor PM. Arthroscopic knot tying: the role of instrumentation in achieving knot security. *Arthroscopy.* 2005;21:69-76.
6. Lo IKY, Burkhart SS, Chan C, et al. Arthroscopic knots: determining the optimal balance of loop security and knot security. *Arthroscopy.* 2004;20(5):489-502.
7. Altchek DW, Warren RF, Wickiewicz TL, et al. Arthroscopic acromioplasty: technique and results. *J Bone Joint Surg Am.* 1990;72:1198-1207.
8. Burkhart SS, Wirth MA, Simonich M, et al. Knot security in simple sliding knots and its relationship to rotator cuff repair: how secure must the knot be? *Arthroscopy.* 2000;16:202-207.

9. Chan KC, Burkhart SS, Thiagarajan P, et al. Optimization of stacked half-hitch knots for arthroscopic surgery. *Arthroscopy*. 2001;17:752-759.

10. Chan KC, Burkhart SS. How to switch posts without rethreading when tying half-hitches. *Arthroscopy*. 1999;15:444-450.

11. Lo IKY, Burkhart SS. Current concepts in arthroscopic rotator cuff repair. *Am J Sports Med*. 2003;31(2): 308-324.

12. Kim S-H, Yoo JC, Wang JH, et al. Arthroscopic sliding knot: how many additional half-hitches are really needed? *Arthroscopy*. 2005;2:405-411.

13. Elkousy HA, Sekiya JK, Stabile KJ, et al. A biomechanical comparison of arthroscopic sliding and sliding-locking knots. *Arthroscopy*. 2005;21:204-210.

14. Elkousy H, Hammerman SM, Edwards TB, et al. The arthroscopic square knot: a biomechanical comparison with open and arthroscopic knots. *Arthroscopy*. 2006;22: 736-741.

Chapter 4

Suture Anchor Fixation for Anterior Shoulder Instability

Jay B. Cook and Craig R. Bottoni

Chapter Synopsis
- This chapter describes the use of suture anchors in the glenohumeral joint for labral repair and stabilizing operations, both open and arthroscopic. The techniques of anterior and posterior stabilization, including anchor insertion, are described in detail. The use of suture anchors has become the standard for soft tissue repairs in the shoulder.

Important Points
- Suture anchors and their proper insertion are paramount to performing most types of instability surgery.
- The shoulder surgeon must be familiar with their use, insertion, and complications.
- Disastrous complications can result from improper use of suture anchors.

Clinical and Surgical Pearls
- The steps in the technique of labral repair and capsular plication require careful planning, a stepwise process, and suture limb management.
- Knowledge of arthroscopic knot tying is a prerequisite for most suture anchors, although knotless anchors are available that obviate the need for arthroscopic knots.

Clinical and Surgical Pitfalls
- Appropriate diagnosis, patient positioning, and surgical technique are paramount to success in arthroscopic or open shoulder surgery.

Recurrent anterior glenohumeral instability is a common sequela of a traumatic glenohumeral dislocation or recurrent subluxation episodes. The major patho-anatomic features of a traumatic dislocation are the capsulolabral avulsion of the inferior glenohumeral ligament (Bankart-Perthes lesion) and capsular redundancy, which typically worsens with repeated injuries.[1-5] Once recurrent instability affects activities of daily living or precludes return to sports, operative stabilization is recommended. Although there is still considerable debate about whether to proceed with surgery after the first traumatic dislocation, the orthopedic literature supports early acute arthroscopic stabilization after a traumatic dislocation in a select group of young athletes who are at high risk for repeated shoulder injuries.[6-11] However, patient issues such as player position, time remaining in a season, and time available for rehabilitation may affect the decision of when to undergo surgery. Immediate stabilization is recommended in athletes who participate in activities or sports in which a subsequent dislocation could be life-threatening (e.g., parachuting or rock climbing).

Before the introduction of arthroscopic techniques in the mid-1980s, shoulder stabilization surgery required a formal deltopectoral approach, through which the subscapularis was either released from its humeral insertion or split longitudinally for access to the glenohumeral joint. The initial technique to reattach the avulsed labrum to bone was done through bone tunnels; however, after their introduction in the 1980s, suture anchors quickly became the most commonly used soft tissue repair devices. With the advancement of arthroscopic shoulder techniques in the 1990s, the number as well as the variety of fixation devices increased dramatically. The introduction of bioabsorbable and then reinforced plastic (PEEK) suture anchors allowed for postoperative imaging without interference from metallic anchors. In addition, revisions, when necessary, were not hindered by retained metallic implants.

Arthroscopic shoulder stabilization offers a number of advantages over traditional open repairs. These include smaller incisions, less muscle dissection, less postoperative pain, and better visualization of the entire glenohumeral joint.[12] The first arthroscopic Bankart repairs were performed by transglenoid suture fixation. Sutures were passed across the glenoid and tied over the posterior fascia. As bioabsorbable polymers were introduced for use in the shoulder, soft tissue fixation with tacks became popular. The tacks were inserted arthroscopically over a guidewire to ensure correct placement. Tacks have been shown to have limited pull-out strength and have, for the most part, been abandoned for shoulder stabilization. The success of metallic suture anchors in open shoulder surgery led to the development of arthroscopic deployment techniques. Development of longer-lasting polymers and high-strength suture made bioabsorbable anchors the most popular choice for soft tissue repair. The goals of any suture anchor are to repair soft tissue to bone and to be able to withstand the forces required for rehabilitation until the normal bone-tissue interface is restored. The focus of this chapter is on the technique of arthroscopic anterior shoulder stabilization with use of suture anchors.

PREOPERATIVE CONSIDERATIONS

History

It is essential to establish an accurate diagnosis. Important information to elicit includes mechanism of initial injury, frequency and direction of dislocation or subluxation episodes, presence of instability during activities of daily living, and prior surgeries.

Recurrent anterior instability typically manifests with a limitation of shoulder function caused by a subjective feeling that the shoulder is "slipping out of the joint." For anterior instability, shoulder abduction with increasing external rotation typically reproduces these symptoms.

Physical Examination

Many shoulder dislocations are reduced by athletic trainers, coaches, or emergency department personnel. The on-field reduction is typically easier and less traumatic than a delayed reduction because of the absence of muscle spasm. Crepitation or pain at the upper arm may be indicative of a proximal humerus fracture. If any question exists, reduction should be delayed until sufficient radiographs have been obtained. Plain radiographs will confirm a shoulder dislocation and can assist in identifying any concomitant fractures before a reduction is performed. Before and after reduction is performed, a physical evaluation is repeated to document any neurologic injury or weakness. A radiographic examination is required to confirm reduction and to evaluate the joint for associated injuries. It is important to determine the presence of an axillary nerve injury, which can be associated with anterior dislocations. It is also imperative to assess the integrity of the rotator cuff, especially in older patients.

Recurrent instability causes apprehension when the shoulder is in the abducted, externally rotated position. Relief of the apprehension with posteriorly directed pressure on the proximal humerus, the relocation sign, is often present. Glenohumeral patholaxity can be assessed and graded in comparison with the contralateral side. This examination should be repeated with use of anesthesia, when a better comparison with the normal side can be achieved. The examination under anesthesia includes the supine load-shift test with the arm abducted at 70 to 90 degrees to document and to quantify the degree of anterior instability of the glenohumeral joint compared with the contralateral side. This test can be performed with the patient supine or sitting upright. Another sign of anterior instability is the scapular protraction sign described by Bottoni.[13] In the seated position, as the abducted arm is slowly externally rotated, the patient may involuntarily protract the scapula to keep the glenoid articulating with the humeral head. This will be identified as a winging appearance of the scapula with increasing external rotation of the shoulder.

Imaging

- A standard anteroposterior view with the arm in slight internal rotation is used to identify fractures of the greater tuberosity and Hill-Sachs lesions (Fig. 4-1).

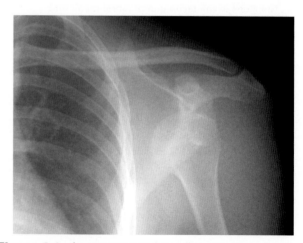

Figure 4-1. An anteroposterior radiograph demonstrating anterior shoulder dislocation.

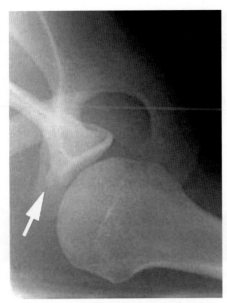

Figure 4-2. A West Point axillary radiograph, best used to evaluate the glenoid. This radiograph reveals an avulsion of the anteroinferior corner of the glenoid (bony Bankart lesion; *arrow*).

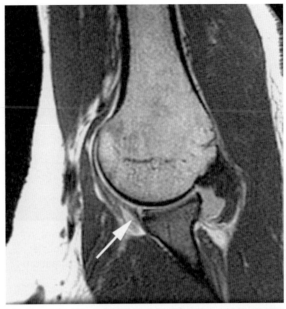

Figure 4-3. Magnetic resonance arthrogram with patient's shoulder in an abducted, externally rotated (ABER) position to tighten the anterior band of the inferior glenohumeral ligament complex. Note the Bankart lesion (*arrow*).

- The trans-scapular Y view can assist with the direction of dislocation before reduction and confirm successful reduction.
- The West Point axillary view can be used to assess glenoid rim fractures (bony Bankart lesion; Fig. 4-2).

Other Modalities

- Computed tomography (CT) is occasionally used to assess the extent of bone injuries of the humerus or glenoid. In addition, CT can be used to evaluate the glenoid version.
- Magnetic resonance imaging is the gold standard for evaluation of intraarticular pathoanatomy. For evaluation of recurrent instability, we prefer magnetic resonance arthrography (MRA) because the addition of intraarticular gadolinium distends the shoulder joint and improves the visualization of the pathoanatomy (Fig. 4-3). After an acute dislocation or subluxation, the hemarthrosis serves to distend the joint and obviates the need for contrast agent.

Indications and Contraindications

The primary operative indication for a stabilization procedure is shoulder instability that interferes with activities of daily living or recreational sports. Recurrent dislocation or subluxation episodes can result in additional chondral or osteochondral damage. Contraindications to surgery include habitual or voluntary dislocators and unwillingness or inability of a patient to comply with the obligatory postoperative restrictions and rehabilitation program. Bone defects such as a large bony Bankart or an engaging Hill-Sachs lesion are best treated with open surgical techniques. A relative contraindication to arthroscopic stabilization includes recurrent instability in athletes involved in contact sports.[14]

SURGICAL TECHNIQUE

Anesthesia and Positioning

Anterior stabilization is typically performed with the patient under general anesthesia. An adjunctive regional (interscalene) block may be performed to provide postoperative analgesia. Positioning of the patient is based on the surgeon's preference. Many surgeons believe that the lateral decubitus position allows better visualization and ease of instrumentation with a shoulder distraction system (STaR Sleeve and 3-Point Shoulder Distraction System, Arthrex, Naples, FL; Fig. 4-4). However, the beach chair position may allow greater control of the entire arm, especially internal and external rotation. This position also facilitates easier conversion to a traditional open approach.

Surgical Landmarks, Incisions, and Portals

The bone landmarks may be identified with a skin marker to assist in portal position (Fig. 4-5). The

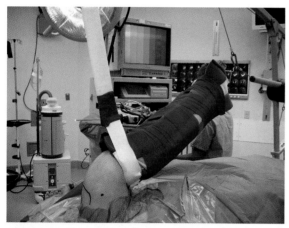

Figure 4-4. Intraoperative photograph of patient in the lateral decubitus position. Excellent intraarticular arthroscopic visualization results from the distraction provided by the axillary strap.

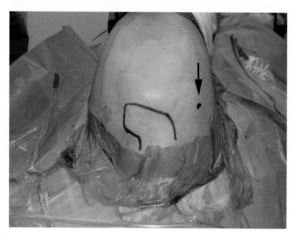

Figure 4-5. Anatomic landmarks identified on skin before arthroscopy. The standard posterior viewing portal is made approximately 2 cm inferior and 2 cm medial to the posterolateral corner of the acromion *(arrow)*.

standard posterior viewing portal is established approximately 2 cm medial and 2 cm inferior to the posterolateral edge of the acromion.

The anterosuperior portal is established by an outside-in technique. An 18-gauge spinal needle is inserted 1 cm anterior to the acromion and 2 cm lateral to the coracoid close to the anterolateral edge of the acromion. The needle should enter the joint high and just medial to the biceps tendon near the root attachment as visualized arthroscopically. A clear 6.5-mm cannula (Stryker Endoscopy, San Jose, CA) is used for instrumentation.

An anteroinferior portal is established just above the superior edge of the subscapularis and as lateral as possible to obtain the best angle toward the glenoid when suture anchors are inserted. Because of the required instrument passage, a larger 8.25-mm twist-in cannula (Arthrex) is used to establish and maintain this portal.

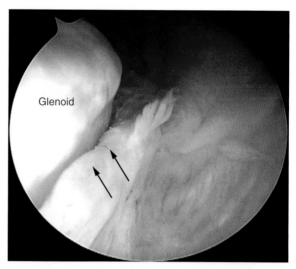

Figure 4-6. Arthroscopic image of a left shoulder with an anterior labral periosteal sleeve avulsion (ALPSA lesion; *arrow*) visualized from the anterosuperior portal.

Arthroscopic Examination

A systematic diagnostic arthroscopy is performed. The superior and posterior labral attachments are inspected. If they are torn, arthroscopic repair is performed as described in Chapters 9 and 26 before anterior stabilization is completed. With anterior instability, the anteroinferior labral attachment is often disrupted (Bankart lesion). Chronic instability often results in a medialized capsulolabral complex (anterior labral periosteal sleeve avulsion [ALPSA lesion]; Fig. 4-6). When it is present, this labral attachment must be sharply reflected from the glenoid and then reattached to the articular margin. The anteroinferior glenoid is evaluated for bone and cartilage loss, and the posterosuperior humeral head for a bony or cartilaginous Hill-Sachs defect (Fig. 4-7).

Specific Steps

For arthroscopic stabilizations to be successfully performed, a reproducible sequence of steps allows the surgeon to properly address the pathoanatomy and avoid the myriad pitfalls that can complicate the procedure (Box 4-1).

1. Positioning and Portal Placement

The correct patient positioning and portal placement are critical to allow access to the entire shoulder. For lateral decubitus positioning, the patient's position is maintained with a deflatable beanbag. It is important to ensure that the patient is well secured to prevent the patient from leaning during the surgery, precluding adequate visualization. The three-point shoulder system (STaR Sleeve and 3-Point Shoulder Distraction System) incorporates a strap that wraps under the proximal

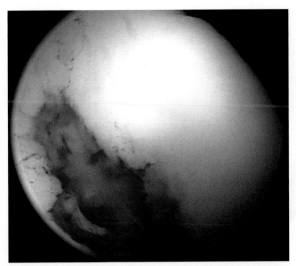

Figure 4-7. An arthroscopic image of a Hill-Sachs lesion of the left shoulder. Note the articular cartilage on both sides of the compression fracture that differentiates it from the normal "bare area" of the posterolateral humeral head.

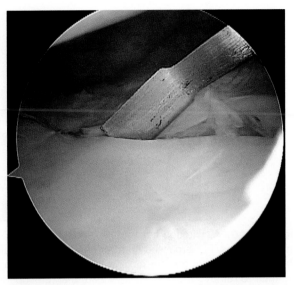

Figure 4-8. A sharp arthroscopic elevator knife is used to mobilize the labrum from the anterior glenoid before repair.

BOX 4-1 Surgical Steps
1. Positioning and portal placement
2. Labral preparation
3. Shuttle wire passage
4. Suture anchor insertion and suture shuttling
5. Knot tying

humerus and allows lateral distraction to improve joint visualization (see Fig. 4-4).

2. Labral Preparation

The labral preparation step is crucial to prepare the capsulolabral tissue for repair. A sharp arthroscopic elevator (Liberator, ConMed Linvatec, Largo, FL) is used to mobilize the capsulolabral tissue from the glenoid attachment (Fig. 4-8). Elevation should be performed until muscle fibers of the subscapularis are visible along the anterior glenoid neck. After mobilization, the capsulolabral tissue will be completely free, thus allowing superior translation for subsequent repair of the articular margin of the glenoid. A mechanical shaver or bur is used to abrade the anterior glenoid and to stimulate a bleeding bed to which the capsulolabral tissue will be reattached (Fig. 4-9). For better visualization of the anterior glenoid during preparation, a 70-degree arthroscope may be used from the posterior portal to "look over the edge," or the standard 30-degree arthroscope can be inserted down the anterosuperior portal with instrumentation through the anteroinferior portal.

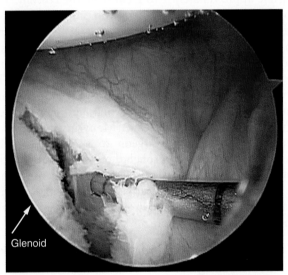

Glenoid

Figure 4-9. Arthroscopic image of a left shoulder visualized from the anterosuperior portal. A mechanical shaver is used to abrade the anterior glenoid in preparation for repair.

3. Shuttle Passage

The next step is to pass a braided wire that will be used subsequently to shuttle one limb of the permanent suture from the anchor through the tissue and labrum, which will secure the capsulolabral tissue back to the glenoid. Several arthroscopic instruments are commercially available to facilitate this step. We prefer to use a 45-degree curved suture shuttle device (SutureLasso SD, Arthrex) through which a braided wire is passed (Fig. 4-10). It is important to pass this shuttle wire as inferior as possible to allow superior translation and retensioning of the capsulolabral complex onto the articular margin. The SutureLasso is passed first through the

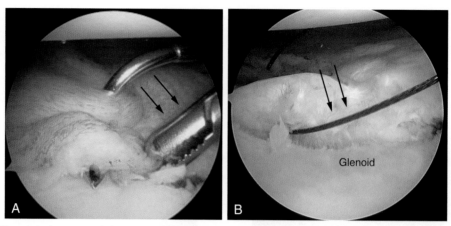

Figure 4-10. A, Through the anteroinferior portal, a curved suture-passing instrument (45-degree, left SutureLasso SD; Arthrex, Naples, FL) is passed first through the capsule and then separately through the interval between the glenoid and labrum. A soft tissue grasper *(double arrows)* is used through the anterosuperior portal to maintain tension on the tissue and then to retrieve the braided wire via the anterosuperior portal once it is passed. **B,** The wire has been passed through the tissue; one limb exits the anterosuperior portal, and the other exits the anteroinferior portal.

capsule approximately 1 to 2 cm from the labrum. The hook is then passed through the interval between the labrum and glenoid (see Fig. 4-10A). The first passage will produce a capsular plication as it forms a pleat in the capsule. The second pass facilitates anatomic repair of the labrum back to the glenoid. The primary purpose of the wire is to serve as a temporary shuttle that will be used to pass one limb of the Fiber-Wire suture through the tissue. Many instruments are available to allow the surgeon to skip this step by passing the instrument through the tissue to retrieve the suture from the previously placed anchor. However, use of a shuttle suture as described allows more precise placement of the sutures through the tissue and produces a capsular plication.

4. Suture Anchor Insertion and Suture Passage

Through the anterosuperior portal, a grasper is used to retrieve the shuttle stitch and pull it out the anterosuperior portal (see Fig. 4-10B). At this time, upward retraction of this shuttle wire will allow a determination of how much superior shifting of the capsulolabral tissue is possible and therefore where the suture anchor should be correctly placed. Excessive tension on this first stitch will increase the likelihood of a knot's loosening. We prefer the 3-mm BioComposite SutureTak suture anchor preloaded with a high-strength suture (No. 2 FiberWire, Arthrex). The primary advantage of this suture anchor is that the implant is bioabsorbable and has a unique suture eyelet, which allows the suture limbs to slide easily. The pilot hole is created with an arthroscopic drill passed through the obturator. The drill and suture anchor are passed through the antero-inferior portal and placed 1 to 2 mm onto the articular margin (Fig. 4-11). After anchor insertion the suture

tails must be separated and cleared of any twists. A knot pusher may be placed on one strand of the suture and passed down the cannula. While the knot pusher is inserted, the more inferior or anterior limb is identified. This limb is then retrieved through the anterosuperior portal with a ringed grasper (Fig. 4-12). It is imperative to clamp or to hold the opposite limb that is exiting the anteroinferior portal to prevent "unloading" of the suture from the anchor. If this does occur, another anchor must be inserted over the first.

At this point, one limb of the shuttle wire and one limb of the permanent suture are exiting out of each cannula. Outside the anterosuperior cannula, the Fiber-Wire suture is passed through the loop in the braided shuttle wire. The shuttle wire and the attached permanent suture are pulled through the tissue and out the anteroinferior portal (Fig. 4-13). Arthroscopic visualization of this maneuver is important to ensure that the sutures do not become entangled during passage through the tissue. Both limbs of the permanent suture are now exiting the anteroinferior portal, with one limb now through the capsular tissue.

5. Knot Tying

The knot pusher is again passed down one limb to ensure that the tails are not twisted around each another. An arthroscopic knot is now tied to secure the capsulo-labral tissue back to the glenoid (Fig. 4-14). Many arthroscopic knots have been described; however, the surgeon should become proficient with one sliding-locking knot so it can be tied quickly and reproducibly with little effort. We prefer to use a modified Roeder knot that allows a strong suture buttress. This is backed up with three half-hitches to secure the knot. To reduce the tension on the tissue during tying, a serrated grasper can be passed through the anterosuperior portal to pull

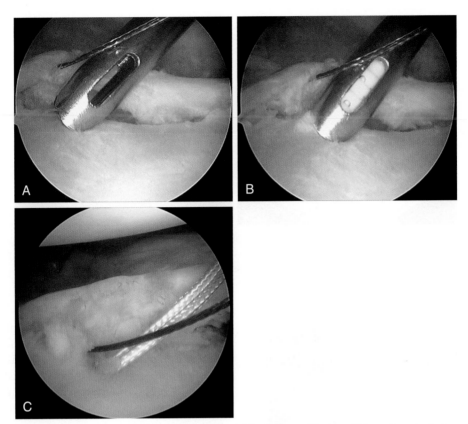

Figure 4-11. The bioabsorbable suture anchors (Bio-Suture Tak; Arthrex, Naples, FL) are inserted along the articular margin of the glenoid following the shuttle wire passage. After the obturator is seated on the edge of the cartilage **(A)**, the drill is passed through the obturator to create the hole **(B)**, and then the press-fit anchor is inserted **(C)**. Note that the suture anchor is placed 1 to 2 mm onto the articular surface just superior to the point where the shuttle wire exits the labral-glenoid interval.

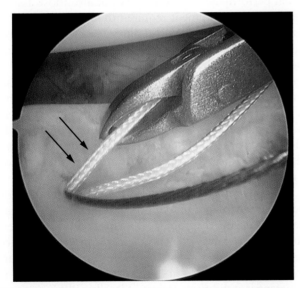

Figure 4-12. A ringed grasper is passed through the anterosuperior portal to pull the inferior limb of the suture through the anterosuperior cannula. Now each cannula has one suture limb and the ends of the shuttle wire and a permanent limb from the suture anchor.

the labrum superiorly while this first knot is tied. The tails of the completed knot are cut with the arthroscopic scissors passed through either the anterosuperior portal or the anteroinferior portal, depending on the optimal angle. This entire process is repeated two or three times to restore the tissue back to the glenoid. The knots should be secure and induce a dimpling effect on the capsulolabral tissue (Fig. 4-15).

POSTOPERATIVE CONSIDERATIONS

Follow-up

Instability surgery is typically performed on an outpatient basis. A standard sling can be applied postoperatively. We prefer the Cryo/Cuff cooling device (DJO Global, Vista, CA) for additional pain relief. The patients are then seen several days after the procedure for their first dressing change.

Rehabilitation

The arthroscopic repair, like its open counterpart, requires that the capsulolabral tissue heal back to the

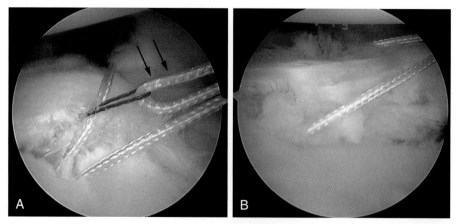

Figure 4-13. The shuttle wire is used to pull the one limb of the FiberWire through the tissue (**A**, *arrows*). This step should be done slowly to ensure that the limbs pass freely without entanglement. Once passed, both limbs of the FiberWire will exit the anteroinferior portal, with one limb passing through the capsule and labrum (**B**).

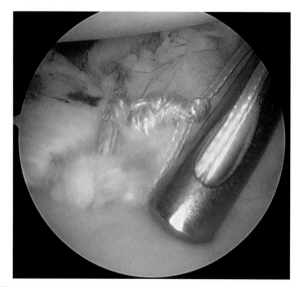

Figure 4-14. A sliding arthroscopic knot is tied outside the cannula and pushed down to abut the tissue. Several half-hitches, while switching the post limb, are then tied to secure the knot.

glenoid. We have adopted a four-phase rehabilitation program. Each phase lasts approximately 4 to 6 weeks but is modified according to the patient's individual progress. The first phase consists of immobilization in a standard arm sling with gentle range-of-motion (Codman pendulum) exercises, wrist and elbow motion, and low-resistance isometrics during supervised physical therapy. The sling is worn at all times during this phase except during physical therapy sessions. The second phase consists of progressive resistive exercises and neuromuscular training. We recommend continued sling use during this period. Abduction with external rotation of the shoulder is avoided, but forward elevation with extension is encouraged. The third phase consists of progressive range-of-motion exercises as

tolerated, increased resistance, neuromuscular training, and aerobic conditioning. Rubber-band resistance exercises and high-repetition sets are used to regain muscle conditioning. The final phase consists of a gradual return to preinjury function including contact sports, and activities requiring overhead or heavy lifting.

Complications

The complications associated with arthroscopic stabilization include not only problems associated with the actual performance of the surgery but also those associated with the equipment required to maintain adequate visualization during the procedure. The camera, arthroscope, and electronic equipment may malfunction, and specialized knowledge by the operating room staff is necessary to troubleshoot problems that inevitably occur. Replacement parts should be readily available to permit continuation of the procedure in the event that some of the equipment becomes damaged. In addition, the surgeon should have the requisite knowledge and ability to convert to an open stabilization if necessary.

Complications associated with anterior stabilization include inadequate tissue preparation leading to an inability to properly mobilize the capsulolabral complex. Medialized repairs often result in recurrent instability. Inadequate tensioning of the tissue can lead to suture breakage or excessive laxity in the tissue, resulting in recurrent instability or failure. Metallic, PEEK, or even bioabsorbable suture anchors, if left protruding above the articular cartilage, can result in disastrous consequences for the humeral articular surface. Even slight prominence can result in a destruction of the humeral cartilage as the shoulder abrades on the metallic edge. In addition, insecurely placed suture anchors can dislodge and become loose bodies that cause destruction

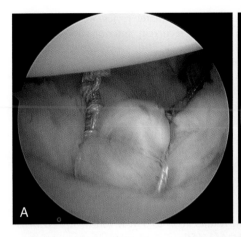
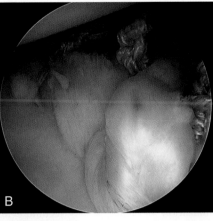

Figure 4-15. The completed repair visualized from posterior **(A)** and anterosuperior **(B)** portals.

TABLE 4-1. Clinical Results of Arthroscopic Bankart Repair with Suture Anchors

Author	Mean Follow-up	Outcome
Warme et al[16] (1999)	25 months	38 shoulders Mean Rowe score: 94 3 (8%) recurrence
Kandziora et al[17] (2000)	38 months	55 shoulders Mean Rowe score: 85 9 (16%) recurrence
Tauro[18] (2000)	39 months	29 shoulders Mean Rowe score: 92 2 (7%) recurrence
Kim et al[19] (2002)	39 months	59 shoulders Mean Rowe score: 93 2 (3%) recurrence
Kim et al[20] (2003)	44 months	167 shoulders Mean Rowe score: 92 7 (4%) recurrence
Fabbriciani et al[21] (2004)	24 months	30 shoulders Mean Rowe score: 91 No recurrence
Mazzocca et al[22] (2005)	37 months	18 shoulders Mean ASES score: 90 2 (11%) recurrence
Bottoni et al[9] (2006)	32 months	32 shoulders Mean Rowe score: 89 11 (11%) recurrence 91% ASES good/excellent
Ozbaydar et al[23] (2008)	47-month average	93 shoulders Mean Rowe score: 86.8 10 (11%) recurrence 85% good/excellent

ASES, American Shoulder and Elbow Surgeons.

of articular cartilage. Some older bioabsorbable fixation devices have been associated with a reactive synovitis as they are hydrolyzed. This may manifest clinically as an increase in shoulder pain 4 to 6 weeks after surgery and a loss of shoulder motion.

RESULTS

Several recent comparisons of arthroscopic and open techniques for recurrent instability have demonstrated comparable outcomes. Godin and Sekiya, in a systematic review, found no statistically significant difference in all clinical factors except postoperative range of motion, which was marginally better in the arthroscopic group.[15] The use of transglenoid fixation, tacks, and nonanatomic repairs results in unacceptably high recurrence rates and therefore should not be used. However, with advanced arthroscopic techniques and implants, the results of arthroscopic instability repair have been equivalent to or even surpassed those of open techniques (Table 4-1). With comparable rates for recurrent dislocation, arthroscopic stabilization is rapidly becoming the technique of choice. A careful and diligent approach to arthroscopic stabilization can lead to success rates greater than 90%.

REFERENCES

1. Arciero RA, St Pierre P. Acute shoulder dislocation. Indications and techniques for operative management. *Clin Sports Med.* 1995;14:937-953.
2. Baker CL, Uribe JW, Whitman C. Arthroscopic evaluation of acute initial anterior shoulder dislocations. *Am J Sports Med.* 1990;18:25-28.
3. Bottoni CR, Arciero RA. Arthroscopic repair of primary anterior dislocations of the shoulder. *Tech Shoulder Elbow Surg.* 2001;2:2-16.
4. Taylor DC, Arciero RA. Pathologic changes associated with shoulder dislocations. Arthroscopic and physical examination findings in first-time, traumatic anterior dislocations. *Am J Sports Med.* 1997;25:306-311.
5. Wheeler JH, Ryan JB, Arciero RA, et al. Arthroscopic versus nonoperative treatment of acute shoulder dislocations in young athletes. *Arthroscopy.* 1989;5:213-217.
6. Arciero RA, Taylor DC. Primary anterior dislocation of the shoulder in young patients. A ten-year prospective study. *J Bone Joint Surg Am.* 1998;80:299-300.

7. Arciero RA, Taylor DC, Snyder RJ, et al. Arthroscopic bioabsorbable tack stabilization of initial anterior shoulder dislocations: a preliminary report. *Arthroscopy*. 1995;11:410-417.

8. Arciero RA, Wheeler JH, Ryan JB, et al. Arthroscopic Bankart repair versus nonoperative treatment for acute, initial anterior shoulder dislocations. *Am J Sports Med*. 1994;22:589-594.

9. Bottoni CR, Smith EL, Berkowitz MJ, et al. Arthroscopic versus open shoulder stabilization for recurrent anterior instability: a prospective randomized clinical trial. *American Journal of Sports Medicine*. 2006;34(11): 1730-1737.

10. DeBerardino TM, Arciero RA, Taylor DC, et al. Prospective evaluation of arthroscopic stabilization of acute, initial anterior shoulder dislocations in young athletes: Two- to five-year follow-up. *Am J Sports Med*. 2001;29: 586-592.

11. Kirkley A, Werstine R, Ratjek A, et al. Prospective randomized clinical trial comparing the effectiveness of immediate arthroscopic stabilization versus immobilization and rehabilitation in first traumatic anterior dislocations of the shoulder: long-term evaluation. *Arthroscopy*. 2005;21:55-63.

12. Green MR, Christensen KP. Arthroscopic versus open Bankart procedures: a comparison of early morbidity and complications. *Arthroscopy*. 1993;9:371-374.

13. Bottoni CR. Clinical Sports Medicine. In: Johnson DL, Mair SD, eds. *Anterior Shoulder Instability*. Philadelphia: Elsevier, Inc.; 2006.

14. Uhorchak JM, Arciero RA, Huggard D, et al. Recurrent shoulder instability after open reconstruction in athletes involved in collision and contact sports. *Am J Sports Med*. 2000;28:794-799.

15. Godin J, Sekiya JK. Systematic review of arthroscopic versus open repair for recurrent anterior shoulder dislocations. *Sports Health: A Multidisciplinary Approach*. 2011;3(4):396-404.

16. Warme WJ, Arciero RA, Savoie 3rd FH, et al. Nonabsorbable versus absorbable suture anchors for open Bankart repair. A prospective, randomized comparison. *Am J Sports Med*. 1999;27:742-746.

17. Kandziora F, Jäger A, Bischof F, et al. Arthroscopic labrum refixation for post-traumatic anterior shoulder instability: suture anchor versus transglenoid fixation technique. *Arthroscopy*. 2000;16:359-366.

18. Tauro JC. Arthroscopic inferior capsular split and advancement for anterior and inferior shoulder instability: technique and results at 2- to 5-year follow-up. *Arthroscopy*. 2000;16:451-456.

19. Kim SH, Ha KI, Kim SH. Bankart repair in traumatic anterior shoulder instability: open versus arthroscopic technique. *Arthroscopy*. 2002;18:755-763.

20. Kim SH, Ha KI, Cho YB, et al. Arthroscopic anterior stabilization of the shoulder: two to six-year follow-up. *J Bone Joint Surg Am*. 2003;85:1511-1518.

21. Fabbriciani C, Milano G, Demontis A, et al. Arthroscopic versus open treatment of Bankart lesion of the shoulder: a prospective randomized study. *Arthroscopy*. 2004;20: 456-462.

22. Mazzocca AD, Brown Jr FM, Carreira DS, et al. Arthroscopic anterior shoulder stabilization of collision and contact athletes. *Am J Sports Med*. 2005;33: 52-60.

23. Ozbaydar M, Elhassan B, Diller D, et al. Results of arthroscopic capsulolabral repair: bankart lesion versus anterior labroligamentous periosteal sleeve avulsion lesion. *Arthroscopy*. 2008;24:1277-1283.

Chapter 5

Arthroscopic Instability Repair with Knotless Suture Anchors

Laith Al-Shihabi, Geoffrey S. Van Thiel, and Brian J. Cole

Chapter Synopsis
- Arthroscopic Bankart repair with suture anchors has shown outcomes equivalent to those of open Bankart repair for traumatic shoulder instability without the morbidity of an open approach. Knotless suture anchors allow for a technically easier and faster surgery with comparable clinical outcomes when compared with repair with traditional anchors.

Important Points
- Arthroscopic Bankart repair is indicated for patients with recurrent unidirectional instability after a traumatic glenohumeral dislocation or subluxation.
- Knotless suture anchors allow for a faster Bankart repair without the technical difficulty of arthroscopic knot tying.
- Most studies demonstrate similar clinical and biomechanical results when comparing traditional and knotless anchors.

Clinical and Surgical Pearls
- Proper patient selection is key to good outcomes. Patients should have a history of recurrent unidirectional instability after a traumatic event that is associated with evidence of a Bankart lesion on imaging studies.
- Techniques of application and philosophies of fixation may vary considerably among different knotless suture anchors. Surgeons should be familiar with these details to ensure optimal function of their anchors.

Clinical and Surgical Pitfalls
- Some studies have suggested that knotless anchors may be subject to failure at lower loads versus traditional anchors.
- Anchors should be positioned such that they are anchored in dense subchondral bone to minimize displacement.
- Displacement of anchors has been reported to cause rapid chondrolysis and joint degeneration.

Of the numerous surgical techniques introduced for performance of successful arthroscopic Bankart repair, fixation of the avulsed labrum with suture anchors has most consistently shown results comparable with those of open repair.[1,2] This has often been attributed to the ability of suture anchors to achieve an anatomically reduced labrum and capsule while also providing a more secure construct when compared with other techniques such as bioabsorbable tacks. Traditional suture anchors, however, require proficiency with technically demanding knot designs and techniques, which are time-consuming and provide the surgeon little room for error. Furthermore, the completed knot may be bulky, and this has been reported to pose a threat to the glenohumeral cartilage via knot abrasion.[3] In an attempt to simplify suture anchor placement, in 2001 Thal introduced the Mitek Knotless Suture Anchor (Mitek, Norwood, MA) and presented its use in the repair of Bankart lesions.[4] The proposed advantages of this suture anchor were faster anchor placement and use, elimination of the arthroscopic knot as a source of failure, technical ease, and superior capsular shift compared with traditional anchors. Since its development, a number of other knotless anchors have been developed that offer the surgeon different options with regard to size, material, and method of fixation. In this chapter we discuss the functional characteristics of knotless anchors, the results of studies that have used such anchors for traumatic Bankart repair (Table 5-1), and the risks and benefits of use of such anchors versus traditional designs.

KNOTLESS ANCHOR DESIGN AND BIOMECHANICAL STUDIES

Since introduction of the Mitek Knotless Suture Anchor, many anchor designs have been introduced that differ

TABLE 5-1. Results of Knotless Suture Anchor Fixation in Shoulder Instability

Author	Follow-up	Outcome
Clinical Results		
Thal[9] (2001)	Average 29 months	27 of 27 (100%) successful
Thal et al[10] (2007)	Minimum 2 years (range: 2-7 years)	67 of 72 (93%) successful
Garofalo et al[11] (2005)	43 months (range: 36-48 months)	18 of 20 (90%) successful
Hayashida et al[12] (2006)	Minimum 2 years	41 of 47 (87%) successful
Oh et al[13] (2009)	Minimum 1 year	Clinical and radiographic—37 patients 100% good or excellent clinical results 23 CT arthrogram—all bone-to-labrum healing
Kocaoglu et al[14] (2009)	40 months	Compared knotless with standard—38 patients (18 standard, 20 knotless) No differences between groups
Author	**Parameters Tested**	**Results**
Biomechanical Results		
Thal[9] (2001)	Suture breakage	Knotless anchor with statistically higher failure load ($P < .0001$)
	Bone pull-out of anchor	Increased anchor pull-out force in knotless anchor not significant ($P < .195$)
	Average capsular shift	Bankart repair: 4.33 mm Barrel stitch repair: 6.04 mm Plication repair: 6.50 mm* Knotless repair: 6.79 mm*
Nho et al[8] (2010)	Compared force-fit type knotless PushLock anchor with SutureTak Noncyclic load-to-failure testing as well as cyclic load-to-failure testing	Ultimate load-to-failure and methods of failure were not significantly different between the two suture anchor constructs

*Statistically significant increase in capsular shift versus Bankart repair with standard suture anchors.

CT, Computed tomography.

in material, method of fixation, and technique of application. Knotless anchors have been demonstrated to similarly restore labral height when compared with traditional suture anchors,[5] but fundamental to their clinical performance is how the anchors will resist displacement once placed, because displacement of the anchor will result in displacement of the labrum and captured tissue from its appropriate position on the glenoid.[6] Broadly, knotless anchors can be grouped based on their method of fixation into bone as either form-fit or force-fit. Form-fit anchors function by changing their original shape once deployed in such a way that they become wedged within the bone. The original Knotless Suture Anchor is an example of this, where nitinol arcs spread after insertion to increase resistance to pullout. Force-fit anchors rely on the friction of the anchor-to-bone interface created by the anchor's design to resist pull-out; screw-type anchors are an example of this.

Initial biomechanical testing of the Mitek Knotless Anchor was done by Thal, who compared maximal pull-out strength of the Knotless Anchor with that of the Mitek GII anchor, on which its design was based.[7] Results from these studies were encouraging—failure by suture breakage occurred at considerably higher loads in the Knotless Anchor group (55.6 pounds vs. 24.3 pounds with use of No. 1 Ethibond), and there was no significant difference in bone pull-out strength. As other designs have been introduced they have also undergone biomechanical and in vitro testing. Nho and colleagues compared the force-fit type knotless PushLock anchor with the SutureTak anchor (both from Arthrex, Naples, FL) with regard to both noncyclic load-to-failure testing and cyclic load-to-failure testing with use of simple, horizontal mattress, and double-loaded simple stitch patterns.[8] This anchor has the proposed advantage of making final tissue tension independent of anchor depth, which would allow the anchor to be wedged more consistently in subchondral bone. Ultimate load-to-failure and methods of failure were not significantly different between the two suture anchor constructs. Overall, knotless suture anchors have provided good results in both clinical and biomechanical studies.

PREOPERATIVE CONSIDERATIONS

History

In assessing a patient with shoulder instability, it is essential to obtain an understanding of the patient's mechanism of injury and direction of instability (e.g., unidimensional versus multidimensional), chronicity, associated injuries, and current level of disability. In addition, the patient's age, activity level, and history of prior treatment should be taken into account for assessment of the need for a potential surgical repair. Patients often report a history of traumatic subluxation or dislocation that results in recurrent unidirectional instability despite attempts at rehabilitation. Patients who sustained their initial injury at a younger age and competitive athletes are also more likely to experience recurrent symptoms.

Physical Examination

Patients typically demonstrate preserved strength and range of motion at the shoulder joint despite their history of instability; absence of these should raise flags for the presence of alternative or additional pathology contributing to the symptoms. A sense of apprehension and discomfort can be elicited by placing the patient in a position of instability, classically at 90 degrees of abduction and external rotation (the apprehension test). Conversely, a sense of relief and stability are achieved by placement of a counterforce on the humeral head in the position of instability (the Jobe relocation test). Patients may also exhibit a sulcus sign in association with inferior instability, in which downward traction on the arm produces a depression between the acromion and humeral head that is greater on the affected side than on the unaffected side.

Imaging

Preoperative imaging should include a full series of shoulder radiographs, including true anteroposterior (AP), scapular-Y, and axillary films of the affected shoulder. Specialized views, such as the West Point axillary or Stryker notch view, can help assess for bony Bankart or Hill-Sachs lesions, respectively. Magnetic resonance imaging of the shoulder with or without intra-articular contrast is valuable to assess the glenoid labrum and rotator cuff and assess for associated pathology such as a humeral avulsion of the glenohumeral ligament (HAGL) lesion that may also be contributing to instability. If glenoid bone loss or fracture is suspected, computed tomography of the shoulder can help quantify its location and extent.

Surgical Indications and Contraindications

Indications for arthroscopic Bankart repair include a history of traumatic subluxation or dislocation with recurring instability that is refractory to conservative treatment such as physical therapy. Examination should reveal apprehension when the arm is placed in a position of instability, and relief of symptoms when a counteracting force is applied. Patients should retain full range of motion and strength to both the deltoid and rotator cuff. Preoperative imaging should demonstrate either a bony or soft tissue Bankart lesion; associated pathology, such as rotator cuff tears, capsular tears, or superior labral anterior-posterior (SLAP) tears, can also be addressed at the time of surgical repair if necessary. In addition, as with any surgery, patients must be willing and able to comply with the surgeon's postoperative rehabilitation protocol to ensure a successful outcome. Contraindications to surgery include degenerative joint disease of the glenohumeral joint, glenoid bone loss (which may be more amenable to bone-restoring reconstructions such as the Latarjet procedure), and atraumatic multidirectional instability.

SURGICAL TECHNIQUE

Anesthesia and Positioning

Bankart repair can be performed with either general or regional anesthesia and in either the beach chair or the lateral decubitus position. Regardless of the chosen technique, an examination under anesthesia should always be performed before final positioning to confirm the direction and magnitude of instability. We prefer to use a combination of an interscalene block along with general anesthesia, with the patient placed in the lateral decubitus position in a combination of light traction (10 pounds) and abduction. If necessary, additional distraction of the glenohumeral joint can be accomplished by lifting the humerus laterally relative to the patient's body. After positioning, the key anatomic landmarks of the acromion, coracoid process, and posterior soft spot should be identified and marked.

Portals

Posterior Portal

The posterior portal (Fig. 5-1) is placed at the posterior soft spot, approximately 2 to 3 cm inferior and 1 to 2 cm medial to the posterolateral corner of the acromion, directed toward the coracoid process and into the glenohumeral joint. Care should be taken not to use excess force in establishing this portal, to avoid inadvertent damage to either the glenoid or the humeral

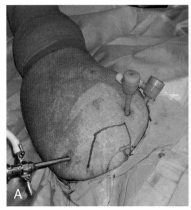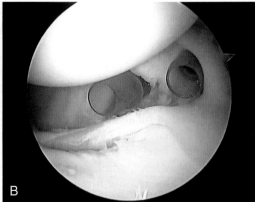

Figure 5-1. Arthroscopic portals for knotless fixation. Outside **(A)** and arthroscopic **(B)** views.

head. Ideally placed, this portal will lie in the interval between the infraspinatus and teres minor muscles. This is the primary viewing portal for the arthroscope.

Anterosuperior Portal

Under direct visualization, a second portal is established anteriorly, starting just lateral to the coracoid process and entering the joint through the rotator interval. An 18-gauge spinal needle is used as a guide to help determine ideal orientation for this portal, followed by placement of an arthroscopic cannula with the aid of a trocar. This portal is placed high in the rotator interval to allow placement of a second anteroinferior portal.

Anteroinferior Portal

This portal is placed with use of spinal needle localization just above the subscapularis in the rotator interval.

Additional Anteroinferior or Posteroinferior Portal

Depending on the need for anchor placement, a 5-o'clock or 7-o'clock portal or both are established under direct visualization with a spinal needle. The 5-o'clock portal is typically through the subscapularis tendon and is only created if absolutely required. These portals allow for anchor placement to the anterior and anteroinferior or posterior and posteroinferior glenoid, respectively.

Diagnostic Arthroscopy

In addition to characterization of the type and extent of the Bankart lesion present, careful and thorough diagnostic arthroscopy should always be performed; this is typically done with the arthroscope in the posterior portal and instrumentation (such as a hooked probe) in the anterosuperior portal. This allows the surgeon to evaluate the condition of the cartilage, biceps tendon, rotator cuff, glenohumeral ligaments, and capsule. Hill-Sachs lesions are frequently present, but large lesions in

BOX 5-1 Surgical Steps in Bankart Repair
1. Labral and capsular preparation
2. Glenoid preparation
3. Tissue capture
4. Anchor placement

particular should be evaluated for "engaging" on the glenoid, which may contribute to the patient's instability by levering the humeral head out of position.

Surgical Steps of Bankart Repair

See Box 5-1.

1. Labral and Capsular Preparation

With either simple visualization or gentle probing, the extent of labral avulsion can be identified. Use an elevator to lift the avulsed labrum and anterior inferior glenohumeral ligament (AIGHL) free from the glenoid and/or subscapularis. Alternatively, if an anterior labroligamentous periosteal sleeve avulsion is encountered (Figs. 5-2 and 5-3), the periosteum can be cut and the AIGHL released from the glenoid; this will allow the repair to continue as with a Bankart repair. If necessary, the labral edge can be lightly debrided with the shaver to help promote healing to bone after repair. The degree of capsular laxity is assessed, as well, and the amount of capsular shift needed to restore proper tension is determined by use of a grasper to tension the labrum and the capsule (Fig. 5-4).

2. Glenoid Preparation

With a bur, a rasp, or the shaver, the labral footprint on the glenoid corresponding to the area of the avulsed glenoid is decorticated to a bleeding bone bed. This

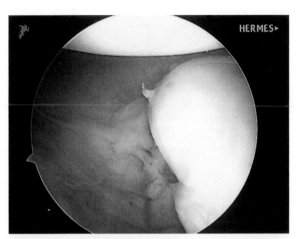

Figure 5-2. Anterior labral periosteal sleeve avulsion lesion *(anterior view). (From Thal R: Knotless suture anchor fixation for shoulder instability. In: Miller MD, Cole BJ, eds.* Textbook of Arthroscopy. *Philadelphia: Elsevier; 2004.)*

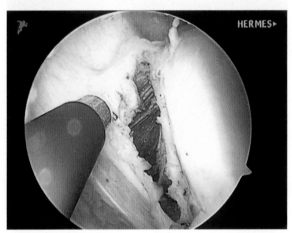

Figure 5-3. Anterior labral periosteal sleeve avulsion lesion during mobilization *(anterior view). (From Thal R: Knotless suture anchor fixation for shoulder instability. In: Miller MD, Cole BJ, eds.* Textbook of Arthroscopy. *Philadelphia: Elsevier; 2004.)*

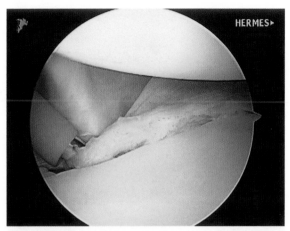

Figure 5-4. A grasper is used to pull the ligament superiorly to the articular margin while capsular tension and mobility are evaluated. The degree of capsular laxity can also be assessed at this time *(posterior view). (From Thal R: Knotless suture anchor fixation for shoulder instability. In: Miller MD, Cole BJ, eds.* Textbook of Arthroscopy. *Philadelphia: Elsevier; 2004.)*

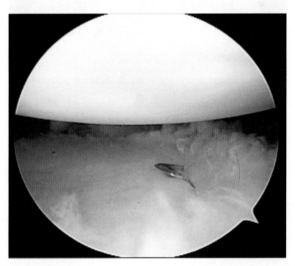

Figure 5-5. A suture-passing device is brought in through one of the portals, and the labrum and capsule are captured for an anatomic repair.

improves healing of the labrum to the bone by eliminating scar tissue or sclerotic bone that may otherwise be interposed between the two structures.

3. Tissue Capture

Multiple knotless anchor options are currently available, and no matter which is chosen, surgeons should be familiar with the technical specifications and technique of application for their chosen anchor. Our preferred anchor is the Arthrex PushLock, and the following sections describe its use, but other anchors can readily be used in its place as surgeon preference dictates. Once the labrum has been adequately elevated and prepared, a curved SutureLasso (Arthrex) is placed through either the anteroinferior or the posteroinferior (7-o'clock) cannula and passed through the capsulolabral tissue

(Fig. 5-5). The nitinol wire or Prolene suture is advanced, captured, and pulled through the anterosuperior cannula (Fig. 5-6). Place 4 cm of FiberWire (Arthrex) No. 2 suture through the nitinol wire or Prolene suture. Retract the wire or suture, then the SutureLasso from its cannula; this should result in a shuttling of the FiberWire around the tissue (Fig. 5-7). Retrieve the second FiberWire tail and pull it through the same portal as the first.

4. Anchor Placement

With the step-drill used through the anteroinferior cannula, drill at the desired site of the first anchor to establish a bony socket (Fig. 5-8). Depending on the degree of capsular shift needed, multiple anchor holes

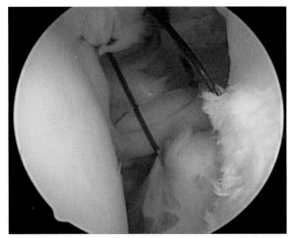

Figure 5-6. A Prolene suture is passed through the passing device and retrieved from the other anterior portal.

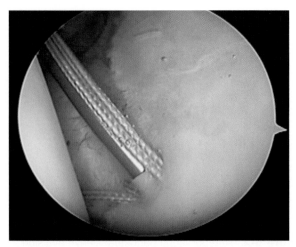

Figure 5-9. The PushLock anchor is loaded and brought in through the anteroinferior portal.

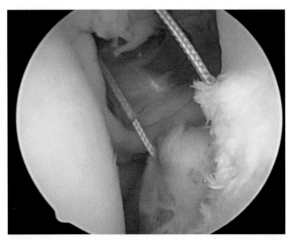

Figure 5-7. The Prolene suture is then used to shuttle a FiberWire (Arthrex, Naples, FL) suture through the capsule and labrum.

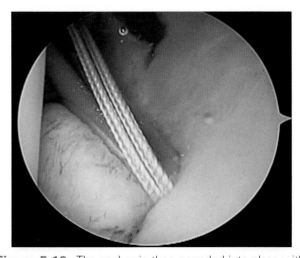

Figure 5-10. The anchor is then pounded into place with resultant tension on the sutures. The "bumper" for the anterior labrum has been re-created.

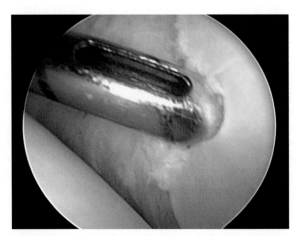

Figure 5-8. A drill guide is brought in through the anteroinferior portal and the drill for the 2.9-mm PushLock (Arthrex, Naples, FL). The sutures are retrieved from this portal and loaded into the PushLock anchor.

may be drilled immediately because visualization may be more difficult afterward. Take care to direct the drill bit medially at least 15 degrees to prevent fracture of the glenoid. Thread the two FiberWire ends into the PushLock eyelet, and pull to establish tissue tension, then advance the PushLock into the bone socket again from one of the inferior cannulas (Fig. 5-9). Release the FiberWire tails as needed to help establish tissue tension; if it is too tight, the driver can be backed out and the tensions readjusted. Tap the proximal end of the driver handle to complete the advancement of the anchor into the bone, then release the handle from the anchor by turning it counterclockwise (Fig. 5-10). The free FiberWire sutures can be cut, completing the Bankart repair (Fig. 5-11). Typically, a minimum of three suture anchors should be used to fix the Bankart lesion. Repeat these steps as necessary to complete full glenoid repair (Fig. 5-12).

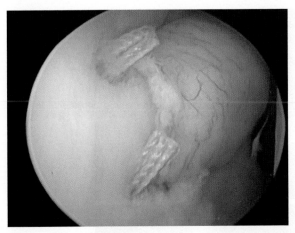

Figure 5-11. Final construct with two knotless anchors.

POSTOPERATIVE CONSIDERATIONS

Patients are discharged to home on the same day. For weeks 0 to 4, patients are instructed on active and active-assisted stretching of the shoulder to 40 degrees of external rotation, 140 degrees of forward flexion, and internal rotation as tolerated, but strengthening is reserved for the muscles below the elbow. The sling is continued at all times. After 4 weeks the sling is removed, shoulder range of motion is increased to full, and strengthening motions distally are slightly expanded. At 6 weeks, patients are allowed full active range of motion of the shoulder, and specific strengthening activities are incorporated into the rehabilitation protocol. After 12 weeks, patients may begin aggressive strength exercise programs along with functional evaluations for work or sports, if applicable.

CLINICAL RESULTS OF KNOTLESS BANKART REPAIR

Since the introduction of the Knotless anchor, several studies have examined the results of the use of these anchors in repair of traumatic Bankart lesions. In 2001 Thal briefly described his initial experience in treating 27 patients with traumatic shoulder instability caused by Bankart lesions, reporting satisfaction among all patients at a mean follow-up of 29 months.[9] One patient had recurrent instability attributed to a traumatic redislocation, which was treated successfully with a revision arthroscopic repair with Knotless anchors. In 2007 a more complete retrospective review of his experience with Mitek Knotless and BioKnotless anchors was published, reporting similarly positive results.[10] Seventy-three patients with a history of traumatic dislocation or subluxation resulting in recurrent instability underwent

arthroscopic repair, with use of the Knotless anchor in the first 45 patients and BioKnotless anchor in the following 27. Failure, defined as redislocation-subluxation or a positive apprehension test result, occurred in five patients, all males younger than 22 years and within 2 years of surgery. Four failures were attributed to recurrent traumatic events, and one to patient noncompliance with postoperative restrictions; three of the four traumatic redislocations were successfully treated with revision arthroscopic Bankart repair with use of BioKnotless anchors without recurrent instability, and the fourth required a Latarjet repair for bony deficiency.

Other authors have also reported positive results with use of knotless anchors for instability. Garofalo retrospectively reviewed 20 patients treated with arthroscopic Bankart repair for traumatic instability with the Mitek Knotless anchor at a mean follow-up of 43 months.[11] Ninety percent of patients reported satisfaction with their surgery, with 80% of patients returning to their preinjury athletic level. Hayashida reviewed 47 patients treated arthroscopically with knotless anchors for traumatic anterior instability at a minimum follow-up of 2 years, with a success rate of 87%.[12] Oh and Lee assessed both clinical and radiologic outcomes of arthroscopic repair with the BioKnotless Suture Anchor for 37 patients with instability, and found all patients to have either a good or an excellent functional result.[13] Twenty-three of these patients consented to reimaging via CT arthrogram at a minimum of 1 year after surgery, and all demonstrated good labrum-to-bone healing. All authors argued that the Knotless or BioKnotless anchor offered a viable and reliable alternative to traditional anchors. Oh and Lee further felt that these anchors may offer improved capsulolabral repair by compressing the repaired tissue to bone to a greater extent than traditional anchors, which would lead to more secure fixation. They did note, however, that the technical difficulty of knot tying with traditional anchors was replaced by a need to more precisely capture the correct amount of tissue to achieve proper tissue tension owing to the fixed length of the anchor loop with this anchor. Kocaoglu prospectively compared the results of 20 arthroscopic Bankart repairs with knotless PushLock (Arthrex) anchors with 18 repairs with traditional knotted anchors and found no significant differences between the two groups.[14]

CONCLUSIONS

Knotless suture anchors offer a technically easier and faster method of use of suture anchors when compared with traditional knotted anchors, and most clinical studies demonstrate good outcomes for Bankart repair performed with knotless anchors. Knotless anchors eliminate the suture knot as the most technically demanding step and the weak link in anchor repairs,

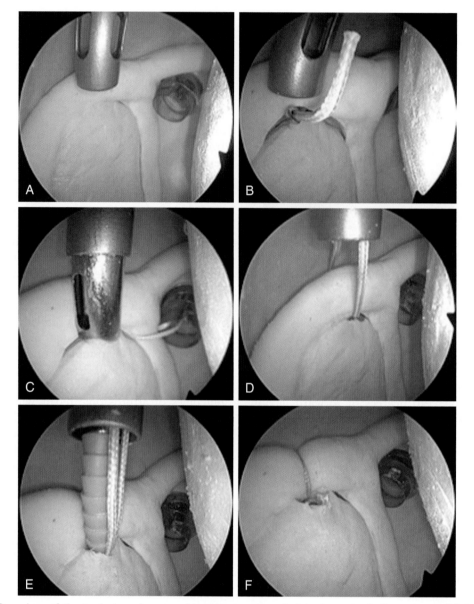

Figure 5-12. Overview of the technique for use of knotless anchors in labral repair. **A,** Cannula established. **B,** Suture passed through anterior portal. **C,** Hole drilled in the glenoid. **D,** Suture retrieved through cannula. **E,** Anchor loaded and placed in glenoid hole. **F,** Anchor impacted into place and sutures cut.

but they are replaced by new challenges such as obtaining proper tissue tensioning and the potential for loosening of the repair construct at lower loads if poorly applied. Given the variety of anchors available for use, the surgeon should be familiar with the biomechanical and clinical data available for his or her selected anchor to maximize its effectiveness in clinical practice.

REFERENCES

1. Kim JM, Kim YS, Ha KY, et al. Arthroscopic stabilization for traumatic anterior dislocation of the shoulder: suture anchor fixation versus transglenoid technique. *J Orthop Sci.* 2008;13(4):318-323.

2. Lenters TR, Franta AK, Wolf FM, et al. Arthroscopic compared with open repairs for recurrent anterior shoulder instability. A systematic review and meta-analysis of the literature. *J Bone Joint Surg Am.* 2007;89(2):244-254.

3. Rhee YG, Ha JH. Knot-induced glenoid erosion after arthroscopic fixation for unstable superior labrum anterior-posterior lesion: case report. *J Shoulder Elbow Surg.* 2006;15(3):391-393.

4. Thal R. A knotless suture anchor: technique for use in arthroscopic Bankart repair. *Arthroscopy.* 2001;17(2):213-218.

5. Slabaugh MA, Friel NA, Wang VM, et al. Restoring the labral height for treatment of Bankart lesions: a comparison of suture anchor constructs. *Arthroscopy.* 2010;26(5):587-591.

6. Leedle BP, Miller MD. Pullout strength of knotless suture anchors. *Arthroscopy.* 2005;21(1):81-85.

7. Thal R. A knotless suture anchor. Design, function, and biomechanical testing. *Am J Sports Med.* 2001;29(5):646-649.

8. Nho SJ, Frank RM, Van Thiel GS, et al. A biomechanical analysis of anterior Bankart repair using suture anchors. *Am J Sports Med.* 2010;38(7):1405-1412.

9. Thal R. Knotless suture anchor: arthroscopic Bankart repair without tying knots. *Clin Orthop Relat Res.* 2001;390:42-51.

10. Thal R, Nofziger M, Bridges M, et al. Arthroscopic Bankart repair using Knotless or BioKnotless suture anchors: 2- to 7-year results. *Arthroscopy.* 2007;23(4):367-375.

11. Garofalo R, Mocci A, Moretti B, et al. Arthroscopic treatment of anterior shoulder instability using knotless suture anchors. *Arthroscopy.* 2005;21(11):1283-1289.

12. Hayashida K, Yoneda M, Mizuno N, et al. Arthroscopic Bankart repair with knotless suture anchor for traumatic anterior shoulder instability: results of short-term follow-up. *Arthroscopy.* 2006;22(6):620-626.

13. Oh JH, Lee HK, Kim JY, et al. Clinical and radiologic outcomes of arthroscopic glenoid labrum repair with the BioKnotless suture anchor. *Am J Sports Med.* 2009;37(12):2340-2348.

14. Kocaoglu B, Guven O, Nalbantoglu U, et al. No difference between knotless sutures and suture anchors in arthroscopic repair of Bankart lesions in collision athletes. *Knee Surg Sports Traumatol Arthrosc.* 2009;17(7):844-849.

Chapter 6

Arthroscopic Rotator Interval Capsule Closure*†

Rachel M. Frank and Matthew T. Provencher

Chapter Synopsis

- The rotator interval (RI) is a triangular space of the anterosuperior shoulder between the supraspinatus and subscapularis tendons. The function of the RI in maintaining overall shoulder stability remains under debate, but surgical closure of the RI has been advocated in specific cases of shoulder instability. In the past, RI closure was commonly performed via open surgical techniques; however, recent all-arthroscopic techniques for RI closure have been described. The purpose of this chapter is to describe the arthroscopic treatment for RI closure.

Important Points

- The components of the RI include the coracohumeral ligament (CHL), the superior glenohumeral ligament (SGHL), the long head of the biceps (LHB) tendon, and a thin layer of joint capsule.
- The RI is a triangular space between the supraspinatus (SS) and subscapularis (SSc).
- The RI shape changes with internal and external rotation of the glenohumeral (GH) joint.
- A competent RI contributes to inferior shoulder stability via the CHL and an intact shoulder capsule (maintains negative intraarticular pressure).
- A sulcus sign that persists in external rotation (ER) is an indicator of RI insufficiency (of the CHL).
- Hyper-ER of the arm at the side (more than 90 degrees) also suggests incompetent anterior stabilization structures (possibly the RI).

- An open RI closure imbricates the CHL better than an arthroscopic closure; thus an open RI closure does not perform the same biomechanically as an arthroscopic RI closure, as both techniques generally repair different tissues in a different vector of closure.
- Volumetric reduction of the GH joint capsule may be achieved with adequate RI closure.

Clinical and Surgical Pearls

Surgical Indications

- Arthroscopic RI closure may be indicated in certain cases of anterior instability, revision anterior instability (to increase the anterior bumper effect), multidirectional instability with laxity and sulcus sign, and possibly posterior or anterior instability in the setting of hyperlaxity.

Surgical Pearls

- Adequate visualization from posterior portal.
- Arthroscopic closure medially and laterally (two separate stitches) in robust tissue of SGHL and middle glenohumeral ligament (MGHL).
- Penetrator device or suture passer may be used to accomplish repair—generally a 1-cm imbrication of the capsular tissues.
- Some advocate SS to SSc closure to obtain more robust tissue closure.
- Tie the sutures over the capsule blindly through a cannula that is pulled out just anterior to the capsule before tying.

Continued

*The views expressed in this article are those of the authors and do not reflect the official policy or position of the Department of the Navy, Department of Defense, or the United States Government.
†Funding: No sources of support in the forms of grants, equipment, or other items were received for this study. The authors report no conflict of interest.

- Imbrication of the CHL medially to laterally is difficult to achieve with arthroscopic methods.

Clinical and Surgical Pitfalls
- Closing the RI in neutral will result in ER losses, especially at the side; close the RI in 30 to 45 degrees of ER to avoid loss of ER postoperatively.
- Avoid suturing the LHB tendon so as not to imbricate the biceps.
- For inadequate shift of tissue, use two stitches—one medially and one laterally based—to obtain an adequate shift.

- Performing RI closure when not indicated will not improve stability and possibly will lead to large losses in motion.

 Video

Video 6-1: Rotator interval closure after Bankart repair

Video 6-2: Rotator interval suture passing

The rotator interval (RI) is a triangular space of the anterosuperior shoulder between the supraspinatus (SS) and subscapularis (SSc) tendons, containing both the coracohumeral ligament (CHL) and the superior glenohumeral ligament (SGHL) (Figs. 6-1 and 6-2). Although injuries to the RI capsule have been associated with increased glenohumeral translation and subsequent instability,[1,2] its contribution to overall shoulder stability remains under debate. Several reports have suggested that RI capsular structures contribute to stability by resisting inferior and posterior glenohumeral translation[3-6] and/or maintaining negative intraarticular pressure,[7]

whereas others have shown that surgical imbrication of the RI augments surgical correction of multidirectional and posterior instability.[3,4,6,8-12] Previously, RI closure was commonly performed via open surgical techniques; however, recent all-arthroscopic techniques for RI closure have been described.[13,14]

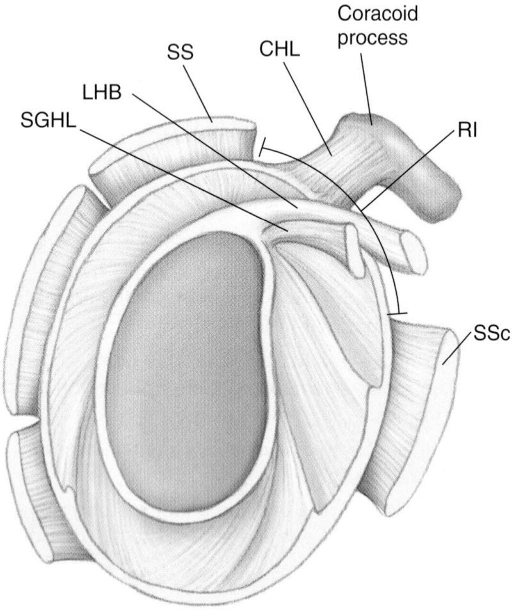

The debate regarding RI closure is centered around the "circle concept" of the shoulder,[15] which states that if the humerus is posteriorly subluxed, there must be an opposite and obligate injury to the anterior superior structures of the glenohumeral joint (the RI). However, several studies have refuted the circle concept theory,[16] indicating no injury to the RI after posterior dislocation.

In addition, the premise of an open RI closure is not the same concept as an arthroscopic RI closure.[3,14,17] As described by Harryman,[3] open RI closure consistently imbricates the CHL from medial to lateral, which adequately restores inferior and posterior stability of the shoulder; however, this occurs at the expense of significant (30- to 40-degree) losses of external rotation (ER) at the side (Fig. 6-3). All-arthroscopic techniques have evolved to address the RI; however, the arthroscopic closure is fundamentally different from the open closure in direction of closure (arthroscopic: superior to inferior; open: medial to lateral and/or superior to inferior), in addition to differences in tissue imbricated (arthroscopic: RI capsule, SGHL to middle glenohumeral ligament [MGHL]; open: CHL or SS to SSc). Based on biomechanical evidence,[12,14,17-19] there are certain indications for an arthroscopic RI closure, including certain cases of anterior instability (in the setting of hyperlaxity) and revision anterior instability (to increase the bumper effect anteriorly), multidirectional instability with laxity and sulcus sign, and possible posterior or anterior instability in the setting of hyperlaxity. The purposes of this chapter are to review the operative indications and surgical technique for arthroscopic RI capsule closure in the setting of glenohumeral instability.

Figure 6-1. The rotator interval (RI) is a triangular structure between the supraspinatus (SS) and subscapularis (SSc) and contains the long head of the biceps (LHB) tendon, the superior glenohumeral ligament (SGHL), the coracohumeral ligament (CHL), and a thin layer of capsule demonstrated in the sagittal oblique orientation.

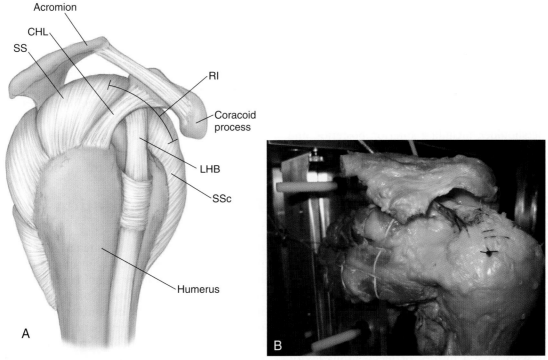

Figure 6-2. A, Coronal view of the rotator interval *(RI)* demonstrating the supraspinatus *(SS)*, subscapularis *(SSc)*, long head of the biceps *(LHB tendon)*, superior glenohumeral ligament *(SGHL)*, coracohumeral ligament *(CHL)*, and capsule. **B,** A cadaveric image outlining the CHL, which originates at the base of the coracoid process and inserts on the lesser tuberosity of the humerus.

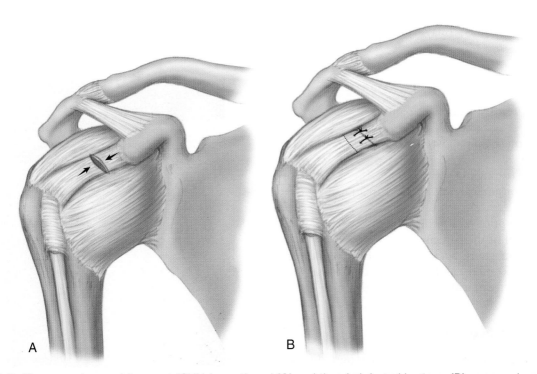

Figure 6-3. The coracohumeral ligament (CHL) is sectioned **(A)** and then imbricated by 1 cm **(B),** as was demonstrated by Harryman[3] in an open rotator interval closure that shortened the CHL to improve inferior and posterior stability of the shoulder. This technique resulted in significant (30- to 45-degree) losses of external rotation at the side.

PREOPERATIVE CONSIDERATIONS

History

A thorough history is necessary in the evaluation of every patient with suspected RI pathology. RI pathology is most often seen with concomitant instability conditions of the shoulder, including anterior, posterior, and multidirectional instability. Therefore questions regarding baseline shoulder stability, including any history of traumatic instability events and/or chronic subluxation or dislocation events, should be asked. Information about any previous shoulder operations, especially stabilization procedures, should be noted. Given the complex anatomy of the RI, several concomitant structures may also be injured with an RI capsular lesion, and patients may report symptoms related to the labrum, CHL, biceps tendon, and rotator cuff. The diagnosis of any pathology in addition to lesions of the RI is thus crucial for preoperative planning and appropriate surgical management. The RI may be suspected to be involved in patients who have a history of ligamentous laxity, multiple recurrences of instability, and history of multidirectional instability or either anterior or posterior instability in the setting of hyperlaxity. Specifically, during the initial clinic visit, the clinician should inquire about the following:

- Original mechanism of injury (traumatic versus insidious onset)
- Current symptoms (may point to alternative diagnosis)
- Locking
- Clicking
- Crepitus
- Pain (e.g., rest pain vs. night pain)
- Stiffness
- Inability to use arm above head
- Instability
- Numbness or tingling
- Previous nonsurgical and surgical treatment of the shoulder
- Response to prior treatment
- Activity level of the patient
- Posttreatment goals; allows the surgeon to address patient expectations and to ensure that these are aligned with treatment options and outcomes

Signs and Symptoms

Patients with RI capsular lesions often report diffuse shoulder pain, night pain, and the sensation of instability. RI pathology is often associated with the finding of shoulder instability, especially in the setting of hyperlaxity. Sensation of subluxation and/or dislocation,

especially in the provocative position of abduction (ABD), and ER may be present. Hallmark symptoms that may be present include pain while carrying objects at the side (gallon of milk), paresthesias, and other findings suggestive of a sulcus sign or inferior laxity of the glenohumeral joint. Swelling is not commonly seen with these injuries and if present warrants a workup for other possible injuries, including articular cartilage defects. Similarly, strength and sensation are typically normal even in patients with significant RI capsule lesions, though limitations resulting from pain may be present.

Physical Examination

Isolated pathology of the RI is difficult to assess on examination, as findings are often vague and representative of anterior, posterior, and/or multidirectional instability. As in any shoulder examination, the appearance, strength, sensation, and range of motion (ROM) of the injured shoulder should be compared with those of the opposite shoulder in every patient with suspected RI capsule pathology. Particular attention should be paid to special tests for shoulder stability, because, as previously mentioned, RI lesions usually occur in the setting of shoulder instability. Physical examination findings suggestive of RI capsule lesions include the following:

- Sulcus sign—downward traction of the arm causes inferior subluxation of the humeral head that does not resolve with ER of the shoulder (Fig. 6-4).
- Sulcus sign that persists in ER at the side—when the RI is intact, ER with the arm at the side will allow for resolution of the sulcus sign as the CHL becomes

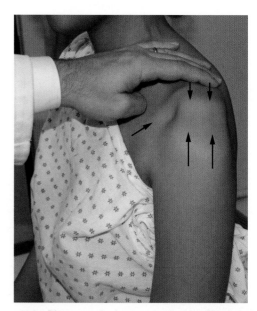

Figure 6-4. Photograph demonstrating a patient with a positive sulcus sign with the arm at neutral demonstrating a gap of greater than 1 cm between the acromion and the top of the humeral head.

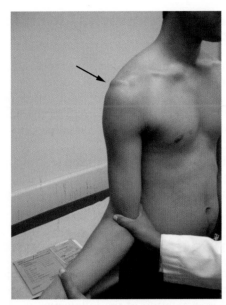

Figure 6-5. Photograph demonstrating a patient with a sulcus sign that persists in external rotation, indicative of insufficiency of the rotator interval; this patient also had hyperlaxity of the glenohumeral joint.

taught. A sulcus that persists in ER is suggestive of RI insufficiency (Fig. 6-5).

- Hyper-ER of the arm at the side (more than 90 degrees) also suggests incompetent anterior stabilization structures (possibly the RI).
- Pain in the bicipital groove—suggests involvement of the long head of the biceps (LHB) tendon.
- Anterior instability in the setting of hyperlaxity (sulcus sign inferiorly).
- Multidirectional instability findings with sulcus sign or inferior laxity.

Imaging

Various imaging modalities are helpful in confirming the diagnosis of RI capsule lesions, including radiographic studies, magnetic resonance imaging (MRI), and magnetic resonance arthrography (MRA). A standard radiographic shoulder series, including anteroposterior, scapular-Y, and axillary views, is helpful in the global evaluation of the shoulder joint; however, there are no specific radiographic findings for RI capsule lesions. MRI is the diagnostic modality of choice for the evaluation of soft tissue structures surrounding the glenohumeral joint, including the labrum and capsular complex, and is useful in evaluating the pathology associated with the RI. MRA is the most sensitive of all imaging studies for RI lesions, with several specific findings, as follows:

- Radiopaque dye in the subacromial and/or subdeltoid bursa through the RI.
- Radiopaque dye under the coracoid on the oblique sagittal images.

- Of note, improper MRA technique can result in dye being injected into the soft tissues as opposed to intraarticularly; can give a false-positive result.
- A widened RI (distance between the SS and SSc), as well as anterior displacement of the LHB tendon relative to the SS on the sagittal oblique images.[20]

Indications and Contraindications

The decision to perform arthroscopic RI capsule closure can be difficult, as the clinical role of the RI in maintaining shoulder stability is still not fully understood. Currently there have been no long-term clinical studies regarding the outcomes of RI closure, and the biomechanical data regarding the benefits of arthroscopic RI closure are controversial. In addition, although clinical and biomechanical studies show improvement in anterior stability when arthroscopic RI closure is performed, the outcomes are not as clear regarding posterior and/or inferior stability. Finally, after RI repair there is a potential for significant loss of ER at the side, which can negatively affect the patient's quality of life; therefore careful preoperative planning and patient selection are crucial for a successful outcome. Although there are no clear absolute indications for arthroscopic RI capsule closure, the following relative indications can be used as a guide:

- Anterior instability with an incompetent sulcus (persistent sulcus sign in ER)
- Anterior instability with hyperlaxity
- Failed anterior instability surgery to increase the stable bumper effect anteriorly
- Significant laxity and a large sulcus in the setting of multidirectional instability
- Patients with posterior instability who have an incompetent RI and hyperlaxity
- Failed nonoperative treatment

Relative contraindications include the following:

- Infection
- Significant glenoid version or structural abnormalities
- Untreated concomitant injuries (e.g., chondral defects, rotator cuff)
- Unrealistic postoperative goals
- Unwillingness to comply with postoperative rehabilitation regimen
- Sports or activities that may be affected by ER losses (e.g., pitching, javelin, volleyball)

SURGICAL TECHNIQUE

Box 6-1 outlines the surgical technique.

BOX 6-1 Surgical Steps

1. Complete appropriate capsulolabral repair.
2. Ensure proper arm positioning—30 to 45 degrees of ER.
3. Penetrate tissue adjacent to MGHL or MGHL proper with sharp crescent hook (loaded with No. 1 monofilament suture).
4. Place first stitch medially, near level of glenoid face.
5. Shuttle the No. 1 monofilament suture into joint.
6. Remove crescent hook.
7. Use penetrator to retrieve the No. 1 monofilament suture.
8. Change suture to No. 2 nonabsorbable suture.
9. Take suture outside the cannula.
10. Remove then replace cannula to place suture external to cannula.
11. Place second stitch if necessary.
12. Replace cannula just anterior to capsule after the two medially based sutures have been placed.
13. Tie a nonsliding knot with aid of knot pusher; ensure that knot is "all inside."
14. Use blind knot cutter to cut knot.
15. Repeat for second stitch.
16. Release arm from the 30 degrees of ER.

ER, External rotation; *MGHL,* middle glenohumeral ligament.

Anesthesia and Positioning

Depending on surgeon and anesthesiologist preference, the majority of arthroscopic shoulder stabilization procedures incorporating RI capsule closure are performed with the patient under general anesthesia with an interscalene block. Alternatively, sedation with interscalene block can also be used. Depending on the procedure being performed as well as surgeon preference and experience, the patient can be positioned in either the beach chair or lateral decubitus position. After the patient is adequately positioned, skin preparation and draping can be performed according to the surgeon's preference. The patient can be in either the beach chair or lateral decubitus position, and the position of the glenohumeral joint adjusted to 30 degrees of ER with an assistant positioning the arm holder. It is crucial to place the shoulder in some level of ER to avoid overtightening and potential postoperative loss of ER. Alternatively, the main part of the instability case may be performed and then the arm removed from the arm holder device to be externally rotated while the RI repair is done. The lateral decubitus position allows for ease of visualization of the RI with the arthroscope from the posterior portal.

Surgical Landmarks, Incisions, and Portals

- Landmarks include the coracoid process, acromion, deltoid insertion, and axillary crease.
- The arthroscope is inserted from posterior, and a small (5-mm) cannula is inserted in the midglenoid portal, just lateral to the coracoid process, through the RI.
- Standard arthroscopy portals for arthroscopic techniques are used.
- At-risk structures include the musculocutaneous nerve and axillary nerve.

Examination Under Anesthesia

The examination under anesthesia (EUA) should be performed before the beginning of arthroscopy and is helpful in evaluation of the following:

- ROM.
- Stability—anterior, posterior, and inferior. Assess sulcus sign with the arm in neutral and externally rotated to determine RI competence.

Specific Surgical Techniques and Steps

Once the capsulolabral repair is completed as deemed appropriate, the authors' preferred technique for arthroscopic RI capsule closure involves a modification of the method described by Taverna.[21] This "all-inside" technique allows direct visualization of the extent of RI repair while preserving the deltoid (Figs. 6-6 through 6-9).

1. A sharp crescent hook device (ConMed, Linvatec, Largo, FL) is loaded with No. 1 monofilament suture. This is brought in through the cannula, and then the tissue adjacent to the MGHL or the MGHL proper is penetrated with the sharp crescent needle.
2. A 5- to 7-mm cannula is placed back into the middle aspect of the RI (where it was previously placed in the beginning of the case), and then backed out such that it is just anterior to the capsule.
3. *Pearl:* If the MGHL is small, the superior aspect of the SSc or other tissues just superior to the SSc can be grasped.
4. The first stitch is placed medially, near the level of the glenoid face; one additional and separate stitch will be placed more laterally if necessary.
5. The No. 1 monofilament suture is shuttled into the joint, and then the crescent hook is removed.
6. *Pearl:* The cannula is maintained in position just anterior to the capsule but is shifted slightly superior so that a sharp penetrator device can pierce the

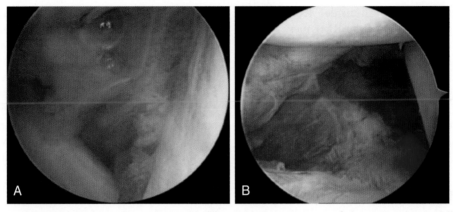

Figure 6-6. A, An arthroscopic image of a patient with fibrosis and contracture of the rotator interval (RI) (frozen shoulder syndrome) and adhesive capsulitis. The RI is often affected in adhesive capsulitis and causes predictable losses of external rotation (ER) at the side. In this case the RI is released arthroscopically. **B,** After a partial release of the RI capsule in a patient with frozen shoulder syndrome (adhesive capsulitis), improved ER of the shoulder at the side is seen in this arthroscopic image.

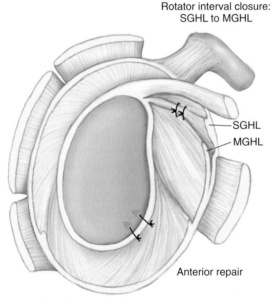

Rotator interval closure: SGHL to MGHL

SGHL
MGHL

Anterior repair

Figure 6-7. A typical rotator interval (RI) closure patient with anterior instability and hyperlaxity with a symptomatic sulcus sign and inferior instability of the shoulder in the setting of anterior instability. The anterior-inferior capsulolabral structures are repaired with anchors, and a two-stitch arthroscopic RI closure is performed.

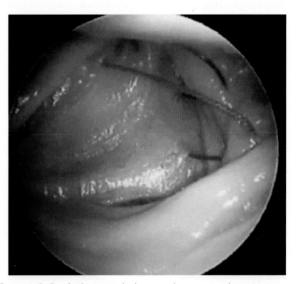

Figure 6-8. Arthroscopic image demonstrating a two-stitch configuration for rotator interval (RI) closure (one medial and one lateral), allowing for a typical shift of the superior glenohumeral ligament to the middle glenohumeral ligament of the RI capsule. This arthroscopic RI closure shifts the tissues in a superior-to-inferior direction.

SGHL and tissues immediately inferior to the SS, again a few millimeters lateral to the glenoid face.

7. The penetrator retrieves the No. 1 monofilament suture and is brought out through the cannula.

8. This is changed to a No. 2 nonabsorbable suture (Ethibond; Ethicon, Somerville, NJ).

9. *Note:* Absorbable sutures may also be used.

10. The No. 2 nonabsorbable suture is taken outside the cannula, and then the cannula is removed and replaced such that the sutures are now external to the cannula.

11. *Note:* A second stitch that is more laterally placed in the tissues may be passed at this point in similar fashion.

12. The cannula is then replaced, just anterior to the capsule, after the two medially based sutures are placed inside the cannula while it is external to the body.

13. The glenohumeral joint is externally rotated 30 to 45 degrees to avoid inadvertent RI contracture and loss of ER. Once down on the capsule, a knot pusher is used to tie a nonsliding knot while the

closure is watched in an "all-inside" technique to ensure adequate plication of the RI tissues.

14. A blind knot cutter is then used, and the process is repeated for the second stitch.
15. The second stitch is placed more lateral to the medially based first stitch. Thus a medial and a lateral RI repair are performed.
16. The arm is then released from 30 to 45 degrees of ER, and stability and postoperative ROM are assessed.

Rehabilitation

Our postoperative protocol for arthroscopic RI capsule closure is guided by any procedures performed in addition to the RI closure (usually an anterior, posterior, or multidirectional stabilization). Most commonly, the dominating procedure will be arthroscopic shoulder stabilization (e.g., anterior shoulder capsulolabral

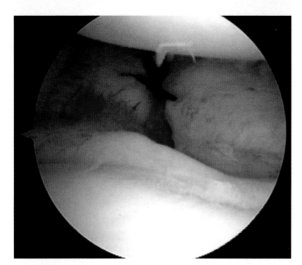

Figure 6-9. Arthroscopic image showing final arthroscopic rotator interval (RI) closure.

plication or suture anchor repair). Patients will be placed into a sling for 4 to 6 weeks, and the primary procedure (as opposed to the RI closure) is allowed to dictate the postoperative regimen. Regardless of the primary procedure, it is advised to avoid more than 30 degrees of ER for the first 5 to 6 weeks after arthroscopic RI capsule closure. After the sling has been removed, active and active-assisted exercises and terminal ROM stretching are begun. Gradual return to activity is then begun with a goal of full activity at 6 months.

Complications

Complications associated with arthroscopic RI capsule closure are rare; however, if they occur, they can be problematic. Known complications include the following:

- Loss of ER, especially at the side
- Postoperative pain caused by excessive constraint
- Skin irritation anteriorly and subacromial irritation from sutures

RESULTS

Arthroscopic RI capsule closure as an augmentation to stability has been described in cases of anterior, posterior, and multidirectional instability; however, the long-term outcomes remain largely unknown. Several studies are summarized in Table 6-1, grouped into direction of shoulder instability and whether or not RI closure was performed. Overall, with regard to anterior shoulder instability, the use of RI closure augmentation has been shown to improve recurrence rates; however, this has not been fully tested with long-term studies, and concerns regarding postoperative loss of ER remain.

With regard to arthroscopic posterior shoulder instability surgery, the role of adjuvant RI capsule closure is

TABLE 6-1 Selected Outcomes Studies

Author	Year	Type of Instability	Method	Position of Shoulder	Results (if Given)
Chiang et al[26] (n = 45 shoulders)	2010	Anterior	Arthroscopic anteroinferior stabilization followed by suture repair of RI and posteroinferior capsular plication	Lateral decubitus position, traction sleeve in 45 degrees ABD with approximately 10 pounds traction	Average follow-up of 77 months
					Improvements in ASES, UCLA, Rowe scores (*P* < .0001) and average ROM deficit compared with healthy shoulder not significant (*P* > .05).
					All returned to preinjury activity level.

TABLE 6-1 Selected Outcomes Studies—cont'd

Author	Year	Type of Instability	Method	Position of Shoulder	Results (if Given)
Chechik et al[25] (n = 83 shoulders)	2010	Anterior	Arthroscopic Bankart repair with or without suture repair of RI (37/83)	Beach chair position, arm in 30 degrees ER for RI portion of case RI decision based on MDI, systemic factors, RI laxity	Average f/u of 46 m.
					Overall recurrent dislocation rate of 11% (instability rate 19%); authors suggest RI closure in patients with shoulder laxity and systemic joint hyperlaxity.
Lino et al[29] (n = 27 shoulders)	2006	Anterior	Arthroscopic labrum repair, thermal capsulorrhaphy, and suture repair of RI (SSc to SS with No. 5 Ethibond, average 2.8 stitches)	Lateral decubitus position with cutaneous traction	Average f/u 32 m.
					All shoulders without recurrent instability; all with improvements in UCLA, Rowe, and ASES scores.
Garofalo et al[27] (n = 20 shoulders)	2005	Anterior	Arthroscopic anterior instability repair with knotless suture anchors, three with RI closure (specific technique not described)	Lateral decubitus position, arm in 30-45 degrees of ABD and 15 degrees of anterior flexion with 3-4 kg traction	Average f/u 43 m.
					Return to sport: 80%; 90% satisfied, 5% re-dislocation, 5% instability.
Mazzocca et al[30] (n = 18 shoulders)	2005	Anterior	Arthroscopic shoulder instability repair with or without suture repair of RI (1/18 only, technique not described)	Not described	Average f/u 37 m.
					Return to sport: 100%; 11% recurrence (collision athletes).
Savoie et al[31] (n = 92 shoulders)	2008	Posterior	Arthroscopic posterior shoulder instability repair RI closed in all patients via "wide-based technique"	Lateral decubitus position rolled 30 degrees posteriorly	Average f/u of 28 m.
					Of treated shoulders, 97% stable and surgery successful (Neer-Foster rating scale).
Kim et al[28] (n = 31 shoulders)	2004	MDI	Arthroscopic MDI repair with arthroscopic RI closure	Lateral decubitus position, arm in 30 degrees ABD and 10 degrees FF with lateral traction	Average f/u 51 m.
					Of treated patients, 30 had stable shoulders, 1 had recurrent instability; 21 had excellent and 9 had good Rowe scores.

ABD, abduction; *ASES,* American Shoulder and Elbow Surgeons scale; *ER,* external rotation; *FF,* forward flexion; *f/u,* follow-up; *MDI,* multidirectional instability; *RI,* rotator interval; *ROM,* range of motion; *SS,* supraspinatus; *SSc,* subscapularis; *UCLA,* University of California at Los Angeles shoulder rating scale.

even less understood. Studies by Bradley (100 patients, no RI closure)[22] and Provencher (33 patients, two with RI closure)[23] did not routinely use RI closure with overall very good to excellent rates of success, although a recent report by Savoie has shown successful outcomes (92 patients, 87 with RI closure).[24] The adjunctive use of RI closure remains to be defined in various forms on shoulder instability, and both further biomechanical studies analyzing advanced surgical techniques as well as further clinical studies are necessary to clearly define its role.

REFERENCES

1. Hunt SA, Kwon YW, Zuckerman JD. The rotator interval: anatomy, pathology, and strategies for treatment. *J Am Acad Orthop Surg.* 2007;15(4):218-227.
2. Nobuhara K, Ikeda H. Rotator interval lesion. *Clin Orthop Relat Res.* 1987;223:44-50.
3. Harryman DT, 2nd, Sidles JA, Harris SL, et al. The role of the rotator interval capsule in passive motion and stability of the shoulder. *J Bone Joint Surg Am.* 1992;74(1):53-66.
4. Jost B, Koch PP, Gerber C. Anatomy and functional aspects of the rotator interval. *Journal of Shoulder & Elbow Surgery.* 2000;9(4):336-341.
5 Pradhan RL, Itoi E. Rotator interval lesions of the shoulder joint. *Orthopedics.* 2001;24(8):798-801.
6. Van der Reis W, Wolf E. Arthroscopic rotator cuff interval capsular closure. *Orthopedics.* 2001;24(7):657-661.
7. Itoi E, Berglund LJ, Grabowski JJ, et al. Superior-inferior stability of the shoulder: role of the coracohumeral ligament and the rotator interval capsule. *Mayo Clinic Proceedings.* 1998;73(6):508-515.
8. Cole BJ, Mazzocca AD, Meneghini RM. Indirect arthroscopic rotator interval repair. *Arthroscopy.* 2003; 19(6):E28-E31.
9. Field LD, Warren RF, O'Brien SJ, et al. Isolated closure of rotator interval defects for shoulder instability. *American Journal of Sports Medicine.* 1995;23(5):557-563.
10. Millett P, Clavert P, Warner J. Arthroscopic management of anterior, posterior, and multidirectional shoulder instability: pearls and pitfalls. *Arthroscopy.* 2003;19(10 (Suppl 1)):86-93.
11. Plausinis D, Bravman JT, Heywood C, et al. Arthroscopic rotator interval closure: effect of sutures on glenohumeral motion and anterior-posterior translation. *Am J Sports Med.* 2006;34(10):1656-1661.
12. Yamamoto N, Itoi E, Tuoheti Y, et al. Effect of rotator interval closure on glenohumeral stability and motion: a cadaveric study. *J Shoulder Elbow Surg.* 2006;15(6): 750-758.
13. Farber AJ, Elattrache NS, Tibone JE, et al. Biomechanical analysis comparing a traditional superior-inferior arthroscopic rotator interval closure with a novel medial-lateral technique in a cadaveric multidirectional instability model. *Am J Sports Med.* 2009.
14. Mologne TS, Zhao K, Hongo M, et al. The addition of rotator interval closure after arthroscopic repair of either anterior or posterior shoulder instability: effect on glenohumeral translation and range of motion. *Am J Sports Med.* 2008;36(6):1123-1131.
15. Warren R, Kornblatt I, Marchand R. Static factors affecting posterior shoulder stability. *Orthop Trans.* 1984;8:89.
16. Weber SC, Caspari RB. A biomechanical evaluation of the restraints to posterior shoulder dislocation. *Arthroscopy.* 1989;5:115-121.
17. Provencher MT, Mologne TS, Hongo M, et al. Arthroscopic versus open rotator interval closure: biomechanical evaluation of stability and motion. *Arthroscopy.* 2007; 23(6):583-592.
18. Ozsoy MH, Bayramoglu A, Demiryurek D, et al. Rotator interval dimensions in different shoulder arthroscopy positions: a cadaveric study. *J Shoulder Elbow Surg.* 2008;17(4):624-630.
19. Shafer BL, Mihata T, McGarry MH, et al. Effects of capsular plication and rotator interval closure in simulated multidirectional shoulder instability. *J Bone Joint Surg Am.* 2008;90(1):136-144.
20. Provencher MT, Dewing CB, Bell SJ, et al. An analysis of the rotator interval in patients with anterior, posterior, and multidirectional shoulder instability. *Arthroscopy.* 2008;24(8):921-929.
21. Taverna E, Sansone V, Battistella F. Arthroscopic rotator interval repair: the three-step all-inside technique. *Arthroscopy.* 2004;20(6):105-109.
22. Bradley JP, Baker CL, 3rd, Kline AJ, et al. Arthroscopic capsulolabral reconstruction for posterior instability of the shoulder: a prospective study of 100 shoulders. *Am J Sports Med.* 2006;34(7):1061-1071.
23. Provencher MT, Bell SJ, Menzel KA, et al. Arthroscopic treatment of posterior shoulder instability: results in 33 patients. *Am J Sports Med.* 2005;33(10):1463-1471.
24. Savoie FH 3rd, Holt MS, Field LD, et al. Arthroscopic management of posterior instability: evolution of technique and results. *Arthroscopy.* 2008;24(4):389-396.
25. Chechik O, Maman E, Dolkart O, et al. Arthroscopic rotator interval closure in shoulder instability repair: a retrospective study. *J Shoulder Elbow Surg.* 2010;19(7): 1056-1062.
26. Chiang ER, Wang JP, Wang ST, et al. Arthroscopic posteroinferior capsular plication and rotator interval closure after Bankart repair in patients with traumatic anterior glenohumeral instability: a minimum follow-up of 5 years. *Injury.* 2010;41(10):1075-1078.
27. Garofalo R, Mocci A, Moretti B, et al. Arthroscopic treatment of anterior shoulder instability using knotless suture anchors. *Arthroscopy.* 2005;21(11):1283-1289.
28. Kim SH, Kim HK, Sun JI, et al. Arthroscopic capsulolabroplasty for posteroinferior multidirectional instability of the shoulder. *Am J Sports Med.* 2004;32(3):594-607.
29. Lino W Jr, Belangero WD. Labrum repair combined with arthroscopic reduction of capsular volume in shoulder instability. *Int Orthop.* 2006;30(4):219-223.
30. Mazzocca AD, Brown FM Jr, Carreira DS, et al. Arthroscopic anterior shoulder stabilization of collision and contact athletes. *Am J Sports Med.* 2005;33(1): 52-60.
31. Savoie FH 3rd, Holt MS, Field LD, et al. Arthroscopic management of posterior instability: evolution of technique and results. *Arthroscopy.* 2008;24(4):389-396.

SUGGESTED READINGS

Farber AJ, Elattrache NS, Tibone JE, et al. Biomechanical analysis comparing a traditional superior-inferior arthroscopic rotator interval closure with a novel medial-lateral technique in a cadaveric multidirectional instability model. *Am J Sports Med.* 2009.

Harryman DT 2nd, Sidles JA, Harris SL, et al. The role of the rotator interval capsule in passive motion and stability of the shoulder. *J Bone Joint Surg Am.* 1992;74(1):53-66.

Mologne TS, Zhao K, Hongo M, et al. The addition of rotator interval closure after arthroscopic repair of either anterior or posterior shoulder instability: effect on glenohumeral translation and range of motion. *Am J Sports Med.* 2008;36(6):1123-1131.

Provencher MT, Mologne TS, Hongo M, et al. Arthroscopic versus open rotator interval closure: biomechanical evaluation of stability and motion. *Arthroscopy.* 2007;23(6): 583-592.

Taverna E, Sansone V, Battistella F. Arthroscopic rotator interval repair: the three-step all-inside technique. *Arthroscopy.* 2004;20(6):105-109.

Chapter 7

Management of the Throwing Shoulder

John M. Tokish and Jay B. Cook

Chapter Synopsis

- The disabled throwing shoulder remains a unique surgical challenge. Few other shoulder conditions so blur the line between pathology and adaptive change. Our understanding of the underlying pathology continues to evolve, with the theories of internal impingement and glenohumeral internal rotation deficit (GIRD) guiding treatment approaches. The cornerstone of nonoperative management remains posterior capsular stretching and dynamic strengthening, which are often effective. Surgical treatment must be individualized and approached with respect for treatment of pathology balanced with an understanding of the normal adaptive changes seen in throwers, as well as the demands inherent to returning to throw.

Important Points

- The throwing shoulder undergoes normal adaptive change.
- Examination findings often include decreased internal rotation and rotator cuff symptoms.
- Nonoperative therapy has shown good results and should always be performed as first-line treatment.
- Operative intervention should address pathology noted.
- Labral pathology, partial-thickness rotator cuff tears, and posterior capsular contracture must all be recognized and carefully approached if nonoperative measures fail.
- Even with successful treatment, returning to the same level of throwing means returning to the same level of stresses that caused the pathology in the first place.

Clinical and Surgical Pearls

- A thorough history and physical examination must be performed, including gathering pertinent input from the thrower's coach and trainer.

- Core strengthening, dynamic scapular stabilization, and posterior capsular stretching should be part of all maintenance and rehabilitation programs.
- Surgical intervention should occur only after failure of prolonged nonoperative management.
- Thorough diagnostic arthroscopy should be performed, including a dynamic evaluation of the joint with the arm throughout the simulated pitching motion.
- Particular attention should be paid to the articular side of the rotator cuff, posterior superior labrum, and posterior capsule.
- Posterior capsular release, if performed, can be expected to restore internal rotation, and frequent intraoperative evaluation should be conducted to ensure adequate release with protection of the cuff and neurovascular structures.
- Postoperative therapy must treat the entire kinetic chain for successful return to throwing.

Clinical and Surgical Pitfalls

- The axillary nerve lies in close proximity to the inferior capsule, and the capsule should be released medially to avoid damage to rotator cuff tendons.
- Overtightening of labral pathology may result in a poor outcome.
- Conversion of partial-thickness tears to full tears with subsequent repair has not been shown effective for returning to throw.

The throwing shoulder continues to be a challenge to manage and treat. The demands placed on the shoulder by overhead athletes produce a unique pathophysiology most evident in elite throwers. The throwing shoulder exerts up to 7000 degrees/sec rotational velocity, reportedly the fastest movement in sports.[1] As a result, throwing shoulders have been noted to exhibit adaptations including increased external rotation, decreased internal rotation, increased humeral and glenoid retroversion, and anterior capsular laxity. The combination of these demands and adaptations has created common pathologic lesions in the shoulder such as partial-thickness articular rotator cuff tears, anterior capsular laxity and pseudolaxity, posterior-inferior capsular contracture, posterior and posterosuperior labral injury, biceps tendon pathology, and scapular dyskinesis.[2]

One of the most difficult challenges in treating the disabled throwing shoulder is understanding the difference between pathologic entity and required adaptation. A "fix everything" approach may well lead to a shoulder that cannot return to the same level of throwing. It is therefore critical that the surgeon use a cautious approach to preoperative evaluation, meticulous surgical technique, and a comprehensive postoperative rehabilitation program in the athlete who hopes to return to such a demanding activity.

PATHOLOGY

Multiple theories about the cause of the dysfunctional throwing shoulder have been presented throughout the years. In 1959, Bennett described a posteroinferior glenoid exostosis as the inciting pathology for pain in the professional pitcher secondary to repetitive traction on the posterior capsule and triceps tendon.[3] This theory has since fallen out of favor, although his focus on the posterior capsule would lay the foundation for future work in treating the throwing shoulder.

Neer described impingement syndrome in 1972, and for a time this was considered a likely cause of the dysfunctional throwing shoulder.[4] The patient's complaints and physical examination findings had much overlap with those of impingement, and it was clear that the rotator cuff was often involved. However, Tibone and colleagues in 1985 reported on a series of shoulders treated with acromioplasty for impingement, including the shoulders of 18 throwers. Despite good pain relief, only 4 of the 18 returned to throwing.[5]

In the 1990s, Jobe introduced the concept of secondary impingement, which proposed that anterior shoulder instability brought on by repetitive stretching of the anterior capsule was the cause of the impingement. Jobe's 1991 article[6] was associated with excellent pain relief, but return to throwing remained elusive.

By the late 1990s, arthroscopy had become an important adjunctive tool in evaluating the throwing shoulder. At that time both Jobe and Walch separately described impingement of the cuff on the posterosuperior glenoid or "internal impingement." Jobe continued to attribute it to anterior laxity or "microinstability" as a result of repetitive forces in an abducted and maximally externally rotated position. Paley and colleagues[7] and Conway[8] both demonstrated that anterior instability was very common in throwers and contributed to internal impingement.

However, Walch reported on arthroscopic examination of 16 throwers with internal impingement but no instability, and described the visualization of the rotator cuff impinging in an abducted and externally rotated position leading to partial-thickness cuff tears and posterior capsular lesions.[9] Other studies have confirmed symptomatic internal impingement without anterior instability and a lack of laxity between throwing and nonthrowing shoulders in pitchers.[10]

In 2003, Burkhart and colleagues reported that internal impingement is actually a physiologic occurrence and that contracture of the posteroinferior capsule shifting the humerus posterosuperiorly is the primary pathology in the disabled throwing shoulder.[2] The authors noted that the resulting glenohumeral internal rotation deficit (GIRD) is the hallmark of the at-risk throwing shoulder. Other studies have confirmed the high prevalence of GIRD in throwing shoulders, its increased association with shoulder pathology, and resolution of symptoms with correction of GIRD.[2,11,12] However, there is evidence contrary to this idea as well. Huffman and colleagues, the same group that performed the biomechanical study that initially supported GIRD, revised their model in 2006 and showed that obligate translation with simulated posterior capsular contracture was in fact anterior and inferior and occurred during follow-through and not cocking.[13] In addition, GIRD has been noted to be present in 40% of asymptomatic throwers.[14] In fact, the disabled throwing shoulder may well be caused by a spectrum of conditions resulting from the adaptations required when variable anatomy and physiology are subjected to the extreme demands of throwing an object beyond physiologic limits.

PREOPERATIVE CONSIDERATIONS

History and Physical Examination

The dysfunctional throwing shoulder may manifest classically with posterior shoulder pain at the cocking phase of the throwing motion or during follow-through. Some patients, however, may describe a loss of control or velocity or the feeling of a "dead arm." The physical examination may reveal tenderness to palpation, increased external rotation with decreased internal

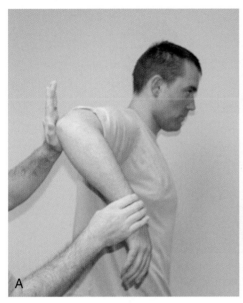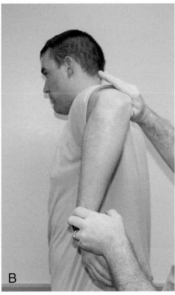

Figure 7-1. Dominant **(A)** and nondominant **(B)** arms in a thrower with loss of internal rotation. Note the difference in internal rotation of 25 degrees.

rotation,[15] instability or laxity, and positive posterior impingement test results,[16] as well as more traditional impingement signs. Decreased internal rotation of more than 20 degrees compared with the contralateral side, especially in the setting of a decreased total arc of motion, is suggestive of GIRD (Fig. 7-1) and should raise the suspicion for the examiner. With this increased suspicion, the examiner must pay particular attention to the core strength of the athlete, the scapula, and associated shoulder pathology. SICK scapula syndrome (scapular malposition, inferior medial border prominence, coracoid pain and malposition, and dyskinesis of scapular movement), or scapular dyskinesia, usually manifests with static and dynamic scapular malposition evident when the patient is asked to repeatedly raise and lower the arms or engage the dynamic stabilizers of the scapula.[17] Associated pathology such as shoulder microinstability, as evidenced by a positive result on relocation test for pain, superior labral tears suspected with a positive active compression test result, and pain with a sleeper stretch are all keys to the physical examination.

Imaging

Although standard radiographs should be included in the workup of the disabled throwing shoulder, they are usually normal. The cornerstone of radiographic evaluation remains magnetic resonance imaging (MRI) or even magnetic resonance arthrography (MRA), which can increase the study's accuracy in detecting labral pathology, rotator cuff and biceps pathology, capsular thickening, bursal pathology, and bony edema (Fig. 7-2). Computed tomography is not a standard method of examination but may be indicated if there is an abnormality on initial radiographic evaluation.

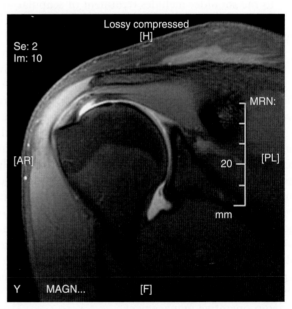

Figure 7-2. Magnetic resonance arthrogram in thrower demonstrating partial articular-sided cuff tear and anterior laxity.

NONOPERATIVE MANAGEMENT

Throwing is the culmination of multiple energy transfers from the proximal to distal kinetic chain. Deficits anywhere along this chain can be translated to more distal injury. Therefore, nonoperative management of the disabled throwing shoulder must address all aspects of the kinetic chain, as well as the shoulder itself, to be successful. Hip and leg strength must be maintained, and core strengthening cannot be overemphasized. The scapular platform must be optimized, as it forms the critical transfer between the power created in the core

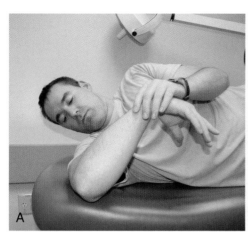
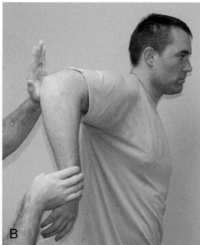

Figure 7-3. Sleeper stretches **(A)** are a cornerstone to treatment of glenohumeral internal rotation deficit (GIRD) in the thrower. Restoration **(B)** of internal rotation in thrower in Figure 7-1, after treatment for GIRD.

and the speed generated in the shoulder. Specific attention to the shoulder includes treatment of scapular and dynamic stabilizers as well as posterior capsular stretching. SICK scapula syndrome is the manifestation of a dyskinetic platform but can be effectively rehabilitated with retraining of scapular mechanics.[17] Rotator cuff weakness is common in the painful throwing shoulder, and cuff strengthening is a mainstay of any nonoperative approach to throwers. Posterior capsular tightness is among the most detrimental adaptations in the thrower but can be effectively treated with stretching techniques such as sleeper stretches, leading to resolution of symptoms (Fig. 7-3). Fortunately, most disabled throwing shoulders respond to this comprehensive approach. Wilk and colleagues[12] recently reported on their experience with one Major League Baseball team over 3 years. Although many of the pitchers exhibited GIRD, the vast majority of these cases resolved with a supervised athletic training program. Of the 33 pitchers who sustained shoulder injuries, only seven went on to undergo operative management.

OPERATIVE MANAGEMENT

Surgical intervention is indicated when the diagnosis is consistent with a pathologic throwing shoulder that has failed to respond to an adequate trial of nonoperative management.

Anesthesia and Positioning

Shoulder arthroscopy is typically performed with the patient under general anesthesia. Both lateral decubitus and beach chair positions can be used based on surgeon preference. It is important that the arm be draped in such a way as to allow a dynamic arthroscopic examination to include a simulated thrower's position. For

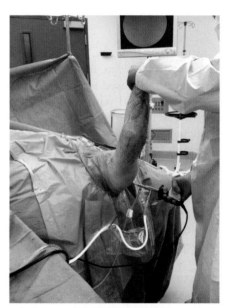

Figure 7-4. Dynamic arthroscopic examination of shoulder. The arm is taken out of traction and can be taken through a simulated throwing motion.

lateral positioning, this means removal from the arm traction device (Fig. 7-4). Abduction of the arm can assist in access to the articular insertion of the rotator cuff, a common location of pathology.

Surgical Landmarks, Incisions, and Portals

A detailed description of portal anatomy for the shoulder can be found elsewhere in this text. We have found it rare to need to modify portals from standard positions to access the pathologies seen in the treatment of the throwing shoulder.

Examination Under Anesthesia and Diagnostic Arthroscopy

Examination with the patient under anesthesia should be performed on both the affected and unaffected shoulders before preparation and draping protocols. Care should be taken to note differences in laxity as well as range of motion. Of particular interest is internal and external rotation at 90 degrees of abduction, as one should note the presence of GIRD on this examination. Once the examination is complete, the patient is positioned and the shoulder is prepared and draped.

A standard posterior portal is placed approximately 2 cm inferior and medial to the posterolateral border of the acromion. A standard anterior portal is established under direct visualization in the rotator interval. Placement of this portal high in the interval allows greater ease of access to the posterior superior glenoid and the rotator cuff. A probe inserted through the anterior portal is used to provide direct palpable feedback while a complete diagnostic arthroscopic procedure is performed. Particular attention is paid to pathology often seen in the throwing shoulder. The biceps tendon and its attachment are noted in addition to the superior labrum. One should take care to differentiate between the labral recess and a superior labral tear. The anterior and posterior labrum should be inspected if instability is suspected. The undersurface of the supraspinatus and infraspinatus should be carefully inspected for signs of rotator cuff tearing, one of the hallmarks of the disabled throwing shoulder. It is critical to repeat this evaluation in the abducted, externally rotated position, as this is the position of internal impingement. Contact between the posterior superior glenoid and the posterior aspect of the rotator cuff is often pathologic, and the so-called peel-back effect of the biceps off the posterior superior labrum should be carefully evaluated. These hallmarks of internal impingement can be treated with debridement or repair depending on the extent of the lesion. The posterior capsule is also carefully inspected for signs of capsular thickening, and this can be watched while the arm is brought into internal rotation. Viewing from the anterior portal lends particular insight here. If additional pathology is suspected in the subacromial space, the camera should be moved to assess the bursal side of the rotator cuff as well as the subacromial bursa, acromioclavicular joint, and extra-articular portion of the biceps tendon.

Surgical Decision Making

Surgical treatment of the disabled throwing shoulder is unique in that the condition is not a single entity but may represent a spectrum of pathologic findings. Most commonly these include partial-thickness rotator cuff tears in the posterior aspect of the supraspinatus; labral

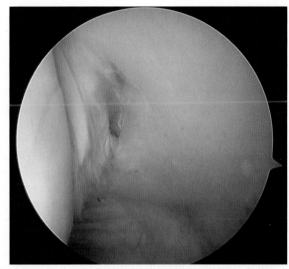

Figure 7-5. View of rotator cuff partial-thickness tear, in a right shoulder from anterior superior portal. Note the more posterior location of the cuff tear compared with the more classic tear directly behind the biceps.

pathology, especially in the posterior and superior quadrants; and posterior capsular tightness. Recognition of each of these conditions and its proper treatment is as follows:

1. Partial articular-sided rotator cuff tear (Fig. 7-5): In general, this tear is more posterior than the classic rotator cuff tear and can be localized by bringing the arm out of traction and into an abducted, externally rotated position. Pathology where the cuff contacts the posterior superior labrum is a hallmark of this condition (Fig. 7-6). Treatment most likely includes debridement, but one study[8] noted that in situ repair reported good results in returning athletes to throwing. Repair of full-thickness tears has not been shown to be effective in returning pitchers to throwing, and therefore caution should be exercised against overly aggressive debridement or conversion of partial- to full-thickness repair.

2. Superior labral anterior-posterior (SLAP) tears (Fig. 7-7): Superior labral tears that extend posterior to the biceps root are often seen in disabled throwing shoulders. Care must be taken to differentiate between labral separation that occurs as an adaptive change with peel-back versus a true pathologic SLAP tear. Although the genesis of such tears is still under debate, their presence can cause pain, create a sense of instability, and affect a thrower's speed and accuracy. Unstable SLAP tears should be repaired, but incarceration of the biceps must be avoided, and knot placement should be well planned to avoid damage to the humeral articular surface (Fig. 7-8). and rates of successful return to throwing have been mixed.

3. Posteroinferior capsular thickening (Fig. 7-9): If a patient has a preoperative diagnosis of GIRD that has not responded to nonoperative management, the posterior capsule should be carefully evaluated at arthroscopy for thickening. A posterior capsular release can be expected to restore the internal rotation of the shoulder. We recommend a thermal hooked device (Fig. 7-10) for this procedure for two main reasons. The first is that thermal capsulotomy will cauterize as it releases tissue and should result in less bleeding and less scar than shaving or incising with a blade. Second, given the proximity to the axillary nerve with the posterior inferior portion of the release, the nerve may contract the shoulder musculature and serve as a warning that the device is getting close, which may provide a margin of protection not provided by mechanical or sharp release. Regardless of the method of release, it should be done close to the glenoid; this has been shown to offer the safest buffer away from the axillary nerve (Fig. 7-11). By using posterior capsular release for GIRD, Yoneda and colleagues[18] demonstrated reliable pain relief though less successful return-to-throwing rates with this approach.

Surgical Pearls

- Abduction of the arm provides easier access and improved visualization of the rotator cuff insertion as it contacts the posterior superior glenoid (see Fig. 7-6).

- No attempt should be made to bring the biceps anchor onto the face of the glenoid, as one might do with other labral repairs. Especially in the thrower, the repair should be made off of the face, with low-profile techniques such as knotless systems and mattress repairs. Failure to follow these principles may result in contact between suture material and the rotator cuff insertion (see Fig. 7-8).

- Release the capsule (see Fig. 7-11) medially, near the glenoid to a depth that exposes the muscle fibers of the cuff. This ensures an adequate release and protects the tendinous portion of the rotator cuff musculature.

POSTOPERATIVE CONSIDERATIONS

Rehabilitation

The postoperative program for the throwing shoulder must be tailored to the surgical procedure. Communication between the surgeon and the athletic trainer is of paramount importance to ensure protection of tissues, with early motion and re-engagement of muscular rhythm and strength. The core strengthening program that is maintenance for these throwers should continue unaffected by the surgery. Scapular platform retraining is begun immediately as well. This includes a program of scapular "six packs," including protraction and retraction, elevation and depression, and inward and outward rotation. If the surgical correction does not include repair, then the patient is encouraged to move

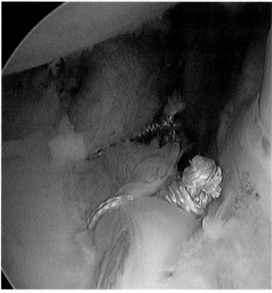

Figure 7-7. Right shoulder superior labral anterior-posterior (SLAP) repair in a 20-year-old collegiate baseball player. Patient continued to have pain in late cocking position and had second surgery to remove suture.

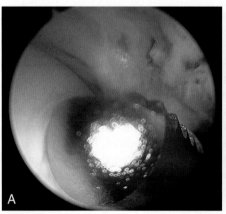 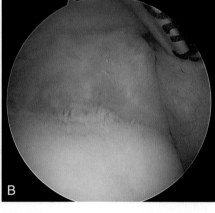

Figure 7-6. Adducted **(A)** and abducted **(B)** views of the rotator cuff insertion in a left-handed pitcher. Note the improvement in visualization of the rotator cuff footprint with the arm brought into abduction.

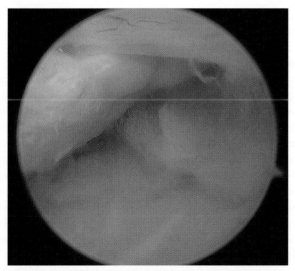

Figure 7-8. Pitcher from Figure 7-7 at third surgery in internal impingement position. Note damage to articular cartilage of humeral head adjacent to where suture was (frayed suture still visible).

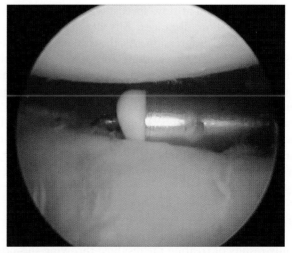

Figure 7-10. Technique of capsular release with hook probe. Posterior inferior capsule of a right shoulder being released near the glenoid allows increased safety margin. If the probe gets near the axillary nerve, a musculature contraction may result and can serve as a warning.

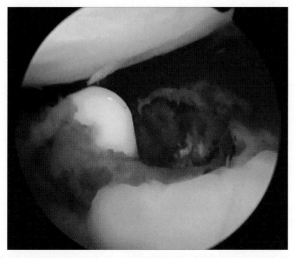

Figure 7-9. View from anterior superior portal in right shoulder of patient with glenohumeral internal rotation deficit (GIRD). The capsule has been released with a radiofrequency probe, and the cross-sectional thickness of the capsule can be viewed in the depth of the image (glenoid to left).

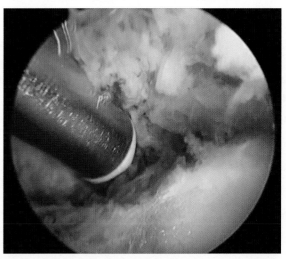

Figure 7-11. Posterior capsular release in left shoulder adjacent to the glenoid. This has been shown to be a safe position away from neurovascular structures.

the arm back to full range of motion as quickly as possible. This includes both active and passive motion, which is supervised to ensure that this motion is done with proper stabilization of the scapular musculature. Once early motion in the correct rhythm has been achieved, progression is begun to increase loads and speeds and to reestablish the link between the central core and the scapular platform. The progression goes from low loads at low speeds with a stable platform in one plane of motion, to higher faster loads in multiple planes that eventually simulate the sport-specific environment. Endurance must not be neglected, as

fatigue can lead to poor mechanics and be detrimental to return.

Once the athlete has regained a solid core, full range of motion, functional strength, and proper scapular rhythm, a return-to-throwing program is begun under the supervision of the athletic training staff. To begin progression the athlete must demonstrate the ability to simulate a pitch at slow speed, to ensure he or she has attained the proper functional range of motion, core strength, and scapular stability.

The return-to-throwing program embodies the same principles of progression stressed in the earlier phases.

Throwing is begun at slow speeds, with a light ball that is tossed for short distances. Any deficits displayed in mechanics halt progression. As the athlete progresses, distance, speed, and repetitions are increased until the athlete has regained the ability to perform his or her specific sport mechanics. Once this has been accomplished, repetitions are increased until the athlete is ready to return to competition. This program must be individualized, and any repair (labral or rotator cuff) must be protected until healed; therefore the postoperative program must be altered to accommodate these considerations.

RESULTS

Study results of treating the disabled throwing shoulder are summarized in the Table 7-1. Results from these studies reveal how difficult it is for surgical approaches to return these athletes to throwing. Furthermore, because of the spectrum of pathologies seen in this population, outcomes studies are not clean, often reporting on multiple surgical techniques. Because pitchers often show a combination of internal impingement and posterior capsular tightness, surgical treatment of the throwing shoulder does not lend itself easily to well-controlled trials. Fortunately, nonoperative management is successful in preventing the need for surgery in many of these athletes.

Burkhart and colleagues demonstrated that nonoperative management focused on sleeper stretches and scapulothoracic rehabilitation was effective in returning 96 shoulders to throwing.[17] Similarly, Kibler randomized high-level tennis players noted to have GIRD to posteroinferior capsular stretches versus no stretching and followed them for 2 years. Those who stretched increased internal rotation and had a 38% decrease in shoulder problems.[19] More recently, Wilk and colleagues[6] followed 40 professional pitchers with GIRD and found that only 3 of 40 eventually required arthroscopy for treatment.

In considering posterior capsular release as an operative treatment, few studies are in the literature. Yoneda and colleagues reported on 16 overhead athletes treated with posterior capsular release. Eleven (69%) of 16 returned to their preinjury performance level. Of the 16, only four patients had isolated posteroinferior capsular tightness, highlighting the complexity of the pathology of the throwing shoulder.[18]

TABLE 7-1. Summary of Treatment Outcomes in the Throwing Shoulder

Study	Year	Treatment	Group	Outcomes	Comments
Nonoperative Treatment					
Burkhart et al[3]	2003	Posterior capsular stretching and scapular rehabilitation	96 Overhead athletes	100% returned to preinjury throwing by 4 months	
Kibler[19]	1998	Posterior capsular stretching vs. regular exercise regimen	Prospective study of tennis players	38% in stretching group had decrease in shoulder problems	
Wilk et al[12]	2011	Postcapsular stretching, dynamic maintenance	3-Year study of one Major League Baseball team	Of 40 patients with GIRD, three underwent surgery	
Rotator Cuff Pathology					
Ferrari et al[26]	1994	Debridement of labrum cuff	Seven competitive pitchers	85% returned to premorbid activity level	
Reynolds et al[27]	2008	Debridement of small cuff tears	82 Competitive pitchers	55% returned to previous level of play	
Levitz et al[29]	2001	Debridement with or without thermal therapy	82 Throwers	Competing at same level: 31/51 (61%) without thermal therapy, 27/31 (87%) with thermal therapy	Thermal therapy group maintained good results better than the nonthermal group
Andrews et al[30]	1985	Debridement of PTaRCT	36 Patients (23 pitchers)	85% returned to play, 76% back to previous level of play	Paper described SLAP tears before the term was coined
Conway[8]	2001	Repair of intratendinous rotator cuff tears in baseball players	Nine baseball players	89% to same or higher level of play	

TABLE 7-1. Summary of Treatment Outcomes in the Throwing Shoulder—cont'd

Study	Year	Treatment	Group	Outcomes	Comments
SLAP Repair					
Morgan et al[31]	1998	Repair of SLAP	44 Pitchers, 37 competitive	87% returned to previous level of play	
Radkowski et al[32]	2008	Posterior capsulolabral repair in throwers vs. nonthrowers	27 Throwers	89% good and excellent; 55% returned to previous level of play	
Kim et al[21]	2002	SLAP repair	18 Overhead athletes	Only 22% returned to previous level of play	
Andrews et al[23]	2003	Repair with or without thermal therapy in throwers	130 Athletes (105 pitchers)	87% returned to previous level of play	Better results with thermal therapy and repair than with repair alone
Ide et al[22]	2005	SLAP repair	19 Pitchers	63% returned to previous level of play	Results worse in baseball players than in other overhead athletes
Instability Treatment for Throwing Shoulder					
Jobe et al[6]	1991	Anterior capsulolabral reconstruction	25 Throwers	92% good or excellent, but only 68% returned to throwing	
Montgomery et al[24]	1994	Anterior capsulolabral repair in athletes	32 Athletes	97% good or excellent; 81% returned to previous level of play	
Bigliani et al[25]	1994	Inferior capsular shift in athletes	63 Athletic patients, including 10 elite pitchers	Of elite pitchers, 5 of 10 returned to play	
Posterior Capsule Tightness					
Yoneda et al[18]	2006	Posterior capsular release	16 Throwers	68% returned to preinjury level of play	4/4 (100%) of those with isolated posterior capsular tightness returned to preinjury level

GIRD, Glenohumeral internal rotation deficit; *PTaRCT*, partial thickness articular-sided rotator cuff tear; *SLAP*, superior labral anterior-posterior.

SLAP repairs have sparsely been reported in an isolated overhead athlete population. Whereas initial reports showed success,[20] most studies have demonstrated only modest return to throwing. Kim and colleagues reported a 22% return-to-throwing rate in SLAP repairs in overhead athletes,[21] and Ide and colleagues found SLAP repair successful in 63% of overhead athletes.[22] Other studies that address combined pathology with SLAP repair have shown improved results.[23]

Instability treated with capsulolabral reconstruction has had similar challenges. Jobe and colleagues reported 92% good and excellent outcomes of 25 throwers, but only 68% returned to throwing at the previous level of competition.[6] Montgomery and colleagues reported on 32 patients who underwent anterior labral repair with slightly better results—97% good and excellent and 81% return to same level of sport.[24] Bigliani and

colleagues, however, performed inferior capsular shift in 10 elite throwers with only 50% return to play.[25]

Rotator cuff damage is perhaps the most common pathology seen in the throwing shoulder. It remains unclear whether it is a primary pathology or secondary to other processes such as internal impingement or GIRD, but addressing its pathology is a cornerstone of treatment. Several studies have reported return-to-throwing rates of 55% to 87%, again with improved results demonstrated when combined pathology was treated.[8,26-30]

CONCLUSION

In conclusion, the throwing shoulder is yet to be fully understood. Multiple pathologies commonly include labral and rotator cuff tears, posterior capsular tightness, and instability. Nonoperative management remains effective in most cases, but when surgical treatment is necessary, the surgeon must be fully prepared, as treatment of the throwing shoulder must be individualized. Obtaining the right balance of debridement, repair, and release is a delicate art in a patient who expects to return to the less-than-delicate forces required for competitive throwing.

REFERENCES

1. Fleisig GS DC, Andrews JR. Biomechanics of the shoulder during throwing. In: Andrews JR WK, ed. *The athlete's shoulder*. New York: Churchill Livingstone; 1994: 360-365.
2. Burkhart SS, Morgan CD, Kibler WB. The disabled throwing shoulder: spectrum of pathology Part I: pathoanatomy and biomechanics. *Arthroscopy*. 2003;19(4): 404-420.
3. Bennett G. Elbow and shoulder lesions of baseball players. *Am J Surg*. 1959;98:484-492.
4. Neer 2nd CS. Anterior acromioplasty for the chronic impingement syndrome in the shoulder: a preliminary report. *J Bone Joint Surg Am*. 1972;54(1):41-50.
5. Tibone JE, Jobe FW, Kerlan RK, et al. Shoulder impingement syndrome in athletes treated by an anterior acromioplasty. *Clin Orthop Relat Res*. 1985;(198):134-140.
6. Jobe FW, Giangarra CE, Kvitne RS, et al. Anterior capsulolabral reconstruction of the shoulder in athletes in overhand sports. *Am J Sports Med*. 1991;19(5):428-434.
7. Paley KJ, Jobe FW, Pink MM, et al. Arthroscopic findings in the overhand throwing athlete: evidence for posterior internal impingement of the rotator cuff. *Arthroscopy*. 2000;16(1):35-40.
8. Conway JE. Arthroscopic repair of partial-thickness rotator cuff tears and SLAP lesions in professional baseball players. *Orthop Clin North Am*. 2001;32(3): 443-456.
9. Walch G, Boileau P, Noel E, et al. Impingement of the deep surface of the supraspinatus tendon on the posterosuperior glenoid rim: an arthroscopic study. *J Shoulder Elbow Surg*. 1992;1:238-245.
10. Sonnery-Cottet B, Edwards TB, Noel E, et al. Results of arthroscopic treatment of posterosuperior glenoid impingement in tennis players. *Am J Sports Med*. 2002;30(2):227-232.
11. Verna C. *Shoulder flexibility to reduce impingement*. Paper presented at: 3rd PBATS (Professional Baseball Athletic Trainer Society), 1991; Mesa, Arizona.
12. Wilk KE, Macrina LC, Fleisig GS, et al. Correlation of glenohumeral internal rotation deficit and total rotational motion to shoulder injuries in professional baseball pitchers. *Am J Sports Med*. 2011;39(2):329-335.
13. Huffman GR, Tibone JE, McGarry MH, et al. Path of glenohumeral articulation throughout the rotational range of motion in a thrower's shoulder model. *Am J Sports Med*. 2006;34(10):1662-1669.
14. Tokish J, Curtin MS, Kim YK, et al. Glenohumeral internal rotation deficit in the asymptomatic professional pitcher and its relationship to humeral retroversion. *J Sports Sci Med*. 2008;7:78-83.
15. Myers JB, Laudner KG, Pasquale MR, et al. Glenohumeral range of motion deficits and posterior shoulder tightness in throwers with pathologic internal impingement. *Am J Sports Med*. 2006;34(3):385-391.
16. Meister K, Buckley B, Batts J. The posterior impingement sign: diagnosis of rotator cuff and posterior labral tears secondary to internal impingement in overhand athletes. *Am J Orthop (Belle Mead NJ)*. 2004;33(8): 412-415.
17. Burkhart SS, Morgan CD, Kibler WB. The disabled throwing shoulder: spectrum of pathology Part III: the SICK scapula, scapular dyskinesis, the kinetic chain, and rehabilitation. *Arthroscopy*. 2003;19(6):641-661.
18. Yoneda M, Nakagawa S, Mizuno N, et al. Arthroscopic capsular release for painful throwing shoulder with posterior capsular tightness. *Arthroscopy*. 2006;22(7):801 e801-805.
19. Kibler WB. *The relationship of glenohumeral internal rotation deficit to shoulder and elbow injuries in tennis players: a prospective evaluation of posterior capsular stretching*. Paper presented at: Annual closed meeting of the American Shoulder and Elbow Surgeons, 1998; New York.
20. Burkhart SS, Morgan CD. The peel-back mechanism: its role in producing and extending posterior type II SLAP lesions and its effect on SLAP repair rehabilitation. *Arthroscopy*. 1998;14(6):637-640.
21. Kim SH, Ha KI, Choi HJ. Results of arthroscopic treatment of superior labral lesions. *J Bone Joint Surg Am*. 2002;84-A(6):981-985.
22. Ide J, Maeda S, Takagi K. Sports activity after arthroscopic superior labral repair using suture anchors in overhead-throwing athletes. *Am J Sports Med*. 2005;33(4): 507-514.
23. Reinold MM, Wilk KE, Hooks TR, et al. Thermal-assisted capsular shrinkage of the glenohumeral joint in overhead athletes: a 15- to 47-month follow-up. *J Orthop Sports Phys Ther*. 2003;33(8):455-467.
24. Montgomery 3rd WH, Jobe FW. Functional outcomes in athletes after modified anterior capsulolabral reconstruction. *Am J Sports Med*. 1994;22(3):352-358.
25. Bigliani LU, Kurzweil PR, Schwartzbach CC, et al. Inferior capsular shift procedure for anterior-inferior shoulder instability in athletes. *Am J Sports Med*. 1994;22(5): 578-584.
26. Ferrari JD, Ferrari DA, Coumas J, et al. Posterior ossification of the shoulder: the Bennett lesion. Etiology, diagnosis, and treatment. *Am J Sports Med*. 1994;22(2):171-175; discussion 175-176.
27. Reynolds SB, Dugas JR, Cain EL, et al. Débridement of small partial-thickness rotator cuff tears in elite overhead throwers. *Clin Orthop Relat Res*. 2008;466(3):614-621.
28. Reference deleted in proofs.
29. Levitz CL, Dugas J, Andrews JR. The use of arthroscopic thermal capsulorrhaphy to treat internal impingement in baseball players. *Arthroscopy*. 2001;17(6):573-577.
30. Andrews JR, Broussard TS, Carson WG. Arthroscopy of the shoulder in the management of partial tears of

the rotator cuff: a preliminary report. *Arthroscopy*. 1985;1(2):117-122.

31. Morgan CD, Burkhart SS, Palmeri M, et al. Type II SLAP lesions: three subtypes and their relationships to superior instability and rotator cuff tears. *Arthroscopy*. 1998;14(6): 553-565.

32. Radkowski CA, Chhabra A, Baker 3rd CL, et al. Arthroscopic capsulolabral repair for posterior shoulder instability in throwing athletes compared with non-throwing athletes. *Am J Sports Med*. 2008;36(4): 693-699.

Chapter 8

Arthroscopic Management of Rare Intra-articular Lesions of the Shoulder

Felix H. Savoie III, Michael O'Brien, and Wendell Heard

Chapter Synopsis
- The shoulder's wide variety of "normal" characteristics and its incredible range of motion and function allow for a wide variety of pathology. This chapter illustrates rare lesions and contrasts them with normal but unusual anatomy.

Important Points
- The superior labrum has a wide variety of normal anatomy, and the understanding of what really constitutes a pathologic process is critical to know when repair is indicated.
- Synovitis of the shoulder may be commonly encountered, but an understanding of areas in which it may extend extra-articularly, as in the axillary and rotator interval, is useful.
- Extra-articular fractures may extend into the glenoid surface, necessitating arthroscopic monitoring of the reduction to ensure adequate joint restoration.
- Instability lesions are often complex, with multiple areas of damage. A complete and thorough inspection of the entire capsulolabral complex, including both humeral and glenoid attachments, should be considered essential in evaluating and correcting these injuries.

Clinical and Surgical Pearls
- Avoid making holes in the tendons of the rotator cuff.
- Complete the diagnostic arthroscopy before establishing accessory portals.
- Use K-wires placed via fluoroscopy into the mobile fragments before beginning arthroscopic fracture management.
- Repair instability by beginning inferiorly and medially, progressing to the lateral inferior, and then moving front to back while slowly progressing toward the superior aspect of the shoulder.

Clinical and Surgical Pitfalls
- The primary problem in rare lesions is the differentiation from what is normal.
- The simplest way to avoid problems is to familiarize oneself with the multiple variations via viewing, reading, and watching videos of arthroscopy.

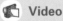 **Video**

- Video 8-1

In no other joint is there as much variability in normal anatomy as in the shoulder. Unusual conditions of the shoulder must be differentiated from normal variants. Although most pathologic processes are covered in other chapters, rare lesions such as pigmented villo-nodular synovitis (PVNS), osteochondritis dissecans of the glenoid and humerus, traumatic chondral fracture, chondrolysis, synovial osteochondromatosis, ganglion and synovial cysts, blending or bifurcation of the biceps and tearing of the attachment of a Buford complex, reverse humeral avulsion of the glenohumeral ligament with infraspinatus tear, coracoid fracture with extension into the joint, and floating anterior capsule (combined Bankart lesion and humeral avulsion of the glenohumeral ligament) are not commonly encountered within the shoulder.

Each of these entities may require different management. The rarity of these problems complicates diagnosis, preparation, and management. Many are encountered only on entering the joint. It is the goal of this chapter to discuss diagnostic studies and tests that can help to preoperatively identify these conditions correctly and assist with their management.

PREOPERATIVE CONSIDERATIONS

History

Most patients with rare intra-articular shoulder lesions have a history of either no trauma or only minor trauma. The exception is the patient with an articular fracture, who often has a clear history of a traumatic event, often a dive to the floor during an athletic event, after which pain and limitation of activity occur. However, in all of these conditions, symptoms frequently are not associated with a specific activity. Unlike with rotator cuff disease, the pain and feelings of swelling are not worse at night. Unlike with shoulder instability, the symptoms are not associated with a particular movement or arm position. Unlike with adhesive capsulitis, there is no consistent loss of motion or pain on inferior glide testing.

Physical Examination

Examination usually reveals palpable swelling within the glenohumeral joint, most easily felt in the area of the rotator interval. There is usually some loss of motion, primarily in internal and external rotation. Crepitation is noted with rotational movements of the glenohumeral joint. When the Buford complex has been avulsed, results of the anterior superior load and shift examination and the dynamic labral shear test result will be positive.

Imaging

Radiographs are usually normal except in synovial osteochondromatosis, in which multiple loose bodies are noted (Fig. 8-1). Magnetic resonance imaging (MRI) is helpful for osteochondritis dissecans lesions, synovial cysts (Fig. 8-2), and chondrolysis. Avulsions of a Buford complex, PVNS, and articular cartilage fractures will not show up on most radiographic tests. Glenohumeral avulsions are visualized by arthrography, and the coracoid fracture is best noted on computed tomographic scans.

Indications and Contraindications

Each of these various entities may be managed by arthroscopy. The main contraindications to arthroscopic surgery are PVNS and in some fractures. Complete excision of PVNS may require open surgery, especially in the axilla, whereas fractures may necessitate a combined approach.

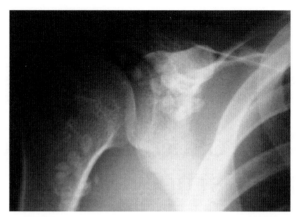

Figure 8-1. Radiologic view of multiple loose bodies in the glenohumeral joint arising from the synovium of the subcoracoid bursa.

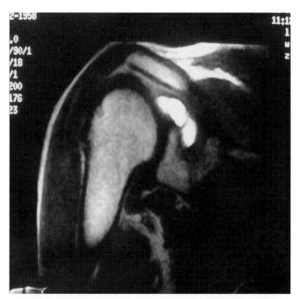

Figure 8-2. Magnetic resonance image of a synovial cyst.

SURGICAL TECHNIQUE

Anesthesia and Positioning

Most of these patients require general anesthesia, although experienced regional anesthesiologists may certainly use interscalene block anesthesia. We prefer the lateral decubitus position because of its ability to allow easier access to all areas of the shoulder joint, but the surgeon's preference is usually the rule in these procedures.

Surgical Landmarks, Incision, and Portals

A standard posterior portal is made in line with the equator of the joint, placed through the raphe in the infraspinatus muscle belly. Additional portals are added

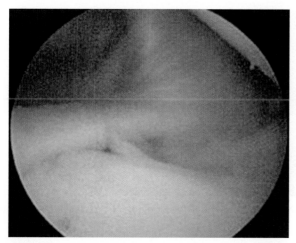

Figure 8-3. A normal Buford complex (cordlike middle glenohumeral ligament) with tearing at the attachment to the glenoid.

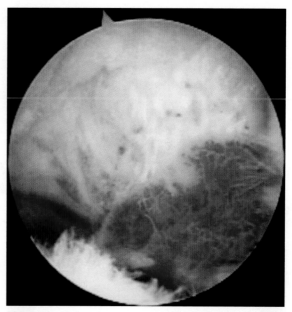

Figure 8-4. Pigmented villonodular synovitis of the shoulder.

under direct visualization, with each one tested with a spinal needle, and are made only after the diagnostic arthroscopy has been completed and the surgical procedure defined.

Examination: Diagnostic Arthroscopy and Specific Steps per Rare Entity

Diagnostic arthroscopy usually reveals the pathologic process. Most of these processes are readily apparent once the arthroscope has been placed within the joint.

1. Avulsion of the Buford Complex Attachment

Avulsion of the Buford complex attachment is the most difficult to differentiate from normal variants. It is thought that the presence of the Buford complex has an incidence of 1.5% to 6.5%,[1,2] but the frequency with which it is avulsed is unknown. Chondromalacia of the glenoid and fraying of the undersurface of the labrum and outer surface of the glenoid isolated to that area alone and not farther inferior on the glenoid are key findings (Fig. 8-3).

2. Pigmented Villonodular Synovitis

In all joints, PVNS has an incidence of approximately 1.8 cases per 1 million people.[3] Eighty percent of cases occur in the knee. PVNS is rare in the shoulder and has the characteristic appearance seen in other joints.[3] However, it is not readily resected because it penetrates through the lining of the joint and expands outward into the surrounding structures (Fig. 8-4). Especially in inferior lesions, the synovial growth may envelope the axillary nerve, necessitating its dissection either through open surgery or by arthroscopic identification of the nerve and protection of it.

3. Synovial Cysts

Synovial cysts (Fig. 8-5) have frequently been documented as a cause of shoulder pain. Cysts have been reported in the acromioclavicular joint,[4] spinoglenoid notch,[5-7] suprascapular notch,[8,9] inferior glenoid beneath the subscapularis muscle,[10] quadrilateral space,[11] and subcoracoid space[12] and intramuscularly.[13] Patients typically have diffuse, nonspecific, generalized pain. Shoulder weakness can occur if the cyst compresses the suprascapular nerve or its branch to the infraspinatus muscle. Synovial cysts are often associated with labral tears and are frequently in contact with the scapula or distal clavicle.[5-7,14-18] The cyst should be resected, and the associated pathologic lesion repaired or removed. We have seen an increase in suture-anchor–related cyst formation. In these situations it is important to remove all the suture material and excavate any component of the cyst within the bone to completely eradicate the problem.

4. Synovial Chondromatosis

Synovial chondromatosis (Fig. 8-6) can affect any synovium-lined cavity. It is typically monoarticular and is characterized by the presence of osteocartilaginous loose bodies. It has been reported in tendon sheaths, bursae, and a number of diarthrodial joints.[19] In the shoulder, synovial chondromatosis has been described in the subacromial bursa, in the acromioclavicular joint, and in the glenohumeral joint with involvement of the long head of the biceps tendon sheath.[19] Milgram[20] classified synovial chondromatosis into three categories. The first category consists of loose bodies arising from osteochondral fractures. The second is caused by

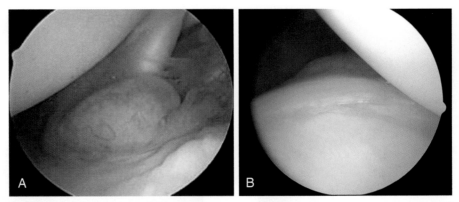

Figure 8-5. A, Arthroscopic view of a synovial cyst arising from a foreign body near the coracoid. **B,** Synovial cyst within the posterior inferior glenohumeral ligament with lobulations.

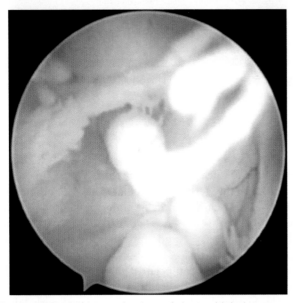

Figure 8-6. Arthroscopic view of the multiple loose bodies of synovial chondromatosis arising from the subcoracoid bursa.

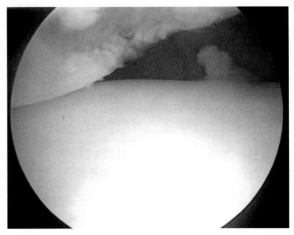

Figure 8-7. Traumatic chondral defect of the humeral head.

degenerative arthritis or avascular necrosis causing fragmentation of the joint. The third category is primary osteochondromatosis in which primary metaplasia of the synovial membrane produces cartilage-forming chondrocytes.[19,20] Milgram[20] also described the three phases of the metaplasia. Initially it is confined to the synovium, and then it progresses to an active synovium with loose-body production. Finally, the late stage shows an inactive synovium with residual intra-articular loose bodies.[20] Unfortunately it is not possible to determine when the synovium has become inactive, and recurrence rates vary from 0 to 31%.[19] Typically the multiple loose bodies are readily apparent. It may be useful to place a much larger cannula, such as that used in urologic procedures, to allow the loose bodies to be removed. It is important to find the area of synovium producing the lesions and to excise it. The most common areas in which to find this synovium in our experience are the subcoracoid bursa and the bicipital groove.

5. Traumatic Chondral Defects and Osteochondritis

Traumatic chondral defects and osteochondritis of the humeral head or glenoid are rare entities that result in irritation and swelling within the glenohumeral joint. The cause of osteochondritis dissecans is unknown, but it is thought that trauma, ischemia, abnormal ossification, or a combination of these factors plays a role in the development of the disease. Finding these loose articular pieces within the shoulder joint and removing them will help decrease symptoms (Fig. 8-7). The injured bed in the articular surface should also be located and debrided, and marrow stimulation at least should be performed.

6. Chondrolysis

The most difficult to manage of these various lesions is chondrolysis of the glenohumeral joint. Although this has been described to follow thermal surgery, the exact cause has yet to be elucidated. The multiple potential etiologic contributors to chondrolysis can generally be classified into three categories: mechanical, chemical, and thermal. Mechanical causes include trauma, surgical insult, and placement of implants. Chemical causes include the use of intra-articular pain pumps that deliver local anesthetics in postoperative settings. Thermal causes include the use of radiofrequency devices during surgical procedures. Arthroscopy reveals an aggressive destruction of the entire articular surface of the humeral head and glenoid, severe synovitis and capsular damage, and almost an avascular necrosis type of destruction of the humeral head (Fig. 8-8). Biologic glenoid resurfacing with or without humeral head replacement seems to provide the best relief.

7. Floating Capsule

Floating capsule is a rare lesion in instability that consists of a Bankart lesion with humeral avulsion of the glenohumeral ligaments. Humeral avulsions of the anterior glenohumeral ligaments are covered elsewhere in this text. However, one may occasionally find this lesion in conjunction with a Bankart lesion (Fig. 8-9); the Bankart lesion is repaired first, and then the humeral avulsion is repaired. This also is an excellent indication for open surgery by the Matsen approach to elevate the lateral subscapularis and use the humeral avulsion to access the Bankart lesion. The capsulolabral complex is repaired to the glenoid, and the humeral avulsion is repaired as part of the reattachment of the lateral capsule and subscapularis tendon.

8. Reverse Humeral Avulsion of the Glenohumeral Ligament

Reverse humeral avulsion of the glenohumeral ligament is an even more uncommon cause of posterior shoulder instability. Careful physical examination can indicate involvement of the infraspinatus. In high-energy trauma, the lateral capsule and the infraspinatus tendon may both be involved, necessitating repair of both the capsule and the tendon with anchors and sutures (Fig. 8-10).[21]

9. Coracoid Fractures

Coracoid fractures are relatively rare lesions in which the fracture may extend into the articular surface of the glenoid. The symptoms are pain, tenderness around the coracoid, and swelling. The fracture is readily visualized on MRI or computed tomographic scans. Although immobilization often results in union, active individuals may require stabilization. Arthroscopy of the glenohumeral joint may allow monitoring of the articular extension while also allowing reduction and fixation (Fig. 8-11).

10. Isolated Avulsion of the Lesser Tuberosity

Isolated avulsion of the lesser tuberosity may also occur in both youths and adults. Standard imaging often fails to reveal the injury without a high index of suspicion from the physical examination. A positive lift off test or

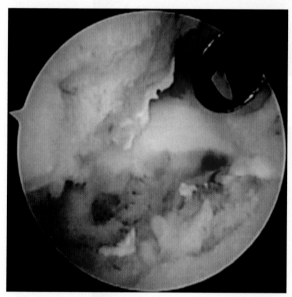

Figure 8-8. Postsurgical avascular necrosis caused by thermal chondrolysis.

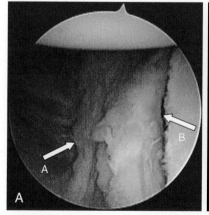 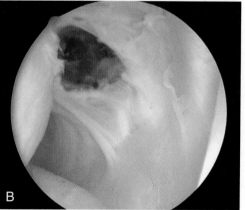

Figure 8-9. Floating anterior capsule; both the Bankart lesion and the humeral avulsion are pictured. **A,** Lateral edge of capsule. **B,** Labrum and medial capsule. **C,** Capsular split.

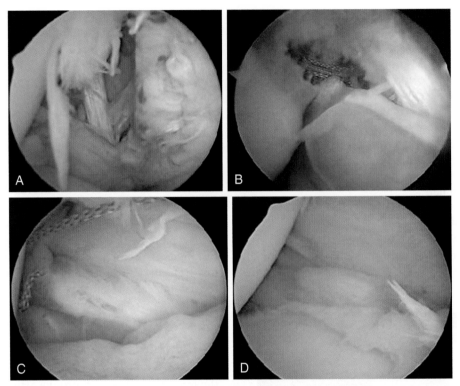

Figure 8-10. Reverse humeral avulsion of the glenohumeral ligament. **A,** Arthroscopic view of the capsule and tendon injury. **B,** Anchor placement in preparation for repair. **C,** First set of sutures tied. **D,** Final view of repaired capsule.

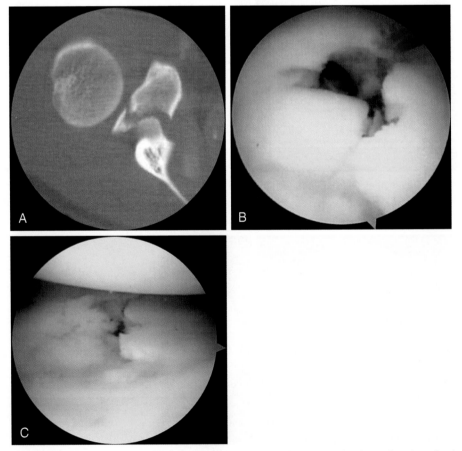

Figure 8-11. A, Coracoid fracture on computed tomographic scan. **B,** Arthroscopic view showing the intra-articular extension. **C,** Arthroscopic view of repaired coracoid.

belly push test is positive but often neglected in these young athletes. Arthroscopic visualization (Fig. 8-12) reveals the injury, which can then be repaired with either suture anchors or screws via arthroscopic techniques and a low anterior portal.

11. Calcific Tendonitis

Calcific tendonitis is a relatively common disorder that becomes painful as the calcification undergoes resorption. However, in the unusual instance in which the lesion is on the underside of the rotator cuff or of the biceps, it is often obscured on plain radiographs and not visualized on many routine MRI scans. The rare lesion of the underside of the supraspinatus tendon, termed *calcium-induced subchondral chondromalacia* by Ellman, can cause chondral erosion and synovitis. In the biceps or labrum the calcium can produce the same painful symptoms as it does in other tendons, often necessitating both excision of the calcium and resection of the damaged part of the tendon with tenodesis of the remaining normal tendon (Fig. 8-13).

SUMMARY

There are many more unusual lesions of the shoulder that may or may not require stabilization. Incorporation of all or part of the biceps into the rotator cuff is a normal variant (Fig. 8-14), just as the Buford complex, hypermobile superior labrum, and absent anterior labrum are.

Recent reports of rare lesions include synovitis from an osteoid osteoma of the coracoid, a collagenous fibroma of the bursa producing impingement, and a prolonged pectoralis minor tendon with absence of the coracohumeral ligament. One can be sure that many more normal and abnormal variants exist than are shown in this chapter.

Before a lesion is repaired, it is incumbent on the surgeon to review the injury, the symptoms, and the physical examination findings to see whether they match the pathologic process that is being viewed. If the mechanism is sufficient to produce the pathologic process being visualized, and the pathologic lesion can produce

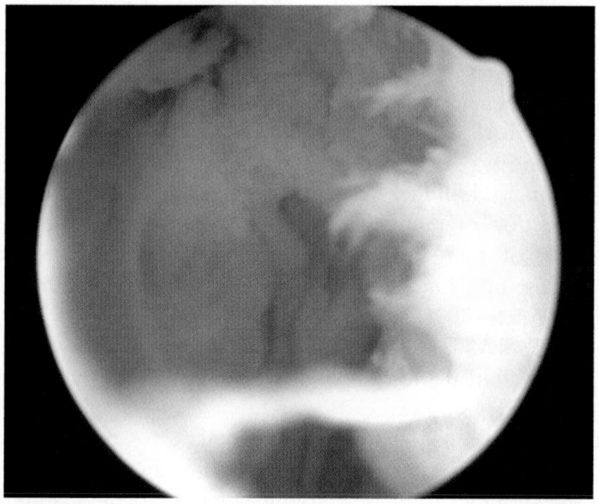

Figure 8-12. Lesser tuberosity fracture in a right shoulder with the avulsed lesser tuberosity to the left and the bone bed of the humerus to the right.

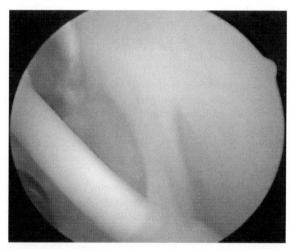

Figure 8-14. Normal variant of the biceps with sling and incorporation into the rotator cuff.

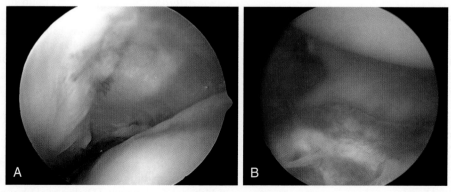

Figure 8-13. A, Calcific tendonitis on the underside of the supraspinatus tendon, termed a calcium-induced subchondral chondromalacia lesion by Harvard Ellman. **B,** Calcifications with the labrum and biceps with associated synovitis.

the symptoms the patient reports, repair is warranted. Elimination of the symptoms after repair may be the only confirmation that the surgeon has performed the correct operation.

REFERENCES

1. Ilahi OA, Labbe MR, Cosculluela P. Variants of the anterosuperior glenoid and associated pathology. *Arthroscopy.* 2002;18:882-886.
2. Williams MM, Snyder SJ, Buford Jr D. The Buford complex—the "cord-like" middle glenohumeral ligament and absent anterosuperior labrum complex: a normal anatomic capsulolabral variant. *Arthroscopy.* 1994;10:241-247.
3. Myers BW, Masi AT. Pigmented villonodular synovitis and tenosynovitis: A clinical epidemiologic study of 166 cases and literature review. *Medicine (Baltimore).* 1980;59:223-238.
4. Craig EV. The acromioclavicular joint cyst. An unusual presentation for a rotator cuff tear. *Clin Orthop Relat Res.* 1986;202:189-192.
5. Aiello I, Serra G, Traina GC, et al. Entrapment of the suprascapular nerve at the spinoglenoid notch. *Ann Neurol.* 1982;12:314-316.
6. Chen AL, Ong BC, Rose DJ. Arthroscopic management of spinoglenoid cysts associated with SLAP lesions and suprascapular neuropathy. *Arthroscopy.* 2003;19:e17-e23.
7. Tirman PFJ, Feller JF, Janzen DL, et al. Association of glenoid labral cysts with labral tears and glenohumeral instability: radiologic findings and clinical significance. *Radiology.* 1994;190:653-658.
8. Iannotti JP, Ramsey ML. Arthroscopic decompression of a ganglion cyst causing suprascapular nerve compression. *Arthroscopy.* 1996;12:739-745.
9. Thompson RC, Schneider W, Kennedy T. Entrapment neuropathy of the inferior branch of the suprascapular nerve by ganglia. *Clin Orthop Relat Res.* 1982;166:185-187.
10. Dietz SO, Lichtenberg S, Habermeyer P. Non-traumatic shoulder instability in an athletic patient with a periglenoid cyst and a glenoid labral tear. *Acta Orthop Belg.* 2003;69:373-376.
11. Sanders TG, Tirman PFJ. Paralabral cyst: an unusual cause of quadrilateral space syndrome. *Arthroscopy.* 1999;15:632-637.
12. Steiner E, Steinbach LS, Schnarkowski P, et al. Ganglia and cysts around joints. *Radiol Clin North Am.* 1996;34:395-425.
13. Tan EW, Dharamsi FM, McCarthy EF, et al. Intramuscular synovial cyst of the shoulder: A case report. *J Shoulder Elbow Surg.* 2010;19(3):e20-e24.
14. Fehrman DA, Orwin JF, Jennings RM. Suprascapular nerve entrapment by ganglion cysts: A report of six cases with arthroscopic findings and review of the literature. *Arthroscopy.* 1995;11:727-734.
15. McCluskey L, Feinberg D, Dolinskas C. Suprascapular neuropathy related to a glenohumeral joint cyst. *Muscle Nerve.* 1999;22:772-777.
16. Moore TP, Fritts HM, Quick DC, et al. Suprascapular nerve entrapment caused by supraglenoid cyst compression. *J Shoulder Elbow Surg.* 1997;6:455-462.
17. Piatt BE, Hawkins RJ, Fritz RC, et al. Clinical evaluation and treatment of spinoglenoid notch ganglion cysts. *J Shoulder Elbow Surg.* 2002;11:600-604.
18. Winalski CS, Robbins MI, Silverman SG, et al. Interactive magnetic resonance image–guided aspiration therapy of a glenoid labral cyst. A case report. *J Bone Joint Surg Am.* 2001;83:1237-1242.
19. Lunn JV, Castellanos-Rosas J, Walch G. Arthroscopic synovectomy, removal of loose bodies and selective biceps tenodesis for synovial chondromatosis of the shoulder. *J Bone Joint Surg Br.* 2007;89:1329-1335.
20. Milgram JW. Synovial osteochondromatosis: a histopathological study of thirty cases. *J Bone Joint Surg Am.* 1977;59:792-801.
21. Brown T, Barton S, Savoie 3rd FH. Reverse humeral avulsion glenohumeral ligament and infraspinatus rupture with arthroscopic repair: a case report. *Am J Sports Med.* 2007;35:2135-2139.

SUGGESTED READINGS

Audenaert EA, Barbaix EJ, Van Hoonacker P, et al. Extraarticular variants of the long head of the biceps brachii: a reminder of embryology. *J Shoulder Elbow Surg.* 2008;17:114S-117S.

Bents RT, Skeete KD. The correlation of the Buford complex and SLAP lesions. *J Shoulder Elbow Surg.* 2005;14:565-569.

Chiffolot X, Ehlinger M, Bonnomet F, et al. Arthroscopic resection of pigmented villonodular synovitis pseudotumor of the shoulder: a case report with three year follow-up. *Rev Chir Orthop Reparatrice Appar Mot.* 2005;91:470-475.

Debeer P, Brys P. Osteochondritis dissecans of the humeral head: clinical and radiological findings. *Acta Orthop Belg.* 2005;71:484-488.

Hamada J, Tamai K, Koguchi Y, et al. Case report: a rare condition of secondary synovial osteochondromatosis of the shoulder joint in a young female patient. *J Shoulder Elbow Surg.* 2005;14:653-656.

Jerosch J, Aldawoudy AM. Chondrolysis of the glenohumeral joint following arthroscopic capsular release for adhesive capsulitis: a case report. *Knee Surg Sports Traumatol Arthrosc.* 2007;15:292-294. Epub June 24, 2006.

Ji J-H, Shafi M, Kim WY. Calcific tendinitis of the biceps-labral complex: A rare cause of shoulder pain. *Acta Orthop Belg.* 2008;74:401-404.

Levine WN, Clark Jr AM, D'Alessandro DF, et al. Chondrolysis following arthroscopic thermal capsulorrhaphy to treat shoulder instability. A report of two cases. *J Bone Joint Surg Am.* 2005;87:616-621.

Mahirogullari M, Chloros GD, Wiesler ER, et al. Osteochondritis dissecans of the humeral head. *Joint Bone Spine.* 2008;75:226-228.

Mankin H, Trahan C, Hornicek F. Pigmented villonodular synovitis of joints. *J Surg Oncol.* 2011;103:386-389.

Milnes LK, Tennent TD, Pearse EO. An unusual cause of subacromial impingement: A collagenous fibroma in the bursa. *J Shoulder Elbow Surg.* 2010;19:e15-e17.

Chapter 9

Arthroscopic Repair of Posterior Shoulder Instability

Steven B. Cohen, Sam G. Tejwani, and James P. Bradley

Chapter Synopsis

- Posterior instability when compared with anterior instability of the shoulder is relatively uncommon. To diagnose posterior instability, the clinician must take a thorough history and perform a thorough physical examination, in addition to maintaining a high index of suspicion. Nearly 70% of patients will improve with an appropriate rehabilitation protocol. Indications for arthroscopic posterior stabilization include patients with continued disabling isolated posterior subluxation after a rehabilitation program, subluxation with a posterior labral tear, multidirectional instability with a primary posterior component, and voluntary positional posterior instability. Arthroscopic techniques have proven to be 80% to 90% effective at midterm follow-up. Throwing athletes and power athletes are generally able to return to full competition within 9 to 12 months postsurgery. Nonathletes are generally able to return to full activity within 6 to 9 months postsurgery.

Important Points

- Good success rates can be gained by a prolonged course of physical therapy with avoidance of activities in the provocative position.
- Patients with recurrent posterior instability resulting from chronic, repetitive microtrauma or generalized ligamentous laxity tend to respond best to a rehabilitation program.
- Patients in whom conservative measures have failed should be considered for surgical reconstruction.
- Arthroscopic techniques have proven to be 80% to 90% effective at midterm follow-up.

Clinical and Surgical Pearls

- The lateral decubitus position for arthroscopy allows better access to both the anterior and the posterior aspects of the shoulder.
- Placing the shoulder in 10 pounds of traction in the position of 45 degrees of abduction and 20 degrees of forward flexion in effect displaces the humeral head anteriorly and inferiorly, bringing the posterior labrum into clear view.
- The posterior portal is placed approximately 1 cm inferior and 1 cm lateral to the standard posterior portal in patients with demonstrable posterior instability on examination with the patient under anesthesia (EUA).
- We recommend performing rotator interval closure in patients with an inferior component to their instability, as defined by a 2+ or greater sulcus sign that does not improve in external rotation.

Clinical and Surgical Pitfalls

- The use of suture anchors for capsulolabral reconstruction is preferred over suture capsulorraphy alone because it results in a more stable repair.
- Difficulty in the placement of suture anchors can be encountered if the posterior portal is located too far superior or medial in the posterior capsule.
- A spinal needle can be used in positioning the auxiliary portal at the 7-o'clock position on the glenoid and approximately 1 cm lateral to the glenoid rim on the posterior capsule for approach to the posteroinferior glenoid at a 30- to 45-degree angle in the sagittal plane.

Posterior instability, when compared with anterior instability of the shoulder, is relatively uncommon. Reports in the literature state that posterior shoulder instability represents approximately 2% to 10% of shoulder instability cases.[1,4,16] Initial attempts to clarify the distinctions of posterior instability were made in 1952 when McLaughlin recognized that differences exist between "fixed and recurrent subluxations of the shoulder," suggesting that the etiology and treatment of the two are distinctly different.[4] More than 20 years later, Hawkins reiterated the difference between true dislocations and subluxations and noted that true recurrent posterior dislocations are rare compared with recurrent posterior subluxation (RPS) episodes.[5] Since that time, additional knowledge has been gained regarding the differences between unidirectional versus multidirectional, traumatic versus atraumatic, acute versus chronic, and voluntary versus involuntary posterior instability. In many respects each of these may represent a distinct form of posterior instability with its own underlying predispositions, anatomic abnormalities, and treatment algorithms.[6-8] Our collective understanding of posterior shoulder instability continues to evolve.

PATHOANATOMY

Our understanding of the spectrum of posterior instability has evolved more recently through the study of shoulder injuries in athletes, patients with generalized ligamentous laxity, and patients with posttraumatic injuries. These athletes typically have posterior shoulder instability secondary to repetitive microtrauma, which can occur in multiple arm positions and under a variety of loading conditions. RPS has been observed in overhead throwers, baseball hitters, golfers, tennis players, butterfly and freestyle swimmers, paddling sport athletes, weightlifters, rugby players, and football lineman, among others.[9,10] The more common cause of RPS is repetitive microtrauma, most commonly resulting from posterior capsular attenuation and posterior labral tears. Regardless of the type of athlete, patients with RPS often have somewhat ambiguous complaints of diffuse pain and shoulder fatigue without a distinct complaint of instability, often making it tricky to expose the underlying diagnosis and thus the associated pathology.

Acute posterior dislocations typically occur as a result of a direct blow to the anterior shoulder or indirect forces that couple shoulder flexion, internal rotation, and adduction.[8] The most common indirect causes are accidental electric shock and convulsive seizures, although these are relatively uncommon in the general population. However, recurrent or locked posterior shoulder dislocations from macrotrauma are exceedingly rare in the athletic population.[4,5] The treating physician, because of incomplete radiographic studies and a failure to recognize the posterior shoulder prominence and mechanical block to external rotation, may overlook up to 80% of locked posterior dislocations. Additional pathologic conditions to look for include the following:

- Reverse Hill-Sachs lesion
- Reverse bony Bankart lesion
- Posterior capsular laxity
- Excessive humeral head retroversion or chondrolabral retroversion
- Glenoid hypoplasia

DIAGNOSIS

To diagnose posterior instability, the clinician must take a thorough history and perform a thorough physical examination in addition to maintaining a high index of suspicion. A history of a posterior dislocation requiring formal reduction is more obvious; however patients with RPS may have more subtle findings. The majority of patients with RPS primarily report pain with specific activities, particularly in the provocative position (90 degrees of forward flexion, adduction, and internal rotation),[8] more often than instability. Knowledge of the athlete's sport, position, and training regimen is critical in deducing the pathogenesis and specific pathology associated with RPS. Pollock and Bigliani noted that two thirds of athletes who ultimately required surgery had presenting symptoms of difficulty using the shoulder outside of sports, particularly with arm above the horizontal.[7] An inquiry should also be made regarding mechanical symptoms; one study found that 90% of patients with symptomatic RPS noted clicking or crepitation with motion.[11] Often this crepitus can be reproduced during examination and is caused by discrete posterior capsulolabral pathology.

Clinical Examination

- Inspection for skin dimpling, atrophy, and scapular motion
- Active and passive range of motion
- Palpation for tenderness (especially posterior glenohumeral joint)
- Strength testing
- Evaluation for impingement
- Assessment for generalized ligamentous laxity (9-point Beighton scale)
- Stability testing
  - Load and shift test for anterior and posterior translation (Fig. 9-1)
  - Sulcus sign (both in neutral and external rotation) for inferior translation
  - Sulcus sign graded as 3+ that remains 2+ in external rotation is pathognomonic for multidirectional instability (MDI)
- Specific tests
  - Jerk test (Fig. 9-2)
  - Kim test (Fig. 9-3)
  - Circumduction test
  - Active compression or O'Brien test

Radiographs

- Plain radiographs including an axillary view, anteroposterior view, and scapular-Y view
  - Reverse Hill-Sachs lesions (Fig. 9-4) of the humeral head
    ○ Lesser tuberosity fracture

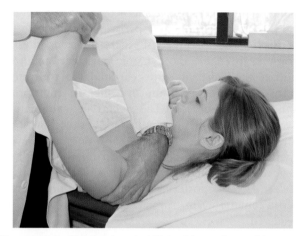

Figure 9-1. The load and shift test is performed by placing the thumb and index or long finger around the humeral head, which is then shifted anteriorly and posteriorly.

- Glenoid pathology (retroversion, rim fractures, and hypoplasia)
  ○ Additional West Point axillary view can be useful
  - Bony humeral avulsion of the glenohumeral ligaments (HAGL)
- Magnetic resonance arthrography (MRA)
  - Labrum (Fig. 9-5)
    ○ Kim classification is used to specifically describe posterior labral tear morphology[12]
      ■ Type I, incomplete detachment
      ■ Type II (the "Kim lesion"), a concealed complete detachment
      ■ Type III, chondrolabral erosion
      ■ Type IV, flap tear of the posteroinferior labrum
  - Capsule, biceps tendon, subscapularis integrity
  - Soft tissue reverse HAGL lesion
  - Posterior labrum periosteal sleeve avulsion (POLPSA)
- Dynamic MRA
  - Demonstrate labral peel-back in the abduction and external rotation (ABER) position, consistent with posterosuperior labral tear (or type VIII superior labral anterior-posterior [SLAP] tear)[13]
- Computed tomography (CT)
  - Glenoid version, locked posterior dislocation (Fig. 9-6)

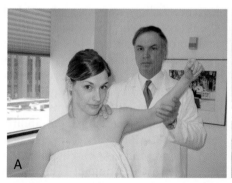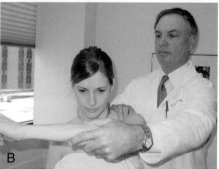

Figure 9-2. The jerk test for posterior instability. **A,** The arm is forward flexed and internally rotated. **B,** Posteriorly directed force subluxes the shoulder. Slow abduction of the arm results in a palpable jerk as the joint is reduced. This test has also been performed in reverse by moving the arm from an abducted position forward.

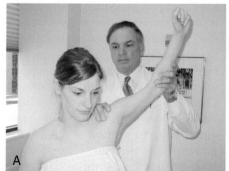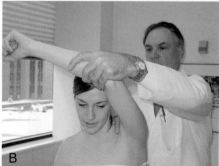

Figure 9-3. The Kim test for the detection of posteroinferior labral lesions is performed by applying axial compression to the 90-degree abducted arm **(A),** which is then elevated and forward flexed in a diagonal direction **(B),** resulting in pain and a possible clunk.

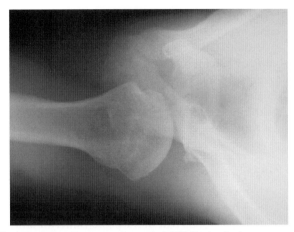

Figure 9-4. A reverse (anterior) Hill-Sachs lesion as demonstrated on an axillary radiograph.

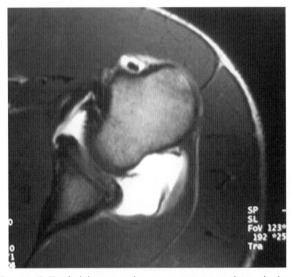

Figure 9-5. Axial magnetic resonance scan through the glenohumeral joint obtained with the intra-articular administration of contrast material demonstrating a capacious posterior capsule.

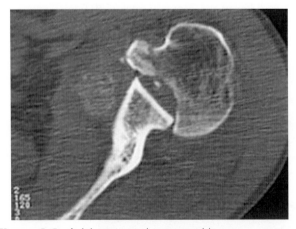

Figure 9-6. Axial computed tomographic scan demonstrating a locked posterior dislocation with large reverse Hill-Sachs lesion and destruction of a significant portion of the articular surface.

TREATMENT

Many patients with RPS can be managed successfully without surgery. Numerous authors have proposed a period of no less than 6 months of physical therapy before consideration of surgical treatment.[5,14] Effective rehabilitation includes avoidance of aggravating activities, restoration of a full range of motion, and shoulder strengthening. Strengthening of the rotator cuff, posterior deltoid, and periscapular musculature is critical. The premise of such directed physical therapy is to enable the dynamic muscular stabilizers to offset the deficient static capsulolabral restraints. Nearly 70% of patients improve after an appropriate rehabilitation protocol. The recurrent subluxation, however, is generally not eliminated, but the functional disability is diminished enough that it does not prevent activities.[15] If the disability fails to improve with an extended 6-month period of directed rehabilitation, or in select cases of posterior instability resulting from a macrotraumatic event, surgical intervention should be considered.

Indications and Contraindications

Patients failing extensive physical therapy protocols should receive surgical consideration. Interval plication and suture capsulorrhaphy techniques have improved arthroscopic results, making them comparable to open procedures.[10,16-18] Advantages of arthroscopic techniques over traditional open techniques include less disruption of normal shoulder anatomy; better visualization of intra-articular landmarks; the ability to perform concomitant SLAP repairs, capsular tear or rent repairs, and anterior and posterior stabilization procedures; and complete visualization of both the intra-articular and subacromial spaces. The surgeon's transition from open to arthroscopic techniques can be difficult. Arthroscopic techniques require the surgeon to be familiar with anchor placement, suture management, and arthroscopic knot tying. A thorough understanding of arthroscopic anatomy is vital to the success of arthroscopic stabilization procedures. Open techniques require larger incisions, a deltoid-splitting approach, and either splitting the bipennate infraspinatus muscle or developing the interval between the infraspinatus and the teres minor. On the other hand, open techniques allow complete visualization of the posterior capsule and offer the opportunity to perform a reliable capsular shift and/or posterior labral repair.

Indications for arthroscopic posterior stabilizations include patients with continued disabling isolated RPS after a rehabilitation program, RPS with a posterior labral tear, MDI with a primary posterior component, and voluntary positional posterior instability. Relative indications include patients with an antecedent macro-traumatic injury. Contraindications include patients not having completed a reasonable rehabilitation program, a surgeon preference for traditional open techniques, a large engaging reverse Hill-Sachs lesion requiring sub-scapularis transfer or an osteochondral allograft, a large reverse bony Bankart lesion, patients with muscular voluntary instability and underlying psychogenic disorders, and patients unable or unwilling to comply with postoperative limitations. Relative contraindications may include chronic instability resulting in compromised capsulolabral tissue, and patients who have undergone previous open surgery. Because successful results have been achieved with arthroscopic treatment of posterior labral tears in contact athletes,[10,19] arthroscopic reconstruction is not contraindicated in this population.[9] As arthroscopic techniques continue to evolve, the surgical indications will likely broaden.

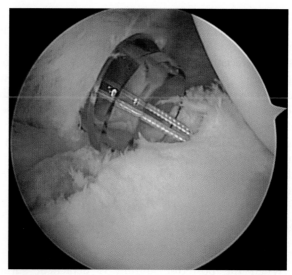

Figure 9-7. Accessory posterior portal for anchor placement.

ARTHROSCOPIC SURGICAL TECHNIQUE

Anesthesia

The procedure can be performed with use of the inter-scalene block or with general endotracheal anesthesia with an interscalene block for postoperative pain control.

Examination Under Anesthesia

EUA is performed on a firm surface with the scapula relatively fixed and the humeral head free to rotate. A load and shift maneuver, as described by Murrell and Warren, is performed with the patient supine.[6] The arm is held in 90 degrees of abduction and neutral rotation while a posterior force is applied in an attempt to trans-late the humeral head over the posterior glenoid. A sulcus sign is elicited with the arm adducted and in neutral rotation to assess whether the instability has an inferior component. A 3+ sulcus sign that remains 2+ or greater in external rotation is considered pathogno-monic for MDI. Testing is completed on both the affected and unaffected shoulders, and differences between the two are documented.

Patient Positioning, Landmarks, and Portals

The patient is placed in the lateral decubitus position with the affected shoulder positioned superiorly. An inflatable beanbag and kidney rests hold the patient in position. Foam cushions are placed to protect the pero-neal nerve at the neck of the fibula on the down leg. An axillary roll is placed. The operating table is placed in a slight reverse Trendelenburg position. The full upper extremity is prepared to the level of the sternum anteri-orly and the medial border of the scapula posteriorly. The operative shoulder is placed in 10 pounds of trac-tion and is positioned in 45 degrees of abduction and 20 degrees of forward flexion. The bony landmarks, including the acromion, distal clavicle, and coracoid process, are demarcated with a marking pen.

After preparation and draping, the glenohumeral joint is injected with 50 mL of sterile saline through an 18-gauge spinal needle to inflate the joint. A posterior portal is established 1 cm distal and 1 cm lateral to the standard posterior portal to allow access to the rim of the glenoid for anchor placement (Fig. 9-7). An anterior portal is then established high in the rotator interval via an inside-to-outside technique with a switching stick. Alternatively, it can also be established via an outside-to-inside technique with the assistance of a spinal needle. Typically, only anterior and posterior portals are required for the procedure. An accessory 7-o'clock portal has been described but is not frequently used in our technique.

Diagnostic Arthroscopy

A diagnostic arthroscopy of the glenohumeral joint is then undertaken. The labrum, capsule, biceps tendon, subscapularis, rotator interval, rotator cuff, and articu-lar surfaces are visualized in systematic fashion. This ensures that no associated lesions will be overlooked by poorly directed tunnel vision. Lesions typically seen in posterior instability include a patulous posterior capsule, posterior labral tear, labral fraying and splitting, widen-ing of the rotator interval, and undersurface partial-thickness rotator cuff tears. After the glenohumeral joint has been viewed from the posterior portal, the arthroscope is switched to the anterior portal to allow improved visualization of the posterior capsule and labrum. Recently we have been using a 70-degree arthroscope from the anterior portal, which allows enhanced visualization of the inferior labrum at the 6-o'clock position. A switching stick can then be used in replacing the posterior cannula with an 8.25-mm distally threaded clear cannula (Arthrex, Naples, FL), thus allowing passage of an arthroscopic probe and other instruments through the clear cannula to explore the posterior labrum for evidence of tears.

Specific Steps

1. Preparation for Repair

- When the posterior labrum is detached, suture anchors are employed in performing the repair. The posterior labrum is visualized from both the posterior and anterior portals to appreciate the full extent of the tear (Fig. 9-8).
- The arthroscope then remains in the anterior portal, and the posterior portal serves as the working portal for the repair.
- An arthroscopic rasp or chisel is used to mobilize the torn labrum from the glenoid rim (Fig. 9-9).
- A motorized synovial shaver or meniscal rasp is used to abrade the capsule adjacent to the labral tear and to debride and decorticate the glenoid rim to achieve a bleeding surface.

2. Placement of Suture Anchors

- Suture anchors are placed at the articular margin of the glenoid rim, rather than down on the glenoid neck, for performance of the labral repair (Fig. 9-10).

- A posterior labral tear extending from the 6-o'clock to 9-o'clock positions on a right shoulder is typically repaired with suture anchors at the 6:30, 7:30, and 8:30 positions.
- We prefer the 2.4-mm BioComposite SutureTak suture anchor with No. 2 FiberWire (Arthrex) because of the ease of placing the anchor on the glenoid surface, but a number of other commercially available anchors are also adequate.
- The suture anchor is placed with the sutures oriented perpendicular to the glenoid rim to facilitate passage of the most posterior suture through the torn labrum.
- Avoid inadvertent injury to the articular cartilage.

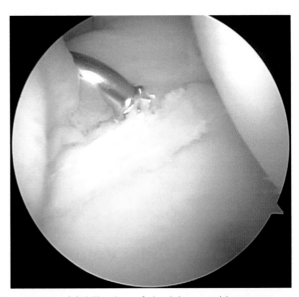

Figure 9-9. Mobilization of the labrum with a rasp.

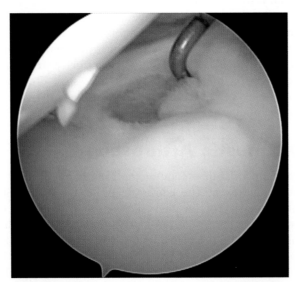

Figure 9-8. Posterior labral tear as viewed through the standard posterior viewing portal; the probe is placed through the accessory posterior portal.

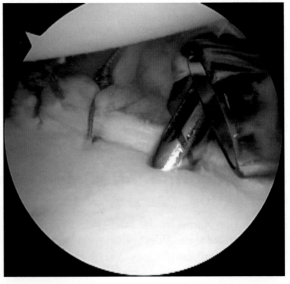

Figure 9-10. Arthroscopic anchor placement on the glenoid rim.

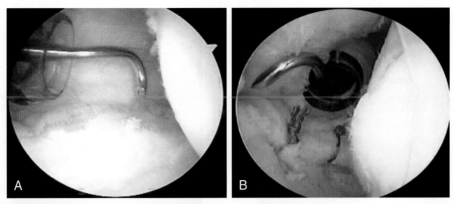

Figure 9-11. A suture-passing device penetrating the labrum and reentering the joint at the edge of the glenoid articular cartilage.

3. Labral Repair

- After placement of the suture anchors, a 45-degree Spectrum suture hook (Linvatec, Largo, FL) is then loaded with a No. 0 polydioxanone (PDS) suture (Ethicon, Somerville, NJ), or a 45-degree Suture-Lasso (Arthrexis) used to pass the suture through the capsule and labrum. Alternatively, there are other commercially available suture passers and suture relays that will also suffice.
- The suture passer is delivered through the torn labrum and advanced superiorly, reentering the joint at the edge of the glenoid articular cartilage (Fig. 9-11).
- Tension must be restored into the posterior band of the inferior glenohumeral ligament (IGHL) to reestablish posterior stability.
- Patients with acute injuries and less evidence of capsular stretching do not require the same degree of capsular advancement as those with more chronic instability.
- In the setting of a labral tear with some capsular laxity, the suture passer is advanced through the posterior capsule approximately 1 cm lateral to the edge of the labral tear and then is advanced underneath the labral tear to the edge of the articular cartilage, the so-called pleat stitch (Fig. 9-12).
- Placement of as many pleat stitches as necessary in the face of a patulous shoulder capsule can reduce capsular redundancy.
- The PDS is then fed into the glenohumeral joint and the suture passer is withdrawn through the posterior clear cannula.
- An arthroscopic suture grasper is used to withdraw both the most posterior suture in the suture anchor and the end of the PDS suture that has been advanced through the torn labrum. This move detangles the sutures in the cannula.
- The PDS is then fashioned into a single loop and tightly tied over the end of the braided suture.

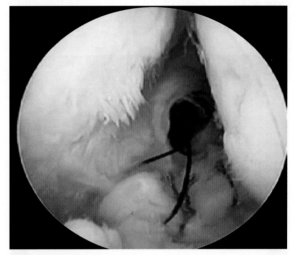

Figure 9-12. Capsular plication (pleat stitch, capsulorrhaphy stitch) can be performed to address capsular redundancy.

- The most lateral PDS suture, which has not been tied to the braided suture, is then pulled through the clear cannula (Fig. 9-13).
- This advances the most posterior suture in the suture anchor behind the labral tear (Fig. 9-14).
- A labral tear at the 7-o'clock position is advanced to the 7:30 suture anchor, and the 8-o'clock labral tear position is advanced to the 8:30 suture anchor. Additional sutures are then placed in similar fashion to complete the labral repair.
- If the capsule requires further tension, suture capsulorrhaphies can be performed in the intervals between the suture anchors directly to the newly secured labrum.
- Knots are tied after passage of each suture, which allows continued assessment of the repair and the degree of the capsular shift achieved by each suture.

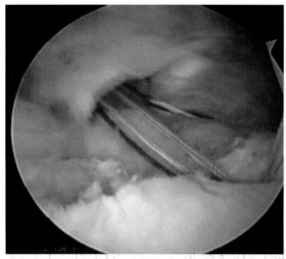

Figure 9-13. Shuttling of the anchor suture through the labrum.

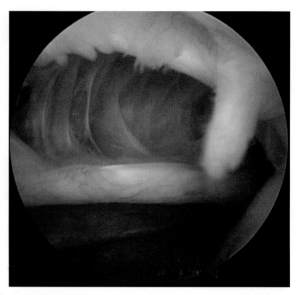

Figure 9-15. Mid posterior capsular rent/tear resulting in posterior instability.

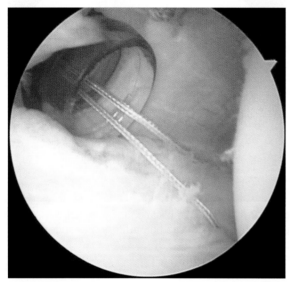

Figure 9-14. Sutures passed through the labrum, before tying.

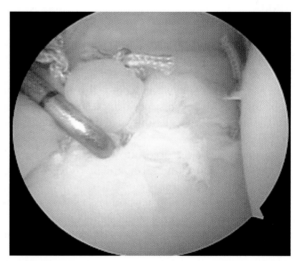

Figure 9-16. Final appearance after capsular advancement.

4. Posterior Capsular Shift

- The majority of patients with unidirectional posterior instability and primary posterior MDI do not have a posterior labral tear and will typically display significant capsular laxity at arthroscopy (Fig. 9-15). An isolated posterior capsulorrhaphy is performed. Occasionally a mid-capsular rent or tear may occur (see Fig. 9-15).
- Suture capsulorrhaphies are placed from inferior (6-o'clock position) to superior (10-o'clock position).
- The 6:30 capsular suture is typically advanced to the 7:30 position, and the reduction in capsular volume is assessed.
- Restoration of adequate tension in the posterior band of the IGHL is critical.

- Additional sutures are then placed at the 7:30, 8:30, and 9:30 positions on the capsule, advancing to the 8:30, 9:30, and 10:30 positions on the glenoid (Fig. 9-16).
- Sutures are tied after each has been passed. If the sutures are not tied until the end, one errant suture may necessitate removal of all other sutures to achieve correction.

5. Arthroscopic Knot Tying

- We prefer the sliding, locking Weston knot because of its low profile, but a number of arthroscopic knot-tying techniques work well.
- What is most important is that the surgeon be familiar with the knot used and be skilled in using it.

- The posterior braided suture exiting through the capsule is threaded through a knot-pusher, and the end is secured with a hemostat.
- This suture serves as the post, which in effect will advance the capsule and labrum to the glenoid rim when the knot is tightened.
- The knot should be secured posteriorly on the capsule and not on the rim of the glenoid to prevent humeral head abrasion from the knot.
- Each half hitch must be completely seated before the next half hitch is thrown.
- Placing tension on the nonpost suture and advancing the knot pusher "past point" will lock the Weston knot.
- Three alternating half hitches are placed to secure the Weston knot.

6. Completion of the Repair

- An arthroscopic awl is used to penetrate the bare area of the humerus, under the infraspinatus tendon, in an effort to achieve some punctate bleeding to augment the healing response.
- The posterior capsular portal incision is then closed by passage of a PDS suture through the crescent Spectrum suture passer and retrieval of the suture with an arthroscopic penetrator.
- Varying the distance of the suture from the portal incision allows titration of the capsulorrhaphy.
- The PDS is then tied blindly in the cannula, closing the posterior capsular incision (Fig. 9-17).

7. Rotator Interval Closure

- In the setting of MDI with a primary posterior component, the rotator interval requires closure (defined by a 2+ or greater sulcus sign that does not improve in external rotation).

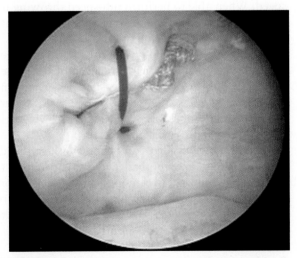

Figure 9-17. Closed posterior portal after cannula removal (as viewed from anterior).

- The rotator interval is viewed with the arthroscope in the posterior portal.
- A crescent suture passer is advanced from the anterior portal through the anterior capsule just above the superior border of the subscapularis tendon 1 cm lateral to the glenoid.
- It is then passed through the middle glenohumeral ligament (MGHL) at the inferior border of the rotator interval. This makes up the inferior aspect of the rotator interval closure.
- A No. 0 PDS suture is then fed into the joint and retrieved with a penetrator through the superior glenohumeral ligament (SGHL).
- The PDS suture is then withdrawn out the anterior cannula and the knot is tied blindly in the cannula as the closure is visualized through the posterior portal.

Technical Alternatives and Pitfalls

There is open debate regarding whether the lateral decubitus or beach chair position better facilitates shoulder arthroscopy. We prefer the lateral position because we feel it allows better access to both the anterior and posterior aspects of the shoulder. Placement of the shoulder in 10 pounds of traction in the position of 45 degrees of abduction and 20 degrees of forward flexion in effect displaces the humeral head anteriorly and inferiorly, bringing the posterior labrum into clear view. We have not been able to achieve such an unimpeded approach to the posteroinferior shoulder capsule in the beach chair position without imparting injury to the articular cartilage of the humeral head in the process.

We prefer to inject the glenohumeral joint with 40 to 50 mL of sterile saline before placement of the cannula into the glenohumeral joint. It inflates the joint to allow safer insertion of the cannula, limiting risk to the articular cartilage of the humeral head and glenoid.

After a determination of posterior labral pathology or capsular laxity is made, a posterior working portal must be established. Placement of an 8.25-mm distally threaded clear cannula (Arthrex) over a switching stick into the posterior portal will allow passage of both the crescent and 45-degree suture hooks. Smaller cannulas will not accommodate the 45-degree suture hook. We also recommend the use of suture anchors for capsulolabral reconstruction instead of suture capsulorrhaphy alone, as it results in a more stable repair.

Difficulty in the placement of suture anchors can be encountered if the posterior portal is located too far superior or medial in the posterior capsule. The conventional posterior portal is located near the 10-o'clock position on the right glenoid, which makes approach to the posteroinferior glenoid difficult for the placement of suture anchors. We therefore place the posterior portal approximately 1 cm inferior and 1 cm lateral to the standard posterior portal in patients with demonstrable posterior instability on EUA. When the posterior portal has been made too far superior, an auxiliary posterior portal can then be made inferior and lateral to the existing posterior portal. A spinal needle can be used in positioning the auxiliary portal at the 7-o'clock position on the glenoid and approximately 1 cm lateral to the glenoid rim on the posterior capsule for approach to the posteroinferior glenoid at a 30- to 45-degree angle in the sagittal plane. Cadaveric studies by Davidson and Rivenburgh[20] have shown the 7-o'clock portal to be located a safe distance from the axillary nerve and posterior humeral circumflex artery (39 ± 4 mm) and the suprascapular nerve and artery (29 ± 3 mm). The use of blunt trocars in the placement of the portal further decreases the risk of neurovascular injury.

We do not routinely close the rotator interval in patients with unidirectional posterior instability. This practice is supported by several studies in the literature.[10,18] Harryman and colleagues[21] sectioned the rotator interval and found that in a position of 60 degrees of flexion and 60 degrees of abduction a significant increase in posterior translation occurred. However, in posterior instability's provocative position of 60 degrees of flexion and 90 degrees of internal rotation, no significant increase in posterior translation occurred after sectioning of the rotator interval. Furthermore, although imbrication of the rotator interval significantly decreased posterior translation at a position of 60 degrees of flexion and 60 degrees of abduction, it did not have a similar effect in the provocative position. A sectioned rotator interval did lead to a significant increase in inferior translation, which was corrected by imbrication of the rotator interval tissue. This was reinforced by a more recent biomechanical study by Mologne and colleagues,[22] which found that posterior stability was not improved with the addition of a rotator interval closure. We do, however, perform rotator interval closure in patients with an inferior component to their instability, as defined by a 2+ or greater sulcus sign that does not improve in external rotation.[21]

Rehabilitation and Return-to-Play Recommendations

The rehabilitation program consists of a series of phases. Initially the posterior capsule must be protected by avoidance of extremes of internal rotation.

- Immobilization in an UltraSling (DonJoy, Carlsbad, CA) for 6 weeks, abducting the shoulder approximately 30 degrees.
- Immobilization is removed for gentle passive painfree range-of-motion exercises. We allow 90 degrees of forward flexion and external rotation to 0 degrees by 4 weeks postsurgery.
- The UltraSling is discontinued 6 weeks postsurgery; active-assisted range-of-motion exercises and gentle passive range-of-motion exercises are progressed, and pain-free gentle internal rotation is instituted.
- At 2 to 3 months postsurgery, range of motion and mobilization are progressed to achieve full passive and active motion. Stretching exercises for the anterior and posterior capsule are instituted.
- By 4 months postsurgery the shoulder should be pain free and concentration on eccentric rotator cuff strengthening is begun.
- At 5 months postsurgery, isotonic and isokinetic exercises are advanced.
- At 4 to 6 months postsurgery, throwing athletes undergo isokinetic testing. When patients are able to achieve at least 80% strength and endurance compared with the uninvolved side, an integrated throwing protocol and/or sport-specific rehabilitation protocol is instituted.
- Throwers begin an easy-tossing program at a distance of 20 feet without a wind-up. Stretching and the application of heat to increase circulation before throwing sessions are critical.
- By 7 months, light throwing with an easy wind-up to 30 feet is allowed 2 or 3 days per week for 10 minutes per session.
- By 9 months postsurgery, long, easy throws from the mid-outfield (150 to 200 feet) are allowed.
- By 10 months, stronger throws from the outfield are allowed, reaching home plate on only one or two bounces.
- At 11 months, pitchers are allowed to throw at half to three-quarter speed from the mound, with emphasis on technique and accuracy.
- By 12 months postsurgery, throwers are allowed to throw from their position at three-quarter to full speed. When able to perform full-speed throwing for 2 consecutive weeks, the throwing athlete is permitted to return to full competition.
- Nonthrowing athletes and nonathletes are managed by different criteria than throwing athletes. When patients are able to achieve at least 80% strength and endurance at the 6-month isokinetic testing compared with the uninvolved side, nonthrowing athletes begin a sport-specific program.
- In general, power athletes and contact athletes, such as weightlifters and football players, can return to full competition by 6 to 9 months postsurgery. Noncontact athletes such as golfers, basketball players, swimmers, and cheerleaders can generally return to full competition by 6 to 8 months.

Results of arthroscopic treatment are given in Table 9-1.

TABLE 9-1. Results of Arthroscopic Treatment.

Study	Follow-up	Outcome
Papendick and Savoie[23] (1995)	10 mo	39 of 41 (95%) successful
McIntyre et al[3] (1997)	31 mo	15 of 20 (75%) successful
Savoie and Field[24] (1997)	34 mo	55 of 61 (90%) successful
Wolf and Eakin[18] (1998)	33 mo	12 of 14 (86%) successful
Mair et al[10] (1998)	2 yr minimum	9 of 9 (100%) successful
Antoniou et al[1] (2000)	28 mo	35 of 41 (85%) successful
Williams et al[19] (2003)	5.1 yr	24 of 26 (92%) successful
Kim et al[12] (2003)	39 mo	26 of 27 (96%) successful
Fluhme et al[17] (2004)	34 mo	15 of 18 (83%) successful
Bottoni et al[16] (2005)	40 mo	16 of 18 (89%) successful
Provencher et al[25] (2005)	39 mo	26 of 33 (79%) successful
Bradley et al[9] (2006)	27 mo	91 of 100 (91%) successful
Seroyer et al[26] (2007)	24 mo	9 of 13 (69%) successful
Radkowski et al[27] (2008)	27 mo	24 of 27 (89%) throwers successful 74 of 80 (93%) nonthrowers successful
Savoie et al[28] (2008)	28 mo	89 of 92 (97%) successful
Bradley et al[29] (2009)	32 mo	145 of 161 (90%) successful

SUMMARY

Posterior shoulder instability is a broad entity ranging from RPS to locked posterior dislocation. It is much less common than anterior shoulder instability but probably occurs more frequently than suggested in the literature. Traditionally confusion existed in the distinction between the different forms of posterior instability, but a much greater understanding has been gained more recently. Good success rates can be achieved with a prolonged course of physical therapy with avoidance of activities in the provocative position. Patients with RPS resulting from chronic, repetitive microtrauma or generalized ligamentous laxity tend to respond best to a rehabilitation program. Patients failing conservative measures should be considered for surgical reconstruction. Arthroscopic techniques have proven to be 80% to 90% effective at midterm follow-up. Arthroscopic methods afford the ability to perform simultaneous anterior and posterior reconstructions, avoid splitting the deltoid and rotator cuff, and offer excellent visualization of both the glenohumeral joint and subacromial space. A directed physical therapy program postsurgery is vital to a successful outcome. Throwing athletes and power athletes are generally able to return to full competition within 9 to 12 months postsurgery. Nonathletes are generally able to return to full activity within 6 to 9 months postsurgery.

REFERENCES

1. Antoniou J, Duckworth DT, Harryman II DT. Capsulolabral augmentation for the management of posteroinferior instability of the shoulder. *J Bone Joint Surg Am.* 2000;82(9):1220-1230.
2. Boyd HB, Sisk TD. Recurrent posterior dislocation of the shoulder. *J Bone Joint Surg Am.* 1972;54:779.
3. McIntyre LF, Caspari RB, Savoie III FH. The arthroscopic treatment of posterior shoulder instability: two-year results of a multiple suture technique. *Arthroscopy.* 1997;13:426-432.
4. McLaughlin HL. Posterior dislocation of the shoulder. *J Bone Joint Surg Am.* 1952;34:584.
5. Hawkins RJ, Koppert G, Johnston G. Recurrent posterior instability (subluxation) of the shoulder. *J Bone Joint Surg Am.* 1984;66:169.
6. Murrell GA, Warren RF. The surgical treatment of posterior shoulder instability. *Clin Sports Med.* 1995;14:903.
7. Pollock RG, Bigliani LU. Recurrent posterior shoulder instability. Diagnosis and treatment. *Clin Orthop Relat Res.* 1993;291:85.
8. Tibone JE, Bradley JP. The treatment of posterior subluxation in athletes. *Clin Orthop Relat Res.* 1993;291:124-137.
9. Bradley JP, Chhabra A, Baker CL, et al. Arthroscopic capsulolabral reconstruction for posterior instability of the shoulder: A prospective study of 100 shoulders. *Am J Sports Med.* 2006;34(7):1061-1071.

10. Mair SD, Zarzour RH, Speer KP. Posterior labral injury in contact athletes. *Am J Sports Med.* 1998;26:753-758.

11. Cyprien JM, Vasey HM, Burdet A, et al. Humeral retrotorsion and glenohumeral relationship in the normal shoulder and in recurrent anterior dislocation (scapulometry). *Clin Orthop Relat Res.* 1983;175:8-17.

12. Kim SH, Ha KI, Park JH, et al. Arthroscopic posterior labral repair and capsular shift for traumatic unidirectional recurrent posterior subluxation of the shoulder. *J Bone Joint Surg Am.* 2003;85:1479-1487.

13. Borrero CG, Casagranda BU, Towers JD, et al. Magnetic resonance appearance of posterosuperior labral peel back during humeral abduction and external rotation. *Skeletal Radiol.* 2010;39(1):19-26.

14. Burkhead Jr WZ, Rockwood Jr CA. Treatment of instability of the shoulder with an exercise program. *J Bone Joint Surg Am.* 1992;74:890-896.

15. Hurley JA, Anderson TE, Dear W, et al. Posterior shoulder instability: surgical versus conservative results with evaluation of glenoid version. *Am J Sports Med.* 1992;20: 396-400.

16. Bottoni CR, Franks BR, Moore JH, et al. Operative stabilization of posterior shoulder instability. *Am J Sports Med.* 2005;33:996-1002.

17. Fluhme DJ, Bradley JP, Burke CJ, et al. *Open versus arthroscopic treatment for posterior glenohumeral instability.* Presented at AOSSM Annual Meeting. June 24-27, 2004; Quebec City, Canada.

18. Wolf EM, Eakin CL. Arthroscopic capsular plication for posterior shoulder instability. *Arthroscopy.* 1998;14: 153-163.

19. Williams III RJ, Strickland S, Cohen M, et al. Arthroscopic repair for traumatic posterior shoulder instability. *Am J Sports Med.* 2003;31:203-209.

20. Davidson PA, Rivenburgh DW. The 7-o'clock posteroinferior portal for shoulder arthroscopy. *Am J Sports Med.* 2002;30:693-696.

21. Harryman DT, Sidles JA, Harris SL, et al. The role of the rotator interval capsule in passive motion and stability of the shoulder. *J Bone Joint Surg Am.* 1992;74:53-66.

22. Mologne TS, Zhao K, Hongo M, et al. The addition of rotator interval closure after arthroscopic repair of either anterior or posterior shoulder instability. *Am J Sports Med.* 2008;36:1123-1131.

23. Papendick LW, Savoie III FH. Anatomy-specific repair techniques for posterior shoulder instability. *J South Orthop Assoc.* 1995;4:169-176.

24. Savoie III FH, Field LD. Arthroscopic management of posterior shoulder instability. *Oper Tech Sports Med.* 1997;5:226-232.

25. Provencher MT, Bell SJ, Menzel KA, et al. Arthroscopic treatment of posterior instability: Results in 33 patients. *Am J Sports Med.* 2005.

26. Seroyer S, Tejwani SG, Bradley JP. Arthroscopic capsulolabral reconstruction of the type VIII superior labrum anterior posterior lesion: mean 2-year follow-up on 13 shoulders. *Am J Sports Med.* 2007;35(9):1477-1483.

27. Radkowski CA, Chhabra A, Baker III CL, et al. Arthroscopic capsulolabral repair for posterior shoulder instability in throwing athletes compared with nonthrowing athletes. *Am J Sports Med.* 2008;36(4):693-699.

28. Savoie 3rd FH, Holt MS, Field LD, et al. Arthroscopic management of posterior instability: evolution of technique and results. *Arthroscopy.* 2008;24(4):389-396.

29. Bradley JP, Lesniak BP, McClincy M. Arthroscopic capsulolabral reconstruction for posterior shoulder instability in athletes: a prospective study of 161 shoulders. Presented at the annual closed meeting of the American Shoulder and Elbow Society, New York, NY, September 2009.

Chapter 10

Arthroscopic Repair of Multidirectional Instability of the Shoulder

Matthew Craig and Jon K. Sekiya

Chapter Synopsis
- Multidirectional instability of the shoulder is a complex pathology currently treated arthroscopically.
- Multipleated capsular plication with glenoid suture anchors is used to decrease capsular volume and restore stability. This technique is ideal because it offers excellent results with minimal risk of complications.

Important Points
- *Indications:* Persistent shoulder instability in multiple directions; unable to be resolved by physical therapy
- *Contraindications:* Volitional instability with secondary gain; Hill-Sachs or other bony defects; inability to follow rehabilitation protocol
- *Symptoms:* Instability in multiple directions; shoulder pain, clicking, numbness, or grinding; difficulty with overhead activities
- *Classification:* Atraumatic, traumatic
- *Surgical technique:* Arthroscopic multipleated capsular plication

Clinical and Surgical Pearls
- Patient in lateral decubitus position with axillary bump
- Anterior and posterior portal creation
- Suture anchor placement on glenoid
- Creation of multipleat—passing suture through labrum and capsule multiple times
- Locking sliding Weston knot backed with three half hitches, tied
- Additional anterior and posterior anchor placement on glenoid until sufficient stability achieved
- Rotator interval closure rarely needed

Clinical and Surgical Pitfalls
- Risk of surgical complications is quite low.
- Patients in postoperative rehabilitation must be closely monitored so range-of-motion exercises can be slowed or accelerated.

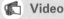 Video
- Video 10-1: Arthroscopic Management of Multidirectional Instability of the Shoulder

---

Multidirectional instability, first described by Neer and colleagues in 1980,[1] is currently defined as instability in at least two of the following directions: anterior, posterior, and inferior. Most cases of instability are thought to be a result of nontraumatic processes—for example, microtrauma caused by repetitive overhead actions such as those common in swimmers and throwers. More recently, though, the disease paradigm has expanded to encompass Pagnani and Warren's circle theory, which states that an anterior dislocation results in the stretching or tearing of both the anterior and posterior capsular ligaments.[2] The stretching of both ligaments then creates variable degrees of multidirectional symptoms in patients with purely anterior dislocations. This has led to the need for posterior repair with anterior dislocations. Clinical experiences have shown that neglecting the posterior band in these patients leaves them still experiencing instability. Biologically, several pathologic processes are thought to be responsible for multidirectional instability: capsular laxity, labral detachment, rotator interval defects, and changes in quality and type of collagen.[3]

Early surgical techniques included open approaches that were aimed at decreasing capsular laxity, especially inferiorly. As arthroscopic techniques have improved, they have become the favored way to treat instability. Prior techniques have included capsular shift by transglenoid sutures, Bankart repair and shift with biodegradable suture anchors, thermal capsulorrhaphy, rotator interval repair, and capsular plication. Currently, our preferred method of surgical treatment of multidirectional instability in which nonoperative attempts at rehabilitation have failed is an arthroscopic capsular shift that reduces glenohumeral joint volume with a multipleated capsular plication.

PREOPERATIVE CONSIDERATIONS

History

Typically, multidirectional instability is a result of microtrauma caused by repetitive overhead actions that lead to global capsular laxity. Less commonly, a traumatic shoulder dislocation may be the inciting event. Additional causes include generalized ligamentous laxity or Ehlers-Danlos syndrome, a disease that causes defects in collagen synthesis. A typical patient is young, is active, and has shoulder pain that may be accompanied by popping, clicking, and grinding in addition to reports of shoulder shifting, instability while sleeping, pain or numbness while carrying heavy objects, difficultly with overhead activity, and feelings of instability during pushups or bench-presses. Often, he or she is no longer able to participate in sports and may report prior physical therapy that was unsuccessful.[4] A subset of patients also report being able to voluntarily dislocate the shoulder. With these individuals, it is imperative to distinguish between those who are able to voluntarily dislocate and those who are dislocating for secondary gain. The former can be a challenging candidate for surgery and scapular retraining in addition to needing evaluation for

potential psychological or psychosocial issues, whereas the latter make poor surgical candidates.

Physical Examination

A thorough physical examination is necessary for an accurate diagnosis of multidirectional instability and prevention of unnecessary surgery. It is important to understand that the amount of instability should always be based on comparison with the patient's unaffected side and not with other patients. For example, a gymnast and a football player both report instability in the left shoulder. The left shoulder of the gymnast will be more unstable than her normal right side. However, owing to the nature of her sport, the normal right side of the gymnast will likely be more lax than the unstable left shoulder of the football player. Although the football player is experiencing less total instability, both athletes have an equal need for treatment. Remember that instability is relative, not absolute.

Throughout the examination, it is important to ask patients to report when they begin to feel instability as well as to note any apprehension, as this will help give an accurate impression of the severity and direction of instability. A complete examination will include inspection for atrophy, scapulothoracic and glenohumeral active and passive range-of-motion testing, strength testing, palpation for tenderness, evaluation of ligamentous laxity, and evaluation for impingement and instability. Anterior instability is best evaluated with the anterior drawer, load and shift, anterior release, and anterior relocation and apprehension tests, whereas posterior instability is evaluated with the posterior drawer, load and shift, and stress and jerk tests. The hallmark finding in multidirectional instability is a positive sulcus sign in neutral rotation (Fig. 10-1). A sulcus sign that remains positive with 30 degrees of external rotation indicates likely rotator interval pathology. The O'Brien, Kim, circumduction, and speed tests are also performed. Examination under anesthesia may be needed to confirm clinical findings before progressing to surgery.

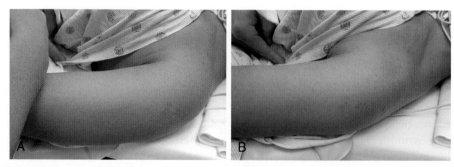

Figure 10-1. A, Sulcus sign test. Patient's arm is relaxed and in neutral rotation. **B,** After application of inferior traction, a depression is visible beneath the acromion—positive sulcus sign.

Imaging

Plain radiographs in the anteroposterior, axillary, outlet, Stryker notch, and West Point views should be obtained and evaluated for Hill-Sachs and reverse Hill-Sachs lesions as well as glenoid bone defects. These lesions may offer clues to the direction of instability but are rare in atraumatic multidirectional instability. Plain film findings of bony defects should be followed up with computed tomography (CT) for further evaluation. Magnetic resonance arthrography (MRA) should be used to evaluate soft tissue pathology including labral and rotator cuff tears, biceps tendon disease, and capsular laxity.

Indications and Contraindications

In many patients with atraumatic multidirectional instability, dynamic neuromuscular control of glenohumeral stability is lost. Before surgical treatment is considered, patients should begin a physical therapy regimen (conservative treatment) that focuses on strengthening rotator cuff muscles and scapular stabilizers as well as improving proprioception. If instability persists after physical therapy, individuals should progress to surgery, especially if there is difficulty with day-to-day activities. Considering that after an acute shoulder dislocation the risk of recurrence can be as high as 80% in young athletic individuals, surgical intervention is highly warranted once physical therapy has failed.[5]

Patients with a history of multidirectional instability who experience glenoid erosion or fractures of the glenoid or humeral head with a dislocation generally require surgery. Those with large Hill-Sachs or glenoid bone lesions from multiple dislocations may require allograft bone placement done nonarthroscopically in addition to tightening of the glenohumeral capsule.

Although not a contraindication to surgery, seizure disorders require that the patient consult with his or her neurologist to make sure neurologic issues are under appropriate control before surgery. Contraindications to surgical intervention include voluntary instability with secondary gain, lack of participation in a formal physical therapy program, and inability or unwillingness of the patient to comply with the planned postoperative rehabilitation program.

Surgical Planning

Educating patients about the goal, complications, and risks associated with surgical intervention is critical. They should be aware that the goal of the surgery is to decrease capsular volume and restore glenoid concavity with capsulolabral augmentation to help stabilize the shoulder and reduce symptoms. It is important that the individual understand that although it is an outpatient procedure, at least a 6-month period of physical rehabilitation will be required before full return to all activities.

One complication that requires extensive discussion is the potential for decreased range of motion after surgery. Although this may be acceptable to older or less active patients, athletes, especially throwers and gymnasts, may have much lower tolerances for loss of motion. Arthroscopic treatment of athletes with multidirectional instability has been successful, with 91% of athletes reporting full or satisfactory range of motion after surgery and 86% returning to their sport with little or no limitation.[6] In addition, although athletes should always participate in a physical therapy program before progressing to surgery, surgical options may be presented earlier if the individual is not making significant progress and is losing valuable playing time. Ideally, physical therapy would begin early in the season to midseason followed by end-of-season surgery, allowing postoperative rehabilitation to take place during the off-season.

Additional complications of surgery include infection, bleeding, pain, neurovascular injury, adhesive capsulitis, recurrence of instability, loss of function, need for follow-up examination and manipulation under anesthesia, and future reoperation.

Surgical planning continues with the examination under anesthesia and diagnostic arthroscopy. This may alter the plan to include rotator interval closure, anterior posterior labral repair, superior labral anterior-posterior repair, and biceps tenodesis or tenotomy. Because the multipleated plication technique is as effective in decreasing capsular volume as an open capsular shift, conversion to an open procedure should not be needed.[7]

SURGICAL TECHNIQUE
Anesthesia, Examination, and Positioning

The procedure is performed with an interscalene block for postoperative pain control and general endotracheal anesthesia with administration of prophylactic antibiotics. The examination under anesthesia is performed on a firm surface with the scapula relatively fixed and the humeral head free to rotate. The degree and direction of instability should be noted. A load and shift test is performed with the arm held in 90 degrees of abduction and neutral rotation while an anterior or posterior force is applied in an attempt to translate the humeral head over the anterior or posterior glenoid. A sulcus sign test is also needed. The arm is adducted and placed in neutral rotation and pulled inferiorly (see Fig. 10-1A). The test result is positive if a dimple appears in the

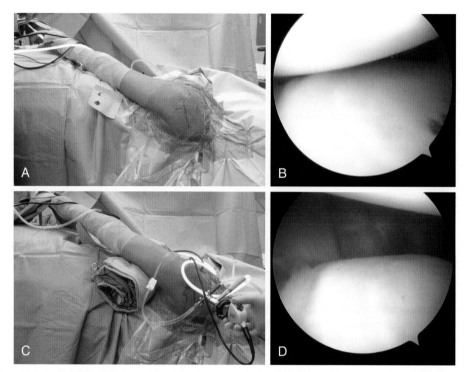

Figure 10-2. Placement of axillary bump greatly improves arthroscopic visualization inferiorly. **A,** No bump. **B,** Corresponding arthroscopic view. **C,** Axillary bump in place. **D,** Corresponding arthroscopic view. Visualization is significantly improved, aiding in precise placement of capsular plication stitches.

subacromial region as the humeral head translates inferiorly (see Fig. 10-1B). Testing should be done on both the affected and unaffected shoulder.[8]

The table should be in a slight reverse Trendelenburg position with the patient in the lateral decubitus position with the operative shoulder facing superiorly. This position offers excellent views of the inferior and posterior capsular regions. Three layers of tape are placed over the greater trochanter, stomach, and chest area to secure the patient. An inflatable beanbag is used for stabilization. Pillows should be placed underneath the down leg and between the legs to keep pressure off the peroneal nerves. The operative adducted arm is then propped up with an axillary bump, which allows for better views of the glenohumeral joint (Fig. 10-2). The arm is then prepared and draped in standard sterile fashion.

Landmarks and Portals

The following bony landmarks should be marked: acromion, coracoid, distal clavicle, acromioclavicular joint, and scapular spine (Fig. 10-3).[9] The location of the posterior portal, 1 to 2 cm distal and medial to the posterolateral edge of the acromion, is then marked. This position facilitates visualization and access to the posterior glenoid, labrum, and capsule. An 18-gauge spinal needle is used to enter the joint through the posterior portal, and a total of 10 to 20 mL of saline is

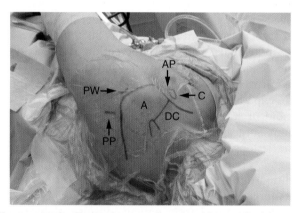

Figure 10-3. Patient's operative shoulder marked for surgery. *A,* Acromion; *AP,* anterior portal; *C,* coracoid; *DC,* distal clavicle; *PP,* posterior portal; *PW,* Port of Wilmington.

injected to inflate the joint. Saline and joint fluid are withdrawn to confirm position. A No. 11 blade is then used to make a small posterior incision, and the trocar and cannula are passed through the incision on the same trajectory as the spinal needle. Once in the joint, the spinal needle is removed, and the camera is introduced.

Next, the anterior portal is created at the level just superior to the subscapularis lateral to the coracoid, at approximately the 5-o'clock position. It is important to ensure that the subscapularis is not pierced when this

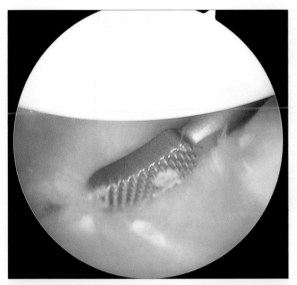

Figure 10-4. Capsular abrasion with a rasp.

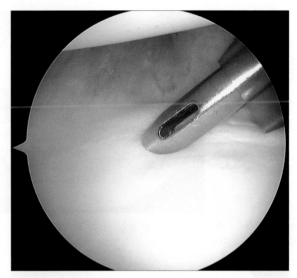

Figure 10-5. Placement of drill on glenoid.

portal is being created. Under direct visualization, an 18-gauge spinal needle is passed through the previously marked anterior skin area and into the joint. The needle is removed, and a small incision is made with a No. 11 blade. A switching stick is then used to enter the joint. The tissue is dilated with a cannulated inserter, and a minimum 8.25-mm cannula is then placed over the switching stick. The switching stick is removed and used to mark the posterior portal, and the trocar and camera are inserted into the anterior portal.

Diagnostic Arthroscopy

After portal creation, a diagnostic arthroscopy is performed. The labrum, capsule, biceps tendon, subscapularis, rotator interval, rotator cuff, and articular surfaces should be visualized via the posterior portal. The camera can then be switched to the anterior portal to aid in assessment of the posterior capsule and labrum as well as for visualization of anterior inferior glenoid bone loss. A complete arthroscopy will prevent the missing of previously unknown pathology. Arthroscopic findings typically include a patulous inferior capsule, labral fraying and splitting, widening of the rotator interval, and undersurface partial thickness rotator cuff tears. A positive drive-through sign is often present. Labral tears, significant cuff pathology, and Bankart or Hill-Sachs lesions are usually not present.[4]

Specific Steps

1. Preparation for Repair

During anterior repair, the arthroscope remains in the posterior portal, and the anterior portal becomes the working portal. During posterior repair, the arthroscope remains in the anterior portal, and the posterior portal becomes the working portal. At the beginning of the

procedure, a rasp or motorized synovial shaver is used to debride any torn labrum from the glenoid rim. If necessary, arthroscopic scissors are used to cut the biceps tendon. The rasp and shaver are then used to debride and decorticate the glenoid rim and capsule, providing a roughened and bleeding surface to encourage healing (Fig. 10-4).

2. Multipleated Plication

The most symptomatic side should always be worked on first. For anterior repair, a 3-mm suture anchor loaded with No. 2 braided nonabsorbable suture (anchor suture) is drilled into the glenoid at the 5-o'clock position (right shoulder) (Fig. 10-5).[7,9,10] For posterior repair, the first anchor is placed at the 7-o'clock position (right shoulder). After placement, sutures are brought out through the working portal (Fig. 10-6). A soft tissue penetrator, such as a suture hook or a crescent suture passer, is inserted into the working portal and passed through the labrum directly adjacent to the anchor, and the inferior anchor suture is pulled through the labrum (Fig. 10-7). The penetrator is then used to pierce the capsule in the most anterior inferior and lateral point during anterior repair or the most posterior inferior and lateral point during posterior repair.

After the capsule has been pierced, a No. 1 absorbable monofilament suture (shuttle suture) is shuttled into the joint, and the penetrator is removed (Fig. 10-8). A suture grasper is then used to grasp both the shuttle suture and the anchor suture that was passed through the labrum. The shuttle suture is then tied with a simple knot to the anchor suture and is used to shuttle the anchor suture through the inferior tuck of the capsule (Fig. 10-9). This process is repeated two or three times, creating multiple pleats or tucks of capsule, working superiorly up the capsule until sufficient tightening has been achieved (Fig. 10-10). The suture is checked to

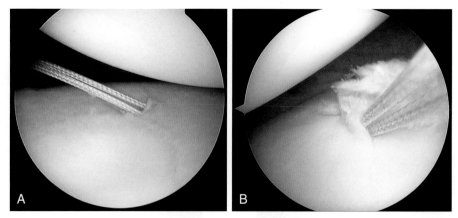

Figure 10-6. A, Placement of anchor on the rim of the glenoid with intact labrum. **B,** Placement of anchor on the rim of the glenoid with torn labrum.

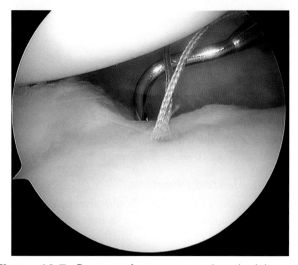

Figure 10-7. Passage of suture passer into the joint.

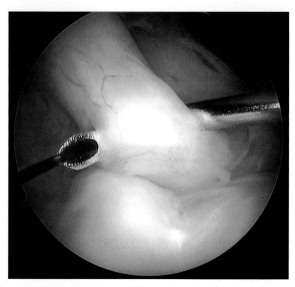

Figure 10-8. Passage of No. 1 absorbable monofilament suture (shuttle suture) into the joint.

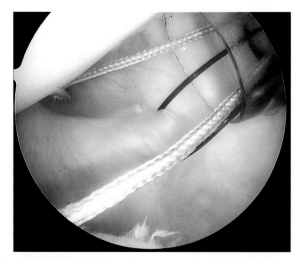

Figure 10-9. Shuttle of No. 1 shuttle suture through capsulolabral tissue.

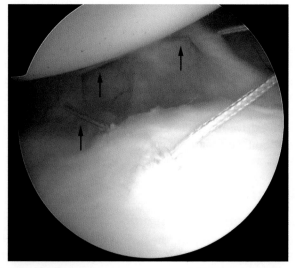

Figure 10-10. Repeated passage of No. 1 shuttle suture and braided nonabsorbable suture (anchor suture) to create the multipleat.

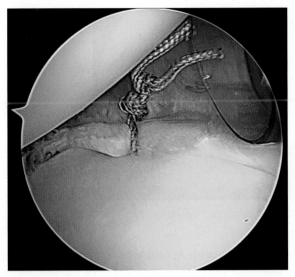

Figure 10-11. Completed Weston sliding locking knot backed with three half hitches after plication.

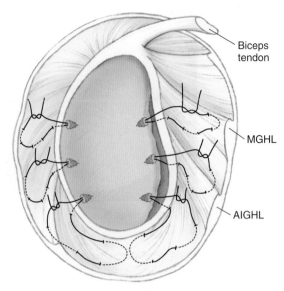

Figure 10-12. Drawing of a completed multipleated plication. *AIGHL,* Anterior inferior glenohumeral ligament; *MGHL,* middle glenohumeral ligament. *(Modified from Sekiya JK. Arthroscopic labral repair and capsular shift of the glenohumeral joint: technical pearls for a multiple pleated plication through a single working portal.* Arthroscopy. *2005;21:766.)*

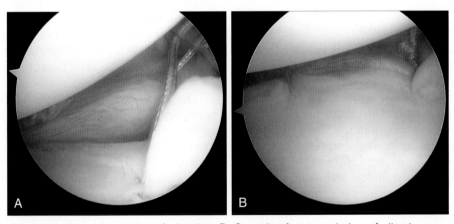

Figure 10-13. A, Capsule before completion of plication. **B,** Capsule after completion of plication.

make sure that it still slides. A locking sliding Weston knot backed with three half hitches is then tied and cut (Fig. 10-11). A cadaveric study found that a 1-cm capsular plication stitch results in approximately a 10% decrease in volume of the glenohumeral joint.[11]

Additional anchors should be placed superiorly (Fig. 10-12). For example, in working anteriorly, anchors may be placed at the 5-o'clock, 3-o'clock, and 1-o'clock positions. Placement will depend on direction and severity of instability. After the most symptomatic side has been addressed, work can begin on the opposite side. The capsule should be considered slightly overtightened at the completion of plication (Fig. 10-13).

This multipleated technique has several advantages. Labral tear repair and capsular plication are not linked in the same grasp of tissue. Multiple pleats evenly distribute the forces and decrease the risk of failure or anchor pullout. Only two portals are needed. The method is also easier to learn and perform than many traditional arthroscopic procedures.

3. Arthroscopic Knot Tying

Although we prefer the locking sliding Weston knot, a number of arthroscopic knot-tying techniques will work well. More important than the type of knot used is that the surgeon be skilled and highly familiar with the tying technique. First, the posterior anchor suture exiting the capsule is threaded through a knot pusher, and the end is secured with a hemostat. This suture serves as the post, which in effect will advance the capsule and

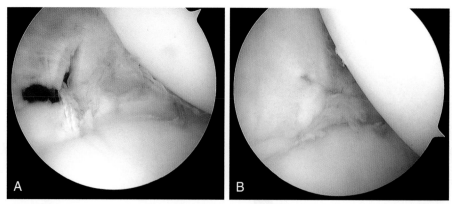

Figure 10-14. A, Posterior portal closure with the anchor method. **B,** Completed posterior portal closure.

labrum to the glenoid rim when tightened. The knot should be secured posteriorly on the capsule and not on the rim of the glenoid, to prevent humeral head abrasion. Each half hitch must be completely seated before the next half hitch is thrown. Placing tension on the nonpost suture and advancing the knot pusher "past point" will lock the Weston knot. In total, three alternating half hitches are placed to secure the Weston knot. This knot is biomechanically similar to an open square knot.[12]

4. Rotator Interval Closure

This procedure is rarely needed but is indicated when the patient has a positive sulcus sign in neutral rotation that does not decrease with 30 degrees of external rotation. Preprocedure diagnostic arthroscopy should be used to confirm this finding. If rotator interval closure is required, the camera is placed in the posterior portal, and the anterior portal serves as the working portal. A crescent suture passer is advanced through the anterior portal to the capsule at the middle glenohumeral ligament, just above the superior border of the subscapularis tendon 1 cm lateral to the glenoid. The suture passer then pierces the middle glenohumeral ligament at the inferior border of the rotator interval. If the middle glenohumeral ligament is deficient, the superior border of the subscapularis may be used, but this may significantly constrain external rotation and should be used with caution. A No. 0 shuttle suture is fed into the joint and then retrieved with a suture-grasping penetrator through the superior glenohumeral ligament. The shuttle suture is then withdrawn out the anterior cannula and switched for an anchor suture. The knot is tied blindly in the cannula as the closure is visualized through the posterior portal. In most cases no more than two sutures are needed to achieve closure of the interval.

5. Posterior Portal Closure

Two techniques are used for posterior portal closure. The more commonly used technique is begun by pulling the posterior cannula out of the glenohumeral joint but not out of the skin. A suture passer is passed through the posterior portal and used to pierce the inferior leaf of the capsule where the portal had previously made a defect. A No. 0 shuttle suture is then fed into the joint. A suture-grasping penetrator is then passed through the superior leaf of the capsule to grab the working end of the shuttle suture and pull it out through the cannula. The shuttle suture is then tied with a simple knot to a No. 2 anchor suture, and the shuttle suture is exchanged for the anchor suture. After exchange, the anchor suture will be coming out of the posterior cannula. It is tied blindly in the back of the capsule with a locking sliding knot backed with three half hitches and then cut. This process is repeated several times to completely close the posterior portal.

The alternative method, which offers increased stability, begins with placement of a 3-mm suture loaded anchor on the glenoid rim at the level of the portal. After anchor placement, the cannula is partially withdrawn, and the inferior anchor suture is passed through the labrum and inferior leaf of the capsule (Fig. 10-14A). A suture-grasping penetrator is passed through the superior leaf of the capsule, and the superior anchor suture is grasped and pulled out the cannula. The sutures are then tied on the back of the capsule with a locking sliding knot backed with three half hitches (Fig. 10-14B).

For completion of the procedure, the cannulas are removed and excess fluid is collected via suction. The two scope portals are then closed with a single subcutaneous stitch of 3-0 absorbable suture. The skin is then closed with two 3-0 Prolene interrupted sutures and covered with Steri-Strips. A cryotherapy sleeve is placed over the shoulder, and the arm is put into an UltraSling.

POSTOPERATIVE CARE

Follow-up

The patient is discharged on the day of surgery and begins an aggressive physical therapy protocol on postoperative day 1. A 1-week follow-up appointment is necessary for suture removal. Patients should be seen in the clinic at 1, 2, 3, and 6 months after surgery for examination and evaluation of progress.

Rehabilitation

Physical therapy should begin on postoperative day 1, with active and passive range of motion of the neck, elbow, wrist, and hand performed five times per day. Gentle passive pendulums should be used beginning on the first postoperative day. Passive and active-assisted range-of-motion exercises with limits can begin 1 month after surgery. Removal of the sling must wait until 6 weeks after surgery, and early removal can have debilitating effects on recovery. From 1 to 2 months, passive, active-assisted, and active range of motion can slowly increase to full motion. Range of motion should be normal by 2 to 3 months. From 3 to 5 months, rehabilitation should focus on restoring full strength. Overhead sports can begin at 5 months, but a full return to contact sports should wait until 6 months after surgery, provided the patient has full range of motion, no pain or tenderness, and satisfactory clinical examination findings.

An active relationship with the physical therapy team, close monitoring, and the setting of specific milestones are essential to a full recovery. Communication with the rehabilitation team also helps ensure that each patient's protocol can be individually modified to suit his or her current level of progress and needs.

Special attention must be paid to patients who were previously able to voluntarily dislocate without secondary gain. These individuals may be tempted to test the strength and integrity of the repair by trying to dislocate the shoulder. It is highly important for the physician to emphasize that multiple attempts to dislocate will stretch and erode the soft tissue repair. We recommend having the patient attempt to dislocate at 2 and 6 months under the supervision of a physician (the successful repair should make this impossible). This failure to dislocate should help individuals feel confident in the strength of the repair, so he or she will hopefully avoid future volitional instability attempts.

Complications

The risk of severe complications is quite low. Physical therapy may be unable to fully restore motion, so a manipulation under anesthesia would be required.

There is a small risk of permanent loss of motion. Instability may recur owing to surgical failure or failure to address the underlying causes of instability such as Hill-Sachs lesions or other bony defects.[13] Additional surgeries may be needed to correct these problems. Finally, there is a small risk of neurovascular injury.

Pearls and Pitfalls

- Patient history and physical examination including instability and sulcus sign tests are essential.
- Radiographic studies are needed to rule out bony defects, a contraindication to a purely arthroscopic technique.
- Patients with volitional instability with secondary gain are not good candidates for surgery.
- Participation in physical rehabilitation is a must before the patient progresses to surgery.
- Lateral decubitus position with axillary bump offers improved views and access to the glenohumeral joint.
- The surgical technique is multipleated plication.
- The aggressive rehabilitation protocol begins day 1 postoperatively.
- Full return to function and sports is achieved at around 6 months.
- Surgical failure is possible if underlying causes of instability are not found and addressed.
- Significant overplication will cause loss of motion.

RESULTS

Clinical Studies

The details of clinical studies of multidirectional shoulder instability repair are presented in Table 10-1.

In Vitro Capsular Volume Studies

Multiple studies have investigated the effect of surgical intervention on capsular volume. Comparisons have been made among open capsular shifts, arthroscopic thermal plication, and arthroscopic suture capsular plication by comparing capsular volume in cadaveric specimens before and after procedures. Table 10-2 summarizes the types of shifts performed in these studies and their results.

TABLE 10-1. Clinical Studies of Multidirectional Shoulder Instability Repair.

Author	Procedure Performed	Follow-up	Outcome
Duncan and Savoie[14] (1993)	Scope inferior capsular shift	1-3 yr	100% satisfactory
Pagnani et al[15] (1996)	Scope stabilization by transglenoid sutures	Average: 4.6 yr (range, 4-10 yr)	74% good-excellent
McIntyre et al[16] (1997)	Scope capsular shift	Average: 34 mo	95% good-excellent
Treacy et al[17] (1999)	Scope capsular shift	Average: 5 yr	88% satisfactory
Gartsman et al[18] (2000)	Scope labral repair and laser capsulorrhaphy	Average: 33 mo (range, 26-63 mo)	92% good-excellent
Tauro[19] (2000)	Scope inferior capsular split and advancement	2-5 yr	88% satisfactory
Fitzgerald et al[20] (2002)	Scope thermal capsulorrhaphy	Average: 3 yr (range, 24-40 mo)	76% satisfactory
Favorito et al[21] (2002)	Scope laser assisted capsular shift	Average: 28 mo	81.5% successful
Frostick et al[22] (2003)	Scope laser capsular shrinkage	Average: 26 mo (range, 24-33 mo)	83% satisfactory
D'Alessandro et al[23] (2004)	Scope thermal capsulorrhaphy	Average: 38 mo (range, 2-5 yr)	63% satisfactory
Hawkins et al[24] (2007)	Scope electrothermal capsulorrhaphy	Average: 4 yr (range, 2-6 yr)	41% very satisfied
Alpert et al[25] (2008)	Scope minimum 270-degree labral repair and anchor capsulorrhaphy	Average: 56 mo (range, 29-72 mo)	69% completely satisfied
Baker et al[6] (2009)	Scope capsular plication	Average: 33.5 mo (range, 24-65 mo)	ASES average: 91.37 (range, 59.86-100)

ASES, American Shoulder and Elbow Surgeons scale.

TABLE 10-2. In Vitro Capsular Volume Studies.

Author	Type of Capsular Shift	Amount of Volume Reduction
Miller et al[26] (2003)	Three open (medial, lateral, vertical)	Medial: 37% Lateral: 50% Vertical: 40%
Karas et al[27] (2004)	Three arthroscopic (thermal, suture plication, combined)	Scope thermal: 33% Scope plication: 19% Scope combined: 41%
Victoroff et al[28] (2004)	Arthroscopic thermal	Scope thermal: 37%
Luke et al[29] (2004)	Open inferior vs. arthroscopic thermal	Open inferior: 50% Scope thermal: 30%
Cohen et al[30] (2005)	Open lateral vs. arthroscopic plication	Open lateral: 50% Scope plication: 23%
Sekiya et al[7] (2007)	Open inferior vs. arthroscopic multipleated plication	Open inferior: 45% Scope multipleated: 58%
Ponce et al[11] (2011)	Suture-based simple plication stitches vs. suture anchor simple plication stitches	Suture only: 50.6% Suture anchor: 58.1%

REFERENCES

1. Neer 2nd CS, Foster CR. Inferior capsular shift for involuntary inferior and multidirectional instability of the shoulder. A preliminary report. *J Bone Joint Surg Am.* 1980;62:897-908.
2. Pagnani MJ, Warren RF. Stabilizers of the glenohumeral joint. *J Shoulder Elbow Surg.* 1994;3:173-190.
3. Rodeo SA, Suzuki K, Yamauchi M, et al. Analysis of collagen and elastic fibers in shoulder capsule in patients with shoulder instability. *Am J Sports Med.* 1998;26:634-643.
4. Bahu MJ, Trentacosta N, Vorys GC, et al. Multidirectional instability: evaluation and treatment options. *Clin Sports Med.* 2008;27:671-689.
5. DeBerardino TM, Arciero RA, Taylor DC. Arthroscopic stabilization of acute initial anterior shoulder dislocation: the West Point experience. *J South Orthop Assoc.* 1996;5:263-271.
6. Baker 3rd CL, Mascarenhas R, Kline AJ, et al. Arthroscopic treatment of multidirectional shoulder instability in athletes: a retrospective analysis of 2- to 5-year clinical outcomes. *Am J Sports Med.* 2009;37:1712-1720.
7. Sekiya JK, Willobee JA, Miller MD, et al. Arthroscopic multi-pleated capsular plication compared with open inferior capsular shift for reduction of shoulder volume in a cadaveric model. *Arthroscopy.* 2007;23:1145-1151.
8. Tzannes A, Murrell GA. Clinical examination of the unstable shoulder. *Sports Med.* 2002;32:447-457.
9. Sekiya JK. Arthroscopic labral repair and capsular shift of the glenohumeral joint: technical pearls for a multiple pleated plication through a single working portal. *Arthroscopy.* 2005;21:766.
10. Caprise Jr PA, Sekiya JK. Open and arthroscopic treatment of multidirectional instability of the shoulder. *Arthroscopy.* 2006;22:1126-1131.
11. Ponce BA, Rosenzweig SD, Thompson KJ, et al. Sequential volume reduction with capsular plications: relationship between cumulative size of plications and volumetric reduction for multidirectional instability of the shoulder. *Am J Sports Med.* 2011;39:526-531.
12. Elkousy HA, Sekiya JK, Stabile KJ, et al. A biomechanical comparison of arthroscopic sliding and sliding-locking knots. *Arthroscopy.* 2005;21:204-210.
13. Shah AS, Karadsheh MS, Sekiya JK. Failure of operative treatment for glenohumeral instability: etiology and management. *Arthroscopy.* 2011;27:681-694.
14. Duncan R, Savoie 3rd FH. Arthroscopic inferior capsular shift for multidirectional instability of the shoulder: a preliminary report. *Arthroscopy.* 1993;9:24-27.
15. Pagnani MJ, Warren RF, Altchek DW, et al. Arthroscopic shoulder stabilization using transglenoid sutures. A four-year minimum followup. *Am J Sports Med.* 1996;24:459-467.
16. McIntyre LF, Caspari RB, Savoie 3rd FH. The arthroscopic treatment of posterior shoulder instability: two-year results of a multiple suture technique. *Arthroscopy.* 1997;13:426-432.
17. Treacy SH, Savoie 3rd FH, Field LD. Arthroscopic treatment of multidirectional instability. *J Shoulder Elbow Surg.* 1999;8:345-350.
18. Gartsman GM, Roddey TS, Hammerman SM. Arthroscopic treatment of anterior-inferior glenohumeral instability. Two to five-year follow-up. *J Bone Joint Surg Am.* 2000;82:991-1003.
19. Tauro JC. Arthroscopic inferior capsular split and advancement for anterior and inferior shoulder instability: technique and results at 2- to 5-year follow-up. *Arthroscopy.* 2000;16:451-456.
20. Fitzgerald BT, Watson BT, Lapoint JM. The use of thermal capsulorrhaphy in the treatment of multidirectional instability. *J Shoulder Elbow Surg.* 2002;11:108-113.
21. Favorito PJ, Langenderfer MA, Colosimo AJ, et al. Arthroscopic laser-assisted capsular shift in the treatment of patients with multidirectional shoulder instability. *Am J Sports Med.* 2002;30:322-328.
22. Frostick SP, Sinopidis C, Al Maskari S, et al. Arthroscopic capsular shrinkage of the shoulder for the treatment of patients with multidirectional instability: Minimum 2-year follow-up. *Arthroscopy.* 2003;19:227-233.
23. D'Alessandro DF, Bradley JP, Fleischli JE, et al. Prospective evaluation of thermal capsulorrhaphy for shoulder instability: indications and results, two- to five-year follow-up. *Am J Sports Med.* 2004;32:21-33.
24. Hawkins RJ, Krishnan SG, Karas SG, et al. Electrothermal arthroscopic shoulder capsulorrhaphy: a minimum 2-year follow-up. *Am J Sports Med.* 2007;35:1484-1488.
25. Alpert JM, Verma N, Wysocki R, et al. Arthroscopic treatment of multidirectional shoulder instability with minimum 270 degrees labral repair: minimum 2-year follow-up. *Arthroscopy.* 2008;24:704-711.
26. Miller MD, Larsen KM, Luke T, et al. Anterior capsular shift volume reduction: an in vitro comparison of 3 techniques. *J Shoulder Elbow Surg.* 2003;12:350-354.
27. Karas SG, Creighton RA, DeMorat GJ. Glenohumeral volume reduction in arthroscopic shoulder reconstruction: a cadaveric analysis of suture plication and thermal capsulorrhaphy. *Arthroscopy.* 2004;20:179-184.
28. Victoroff BN, Deutsch A, Protomastro P, et al. The effect of radiofrequency thermal capsulorrhaphy on glenohumeral translation, rotation, and volume. *J Shoulder Elbow Surg.* 2004;13:138-145.
29. Luke TA, Rovner AD, Karas SG, et al. Volumetric change in the shoulder capsule after open inferior capsular shift versus arthroscopic thermal capsular shrinkage: a cadaveric model. *J Shoulder Elbow Surg.* 2004;13:146-149.
30. Cohen SB, Wiley W, Goradia VK, et al. Anterior capsulorrhaphy: an in vitro comparison of volume reduction–arthroscopic plication versus open capsular shift. *Arthroscopy.* 2005;21:659-664.

Chapter 11

Arthroscopic Treatment of the Disabled Throwing Shoulder

Matthew T. Boes, James A. Thiel, and Craig D. Morgan

Part 1 Arthroscopic Treatment of Internal Impingement

The term *internal impingement* was initially used by Walch[1] to describe contact of the undersurface of the rotator cuff with the posterior superior labrum in the abducted and externally rotated position. Jobe[2] described progressive internal impingement caused by repetitive stretching of anterior capsular structures as the primary cause of shoulder pain in overhead athletes. Our treatment of disability in the throwing shoulder is predicated on the inciting lesion being an acquired contracture of the posteroinferior capsule.[3] The posteroinferior capsular contracture alters the biomechanics of the joint and leads to a progressive pathologic cascade observed in the disabled throwing shoulder.

Because of repetitive overuse, throwers are susceptible to the development of posterior shoulder muscle fatigue and weakness, including fatigue and weakness of the scapular stabilizers and rotator cuff. Posterior muscle weakness leads to failure to counteract the deceleration force of the arm during the follow-through phase of throwing. In the healthy throwing shoulder, a glenohumeral distraction force of up to 1.5 times body weight is generated during the deceleration phase of the throwing motion. This distraction force is counteracted by violent contraction of the posterior shoulder musculature at ball release, which protects the glenohumeral joint from abnormal forces and prevents development of pathologic changes in response to these forces. In the presence of posterior muscle weakness, as seen initially in the disabled thrower, the distraction force becomes focused on the area of the posterior inferior glenohumeral ligament (PIGHL) complex because of the position of the arm in forward flexion and adduction during the follow-through phase of throwing. Fibroblastic thickening and contracture of the PIGHL zone occur as a response to this distraction stress (Fig. 11-1A and B). PIGHL contracture causes a shift of the glenohumeral contact point posteriorly and superiorly in the abducted and externally rotated position[4] (Fig. 11-1C). This shift allows clearance of the greater tuberosity over the posterosuperior glenoid rim, enabling hyperexternal rotation (unlike normal internal impingement). In addition, the posterosuperior shift causes a relaxation of the anterior capsular structures, which manifests as anterior pseudolaxity and allows even further hyperexternal rotation around the new glenohumeral rotation point (Fig. 11-1D).

High-level throwing athletes need to achieve extreme external rotation (ER) of the humerus in the late cocking phase to maximize the throwing arc to generate maximal velocity at ball release. This maneuver creates an abnormal and posteriorly directed force vector on the superior labrum through the long head of the biceps tendon as well as torsion at the biceps anchor. With repetitive stress in the hyperexternally rotated position, the labrum fails and "peels back" from the glenoid rim medially along the posterior superior scapular neck. Failure of rotator cuff fibers in this position can occur through abrasion but also, more important, from twisting and shear failure, which is most pronounced on the articular side of the cuff tendons. Tension failure may ultimately occur in the anterior capsule, causing anterior instability that in our view is a tertiary event and has been

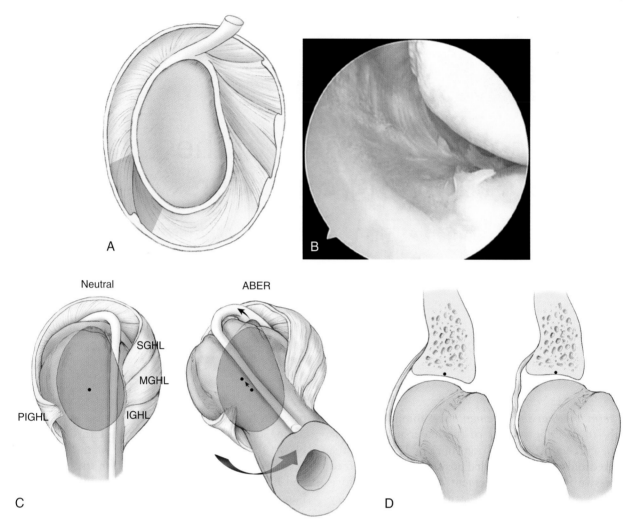

Figure 11-1. A, Diagram showing location of posterior inferior capsular contracture in the area of the posterior inferior glenohumeral ligament *(PIGHL)* complex. **B,** Arthroscopic image from the posterior portal with the camera directed inferior to view posterior inferior capsular contracture. **C,** Diagram showing biomechanical effect of posterior inferior capsular contracture. In the abduction and external rotation *(ABER)* position, the glenohumeral *(GH)* contact point is shifted posterosuperiorly, causing tension on the biceps anchor. **D,** Diagram showing relative anterior laxity as a result of the posterosuperior shift of the glenohumeral contact point. *IGHL,* Inferior glenohumeral ligament; *MGHL,* middle glenohumeral ligament; *SGHL,* superior glenohumeral ligament.

erroneously identified as the primary lesion in the disabled thrower.

The collection of symptoms observed in the disabled throwing shoulder has been termed the *dead arm syndrome*. Essentially, the athlete is unable to throw with premorbid velocity and control because of pain and subjective discomfort in the shoulder. Five pathologic components contribute to symptoms in the dead arm syndrome:

1. Posterior muscle weakness, demonstrated by scapular asymmetry

2. PIGHL contracture, the inciting lesion—manifests as a glenohumeral internal rotation deficit (GIRD) in the throwing shoulder versus the nonthrowing shoulder

3. Superior labral anterior-posterior (SLAP) tear, type II—typically the anterior and posterior or posterior subtype (the "thrower's SLAP")[5]

4. Rotator cuff failure—generally partial undersurface and occasionally full-thickness tearing in the posterosuperior cuff

5. Anterior instability (anterior capsular attenuation or capsulolabral injury)—in approximately 10% of cases

PREOPERATIVE CONSIDERATIONS

History

Typical History
- Vague "tightness" in the shoulder
- "Difficulty getting loose"
- Loss of throwing velocity over previous season
- Pain with throwing, particularly in late cocking phase, when the peel-back phenomenon occurs

Symptoms
- Pain, usually posterior superior; described as "deep" in the shoulder.
- Mechanical symptoms: painful clicking and popping. These occur after actual injury to the superior labrum or the "SLAP event."

Physical Examination

Inspection
- Both exposed shoulder girdles are inspected from behind.
- Note asymmetry in both shoulder height and scapular position.
- The superior and inferior medial scapular angles are marked as a visual reference.
- Dropped position of the acromion and elevation of the inferomedial angle of the scapula from the chest wall signify scapular protraction and antetilt and are evidence of scapular muscle weakness (Fig. 11-2).

Palpation
- Posterosuperior joint line—superior labral pathology.
- Coracoid—Protraction of the scapula forces the coracoid into a more lateral position and places tension on the pectoralis minor tendon, causing tenderness at its insertion.

- Superior scapular angle—Scapula infera places tension on the levator scapula muscle insertion, causing similar tenderness.

Range of Motion
- Measurements are made with the patient in the supine position with the scapula stabilized by anterior pressure on the shoulder against the examining table. A goniometer is used with carpenter's level bubble chamber attached.
- The arm is abducted 90 degrees to the body, scapular plane; internal rotation and ER are measured from a vertical reference point (perpendicular to floor) (Fig. 11-3).
- The throwing shoulder is compared with the non-throwing shoulder.
- Internal rotation, ER, total motion arc (TMA), and GIRD of the throwing shoulder versus the non-throwing shoulder are recorded.

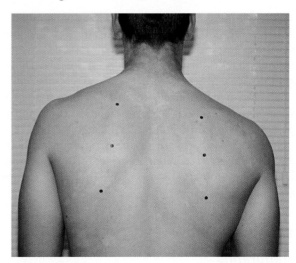

Figure 11-2. Right-hand dominant thrower with significant posterior scapular muscle weakness and resultant scapular asymmetry. Corresponding superior and inferior scapular angles and medial scapular border are marked for comparison.

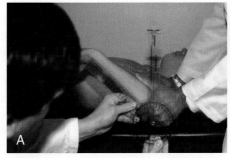 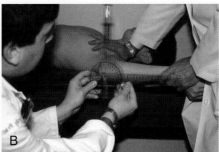

Figure 11-3. Measurement of glenohumeral rotation. The scapula is stabilized with posteriorly directed pressure by the examiner against the table to prevent scapulothoracic motion. True glenohumeral internal **(A)** and external **(B)** rotation is recorded from a vertical reference point.

- Specificity of clinical tests for type II SLAP tears in these athletes has been determined.[5]
  - Modified Jobe relocation test: specific for posterior SLAP lesions (the thrower's SLAP)
  - Speed test and O'Brien test: specific for anterior SLAP tears

The Jobe relocation test is performed by placing the arm in maximal abduction and ER. Throwers with a posterior SLAP tear will experience pain in this position as a result of the unstable biceps anchor falling into the peel-back position. The discomfort is relieved with a posteriorly directed force to the front of the shoulder, which has been shown under direct arthroscopic visualization to reduce the labrum into the normal position.[6]

Factors Affecting Surgical Planning

Patients with long-standing GIRD may require a selective posteroinferior quadrant capsulotomy. As outlined later, response to a period of focused internal rotation stretches determines the need for a posterior capsulotomy.

Extreme hyperexternal rotation (more than 130 degrees) is associated with attenuation of anterior capsuloligamentous structures. This finding occurs in approximately 10% of all disabled throwers. Patients with this amount of scapular stabilized ER require anterior capsular suture plication. We do not perform thermal capsulorrhaphy.

Imaging

Radiographs

- Anteroposterior, scapular lateral, and axillary views to reveal bone abnormalities (e.g., Bennett lesion)

Magnetic Resonance Arthrography

- The intra-articular administration of contrast material allows better resolution of labral pathology and partial-thickness tearing of the rotator cuff.
- Abduction-ER views are best for visualization of undersurface rotator cuff tears in throwers.

Indications and Contraindications

Arthroscopic evaluation and treatment are indicated for throwing athletes with a history of pain and mechanical symptoms as described earlier with pathologic findings on magnetic resonance arthrography. Once the pathologic cascade has progressed to actual injury to labral

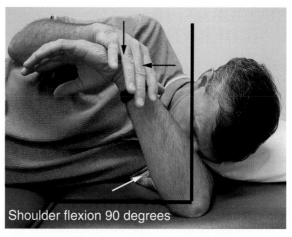

Shoulder flexion 90 degrees

Figure 11-4. Glenohumeral internal rotation or sleeper stretches. The patient lies on the involved side to minimize scapulothoracic motion. The opposite hand provides steady internal rotation pressure.

and cuff structures, the regaining of premorbid function is not possible without surgical repair of these structures.

Patients start internal rotation "sleeper stretches" preoperatively for assessment of the extent of PIGHL contracture (Fig. 11-4). In general, 90% of patients with severe GIRD (more than 25 degrees) are able to decrease their internal rotation deficit to less than 20 degrees with 10 to 14 days of focused stretching. The remaining 10% are stretch "nonresponders" and are generally older athletes with long-standing GIRD and substantial thickening of the posteroinferior capsule. In these patients a posteroinferior capsulotomy is indicated to increase internal rotation at the time of surgery.

Contraindications to the procedure are similar to those for other elective arthroscopic shoulder procedures, such as infection and concomitant medical illness.

Surgical Planning

Before the procedure is begun, it is important to have all anticipated instruments and materials needed for the surgery available and on the surgical field so that the procedure can be performed without unnecessary intraoperative delays (Table 11-1). Efficient performance of the procedure will avoid the dreaded scenario of attempting an arthroscopic repair in the distended, "watermelon" shoulder that can severely compromise the quality of the surgery. This cannot be overemphasized. As a general guideline, the type of repair described here should be accomplished in 20 to 40 minutes, depending on the associated pathologic processes. Superior labral tears in throwers may be associated with rotator cuff and anterior capsulolabral pathology. Treatment of these associated pathologic processes must be anticipated at the time of surgery.

TABLE 11-1. Recommended Instruments for Arthroscopic Treatment of Pathologic Processes in the Throwing Shoulder

Instrument	Use
Camera	
30-Degree lens	
Shoulder arthroscopy set (Arthrex)	
Arthroscopic rasp	Labral detachment
Arthroscopic elevator	
Arthroscopic cannulas	
8 mm	Anterior working portal
5 mm	Anterior accessory portal
Motorized shaver	Debridement
Full-radius blade (Stryker)	
Motorized bur	Preparation of glenoid rim
Protective hood; SLAP bur (Stryker)	
Arthroscopic bovie	Posterior capsulotomy
Long handle, hook tip (Linvatec)	
Bio-Suture Tak anchors (Arthrex)	Labral fixation
No. 1 PDS suture	SLAP fixation
	Free suture: capsular plication
SutureLasso passer device (Arthrex)	Suture passage: superior labrum
Right-angled	
Birdbeak suture retrievers (Arthrex)	Suture passage
45-Degree	Posterior superior labrum
22-Degree	Anterior superior labrum
Suture-passer set (e.g., Spectrum)	Suture passage
Straight	Longitudinal rotator cuff tear
45-Degree curved hook (left and right)	Capsular plication

PDS, polydioxanone; *SLAP,* superior labral anterior-posterior.

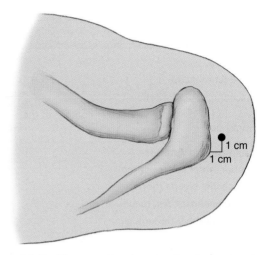

Figure 11-5. Diagram showing location for posterolateral portal or portal of Wilmington. A spinal needle is used for specific localization.

SURGICAL TECHNIQUE
Anesthesia and Positioning

Patients are administered general anesthesia after placement of an intrascalene nerve block, which greatly assists with postoperative pain control.

We perform all arthroscopic repairs with the patient in the lateral decubitus position. Positioning is controlled with a beanbag brought to the level of the axilla. The operative extremity is secured in 30 to 40 degrees of abduction by a pulley device with 10 pounds hung to counterweight the arm. The patient is administered antibiotic prophylaxis for skin flora, and the skin is painted with povidone-iodine (Betadine).

Surgical Landmarks, Incisions, and Portals

Repairs in throwing athletes are performed through the following portals:

- Posterior: viewing portal
- Anterior: main working portal; anchor placement in anterior labrum, knot tying
- Posterolateral (portal of Wilmington): anchor placement and suture passage in posterior labrum (Fig. 11-5)
- Anterosuperior: accessory portal; viewing and suture passage in anterior labrum or capsule (depending on associated pathologic changes)

The posterolateral border of the acromion is marked, and a posterior portal is established approximately 2 cm medial and 2 or 3 cm inferior to the corner of the acromion. The blunt camera trocar is directed through the posterior capsule just above the level of the equator of the humeral head. Both the anterior portal and the portal of Wilmington are established by an outside-in technique with an 18-gauge spinal needle.

BOX 11-1 Arthroscopic Findings Consistent with Labral Injury or an Unstable Biceps Anchor

Labral Injury

- Frayed labral edge
- Adjacent capsular irritation
- Disruption of the smooth articular contour of the glenoid rim

Unstable Biceps Anchor

- Superior labral sulcus >5 mm
- Displaceable biceps root
- Positive peel-back test result
- Presence of drive-through sign

BOX 11-2 Recommended Sequence for Arthroscopic Repairs in Throwing Shoulders with Multiple Pathologic Sites

1. Anterior inferior capsulolabral disruption (if present)
2. Posterior portion SLAP tear
3. Anterior portion SLAP tear
4. Anterior inferior capsular attenuation (if present)
5. PIGHL contracture (if present)
6. Rotator cuff tear (if present)

PIGHL, Posterior inferior glenohumeral ligament; *SLAP,* superior labral anterior-posterior.

BOX 11-3 Surgical Steps

1. Placement of secondary portals
2. Probing of intra-articular structures
3. Intra-articular debridement
4. Preparation of superior labral bone bed
5. Anchor placement, suture passage, and knot tying
6. Dynamic assessment of repair
7. Treatment of associated pathology

Examination

Diagnostic Arthroscopy and Surgical Techniques

Routine diagnostic arthroscopy is performed to ensure that all portions of the joint are inspected and no pathologic lesion is overlooked. In the disabled throwing shoulder, areas requiring particular attention include the following:

- Superior labrum and biceps anchor
- Rotator cuff insertion
- Anterior labrum and capsuloligamentous structures
- Posterior capsule

Evidence of labral injury must be assessed carefully, as findings may be subtle (Box 11-1). An assessment is quickly made of the pathologic areas to be addressed, and a plan is made for the completion of the repair (Box 11-2).

Provocative Tests

Drive-Through Sign

Before other cannulas or instruments are introduced, an assessment is made of laxity in the joint by testing for the drive-through sign. In a normal shoulder, capsular restraints prevent passage of the arthroscope from posterior to anterior at the midlevel of the humeral head or sweeping of the scope from superior to inferior along the anterior glenoid rim. The drive-through sign may be present in patients with a SLAP tear because of pseudolaxity from the loss of labral continuity around the glenoid rim.[7]

Peel-Back Test

The peel-back test is performed by removing the arm from traction and placing it into the abducted and externally rotated position. With a posterior SLAP lesion, the labrum can be observed to fall medially along the glenoid neck during this maneuver (Fig. 11-6). Anterior SLAP lesions will have a negative result for the peel-back test. After assessment of the biceps anchor, the probe is used to assess the undersurface of the rotator cuff and to estimate depth of partial-thickness tears, to determine the stability of the anterior inferior labrum, and to identify any redundancy in the anterior capsule.[8]

Specific Steps

Specific steps are outlined in Box 11-3.

1. Placement of Secondary Portals

An 8-mm cannula is used as a primary anterior working portal. An 18-gauge spinal needle is used to localize the cannula so that it can accommodate all necessary repairs, including anterosuperior anchor placement in the labrum and tying of posterosuperior anchor sutures. The cannula is readied near the skin surface, the spinal needle is used as a guide to the proper insertion angle, the spinal needle is withdrawn, and the cannula is inserted. An accessory 5-mm anterior portal may be placed, depending on the location of associated pathologic lesions requiring treatment.

2. Probing of Intra-articular Structures

A probe is introduced in the anterior cannula for more careful assessment of stability of intra-articular structures. Normally, a sublabral sulcus with healthy-appearing articular cartilage can be seen extending up

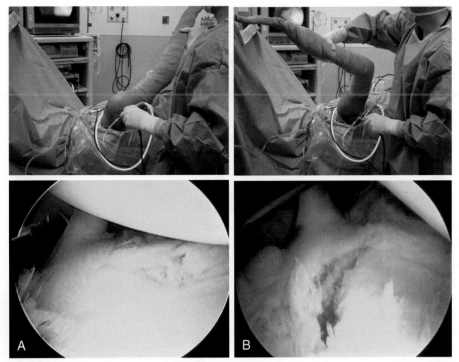

Figure 11-6. Images and corresponding arthroscopic views during dynamic peel-back test. **A,** The superior labrum is reduced in neutral position. **B,** When the shoulder is placed in abduction-external rotation, superior labral instability is revealed, with the labrum falling posteriorly and medially along the scapular neck.

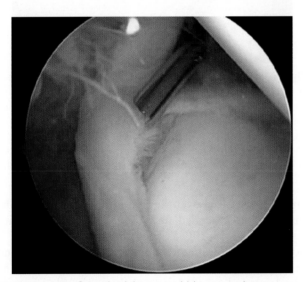

Figure 11-7. Superior labrum and biceps anchor are gently probed to identify evidence of injury or instability.

to 5 mm beneath the labrum. An unstable biceps root can easily be displaced with the probe medially along the glenoid neck[8] (Fig. 11-7; see also Box 11-1).

3. Intra-articular Debridement

A full-radius blade motorized shaver is used to gently debride loose and frayed tissue to prevent snagging of tissue with joint motion or potential loose bodies.

4. Preparation of Superior Labral Bone Bed

An arthroscopic rasp is used to completely separate any remaining attachments in the injury area. A rasp is used because there is less risk of causing intrasubstance injury in the labrum than with an elevator. On occasion, some tenuous attachments from the labrum may be present medially, but the biceps anchor is still unstable. In these cases we routinely complete the lesion by removing these loose attachments before repair. All loose soft tissue is removed from the repair site carefully with the shaver.

An arthroscopic bur is then used to remove cartilage along the superior glenoid rim to make a bleeding bone bed for labral repair (Fig. 11-8). This step is crucial to allow subsequent healing of the labrum back to the glenoid rim. We prefer a bur with a protective hood that is specifically designed to prevent damage to labral tissue during this step (SLAP bur, Stryker Endoscopy, San Jose, CA). No suction is used while the bur is on to ensure that tissue is not inadvertently sucked into the instrument.

5. Anchor Placement, Suture Passage, and Knot Tying

The portal of Wilmington is used for posterior anchor placement. Only small-diameter instruments are passed through this portal. No cannulas are placed in this portal to prevent damage to the rotator cuff tendons. A

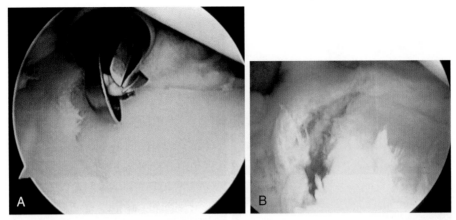

Figure 11-8. An arthroscopic bur with protective hood to prevent inadvertent damage to the labrum is used to remove a small amount of cortical bone on the superior glenoid to make a bleeding bone bed for subsequent repair.

spinal needle again is used to localize the portal, which is approximately 1 cm anterior and 1 cm lateral to the posterolateral acromial margin (see Fig. 11-5). The angle of approach for the portal must provide for orientation of the anchor insertion device at 45 degrees to the glenoid rim to ensure solid anchor placement. We prefer to use a biodegradable, tap-in type anchor for superior labral repair (Bio-Suture Tak, Arthrex, Naples, FL).

After skin incision, the Spear guide (3.5 mm; Arthrex) is brought into the joint through the portal of Wilmington as described previously for anterior cannula placement. The guide enters medial to the musculotendinous junction of the infraspinatus with minimal damage given its small diameter. The number of anchors to be placed is somewhat subjective but must be sufficient to neutralize peel-back forces.[8] The Spear guide is brought immediately onto the glenoid rim in the area of the previously prepared bone bed. The sharp obturator is removed after proper localization, and a hole is drilled for anchor insertion. The angle of approach of the Spear guide must be meticulously maintained during drilling and subsequent anchor placement to ensure adequate fixation in the bone. We insert anchors until the hilt of the anchor insertion handle abuts the handle of the Spear guide. Gentle twisting in line with the anchor is often needed to remove the insertion handle in dense bone (Fig. 11-9). The Spear guide is removed, and both ends of the suture are brought through the anterior cannula with a looped grasper instrument.

For passage of a suture limb through the labrum, we use a small-diameter, pointed suture-passing device with a wire loop (SutureLasso suture passer, Arthrex). The passing device is brought through the portal of Wilmington without a cannula (again to minimize cuff damage) and into the joint through the muscle rent made by the Spear guide (Fig. 11-10A and B). The passer is brought through the labrum from superior to inferior, achieving a solid bite of labral tissue, and

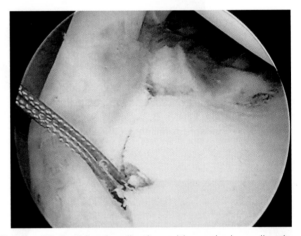

Figure 11-9. After localization with a spinal needle, the Spear guide is introduced into the shoulder through the portal of Wilmington for anchor placement on the posterior superior glenoid rim. The Spear guide is introduced into the joint medial to the rotator cable and in the muscular portion of the cuff. Because of its relatively small diameter (3.5 mm), this causes minimal damage to the rotator cuff.

carefully advanced over the rim to the glenoid face. The wire loop is extended and brought out the anterior cannula (Fig. 11-10C). Next, the suture limb that is closest to the labrum at the anchor site is identified and passed through the wire loop outside the cannula. The wire loop and suture lasso are then carefully removed from the portal of Wilmington, and one of the suture limbs is brought through the labrum and out the portal (Fig. 11-11A). The suture limbs around the anchor are carefully observed as the suture is passed to ensure that no tangling has occurred. Next, the suture that has been passed through the labrum and is now out the portal of Wilmington is brought out the anterior cannula and becomes the post limb of the arthroscopic knot (Fig. 11-11B). Posterior anchors are tied through the anterior portal either medial or lateral to the biceps tendon. Additional suture anchors are placed posterior or

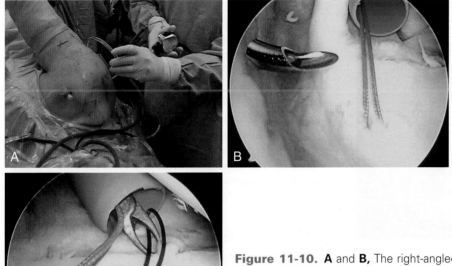

Figure 11-10. A and **B,** The right-angled suture-passing device, which is also small diameter, is brought along the same trajectory and through the same muscle rent made by the Spear guide. **C,** The superior margin to the labrum is pierced with the device, a firm bite of labral tissue is captured, and the pointed device is gently advanced onto the glenoid face. The wire loop is deployed and retrieved from the anterior cannula for passage of the labral post suture.

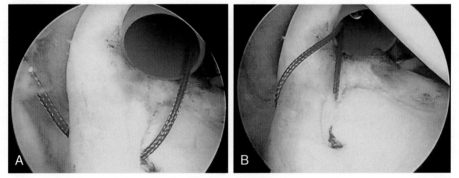

Figure 11-11. A, The wire loop is carefully retracted to pass a suture limb through the labrum and out the portal of Wilmington. **B,** A looped suture grasper is then used to retrieve this suture limb out the anterior cannula, where it becomes the post limb for the arthroscopic knot. To prevent "snagging" or capturing of the biceps tendon with suture, all passage, retrieval, and tying of sutures are performed on one side of the biceps or the other.

anterior to the biceps anchor until it is secure. Posterior anchors are most easily placed through the portal of Wilmington as described before. Anterior anchors may be placed through the anterior cannula. Although we prefer the lasso suture passer for passing sutures, Bird-beak suture retrievers (Arthrex) may alternatively be used, depending on the surgeon's preference. The 45-degree Birdbeak is ideal for passing sutures in the posterior labrum through the anterior superior cannula; the 22-degree Birdbeak works well for the anterior labrum.

6. Dynamic Assessment of Repair

After labral repair, the peel-back and drive-through signs are again assessed to confirm that they are negative and that the pathologic process has been corrected. The

peel-back maneuver can be performed for dynamic assessment of whether forces at the biceps anchor have been neutralized (Fig. 11-12). The drive-through sign is performed to assess for additional anterior laxity that may require correction by capsular plication techniques.

7. Treatment of Associated Pathology

We generally perform a miniplication in the anterior capsule when there is a persistent drive-through sign, evidence of anterior capsular tissue attenuation, or more than 130 degrees of ER in the 90-degree abducted position. The anterior capsular tissue to be plicated is first abraded with a rasp or "whisker" shaver. Capsular redundancy is then obliterated by suturing a lateral portion of the capsule to the glenoid labrum. The

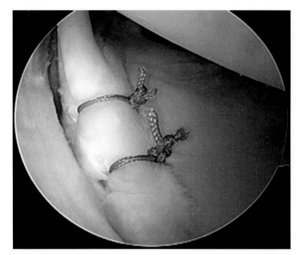

Figure 11-12. After anchor placement and knot tying, the dynamic peel-back maneuver is performed again to confirm stable fixation of the biceps anchor.

amount of tissue plicated depends on the amount of redundancy observed on arthroscopic examination (Fig. 11-13). Rarely, a discrete capsulolabral avulsion in the anteroinferior glenoid needs to be repaired as described elsewhere in this text.

A posteroinferior capsulotomy is performed in patients who are selective stretch nonresponders. The response to stretching is assessed preoperatively as outlined earlier. A posterior capsular release is rarely required as part of the treatment of the disabled throwing shoulder. However, for restoration of full motion, the procedure is indicated for patients who display little or no response to stretching. Arthroscopic findings consistent with a pathologic posteroinferior capsular contracture include inferior recess restriction and a thickened PIGHL complex, which can be up to ½ inch thick in some cases (Fig. 11-14). Biopsy of the capsule in these cases reveals hypocellular and disorganized fibrous scar tissue similar in appearance to end-stage adhesive capsulitis.

Posteroinferior capsular release may be performed by one of two methods:

1. Scope in the anterior portal and instrumentation in the standard posterior portal
2. Scope in the standard posterior portal and instrumentation in the posterosuperior portal (portal of Wilmington)

We prefer method 2 because it allows better direct visualization of the capsule during release.

The procedure is performed with electrocautery in a nonparalyzed patient. During the capsulotomy, any twitching of the shoulder musculature will alert the surgeon that the procedure is being performed too close to the axillary nerve, thus placing the nerve at risk for injury. If this occurs, the capsulotomy should be moved to a more superior or medial portion of the capsule or abandoned altogether if no safe zone can be found. A hooked-tip arthroscopic bovie (meniscal bovie; Linvatec, Largo, FL) with a long shaft is used. The capsulotomy is full thickness and is made ¼ inch peripheral to the labrum in the posterior inferior quadrant (6-o'clock to 3- or 9-o'clock position). A sweeping technique is used to gently section progressively deeper layers of the capsule under direct visualization (Fig. 11-15). The capsulotomy typically results in a 50- to 60-degree increase in internal rotation immediately (Fig. 11-16).

POSTOPERATIVE CONSIDERATIONS

Follow-up

All procedures are performed on an outpatient basis. Patients are typically seen 1 day after surgery for dressing change. At 1 week, sutures are removed, and self-directed range of motion is begun under specific guidelines. Patients are seen at regular intervals during the rehabilitation phase to monitor progress with motion and to advance therapy as appropriate.

Rehabilitation

- *Immediate:* Passive ER with arm at the side (not in abduction); flexion and extension of the elbow. Patients undergoing posterior inferior capsulotomy begin internal rotation sleeper stretches on postoperative day 1.
- *Weeks 1 to 3:* Pendulum exercises. Passive range of motion is begun with a pulley device in forward flexion and abduction to 90 degrees. Shoulder shrugs and scapular retraction exercises are begun in the sling. The sling is worn when the arm is not out for exercises.
- *Weeks 3 to 6:* The sling is discontinued after 3 weeks. Passive range of motion is advanced to full motion in all planes. Sleeper stretches are started in patients not undergoing capsulotomy.
- *Weeks 6 to 16:* Stretching and flexibility exercises are continued. Passive ER stretching in abduction is begun. Strengthening for rotator cuff, scapular stabilizers, and deltoid is initiated at 6 weeks. Biceps strengthening is begun at 8 weeks. Daily sleeper stretches are continued indefinitely.
- *At 4 months:* Interval throwing program is started on level surface. Stretching and strengthening are continued with emphasis on posterior inferior capsular stretching.
- *At 6 months:* Pitchers start throwing at full speed, depending on progression in interval throwing

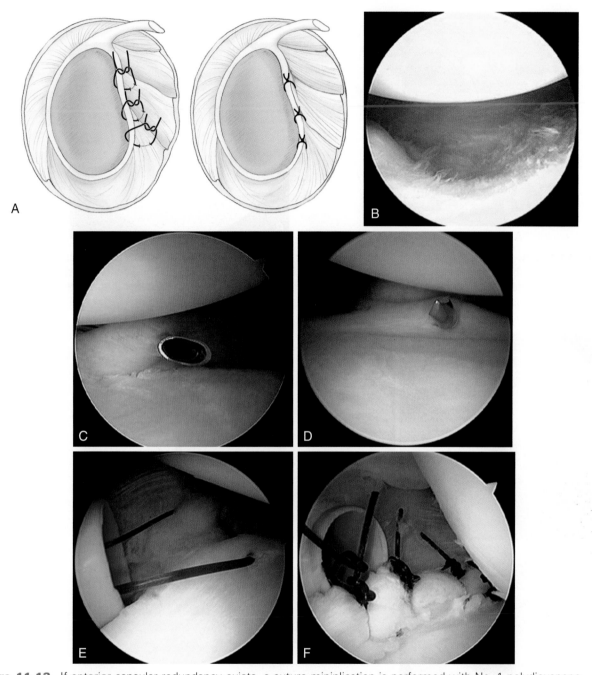

Figure 11-13. If anterior capsular redundancy exists, a suture miniplication is performed with No. 1 polydioxanone suture. **A,** Diagram of miniplication technique. **B,** The tissue is gently abraded to promote healing. **C,** Starting inferiorly, a lateral bite of capsular tissue is captured with the suture device. **D,** The capsular tissue is advanced medially up onto the glenoid rim and secured to the anterior labrum. **E,** Once the suture has been passed, the amount of capsular redundancy is assessed before knot tying, and adjustments are made as needed. **F,** Subsequent sutures are placed, advancing superiorly along the anterior labrum until the anterior capsular redundancy has been obliterated.

program. Daily sleeper stretches are continued indefinitely.

- *At 7 months:* Pitchers are allowed full-velocity throwing from the mound. Daily sleeper stretches are continued indefinitely.

Complications

Complications are similar to those of other procedures involving arthroscopic shoulder reconstruction, including a rare incidence of infection, failed repair, painful adhesion formation, and stiffness. Physicians

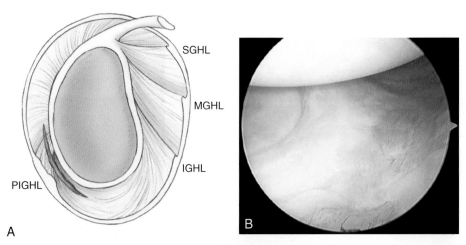

Figure 11-14. A, Diagram showing location of the posterior inferior capsulotomy. **B,** Arthroscopic photograph from the posterior portal with the camera directed inferiorly shows thickening around the PIGHL and inferior recess restriction. *IGHL,* Inferior glenohumeral ligament; *MGHL,* middle glenohumeral ligament; *PIGHL,* posterior inferior glenohumeral ligament; *SGHL,* superior glenohumeral ligament.

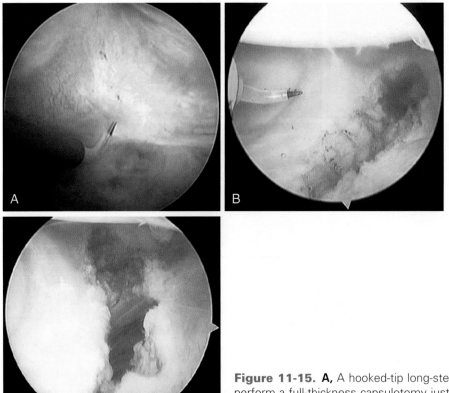

Figure 11-15. A, A hooked-tip long-stem arthroscopic bovie is used to perform a full-thickness capsulotomy just adjacent to the posterior inferior labrum. **B,** Gentle sweeping motions divide the capsule under direct vision. **C,** Completed posterior inferior capsulotomy.

and therapists working with throwing athletes must be vigilant for the development of postoperative shoulder stiffness through regular follow-up and a directed therapy program. All athletes are instructed to continue daily internal rotation stretches indefinitely to prevent recurrence of the pathologic cascade that will place stress on the repair.

RESULTS

In 182 baseball pitchers (one third professional, one third college, one third high school) treated during an 8-year period, 92% resumed pitching at the preinjury performance level or better. University of California at Los Angeles shoulder rating scale (UCLA) scoring

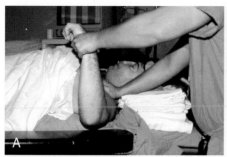
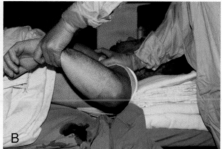

Figure 11-16. A, Preoperative internal rotation. **B,** Internal rotation immediately after posterior inferior capsulotomy. A gain of 50 to 60 degrees of internal rotation can be expected immediately intraoperatively.

TABLE 11-2. GIRD Reduction SLAP Repair with Posteroinferior Capsular Stretching*

	Preoperative	1 Year	2 Years
GIRD (average degrees)	46	13	15
TMA (throwing shoulder)	120	148	146
TMA (nonthrowing shoulder)	158	160	159

*In 164 baseball pitchers.
GIRD, Glenohumeral internal rotation deficit; SLAP, superior labral anterior-posterior; TMA, total motion arc.

TABLE 11-3. GIRD Reduction of SLAP Repair with Posteroinferior Capsulotomy*

	Preoperative	1 Year	2 Years
GIRD (average degrees)	42	12	12
TMA (throwing shoulder)	114	147	147
TMA (nonthrowing shoulder)	158	160	157

*In 18 baseball pitchers.
GIRD, Glenohumeral internal rotation deficit; SLAP, superior labral anterior-posterior; TMA, total motion arc.

TABLE 11-4. UCLA Scores for Results of SLAP Repair with Capsular Stretching or Capsulotomy*

	1 Year (n = 182)	2 Years (n = 124)	3 Years (n = 86)
Excellent	92%	90%	87%
Good	8%	10%	13%
Fair	0%	0%	0%
Poor	0%	0%	0%

*In 182 baseball pitchers.
SLAP, Superior labral anterior-posterior; UCLA, University of California at Los Angeles shoulder rating scale.

averaged 92% excellent results at 1 year and 87% excellent results at 3 years. Pitchers undergoing posteroinferior capsulotomy had an average GIRD reduction of 31 degrees at 6 months and 30 degrees at 2 years and an average increase in fastball velocity of 11 mph at 1 year after the procedure. Results of GIRD reduction for patients treated with SLAP repair with capsular stretching and SLAP repair with capsulotomy are shown with combined UCLA scores in Tables 11-2 to 11-4.

Part 2 Throwing Acquired Superior Glenohumeral Ligament Injury with Biceps Pulley Disruption and Biceps Outlet Instability

The anatomy and function of the soft tissue biceps pulley and outlet are important parts of the anterior rotator interval of the shoulder and have been reported previously.[9-11] The medial wall is a reflection of the superior glenohumeral ligament (SGHL) portion of the anterior superior capsule, the lateral wall is the anterior margin of the supraspinatus tendon, and the roof is the coracohumeral ligament (CHL) (Fig. 11-17).[10,11] The soft tissue pulley functions as a sling to contain and stabilize the distal portion of the intra-articular long head of the biceps tendon through shoulder range of motion.[10,11] The intra-articular long head of the biceps tendon may become symptomatic and unstable owing to trauma either proximally, at its supraglenoid tubercle

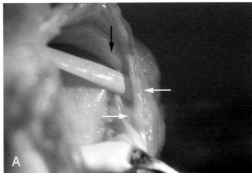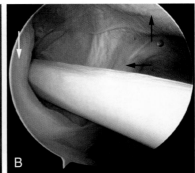

Biceps soft tissue pulley/outlet – left shoulder
Anterior wall = SGHL
Posterior wall = SS tendon
Roof = CHL

Normal biceps pulley/outlet –
arthroscopic view left shoulder
Medial wall = SGHL
Lateral wall = Supraspinatous tendon
Roof = Coracohumeral ligament

Figure 11-17. A, Biceps soft tissue pulley and outlet, left shoulder. Medial wall = superior glenohumeral ligament (SGHL; *blue arrow*); lateral wall = supraspinatus tendon *(yellow arrow)*; roof = coracohumeral ligament *(green arrow)*. **B,** Normal biceps pulley and outlet, left shoulder, arthroscopic view. Medial wall = SGHL *(blue arrow)*; lateral wall = supraspinatus tendon *(yellow arrow)*; roof = coracohumeral ligament *(green arrow)*.

attachment as a SLAP lesion, or distally at the biceps intra-articular outlet secondary to pulley injury.[12-17] In 1994, Walch described rotator interval pathology associated with supraspinatus rotator cuff tears as "hidden" lesions of the rotator interval.[18] Subsequently others have reported traumatic tears of the biceps pulley portion of the rotator interval associated with rotator cuff pathology.[8,12-14,17] In 2004, Habermeyer reported arthroscopic findings of biceps pulley injury associated with rotator cuff tears in a clinical series.[13] In a preliminary report in 2000, Gerber and Sebesta proposed a forward flexion, adduction, internal rotation mechanism of injury creating injury to the SGHL portion of the pulley and the upper subscapularis portion of the rotator cuff owing to what they termed "anterosuperior impingement" of these soft tissue structures on the anterosuperior glenoid margin in this position.[9]

Forceful repetitive forward flexion, adduction, and internal rotation of the shoulder occur during the follow-through phase of the throwing cycle in overhead and throwing athletes.[18] Throwing athletes with throwing-acquired anterosuperior shoulder pain often demonstrate injury to the SGHL portion of their biceps pulley and outlet, as described by Gerber and Sebesta.[9] This is especially seen in throwers with mechanical flaws who "throw across the body" with the arm more horizontal to the ground. This forward-flexed and adducted position leads to anterosuperior glenohumeral internal impingement, SGHL injury with widening of the biceps pulley, and biceps outlet instability, resulting in anterosuperior shoulder pain and pain in the upper bicipital groove (Figs. 11-18 and 11-19). Biceps pulley lesions can also be caused by trauma or degenerative change.[13,14] Le Huec described the mechanism of a fall on the outstretched arm in combination with full external or

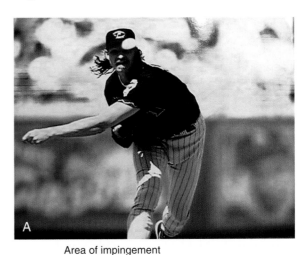

Area of impingement

Figure 11-18. In throwers who "throw across the body," superior glenohumeral ligament (SGHL) injury is caused by SGHL anterosuperior glenoid impingement during the follow-through phase of the throwing cycle. This is especially prevalent if the athlete has the mechanical flaw of following through with the shoulder forward flexed and more horizontal to the ground during follow-through.

internal rotation or a fall backward on the hand or elbow leading to a biceps pulley lesion.[14]

This section reviews physical examination findings, imaging characteristics, and arthroscopic findings in patients with SGHL injury, biceps pulley disruption, and biceps outlet instability. Specific arthroscopic steps to close the anterior rotator interval and restore the biceps outlet to a normal size are presented.

PREOPERATIVE CONSIDERATIONS

History

Typical History

- Decreased throwing velocity and performance

Symptoms

- Isolated anterior superior shoulder pain with throwing and overhead activities

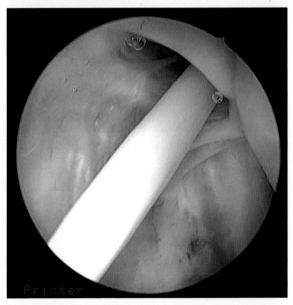

Figure 11-19. Widening of biceps pulley and outlet.

Physical Examination

Inspection

- Inspect bilateral shoulders and scapulae as described in Part 1.

Palpation

- Reproducible anterior superior shoulder pain in abduction and ER reduced by Jobe relocation maneuver
- Digital pain over the anterior rotator interval and upper bicipital groove
- Increased asymmetrical sulcus sign on the symptomatic versus the asymptomatic shoulder in neutral and maximal ER of the shoulder (Fig. 11-20)

Range of Motion

- Increased scapular stabilized glenohumeral ER and TMA of the symptomatic versus the asymptomatic shoulder by more than 10 degrees (Fig. 11-21)

Factors Affecting Surgical Planning

- Perform all concomitant procedures (e.g., SLAP repair, anterior or posterior Bankart repair, capsular plication) before anterior rotator interval closure.

Imaging

Radiography

- Anteroposterior, scapular lateral, and axillary views to reveal bone abnormalities

Magnetic Resonance Imaging Arthrography

For quantification of the rotator interval size in the area of the biceps soft tissue pulley and outlet, the sagittal rotator interval angle (SRIA) is measured on sagittal oblique images through the center of the biceps pulley. This is measured goniometrically between a line drawn from the anterior margin of the supraspinatus tendon

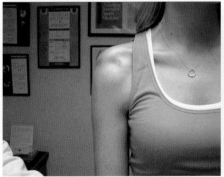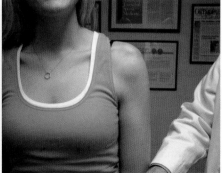

Figure 11-20. Positive asymmetrical sulcus sign in right shoulder. Sulcus sign is present in both shoulders but increased in symptomatic shoulder.

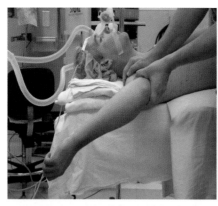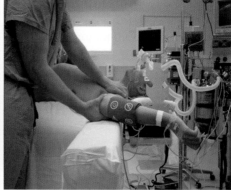

Figure 11-21. Increased passive external rotation in symptomatic shoulder with scapula stabilized.

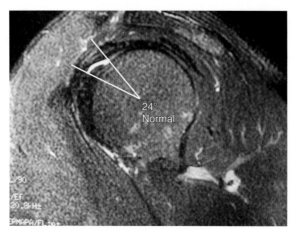

Sagittal oblique arthrogram MRI
Normal biceps pulley/outlet
Normal sagittal rotator interval angle

Figure 11-22. Sagittal oblique magnetic resonance arthrogram. Normal biceps pulley and outlet. Normal sagittal rotator interval angle.

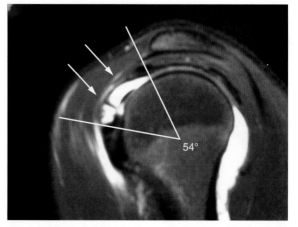

Figure 11-23. Sagittal oblique magnetic resonance arthrogram of a superior glenohumeral ligament–injured biceps outlet and pulley. Sagittal rotator interval angle is 54 degrees.

to a point central in the humeral head and a line drawn from the superior margin of the subscapularis tendon to the same central humeral head point (Fig. 11-22). In an ongoing prospective study correlating magnetic resonance imaging (MRI) findings with arthroscopic findings, we have found that an SRIA of 22 to 30 degrees is normal. An SRIA greater than 50 degrees has been found to correlate with arthroscopic findings of an anterior rotator interval lesion (Fig. 11-23).

On the same sagittal oblique image used to measure the SRIA, the location of the biceps tendon in the pulley portion of the rotator interval is noted to be central (normal) or subluxed inferomedially in a widened pulley (SGHL injured). We have termed this subluxation the biceps "drop-out sign." In addition, injury to the SGHL is noted on these images. Commonly the SGHL demonstrates a substance tear of the medial wall portion of the biceps pulley that we call the "chandelier sign" (Fig. 11-24).

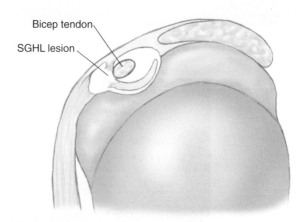

Bicep tendon

SGHL lesion

Figure 11-24. Line drawing illustrating a superior glenohumeral ligament (SGHL)–injured biceps pulley with a widened biceps outlet and pulley, biceps drop-out sign, and SGHL chandelier sign.

Indications and Contraindications

Arthroscopic evaluation and treatment are indicated for throwing and overhead athletes with a history of pain and symptoms as described earlier with MRI findings of SRIA greater than 50 degrees.

Contraindications to the procedure are similar to those for other elective arthroscopic shoulder procedures, such as infection and concomitant medical illness.

SURGICAL TECHNIQUE

Anesthesia and Positioning

Anesthesia and positioning information is given in Part 1.

Surgical Landmarks, Incisions, and Portals

Anterior rotator interval closure is performed through two portals:

- Posterior: viewing portal
- Anterior: main working portal; suture passage through middle glenohumeral ligament (MGHL) and SGHL, knot tying

Examination

Arthroscopic Findings

- Focal hyperemic synovitis on the dorsal aspect of the biceps tendon as it exits the biceps pulley and outlet (Fig. 11-25)
- Focal hyperemic synovitis of the upper MGHL and SGHL capsule (Fig. 11-26)
- Markedly widened biceps outlet and pulley (Fig. 11-27)
- Biceps drop-out sign (biceps located inferomedial from its normal central location within a widened pulley) (Fig. 11-27)
- A visible tear of the SGHL portion on the pulley (Figs. 11-27 and 11-28)
- MGHL laxity to probing
- Biceps outlet instability with moving the shoulder from neutral to abduction ER (Fig. 11-29)

Specific Steps

1. Performance of all associated procedures first as described in Part 1 of this chapter and elsewhere in this text.
2. Placement of posterior viewing portal and arthroscopic examination are performed. Arthroscopic findings as described previously (Fig. 11-30).

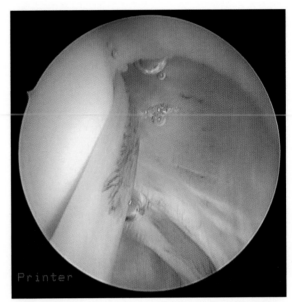

Figure 11-25. Superior glenohumeral ligament–injured left shoulder. Arthroscopic findings: focal dorsal biceps hyperemic synovitis.

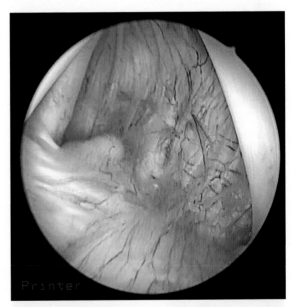

Figure 11-26. Left shoulder. Focal hyperemic synovitis over middle glenohumeral ligament and superior glenohumeral ligament.

3. Placement of anterior working portal with an 18-gauge spinal needle to localize the cannula so that all intra-articular structures can be probed and sutures placed through the MGHL and SGHL. An 8-mm plastic cannula is used in the anterior portal. Diagnosis of SGHL injury with biceps pulley disruption and biceps outlet instability confirmed as described earlier and demonstrated in Figures 11-25 to 11-29.
4. With a crescent SutureLasso, a No. 1 polydioxanone (PDS) suture is placed through the upper MGHL just

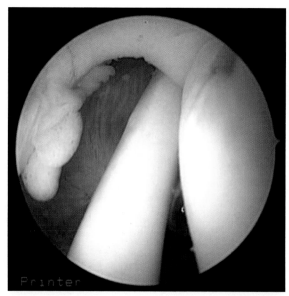

Figure 11-27. Right shoulder. Biceps drop-out in widened outlet and pulley. Obvious superior glenohumeral ligament (SGHL) tear with SGHL visible stump.

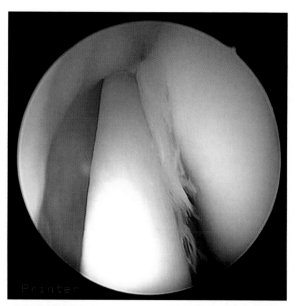

Figure 11-29. Right shoulder. Biceps dynamic relocation in abduction and external rotation shoulder position. Same shoulder as in Figure 11-25.

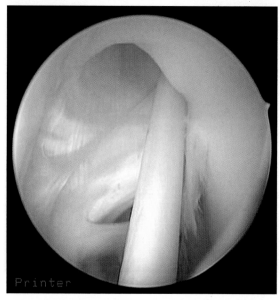

Figure 11-28. Right shoulder. Biceps inferomedial subluxation in neutral shoulder position. Obvious superior glenohumeral ligament (SGHL) tear.

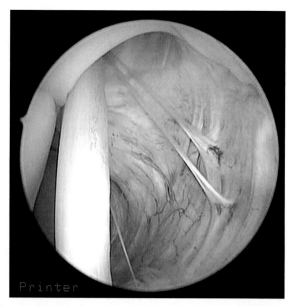

Figure 11-30. Superior glenohumeral ligament (SGHL)–injured, widened biceps pulley. Right shoulder prerepair.

lateral to the labrum (Fig. 11-31). The crescent SutureLasso is then removed, leaving the suture in place through the MGHL and exiting the anterior cannula. The cannula is then withdrawn slightly to an extracapsular position. With the same anterior cannula, a Birdbeak suture retriever (Arthrex) is then used to pierce the SGHL just lateral to the labrum. The suture is then retrieved through the SGHL with the Birdbeak (Fig. 11-32). At this point the suture is

looped around the MGHL and SGHL with the suture tails extracapsular and exiting through the anterior cannula. The suture is tied extracapsularly with a two-hole knot pusher (Fig. 11-33). These steps are then repeated in a slightly more lateral position to place a second suture (Fig. 11-34).

5. This procedure restores the widened biceps pulley to a normal size, resolving biceps tendon subluxation (Fig. 11-34).

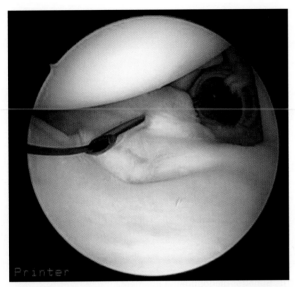

Figure 11-31. Suture passed through the upper middle glenohumeral ligament just lateral to the labrum.

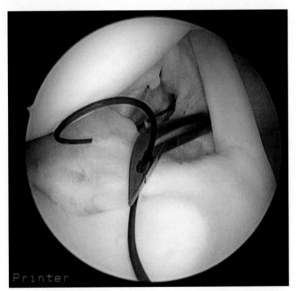

Figure 11-32. Superior glenohumeral ligament (SGHL)–injured right shoulder. Suture on left side of image is through middle glenohumeral ligament (MGHL). The Birdbeak is placed through the anterior cannula (which is now extracapsular), piercing the SGHL. The Birdbeak retrieves the end of suture that has been placed through the MGHL and brings it through the SGHL and out of the anterior cannula.

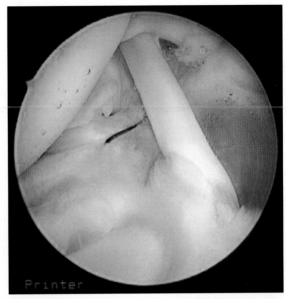

Figure 11-33. Sutures tied extracapsularly with two-hole knot pusher.

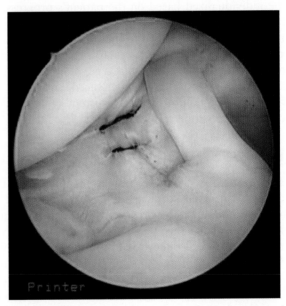

Figure 11-34. Completed suture repair. Restoration of biceps pulley and outlet to normal size.

POSTOPERATIVE CONSIDERATIONS

Follow-up

All procedures are performed on an outpatient basis. Patients are typically seen approximately 8 days after surgery for wound check and suture removal. Patients are seen at regular intervals during the rehabilitation phase to monitor progress with motion and to advance therapy as appropriate.

Rehabilitation

- Sling immobilization for 4 weeks, avoiding ER.
- At 4 weeks, passive and active range of motion and scapular stabilization muscle strengthening are started.
- At 8 weeks, rotator cuff strengthening and total body conditioning are added.
- At 4 months, a progressive distance interval throwing program is initiated.

- At 6 months, throwing from the mound and return to sport are allowed.

Complications

Complications are similar to those of other procedures involving arthroscopic shoulder reconstruction, including a rare incidence of infection, failed repair, painful adhesion formation, and stiffness. Previous studies have reported decreased ER after anterior rotator interval closure, but we have not experienced this complication.[19] In fact, we have noted that preoperative excessive ER returns to a more normal and symmetrical level after surgery. Physicians and therapists working with throwing athletes must be vigilant for the development of postoperative shoulder stiffness through regular follow-up and a directed therapy program.

We use PDS for our anterior rotator interval closure, as this is a resorbable suture, allowing postoperative therapy to be modified if necessary. We have found that use of a resorbable suture allows each patient's therapy to be individualized based on the patient's progress. If the patient begins to show signs of loss of ER, his or her therapy can be changed to increase this motion. In our experience, the use of permanent suture for this procedure does not allow this type of modification. Accordingly, we have not experienced any signs of suture or repair failure such as recurrent symptoms or excessive ER postoperatively.

RESULTS

Based on history, clinical examination findings, MRI, and diagnostic arthroscopic parameters, 32 overhead or throwing athletes were prospectively diagnosed and treated for isolated throwing-acquired rotator interval lesions of the biceps pulley (SGHL-injured group) over a 3-year period. During the same period and with use of the same clinical and MRI parameters used for the SGHL-injured group, an age-matched control group of 31 overhead or throwing athletes were prospectively diagnosed with either GIRD or scapular dyskinesis[20-22] without intra-articular pathology on MRI and treated nonoperatively. Patient demographics for each group at the time of presentation are listed in Boxes 11-4 and 11-5. After arthroscopic confirmation of pathology in the biceps pulley and outlet portion of the rotator interval in the SGHL-injured group, an arthroscopic anterior rotator interval capsular repair (closure) was done as described previously. All patients in the control group were treated nonoperatively with corrective posterior capsular and muscle stretches for their GIRD and scapular stabilizer muscle-strengthening exercises for their scapular dyskinesis.[20-22]

All patients in the SGHL-injured group were clinically scored on a disabled throwing shoulder rating

---

BOX 11-4 Patient Demographics: SGHL-Injured Group (32 Patients)

Age
  o Average: 19 years
  o Range: 14-29 years
Sex
  o Males: 24 years
  o Females: 8 years
Baseball: 22 patients
  o 18 Pitchers
  o 4 Position players
  o 4 High school
  o 10 College
  o 8 Professional

Softball: 3 patients
  o All pitchers
  o 1 High school
  o 2 College
Lacrosse: 4 patients
  o All college
Tennis: 2 patients
  o 1 College
  o 1 Professional
Golf : 1 patient
  o Professional

SGHL, Superior glenohumeral ligament.

BOX 11-5 Patient Demographics: Control Group (31 Patients)

Age
  o Average: 22 years
  o Range: 14-34 years
Sex
  o Males: 27
  o Females: 4
Baseball: 16 patients
  o All pitchers
  o 6 High school
  o 8 College
  o 2 Professional
Tennis: 4 patients
  o 1 High school
  o 2 College
  o 1 Recreational

Football: 3 patients
  o All quarterbacks
  o All college
Golf: 2 patients
  o 1 College
  o 1 Recreational
Boxers: 2 patients
  o All professional
Basketball: 1 patient
  o Professional
Weightlifters: 3 patients

---

scale that was developed to address the unique signs and symptoms related to throwing-acquired SGHL biceps pulley injury and instability (Box 11-6). With this rating system, SGHL-injured patients were scored prospectively at presentation and at 1 and 2 years after arthroscopic capsular biceps pulley repair.

All 32 patients in the SGHL-injured group met all clinical parameters, and none of the 31 control group patients had positive clinical parameters except for painless decreased velocity in 27 (87%) caused by GIRD or scapular dyskinesis (Table 11-5). At 2-year prospective follow-up, all 31 SGHL-injured patients who underwent arthroscopic capsular rotator interval closure had absence of all clinical parameters that had been present preoperatively (Table 11-6).

BOX 11-6 Clinical Parameters Evaluated in Both Groups at Presentation

1. Complaints of anterior superior shoulder pain with throwing
2. Complaints of decreased throwing velocity and performance
3. Reproducible anterior superior shoulder pain in ABER reduced by Jobe relocation maneuver
4. Upper bicipital groove pain on digital pressure
5. Asymmetrical increased sulcus sign in dominant shoulder in neutral and ER
6. Asymmetrical increased scapular stabilized ER and TMA of the dominant versus the nondominant shoulder of more than 10 degrees

ABER, Abduction and external rotation; *ER,* external rotation; *TMA,* total motion arc.

TABLE 11-5. Disabled Throwing Shoulder Clinical Rating Scale (100 Points)

Parameter	Yes	No
Pain-free throwing	20	0
Preinjury velocity and performance	10	0
ER and TMA dominant shoulder within 10 degrees of nondominant shoulder	20	0
Symmetrical sulcus sign in neutral and ER	20	0
Pain-free ABER test	20	0
Pain-free bicipital groove	10	0
TOTAL	100	0

ABER, Abduction and external rotation; *ER,* external rotation; *TMA,* total motion arc.

TABLE 11-6. Results: Clinical Parameters, Both Groups

Signs or Symptoms	SGHL Injured at Presentation (n = 32)	Control Group at Presentation (n = 31)	SGHL Injured 2 Years Postoperatively (n = 32)
Anterior-superior pain	32	0	0
Decreased velocity	32	27	0
Positive pain on ABER test	32	0	0
Upper bicipital groove pain	32	0	0
Asymmetrical increased sulcus sign	32	0	0
Asymmetrical increased ER and TMA	32	0	0

ABER, Abduction and external rotation; *ER,* external rotation; *TMA,* total motion arc.

TABLE 11-7. Results: Disabled Throwing Shoulder Clinical Rating in SGHL-Injured Group Preoperatively and 2 Years Postoperatively

	Score (Points)
SGHL-injured patients at presentation	0
SGHL-injured patients 2 years postoperatively	100

SGHL, superior glenohumeral ligament.

At presentation, all members of the SGHL-injured group had extremely disabled throwing shoulder rating scale scores of 0, whereas the control group had an average score of 90. At 2 years after arthroscopic anterior rotator interval closure, all patients in the SGHL-injured group had scores of 100 and had resumed pain-free throwing at or better than their preinjury level of performance (Table 11-7).

At presentation, all patients in the SGHL-injured group had asymmetrical dominant shoulder increased ER and TMA of more than 20 degrees. The average was 26 to 27 degrees (range, 20 to 36 degrees), which was significantly statistically different ($P < .05$) when compared with the control group, in which the average increased ER and TMA of the dominant shoulders was 6 degrees (range, 0 to 12 degrees). At 2-year prospective follow-up after rotator interval closure, in the SGHL-injured group the increased ER and TMA had resolved to an average 7 degrees (range, 0 to 10 degrees) (Table 11-8).

On MRI, SRIA averaged 58 degrees (range, 44 to 68 degrees) in contrast to an average SRIA for the control group of 25 degrees (range, 22 to 30 degrees). The difference in SRIA between these two groups is highly statistically significant ($P < .05$). All patients in the SGHL-injured group had a positive biceps drop-out sign on sagittal oblique arthrogram MRI images through the center of the soft tissue biceps outlet and pulley. In contrast, none of the control group had a biceps drop out sign on similar images, but rather the biceps was seen to be central within the pulley. Of the 32 SGHL-injured patients, 22 (68.8%) had an obvious chandelier sign representing a tear of the SGHL medial wall portion of the biceps outlet and pulley. None of the control group sagittal oblique magnetic resonance arthrogram images had a chandelier sign (Table 11-9).

TABLE 11-8. Results: Scapular Stabilized Glenohumeral Rotation Data: Both Groups

	Internal Rotation		External Rotation				Total Motion Arc	
	T	NT	T	NT	GERG—T	GIRD—T	T	NT
SGHL-Injured Group at Presentation								
Average	51	54	122	88	26	9	170	144
Range	**38-65**	46-67	105-134	85-101	20-35	5-15	151-184	130-162
Control Group at Presentation								
Average	42	55	89	84	6	15	148	154
Range	25-62	45-74	88-109	80-101	0-12	0-25	130-158	128-160
SGHL-Injured Group 2 Years Postoperatively								
Average	53	55	91	87	5	12	152	154
Range	40-65	47-67	85-100	82-102	0-11	0-15	135-154	130-160

GERG, glenohumeral external rotation gain; *GIRD*, glenohumeral internal rotation deficit; *NT*, non-throwing; *SGHL*, superior glenohumeral ligament; *T*, throwing.

TABLE 11-9. Results: Sagittal Oblique Magnetic Resonance Arthrogram

Group	Sagittal Rotator Interval Angle	Drop-out Sign	Chandelier Sign
SGHL injured	Average, 58 degrees	All	70%
	Range, 44-68 degrees		
Control	Average, 25 degrees	None	None
	Range, 22-30 degrees		

SGHL, Superior glenohumeral ligament.

Repetitive overhead throwing athletes with SGHL injury with biceps pulley disruption and biceps outlet instability who are found to have positive clinical, MRI, and arthroscopic findings as presented in this discussion are indicated and best treated by an arthroscopic capsular rotator interval repair between the upper MGHL and the SGHL as described. Two-year prospective clinical outcomes in this specific group of athletes with throwing-acquired SGHL injuries who had this type of capsular repair reveal an extremely high rate of success in returning the athletes their preinjury level of pain-free performance.

REFERENCES

1. Walch G, Boileau J, Noel E, et al. Impingement of the deep surface of the supraspinatus tendon on the posterosuperior glenoid rim: an arthroscopic study. *J Shoulder Elbow Surg.* 1992;1:238-243.
2. Jobe CM. Posterior superior glenoid impingement: expanded spectrum. *Arthroscopy.* 1995;11:530-537.
3. Burkhart SS, Morgan CD, Kibler WB. The disabled throwing shoulder: spectrum of pathology. Part I: Pathoanatomy and biomechanics. *Arthroscopy.* 2003;19:404-420.
4. Grossman MG, Tibone JE, McGarry MH, et al. A cadaveric model of the throwing shoulder: a possible etiology of superior labrum anterior-to-posterior lesions. *J Bone Joint Surg Am.* 2005;87:824-831.
5. Morgan CD, Burkhart SS, Palmeri M, et al. Type II SLAP lesions: three subtypes and their relationships to superior instability and rotator cuff tears. *Arthroscopy.* 1998;14:553-565.
6. Burkhart SS. *Arthroscopically-observed dynamic pathoanatomy in the Jobe relocation test.* Presented at the symposium on SLAP lesions, 18th open meeting of the American Shoulder and Elbow Surgeons; Dallas, Texas; February 16, 2002.
7. Panossian VR, Mihata T, Tibone JE, et al. Biomechanical analysis of isolated type II SLAP lesions and repair. *J Shoulder Elbow Surg.* 2005;14:529-534.
8. Burkhart SS, Morgan CD, Kibler WB. The disabled throwing shoulder: spectrum of pathology. Part II: Evaluation and treatment of SLAP lesions in throwers. *Arthroscopy.* 2003;19:531-539.
9. Gerber C, Sebesta A. Impingement of the deep surface of the subscapularis tendon and the reflection pulley on the anterosuperior glenoid rim: a preliminary report. *J Shoulder Elbow Surg.* 2000;9:483-490.
10. Harryman DT 2nd, Sidles JA, Harris SL, et al. The role of the rotator interval capsule in passive motion and stability of the shoulder. *J Bone Joint Surg Am.* 1992;74(A):53-66.
11. Werner A, Mueller T, Boehm D, Gohlke F. The stabilizing sling for the long head of the biceps tendon in the rotator cuff interval. A histoanatomical study. *Am J Sports Med.* 2000;28:28-31.
12. Braun S, Horan MP, Elser F, Millett PJ. Lesions of the biceps pulley. *Am J Sports Med.* 2011;20:1-6.

13. Habermeyer P, Magosch P, Pritsch M, et al. Anterosuperior impingement of the shoulder as a result of pulley lesions: A prospective arthroscopic study. *J Shoulder Elbow Surg.* 2004;13:5-12.

14. Le Huec JC, Schaeverbeke T, Moinard M, et al. Traumatic tear of the rotator interval. *J Shoulder Elbow Surg.* 1996;5:41-46.

15. Snyder SJ, Karzel RP, Del Pizzo W, et al. SLAP lesions of the shoulder. *Arthroscopy.* 1990;6(4):274-279.

16. Walch G, Nove-Josserand L, Levigne C, et al. Tears of the supraspinatous tendon associated with "hidden" lesions of the rotator interval. *J Shoulder Elbow Surg.* 1994;3: 353-360.

17. Walch G, Nové-Josserand L, Boileau P, et al. Subluxations and dislocations of the tendon of the long head of the biceps. *J Shoulder Elbow Surg.* 1998;7:100-108.

18. Jobe CM, et al. In Jobe FW, ed. *Operative Techniques in Upper Extremity Sports Injuries.* St. Louis: Mosby, 1996: 164-176.

19. Mologne TS, Zhao K, Hongo M, et al. The addition of rotator interval closure after arthroscopic repair of either anterior or posterior shoulder instability: effect on glenohumeral translation and range of motion. *Am J Sports Med.* 2008;36:1123-1131.

20. Morgan C, Burkhart S, Kibler B. The disabled throwing shoulder—part I. *Arthroscopy.* 2003;19(4):404-420.

21. Morgan C, Burkhart S, Kibler B. The disabled throwing shoulder—part II. *Arthroscopy.* 2003;19(5):531-539.

22. Morgan C, Burkhart S, Kibler B. The disabled throwing shoulder—part III. *Arthroscopy.* 2003;19(6):641-661.

Chapter 12

Open Repair of Anterior Shoulder Instability

Michael J. Pagnani

Chapter Synopsis

- Open stabilization techniques continue to have important places in the armamentarium of the shoulder surgeon.
- The results of open stabilization have been uniformly excellent, with postoperative recurrence rates of 0% to 5% generally reported.
- My basic procedure for the open surgical treatment of recurrent anterior instability is a modification of the Bankart procedure and involves repair of the anterior capsule and labrum to the glenoid.

Important Points

- Open stabilization techniques may provide superior results compared with arthroscopic methods in the following patient groups:
  - Contact athletes
  - Patients with bony defects in humeral head or glenoid
  - Patients with humeral avulsion of glenohumeral ligaments
  - Those with rupture of the subscapularis in association with primary dislocation
  - Individuals with failed arthroscopic or open repair
  - Patients with atraumatic instability
- Results suggested that bone-block or grafting procedures do not appear to be necessary in the majority of patients with bone loss.

Clinical and Surgical Pearls

- For optimal cosmesis, mark the skin incision in the preoperative holding area by having the patient internally rotate the shoulder. Identify the skin crease extending from the axilla to a point inferior and 1 to 2 cm lateral to the coracoid. Use this crease for the incision.
- Use two self-retaining retractors to free your assistants. I prefer the Kolbel self-retaining shoulder retractor with detachable blades (Link America, Waldemar Link, Hamburg, Germany). I use the retractors so that the convex side faces the wound. Blades of an appropriate depth are then attached. The first retractor is used to spread the wound from medial to lateral. I place the second retractor so that its base enters from the medial side to spread the wound from inferior to superior. Generally a deeper blade is placed inferiorly than superiorly.
- Pay attention to arm position when tensioning the capsule. Remind the assistant to keep the arm at the 45/45 position for a standard repair.
- Make sure the assistant has the humeral head reduced in the glenoid when capsular suture are being tied. If the shoulder is not reduced, the capsule will not appose the glenoid neck.
- Be meticulous in closing the subscapularis. Consider use of modified Kessler or Mason-Allen sutures for added strength.

Clinical and Surgical Pitfalls

- Dissect medial to the cephalic vein when developing the deltopectoral interval because branches to the vein enter laterally
- Avoid overzealous retraction on the conjoined tendon that attaches to the coracoid to avoid injury to the musculocutaneous nerve.
- Make sure that the subscapularis is not tenotomized too far laterally, or there will not be a stump to sew back to at closure.
- Externally rotate the shoulder as you take down the inferior aspect of the subscapularis to protect the axillary nerve. Expect to encounter branches of the anterior humeral circumflex artery in this area, and be prepared to ligate or coagulate them.

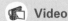 **Video**

- Video 12-1

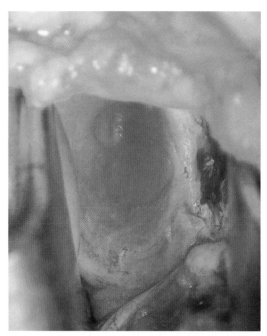

Figure 12-1. The Bankart lesion—detachment of the anteroinferior labrum and the inferior glenohumeral ligament complex insertion from the glenoid.

The shoulder is notable in that it has the greatest range of motion of all the joints in the human body. Osseous restraints to motion are minimal. The surrounding soft tissue envelope is the primary stabilizer that maintains the humeral head on the glenoid.

The shoulder capsule is large, loose, and redundant to allow the large range of shoulder motion. There are three main ligaments in the anterior capsule that help prevent subluxation or dislocation: the superior glenohumeral ligament, the middle glenohumeral ligament, and the inferior glenohumeral ligament complex (IGHLC). Damage to the IGHLC, which supports the inferior part of the shoulder capsule and acts like a hammock, is related to most cases of anterior instability. The Bankart lesion,[1] involving detachment of the IGHLC insertion on the glenoid, is the most common pathologic lesion associated with traumatic anterior instability (Fig. 12-1). Defects or injuries to the superior and middle glenohumeral ligaments may also contribute to instability.[2]

The primary goals of the surgical treatment of shoulder instability are to restore stability and to provide the patient with nearly full pain-free motion. Older techniques of shoulder stabilization tended to limit shoulder range of motion in exchange for providing stability. We now understand that it is probably more important to preserve motion than it is to stabilize the shoulder. Techniques that limit shoulder motion often lead to osteoarthritis, whereas it is unusual for recurrent dislocation itself to lead directly to osteoarthritis. As a result, any method of open stabilization should be designed to provide full functional use of the shoulder as well as normal stability.

PREOPERATIVE CONSIDERATIONS

History

The diagnosis of an anterior dislocation is usually readily apparent.[3] The patient typically gives a history of a specific injury in which the shoulder "popped out." In some cases, dislocation occurs with no history of significant trauma; these patients are frequently noted to have generalized ligamentous laxity and are less likely to demonstrate a Bankart lesion.

The diagnosis of anterior subluxation is often more subtle. The chief complaint may be a sense of movement, pain, or clicking with certain activities. Pain, rather than instability, may be the predominant complaint. In throwers and other overhead athletes, "dead arm" episodes may occur during which the patient experiences a sharp pain followed by loss of control of the extremity.[4] It should also be noted that patients who report multiple dislocations, atraumatic dislocations (in sleep), or continued instability should be evaluated for potential bone loss on the anterior glenoid.

Physical Examination

Apprehension tests are designed to induce anxiety and protective muscle contraction as the shoulder is brought into a position of instability. The anterior apprehension test is performed with the arm abducted and externally rotated. As the examiner progressively increases the degree of external rotation, the patient develops apprehension that the shoulder will slip out. This test result is uniformly positive in patients with anterior instability.

During the relocation test, the examiner's hand is placed over the anterior shoulder of the supine patient. A posteriorly directed force is applied with the hand to prevent anterior translation of the humeral head. The shoulder is then abducted and externally rotated as it is in the apprehension test. A positive result is obtained when this anterior pressure allows increased external rotation and diminishes associated pain and apprehension. The relocation test seems to be more reliable in overhead athletes, and the result may not be positive in all cases of anterior instability.

The belly press and liftoff tests should also be performed to confirm the integrity of the subscapularis tendon in the setting of an anterior dislocation.

Imaging

Routine radiographic examination of the unstable shoulder includes an anteroposterior view (deviated 30 to 45 degrees from the sagittal plane to parallel the glenohumeral joint), a trans-scapular (Y) view, and an axillary view. In the assessment of more chronic instability, West Point and Stryker notch views are helpful in demonstrating bone lesions of the humeral head and glenoid.

Magnetic resonance imaging is not necessarily performed routinely in patients with instability because the findings are usually predictable; however, it may be helpful in preoperative planning. The accuracy of magnetic resonance imaging in determining labral disease is increased with arthrography. Because of the possibility of concomitant rotator cuff injury, magnetic resonance imaging should always be considered in older patients with instability—especially if strength and motion are slow to recover after an episode of dislocation. Lastly, if the patient has a history of multiple dislocations or unidirectional atraumatic dislocations or there is a suggestion of bony deficiency on the radiographs, a CT scan is recommended to evaluate for any bone loss on the anterior glenoid and to assist in the preoperative planning.

Indications and Contraindications

The indications for surgical treatment of recurrent anterior shoulder instability are highly subjective. They include a desire of the patient to avoid recurrent problems with instability (including the necessity of reporting to the emergency department on a frequent basis to have the shoulder reduced), problems with recurrent pain, an inability to perform certain activities because of a fear of further shoulder instability, and the desire to improve athletic performance with improved shoulder stability. Failure of a thorough trial of nonoperative treatment is also an indication for surgical treatment.

There are several relative contraindications to performing a stabilization procedure by an arthroscopic method in patients in whom an operation is deemed advisable. Although there is controversy in this area, reported indications for open stabilization over arthroscopic stabilization include participation in a contact or collision sport, bone defects of the humeral head or glenoid, humeral avulsion of the glenohumeral ligaments, rupture of the subscapularis in association with a traumatic dislocation, failed open or arthroscopic repair, and atraumatic instability.

Contraindications to the open technique include voluntary instability and concomitant psychological issues. Large defects of the humeral head (Hill-Sachs lesions)

or glenoid may require supplemental bone grafting to fill the defects[5]; however, the recent trend toward increased performance of the Latarjet procedure may be an overreaction. The literature has shown consistently high levels of success with conventional *open* techniques of stabilization (*without* bone blocks) in patients with bony defects of the humeral head and/or glenoid. Owing to success with the procedure described later, in my practice the Latarjet procedure is considered only in patients who have glenoid defects involving more that 30% of the glenoid diameter or in patients with humeral head defects involving more than 25% of the head and with a depth of at least 1 centimeter. I seldom perform bone block procedures except in revision cases.

I prefer to use arthroscopic methods of stabilization in throwing athletes. If an open method is used in this group, I recommend the technique of anterior capsulolabral reconstruction described by Jobe,[6] in which the subscapularis tendon is split rather than detached.

SURGICAL TECHNIQUE

The basic procedure for the open surgical treatment of recurrent anterior instability is a modification of the Bankart procedure[1] and involves repair of the anterior capsule and labrum to the glenoid.[11] In most cases the capsular ligaments are stretched as well as detached, and the procedure is also designed to remove any abnormal laxity.

Anesthesia and Positioning

The procedure is performed after placement of an interscalene block. In some cases the block is supplemented with general anesthesia. The patient is positioned supine with the head of the operating table raised 15 to 30 degrees and the involved upper extremity abducted 45 degrees on an arm board. Folded sheets are placed beneath the elbow and taped to the arm board. The sheets maintain the arm in the coronal plane of the thorax and minimize extension of the shoulder.

The surgeon initially stands in the axilla area. Two assistants are used. The first assistant's primary responsibilities are to control arm position and to keep the humeral head reduced during the capsular repair. The first assistant alternates position with the surgeon. When the surgeon is in the axilla area, the first assistant stands lateral to the arm. When the surgeon moves to the lateral aspect of the arm, the first assistant shifts to the axilla. The first assistant also holds the humeral head retractor when it is in position. The second assistant stands on the opposite side of the table and holds the medial (glenoid) retractors. The use of a mechanized arm holder can free the assistants' hands and may facilitate exposure.

Examination Under Anesthesia and Arthroscopic Evaluation

I routinely examine the shoulder with the patient under anesthesia to confirm the presence of abnormal anterior translation. Drawer tests are best performed in 90 degrees of abduction and neutral rotation where translation is greatest. Translation is graded 1+ if there is increased translation compared with the opposite shoulder but neither subluxation nor dislocation occurs. If the head can be subluxated over the glenoid rim but then spontaneously reduces, translation is graded 2+. Frank dislocation without spontaneous reduction constitutes 3+ translation.

I also routinely perform an arthroscopic examination of the shoulder with the patient in the beach chair position before open stabilization. The arthroscopic examination allows identification and treatment of concomitant injuries to the shoulder, including superior labral and rotator cuff disease, that can be difficult to identify through an open approach. In addition, the examination is helpful in planning the specific method of capsular repair.

Specific Steps

Specific steps are outlined in Box 12-1. The skin is incised along the anterior axillary crease (Fig. 12-2) in a longitudinal fashion along Langer's lines. The incision is placed lateral to the coracoid process. The deltopectoral interval is identified (Fig. 12-3), the cephalic vein is retracted laterally, and the interval is developed. The clavipectoral fascia is then incised at the lateral border of the conjoined tendon at its coracoid attachment, and the coracoacromial ligament is divided to facilitate exposure of the superior aspect of the capsule and, particularly, the rotator interval area.

BOX 12-1 Surgical Steps

- Incision along the anterior axillary crease
- Identification of the deltopectoral interval and cephalic vein
- Takedown of the subscapularis tendon
- Closure of the rotator interval
- Horizontal capsulotomy
- Exposure of Bankart lesion after placement of ring (Fukuda) retractor
- Debridement of anterior glenoid neck to bleeding bone with a motorized bur
- Repair of Bankart lesion with inferior capsular flap
- Lateral T-plasty capsular shift in cases with pronounced capsular laxity
- Reattachment of subscapularis tendon

Two self-retaining retractors are then placed in the wound (Fig. 12-4). Placement of these retractors frees the assistants to aid in arm position and shoulder reduction. At this point the surgeon shifts position from the axilla and stands lateral to the arm. If a mechanized arm holder is used, it is attached to the forearm when the surgeon moves from the axilla.

The bicipital groove and the lesser tuberosity are identified. A vertical tenotomy of the subscapularis tendon is performed with electrocautery approximately 1 cm medial to its insertion on the lesser tuberosity (Fig. 12-5). The medial portion of the tendon is tagged with heavy No. 1 nonabsorbable braided polyester (Ethibond) sutures. The interval between the anterior aspect of the capsule and the subscapularis tendon is then carefully

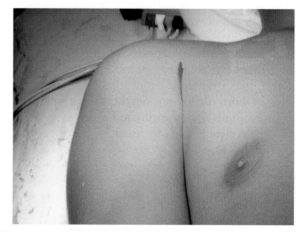

Figure 12-2. Incision along the anterior axillary crease.

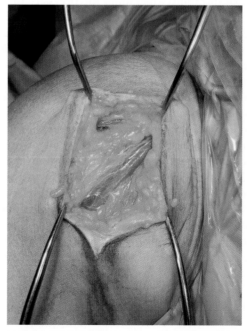

Figure 12-3. Identification of the deltopectoral interval and cephalic vein.

developed with a combination of blunt and sharp dissection.

The laxity and quality of the capsule are then assessed. If there is a lesion in the rotator interval, it is generally closed at this point with No. 1 nonabsorbable braided polyester (Ethibond) sutures (Fig. 12-6). A transverse capsulotomy is then performed (Fig. 12-7), and a ring (Fukuda) retractor is placed intra-articularly. The anterior glenoid neck is explored for evidence of a

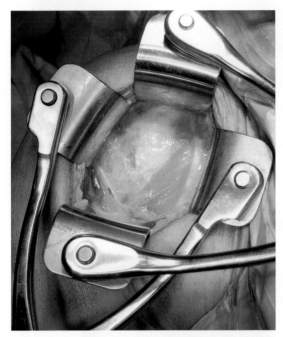

Figure 12-4. Placement of self-retaining retractors.

Bankart lesion. The joint is then irrigated to remove any residual loose bodies.

If a Bankart lesion is noted, the capsulolabral separation at the anteroinferior glenoid neck is extended medially with use of an elevator or knife to allow placement of a retractor along the glenoid neck (Fig. 12-8). The glenoid neck is then roughened with an osteotome or motorized bur to provide a bleeding surface (Fig. 12-9). Two or three suture anchors are placed in the anteroinferior glenoid neck near but not on the articular margin of the glenoid (Fig. 12-10). The arm is placed in 45 degrees of abduction and 45 degrees of external rotation. The inferior capsular flap is then mobilized slightly medially and superiorly. The inferior flap is reattached to the anterior aspect of the glenoid to repair the Bankart lesion with use of the suture anchors (Fig. 12-11). The goal is not to reduce external rotation but to obliterate excess capsular volume and to restore the competency of the IGHLC at its glenoid insertion.

After repair of the Bankart lesion (or in the absence of a Bankart lesion), an anterior capsulorrhaphy is performed to eliminate excess capsular laxity. The arm is maintained in 45 degrees of abduction and 45 degrees of external rotation, and the superior and inferior capsular flaps are reapproximated with forceps. The shoulder is held in a reduced position. If the capsular flaps can be overlapped, the capsule is shifted to eliminate excess capsular volume: if 5 mm (or less) of overlap is present, the capsule is imbricated by shifting the superior flap over the inferior flap and passing the sutures a second time through the superior flap (Fig. 12-12); with more than 5 mm of capsular overlap, the capsulotomy

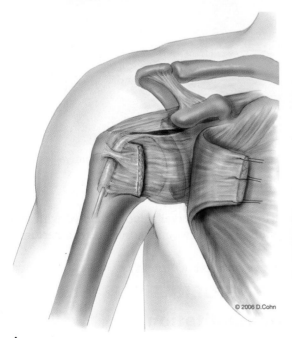

© 2006 D.Cohn

A

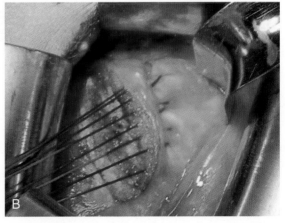

Figure 12-5. Takedown of the subscapularis tendon.

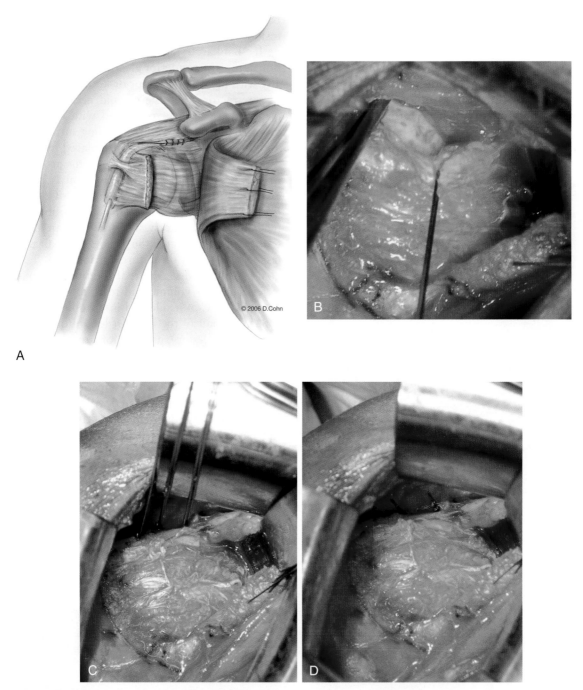

© 2006 D.Cohn

Figure 12-6. A, Closure of the rotator interval. Clinical photographs show identification of rotator interval lesion **(B)** and its closure **(C** and **D).**

is extended in a vertical direction near its lateral insertion on the humeral neck, and a T-plasty capsular shift is performed (Fig. 12-13). The inferior capsular flap is shifted superolaterally, and the superior flap is moved over the inferior flap in an inferolateral direction. The transverse portion of the capsulotomy is then closed.

After the capsule has been addressed satisfactorily, the subscapularis is reapproximated, but not shortened, with nonabsorbable suture (Fig. 12-14). The

deltopectoral interval is loosely closed with absorbable suture. Routine wound closure is then performed.

POSTOPERATIVE CONSIDERATIONS

Rehabilitation

The standard rehabilitation protocol and special situations are described in Box 12-2.

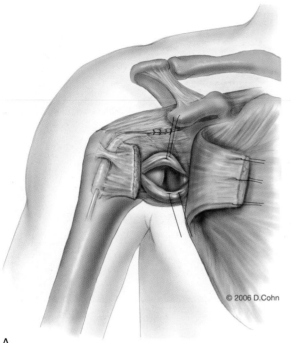

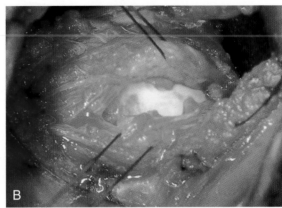

A

Figure 12-7. Horizontal capsulotomy.

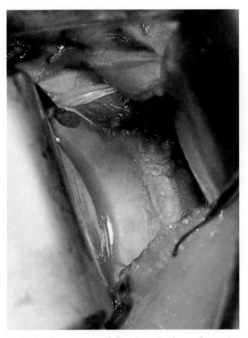

Figure 12-8. Exposure of Bankart lesion after placement of ring (Fukuda) retractor.

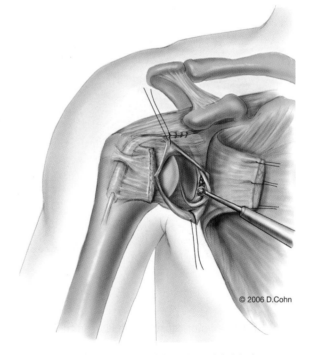

Figure 12-9. Anterior glenoid neck is debrided to bleeding bone with a motorized bur.

Complications

Recurrent instability is the greatest concern after any stabilization procedure. Subcutaneous hematoma formation is the most common complication in my experience (1.5% of cases). If a hematoma forms, it may be observed as long as the wound is not draining. When the hematoma causes persistent wound drainage, surgical evacuation is recommended.

Subscapularis rupture has been reported after open anterior stabilization. Although I have no experience with subscapularis rupture in this setting, I recommend

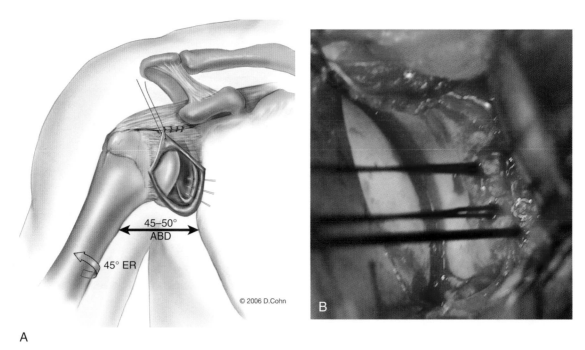

Figure 12-10. Placement of suture anchors. *ABD,* Abduction; *ER,* external rotation.

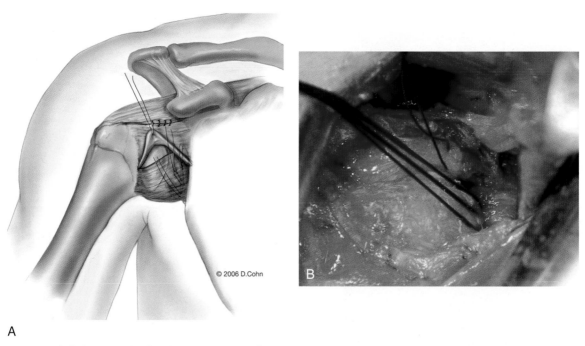

Figure 12-11. Inferior capsular flap is used to repair Bankart lesion.

meticulous reapproximation of the tendon and restriction of external rotation for 3 months postoperatively as prophylactic measures to prevent its occurrence.

RESULTS

The published recurrence rates after open stabilization for anterior instability have generally been low, ranging from 0% to 10% in most series (Table 12-1). However,

one report from West Point described a failure rate of 22% in active cadets, indicating that results are not uniformly and predictably good.[11] The outcome of open stabilization in contact athletes appears to be superior to that reported in similar populations with arthroscopic techniques.[7,10] The reported motion loss with current open techniques is also acceptable; in my experience, 84% of patients regained all or nearly all of their motion. No patient lost more than 15 degrees of

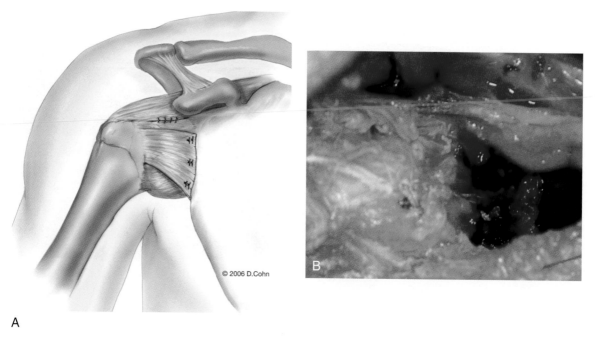

Figure 12-12. Sutures are passed a second time through the superior capsular flap to double the thickness of the repair and to eliminate excess capsular laxity.

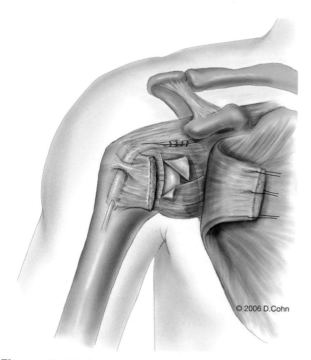

Figure 12-13. Lateral T-plasty capsular shift in cases with pronounced capsular laxity.

external rotation compared with the contralateral side. Finally, when the incision is placed in the anterior axillary crease, the cosmetic result is usually satisfactory (Fig. 12-15).

Clinical and biomechanical studies have led some authors to postulate that conventional capsular repair may be insufficient in selected patients with bony deficiency of the glenoid. Historically, the Bristow, Latarjet, and Trillat coracoid transfer procedures were designed to address instability by creating an anterior bony buttress. Procedures of this type were largely abandoned in North America for a time because of concerns that (1) the concept of a bony buttress did not address excess capsular laxity or capsulolabral separation at the glenoid neck, (2) such procedures carried a high risk of complications from hardware loosening or nonunion, (3) revision surgery was especially difficult owing to extensive scarring of the anterior capsule and subscapularis tendon, and (4) there was a high incidence of postoperative arthrosis.

A review of the published reports of open capsular repair in the face of defects of the glenoid shows that the results have been deemed acceptable. Rowe and colleagues,[13] in their historic 1978 end-result study of open Bankart repairs, found that the postoperative recurrence actually decreased from 3.5% to 2% in patients with defects of the glenoid rim. Bigliani and colleagues,[14] in the study referenced earlier, reported a 12% recurrence rate after open capsular shift in patients with glenoid bone loss. These reports led to questioning regarding the need to perform bone augmentation in patients with glenoid insufficiency except in rare cases.

Rowe and colleagues[13] found a slight increase in recurrence after open Bankart repair in patients with moderate or severe Hills-Sachs lesions (5% vs. 3.5%). Gill and Zarins,[15] in a more recent series of open Bankart repairs, found that the recurrence rate doubled from 3% to 6% in the presence of a large Hill-Sachs lesion.

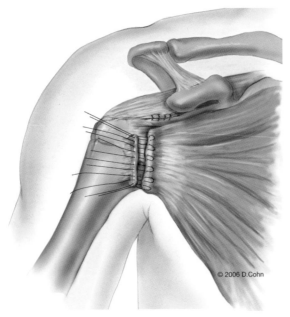

A

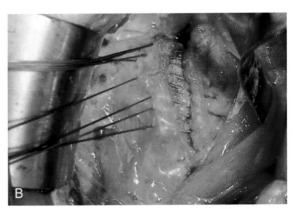

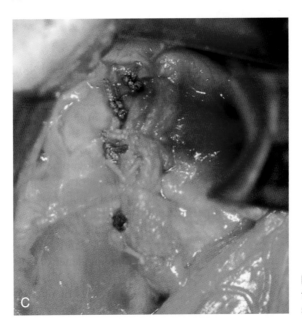

C

Figure 12-14. A, Reattachment of subscapularis tendon. **B** and **C,** Clinical images demonstrate subscapularis reapproximation.

In our series[16] investigating the results of traditional open stabilization in patients with bony defects, no recurrences were found in patients with defects of the glenoid rim, and the risk of postoperative recurrence in patients with humeral head lesions increased slightly but did not achieve statistical significance. Based on the low rates of recurrence in these series, motion loss that is equal to or better than that reported with bone-block procedures, and the seemingly self-evident premise that the complication rate of capsular repair alone should be lower than that of capsular repair combined with bone augmentation, it appears that bone-block or grafting procedures are not necessary in the majority of patients with bony defects of the glenoid or humeral head.

TABLE 12-1. Results of Open Stabilization

Author	N	Recurrence Rate (%)
Cole et al[8] (2000)	24	9
Gill et al[9] (1997)	60	5
Hubbell et al[10] (2004)	20	0
Pagnani and Dome[7] (2002)	58	3
Uhorchak et al[11] (2000)	66	22
Wirth et al[12] (1996)	142	3

BOX 12-2 Standardized Postoperative Rehabilitation Protocol

Weeks 4-8

- Passive and active assisted range of motion.
- Limit external rotation to 45 degrees.
- Deltoid isometrics with arm at low abduction levels.
- When 140 degrees of active forward flexion is achieved, begin the following:
  - Thera-Bands: internal and external rotation cuff strengthening with arm at side
  - No internal rotation strengthening or resistance
- Scapular rehabilitation:
  - Stability exercises:
    - Isometrics
    - Scapular pinch
    - Scapular shrug
  - Closed-chain exercises—hand in contact with wall or ball
  - Perform specific scapular maneuvers:
    - Elevation
    - Depression
    - Retraction
    - Protraction
- Correct strength or flexibility deficit in trunk, back, hip.

Weeks 8-12

- Limit external rotation to 45 degrees.
- Continue internal and external rotation strengthening with bands:
  - If no impingement or cuff symptoms, may slowly increase abduction with time
- Scapular elevation with thumbs up ("full can").
- Prone horizontal abduction in external rotation and 100 degrees of abduction.
- Prone horizontal abduction in neutral.
- Shoulder abduction to 90 degrees.
- Prone rowing.
- *No empty cans.*
- Scapular rotator strengthening:
  - Press-ups
  - Shrugs
  - Horizontal abduction
  - Open can exercises
  - Body blade
- Manual resistance scapular stabilization drills.

Weeks 12-16

- Work on regaining terminal external rotation.
- External rotation at 0 degrees (side-lying dumbbell or tubing) and 90 degrees.

- Internal rotation at 0 and 90 degrees.
- Diagonal pattern extension.
- Diagonal pattern flexion.
- Specific drills to restore neuromuscular control.
  - Rhythmic stabilization.
  - Reciprocal isometric contractions for internal rotation and external rotation muscles.
  - Proprioceptive neuromuscular feedback (PNF) patterns with rhythmic stabilization.
  - Facilitate agonist-antagonist cocontraction to restore balance to force couples.
- Dynamic stabilization.
  - Rhythmic stabilization throwing Plyoball against wall.
  - Push-ups onto ball.
  - Ball throws.
- Plyometrics.
  - Two-handed drills: chest pass, overhead soccer throw, side-to-side throws.
  - Progress to one-handed drills.
- Endurance drills.
  - Wall dribbling with Plyoball
  - Wall arm circles
  - Upper body cycle
  - Low-weight, high-rep isotonic weights
- Scapular rehabilitation.
  - Open chain exercises
  - PNF
  - Diagonals
  - Plyometrics

Week 16 and Beyond

- Conventional weight training.
- Orient for return to sport.
- If indicated, obtain abduction harness (Duke-Wyre vs. Sawa).

Special Situations

- Throwers
  - Perform capsular repair at 60 degrees of external rotation.
  - Try to achieve 60 degrees of external rotation by 8 weeks.
  - Begin throwing program at 6 months.
- Atraumatic instability
  - Immobilize for 6 weeks instead of 4 weeks.
- Older than 40 years
  - Immobilize for 3 weeks instead of 4 weeks.

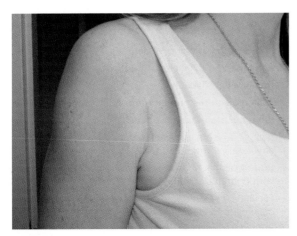

Figure 12-15. Typical cosmetic result.

REFERENCES

1. Bankart ASB. The pathology and treatment of recurrent dislocation of the shoulder-joint. *Br J Surg.* 1938;26:23-29.
2. Pagnani MJ, Warren RF. Stabilizers of the glenohumeral joint. *J Shoulder Elbow Surg.* 1994;3:173-190.
3. Pagnani MJ, Galinat BJ, Warren RF. Glenohumeral instability. In: DeLee JC, Drez D, eds. *Orthopaedic Sports Medicine.* Philadelphia, WB Saunders, 1994:580-622.
4. Rowe CR, Zarins B. Recurrent transient subluxation of the shoulder. *J Bone Joint Surg Am.* 1981;63:863-872.
5. Chen AL, Hunt SA, Hawkins RJ, et al. Management of bone loss associated with recurrent anterior glenohumeral instability. *Am J Sports Med.* 2005;33:912-925.
6. Jobe FW, Giangarra CE, Kvitne RS, et al. Anterocapsulolabral reconstruction of the shoulder in athletes in overhead sports. *Am J Sports Med.* 1991;19:428-434.
7. Pagnani MJ, Dome DC. Surgical treatment of traumatic anterior shoulder instability in American football players: two- to six-year follow-up in fifty-eight athletes. *J Bone Joint Surg Am.* 2002;84:711-715.
8. Cole BJ, L'Insalata J, Irrgang J, et al. Comparison of arthroscopic and open anterior shoulder stabilization: a two- to six-year follow-up study. *J Bone Joint Surg Am.* 2000;82:1108-1114.
9. Gill TJ, Micheli LJ, Gebhard F, et al. Bankart repair for anterior instability of the shoulder. Long-term outcome. *J Bone Joint Surg Am.* 1997;79:850-857.
10. Hubbell JD, Ahmad S, Bezenoff LS, et al. Comparison of shoulder stabilization using arthroscopic transglenoid sutures versus open capsulolabral repairs: a 5-year minimum follow-up. *Am J Sports Med.* 2004;32:650-654.
11. Uhorchak JM, Arciero RA, Huggard D, et al. Recurrent shoulder instability after open reconstruction in athletes involved in collision and contact sports. *Am J Sports Med.* 2000;28:794-799.
12. Wirth MA, Blatter G, Rockwood CA Jr. The capsular imbrication procedure for recurrent anterior instability of the shoulder. *J Bone Joint Surg Am.* 1996;78:246-260.
13. Rowe CR, Patel D, Southmayd WW. The Bankart Procedure: a long-term end-result study. *J Bone Joint Surg.* 1978;60-A:1-16.
14. Bigliani LU, Newton PM, Steinmann SP, et al. Glenoid rim lesions associated with recurrent anterior dislocation of the shoulder. *Am J Sports Med.* 1998;26:41-45.
15. Gill TJ, Zarins B. Open repairs for the treatment of anterior instability. *Am J Sport Med.* 2003;31:142-153.
16. Pagnani MJ. Open capsular repair without bone block of anterior instability in patients with and without bony defects of the glenoid and/or humeral head. *Am J Sports Med.* 2008;36:1805-1812.

Chapter 13

Open Repair of Posterior Shoulder Instability

Patrick M. Birmingham and Mark K. Bowen

Chapter Synopsis
- This chapter describes the background, etiology, diagnosis, treatment, rehabilitation, and outcomes for posterior instability of the glenohumeral joint treated with open surgical repair.

Important Points
- Distinguish type: repetitive microtrauma, traumatic, atraumatic
- Voluntary: positional or muscular
- Symptoms can be similar to those of impingent or biceps pathology
- Jerk and Kim tests on examination
- Open procedure: poor tissue, revision, bony abnormality, 3+ instability

Clinical and Surgical Pearls
- Lateral or beach chair position
- Saber incision
- Deltoid and infraspinatus split
- Determine if augmentation needed

Clinical and Surgical Pitfalls
- Stay less than 15 mm medial to glenoid to avoid suprascapular nerve
- Avoid axillary nerve and posterior humeral circumflex artery inferior to teres minor

Posterior instability accounts for only 2% to 10% of all cases of shoulder instability.[1,2] Posterior glenohumeral instability most commonly arises from acute traumatic instability, atraumatic instability, or repetitive microtrauma.[2,3] Repetitive microtrauma is the most common type and includes things such as bench-press, overhead weightlifting, rowing, swimming, and blocking in football linemen. The repetitive loading causes stretch and injury to the posterior capsule.[3] The second most frequent type is acute trauma and includes injuries sustained by football linemen, bench-press injuries, seizures, and electrocution.[2] The rarest form is atraumatic instability and is most commonly associated with generalized ligamentous laxity. Accurate diagnosis relies on a detailed history, comprehensive physical examination including special tests for posterior instability, appropriate imaging, examination under anesthesia, and intraoperative confirmation of pathology. The posterior capsule is thin in comparison with the anterior capsule, but it does contain the posterior inferior glenohumeral ligament (PIGHL). The PIGHL is the primary restraint to posteroinferior instability; it is under tension with shoulder flexion and internal rotation.[2] This is consistent with the clinical observation that the position of posteroinferior glenohumeral instability is shoulder flexion, internal rotation, and adduction. Other anatomic factors that can contribute to posterior glenohumeral instability include a dysfunctional or torn subscapularis,[4] glenoid or humeral retroversion,[5,6] glenoid hypoplasia,[5] loss of glenoid concavity as a result of labral injury,[6] compromise of the middle and superior glenohumeral ligaments,[7] and possibly a nonfunctional rotator interval.

PREOPERATIVE CONSIDERATIONS

History

Although patients may report discrete episodes of posterior dislocation, the most common presenting complaint is shoulder pain, which may be localized to the deep posterior shoulder. Patients also often describe an inability to perform certain activities, or subjective feeling of weakness.[2]

Signs and Symptoms

Symptoms can appear similar to those of subacromial impingement or biceps tendonitis; therefore, posterior instability should be on the differential diagnosis for such a presentation. Some patients will be able to voluntarily sublux the shoulder. The two types of voluntary subluxation are positional and muscular.[8] The particular type should be carefully distinguished because the surgical outcomes in these two groups are very different. Positional subluxators can reproduce the instability with flexion and internal rotation,[2,9] in the same way that a patient with anterior instability can with flexion, abduction, and external rotation. Voluntary muscular subluxators reproduce instability with the arm in adduction, and this is associated with global laxity or muscular dysfunction.[2] Patients with positional instability do well with surgery, whereas patients with muscular instability usually do poorly.[8,9]

Physical Examination

Physical examination of the shoulder should always begin with examination of the cervical spine. This should include a motor and sensory examination for all nerve roots and a provocative Spurling test for reproducible nerve impingement. Examination should then proceed to the affected shoulder, with examination of the contralateral shoulder for comparison. Anatomic symmetry should be checked first, followed by a comparative range-of-motion examination of both shoulders. Any positions of apprehension should be noted. Scapulothoracic motion should then be checked for any dyskinesis. Some common findings include posterior glenohumeral tenderness, increased external rotation, and mild loss of internal rotation. The presence of a sulcus sign can indicate posterior instability or multidirectional instability. This should be assessed with the arm at the side and in neutral rotation. Loss of the sulcus with external rotation of the arm indicates that it is probably not clinically significant. Posterior instability can be assessed with several provocative tests, which include the jerk test, the Kim test, the posterior stress test, and the load-shift test.[2]

To perform the jerk test, the examiner grasps the elbow in one hand and the clavicle and scapular spine with the other. The patient can be seated or lateral. The arm is flexed and internally rotated, the humerus is axially loaded posteriorly and inferiorly at approximately the 7-o'clock position, and the scapula is translated anteriorly. The test result is positive if a sudden jerk associated with pain occurs as the humeral head relocates.[4]

The Kim test is performed with a patient seated and the arm in 90 degrees of abduction. The elbow is grasped with one hand and the lateral arm is grasped with the

other. The humerus is then axially loaded, and while the arm is elevated to 45 degrees, a posterior force is applied to the arm. Production of pain indicates a positive test result.[10] Positive jerk and Kim test results together indicate 97% sensitivity for posterior glenohumeral instability.

The posterior stress test has been described in the seated position; however, it is sometimes easier to stabilize the scapula with the patient supine and lateralized off the edge of the examining table. The arm is flexed 90 degrees, adducted and internally rotated, and then translated posteriorly. A positive test result is present if dislocation, subluxation, pain, or apprehension occurs.[11]

The load-shift test can be performed with the patient supine or standing. The arm is forward flexed and abducted 20 degrees, and the humeral head is axially loaded and then translated anteriorly and posteriorly while the scapula is stabilized. The test is graded as anterior or posterior and as 1+, 2+, or 3+. A grade of 1+ indicates that the head translates to the glenoid rim but not over it, a grade of 2+ indicates that the head translates over the rim but spontaneously reduces, and a grade of 3+ indicates that the head translates over the rim and stays dislocated.[12]

Imaging

A complete evaluation for posterior instability with diagnostic imaging includes radiographs, magnetic resonance imaging (MRI), and in some cases computed tomography (CT).

Plain radiographs should include a standard anteroposterior view and an axillary view. These are used to assess the glenohumeral articulation. The axillary view is helpful for determining if there is any humeral or glenoid bone loss or if there is any relative retroversion of the glenoid. Findings suggestive of bone loss, abnormal version, or glenoid hypoplasia should lead to obtaining a CT scan for a complete evaluation of the bony architecture.

MRI is used to evaluate the articular cartilage, labrum, capsule, glenohumeral ligaments, rotator cuff, biceps, and bony structures. Partial avulsion injuries to the posterior labrum (Kim lesion) have been described in posterior instability and can appear as a loss of posterior labral height or a marginal labral crack.[6] Magnetic resonance arthrograms can be used; however, if the MRI is performed with a 3-tesla magnet, intraarticular contrast can often be avoided.

Indications and Contraindications

Physical therapy is the first line of treatment for posterior glenohumeral instability. It has been shown to lead to favorable improvement in two thirds of patients.[3,13]

It is most successful in patients with multidirectional instability and repetitive microtrauma.[2] Success rates for nonoperative treatment range from 89% for atraumatic subluxors to 16% for traumatic subluxors.[13] Patients with MRI evidence of a posterior labral tear are also less likely to respond to therapy.[14] A major component of therapy should focus on subscapularis strengthening because the subscapularis is an important dynamic posterior stabilizer.

For patients in whom physical therapy fails, traumatic subluxors, patients with significant posterior labral injury, patients with glenoid or humeral bone loss, and patients with abnormal humeral or glenoid version, surgery is indicated. Voluntary muscular subluxation is a contraindication for surgery because of the poor outcomes.

Arthroscopic stabilization for posterior glenohumeral instability has been described with success rates ranging from 55% to 97%.[15] Arthroscopic stabilizations are indicated as primary procedures for patients with good tissue quality and no bony abnormalities. Open posterior stabilizations should be used for revisions, poor tissue quality, glenoid retroversion, or significant glenoid bone loss. Some authors suggest that laxity graded 3+ is also an indication for open stabilization.[16]

SURGICAL TECHNIQUE

Anesthesia and Positioning

This procedure should be performed with the patient under a general anesthetic. Regional anesthesia (interscalene block with C4 coverage) may be helpful with postoperative pain management. Positioning for arthroscopy is subject to the surgeon's preference; both the lateral decubitus and beach chair positions are acceptable. Open stabilization can be performed with the patient in the beach chair position, but the exposure is difficult, and excellent assistance with retraction is required for adequate visualization, especially in a muscular shoulder. The "floppy" lateral decubitus position with the arm draped free allows easier retraction and manipulation of arm position during the surgical procedure. A mechanical arm positioning device may be helpful in positioning the limb during different portions of the procedure.

Surgical Landmarks, Incisions, and Portals

Landmarks

- Acromion
- Scapular spine
- Axillary crease
- Glenohumeral joint
- Posterolateral corner of scapula
- Posterior portal for shoulder arthroscopy centered over the glenohumeral joint

Structures at Risk

- Approach: axillary nerve, posterior humeral circumflex vessels inferior to teres minor
- Capsulotomy: suprascapular nerve, 15 mm medial to posterior labrum, along the infraspinatus

The most common incisions described for the posterior approach to the shoulder include a horizontal incision along the inferior border of the scapular spine and a "saber" type incision beginning over the acromion and continuing down toward the axillary fold. The saber incision is more common in the literature and is our preferred incision. The posterior portal used for diagnostic arthroscopy is located 1 cm inferior and 2 cm medial to the posterolateral acromial angle. In this position, the portal can be extended proximally and distally to complete the saber incision.

Examination Under Anesthesia and Arthroscopic Examination

After administration of anesthesia, a repeat physical examination including range of motion and provocative tests for posterior instability should be carried out. The degree of posterior instability should be graded if possible via the load-shift test. The presence of a sulcus sign should also be evaluated. The patient should then be draped and prepared, and diagnostic arthroscopy carried out. The joint should be evaluated in a systematic way. Our method is to begin with the superior labrum and biceps; then proceed to the subscapularis, anterior capsule, rotator cuff, humeral head, inferior pouch, posterior capsule, and labrum; and finish with the glenoid. Final determination regarding whether to proceed with an open approach is made according to the arthroscopic appearance of the tissue quality, and bony anatomy. An arthroscopic load shift can also be carried out to confirm the degree of instability.

Specific Steps

Specific steps are outlined in Box 13-1.

BOX 13-1 Surgical Steps

1. Exposure
2. Capsulotomy
3. Capsulorrhaphy
4. Augmentation
5. Closure

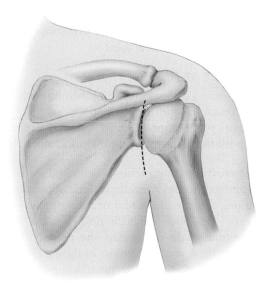

Figure 13-1. Vertical incision over glenohumeral joint.

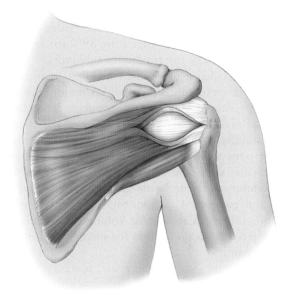

Figure 13-3. Horizontal split through infraspinatus in line with fibers; avoid unnecessary inferior dissection.

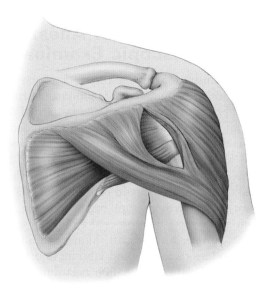

Figure 13-2. Deltoid split in line with fibers.

1. Exposure

A vertical "saber" incision is oriented from the acromial angle to the axillary fold centered over the glenohumeral joint (Fig. 13-1). The posterior portal from diagnostic arthroscopy can be incorporated into the middle of the incision. The orientation of the deltoid muscle fibers is defined, and its fascia is split in line with the fibers between the lateral and posterior heads (Fig. 13-2). The location of the deltoid split is directly over the glenohumeral joint, determined by palpation of the joint between the surgeon's thumb posteriorly and long finger anteriorly. In very muscular individuals some of the posterior deltoid head may need to be released off the scapular spine. Development of the interval in the

deltoid exposes the fascia over the infraspinatus and teres minor. The center of the joint is again reassessed by manual palpation. A yellow fat stripe in the infraspinatus muscle is frequently visible, and the bipennate anatomy of the infraspinatus makes it easy to identify. The overlying fascia is opened horizontally, and a dissection plane is made through the two heads of the infraspinatus muscle (Fig. 13-3). Alternatively, dissection can proceed through the infraspinatus–teres minor interval, but more caution is necessary not to dissect inferior to the teres minor because of the proximity of the axillary nerve. If distinguishing the tendons is difficult laterally, it is often easier to distinguish the interval medially. At this point it is critical to expose the entire posterior capsule, particularly inferiorly and laterally, where the infraspinatus is most adherent to the capsule. In some cases the infraspinatus will need to be taken down laterally for adequate exposure. Patience, blunt dissection, deep right-angled retractors, and good assistants are helpful at this stage (Fig. 13-4). Dissection should be limited to 1 cm medial of the glenoid to avoid injury to the suprascapular nerve, as it usually sits 15 mm medial to the glenoid.

2. Capsulotomy

Once the capsule is completely defined, a horizontal incision centered over the middle of the joint is made from the glenoid extending laterally. A vertical incision is made just lateral to the capsular attachment to the glenoid to make a T-shaped pattern and two mobile flaps of capsule (Fig. 13-5). Complete mobilization of the inferior and superior flaps permits successful capsulorrhaphy (Fig. 13-6).

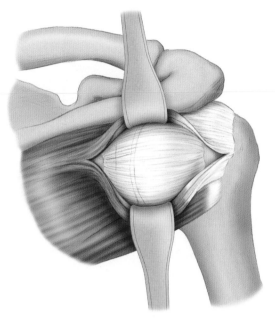

Figure 13-4. Complete exposure of inferior and lateral capsule by blunt dissection and retraction.

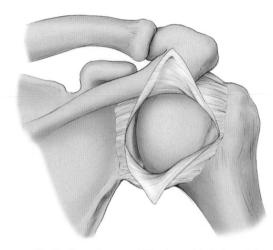

Figure 13-6. Complete mobilization of inferior and superior flaps for proper capsulorrhaphy.

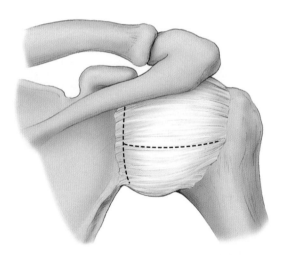

Figure 13-5. T-shaped incision based medially.

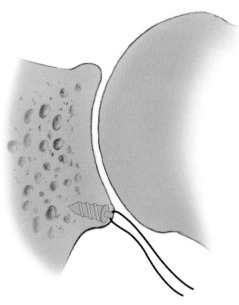

Figure 13-7. Proper placement of suture anchor, if required, at the articular margin.

3. Capsulorrhaphy

A humeral head retractor is used to investigate the posterior aspect of the glenohumeral joint. The condition of the posterior labrum can be difficult to visualize directly and is more accurately confirmed by prior arthroscopy. If the labrum is detached, suture anchors are placed under the labrum, on the posterior glenoid articular margin, after debridement and roughening with a rasp or bur (Fig. 13-7). The sutures are placed through the labrum for repair in situ, and these sutures are tied and then used for the medial repair in the capsulorrhaphy. If the labrum is intact, nonabsorbable sutures can be placed through the labrum for repair of the capsule. The medial-based capsular shift is performed with the arm in 20 degrees of abduction and neutral rotation. The inferior flap is first advanced superiorly (Fig. 13-8), and then the superior flap is shifted inferiorly, overlapping the inferior flap (Fig. 13-9). Excessive capsular redundancy is eliminated by imbricating the horizontal capsulotomy during closure, or by making a second vertical incision laterally for an H-type repair (Figs. 13-10 and 13-11).

4. Augmentation

In the case of severe capsule deficiency, revision surgery, glenoid hypoplasia, or excessive glenoid retroversion, it

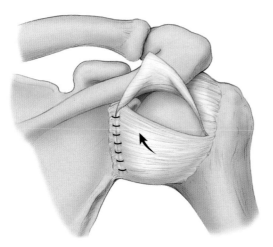

Figure 13-8. Inferior capsular flap is mobilized superiorly first.

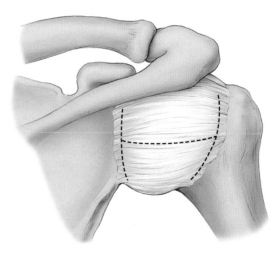

Figure 13-10. H-type incision for excessive capsular laxity.

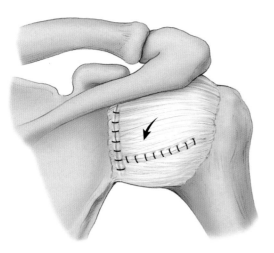

Figure 13-9. Repair is completed with inferior shift of the superior capsular flap.

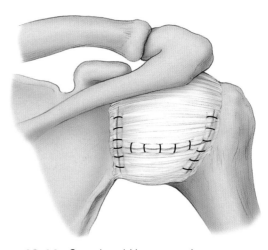

Figure 13-11. Completed H-type repair.

may be necessary to augment the repair. Soft tissue augmentation is accomplished by vertically incising the infraspinatus at the level of the glenoid and securing it to the capsule and glenoid with use of the previously placed capsule repair sutures. Rarely, an extracapsular posterior bone block can be added for cases of glenoid deficiency or at revision when repaired capsule tissue is deficient. A tricortical graft 4 × 2.5 cm may be harvested from the scapular spine. The graft and glenoid neck are predrilled before capsular repair to ensure accurate placement. The graft is placed on the posteroinferior quadrant to increase glenoid depth without impinging on the humeral head. In addition, there are several reports of opening wedge glenoid osteotomy for excessive glenoid retroversion. This is usually reserved for patients with severe instability and glenoid retroversion of more than 10 degrees as determined by CT scan.

5. Closure

Typically, sutures are not necessary in the infraspinatus split or deltoid fascia. The skin incision is closed in a standard fashion.

POSTOPERATIVE CONSIDERATIONS

Rehabilitation

Patients are immobilized in a 30-degree abduction sling or a "gunslinger" sling in neutral rotation and 30 degrees of abduction for 6 weeks. Internal rotation and adduction are restricted for the first 6 weeks. Passive range of motion is initiated on postoperative day 2, including flexion in the plane of the scapula to 120 degrees, abduction to 90 degrees, and external rotation to 30 degrees. Progressive strengthening and motion are started at 6 weeks, and return to full activity usually is achieved at 4 to 6 months. Return to full activity or sport is dependent on isokinetic internal and external rotation strength being equal to that on the unaffected side, and a pain-free shoulder.

Complications

- Recurrent instability.
- Injury to axillary nerve or posterior humeral circumflex vessels.
- Injury to suprascapular nerve and vessels.
- Overtightening of the glenohumeral joint, resulting in decreased range of motion and arthrofibrosis with loss of internal rotation.
- Infection.
- Intra-articular fracture, nonunion, degenerative arthritis, and osteonecrosis of the glenoid are risks unique to glenoid osteotomy.

RESULTS

The available literature on open posterior stabilizations suggests that subjective satisfaction outcomes range from 50% to 93% good to excellent results with mean follow-up of 34 months to 7.6 years. Recurrence rates for instability range from 0% to 30%. One of the larger series in the literature by Wolf and colleagues consisted of 44 shoulders (42 with posterior instability and/or multidirectional instability, 32 with isolated posterior instability) with a mean follow-up of 7.6 years for posterior capsular plication. In this series 76% had good to excellent results, 13% had a recurrence of instability, and 74% were able to return to their previous level of activity. The presence of a chondral injury at the time of surgery was a negative prognostic indicator. Overall, 80% of the shoulders were rated as good or excellent by use of an 8-point rating system based on stability, pain, range of motion, and level of activity, as compared with an overall satisfactory outcome in 84% in the series.[16]

In another series of 26 shoulders by Fuchs and colleagues, 92% of patients had good to excellent subjective outcomes and 23% had a recurrence at a mean of 7.6 years. Recurrence was associated with previous posterior glenohumeral surgery or with new traumatic injury. The average postoperative Constant score was 91%.[9]

REFERENCES

1. Antoniou J, Duckworth DT, Harryman DT 2nd. Capsulolabral augmentation for the management of posteroinferior instability of the shoulder. *J Bone Joint Surg Am.* 2000;82(9):1220-1230.

2. Provencher MT, LeClere LE, King S, et al. Posterior instability of the shoulder: diagnosis and management. *Am J Sports Med.* 2011;39(4):874-886.

3. Fronek J, Warren RF, Bowen M. Posterior subluxation of the glenohumeral joint. *J Bone Joint Surg Am.* 1989;71(2):205-216.

4. Blasier RB, Soslowsky LJ, Malicky DM, et al. Posterior glenohumeral subluxation: active and passive stabilization in a biomechanical model. *J Bone Joint Surg Am.* 1997;79(3):433-440.

5. Inui H, Sugamoto K, Miyamoto T, et al. Glenoid shape in atraumatic posterior instability of the shoulder. *Clin Orthop Relat Res.* 2002;403:87-92.

6. Kim SH, Noh KC, Park JS, et al. Loss of chondrolabral containment of the glenohumeral joint in atraumatic posteroinferior multidirectional instability. *J Bone Joint Surg Am.* 2005;87(1):92-98.

7. O'Brien SJ, Neves MC, Arnoczky SP, et al. The anatomy and histology of the inferior glenohumeral ligament complex of the shoulder. *Am J Sports Med.* 1990;18(5):449-456.

8. Millett PJ, Clavert P, Hatch GF 3rd, et al. Recurrent posterior shoulder instability. *J Am Acad Orthop Surg.* 2006;14(8):464-476.

9. Fuchs B, Jost B, Gerber C. Posterior-inferior capsular shift for the treatment of recurrent, voluntary posterior subluxation of the shoulder. *J Bone Joint Surg Am.* 2000;82(1):16-25.

10. Kim SH, Park JS, Jeong WK, et al. The Kim test: a novel test for posteroinferior labral lesion of the shoulder—a comparison to the jerk test. *Am J Sports Med.* 2005;33(8):1188-1192.

11. Pollock RG, Bigliani LU. Recurrent posterior shoulder instability. Diagnosis and treatment. *Clin Orthop Relat Res.* 1993;291:85-96.

12. Gerber C, Ganz R. Clinical assessment of instability of the shoulder. With special reference to anterior and posterior drawer tests. *J Bone Joint Surg Br.* 1984;66(4):551-556.

13. Burkhead WZ Jr, Rockwood CA Jr. Treatment of instability of the shoulder with an exercise program. *J Bone Joint Surg Am.* 1992;74(6):890-896.

14. Provencher MT, Bell SJ, Menzel KA, et al. Arthroscopic treatment of posterior shoulder instability: results in 33 patients. *Am J Sports Med.* 2005;33(10):1463-1471.

15. Savoie FH 3rd, Holt MS, Field LD, et al. Arthroscopic management of posterior instability: evolution of technique and results. *Arthroscopy.* 2008;24(4):389-396.

16. Wolf BR, Strickland S, Williams RJ, et al. Open posterior stabilization for recurrent posterior glenohumeral instability. *J Shoulder Elbow Surg.* 2005;14(2):157-164.

SUGGESTED READINGS

Bigliani LU, Pollock RG, McIlveen SJ, et al. Shift of the posteroinferior aspect of the capsule for recurrent posterior glenohumeral instability. *J Bone Joint Surg Am.* 1995;77(7):1011-1020.

Fronek J, Warren RF, Bowen M. Posterior subluxation of the glenohumeral joint. *J Bone Joint Surg Am*. 1989;71(2): 205-216.

Fuchs B, Jost B, Gerber C. Posterior-inferior capsular shift for the treatment of recurrent, voluntary posterior subluxation of the shoulder. *J Bone Joint Surg Am*. 2000;82(1): 16-25.

Provencher MT, LeClere LE, King S, et al. Posterior instability of the shoulder: diagnosis and management. *Am J Sports Med*. 2011;39(4):874-886.

Tibone JE, Bradley JP. The treatment of posterior subluxation in athletes. *Clin Orthop Relat Res*. 1993;291:124-137.

Chapter 14

Open Repair of Multidirectional Instability

Pradeep Kodali and Gordon Nuber

Chapter Synopsis

- Multidirectional instability (MDI) is a traumatic or atraumatic condition resulting in the ability to dislocate or subluxate the glenohumeral joint anteriorly, posteriorly, and inferiorly. Patients with atraumatic MDI generally have pathologic laxity contributing to their instability. Treatment is initially conservative. This chapter describes the classic surgical treatment for this problem—the open inferior capsular shift.

Important Points

- Operative treatment is reserved for patients who demonstrate persistent symptoms after a structured rehabilitation program.
- Avoid surgery in voluntary dislocators with psychiatric problems or those for whom pain is the only complaint.
- Open inferior capsular shift is the classic and still gold standard treatment, though arthroscopic techniques are becoming more popular.
- An anterior approach to the inferior capsular shift can provide global stability by decreasing capsular volume. Care should be taken to avoid overtensioning the subscapularis repair.

Clinical and Surgical Pearls

- A standard deltopectoral approach can be used.
- A humeral- or glenoid-based T-shaped capsulotomy is used, with the inferior flap advancement being the key to adequate reduction of capsular volume.
- Confirm adequate T-shaped capsulotomy by placing the index finger in the pouch and assessing for extrusion of the finger as the inferior flap is advanced.
- Close the rotator interval.

Clinical and Surgical Pitfalls

- Always be aware of the location of the axillary nerve; it is the main neurovascular risk in the technique. It can be avoided by making sure to stay on bone while releasing the capsule off the humerus.
- Ensure adequate capsulotomy by using the index finger in the pouch technique.
- Avoid overtensioning the subscapularis. This can be avoided by careful closure of the subscapularis tenotomy or by using a subscapularis split technique.

One of the earliest descriptions of multidirectional instability (MDI) was offered by Neer and Foster in 1980, who described this pathologic entity as the ability to dislocate or subluxate the glenohumeral joint anteriorly, posteriorly, and inferiorly. They also reported that patients were most symptomatic during mid–range of motion while performing activities of daily living.[1] MDI is described as global shoulder laxity that can be congenital, acquired, or both. It is primarily caused by the combination of a redundant inferior capsular pouch, lax ligaments about the shoulder, and weakened musculotendinous structures.[2-4] Congenital laxity often occurs in multiple joints of the body in conditions such as

Marfan syndrome. Acquired laxity is found in competitive athletes, specifically gymnasts and swimmers. The combination of both is found in individuals who have baseline laxity who become symptomatic after mild to moderate trauma. Diagnosis is largely by clinical examination; however, magnetic resonance imaging (MRI) can be helpful to evaluate the presence and extent of a traumatic component. The mainstay of treatment is nonoperative management focusing on physical therapy that involves strength and neuromuscular coordination of the rotator cuff, deltoid, and scapula.[4,5] Operative management is reserved for those refractory to conservative measures. The open inferior capsular shift, as originally described by Neer and Foster,[1] stabilizes the shoulder by decreasing capsular volume and has been the operative treatment of choice. With advances in arthroscopic techniques, the amount of capsular volume reduction is comparable to that with the open technique.[6] The results of arthroscopic techniques have been promising, and as a result the open procedure is used less frequently but remains an option, especially in those in whom arthroscopic treatment has failed.[7,8]

PREOPERATIVE CONSIDERATIONS

History

Most patients are young adults and can have bilateral symptoms. It is important to ascertain a family history of similar complaints to evaluate for congenital causes. A psychiatric history (i.e., in voluntary or intentional dislocators) may preclude individuals from undergoing surgery.[1,4] Pain is the most common presenting complaint and is generally provoked by normal daily activities. Also, a sense of instability is a frequent complaint. It is important to differentiate whether patients have pathologic hyperlaxity with pain versus laxity with pain and instability. Patients with pain and without instability have relatively poor outcomes compared with those who demonstrate instability.[9] Rarely patients may report numbness, tingling, and weakness of the affected extremity.

Physical Examination

The mainstay of diagnosis is physical examination. Basic shoulder examination includes inspection for muscle atrophy, palpation for any point tenderness, and active and passive range of motion to evaluate shoulder biomechanics. As with any complete examination of the shoulder, the physician should evaluate the cervical spine. Signs of global ligamentous laxity including elbow hyperextension, ability to touch the thumb to the forearm (Fig. 14-1), and patellar subluxation are frequently observed. A positive sulcus and/or apprehension sign is common (Fig. 14-2). We also use the load and shift test to quantify both anterior and posterior laxity (Fig. 14-3).[10] This is done by placing the shoulder off the edge of the table in 90 degrees of abduction and applying an anterior and posterior translational force. The result is graded as minimal translation (trace), humeral head translation to the rim (1+), translation over the rim with spontaneous reduction (2+), and

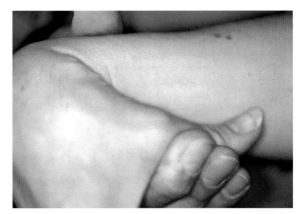

Figure 14-1. Thumb-to-forearm test demonstrating ligamentous laxity.

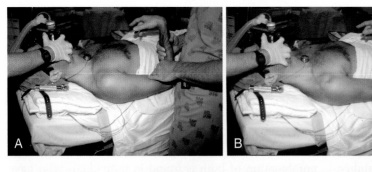

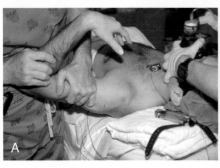
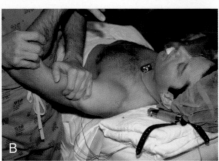

Figure 14-2. A, Shoulder before sulcus test. **B,** Sulcus sign with longitudinal pull on the arm.

Figure 14-3. A, Load-shift test for anterior instability. **B,** Load-shift test for posterior instability.

dislocation (3+). The contralateral shoulder should be evaluated for laxity as well. Additional maneuvers to demonstrate increased translation include the Fukuda test and the jerk test.[4]

Imaging

MDI typically can be diagnosed clinically. However, plain radiographs can be obtained to rule out bony abnormalities such as a bony Bankart or Hill-Sachs lesion. Bone defects are typically present in traumatic cases and less common in atraumatic cases with pathologic capsular laxity causing MDI. Computed tomography (CT) or magnetic resonance arthrography (MRA) can be used to evaluate capsular volume.

Indications and Contraindications

Conservative management remains the treatment of choice. Initial management should include a period of immobilization and anti-inflammatory drugs for an acute exacerbation. It is thought that MDI is caused in part by stretching of the static shoulder stabilizers. Therefore treatment should initially involve strengthening of the shoulder stabilizers including the rotator cuff muscles and deltoid. Conditioning of the upper thoracic muscles and the scapular stabilizers is also important for stability.[2] A change in lifestyle to limit pain-provoking activities such as overhead work is recommended. A formal two-phase rehabilitation program including Thera-Band and lightweight exercises, focused on strengthening of the rotator cuff and deltoid muscles, has also been described.[5] The primary indication for operative treatment is a failure of conservative management with persistent pain.[1,2,4,11,12] Those in whom conservative management is likely to fail include patients with unilateral involvement, difficulties performing activities of daily living, and higher grades of laxity on initial examination.[12] Contraindications to surgical treatment include noncompliance during a trial of conservative management, voluntary dislocation, and the presence of psychiatric abnormalities.[1,13] A poor prognostic indicator, particular in athletes, is bilateral MDI requiring bilateral repair.[13] The risk of limited range of motion compared with the contralateral shoulder and, conversely, persistent patholaxity should be a significant part of any preoperative discussion regarding this problem.

Historically, surgical options have included thermal capsular shrinkage, glenoid osteotomy, or humeral osteotomy.[4,14,15] The open inferior capsular shift, as described by Neer and Foster, has been the most commonly performed open procedure for this problem, with arthroscopic techniques now becoming increasingly common. The inferior capsular shift procedure reduces total capsular volume by releasing the inferior capsule and shifting it superiorly.[1,11]

SURGICAL TECHNIQUE
Anesthesia and Positioning

We prefer an interscalene block in combination with general anesthesia, with regional anesthesia providing excellent postoperative pain control. Local anesthesia with infiltration of the skin and subcutaneous tissue is also used. The patient can be positioned supine or 20 degrees upright. Although some authors state that all inferior capsular shift procedures can be performed through an anterior approach,[11] others believe the approach should be determined by the primary direction of instability, as described by the patient or determined on physical examination.[1,13,16] We use an anterior approach for MDI and feel that a reduction in capsular volume can treat instability in all directions in these patients. For the anterior approach the patient is placed in a supine position with a rolled towel positioned between the thoracic spine and medial border of the scapula.[17] If a posterior approach is chosen, the surgeon must keep in mind that a separate anterior incision may be needed if a Bankart lesion is identified intraoperatively. If a large posterior labral tear is identified on preoperative imaging, a combined arthroscopy to treat the labral tear with an open inferior capsular shift is an option, though most will elect arthroscopic management for the entire problem. An examination under anesthesia is imperative for thorough understanding of the pathology.[1,4,10]

Surgical Landmarks

- Acromion
- Coracoid process
- Axillary fold

Examination Under Anesthesia

An examination under anesthesia should be performed to document motion and direction of instability before surgical stabilization. An assessment of the degree of capsular redundancy can be accomplished by the sulcus test. This is performed by applying downward traction to the adducted arm (see Fig. 14-2) followed by assessing the degree of downward displacement in varying degrees of external rotation.[10] Persistent inferior displacement with downward traction (sulcus sign) with external rotation may suggest a contribution from the rotator interval. The load and shift assesses the relative degree of anterior and/or posterior instability (see Fig. 14-3). Finally, diagnostic arthroscopy can aid in

BOX 14-1 Surgical Steps—Anterior Approach

1. Deltopectoral approach
2. Subscapularis tenotomy
3. T-capsulotomy
4. Preparing the reattachment site
5. Capsular shift
6. Subscapularis repair and closure

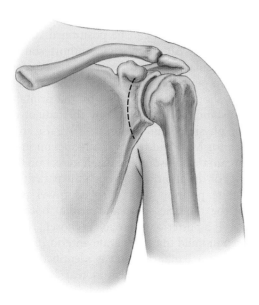

Figure 14-4. Incision for deltopectoral approach.

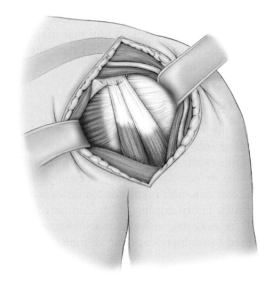

Figure 14-5. The deltopectoral interval is developed, showing the subscapularis.

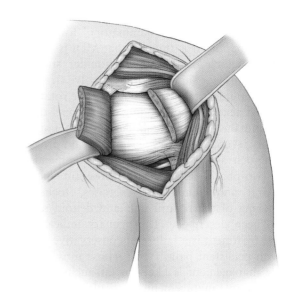

Figure 14-6. Reflect the subscapularis, leaving a stump for reattachment.

identifying associated Bankart or posterior labral lesions before continuation with the open procedure.

Specific Steps

Anterior Approach

The anterior approach is described in Box 14-1.

1. Deltopectoral Approach

The landmark for this approach is the coracoid process. The technique for the inferior capsular shift is very similar to that used in the original series by Neer and Foster.[1] Various modifications have been made since then. The incision should be made from the tip of the coracoid process to the axilla along the deltopectoral groove (Fig. 14-4).[18] The deltopectoral interval is developed medial to the cephalic vein, retracting the deltoid laterally and the pectoralis medially (Fig. 14-5). Divide the clavipectoral fascia and retract the coracobrachialis and the short head of the biceps medially. Identify and ligate the anterior humeral circumflex vessels located at the inferior border of the tendinous portion of the subscapularis. Place the arm in external rotation, and divide the subscapularis 1.0 cm medial to its insertion,

carefully developing a plane between the subscapularis tendon and capsule. Tag the proximal end and retract medially (Fig. 14-6). In athletes who rely heavily on upper extremity function, consider use of a subscapularis splitting approach.[19] It has been shown to result in a higher rate of return to professional level activity. Close the rotator interval between the superior and middle glenohumeral ligaments with absorbable suture if a lesion is present. Identify and protect the axillary nerve as it crosses near the inferior border of the capsule.

2. T-Capsulotomy

Make a T-shaped capsulotomy, starting the horizontal limb medially between the superior and middle

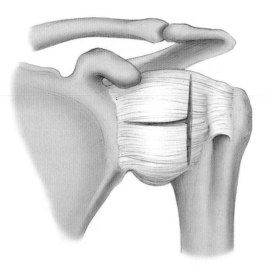

Figure 14-7. The humeral-based T-shaped capsular incision.

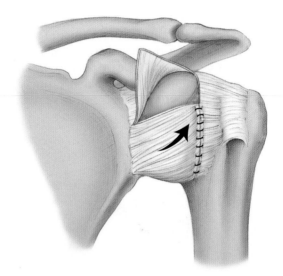

Figure 14-9. The inferior flap is brought up and sutured to the humeral side to decrease the volume of the inferior pouch.

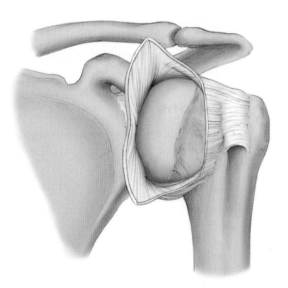

Figure 14-8. The joint is now exposed after the T-shaped capsular incision.

glenohumeral ligaments, extending the incision infero-laterally toward the humeral neck (Fig. 14-7).[10] Place the arm in external rotation and release the inferior capsule from the humeral neck, proceeding posteriorly. Tag the inferior flap at its corner. One technique to assess adequate reduction in capsular volume is to place a finger in the inferior capsular pouch and pull the capsular stitch superiorly until the surgeon's finger is extruded. If it does not extrude, then extend the capsular incision around the humeral neck even further posteriorly.[10,16] Inspect the joint for any loose bodies or labral pathology (Fig. 14-8).

3. Preparing the Reattachment Site

With a curette or high-speed bur, decorticate the anterior and inferior sulcus of the humeral neck to obtain a bleeding bed of bone.

4. Capsular Shift

Suture the capsular flap to the stump of the subscapularis tendon and to the part of the capsule that remains on the humerus. Alternatively, the capsule can be sutured directly into the humerus with the aid of suture anchors. Select the appropriate tension on the flap to eliminate the inferior pouch and reduce the posterior capsular redundancy. Place the arm in 40 degrees of abduction and 40 degrees of external rotation. Advance the inferior flap superiorly such that it is repaired to the bleeding bed of cancellous bone and to the lateral aspect of capsule (Fig. 14-9). Use nonabsorbable sutures in a pants-over-vest fashion.[11] The superior flap is advanced distally and laterally and repaired in a similar fashion to reinforce the anterior capsule (Fig. 14-10). This also allows the middle glenohumeral ligament to reinforce the capsule anteriorly.

5. Subscapularis Repair and Closure

The subscapularis tendon is brought over the capsular shift and repaired to the stump with multiple nonabsorbable sutures, with care taken not to overtension the repair. Close the deltopectoral interval with absorbable sutures and the skin and subcutaneous tissues in usual fashion.

An alternative to the humeral-based capsular incision is the glenoid-based capsulotomy. Similar concepts apply with regard to capsular advancement (Fig. 14-11). However, the flaps are attached to the glenoid margin, commonly with suture anchors.[20-22]

Posterior Approach

In our experience, most cases of MDI can be treated with the anterior approach, as the typical presentation involves anterior instability as the primary component. Cooper and Brems advocate use of the anterior approach for all cases, including those with posterior instability as the primary component.[11] Please refer to the chapter on the posterior approach for instability surgery for further detail on this procedure.

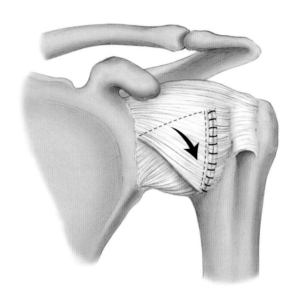

Figure 14-10. After advancement of the inferior flap *(arrow)*, the superior flap is brought down to and sutured to the humeral side.

POSTOPERATIVE CONSIDERATIONS

Rehabilitation

Postoperative care is integral to the healing process. We base our method of immobilization on the primary direction of instability. For anterior instability, patients can typically be discharged in a sling; for posterior instability, we advocate use of a gunslinger brace. After a 6-week period of immobilization, gradual range-of-motion exercises are initiated according to a strict protocol. Overzealous patients doing too much too early can develop recurrent instability. During weeks 6 through 10, below-the-shoulder exercises are conducted, limiting external rotation to 45 degrees. Beginning in week 10 a stretching program is initiated, focusing on forward elevation and external rotation. At weeks 14 to 16, deltoid and rotator cuff strengthening is added, followed by scapular stabilization exercises at weeks 18 to 20. Contact sports are typically allowed only after complete restoration of strength and condition, usually about 6 months after surgery.

Complications

Reported complications include recurrent instability, persistent symptoms of apprehension, axillary nerve neurapraxia, stiffness, and infection.

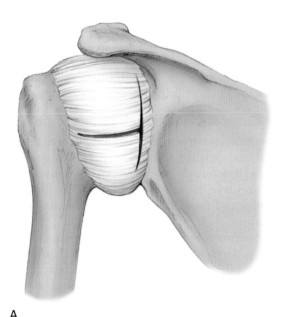

A

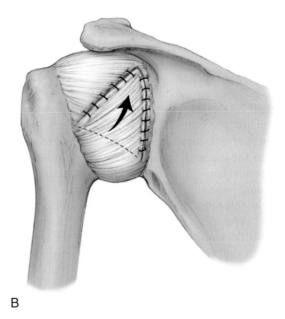

B

Figure 14-11. Glenoid-based capsular shift. *(Modified from Bowen M, Warren R. Surgical approaches to posterior instability of shoulder. In: Operative Techniques in Sports Medicine, vol 1, no 4, Philadelphia: WB Saunders; 1993.)*

TABLE 14-1. Results of Inferior Capsular Shift

Study	Successful Results/Number of Shoulders	Follow-up	Recurrent Instability (%)
Neer and Foster[1] (1980)	39/40	Variable*	3
Cooper and Brems[11] (1992)	39/43	2-6 yr	9
Bak et al[19] (2000)	24/26	Median, 54 mo	8
Pollock et al[16] (2000)	46/49	Average, 61 mo	4
Choi and Ogilvie-Harris[13] (2002)	48/53	Average, 42 mo	9
Tillander et al[9] (1998)	12/14†	9-53 mo	NA
van Tankeren et al[4] (2002)	14/17	Mean, 39 mo	6‡

*Less than 12 months, eight shoulders; 12-24 months, 15 shoulders; longer than 24 months, 17 shoulders.

†Patients with multidirectional laxity and instability did best.

‡Without any associated injuries.

NA, Not available.

RESULTS

Historical results of the open procedure have been good. However, with increasing success of arthroscopic techniques, the role of the open procedure is diminishing. In our practice the arthroscopic approach is used as the primary procedure, with a formal inferior capsular shift reserved for patients in whom arthroscopic measures have failed. In Neer and Foster's original series, 39 of 40 shoulders had good results.[1] Cooper and Brems reported that 39 of 48 shoulders functioned well and without instability after up to 6 years of follow-up.[11] Four shoulders had recurrent instability, and the patients were subjectively dissatisfied. The authors also stated that if failure occurs, it tends to happen early in the postoperative period. van Tankeren and colleagues reported excellent results based on objective scores in 14 of 17 shoulders at a mean follow-up of 39 months.[4] Pollock and colleagues described good or excellent results in 46 of 49 shoulders with an average follow-up of more than 5 years (Table 14-1).[16]

REFERENCES

1. Neer 2nd CS, Foster CR. Inferior capsular shift for involuntary inferior and multidirectional instability of the shoulder. A preliminary report. *J Bone Joint Surg Am.* 1980;62:897-908.
2. An YH, Friedman RJ. Multidirectional instability of the glenohumeral joint. *Orthop Clin North Am.* 2000;31:275-285.
3. Schenk TJ, Brems JJ. Multidirectional instability of the shoulder: pathophysiology, diagnosis, and management. *J Am Acad Orthop Surg.* 1998;6:65-72.
4. van Tankeren E, de Waal Malefijt MC, van Loon CJ. Open capsular shift for multi directional shoulder instability. *Arch Orthop Trauma Surg.* 2002;122:447-450.
5. Burkhead Jr WZ, Rockwood Jr CA. Treatment of instability of the shoulder with an exercise program. *J Bone Joint Surg Am.* 1992;74:890-896.
6. Sekiya JK, Willobee JA, Miller MD, et al. Arthroscopic multi-pleated capsular plication compared with open inferior capsular shift for reduction of shoulder volume in a cadaveric model. *Arthroscopy.* 2007;23:1145-1151.
7. Baker 3rd CL, Mascarenhas R, Kline AJ, et al. Arthroscopic treatment of multidirectional shoulder instability in athletes: a retrospective analysis of 2- to 5-year clinical outcomes. *Am J Sports Med.* 2009;37:1712-1720.
8. Voigt C, Schulz AP, Lill H. Arthroscopic treatment of multidirectional glenohumeral instability in young overhead athletes. *Open Orthop J.* 2009;3:107-114.
9. Tillander B, Lysholm M, Norlin R. Multidirectional hyperlaxity of the shoulder: results of treatment. *Scand J Med Sci Sports.* 1998;8:421-425.
10. Levine WN, Prickett WD, Prymka M, et al. Treatment of the athlete with multidirectional shoulder instability. *Orthop Clin North Am.* 2001;32:475-484.
11. Cooper RA, Brems JJ. The inferior capsular-shift procedure for multidirectional instability of the shoulder. *J Bone Joint Surg Am.* 1992;74:1516-1521.
12. Misamore GW, Sallay PI, Didelot W. A longitudinal study of patients with multidirectional instability of the shoulder with seven- to ten-year follow-up. *J Shoulder Elbow Surg.* 2005;14:466-470.
13. Choi CH, Ogilvie-Harris DJ. Inferior capsular shift operation for multidirectional instability of the shoulder in players of contact sports. *Br J Sports Med.* 2002;36:290-294.
14. Fitzgerald BT, Watson BT, Lapoint JM. The use of thermal capsulorrhaphy in the treatment of multidirectional instability. *J Shoulder Elbow Surg.* 2002;11:108-113.
15. Surin V, Blader S, Markhede G, et al. Rotational osteotomy of the humerus for posterior instability of the shoulder. *J Bone Joint Surg Am.* 1990;72:181-186.
16. Pollock RG, Owens JM, Flatow EL, et al. Operative results of the inferior capsular shift procedure for

multidirectional instability of the shoulder. *J Bone Joint Surg Am*. 2000;82:919-928.

17. Hoppenfeld S, DeBoer P, Buckley R. *Surgical exposures in orthopaedics: the anatomic approach*. Philadelphia: Lippincott Williams & Wilkins; 2009.

18. Leslie J, Ryan T. The anterior axillary incision to approach the shoulder joint. *J Bone Joint Surg Am*. 1962;44: 1193-1196.

19. Bak K, Spring BJ, Henderson JP. Inferior capsular shift procedure in athletes with multidirectional instability based on isolated capsular and ligamentous redundancy. *Am J Sports Med*. 2000;28:466-471.

20. Altchek DW, Warren RF, Skyhar MJ, et al. T-plasty modification of the Bankart procedure for multidirectional instability of the anterior and inferior types. *J Bone Joint Surg Am*. 1991;73:105-112.

21. Cordasco F, Pollock R, Flatow E, et al. Management of multidirectional instability. *Oper Tech Sports Med*. 1993;1:293-300.

22. Marquardt B, Potzl W, Witt KA, et al. A modified capsular shift for atraumatic anterior-inferior shoulder instability. *Am J Sports Med*. 2005;33:1011-1015.

Chapter 15

Treatment of Combined Bone Defects of Humeral Head and Glenoid: Arthroscopic and Open Techniques

Jack G. Skendzel and Jon K. Sekiya

Chapter Synopsis

- Traumatic anterior dislocation of the glenohumeral joint is associated with osteoarticular injury, including glenoid bone loss (bone Bankart lesion) and compression fractures of the posterosuperior humeral head (Hill-Sachs lesion). Recognition of bony lesions is critical to prevent an imbalance of static and dynamic forces that contribute to shoulder stability. Failure to recognize and address bone loss can lead to recurrent instability and poor clinical results. This chapter focuses on anatomic osteoarticular allograft reconstruction for bony Bankart and Hill-Sachs lesions to reduce the risk of recurrent instability and improve postoperative outcomes.

Important Points

- Shoulder instability is often multifactorial; thus a thorough evaluation is warranted to identify all pathologic conditions contributing to instability.
- Plain radiographs often underestimate the size of the glenoid or humeral head defect. Computed tomography scans with three-dimensional reconstruction allow for the best assessment of lesion size and orientation.
- Osteoarticular allograft reconstruction is indicated for patients with symptomatic defects of the glenoid and/or humeral head, engaging lesions, or inverted pear glenoids. Overhead athletes may benefit by prevention of restrictions in postoperative motion.
- Reconstruction is recommended for glenoid defects greater than 25% to 30% of the articular surface, and Hill-Sachs defects encompassing 20% to 40% of the humeral head.
- Contraindications to reconstruction include advanced degenerative glenohumeral osteoarthritis, humeral head avascular necrosis, unaddressed rotator cuff deficiency, and advanced age.

Clinical and Surgical Pearls

- Glenoid reconstruction can be performed through an open deltopectoral approach with takedown of the subscapularis or through an arthroscopic approach without subscapularis takedown via a capsulotomy in the rotator interval.
- Preservation of the subscapularis allows for a more rapid and aggressive postoperative rehabilitation protocol.
- For cases of isolated humeral head defects without anterior pathology, the lesion is best exposed through a limited posterior approach with an infraspinatus split at the tendinous raphe.
- Diagnostic arthroscopy may be performed alone before the definitive procedure to allow for thorough inspection and measurement of the size and orientation of the defects and to evaluate soft tissue and chondral injury.
- Remove remaining anterior soft tissues until a clear view of the glenoid rim is present; measure the size and orientation of the glenoid defect, and fashion the graft with a microsagittal saw, rongeur, and/or motorized bur.
- Nonabsorbable sutures are passed through the peripheral edge of the glenoid allograft articular surface to aid in reduction through the capsulotomy and for later plication of anterior capsulolabral structures.
- Provisional fixation of the glenoid allograft is performed with 0.045 K-wires; definitive fixation is with 4.0-mm partially threaded cortical screws.
- Fix the humeral head allograft with headless compression screws that are countersunk below the articular cartilage surface. Take the shoulder through a range of motion to ensure that the screws are sufficiently countersunk.

Continued

Clinical and Surgical Pitfalls

- Potential complications include graft nonunion, failure of the graft to incorporate to host bone, and hardware failure.
- Certain allografts may be difficult to obtain from tissue banks and thus should be arranged for in advance.
- Be cautious of aggressive capsular shift once the glenoid allograft has been placed; the graft itself takes up considerable volume, and the humeral-based shift may not need to be as extensive as anticipated.

- It is important that the humeral head allograft be obtained from the exact location of the defect so that the graft is matched with respect to radius of curvature to the native humeral head.
- No long-term data are available.

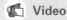 **Video**

- Video 15-1

Traumatic anterior dislocation of the glenohumeral joint is frequently associated with disruption of the anteroinferior capsulolabral structures, the so-called Bankart lesion.[1,2] Surgical treatment of Bankart lesions has demonstrated long-term success in reducing the rate of recurrent instability after first-time anterior shoulder dislocation (10% vs. 58% for 3- to 10-year results) when compared with nonoperative treatment.[3] However, glenohumeral dislocation is also associated with a high prevalence of osteoarticular injury, including glenoid bone loss (bony Bankart lesions) and compression fractures of the posterosuperior humeral head (Hill-Sachs lesion).[2,4] Frequently, recurrent anterior glenohumeral instability is associated with bone loss. Hill-Sachs defects are present in up to 100% of first-time anterior dislocations, and anteroinferior glenoid bone deficiency has been reported in 22% of primary dislocations.[1,2,4-6] Because the glenohumeral joint is minimally constrained, bony defects can significantly alter the balance of static and dynamic forces that contribute to shoulder stability. Therefore recognition of bony Bankart and Hill-Sachs lesions is critical for formulation of a thoughtful treatment plan and prevention of recurrent instability.

Bankart repair with anterior glenoid bone loss can lead to unpredictable outcomes and a high failure rate. Burkhart and de Beer[7] retrospectively reviewed 194 cases of arthroscopic Bankart repair, dividing patients into two groups—those with significant bone defects of the glenoid or humeral head, and those without such defects. If a soft-tissue repair was performed in patients with significant bone defects (inverted-pear glenoid or "engaging" Hill-Sachs lesion), there was a 67% recurrence rate compared with 4% in patients without significant bone defects. Several other authors have demonstrated similar results, suggesting that anterior glenoid bone loss as an important risk factor for recurrent shoulder instability.[8-11]

Hill-Sachs lesions also play a role in recurrent instability. Rowe and colleagues[12] initially reported a 76% incidence of Hill-Sachs lesions in failed instability surgery, and Burkhart and de Beer[7] reported engaging Hill-Sachs lesions to be associated with failed instability

surgery in 100% of cases. Boileau and colleagues[9] reported that 84% of patients with recurrent traumatic anterior shoulder instability had a Hill-Sachs lesion and that large lesions were significantly correlated with recurrent instability. Several cadaveric studies have also demonstrated a decrease in glenohumeral stability after the creation of posterosuperior humeral head bone defects.[13,14] Balg and Boileau[15] developed a preoperative assessment to determine which patients are at risk for recurrent instability after a Bankart repair, identifying the presence of a Hill-Sachs lesion and glenoid bone loss as important factors to consider in planning surgical reconstruction.

Historically, the goal of treatment has been to create a stable glenohumeral joint and prevent recurrent instability. Numerous nonanatomic techniques have been described, including transfer of the coracoid process[16] (Bristow and Latarjet procedures), open capsular shift[17,18] (Putti-Platt and Magnusson-Stack procedures), infraspinatus transfer into the Hill-Sachs defect[19] (Remplissage), and rotational humeral osteotomy.[20] More recently, anatomic reconstruction techniques have also been described to address both glenoid and humeral head bone loss. The use of iliac crest autograft,[21] distal tibia allograft,[22] femoral head allograft,[23] or glenoid allograft[24,25] has been reported to restore normal glenoid contour and glenohumeral biomechanics. Similarly, humeral head convexity can be restored with a humeroplasty,[26,27] arthroscopic mosaicplasty with fresh-frozen allograft plugs,[28] osteoconductive graft plugs,[29] and humeral head allograft reconstruction.[30-32] These anatomic techniques theoretically allow for improved postoperative motion and decrease the risk of recurrent instability while avoiding the complications of nonanatomic techniques.[33,34]

The surgical management of shoulder instability aims to develop techniques that reduce the risk of recurrent instability while promoting postoperative range of motion and strength, especially in overhead athletes. Although no anatomic reconstruction method has proven superior to another, further investigation is required to document their long-term success. In the appropriate setting, combined reconstructive procedures to address both glenoid and humeral head bone loss can be performed. This chapter focuses on osteoarticular allograft reconstruction of significant glenoid and humeral head bone defects.

PREOPERATIVE CONSIDERATIONS

History

A thorough and detailed clinical history is obtained. Shoulder instability is often multifactorial; thus a thorough approach is warranted to properly identify all pathologic conditions contributing to instability. Important points including the mechanism of injury, the frequency of current symptoms, any arm positions that cause pain or recurrent dislocation, and the patient's activity level must be documented. Typically patients dislocate the shoulder after high-energy injury, as in a fall, motor vehicle trauma, or contact sports. Any prior treatments (surgical and nonsurgical) are important for preoperative planning and to help understand why the patient continues to have recurrent instability. Often patients with recurrent glenohumeral instability and bony defects will have already undergone multiple instability procedures without success. The goals of treatment depend on the patient's overall activity level and occupation.

Physical Examination

The physical examination proceeds in a systematic fashion, beginning with inspection. Any previous surgical scars are noted. Active and passive range of motion and rotator cuff strength are tested and compared with the contralateral unaffected arm. Instability is assessed in the anterior, posterior, and inferior directions. Instability is graded on a three-point scale. Typically, patients with soft-tissue Bankart lesions will experience apprehension at 90 degrees of shoulder abduction and 90 degrees of external rotation; in those with bone defects the examiner may note apprehension at lower angles of abduction and external rotation (ABER), termed the *bony apprehension test*.[35] Because pain may limit the in-office examination, all findings are verified later with a complete examination under anesthesia.

Imaging

Radiography

- Anteroposterior view (internal and external rotation)
- True glenohumeral anteroposterior view (Grashey view)
- Axillary lateral view
- Stryker notch view (evaluate Hill-Sachs lesions)
- West Point view (evaluate glenoid rim)

Other Modalities

Plain radiographs often underestimate the size of the glenoid or Hill-Sachs defect. Computed tomography (CT) scans (including three-dimensional reconstructions) offer the best assessment of the size and orientation of the defect. In addition, CT scans are helpful for preoperative measurements to confidently and consistently obtain the proper size-matched glenoid or proximal humeral allograft before surgery.

Magnetic resonance imaging (MRI) with or without intra-articular contrast material is helpful to detect associated soft tissue injury. If possible, the study may be more useful if performed with the arm in the ABER position. This may provide further clues as to the contribution of the bony defect when the arm is in a functional position of instability.

Indications and Contraindications

Individuals with large, symptomatic osseous defects of the glenoid and/or humeral head are candidates for osteoarticular allograft reconstruction. Patients with engaging humeral head lesions or inverted pear glenoids with instability may benefit from osteoarticular reconstruction. Younger patients, particularly those with significant overhead demands such as throwing athletes, are ideal candidates to avoid the often-restricted range of motion after treatment with more traditional methods. Older patients and those with less physical demands may be candidates for coracoid transfer procedures, capsular shifts, or arthroplasty.

The goal of osteoarticular allograft reconstruction is to restore normal shoulder biomechanics. Glenoid bone defects decrease the available articular arc length so that during positions of increasing ABER, the humeral head subluxes or dislocates anteriorly owing to a lessening of the glenoid fossa concavity, a loss of the anteroinferior labrum ("bumper"), and a loss of the concavity-compression mechanism for dynamic support.[36-38] Similarly, large Hill-Sachs lesions decrease the available arc of motion and, if oriented properly, can "engage" on the anterior glenoid rim.[7] In the case of concomitant glenoid and humeral head bone loss, the amount of articular arc length may be further compromised, exacerbating feelings of instability. Although imaging modalities such as CT and MRI can show the size and location of bony defects, diagnostic arthroscopy provides the most comprehensive and dynamic method of evaluation.

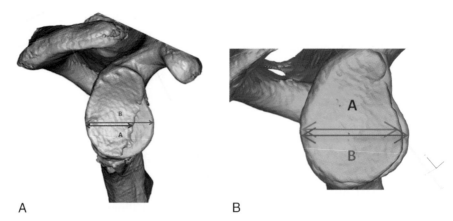

Figure 15-1. Contralateral overlay in large **(A)** and subtle **(B)** glenoid bone loss. The affected glenoid is superimposed on the normal glenoid, and anterior-posterior glenoid width is measured. Bone loss is calculated as (A − B)/B × 100%.

There is no consensus regarding the amount of glenoid or humeral head bone loss required to cause recurrent instability and justify an anatomic reconstruction procedure. Rowe and colleagues[1] originally described glenoid lesions as significant if they involve 30% of the articular surface. On the basis of a biomechanical study, Gerber and Nyffeler[39] found that anteroinferior glenoid defects with a total length greater than half the maximum anterior-to-posterior diameter decreased the resistance to dislocation by 30%. Bigliani and co-workers[8] reported a 12% recurrence rate in patients with glenoid rim fractures after Bankart repair and recommended a coracoid transfer for bone loss greater than 25% of the anteroposterior diameter of the glenoid. Burkhart and de Beer[7,40] suggested that there is a high chance of recurrent instability if the anterior-to-posterior glenoid diameter is less than the diameter above the midglenoid notch, termed the *inverted pear glenoid*. The authors showed that when the glenoid bare spot is used as a reference for arthroscopic measurement, a 6-mm loss of anterior glenoid rim bone results in a 25% deficiency of the glenoid diameter. The consensus of these and other authors is that glenoid bone grafting is recommended for defects greater than 25% to 30% of the articular surface.

Hill-Sachs lesions that engage on the anterior glenoid rim in functional positions should be addressed surgically. Several cadaver studies have evaluated the effect of lesion size on shoulder stability. Sekiya and colleagues[14] reported that defects as small as 12.5% of the humeral head diameter can cause changes in glenohumeral biomechanics that may alter stability. Kaar and co-workers[13] created humeral head defects of varying radii and showed a significant decrease in shoulder stability with defects of 5/8 radius. Furthermore, Yamamoto and colleagues[41] described the concept of a "glenoid track," in which Hill-Sachs lesions that lie medial to this zone can engage as the humeral head overrides the glenoid rim in the presence of humeral head or glenoid bone defects.

Contraindications to anatomic reconstruction include arthroscopic or radiographic evidence of advanced degenerative glenohumeral osteoarthritis, humeral head avascular necrosis, unaddressed rotator cuff deficiency, and advanced age.

Surgical Planning

The size and orientation of the humeral head or glenoid bone defect are determined preoperatively through CT or MRI. We have developed a technique for measuring glenoid bone loss we termed *contralateral overlay*. The patient's normal contralateral glenoid is flipped and superimposed onto the affected glenoid. The anterior-posterior width of the affected glenoid is compared with the normal glenoid width. This technique has the advantage of detecting subtle glenoid bone loss and better quantifying larger bone loss (Fig. 15-1). Fresh-frozen allograft is selected from a tissue bank and is size- and side-matched based on preoperative measurements. A thorough discussion of the potential risks associated with the use of allograft tissue is undertaken with the patient. Informed consent is obtained.

The surgeon must also decide on the surgical approach. Glenoid reconstruction can be performed through an open deltopectoral approach with takedown of the subscapularis, or through an arthroscopic approach without subscapularis takedown. Benefits of an arthroscopic approach include leaving the subscapularis intact, eliminating the risk of failure of tendon repair postoperatively. This also allows for a more aggressive rehabilitation protocol.

We will separately present the techniques of arthroscopic and open osteochondral allograft reconstruction for glenoid bone loss, and open reconstruction of humeral head bone loss; in patients with combined lesions, reconstruction can be performed with a combination of these techniques during the same surgical procedure.

ARTHROSCOPIC OSTEOARTICULAR ALLOGRAFT RECONSTRUCTION OF GLENOID BONE DEFECTS

Anesthesia and Positioning

After general endotracheal anesthesia has been induced, the patient is placed in the beach chair position. A regional block may be placed at the discretion of the surgeon and anesthesiologist for postoperative pain control. The arm is prepared and draped in the standard fashion and securely held by a commercial arm holder during the procedure.

Surgical Landmarks, Incisions, and Portals

Landmarks

- Anterior, lateral, and posterior borders of the acromion
- Coracoid process
- Distal clavicle
- Acromioclavicular joint
- Deltopectoral groove

Portals and Approaches

- Posterior portal
- Anterior portal
- Deltopectoral approach to glenohumeral joint

Examination Under Anesthesia and Diagnostic Arthroscopy

Examination with the patient under anesthesia is performed, and the findings are compared with the contralateral side with specific attention to the degree and position of instability. Instability should be graded in the anterior, posterior, and inferior directions.

Diagnostic arthroscopy is performed through a posterior portal with a 30-degree arthroscope to visualize the bony defect in addition to associated capsulolabral and chondral injury. The size and position of the glenoid or humeral head defect can be thoroughly inspected. In the most common clinical scenario, the surgeon may have underestimated the size of the defect, resulting in incorrectly ordered allograft tissue; therefore it is not uncommon for diagnostic arthroscopy to be performed alone before the definitive procedure.

Specific Steps

1. Creation of Anterior Portal

After diagnostic arthroscopy, if performed through the posterior portal, the anterior portal is created through the rotator interval. A deltopectoral incision is marked on the skin with indelible ink from the tip of the coracoid process directed distally. A skin incision is placed anteriorly in line with the deltopectoral approach for anterior portal placement through the rotator interval (Fig. 15-2).

2. Preparation of the Recipient Glenoid Site

The glenoid is prepared so the dimensions and shape can be measured. With the motorized shaver, the remaining anterior capsulolabral structures are removed until a clear view of the anterior glenoid rim is achieved (Fig. 15-3).

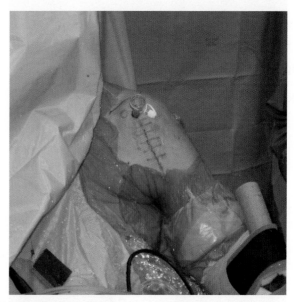

Figure 15-2. The patient is placed in the beach chair position with the arm secured in a commercial holder. A deltopectoral incision is marked from the coracoid process to the deltoid insertion. Diagnostic arthroscopy can be performed before the open portion of the procedure.

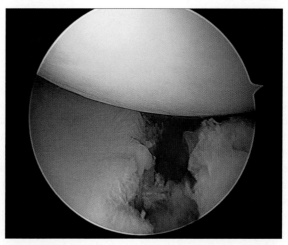

Figure 15-3. Arthroscopic view from the posterior portal demonstrating a large anteroinferior glenoid bone defect. The soft tissues have been removed with the motorized shaver to permit adequate visualization.

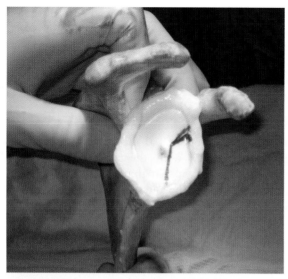

Figure 15-4. Margins of the planned glenoid osteochondral allograft marked on the larger scapular allograft with marker.

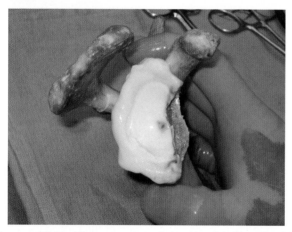

Figure 15-5. After resection of the glenoid allograft with an oscillating saw.

3. Allograft Preparation

The borders of an appropriately sized graft are marked on the fresh-frozen glenoid osteoarticular allograft based on its measured dimensions during diagnostic arthroscopy (Figs. 15-4 and 15-5). A microsagittal saw is then used to fashion the graft. A rongeur and motorized bur can be used to make minor adjustments to the graft. Two braided, nonabsorbable transglenoid sutures (No. 0 Ethibond) are then passed from anterior to posterior through the peripheral edge of the graft articular surface. The purpose of these sutures is twofold: first, to aid in reduction of the allograft through the anterior capsulotomy and into the joint, and second, for plication and tensioning of anterior capsulolabral structures (Fig. 15-6).

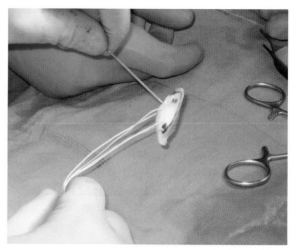

Figure 15-6. The glenoid osteochondral allograft with two No. 2 Ethibond sutures placed from anterior to posterior at the peripheral edge of the articular margin.

4. Allograft Placement

Once the allograft is prepared, the previously placed anterior cannula is removed. The skin incision is then extended approximately 2 cm along the marked deltopectoral incision to accommodate for passage of the allograft. The capsulotomy through the rotator interval only (sparing subscapularis takedown) is enlarged as needed with a knife to facilitate graft passage. The allograft glenoid is then passed into the shoulder and positioned into the defect. With the arthroscope in the posterior portal for visualization, adequate reduction is confirmed. Changes to the shape and contour of the allograft can be made as needed for a precise fit. When a good fit is present between the glenoid allograft and native glenoid, it is provisionally held in place with two 0.045 Kirschner wires placed through the anterior capsulotomy (Fig. 15-7). Fluoroscopy is then used to confirm placement and the graft is secured with two cannulated, partially threaded 4.0-mm screws (Fig. 15-8). The K-wires are then removed.

5. Capsular Plication

The two previously placed Ethibond sutures are then passed from the anterior working portal with an arthroscopic suture passer to shift the anteroinferior capsule and middle glenohumeral ligament. These sutures are placed through the peripheral margin of the allograft to avoid iatrogenic graft damage from suture anchor use. When the plication is complete, the anterior cannula is removed. The shoulder is taken through a complete range of motion to ensure a congruent glenohumeral surface without instability or engagement (Fig. 15-9).

6. Closure

The anterior incision is closed in layers of interrupted absorbable sutures for the joint capsule and

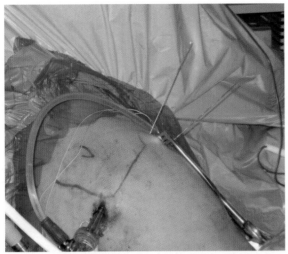

Figure 15-7. The graft is provisionally held in place with two K-wires, as seen here exiting from the anterior skin incision. The arthroscope is placed in the posterior portal to aid with reduction and ensure a congruent fit between the glenoid allograft and native glenoid.

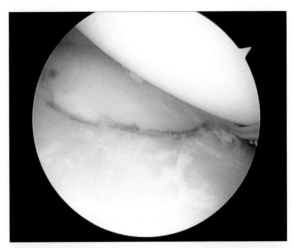

Figure 15-9. After final fixation of the graft with two cortical screws and capsulolabral repair. The allograft is flush with the native glenoid articular cartilage.

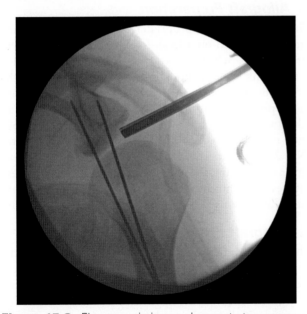

Figure 15-8. Fluoroscopic image demonstrates proper placement of glenoid allograft held in place with K-wires.

subcuticular layers. The posterior arthroscopic incision is closed with interrupted nylon sutures. A sterile dressing is placed.

Postoperative Considerations

Immobilization and Rehabilitation

The patient is placed immediately into a shoulder immobilizer. A modified arthroscopic anterior stabilization physical therapy rehabilitation protocol is used after arthroscopic glenoid osteoarticular allograft reconstruction. If an open posterior approached is performed concomitantly to address Hill-Sachs pathology, a

multidirectional instability protocol is followed. Sling immobilization is maintained for 6 weeks postoperatively; pendulums are allowed to begin 2 weeks postoperatively. Gentle passive elevation of the arm up to 90 degrees in the scapular plane is also allowed at this point. Active-assisted range of motion is started at 4 weeks, including isometric strengthening exercises and periscapular strengthening. Precautions to prevent external rotation are minimal owing to preservation of the subscapularis muscle and tendon.

Radiographs

Radiographs are taken at 2, 6, 12, and 24 weeks postoperatively to monitor appropriate incorporation of the graft. If clinically warranted, a CT scan can be performed to ensure graft healing.

OPEN OSTEOARTICULAR ALLOGRAFT RECONSTRUCTION OF GLENOID BONE DEFECTS

Anesthesia and Positioning

After general endotracheal anesthesia has been induced, the patient is placed in the beach chair position with the head of the bed raised 30 degrees. A bump is placed under the medial border of the scapula. A regional block may be placed at the discretion of the surgeon and anesthesiologist for postoperative pain control. The arm is prepared and draped in the standard fashion and securely held by a commercial arm holder during the procedure.

As detailed in the previous section, a thorough examination with the patient under anesthesia is performed. The findings are compared with the contralateral side. Diagnostic arthroscopy is useful in this setting to evaluate for soft tissue and chondral injury, as well as the size and position of the glenoid bone defect.

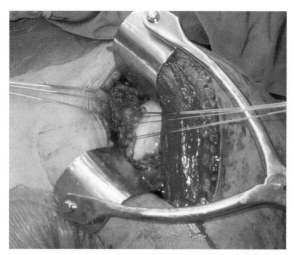

Figure 15-10. Deltopectoral approach with the joint capsule and subscapularis tendon tagged for later repair.

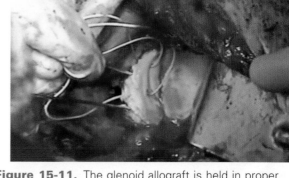

Figure 15-11. The glenoid allograft is held in proper position with two K-wires. Note the previously placed No. 2 Ethibond sutures for capsulolabral repair and the presence of a labrum on the glenoid graft.

Specific Steps

1. Exposure

A 6- to 10-cm skin incision is made in line with the deltopectoral groove from the tip of the coracoid directed distally. Subcutaneous tissue is dissected sharply with meticulous hemostasis down to the level of the deltopectoral fascia. The deltopectoral interval is identified and developed; the pectoralis major is retraced medially and the deltoid laterally. The cephalic vein can be taken medially or laterally, depending on the situation. If it is traumatized, the vein should be tied off before the deep dissection proceeds. The lateral border of the conjoint tendon is identified and retracted medially. The subscapularis tendon is then tagged with stay sutures and incised perpendicular to its fibers approximately 5 mm from its insertion point on the lesser tuberosity, ensuring that adequate tissue is left for later repair; the subscapularis tendon is then incised. It is important to externally rotate the humerus to minimize the risk of iatrogenic injury to the axillary nerve. A lateral humeral-based capsulotomy incision is made, again leaving a small cuff of tissue for later repair (Fig. 15-10).

2. Preparation of the Glenoid Rim

The humeral head is retracted posteriorly with a humeral retractor (Fukuda), and the glenoid rim is exposed. A curved osteotome is used to subperiosteally strip the soft tissues medially off of the anteroinferior glenoid rim. The full extent of the anteroinferior glenoid rim defect is then appreciated. Direct measurements can be made and correlated with the preoperative CT scan estimate of the defect size. The glenoid defect is then prepared with a high-speed bur until a surface of fresh bleeding bone is present.

3. Allograft Preparation

The borders of an appropriately size- and side-matched graft are marked on a fresh-frozen glenoid osteoarticular allograft, which is ordered preoperatively from a tissue bank. The glenoid graft is fashioned from the larger allograft with a microsagittal saw and placed into the appropriate position to check for a good fit; small adjustments are made as needed with a high-speed bur and rongeur. Two braided, nonabsorbable sutures (No. 2 Ethibond) are then passed from anterior to posterior through the articular surface at is periphery. These sutures are technically easier to pass before graft implantation and are used for subsequent capsulolabral shift.

4. Allograft Fixation

The prepared glenoid allograft is then placed into the appropriate anatomic position. When adequate placement has been confirmed, the graft is provisionally fixed to the native glenoid with two 0.045 K-wires, which are sequentially exchanged for two 4.0-mm partially threaded cortical screws (Fig. 15-11).

5. Capsular Shift

The glenohumeral joint is reduced and capsular redundancy is addressed as necessary by capsular shift. The previously placed Ethibond sutures in the glenoid allograft are passed through the intact capsule in a horizontal mattress fashion and tied on the outside of the capsule. This anchors the glenohumeral capsule to the newly secured glenoid allograft. The humeral-based shift is then completed in a standard fashion, with the arm placed in 30 degrees of abduction and external rotation. Often the mere presence of the allograft will greatly reduce the size of the infraglenoid recess, as the void is now filled with graft.

6. Closure

The wound is copiously irrigated. The shoulder is taken through a complete range of motion to ensure smooth articulation among the humeral head, glenoid allograft, and native glenoid. The joint capsule is closed with absorbable suture, and the subscapularis is anatomically repaired back to the remaining cuff of tissue with non-absorbable suture. The conjoint tendon and deltopectoral interval are allowed to fall back into their native position. A 2-0 absorbable subcutaneous suture and running 4-0 absorbable subcuticular suture are used to approximate the skin.

Postoperative Considerations

Immobilization and Rehabilitation

The patient is placed immediately into a shoulder immobilizer. At the first postoperative visit 6 to 8 days later, the dressing is removed and the wound inspected. The patient is then allowed to begin pendulum exercises only. At 1 month postoperatively, active and passive range of motion is initiated under the guidance of an experienced physical therapist. Strengthening begins at 4 to 6 months. The patient is generally not cleared to return to sports or strenuous overhead activity until 7 to 12 months after surgery.

Radiographs

Radiographs are obtained at 2, 6, 12, and 24 weeks postoperatively to ensure proper positioning and healing of the allograft. If it is clinically warranted, a CT scan can be performed to ensure graft incorporation.

OPEN OSTEOARTICULAR ALLOGRAFT RECONSTRUCTION OF HUMERAL HEAD BONE DEFECTS

In cases of concomitant glenoid and humeral head bone defects, allograft reconstruction of both lesions can be performed through an extensive deltopectoral approach, with maximum humeral external rotation required to present the Hill-Sachs defect into the working field. However, in patients with only a soft tissue Bankart and an associated Hill-Sachs defect, often the surgeon will elect to perform an arthroscopic Bankart repair without addressing the large humeral head defect, but we believe that this is a mistake and can lead to failed instability surgery.[7] If the anterior soft tissue reconstruction is intact or if performance of an arthroscopic anterior capsulolabral repair is desired, we believe the humeral head defect can best be addressed through a limited posterior approach with subsequent osteochondral allograft transplantation.[30]

Anesthesia and Positioning

After general anesthesia has been induced, an examination of the affected extremity is performed and findings are compared with the contralateral side. The patient is placed in the beach chair position. Diagnostic arthroscopy is performed, and any pathologic changes are noted. The size and orientation of the humeral head defect are confirmed and correlated with preoperative CT scans. If there is no glenoid bone loss or glenoid erosion, we elect to address the labral injury and capsular laxity arthroscopically. An anterior working portal is then established by needle localization; arthroscopic labral repair and capsular plication are performed from a single working portal.[42]

Specific Steps

1. Exposure

A skin incision is made from the posterolateral corner of the acromion directed distally in line with the deltoid fibers for approximately 6 cm (Fig. 15-12). Superficial dissection is carried down to the deltoid fascia and split in line with its fibers to the level of the upper border of the teres minor. The infraspinatus is split at the level of its tendinous raphe and retracted superiorly and inferiorly to expose the posterior joint capsule. Careful attention is given to protect the axillary nerve inferiorly. A vertical capsulotomy incision is made. The Hill-Sachs lesion is then easily visualized in its posterosuperior location with the need to excessively rotate the humerus (Fig. 15-13).

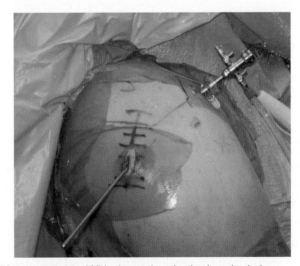

Figure 15-12. With the patient in the beach chair position, a posterior skin incision is marked off the posterolateral corner of the acromion for exposure of the humeral head defect. Diagnostic arthroscopy was carried out with a portal placed within the planned surgical incision.

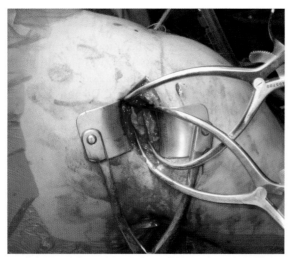

Figure 15-13. The humeral head defect is directly visualized.

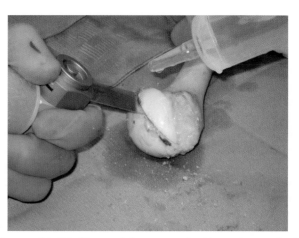

Figure 15-15. The graft is removed with a microsagittal saw.

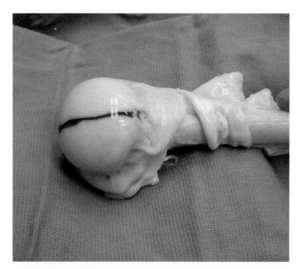

Figure 15-14. The planned cut on the proximal humeral allograft is marked in ink. Care is taken to remove the graft from the same anatomic quadrant as on the recipient humeral head defect to match the radius of curvature.

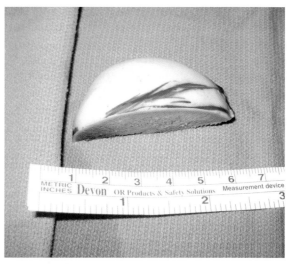

Figure 15-16. The humeral head allograft is wedge shaped. Small adjustments can be made with a rongeur or bur to ensure good fit.

2. Preparation of the Recipient Bed

Once the humeral head has been exposed, the defect and its margins are clearly identified. A motorized bur is used to roughen the edges of the defect.

3. Preparation of the Humeral Head Allograft

The approximate dimensions of the humeral head defect are then marked on the proximal humeral allograft (Fig. 15-14). Care is taken to closely approximate the native radius of curvature of the humeral head. The allograft is then removed with a microsagittal saw and osteotome (Figs. 15-15 and 15-16). Adjustments are then made to

the graft with a bur and rongeur to ensure proper fit into the defect.

4. Placement of the Allograft

After a good fit has been confirmed, the humeral head allograft is placed into the defect and secured with two K-wires (Fig. 15-17). The K-wires are then overdrilled, and two headless compression screws are used to fix the graft to the native humerus.

5. Closure

The posterior capsulotomy is closed with interrupted absorbable sutures. After the capsule has been closed,

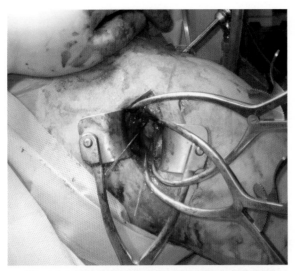

Figure 15-17. The graft is positioned into the defect and held in place with K-wires that are overdrilled, and the graft is fixed with two headless compression screws.

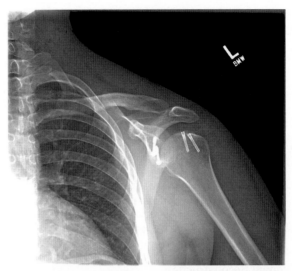

Figure 15-19. Postsurgical radiograph shows screw fixation in a patient who underwent concomitant glenoid and humeral head osteochondral allograft reconstruction.

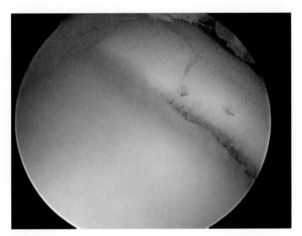

Figure 15-18. Arthroscopic view after graft fixation shows congruent surfaces and restoration of articular convexity.

the arthroscope can then be reinserted through the anterior portal, and in this way the surgeon can directly visualize the congruent glenohumeral surfaces and evaluate for any further engagement or subluxation (Fig. 15-18). The skin and subcutaneous tissue are then closed with absorbable sutures. A sterile dressing is placed.

Postoperative Considerations

Immobilization and Rehabilitation

The patient is placed immediately into a shoulder immobilizer. At the first postoperative visit 6 to 8 days later,

the dressing is removed and the wound inspected. Pendulum exercises begin at 1 week. Passive and active-assisted range of motion begins at 1 to 2 months, avoiding stress on the posterior capsule (no adduction or internal rotation). The sling is discontinued at 2 months. Range of motion is gradually increased; if the patient has full motion at 4 to 5 months, shoulder and periscapular strengthening is initiated. A functional training or throwing program begins at 6 to 7 months. Return to sport or full work duty is allowed when full and functional pain-free motion has been achieved, in addition to reasonable strength.

Radiographs

Radiographs are obtained at 2, 6, 12, and 24 weeks postoperatively to ensure proper positioning and healing of the allograft (Fig. 15-19). If it is clinically warranted, a CT scan can be performed to ensure graft incorporation.

COMPLICATIONS

To date, no long-term follow-up is available for these procedures, making predictions of potential complications difficult. Theoretical complications include those of autograft or allograft procedures, including graft nonunion, failure of the graft to incorporate, and hardware failure. Long-term prospective data are needed to determine the rate of progression to degenerative arthritis.

Pearls and Pitfalls

- A preoperative computed tomography (CT) scan is essential in the workup of patients with suspected bone defects. Plain radiographs and magnetic resonance imaging routinely underestimate the size of these lesions. Include three-dimensional CT scans when indicated. Contralateral overlay can be used to calculate glenoid bone loss.

- Functional diagnostic arthroscopy can be helpful to appreciate the relative contributions of glenoid and humeral head osteoarticular defects in the recurrent instability. With the arm in a functional position of abduction and external rotation, the position and degree of engagement, if present, can be visualized.

- Certain allografts may be difficult to obtain from tissue banks and thus should be arranged for in advance.

Glenoid Reconstruction

- Preservation of the subscapularis allows for a more rapid and aggressive postoperative rehabilitation protocol.

- Before placing the allograft in the native glenoid defect, pass two No. 2 Ethibond sutures through the graft articular surface from anterior to posterior at its periphery. These will be used later for tightening of the

anterior capsulolabral structures. It is significantly easier to place these sutures before fixing the graft and lessens the risk of iatrogenic damage to the allograft.

- Two K-wires from the cannulated screw set can be placed into the glenoid allograft before implantation to facilitate correct placement in a joystick-type maneuver into the native glenoid defect.

- Be cautious of overly aggressive capsular shift once the glenoid allograft is in place. The allograft will restore size to the glenoid and fill the previous void. Once the native capsule is attached to the allograft, redundancy is partially addressed and the humeral-based shift need not be as aggressive as may have been anticipated.

Humeral Head Reconstruction

- It is important to ensure that the humeral head allograft harvest site is obtained from the exact location of the defect so that the graft is matched in terms of radius of curvature to the native humeral head.

- Fix the graft with headless compression screws that are countersunk below the articular cartilage surface. Take the shoulder through a range of motion to ensure the screws are sufficiently countersunk.

TABLE 15-1. Summary of Glenoid Reconstruction Techniques

Study	Procedure	Patients	Mean Follow-up	Capsulolabral Repair	Outcome
Warner et al[21] (2006)	Iliac crest autograft	11	33 mo	Yes	No recurrent instability
Provencher et al[22] (2009)	Distal tibia allograft	3	NR	Yes, if available	NR
Weng et al[23] (2009)	Femoral head allograft	9	4.5 yr	Yes, capsular shift	Two cases of recurrent instability after seizure
Tjoumakaris et al[25] (2007)	Glenoid allograft	1	12 mo	Yes	No recurrent instability
Skendzel and Sekiya[24] (2011)	Glenoid allograft	2	NR	Yes	NR

NR, Not reported.

RESULTS

The treatment of glenohumeral instability with glenoid and humeral head bone loss continues to evolve. Non-anatomic techniques such as the Bristow and Latarjet procedures have demonstrated long-term successful prevention of recurrent glenohumeral instability[43] but are not without complications, including the development of osteoarthritis, hardware failure, and graft nonunion.[34] In response, several anatomic glenoid and humeral head reconstruction methods have been described to recreate the normal glenohumeral anatomy and restore missing bone (Tables 15-1 and 15-2).[21-23,25,28-31]

There are no long-term clinical studies available for anatomic reconstruction of glenoid and humeral head bone loss. In addition, no technique has shown

superiority over another, and most authors have reported only small case series. Despite this, the current clinical results are promising. Osteochondral allograft transplantation allows for restoration of normal shoulder anatomy including the glenoid articular surface, the anteroinferior labrum, and the normal convexity of the humeral head. We theorize that this reduces the risk of development of osteoarthritis and recurrent instability. These techniques do have limitations, including the procurement of fresh glenoid and humeral head allograft from tissue banks as well as the considerable cost of these grafts. We believe that anatomic reconstruction represents a viable and safe alternative to the Bristow and Latarjet procedures in the patient with symptomatic glenohumeral instability caused by large osseous defects of the glenoid and/or humeral head.

TABLE 15-2. Summary of Humeral Head Reconstruction Techniques

Authors	Procedure	Patients	Mean Follow-up	Approach	Outcome
Miniaci and Gish[31] (2004)	Humeral head allograft	18	50 mo	Extended deltopectoral approach	No recurrent instability; 16 of 18 returned to work
Kropf and Sekiya[30] (2007)	Humeral head allograft	1	1 yr	Infraspinatus–teres minor interval	Returned to full active military duty
Tjoumakaris et al[25] (2007)	Humeral head allograft	1	12 mo	Deltopectoral approach	No recurrent instability
Chapovsky and Kelly[28] (2005)	Osteochondral allograft plugs	1	1 yr	Arthroscopic (OATS instrumentation)	No recurrent instability
Yagishita and Thomas[44] (2002)	Frozen femoral head allograft	1	2 yr	Open (not specified)	No recurrent instability
Wahl et al[29] (2010)	Osteoconductive graft plugs	19	17.5 mo	Arthroscopic, plastic delivery tube and tamp	One patient with recurrent instability; 18 of 19 returned to previous activity level

OATS, Osteoarticular Transfer System.

REFERENCES

1. Rowe CR, Patel D, Southmayd WW. Bankart procedure—long-term end-result study. *J Bone Joint Surg Am.* 1978; 60(1):1-16.

2. Taylor DC, Arciero RA. Pathologic changes associated with shoulder dislocations—Arthroscopic and physical examination findings in first-time, traumatic anterior dislocations. *Am J Sports Med.* 1997;25(3):306-311.

3. Brophy RH, Marx RG. The treatment of traumatic anterior instability of the shoulder: nonoperative and surgical treatment. *Arthroscopy.* 2009;25(3):298-304.

4. Owens BD, Nelson BJ, Duffey ML, et al. Pathoanatomy of first-time, traumatic, anterior glenohumeral subluxation events. *J Bone Joint Surg Am.* 2010;92(7): 1605-1611.

5. Calandra JJ, Baker CL, Uribe J. The incidence of Hill-Sachs lesions in initial anterior shoulder dislocations. *Arthroscopy.* 1989;5(4):254-257.

6. Norlin R. Intraarticular pathology in acute, first-time anterior shoulder dislocation: an arthroscopic study. *Arthroscopy.* 1993;9(5):546-549.

7. Burkhart SS, de Beer JF. Traumatic glenohumeral bone defects and their relationship to failure of arthroscopic Bankart repairs: Significance of the inverted-pear glenoid and the humeral engaging Hill-Sachs lesion. *Arthroscopy.* 2000;16(7):677-694.

8. Bigliani LU, Newton PM, Steinmann SP, et al. Glenoid rim lesions associated with recurrent anterior dislocation of the shoulder. *Am J Sports Med.* 1998;26(1):41-45.

9. Boileau P, Villalba M, Hery JY, et al. Risk factors for recurrence of shoulder instability after arthroscopic Bankart repair. *J Bone Joint Surg Am.* 2006;88:1755-1763.

10. Lo IKY, Parten PM, Burkhart SS. The inverted pear glenoid: An indicator of significant glenoid bone loss. *Arthroscopy.* 2004;20(2):169-174.

11. Sugaya H, Moriishi J, Dohi M, et al. Glenoid rim morphology in recurrent anterior glenohumeral instability. *J Bone Joint Surg Am.* 2003;85(5):878-884.

12. Rowe CR, Zarins B, Ciullo JV. Recurrent anterior dislocation of the shoulder after surgical repair—apparent causes of failure and treatment. *J Bone Joint Surg Am.* 1984; 66:159-168.

13. Kaar SG, Fening SD, Jones MH, et al. Effect of humeral head defect size on glenohumeral stability: a cadaveric study of simulated Hill-Sachs defects. *Am J Sports Med.* 2010;38(3):594-599.

14. Sekiya JK, Wickwire AC, Stehle JH, et al. Hill-Sachs defects and repair using osteoarticular allograft transplantation biomechanical analysis using a joint compression model. *Am J Sports Med.* 2009;37(12): 2459-2466.

15. Balg F, Boileau P. The instability severity index score. A simple pre-operative score to select patients for arthroscopic or open shoulder stabilisation. *J Bone Joint Surg Br.* 2007;89(11):1470-1477.

16. Allain J, Goutallier D, Glorion C. Long-term results of the Latarjet procedure for the treatment of anterior instability of the shoulder. *J Bone Joint Surg Am.* 1998;80(6): 841-852.

17. Magnusson BP, Stack JK. Recurrent dislocation of the shoulder. *JAMA.* 1943;123:889-892.

18. Osmond-Clarke H. Habitual dislocation of the shoulder; the Putti-Platt operation. *J Bone Joint Surg Br.* 1948; 30(1):19-25.

19. Connolly JF. Humeral head defects associated with shoulder dislocation—Their diagnostic and surgical significance. *Instr Course Lect.* 1972;1972(21):42-54.

20. Weber BG. Operative treatment for recurrent dislocation of the shoulder. Preliminary report. *Injury.* 1969;1: 107-109.

21. Warner JJP, Gill TJ, O'Hollerhan JD, et al. Anatomical glenoid reconstruction for recurrent anterior glenohumeral instability with glenoid deficiency using an autogenous tricortical iliac crest bone graft. *Am J Sports Med.* 2006;34(2):205-212.

22. Provencher RMT, Ghodadra N, LeClere L, et al. Anatomic osteochondral glenoid reconstruction for recurrent

glenohumeral instability with glenoid deficiency using a distal tibia allograft. *Arthroscopy.* 2009;25(4):446-452.

23. Weng PW, Shen HC, Lee HH, et al. Open reconstruction of large bony glenoid erosion with allogeneic bone graft for recurrent anterior shoulder dislocation. *Am J Sports Med.* 2009;37(9):1792-1797.

24. Skendzel JG, Sekiya JK. Arthroscopic glenoid osteochondral allograft reconstruction without subscapularis takedown: technique and literature review. *Arthroscopy.* 2011;27(1):129-135.

25. Tjoumakaris F, Kropf E, Seikya J. Osteoarticular allograft reconstruction of a large glenoid and humeral head defect in recurrent shoulder instability. *Tech Shoulder Elbow Surg.* 2007;8(2):98-104.

26. Kazel MD, Sekiya JK, Greene JA, et al. Percutaneous correction (humeroplasty) of humeral head defects (Hill-Sachs) associated with anterior shoulder instability: A cadaveric study. *Arthroscopy.* 2005;21(12):1473-1478.

27. Re P, Gallo RA, Richmond JC. Transhumeral head plasty for large Hill-Sachs lesions. *Arthroscopy.* 2006;22(7):798A-U769.

28. Chapovsky F, Kelly JD. Osteochondral allograft transplantation for treatment of glenohumeral instability. *Arthroscopy.* 2005;21(8).

29. Wahl CJ, Wilcox JJ, Merritt AL, et al. Surgical technique: Arthroscopic reconstruction of engaging humeral Hill-Sachs defects using cannulated osteoconductive grafts (COGs). *Tech Shoulder Elbow Surg.* 2010;11(4):101-106.

30. Kropf EJ, Sekiya JK. Osteoarticular allograft transplantation for large humeral head defects in glenohumeral instability. *Arthroscopy.* 2007;23(3).

31. Miniaci A, Gish MW. Management of anterior glenohumeral instability associated with large Hill-Sachs defects. *Tech Shoulder Elbow Surg.* 2004;5(3):170-175.

32. Tjoumakaris FP, Humble B, Sekiya JK. Combined glenoid and humeral head allograft reconstruction for recurrent anterior glenohumeral instability. *Orthopedics.* 2008;31(5):497.

33. Hawkins RJ, Angelo RL. Glenohumeral osteoarthrosis. A late complication of the Putti-Platt repair. *J Bone Joint Surg Am.* 1990;72(8):1193-1197.

34. Young DC, Rockwood CA. Complications of a failed Bristow procedure and their management. *J Bone Joint Surg Am.* 1991;73(7):969-981.

35. Bushnell BD, Creighton RA, Herring MM. The bony apprehension test for instability of the shoulder: A prospective pilot analysis. *Arthroscopy.* 2008;24(9):974-982.

36. Burkhart SS, Danaceau SM. Articular arc length mismatch as a cause of failed Bankart repair. *Arthroscopy.* 2000;16(7):740-744.

37. Itoi E, Lee SB, Berglund L, et al. The effect of a glenoid defect on anteroinferior stability of the shoulder after Bankart repair: A cadaveric study. *J Bone Joint Surg Am.* 2000;82(1):35-46.

38. Lippitt S, Matsen F. Mechanisms of glenohumeral joint stability. *Clin Orthop Relat Res.* 1993;291:20-28.

39. Gerber C, Nyffeler RW. Classification of glenohumeral joint instability. *Clin Orthop Relat Res.* 2002;400:65-76.

40. Burkhart SS, de Beer JF, Tehrany AM, et al. Quantifying glenoid bone loss arthroscopically in shoulder instability. *Arthroscopy.* 2002;18(5):488-491.

41. Yamamoto N, Itoi E, Abe H, et al. Contact between the glenoid and the humeral head in abduction, external rotation, and horizontal extension: A new concept of glenoid track. *J Shoulder Elbow Surg.* 2007;16(5):649-656.

42. Hutchinson JW, Neumann L, Wallace WA. Bone buttress operation for recurrent anterior shoulder dislocation in epilepsy. *J Bone Joint Surg Brm.* 1995;77(6):928-932.

43. Hovelius L, Sandstrom B, Sundgren K, et al. One hundred eighteen Bristow-Latariet repairs for recurrent anterior dislocation of the shoulder prospectively followed for fifteen years: Study I—Clinical results. *J Shoulder Elbow Surg.* 2004;13(5):509-516.

44. Yagishita K, Thomas BJ. Use of allograft for large Hill-Sachs lesion associated with anterior glenohumeral dislocation—A case report. *Injury.* 2002;33(9):791-794.

Chapter 16

Treatment of Recurrent Anterior Inferior Instability Associated with Glenoid Bone Loss: Distal Tibial Allograft Reconstruction

Robert Waltz, Lance LeClere, and Matthew T. Provencher*

Chapter Synopsis

- Glenoid bone loss is frequently present in patients with recurrent anterior shoulder instability. Key factors indicative of significant glenoid bone loss of more than 20% are instability at midranges of abduction (20 to 60 degrees) and progressive ease of subluxation with daily activities. Young, highly active patients, especially contact or overhead athletes, should be considered for glenoid bony augmentation to restore glenoid surface area, articular length, and depth. Use of a distal tibia allograft has the advantages of a near congruent articular surface with the native glenoid, dense corticocancellous bone, and a robust cartilage layer. In addition, it restores the native anatomy without altering mechanical function of surrounding structures and requires no donor site morbidity.

Important Points

- Indicated for highly active, young patients with apprehension or instability in midranges of abduction (20 to 60 degrees) with more than 20% anterior glenoid bone loss measured on three-dimensional (3D) computed tomography (CT).

- Not indicated for older, low-demand patients; those with multidirectional instability; voluntary dislocators; or those unable to comply with postoperative restrictions (including smokers).

- Always perform a CT scan with 3D reconstruction of the glenoid preoperatively with the humeral head digitally subtracted to measure glenoid bone loss on the sagittal oblique images.

- Use fresh distal tibia allograft for optimal bone and cartilage quality.

- Allograft is taken from the lateral aspect of the distal tibia, which is nearly identical to the native anterior glenoid radius of curvature.

Clinical and Surgical Pearls

- Patient positioning: elevate the back and head to only 40 degrees and ensure the back is well supported with two towels along the medial border of the scapula to facilitate adequate anterior glenoid exposure.

- Use of a padded mayo stand allows additional arm and shoulder mobility and additional scapular external rotation to expand exposure.

- Always perform diagnostic arthroscopy first.

- Identify the subscapularis and capsular plane from lateral to medial, taking care to identify the long head of the biceps tendon before the subscapularis horizontal split.

- Remove all capsular and labral tissue from the glenoid neck, and ensure that the glenoid neck is flat and perpendicular to the articular surface before allograft placement.

- The allograft is cut from the lateral third of the distal tibia donor.

Continued

---

*The views expressed in this article are those of the authors and do not necessarily reflect the official policy or position of the Department of the Navy, Department of Defense, or the U.S. Government.

- The medial allograft cut is angled 5 to 10 degrees medially to restore the normal glenoid morphology and fit congruently with a perpendicular cut to the glenoid.
- Lag screws are inserted perpendicular to the glenoid to ensure bicortical purchase and should be 36 to 40 mm in length.

Clinical and Surgical Pitfalls

- Unrecognized anterior glenoid bone loss of 20% to 30% represents a high failure rate with soft tissue stabilization procedures.
- If the medial border of the scapula is not supported, the scapula may not be externally rotated sufficiently to

expose the anterior glenoid. If the glenoid is internally rotated and adequate exposure is not obtained, the pectoralis minor may be released from the coracoid.

- The axillary nerve is at risk during glenoid preparation. It may be protected with a smooth retractor or a gloved finger.
- Ensure that the Kirschner wires used for graft positioning are not in the intended path of the cortical screws.
- If the graft is not drilled perpendicular to the glenoid face, bicortical fixation will not be achieved, which will cause graft migration and inadequate fixation.

A certain degree of anterior inferior glenoid bone loss has been reported in up to 90% of patients with recurrent anterior instability.[1] Bone loss patterns may be traumatic, with a bony fragment present from an acute dislocation, or may be attritional, with erosion of a previous fragment or the anterior glenoid surface.[2,3] In either case, the glenoid morphology changes over time, usually progressing to more significant bone loss with repeated instability events.[4] Glenoid bone loss represents the progressive loss of a key static stabilizer in glenohumeral stability because there is a smaller surface area to resist axial loads, less articular length, and decreased depth of articular conformity.[3,4] All of this contributes to increased instability events. It is well documented that when glenoid bone loss reaches a key threshold level of 20% to 30%, significant instability ensues.[2-6] To adequately reconstitute the glenoid bony arc and restore stability, bony augmentation is required for adequate glenohumeral stability. Options for restoration of glenoid bone traditionally have included coracoid transfer consisting of one of the variants of the Bristow-Latarjet procedure, iliac crest autograft, or allograft glenoid.[1,7-12]

Recently, a novel technique for glenoid bone and cartilage restoration using distal tibia allograft has been proposed.[13] The following technique describes the procedure in detail, as well as preoperative considerations and intraoperative pearls and pitfalls. This technique offers several unique advantages over previous glenoid bone augmentation procedures: no donor site morbidity, abundant availability, and anatomic reconstruction of the glenoid arc with a robust intra-articular chondral surface with a foundation of abundant, dense corticocancellous bone that can be conformed to each individual's degree of bone loss.[13]

PREOPERATIVE CONSIDERATIONS

History

Patients typically report recurrent anterior instability. A detailed history should be taken to determine their activity level as well as the details of their initial dislocation event. Patients with significant glenoid bone loss (15% to 30%) typically have a history of either a high-energy axial load event or low-energy traumatic dislocation with progressive ease of subluxation.[3,4] Instability is usually in the midabduction (20 to 60 degrees) ranges of motion.[4,12] They describe instability with daily activities and inability to participate in athletic activities. Many patients have already undergone a previous soft tissue anterior stabilization and have recurrent instability or dislocation events.

Physical Examination

Examination should begin with a careful inspection of both shoulders for deltoid or rotator cuff atrophy, scapular dyskinesis, pectoralis minor tightness, and deformity. A careful neurologic examination should also be conducted. Active and passive range of motion should be tested along with rotator cuff strength, with any side-to-side asymmetry noted. Special attention should be directed toward subscapularis testing because this may be either split or taken down and repaired during the operative procedure.[4] Provocative testing should evaluate for long head of biceps pathology, labral tears, and subacromial pathology. Instability testing should focus on anterior subluxation or apprehension at the midranges of abduction (20 to 60 degrees) in addition to full abduction and external rotation (the 90-90 position).[4,12] Patients with glenoid bone loss generally do not have multidirectional instability, and this should be carefully evaluated before any surgical procedure is considered.

Imaging

Imaging should begin with plain radiographs of the shoulder to include standard anteroposterior (AP), glenoid profile AP, scapular-Y, and axillary views. Additional views focused on the glenoid face include the West Point, Didiee, and apical oblique views.[4] Plain radiographs are only mildly effective at demonstrating glenoid bone loss; however, they will demonstrate loss of the sharp cortical density at the inferior glenoid, which is replaced by a bony shadow.[14]

Magnetic resonance imaging (MRI) and magnetic resonance arthrography (MRA) are also useful for demonstrating soft tissue pathology including rotator cuff tears and labral degeneration and tears and can demonstrate bone loss with a high-quality 3-tesla magnet on a sagittal oblique cut of the glenoid.[4]

Computed tomography (CT) with three-dimensional reconstruction is the most accurate method for determining glenoid bone loss and should be included in the standard workup for recurrent anterior instability[1] (Fig. 16-1). A best-fit circle is drawn over the inferior two thirds of the glenoid on the glenoid image with the humerus digitally subtracted.[15] The amount of bone loss is then measured as a percent of total surface area of the previously drawn circle.[4] There are multiple techniques described for measuring glenoid bone loss; however, the quickest method is simply measuring the bony deficit anteriorly and dividing by the total circle diameter. Typically a 6- to 7-mm deficit represents approximately 25% glenoid bone loss.[2,5,6] The usual pattern of bone loss is parallel to the long axis of the glenoid and generally occurs between the 2:30 and 4:20 positions with reference to a clock face.[16]

Indications

The two strongest indications for open glenoid bony augmentation are degree of bone loss and activity level.[4] This procedure should be considered for younger (aged 20 to 30 years) individuals with bone loss of more than 20% who are involved in contact or overhead sports or highly demanding physical activities, such as military personnel involved with special forces (e.g., U.S. Navy Sea, Air, and Land Teams [SEALs]) or pilots who cannot afford a dislocation in critical situations.

This procedure should be avoided in older, less active patients; those who are voluntary dislocators; those who have multiple risky comorbidities or who smoke; and those who are unable to comply with the postoperative rehabilitation.[4]

SURGICAL TECHNIQUE

Positioning

After general anesthesia has been induced, the patient is placed in the beach chair position with a head elevation of approximately 40 degrees. Two small towels are placed between the medial border of the operative scapula and the bed to prevent anterior rotation of the glenoid and scapula. This also facilitates anterior glenoid neck exposure to optimize screw trajectory through the allograft by externally rotating the glenoid face. The patient's shoulder and entire arm are then prepared and draped, ensuring a wide surgical field. The arm is left free, supported by a padded mayo stand (Fig. 16-2).

Surgical Landmarks, Incisions, and Portals

Standard shoulder bony landmarks are then drawn out to include the coracoid, acromion, scapular spine, and acromioclavicular joint. A standard deltopectoral approach is used. The skin incision line is marked from the tip of the coracoid to the superior axillary fold along the deltopectoral groove and should be 8 to 10 cm in length.

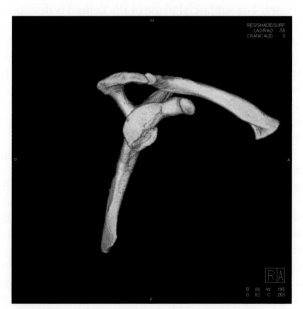

Figure 16-1. Computed tomography with three-dimensional reconstruction and proximal humerus subtraction demonstrates 35% bone loss perpendicular to the long axis of the glenoid.

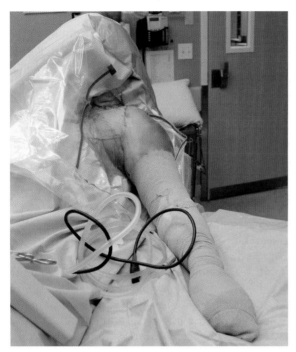

Figure 16-2. The patient is prepared, and incision is marked as a standard deltopectoral approach. The arm is left free on a padded mayo stand for ease of mobility.

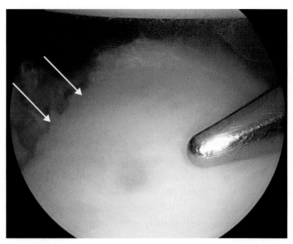

Figure 16-3. Arthroscopic image from the anterior portal demonstrating the typical inverted pear morphology of the glenoid. White arrows indicate anterior inferior glenoid deficiency.

BOX 16-1 Surgical Steps
1. Exposure
2. Glenoid preparation
3. Graft preparation
4. Graft fixation
5. Closure

Examination and Diagnostic Arthroscopy

In preparation for diagnostic arthroscopy, a posterior portal is then marked 1 cm medial and 2 cm inferior to the posterior lateral border of acromion. An anterior midglenoid portal is marked just lateral to the coracoid to facilitate inclusion into the deltopectoral incision. Examination with the patient under anesthesia is conducted, documenting range of motion, instability, and any engaging Hill-Sachs lesions. Diagnostic arthroscopy is then conducted in the standard fashion, ensuring documentation of the glenoid from the anterior midglenoid portal to demonstrate the inverted pear morphology[3,6] (Fig. 16-3).

Specific Steps

Specific steps of this procedure are outlined in Box 16-1.

1. Exposure

The skin incision is made along the previously marked deltopectoral interval from the coracoid tip to the axilla. Full thickness medial and lateral skin flaps are developed through the deltopectoral fascia. The deltopectoral interval is identified, and the cephalic vein is dissected and retracted laterally with the deltoid fascia. The conjoined tendon (short head of biceps laterally, coracobrachialis medially) is identified proximally at the coracoid, and the fascia overlying is released with Metzenbaum scissors. The subfascial plane of the deltoid is developed laterally. Kolbel retractors are placed under the lateral aspect of the conjoined tendon and under the medial aspect of the deltoid and held in place with a towel clamp, securing the finger rings to the stocking over the arm. Take care not to over-retract the conjoined tendon, as the musculocutaneous nerve inserts medially into the coracobrachialis 5 to 8 cm distal to its origin on the coracoid.

The subscapularis tendon is identified, and a tendon-splitting approach is performed. An incision is made in line with the fibers in the middle portion. Start laterally at the medial border of the long head of the biceps over the lesser tuberosity and incise directly to bone. Identify the capsular plane medially and continue dissection with Metzenbaum scissors to the glenoid neck. Place a pointed retractor within the split to allow full capsular access. If this exposure is inadequate, the superior two thirds or the entire subscapularis may be taken down to facilitate better access. Be aware that the axillary nerve lies just inferior to the subscapularis in the interval between the subscapularis and the teres major. The capsule is then incised horizontally as far superiorly as possible to the glenoid neck. The inferior portion is

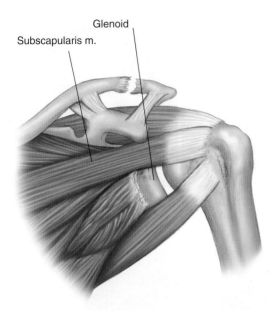

Figure 16-4. Sketch demonstrating the subscapularis split and capsular reflection off of the glenoid neck. Capsule is reflected inferiorly.

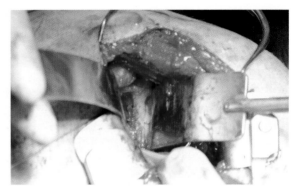

Figure 16-5. Anterior glenoid after preparation with a high-speed bur. The anterior surface is perpendicular to the articular surface.

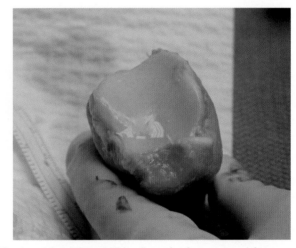

Figure 16-6. Distal tibia allograft after removal from storage medium. The lateral third is used for the graft.

elevated off of the glenoid neck subperiosteally, and reflected inferiorly (Fig. 16-4). Of note, significant scar tissue can form among the capsule, subscapularis, and labrum in patients who have undergone prior Bankart repairs, making this dissection more difficult. The capsule is then tagged with No. 2 nonabsorbable suture and is repaired back to the anterior aspect of the graft under sutures placed in the washers that affix the graft. The glenohumeral joint should now be visible.

2. Glenoid Preparation

The anterior glenoid is inspected to confirm the preoperative level of bone loss. The anterior glenoid is then prepared by first elevating any labral tissue and dissecting medially with a key elevator. This will later be repaired to the anterior aspect of the allograft unless there is a significant soft tissue deficiency not amenable to repair. Take care to protect the axillary nerve by staying on bone throughout the dissection and protecting the nerve with a smooth retractor (Chandler or Darrach) or a gloved finger. Further exposure is facilitated with the use of a humeral head retractor and glenoid neck retractor. A high-speed bur with an oval cutting tip is used to prepare the anterior glenoid bone to create a level surface perpendicular to the glenoid face to couple with the distal tibia allograft (Fig. 16-5). The distance from the glenoid bare spot to the prepared anterior glenoid is measured for final allograft preparation. The sum of the allograft and the remaining anterior glenoid shoulder equals the distance from the bare spot to the posterior glenoid, or on average 12 to 13 mm.

3. Graft Preparation

A fresh distal tibia allograft is obtained from a reliable donor source, and preoperative cultures are obtained. The allograft is stored in a sterile medium and transported to the operating room without freezing. The radius of curvature of the distal tibia is very well matched universally to that of the glenoid and humeral head, and size-matched specimens are not necessary. The lateral third of the distal tibia allograft is used for the graft (Fig. 16-6).

The medial-to-lateral dimensions of the graft are marked based on the preoperative CT measurements and the intraoperative measurements taken after glenoid preparation. This is typically an 8- to 11-mm chondral surface, depending on the size of the defect (Fig. 16-7A). The depth of the graft (lateral to medial) is typically 10 to 13 mm, and the angle of the perpendicular cut is approximately 5 to 10 degrees toward the medial tibia to retrovert the anterior glenoid graft to recreate the normal glenoid morphology (Fig. 16-7B and C). Cuts are made with a 0.5-inch sagittal saw while an assistant

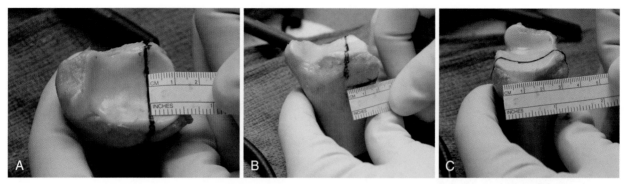

Figure 16-7. A surgical marker is used to mark a 10-mm measurement of the lateral chondral surface **(A)**. An angular cut is marked at 5-10 degrees toward the medial tibia to retrovert the graft **(B)**. View from the lateral graft **(C)**.

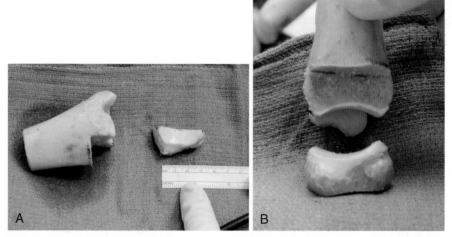

Figure 16-8. Graft after cuts have been made with a sagittal saw. **A,** Chondral surface. **B,** Lateral graft.

holds the graft in place with two towel clamps. Alternatively, a four-prong graft clamp can be used. Irrigation is also used to keep the allograft cool. After the graft has been cut, the superior and inferior aspects of the nonarticular side of the graft can be rounded with the sagittal saw or bur to match the contour of the medial glenoid (Fig. 16-8). Once the graft has been prepared, it is pulse-lavaged with approximately 2 L of lactated Ringer's solution, similar to the process with a fresh osteochondral knee allograft, to remove the bony marrow elements.

4. Graft Fixation

Two 1.6-mm K-wires are placed in the graft at a 45-degree angle to facilitate placement of the graft onto the anterior glenoid to assess fit, conformity, and angle relative to the articular surface (Fig. 16-9). Additional minor cuts may be necessary. Once fit has been confirmed, the K-wires are driven into the native glenoid for provisional fixation. Ensure these are not in the path of intended screw placement. Two 3.5-mm fully threaded cortical screws are then placed through the graft in standard lag technique perpendicular to the prepared anterior glenoid. Screw lengths should be 36 to 40 mm.

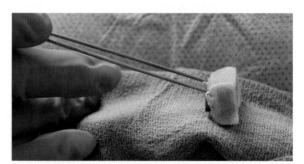

Figure 16-9. Kirchner wires inserted into the graft at a 45-degree angle to facilitate placement of graft. Ensure wires are not in intended screw paths.

Washers may be used (Figs. 16-10 and 16-11). If the capsule and labrum are available for repair, they are sutured to the screw heads before final tightening.

5. Closure

The subscapularis is then reapproximated with No. 2 nonabsorbable suture. The deltopectoral interval is reapproximated with No. 2 nonabsorbable suture to facilitate identification of the interval if needed. The skin is closed with 2-0 monocryl in the dermal layer

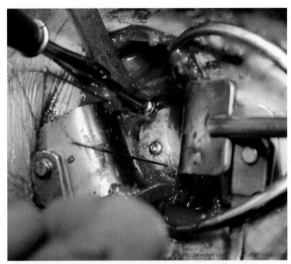

Figure 16-10. Screw fixation of distal tibia allograft to glenoid.

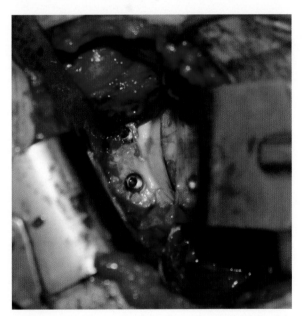

Figure 16-11. Final reconstruction of anterior glenoid. Near anatomic restoration of the glenoid contour is achieved.

and a 3-0 monocryl running subcuticular closure. The wounds are then sealed with acrylic skin glue, and standard dressings are applied. The patient's arm is placed in a padded abduction sling.

POSTOPERATIVE CONSIDERATIONS

Pendulum exercises are started on postoperative day 1, and passive range of motion in the scapular plane is performed for the first 2 weeks. Passive range-of-motion exercises are then progressed with physical therapy guidance. At the 4- to 6-week mark, AP, scapular-Y, and axillary radiographs are obtained, active-assisted exercises are started, and the sling is discontinued. At 8 weeks, strength training is initiated. Anticipated return to full activity is 5 to 6 months.

Complications with this procedure have been few but may include axillary or musculocutaneous nerve traction injury, postoperative stiffness, subscapularis weakness, potential graft partial resorption, and superficial or deep wound infection.

RESULTS

This procedure has been performed in over 20 highly active, active duty military patients over the past 3 years with no episodes of recurrent subluxation or dislocation. There has been one deep infection with *Propionibacterium acnes*, which was treated with removal of the allograft and screws and 6 weeks of antibiotics. The patient underwent revision distal tibia allograft 4 months after the initial presentation with the infection. There is no evidence of graft resorption, advanced osteoarthritis, or nerve palsies. These results have not been formally reported in the literature, and long-term data are still being collected.

REFERENCES

1. Sugaya H, Moriishi J, Dohi M, et al. Glenoid rim morphology in recurrent anterior glenohumeral instability. *J Bone Joint Surg Am.* 2003;85:878-884.
2. Bigliani LU, Newton PM, Steinmann SP, et al. Glenoid rim lesions associated with recurrent anterior dislocation of the shoulder. *Am J Sports Med.* 1998;26:41-45.
3. Burkhart SS, De Beer JF. Traumatic glenohumeral bone defects and their relationship to failure of arthroscopic Bankart repairs: Significance of the inverter-pear glenoid and the humeral engaging Hill-Sachs lesion. *Arthroscopy.* 2000;16:677-694.
4. Piasecki DP, Verma NN, Romeo AA, et al. Glenoid bone deficiency in recurrent anterior shoulder instability: diagnosis and management. *J Am Acad Orthop Surg.* 2009; 17:482-493.
5. Itoi E, Lee SB, Berglund LJ, et al. The effect of a glenoid defect on anterior inferior stability of the shoulder after Bankart repair: a cadaveric study. *J Bone Joint Surg Am.* 2000;82:35-46.
6. Lo IK, Parten PM, Burkhart SS. The inverter pear glenoid: an indicator of significant glenoid bone loss. *Arthroscopy.* 2004;20:169-174.
7. Helfet AJ. Coracoid transplantation for recurring dislocation of the shoulder. *J Bone Joint Surg Br.* 1958;40: 198-202.
8. Hindmarsh J, Lindberg A. Eden-Hybbinette's operation for recurrent dislocation of the humero-scapular joint. *Acta Orthop Scand.* 1967;38:459-478.
9. Hovelius L, Sandstrom B, Sundgren K, et al. One hundred eighteen Bristow-Latarjet repairs for recurrent anterior

dislocation of the shoulder prospectively followed for fifteen years: study I. clinical results. *J Shoulder Elbow Surg.* 2004;13:509-516.

10. Montgomery Jr WH, Wahl M, Hettrich C, et al. Anterior inferior bone-grafting can restore stability in osseous glenoid defects. *J Bone Joint Surg Am.* 2005;87: 1972-1977.

11. Schroder DT, Provencher MT, Mologne TS, et al. The modified Bristow procedure for anterior shoulder instability: 26-year outcomes in Naval Academy midshipmen. *Am J Sports Med.* 2006;34:778-786.

12. Warner JJ, Gill TJ, O'Hollerhan JD, et al. Anatomical glenoid reconstruction for recurrent anterior glenohumeral instability with glenoid deficiency using an autogenous tricortical iliac crest bone graft. *Am J Sports Med.* 2006;34:205-212.

13. Provencher MT, Ghodadra N, LeClere L, et al. Anatomic osteochondral glenoid reconstruction for recurrent glenohumeral instability with glenoid deficiency using a distal tibia allograft. *Arthroscopy.* 2009;25(4):446-452.

14. Edwards TB, Boulahia A, Walch G. Radiographic analysis of bone defects in chronic anterior shoulder instability. *Arthroscopy.* 2003;19:732-739.

15. Huysmans PE, Haen PS, Kidd M, et al. The shape of the inferior part of the glenoid: a cadaveric study. *J Shoulder Elbow Surg.* 2006;15:759-763.

16. Saito H, Itoi E, Sugaya H, et al. Location of the glenoid defect in shoulders with recurrent anterior dislocation. *Am J Sports Med.* 2005;33:889-893.

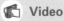

Chapter 17

Arthroscopic Remplissage for Management of Engaging and Deep Hill-Sachs Lesions

Kieran O'Shea and Pascal Boileau

Chapter Synopsis
- Arthroscopic Hill-Sachs remplissage (AHSR) is indicated for patients who are at high risk for recurrence or failure after isolated arthroscopic anterior soft tissue repair and in whom large humeral head defects are contributing significantly to the instability complex.

Important Points
- Indications: Anterior shoulder instability with associated large Hill-Sachs defects as visualized on preoperative plain radiographs, computed tomography (CT) scanning, or magnetic resonance imaging (MRI) or identified as engaging the glenoid surface during diagnostic arthroscopy at the time of instability surgery.
- Contraindications: Isolated glenoid bone loss; other forms of shoulder instability than that in an isolated traumatic anterior direction.
- Surgical technique: AHSR is not indicated as an isolated procedure. It is always performed in combination with an anterior capsulolabral repair.

Clinical and Surgical Pearls
- Adequate preoperative workup is important to fully assess the size and location of osseous deficiency on both the humeral and glenoid sides of the shoulder joint.
- An accessory posterolateral portal is established through which the base of the lesion is debrided and suture anchors are inserted.

- The anterior repair must be prepared before proceeding to the posterior procedure, as the working space within the joint is significantly reduced after remplissage.
- Once the humeral sutures have been placed, repositioning of the arthroscope in the posterior subdeltoid space before knot tying is not necessary. More important is the ability to visualize the quality of reduction of the posterior capsulotenodesis into the defect, from within the joint, as the sutures are being tied.

Clinical and Surgical Pitfalls
- After preparation of the anterior capsulolabral tissues, the humeral head is translated anteriorly and perched on the glenoid rim. The Hill-Sachs defect is prepared, and anchors are inserted into its base via an 8-mm cannula placed through the posterolateral accessory portal. Extreme care should be taken to ensure an optimal trajectory of suture anchor insertion. If a poor line is taken, there is a risk of anchor penetration of the anterior humeral head cartilaginous surface.
- Neither of the two suture limbs exiting via the posterolateral portal should be used as the posts during arthroscopic knot tying, as the resultant knot will end up within the joint and the quality of remplissage will be reduced.

Video
- Video 17-1: Arthroscopic Bankart and Hill-Sachs remplissage

Recurrence rates of up to 15% have been reported after arthroscopic labral repair for anterior shoulder instability.[1] Patient age and activity level, soft tissue quality, and the presence of glenoid or humeral bone loss have been identified as predisposing factors.[2] A number of potential therapeutic options exist for the management of humeral lesions that are contributing significantly to the instability complex. These include open matched osteoarticular allograft transplantation, transhumeral bone grafting, humeroplasty, rotational humeral osteotomy, and partial or complete humeral head resurfacing.[3-7]

In arthroscopic Hill-Sachs remplissage (AHSR), a procedure pioneered by Wolf,[8] adapted from the open technique described by Connolly,[9] the infraspinatus tendon and posterior capsule are used to fill the humeral defect. The term *remplissage* derives from the French verb *remplir,* meaning "to fill." This posterior capsulo-tenodesis is not intended as an isolated procedure, but rather is always performed in combination with an anterior soft tissue repair. Through "filling" of the defect, the defect is rendered extra-articular and thus is prevented from engagement with the glenoid. In addition, the infraspinatus tendon and capsule act as a checkrein, preventing anterior humeral head translation[10] (Fig. 17-1).

PREOPERATIVE CONSIDERATIONS

History and Physical Examination

Because the Hill-Sachs lesion represents a humeral head impaction fracture, the history is typically of joint dislocation rather than repeated episodes of subluxation. The specific sporting activity and level to which it is played should be recorded.

Physical examination is per the standard for anterior instability. The location of the humeral defect will predict the position of apprehension and engagement. Defects with a more vertical orientation will have a tendency to engage with the arm positioned by the side.

Signs of anterior and inferior apprehension and hyperlaxity are sought. Anterior hyperlaxity is present if the examiner can easily subluxate the humeral head out of the socket in the anteroposterior (AP) direction on drawer testing or if passive external rotation is greater than 85 degrees with the patient's arm at his or her side. Inferior hyperlaxity is assessed with sulcus sign testing and the hyperabduction test, the result of which is positive with a minimum of 20 degrees of asymmetrical abduction at the glenohumeral joint.[11] The presence of skin striae can be a subtle but useful finding suggestive of a predisposition toward soft tissue laxity.

Imaging

AP radiographs are obtained with the arm in three different rotations (neutral, external, and internal), as well as a scapular lateral radiograph and an axillary radiograph. The Hill-Sachs lesion may be considered large if it is visible on the AP radiograph performed with the arm in external rotation. Computed tomography (CT) scanning is the senior author's (P.B.) preferred modality to evaluate the location and size of the osseous

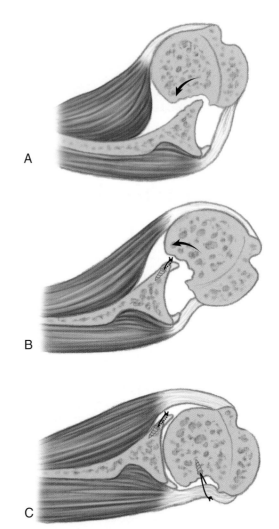

Figure 17-1. Biomechanics of Hill-Sachs lesion and Hill-Sachs remplissage. **A,** Impaction of the posterior humeral head on the anterior glenoid rim (*arrow*) produces the engaging Hill-Sachs lesion. **B,** Recurrence of anterior instability despite anterior Bankart repair because of engagement of the large Hill-Sachs lesion on the anterior glenoid rim (*arrow*). **C,** The transfer (and healing) of the capsule and infraspinatus tendon into the bone defect has the dual effects of (1) placing the humeral bony lesion extra-articularly (exclusion effect), and (2) decreasing anterior translation (checkrein effect).

lesions associated with anterior instability. In patients over the age of 40 years, because of the higher probability of rotator cuff tear, intra-articular contrast is coadministered.

Instability Severity Index Score

To assist in the surgical decision-making process for cases of anteroinferior instability, a preoperative scoring system—the instability severity index score (ISIS)—was developed.[12] It enables selection of patients at high risk for treatment failure after isolated arthroscopic Bankart

TABLE 17-1. Instability Severity Index Score (ISIS) System to Determine Patients at High Risk for Treatment Failure after Isolated Arthroscopic Bankart Repair

	Prognostic Factors		Points
Questionnaire	Age at surgery	≤20 yr	2
		>20 yr	0
	Degree of sport practice	Competition	2
		Recreational or no sports	0
	Type of sports	Contact or forced abduction or external rotation	1
		Other	0
Examination findings	Shoulder hyperlaxity	Shoulder hyperlaxity	1
		Normal laxity	0
Anteroposterior (AP) radiograph	Hill-Sachs lesion on AP radiograph	In external rotation	2
		Not visible in external rotation	0
	Glenoid loss of contour on AP radiograph	Loss of contour	2
		No lesion	0

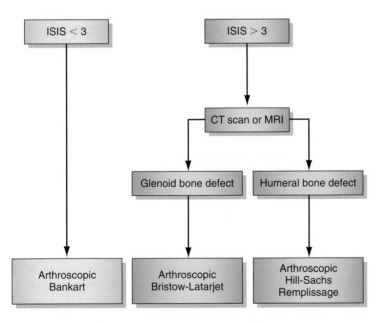

Figure 17-2. Treatment algorithm for anterior shoulder instability. *CT,* Computed tomography; *ISIS,* instability severity index score; *MRI,* magnetic resonance imaging.

repair. Six risk factors, shown to predict an increased recurrence rate after surgery, were integrated into a 10-point scale (Table 17-1). A score of 3 or fewer points correlates with an acceptable postsurgical recurrence risk of 5% and therefore potential suitability for isolated arthroscopic Bankart repair. For a score of 4 to 6, the recurrence risk is 10%; risk of recurrence rises to 70% with a score over 6. The associated soft tissue and osseous defects dictate the supplemental procedure, performed in addition to a Bankart repair, required to minimize recurrence in patients with an ISIS score higher than 3 (Fig. 17-2). In the senior author's practice, a combined arthroscopic Bankart and Hill-Sachs remplissage (BHSR) procedure is performed for

approximately 10% of cases requiring surgical treatment of anterior shoulder instability.

Indications and Contraindications

BHSR is indicated in the primary treatment of recurrent traumatic anteroinferior shoulder instability in the presence of significant Hill-Sachs defects. Significant defects are defined by virtue of their appearance on preoperative plain AP shoulder radiographs, CT scans, or magnetic resonance images or by identification as engaging the glenoid surface during diagnostic arthroscopy at the time of instability surgery. A second, less common indication for BHSR is in the setting of revision surgery for failed prior stabilization. Patients who have undergone previous anterior soft tissue or bony reconstruction and in whom humeral-sided osseous lesions are implicated in the recurrence of instability are suitable candidates for BHSR.

Contraindications to BHSR include untreated glenoid osseous deficiency, which should be treated with anterior bony reconstruction (i.e., Bristow-Latarjet or Eden-Hybinette procedure). The procedure is not indicated for the treatment of forms of instability, such as voluntary instability, posterior instability, or multidirectional instability. Severe preexisting glenohumeral osteoarthritis is a further contraindication.

SURGICAL TECHNIQUE

Anesthesia and Positioning

After administration of upper limb regional anesthetic block, general anesthesia is administered with endotracheal tube intubation. Supplemental muscle relaxation with a cholinesterase inhibiting agent may be helpful. The procedure is performed with the patient in the beach chair position. The upper extremity is draped free. An arm-holding device is not routinely used; rather, the arm is rested on a moveable support so that it can be freely positioned to facilitate arthroscopic access to both the anterior and posterior regions of the joint.

Surgical Landmarks, Incisions, and Portals

The bony landmarks and portals of the shoulder are outlined with a sterile marker, including the distal clavicle, the coracoid, and the acromion. In addition to the standard posterior and anterosuperior portals, an accessory posterolateral portal centered over the Hill-Sachs lesion is created from outside in with use of a spinal needle, enabling preparation and insertion of suture anchors into the defect.

Arthroscopic Examination

The arthroscope is first introduced via the posterior portal, and a systematic evaluation of the joint is performed after syringe insufflation with 20 mL of air. Humeral translation as well as the size, depth, and position of engagement of the Hill-Sachs defect are gauged. The arthroscopic examination then proceeds with use of standard saline irrigation solution. An anterosuperior portal is created under direct visualization with a spinal needle and an outside-in technique. Associated bone and soft tissue lesions on the glenoid and humeral sides of the joint are evaluated.

> **BOX 17-1** Surgical Steps
>
> 1. Glenoid preparation and passage of traction sutures through the anterior labrum and capsule
> 2. Hill-Sachs preparation and humeral anchor insertion
> 3. Suture passage and filling of the humeral defect
> 4. Completion of the anterior capsulolabral reconstruction

Specific Steps

The specific steps of the procedure are outlined in (Box 17-1).

1. Glenoid Preparation and Passage of Traction Sutures Through the Anterior Labrum and Capsule

In this combined procedure the optimal time for preparation of the anterior capsulolabral repair is before the Hill-Sachs lesion has been addressed, because once remplissage has been performed, the working space within the joint is markedly reduced. To allow it to be shifted superiorly and medially, the anterior labrum is mobilized initially with a periosteotome and subsequently a bipolar cautery device (VAPR, Mitek, Johnson & Johnson). The anterior glenoid rim is debrided from the 2- to the 6-o'clock positions. One or two temporary outside traction sutures (TOTSs)[13] are inserted into the capsulolabral tissues before complete detachment of the Bankart lesion (Fig. 17-3). Instead of struggling to try to pass a suture through the detached and mobile anteroinferior capsule, it is easier to pass such a suture when the capsule is still partially attached to the anterior neck of the scapula. In our experience this maneuver allows an easier and more reproducible bidirectional capsular retensioning. The advantages of a TOTS include the ability to (1) decide how much capsular tissue to incorporate in labrum repair ("east-west" shift) and (2) translate the soft tissue proximally and place another, more distal suture through the capsule and labrum ("north-south" shift). To shorten and retension the inferior glenohumeral ligament, a north-south as well as an east-west shift must be performed.

2. Hill-Sachs Preparation and Humeral Anchor Insertion

With the surgeon viewing from the posterior portal, the upper extremity is positioned such that the Hill-Sachs lesion engages the anterior glenoid and becomes perched on the anterior glenoid neck, effectively dislocating the glenohumeral joint in an anterior direction (Fig. 17-4A). Usually this is achieved by positioning the shoulder in internal rotation while an assistant applies

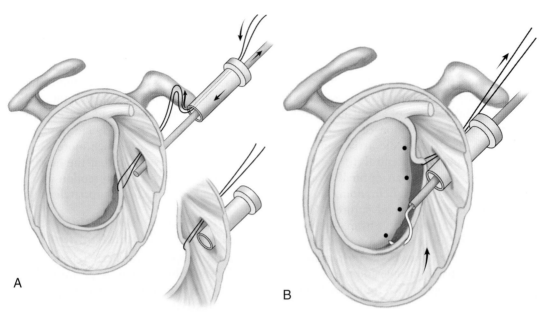

Figure 17-3. The temporary outside traction suture (TOTS). **A,** Placement of a temporary outside traction suture. **B,** The TOTS facilitates a superior shift of the capsulolabral tissue (*arrow*).

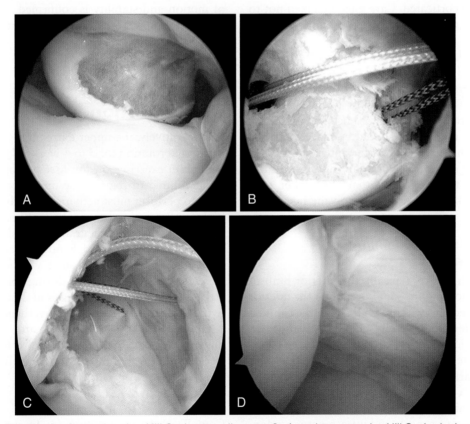

Figure 17-4. Arthroscopic views showing Hill-Sachs remplissage. **A,** At arthroscopy the Hill-Sachs lesion is brought into an engaging position such that it is perched on the anterior glenoid rim. **B,** Intra-articular view from posterior portal. Two suture anchors are introduced into the base of the humeral defect. **C,** The two anchors with the four limbs of sutures are ready to be tied over the infraspinatus tendon and posterior capsule. **D,** Once the sutures have been tied, a capsulotenodesis is created and the Hill-Sachs lesion is filled.

an anteromedially directed translational force on the humeral shaft.

The arthroscope is then transferred to the anterosuperior portal. An accessory posterolateral portal, approximately two fingerbreadths lateral to the posterior portal, is established under direct visualization from the anterosuperior portal with use of an outside-in technique with a spinal needle. Rotation of the humeral head is controlled so that the needle arrives into the joint strictly perpendicular and central to the bone defect. It is important to create an optimal working angle for the posterolateral portal. In doing so, the humeral lesion may be prepared and suture anchors inserted in the correct trajectory to ensure optimum filling of the Hill-Sachs defect. An 8-mm threaded cannula is inserted into the joint via the posterolateral portal, traversing the posterior capsule and the infraspinatus tendon. The arthroscope is then transferred to the posterior portal.

Next, the VAPR is used to clear soft tissue from the base of the humeral defect. Then, with an arthroscopic shaving device, the bony surface in the base of the defect is abraded and decorticated. Care must be taken not to iatrogenically increase the size of the humeral lesion during this step.

Via the cannula situated in the posterolateral portal, two single loaded suture anchors are inserted into the base of the humeral defect, one superiorly and one inferiorly (Fig. 17-4B). Great care must be taken during this step to ensure an appropriate trajectory of anchor insertion. Ideally the anchor should be placed into the deepest part of the defect and as far anteriorly as possible. If the angle of suture anchor insertion is not carefully controlled, there is a risk that the anchor may penetrate the humeral head cartilage on the far side of the defect.

3. Suture Passage and Filling of the Humeral Defect

One limb of each suture, typically the inferior limb of the superior anchor and the superior limb of the inferior anchor, is retrieved and withdrawn through the cannula in the posterolateral portal. The cannula is withdrawn into the subdeltoid bursa. The arthroscope is then transferred to the anterosuperior portal, with direct visualization of the articular side of the posterior capsule and the cannula insertion site. With a penetrating grasper the remaining two suture limbs are retrieved through the posterior capsule and infraspinatus tendon; thus two mattress sutures are formed (Fig. 17-4C). The objective is to capture a 10-mm bridge of posterior capsule and tendon in each of the sutures, which can then be drawn into the defect. At this point the humeral head is allowed to reduce and lie congruent with the glenoid, with the shoulder placed in neutral rotation. Two arthroscopic knots are then tied on the bursal side

of the cuff, creating the capsulotenodesis. It is important not to use the sutures that have exited through the cannula insertion site as posts. If this mistake is made, the knot will end in an intra-articular location and the quality of remplissage will be diminished. While this procedure was being developed, the arthroscope was transferred to the subdeltoid space so that the knots could be visualized during tying; this step is no longer performed. Instead, it is much more useful to maintain an intra-articular view so that the quality of reduction of the posterior capsule and tendon into the lesion can be seen and controlled appropriately (Fig. 17-4D).

4. Completion of the Anterior Capsulolabral Reconstruction

The arthroscope is transferred back to the posterior portal. The labral repair is performed in a standard fashion with use of an average of four suture anchors. The sutures exiting from the more inferiorly positioned anchors are shuttled through the previously placed TOTSs, ensuring satisfactory bidirectional capsular shift. The shoulder is then taken through a passive range of motion and stability is confirmed. Suture closure of the arthroscopic portals is not performed.

POSTOPERATIVE CONSIDERATIONS

Rehabilitation

Postoperatively, the upper extremity is placed in a sling in internal rotation for 3 to 4 weeks. Patients commence pendulum exercises on the first postoperative day and are permitted to remove the upper extremity from the sling to perform most activities of daily living including bathing. Passive and then active range-of-motion exercises are introduced in a graduated fashion. Normal use of the elbow, wrist, and hand is encouraged. Formal physiotherapy is initiated at 4 weeks postoperatively. Heavy lifting is prohibited during the first 2 months. Strengthening work commences at 2 months postoperatively, and return to contact or overhead sports is anticipated to occur at 3 to 6 months after surgery. Patients undergo routine follow-up in the office at 6 and 12 weeks and at 6 months postoperatively.

Complications

Complications are uncommon. In the senior author's (P.B.) clinical series, no infections or nerve injuries have been encountered. At short-term follow-up (mean 24 months), no patient has developed symptoms of radiographic evidence of new or progressive degenerative changes within the shoulder joint. Patients have been able to return to all preinjury activities, including overhead and high-risk sports.

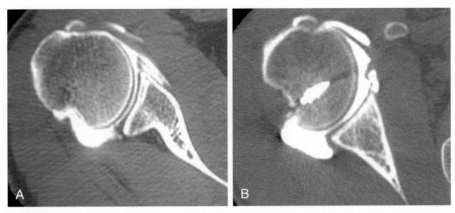

Figure 17-5. Axial images from a representative computed tomography arthrogram before **(A)** and after **(B)** arthroscopic Hill-Sachs remplissage. The lack of contrast within the base of the humeral defect on the postoperative image is indicative of complete filling or remplissage.

TABLE 17-2. Results

Functional results (N = 47)	Rowe score: 91 ± 11 Walch-Duplay score: 89.5 ± 12 Constant score: 94 ± 7				
Range of Motion	**AAE**	**ER 1**	**ER 2**	**IR 1**	**IR 2**
Operated shoulder	175 ± 7	55 ± 16	76 ± 12	9.3 ± 1.1	64 ± 11
Contralateral shoulder	177 ± 5	63 ± 16	85 ± 13	9.8 ± 0.6	69 ± 11
Difference	2 ± 4	8 ± 7	9 ± 7	0.5 ± 0.9	5 ± 6
P value	.002	<.001	<.001	.003	<.001

AAE, Active anterior elevation; *ER 1,* external rotation, arm at side; *ER 2,* external rotation in abduction; *IR 1,* internal rotation, arm at side, expressed in points as per the Constant score; *IR 2,* internal rotation in abduction.

RESULTS

We have reported the results of BHSR in a cohort of 47 patients treated for recurrent traumatic anterior shoulder instability at a mean follow-up of 24 months.[14] On postoperative contrast CT or magnetic resonance imaging (MRI), there was evidence of capsulotenodesis healing in all cases (Fig. 17-5). There were no significant postoperative complications in the treatment group. At latest follow-up, there was a recurrence of instability in only one patient, occurring as a result of a reinjury. The restriction in postoperative external rotation is modest, measuring on average less than 10 degrees. Ninety percent of patients have been able to return to sport postoperatively, with 68% achieving their preinjury level of sporting activity. The clinical outcome and range-of-motion data are presented in Table 17-2.

REFERENCES

1. Voos JE, Livermore RW, Feeley BT, et al. Prospective evaluation of arthroscopic Bankart repairs for anterior instability. *Am J Sports Med.* 2010;38(2):302-307.

2. Boileau P, Villalba M, Hery JY, et al. Risk factors for recurrence of shoulder instability after arthroscopic Bankart repair. *J Bone Joint Surg Am.* 2006;88: 1755-1763.

3. Kazel MD, Sekiya JK, Greene JA, et al. Percutaneous correction (humeroplasty) of humeral head defects (Hill-Sachs) associated with anterior shoulder instability: a cadaveric study. *Arthroscopy.* 2005;21(12):1473-1478.

4. Kropf EJ, Sekiya JK. Osteoarticular allograft transplantation for large humeral head defects in glenohumeral instability. *Arthroscopy.* 2007;23(3):322.e1-5. Epub 2006 Nov 27.

5. Miniaci A, Berlet G. Recurrent anterior instability following failed surgical repair: allograft reconstruction of large humeral head defects. *J Bone Joint Surg Br.* 2001;83 (suppl 1):19-20.

6. Re P, Gallo RA, Richmond JC. Transhumeral head plasty for large Hill-Sachs lesions. *Arthroscopy.* 2006;22(7): 798.e1-4.

7. Weber BG, Simpson LA, Hardegger F. Rotational humeral osteotomy for recurrent anterior dislocation of the shoulder associated with a large Hill-Sachs lesion. *J Bone Joint Surg Am.* 1984;66(9):1443-1450.

8. Purchase RJ, Wolf EM, Hobgood ER, et al. Hill-Sachs "remplissage": an arthroscopic solution for the

engaging Hill-Sachs lesion. *Arthroscopy*. 2008;24:723-726.

9. Connolly J. Humeral head defects associated with shoulder dislocations. In: American Academy of Orthopedics: *Instructional Course Lectures*. St Louis: Mosby; 1972:42-54.

10. Saha AK. *Theories of shoulder mechanism*. Springfield Ill: Charles C Thomas; 1961.

11. Gagey J, Gagey N. The hyperabduction test. An assessment of the laxity of the inferior glenohumeral ligament. *Journal of Bone and Joint Surgery Br*. 2001;83:69-74.

12. Balg F, Boileau P. The instability severity index score: a simple preoperative score to select patients for arthroscopic or open shoulder stabilisation. *J Bone Joint Surg Br*. 2007;89:1470-1477.

13. Boileau P, Ahrens P. The TOTS (temporary outside traction suture): a new technique to allow easy suture placement and improve capsular shift in arthroscopic Bankart repair. *Arthroscopy*. 2003;19(6):672.

14. Boileau P, O'Shea K, Vargas P, et al. Anatomical and functional results after arthroscopic Hill-Sachs remplissage. *J Bone Joint Surg Am*. 2012;94(7):618-626.

Chapter 18

Coracoid Transfer: The Modified Latarjet Procedure for the Treatment of Recurrent Anterior Inferior Glenohumeral Instability in Patients with Bone Deficiency

Patrick J. Denard and Stephen S. Burkhart

Chapter Synopsis

- The majority of anterior instability cases requiring surgery can be successfully managed with arthroscopic Bankart repair. In the setting of significant bone defects, however, recurrence is high with a Bankart repair. The Latarjet procedure reduces recurrence in such cases. The technique has recently been simplified with the development of instruments that facilitate graft harvest and placement.

Important Points

- Recognizing bone defects in anterior instability will reduce the risk of recurrence after surgical stabilization.
- Indications for the Latarjet procedure include glenoid bone loss of more than 25% of the inferior glenoid diameter (inverted-pear glenoid), and/or a deep Hill-Sachs lesion that engages in a position of 90 degrees of abduction plus 90 degrees of external rotation (position of athletic function).
- Placing the inferior aspect of the coracoid flush with the glenoid results in a more anatomic reconstruction with greater extension of the congruent arc.

Clinical and Surgical Pearls

- Aim to harvest a graft of 2.5 to 3 cm.
- Graft placement (flush with the native glenoid articular arc) is the most critical portion of the procedure and is important to avoid glenohumeral arthritis.
- Self-drilling, self-tapping screws minimize the risk of injury to the suprascapular nerve.

Clinical and Surgical Pitfalls

- Avoid an overhanging lateral graft.
- Contact sports are avoided until at least 9 months postoperative and the graft is fully healed.

Recognizing and properly addressing bone defects is crucial to achieving good surgical outcomes in shoulder instability. One of the most important requirements for glenohumeral stability is a long congruent articular arc in which the humerus and glenoid remain in contact throughout motion. Loss of this congruent arc can occur from glenoid bone loss or defects in the posterior humeral head (i.e., Hill-Sachs lesions) (Figs. 18-1 and 18-2). Such lesions are present in up to 95% of patients with recurrent shoulder instability.[1] Examining the glenoid alone, Sugaya and colleagues reported that 90% of patients with recurrent instability have glenoid bone abnormalities (including bone loss or abnormal contour).[2] Glenoid bone loss (distinct from abnormal contour alone) was seen in 50% of cases; in over half, the defect was greater than 5% of the glenoid width. In the setting of glenoid bone loss of greater than 25% of the inferior glenoid diameter, recurrence after arthroscopic Bankart repair is 67% to 75%.[1,3] In such cases, recurrence can be dramatically reduced by the Latarjet procedure, in which the coracoid is transferred to the glenoid (Fig. 18-3). As noted by Patte, the success of the

Latarjet procedure can be attributed to the *triple effect*, which is composed of the following:

1. Lengthening of the articular arc by the bone graft
2. The sling effect of the conjoined tendon
3. Tensioning of the lower subscapularis by means of the conjoined tendon in its new position (draped over the lower subscapularis)

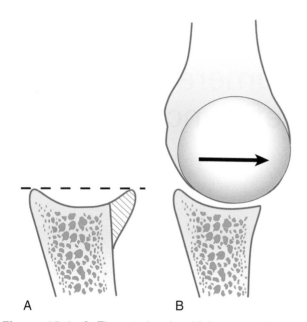

Figure 18-1. **A,** The anterior glenoid rim serves to "deepen the dish" of the glenoid and acts as a buttress to resist dislocation. **B,** A glenoid with bone loss has a decreased congruent arc with less resistance to shear forces and less resistance to obliquely applied off-axis loads. *(From Burkhart SS, Lo IK, Brady PC.* Burkhart's View of the Shoulder: The Cowboy's Guide to Advanced Shoulder Arthroscopy. *Philadelphia: Lippincott Williams & Williams; 2006.)*

PREOPERATIVE CONSIDERATIONS

History

A thorough history is essential and should elicit the mechanism of injury and prior treatments received. Previous operative reports should be obtained and reviewed; they often yield valuable information about areas of bone deficiency, tissue quality, and fixation devices used. Essential components of the history include age, mechanism of dislocations, number of dislocations, position of shoulder during dislocation, reduction efforts (self- or physician-reduced), hand dominance, sport and work requirements, prior treatments, and patient's goals.

Physical Examination

The physical examination determines the position and direction of instability as well as identifying or eliminating factors that contribute to instability:

- Muscle tone or wasting
- Range of motion, active and passive
- Strength assessment (rule out concomitant rotator cuff tear)
- Position of apprehension
- Relocation relief
- Direction of instability (load and shift test)
- Generalized ligamentous laxity
- Neurovascular examination

Imaging

Our evaluation for bone loss is based on preoperative and intraoperative assessments. We routinely obtain

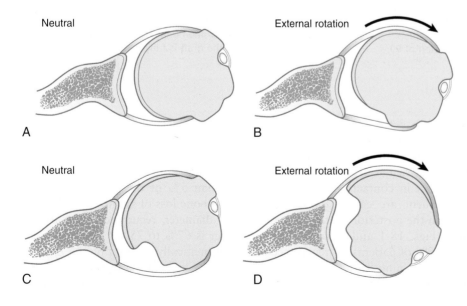

Figure 18-2. **A,** Normal relationship of the glenoid and humeral articular surfaces. **B,** Full external rotation still maintains contact between the humeral and glenoid articular surfaces. **C,** Large Hill-Sachs lesion creates an articular arc length mismatch. **D,** A small amount of external rotation will cause the Hill-Sachs lesion to engage the anterior corner of the glenoid. *(From Burkhart SS, Lo IK, Brady PC.* Burkhart's View of the Shoulder: The Cowboy's Guide to Advanced Shoulder Arthroscopy. *Philadelphia: Lippincott Williams & Williams; 2006.)*

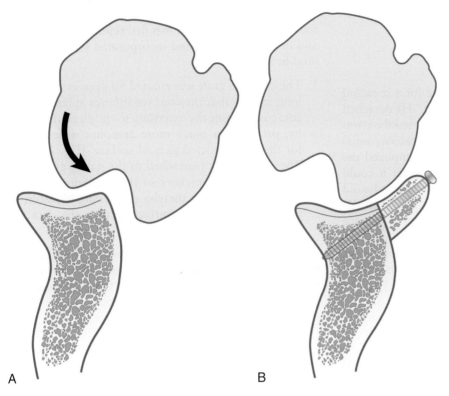

A   **B**

Figure 18-3. Schematic drawing demonstrating the use of a modified Latarjet procedure to lengthen the glenoid articular arc to prevent engagement of an engaging Hill-Sachs lesion. **A,** Engagement of Hill-Sachs lesion with external rotation of the humerus *(arrow)*. **B,** Prevention of engagement by lengthening the glenoid articular arc. *(From Burkhart SS, Lo IK, Brady PC.* Burkhart's View of the Shoulder: The Cowboy's Guide to Advanced Shoulder Arthroscopy. *Philadelphia: Lippincott Williams & Williams; 2006.)*

anterior-posterior, trans-scapular lateral, and axillary radiographs of the glenohumeral joint. Radiographs from all patients are evaluated for the presence of glenoid bone loss or a Hill-Sachs lesion. Whereas plain radiographs can grossly demonstrate bone defects, the severity is often underestimated. We therefore obtain a computed tomography (CT) scan with three-dimensional (3D) reconstructions on all individuals with suspected bone loss. In addition, we have a low threshold for performing CT in patients without plain radiographic evidence of bone loss who otherwise have risk factors for recurrence (e.g., young patients, multiple dislocations). For estimation of glenoid bone loss, bilateral 3D CT scans are obtained. Assuming a normal contralateral shoulder, the percentage of bone loss is easily estimated by comparing the width of the glenoid on the affected side with the width of the glenoid on the normal shoulder in the en face view. In 96% of cases this technique accurately stratifies glenoid bone loss as less than or greater than 25% of glenoid width.[4]

Indications and Contraindications

Our main indications for performing an open Latarjet procedure are the following:

1. Glenoid bone loss of greater than 25% of the inferior glenoid diameter ("inverted pear" glenoid) *or*

2. Deep Hill-Sachs lesion that engages in a position of 90 degrees of abduction plus 90 degrees of external rotation (position of athletic function)

In general, we have found that a large engaging Hill-Sachs lesion usually occurs in combination with an inverted pear glenoid, so such a case satisfies both indications. Also, when a large Hill-Sachs lesion is present, the coracoid bone graft in the Latarjet procedure will lengthen the articular arc to such an extent that the Hill-Sachs lesion will not be able to engage the glenoid rim. In this way, the Latarjet procedure effectively addresses the Hill-Sachs lesion without the need for an additional bone graft to the humeral defect.

One relative indication for the Latarjet reconstruction is in the patient with severe soft tissue loss involving the anterior labroligamentous complex. Such soft tissue deficiency can occur because of thermal capsular necrosis or because of multiple failed soft tissue procedures for instability. Although some authors have recommended soft tissue allografts, we have preferentially done the Latarjet reconstruction without soft tissue augmentation. Alternatively, we have noted that there are occasional cases with partial loss of the capsule (thermal capsular necrosis; multiple failed surgeries) without any significant bone loss. We have found that such cases may be amenable to arthroscopic repair with a flap of the deep surface of the subscapularis to augment or to substitute for the anterior capsule.[5]

The major contraindications to the Latarjet procedure are infection and voluntary instability.

SURGICAL TECHNIQUE

In 1954 Latarjet described his technique for a coracoid bone graft to prevent anterior dislocation.[6] He detached the pectoralis minor from the coracoid, incised the coracoacromial ligament, left a stump of the coracoacromial ligament attached to the coracoid, then completed the osteotomy at the base of the coracoid so that it could be placed as a bone graft against the anterior glenoid neck. The coracoid was passed through a split in the subscapularis and positioned so that its inferior surface was in contact with the anterior glenoid neck, where it was secured with two screws (Fig. 18-4). In doing this, the posterolateral surface of the coracoid was placed adjacent to the glenoid joint surface.

We call our surgical technique the *congruent-arc technique.* This technique was first reported by Burkhart and de Beer[7] in 2000 and incorporated two important modifications:

1. The coracoid graft was rotated 90 degrees around its long axis so that the concave inferior surface of the coracoid became the extension to the glenoid concavity, providing a much more anatomic articular arc for the reconstructed glenoid surface[8] (Fig. 18-5).
2. The capsule was reattached to the native glenoid by means of suture anchors so that the coracoid graft was extra-articular, thereby preventing abrasion of the humeral articular surface against the coracoid graft.

The original congruent arc technique required freehand positioning of the coracoid graft. We now use an instrumented Latarjet guide system (Glenoid Bone Loss

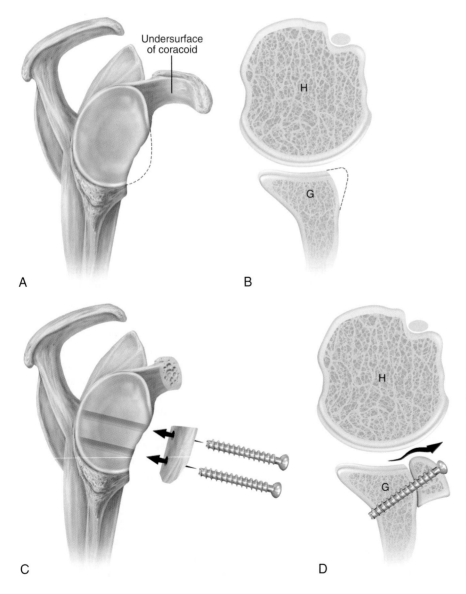

Undersurface of coracoid

A

B

C

D

Figure 18-4. Schematic of the French technique for Latarjet reconstruction. Sagittal (**A**) and axial (**B**) schematics before Latarjet reconstruction. **C** and **D,** The coracoid is osteotomized and the undersurface of the coracoid is fixed directly to the glenoid. The contour of the coracoid graft does not match the contour of the native glenoid. *G,* Glenoid; *H,* humerus. *(From Burkhart SS, Lo IK, Brady PC, Denard PJ. The Cowboy's Companion: A Trail Guide for the Arthroscopic Shoulder Surgeon. Philadelphia: Lippincott Williams & Wilkins; 2012.)*

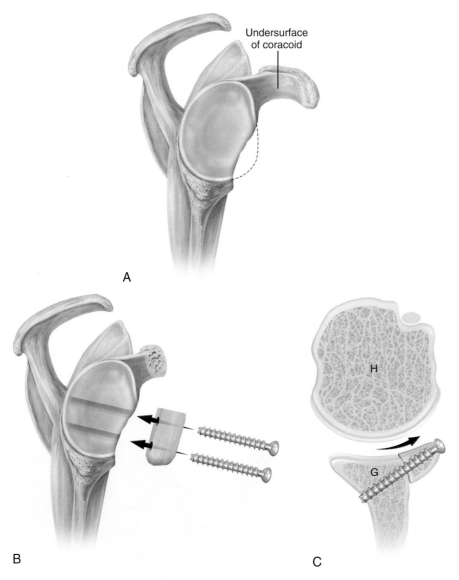

A

B

C

Figure 18-5. Schematic of the Burkhart–de Beer modification of the Latarjet reconstruction. **A,** Sagittal view demonstrates glenoid bone loss. The undersurface of the coracoid is shaded in blue. **B,** After coracoid osteotomy the graft is rotated 90 degrees so the undersurface of the coracoid is flush with the glenoid and forms a continuation of the concave glenoid articular arc. The graft is secured with two screws. **C,** Axial view demonstrates how the orientation change (compared with the original French technique [see Fig. 18-4]) provides a contour that more closely matches the native glenoid concavity and also provides greater length extension of the articular arc. *G,* Glenoid; *H,* humerus. *(From Burkhart SS, Lo IK, Brady PC, Denard PJ. The Cowboy's Companion: A Trail Guide for the Arthroscopic Shoulder Surgeon. Philadelphia: Lippincott Williams & Wilkins; 2012.)*

Set, Arthrex, Naples, FL) to ensure accurate and reproducible positioning of the coracoid graft.

Anesthesia and Positioning

The procedure is usually performed with the patient under general anesthesia. The patient is first positioned in the lateral decubitus position for arthroscopy to confirm the extent of bone loss. The coracoid transfer is best performed with the beach chair position.

Surgical Landmarks, Incisions, and Portals

Diagnostic arthroscopy uses posterior and anterosuperolateral portals. Additional portals are established as necessary if further treatment is required (e.g., superior labral anterior-posterior [SLAP] repair). The coracoid

transfer is performed through a standard deltopectoral approach, which begins at the level of the coracoid and extends distally.

Examination

We perform an arthroscopic assessment of bone loss in all patients with instability who are managed surgically. Through an anterosuperolateral viewing portal the width of the inferior glenoid is assessed with a calibrated probe inserted through the posterior portal.[9] The bare spot of the glenoid marks the center of the glenoid and is used to compare the posterior glenoid width to the anterior width. The posterior proximal humerus is assessed for the presence and severity of a Hill-Sachs lesion. A calibrated probe can be used to estimate the depth of the lesion. The arm is then removed from traction and placed in a position of 90 degrees of abduction and 90 degrees of external rotation to assess for an engaging Hill-Sachs lesion. If either glenoid bone loss of more than 25% or an engaging Hill-Sachs lesion in the 90-90 position is noted, we next address any associated pathology that is amenable to arthroscopic repair. We previously reported a 64% incidence of SLAP lesions in our patients who underwent Latarjet reconstruction.[10] In these cases we perform an arthroscopic SLAP repair using previously described techniques.[5] Then we turn the patient supine and adjust the table to a modified beach chair position, then reprepare and redrape for the open Latarjet.

Specific Steps: Modified Latarjet Procedure

The specific steps of this procedure are outlined in Box 18-1.

Coracoid Osteotomy

A standard deltopectoral incision is used. The coracoid is exposed from its tip to the insertion of the coracoclavicular ligaments at the base of the coracoid. The coracoacromial ligament is sharply dissected from the lateral aspect of the coracoid, and the pectoralis minor tendon insertion on the medial side of the coracoid is also sharply dissected from the bone. The medial surface of the coracoid, from which the pectoralis minor is detached, is the surface that will later be in contact with the anterior glenoid neck when the graft is secured by screws.

Coracoid osteotomy may be performed with an osteotome (Fig. 18-6A) or angled saw blade (Fig. 18-6B). We believe that an osteotome should be used only in thin patients. In a muscular patient with a large deltoid and pectoralis major, the bulk of these muscles may prevent a proper angle of approach anterior to the glenoid, resulting in the possibility of an intra-articular glenoid fracture. Neurovascular structures are protected by retractors medial and inferior to the saw blade or osteotome. With either technique, the osteotomy is made just anterior to the coracoclavicular ligaments to obtain as much length to the coracoid graft as possible. A graft measuring 2.5 to 3.0 cm in length is ideal,

though in small patients a graft of 2.0 cm is adequate for fixation with two screws.

The conjoined tendon is left attached to the coracoid graft to maintain vascularity of the graft and to augment stability of the glenohumeral joint by providing a *sling effect* on completion of the procedure. After mobilization of the coracoid and conjoined tendon, the musculocutaneous nerve is protected by retracting the coracoid medially, thereby preventing any stretch injury to the nerve.

Glenohumeral Joint Exposure and Glenoid Preparation

Once the coracoid has been osteotomized, there is a clear view of the anterior shoulder. The upper half of the subscapularis tendon is detached distally and reflected medially (Fig. 18-7). The insertion of the lower half of the subscapularis is preserved. After detachment of the upper subscapularis tendon, the plane between the lower subscapularis tendon and anterior joint capsule is developed.

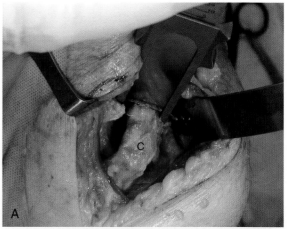

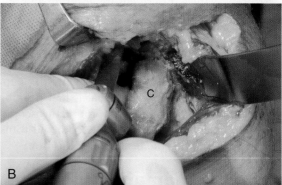

Figure 18-6. Coracoid osteotomy may be performed with **(A)** an osteotome, or **(B)** an angled saw blade. *C,* Coracoid. *(From Burkhart SS, Lo IK, Brady PC, Denard PJ. The Cowboy's Companion: A Trail Guide for the Arthroscopic Shoulder Surgeon. Philadelphia: Lippincott Williams & Wilkins; 2012.)*

BOX 18-1 Surgical Steps

1. Diagnostic arthroscopy
2. Coracoid osteotomy
3. Glenohumeral joint exposure and glenoid preparation
4. Coracoid graft preparation
5. Graft positioning and fixation
6. Closure

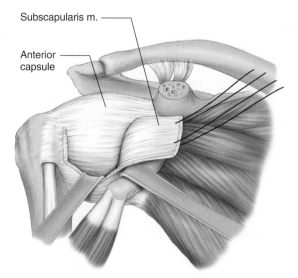

Figure 18-7. Management of the subscapularis tendon. Detach the superior half of the tendon, then develop a plane between the inferior half of the subscapularis and the capsule. *(From Burkhart SS, Lo IK, Brady PC.* Burkhart's View of the Shoulder: The Cowboy's Guide to Advanced Shoulder Arthroscopy. *Philadelphia: Lippincott Williams & Williams; 2006.)*

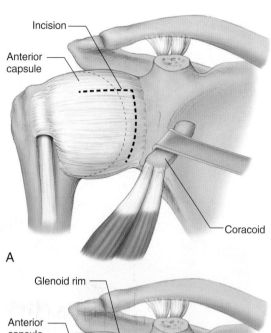

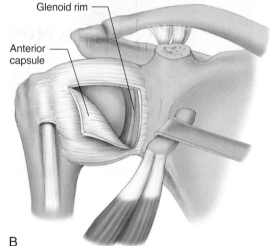

Figure 18-8. A, Outline of capsulotomy. **B,** Dissect the capsule 1 cm medial to the glenoid rim before detaching it from the glenoid neck to preserve as much capsular length as possible for later reattachment. *(From Burkhart SS, Lo IK, Brady PC.* Burkhart's View of the Shoulder: The Cowboy's Guide to Advanced Shoulder Arthroscopy. *Philadelphia: Lippincott Williams & Williams; 2006.)*

Alternatively, the glenoid may be exposed by use of a subscapularis split approach. The subscapularis split is made through the muscular fibers at the junction of the superior and middle thirds of the muscle. The capsule is bluntly dissected from the subscapularis, and then the capsular incision is made. We prefer not to use the subscapularis splitting approach because visualization can be quite limited, and the position of the split severely limits the surgeon's ability to change the position of the graft on the glenoid if needed.

The capsular incision is begun 1 cm medial to the rim of the glenoid by subperiosteal sharp dissection to preserve enough capsular length for later reattachment (Fig. 18-8). The anterior glenoid neck is prepared as the recipient bed for the coracoid bone graft by means of a curette or a bur, with care taken to preserve as much native glenoid bone as possible. "Dusting" of the anterior glenoid neck to a bleeding surface is performed with a high-speed bur without actually removing bone.

Coracoid Graft Preparation

While stabilizing the coracoid with a Kocher grasper, use an oscillating saw to remove a thin sliver of bone from the medial coracoid surface where the pectoralis minor had been inserted. This is the surface that will be in contact with the anterior glenoid neck (Fig. 18-9).

Grasp the coracoid graft with the grasping coracoid drill guide (Arthrex) (Fig. 18-10). Position the guide on the graft so that the elongated clearance slots are on the freshened surface of the coracoid that will eventually be in contact with the glenoid. The coracoid drill guide

allows the surgeon to drill two parallel 4-mm holes through the graft. Care is taken to ensure that the holes are centered on the graft and are perpendicular to the prepared bone surface.

Grafting Positioning and Fixation

Before the development of the Glenoid Bone Loss Set (Arthrex), the coracoid graft had to manually be positioned on the glenoid in a freehand manner. This was technically very difficult and was not easily reproducible. The parallel drill guide (Arthrex) has greatly simplified this part of the procedure and has also made it very reproducible.

The pegs on the parallel drill guide mate with the predrilled holes on the coracoid graft (i.e., those that

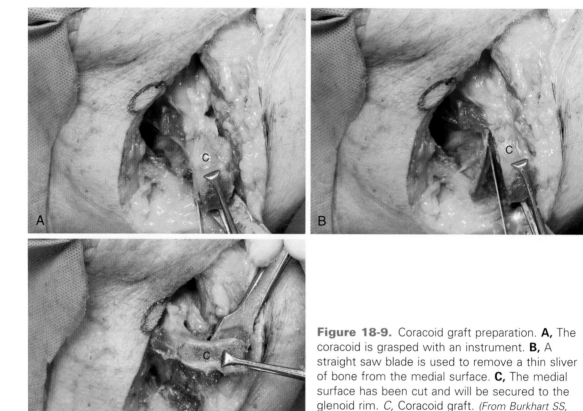

Figure 18-9. Coracoid graft preparation. **A,** The coracoid is grasped with an instrument. **B,** A straight saw blade is used to remove a thin sliver of bone from the medial surface. **C,** The medial surface has been cut and will be secured to the glenoid rim. *C,* Coracoid graft. *(From Burkhart SS, Lo IK, Brady PC, Denard PJ. The Cowboy's Companion: A Trail Guide for the Arthroscopic Shoulder Surgeon. Philadelphia: Lippincott Williams & Wilkins; 2012.)*

were created with the coracoid drill guide) to allow for easy control and positioning of the coracoid graft onto the glenoid (Fig. 18-11A). Three offset sizes are available (4, 6, and 8 mm) to adapt to various graft diameters. Some additional shaping of the graft with a rongeur or a power bur may be required to obtain the best possible fit of the guide against the graft. An optimal fit occurs when the coracoid is flush under the overhanging offset fin once the pegs are fully engaged (Fig. 18-11B).

The glenoid is optimally exposed by placing a Fukuda retractor to lever the humeral head posteriorly and by placing a two-pronged Hohmann retractor medially to retract the medial soft tissues.

Proper position of the coracoid bone graft relative to the glenoid is critical. The graft must be placed so that it serves as an extension of the articular arc of the glenoid (Fig. 18-12). The parallel drill guide is invaluable in placing the graft flush with the articular surface of the glenoid so that it is neither too far medial nor too far lateral. It is important to be sure that the guide is angled slightly medially, toward the face of the glenoid, to achieve the proper screw insertion angle and to avoid any potential screw penetration into the articular cartilage.

Use a pin driver to advance the shorter (6 inch) of the two guidewires directly through the lower hole of the guide and graft, and then into the glenoid neck. The guidewires are not terminally threaded, to allow for better feel when the posterior glenoid cortex is penetrated. Next, advance the longer (7 inch) guidewire through the second guide cannulation (Fig. 18-13A).

Next, remove the parallel drill guide. Hold the graft firmly against the glenoid with an instrument (as the pegs may be tightly wedged into the coracoid drill holes) while the parallel drill guide is withdrawn, leaving both guidewires in place (Fig. 18-13B). Although the 3.75-mm, fully threaded, cannulated titanium screws are self-drilling and self-tapping, it is recommended to use the 2.75-mm cannulated drill to penetrate only the near cortex of the native glenoid before screw insertion. Owing to the potential proximity of the screws to the suprascapular nerve posteriorly, it is advisable to rely on the self-drilling and self-tapping nature of the screws to penetrate the posterior glenoid cortex.

The screw-length depth gauge can then be used to help determine the proper screw length. Screw length is read directly from the back end of the shorter 6-inch guidewire, and from the laser line of the longer 7-inch guidewire. We have found that the most common screw

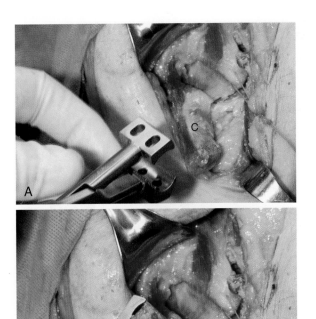

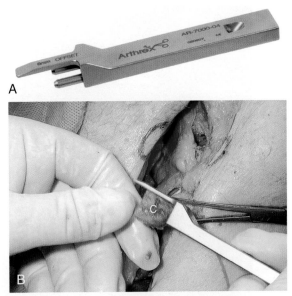

Figure 18-10. Coracoid drill guide. **A,** The coracoid drill guide (Arthrex, Naples, FL) has slots for drilling the coracoid in preparation for Latarjet. **B,** The elongated slots are placed on the medial surface of the coracoid graft (the side that will rest against the glenoid). The guide facilitates placement of two 4-mm parallel drill holes. *C,* Coracoid graft. *(From Burkhart SS, Lo IK, Brady PC, Denard PJ.* The Cowboy's Companion: A Trail Guide for the Arthroscopic Shoulder Surgeon. *Philadelphia: Lippincott Williams & Wilkins; 2012.)*

Figure 18-11. Parallel drill guide (Arthrex, Naples, FL). **A,** Pegs on the guide mate with the predrilled holes in the coracoid graft. Different offsets are available to accommodate grafts of varying thickness. A 6-mm offset guide is pictured. **B,** An optimal fit occurs when the overhanging fin is flush with the coracoid graft. *C,* Coracoid graft. *(From Burkhart SS, Lo IK, Brady PC, Denard PJ.* The Cowboy's Companion: A Trail Guide for the Arthroscopic Shoulder Surgeon. *Philadelphia: Lippincott Williams & Wilkins; 2012.)*

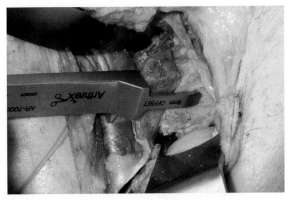

Figure 18-12. Correct placement of the coracoid bone graft occurs when the graft is flush with the glenoid surface so that the arc of the glenoid is effectively extended. The parallel drill guide (Arthrex, Naples, FL) facilitates proper placement of the graft. *(From Burkhart SS, Lo IK, Brady PC, Denard PJ.* The Cowboy's Companion: A Trail Guide for the Arthroscopic Shoulder Surgeon. *Philadelphia: Lippincott Williams & Wilkins; 2012.)*

lengths are 34 mm for the more inferiorly positioned screw and 36 mm for the superior screw.

Each screw is inserted over its guidewire with a cannulated hex driver. One must be careful not to overtighten the screws, as this may crack or damage the graft. Once the screws are almost fully seated, the surgeon double-checks the position of the coracoid graft. If the position is satisfactory, the guide pins are removed and the screws are advanced to their fully seated position (Fig. 18-13C). Intraoperative anteroposterior (AP) and axillary radiographs are taken to confirm satisfactory position of the screws and graft.

At this point the surgeon assesses the stability of the Latarjet construct. One of the most amazing things about this construct is that, with the arm in abduction and external rotation and with a manually applied, anteriorly directed force, the shoulder cannot be dislocated, even though the capsule has not yet been repaired.

Closure

Place three BioComposite SutureTak anchors (Arthrex) into the native glenoid above, between, and below the cannulated screws to repair the capsule. This makes the graft an extra-articular structure and prevents its

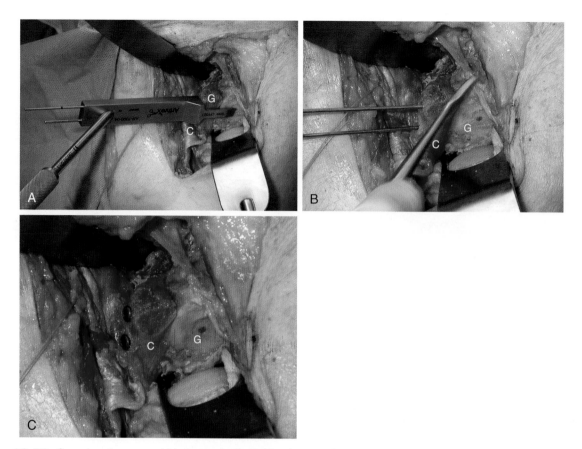

Figure 18-13. Securing the coracoid bone graft. **A,** Guidewires are inserted through the parallel drill guide (Arthrex, Naples, FL) to temporarily hold the graft in place. **B,** The drill guide is removed and the appropriate screw length can be measured. **C,** Final appearance of secured graft after placement of two cannulated 3.75-mm screws. The graft is flush with the glenoid articular surface and extends the native glenoid arc. *C,* Coracoid graft; *G,* glenoid. *(From Burkhart SS, Lo IK, Brady PC, Denard PJ.* The Cowboy's Companion: A Trail Guide for the Arthroscopic Shoulder Surgeon. *Philadelphia: Lippincott Williams & Wilkins, 2012.)*

articulation directly against the humeral head, eliminating any abrasive potential of the graft against the articular cartilage of the humerus (Fig. 18-14).

If a subscapularis split has been used, the upper and lower subscapularis muscle segments will reapproximate themselves once the retractors have been removed, and no sutures are necessary. When the upper subscapularis has been detached and retracted medially during the exposure, it is usually repaired back to its stump with No. 2 FiberWire suture (Arthrex). If the tendon stump is of poor quality, then BioComposite CorkScrew FT suture anchors (Arthrex) are used. After subscapularis repair, a standard skin closure is performed.

It is not necessary to reattach the pectoralis minor to the residual coracoid base or adjacent soft tissues because it does not retract. We have not observed any residual symptoms or cosmetic deformity relative to the unrepaired pectoralis minor.

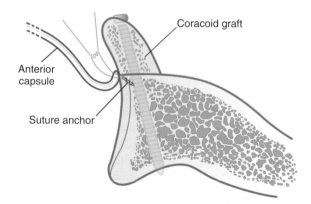

Figure 18-14. Suture anchors are placed at the interface of the graft and the native glenoid arc and used to repair the anterior capsule so that the coracoid graft remains extra-articular. *(From Burkhart SS, Lo IK, Brady PC.* Burkhart's View of the Shoulder: The Cowboy's Guide to Advanced Shoulder Arthroscopy. *Philadelphia: Lippincott Williams & Williams; 2006.)*

TABLE 18-1. Results

Study	No. Patients	Mean Follow-up	Outcomes	Recurrence
Allain et al[16]	58	14 years	88% good and excellent results	1.7%
Burkhart et al[11]	104	59 months	Constant: 94 Walch-Duplay: 92	4.9%

POSTOPERATIVE CONSIDERATIONS

Rehabilitation

The patient uses a sling for 6 weeks, with external rotation restricted to 0 degrees. After 6 weeks, the sling is discontinued and overhead motion is encouraged. Gentle external rotation stretching is begun 6 weeks postoperatively with the goal that at 3 months postoperatively the external rotation on the operated shoulder will be half that on the opposite shoulder. At 3 months postoperatively the patient begins strengthening with elastic bands. At 6 months he or she progresses to weightlifting in the gym if the graft remains in good position and shows early signs of consolidation. Contact sports or heavy labor are generally allowed when the bone graft appears radiographically healed, which is usually 9 to 12 months postoperatively.

Complications

- The majority of the reported complications are related to the coracoid graft harvest and the position of graft fixation along the glenoid.
  - Scapula fracture can occur during graft harvest with the osteotome, and in most cases we prefer the angled saw blade.
  - The tendency is to obtain an undersized graft. The goal is to obtain a graft of 2.5 to 3 cm. A flare of bone at the base of the graft usually indicates an adequate osteotomy.
  - Late graft fracture and recurrent dislocation have occurred after traumatic athletic injury. We recommend avoiding contact sports until 9 to 12 months postoperatively.
  - Fibrous union or nonunion of the graft occurs in less than 1% of cases in our experience.[11] It is minimized by placing two screws in a compression technique, decorticating the coracoid graft, and preparing the glenoid.
  - Significant glenohumeral arthritis has been reported to develop in 20% of shoulders at 14 years of follow-up.[6] However, at long-term follow-up, arthritis is less frequent after surgical stabilization compared with untreated recurrent dislocations.[12] Postoperative arthritis is best avoided by careful attention to graft position.
- The occurrence of postoperative infection and/or hematoma is uncommon.
- Recurrence is less than 5%, and surgical treatment of a failed Latarjet procedure requires an iliac crest autograft[13] or tibia plafond allograft.
- There is evidence that postoperative fatty degeneration is decreased by use of a subscapularis split approach compared with an L-shaped subscapularis incision.[14] However, the subscapularis split exposure is less forgiving, and because we feel that graft position is the most important part of the procedure, we recommend the L-shaped subscapularis incision, particularly for surgeons who perform few Latarjet procedures.
- Suprascapular nerve injury has been described.[15] To avoid injury, we recommend orienting screws within 10 degrees of the face of the glenoid, drilling only the anterior cortex of the glenoid, and inserting self-tapping, self-drilling screws.

RESULTS

There are few reports of the Latarjet procedure in the English language literature (Table 18-1).[11,16] There are many reports of the Bristow procedure (often called the *Latarjet-Bristow procedure*), which is a significantly different procedure that transfers only the coracoid tip to the glenoid neck. Regarding the Latarjet procedure, Burkhart and colleagues reported the results of 102 patients an average of 59 months after reconstruction.[11] There were four recurrent dislocations and one recurrent subluxation (4.9% recurrence rate). All recurrent dislocations were related to violent trauma in the early postoperative period and occurred with graft dislodgement. Patients achieved an average of 180 degrees of forward elevation (2 degrees improved from preoperative range) and an average of 48 degrees of external rotation with the arm at the side (5 degrees less than preoperative range). The mean Constant score was 94, and the mean Walch-Duplay score was 92 at final follow-up. Five complications were reported including two hematomas, two loose screws that did not require removal, and one fibrous union.

Allain and colleagues retrospectively reviewed 58 shoulders at an average of 14 years after the Latarjet procedure for recurrent anterior instability.[16] Although six patients had a positive apprehension sign, there were no cases of postoperative dislocation and only one subluxation. Overall, 20% of the shoulders developed clinically significant glenohumeral arthritis. It is interesting to note that although over 30% of the subscapularis tenotomy repairs were performed by overlapping the subscapularis tendon edges (as opposed to side to side), with an average 29 degrees of external rotation loss, there was no statistically significant association between the type of subscapularis repair and development of glenohumeral arthritis. Significant glenohumeral arthritis was seen in 27% of grafts placed too far laterally, compared with no cases in which the graft was placed perfectly or medially.

REFERENCES

1. Edwards TB, Boulahia A, Walch G. Radiographic analysis of bone defects in chronic anterior shoulder instability. *Arthroscopy*. 2003;19:732-739.
2. Sugaya H, Moriishi J, Dohi M, et al. Glenoid rim morphology in recurrent anterior glenohumeral instability. *J Bone Joint Surg Am*. 2003;85:878-884.
3. Boileau P, Villalba M, Hery JY, et al. Risk factors for recurrence of shoulder instability after arthroscopic Bankart repair. *J Bone Joint Surg Am*. 2006;88:1755-1763.
4. Chuang TY, Adams CR, Burkhart SS. Use of preoperative three-dimensional computed tomography to quantify glenoid bone loss in shoulder instability. *Arthroscopy*. 2008;24:376-382.
5. Burkhart SS, Lo IK, Brady PC, et al. *The Cowboy's Companion: A Trail Guide for the Arthroscopic Shoulder Surgeon*. Philadelphia: Lippincott Williams & Wilkins; 2012.
6. Latarjet M. Treatment of recurrent dislocation of the shoulder [in French]. *Lyon Chir*. 1954;49:994-997.
7. Burkhart SS, de Beer JF. Traumatic glenohumeral bone defects and their relationship to failure of arthroscopic Bankart repairs: significance of the inverted-pear glenoid and the humeral engaging Hill-Sachs lesion. *Arthroscopy*. 2000;16:677-694.
8. Ghodadra N, Gupta A, Romeo AA, et al. Normalization of glenohumeral articular contact pressures after Latarjet or iliac crest bone-grafting. *J Bone Joint Surg Am*. 2010;92:1478-1489.
9. Burkhart SS, de Beer JF, Tehrany AM, et al. Quantifying glenoid bone loss arthroscopically in shoulder instability. *Arthroscopy*. 2002;18:488-491.
10. Arrigoni P, Huberty D, Brady PC, et al. The value of arthroscopy before an open modified latarjet reconstruction. *Arthroscopy*. 2008;24:514-519.
11. Burkhart SS, de Beer JF, Barth JR, et al. Results of modified Latarjet reconstruction in patients with anteroinferior instability and significant bone loss. *Arthroscopy*. 2007;23:1033-1041.
12. Hovelius L, Saeboe M. Neer Award 2008: arthropathy after primary anterior shoulder dislocation—223 shoulders prospectively followed up for twenty-five years. *J Shoulder Elbow Surg*. 2009;18:339-347.
13. Lunn JV, Castellano-Rosa J, Walch G. Recurrent anterior dislocation after the Latarjet procedure: outcome after revision using a modified Eden-Hybinette operation. *J Shoulder Elbow Surg*. 2008;17:744-750.
14. Maynou C, Cassagnaud X, Mestdagh H. Function of subscapularis after surgical treatment for recurrent instability of the shoulder using a bone-block procedure. *J Bone Joint Surg Br*. 2005;87:1096-1101.
15. Maquieira GJ, Gerber C, Schneeberger AG. Suprascapular nerve palsy after the Latarjet procedure. *J Shoulder Elbow Surg*. 2007;16:e13-5.
16. Allain J, Goutallier D, Glorion C. Long-term results of the Latarjet procedure for the treatment of anterior instability of the shoulder. *J Bone Joint Surg Am*. 1998;80:841-852.

Chapter 19

Arthroscopic Latarjet Procedure

Laurent Lafosse, Dipit Sahu, and Wade Andrews

Chapter Synopsis
- Failure of Bankart repair has led many surgeons to perform a Latarjet procedure for recurrent instability. Open Latarjet repair has shown good long-term results. The arthroscopic Latarjet procedure combines the advantages of an open Latarjet procedure with the advantages of an arthroscopic approach.

Important Points
- Indications include instability with bone loss, complex soft tissue injury, humeral avulsion of the glenohumeral ligaments (HAGL lesions), high-risk activity (e.g., in throwing athletes), and revision of failed Bankart repair.

Clinical and Surgical Pearls
- The technique progresses through the following steps:
  - Intra-articular preparation
  - Coracoid exposure
  - Subscapularis split
  - Coracoid harvesting
  - Coracoid transfer
  - Coracoid fixation

Clinical and Surgical Pitfalls
- The pectoralis minor tendon should be completely erased from the coracoid.
- The coracoid graft should be given enough freedom from all adhesions and bursa to allow it to be displaced to the level of the glenoid.
- The subscapularis split should be wide enough to allow easy passage of the graft to the glenoid.
- Final position of the graft should be checked from three different portals.

Several options exist for the surgical treatment of anterior glenohumeral instability. Although the Bankart procedure has been shown to have reliably favorable results, there exist certain conditions (e.g., glenoid fracture, engaging Hill-Sachs lesion, inferior ligament hyperlaxity) that can signal a potentially suboptimal outcome.[1,2] The open Latarjet procedure, transfer of the coracoid such that its inferior surface abuts the anterior glenoid, has been reported by several authors to return a high rate of good to excellent results in long-term follow-up studies.[3-9] Mid-range stability is increased by the additional bone stock increasing the effective surface area of the glenoid. End-range stability is aided by the sling effect of the transferred short head of the biceps; as the arm is brought into increasing abduction, this tendon is brought under increasing tension, resisting anterior translation of the humeral head. The goal of this procedure is to recreate the open Latarjet procedure through an all-arthroscopic approach. This allows not only the reproduction of a reliable procedure, but also enhanced ability to address concomitant pathology, as well as accelerating patient mobility.

PREOPERATIVE CONSIDERATIONS

History

It is important to determine the functional use of the shoulder by the patient's age, sport (type and level), work, and level of danger in case of instability (e.g., climbers, carpenters). It is also desirable to know any modifications to activity or change in level of performance caused by the instability.

Pertinent history includes a description of the initial instability event, including the mechanism of injury and method of reduction. The number and quality (subluxation versus dislocation) of subsequent instability episodes should be investigated, as well as any aggravating factors or positions. Particular attention must be paid to the exact definition of dislocation or instability; this determination is easy when diagnosis is via a radiograph showing a dislocated position, but more difficult if no radiograph was obtained before reduction. Other pertinent details include the exact mechanism of injury, the time elapsed before relocation, and whether the relocation was performed by a physician or by someone else. Occasionally it is not possible to determine if the episode was a subluxation or an actual dislocation, and the final diagnosis of instability will depend on secondary bony or soft tissue lesions from radiologic investigations.

Symptoms

The classic anterior instability patient will report apprehension or frank instability when the affected arm is brought into increasing amounts of abduction and external rotation. Patients may also describe pain, catching sensations, weakness, and inability to perform at previous levels in their sport.

Physical Examination

In the case of an acute injury, it is important to evaluate a radiograph before physical examination, to exclude any fracture (e.g., glenoid fracture, great tuberosity fracture). The physical examination should begin with the patient being asked to demonstrate his or her range of motion and any positions that are known to cause apprehension. Some patients may be able to demonstrate intentional subluxation or even dislocation. With the patient in a standing position, both shoulders are taken through a passive range of motion as comfort allows. End range is measured in flexion, abduction (Gagey test), internal and external rotation, and extension (retropulsion). Apprehension tests are performed at 0, 90, and 140 degrees of abduction. One should remember to perform a complete examination including assessment for other possible pathologies. Posterior instability can be examined with either a jerk or a drawer test. The rotator cuff strength should be examined and the acromioclavicular joint evaluated for tenderness. Finally, one should remember to test for a sulcus sign and look for other signs of ligamentous laxity.

Imaging

High-quality imaging studies are of paramount importance in accurate evaluation of patients with instability.

Plain radiographs with five views of both shoulders are obtained: true anteroposterior (AP) views in neutral and internal and external rotation, Y-lateral view, and Bernageau glenoid profile view or axillary view if fluoroscopy is not available. It is critical that the Bernageau view be performed with the x-ray beam aligned parallel to the long axis of the scapula (from superior to inferior). Furthermore, this relationship must be maintained when the uninvolved shoulder is imaged. This should produce images that show the glenoid in near-identical profiles, allowing an accurate assessment of bone loss in the AP plane. If radiographs show clear proof of dislocation, such as a large Hill-Sachs lesion or an inferior glenoid fracture, further investigation may not be necessary. However, for clear definition of soft tissue to be achieved, radiography is often supplemented with either computed tomography (CT) or magnetic resonance arthrography (MRA). Although magnetic resonance imaging (MRI) does show more soft tissue detail, it is the senior author's (L.L.) preference to obtain a CT arthrogram for increased detail of bony lesions.

Indications

- Instability with glenoid, humeral, or combined bone loss
- Complex soft tissue injury, humeral avulsion of the glenohumeral ligaments (HAGL lesions)
- High-risk activity—for example, in throwing athletes, contact athletes (American football, rugby), overhead athletes (rock climbing, swimming), manual laborers
- Numerous episodes of instability

Contraindications

- Absence of coracoid (previous Latarjet procedure)
- Voluntary and intentional dislocators
- Multidirectional instability with pronounced ligamentous laxity

SURGICAL TECHNIQUE FOR ARTHROSCOPIC LATARJET PROCEDURE AFTER A FAILED BANKART PROCEDURE

Anesthesia and Positioning

General anesthesia with a regional nerve block is the preferred technique.

The patient is prepared as for a normal shoulder arthroscopic procedure, with care taken to have a wider area exposed medially for the most medial portal (Fig. 19-1). The patient is placed in the beach chair position.

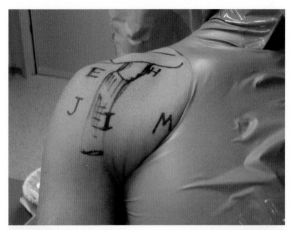

Figure 19-1. Lateral view of portals used in the Latarjet procedure.

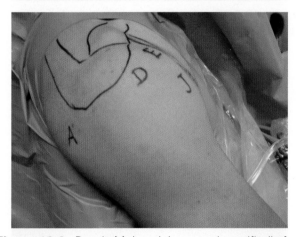

Figure 19-2. Portals M, I, and J are used specifically for the arthroscopic Latarjet procedure.

The following technical tips are important and specific for this procedure:

- The arm should be free (without any traction).
- The medial border of the scapula should be supported by a back support. This helps to act as a hinge on which the scapula can be rotated posteriorly with the help of switching sticks (as described later) to make the glenoid face more laterally. Supporting the shoulder on its back at the level of the spinal edge of the scapula maintains it in an external rotation position and facilitates the fixation of the bone graft to the glenoid.

Surgical Landmarks, Incisions, and Portals

Seven portals are used, denoted by the letters *A, D, E, H, M, I,* and *J* (Figs. 19-1 and 19-2).

Portals A and E are the starting portals, and the rest are introduced as the surgery proceeds.

BOX 19-1 Surgical Steps

1. Intra-articular preparation
   - Inspect the glenohumeral joint through portals A and E
   - Remove the labrum
   - Remove the capsule
2. Coracoid exposure
   - Create the rotator interval opening
   - Conjoint tendon
   - Visualize the axial nerve
3. Subscapularis split
   - Establish the inferior I and inferolateral J portals
   - Determine the level of subscapularis split
   - Create portal M
   - Subscapularis split
4. Coracoid harvesting
   - Create a workspace above the coracoid
   - Release the pectoralis minor tendon
   - Create portal H
   - Coracoid drilling
   - Insert the top hats
   - Coracoid osteotomy
   - Coracoid control
   - Trim the graft
5. Coracoid transfer
6. Coracoid fixation

The three portals that are used specifically in this surgery are as follows:

- Portal M: This is the most medial portal, through which the double-barrel cannula is introduced to control the coracoid graft.
- Portal I: This portal is in direct line with the axis of coracoid.
- Portal J: This is used as a viewing portal for the subscapularis muscle.

Specific Steps

Specific steps for this procedure are outlined in Box 19-1.

1. Intra-articular Preparation

1. The procedure commences with the introduction of the arthroscope through portal A in the soft spot. A probe is then introduced through the rotator interval through portal E. The glenohumeral joint is inspected for soft tissue lesions (e.g., glenoid labral defects, HAGL lesions, bony defects) (Fig. 19-3).

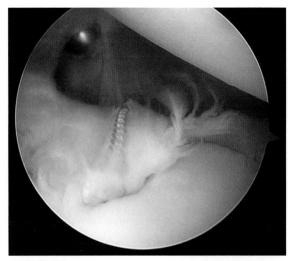

Figure 19-3. Intra-articular view from the posterior portal.

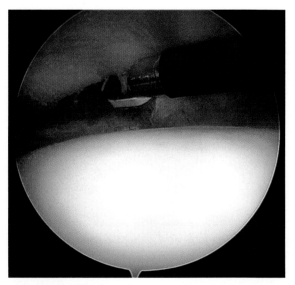

Figure 19-5. Opening of the capsule to expose subscapularis.

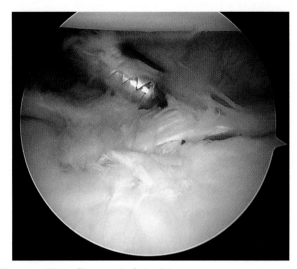

Figure 19-4. Removal of the labrum.

2. Electrocautery is introduced through portal E, and the anteroinferior labrum and middle glenohumeral ligament between the 2- and 5-o'clock positions are resected to expose the glenoid neck. A shaver introduced from portal E may also aid in labrum removal (Fig. 19-4). After exposure of the glenoid neck, the intended graft site is marked with the help of electrocautery. The selected site is usually between the 3-o'clock and 5-o'clock positions.
3. The capsule between the glenoid neck and the subscapularis is removed, or at least opened, to expose the subscapularis muscle (Fig. 19-5).

2. Coracoid Exposure

1. The rotator interval is opened with the help of a shaver, which is introduced from anterolateral portal D (Fig. 19-6). The coracoacromial ligament is located, followed down to the coracoid, and then

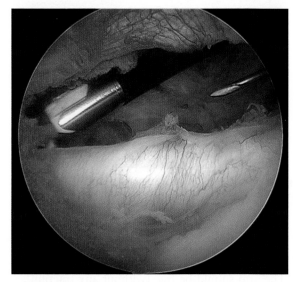

Figure 19-6. Opening of the rotator interval.

excised from the bone. The conjoint tendon is then exposed along its entire length to the upper border of the pectoralis major tendon (Fig. 19-7).
2. Dissection is continued on the anterior and lateral aspect of the conjoint tendon. The purpose of this dissection is to remove the fascia among the deltoid, pectoralis major, and conjoint tendon. Further dissection is carried out posterior to the conjoint tendon, with the arthroscope in portal D, which gives a better view of the tendon and the subscapularis muscle (Fig. 19-8).
3. The medial tissue barrier between the subscapularis and conjoint tendon is removed, and with a gentle medial dissection, axillary nerve is visualized (Fig. 19-9). The fatty tissue under the coracoid process is

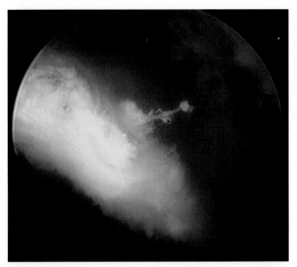

Figure 19-7. View of the conjoint tendon.

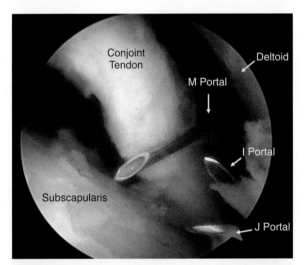

Figure 19-8. View of the subscapularis, conjoint tendon, and needle through the intended portals.

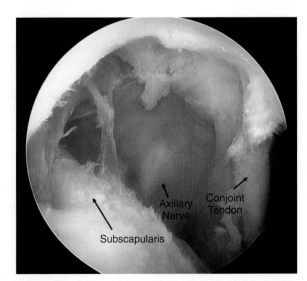

Figure 19-9. View of the axillary nerve, subscapularis, and conjoint tendon.

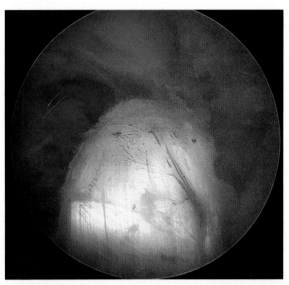

Figure 19-10. Head-on view of the coracoid from portal I.

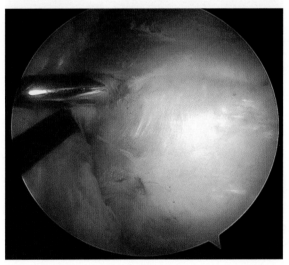

Figure 19-11. Switching stick through the subscapularis at the intended level of split.

removed, and the bleeding vessels are coagulated to perfectly expose the base of the coracoid.

3. Subscapularis Split

1. Portal J is established under vision by the outside-in technique. Portal J is in a direct line with the subscapularis axis and facilitates easy viewing of the entire subscapularis muscle. Portal I is introduced in a direct line with the coracoid axis. This portal gives a head-on view of the entire coracoid (Fig. 19-10).
2. A switching stick is inserted through portal A and is passed across the glenohumeral joint at the level of the glenoid defect. It is then advanced through the subscapularis at the intended level of the split (Fig. 19-11). Particular attention must be paid at this step as the plexus is in line with the glenoid surface and

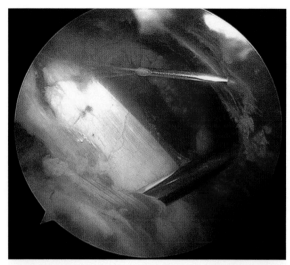

Figure 19-12. Switching stick advancing through the subscapularis and pushing the conjoint tendon medially.

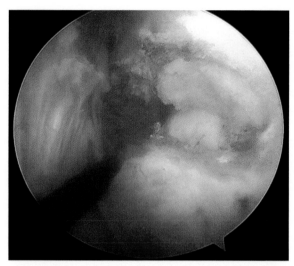

Figure 19-14. Subscapularis split being created by electrocautery.

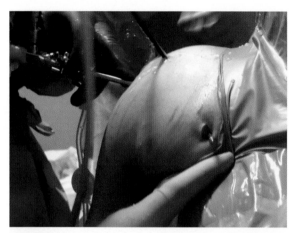

Figure 19-13. Portal M created at the tip of advancing switching stick.

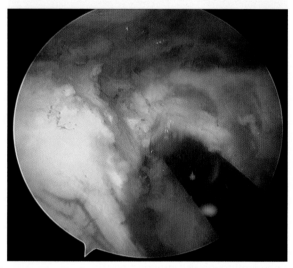

Figure 19-15. Pectoralis minor tendon being removed from the bone.

the switching stick may penetrate and damage the plexus and/or the vessels. It is tremendously important to move the tip of the stick outside the conjoint tendon as soon as the subscapularis muscle as been penetrated, taking care not to harvest the axillary nerve. The shoulder must be placed in adequate position to facilitate this maneuver.

3. The switching stick is advanced anteriorly, with care taken to stay lateral to the conjoint tendon. The conjoint tendon is pushed medially by the advancing stick, thus protecting the brachial plexus (Fig. 19-12). This switching stick is advanced to the level of skin, and portal M is created at the tip of the switching stick through the pectoralis major muscle (Fig. 19-13).

4. Electrocautery is now introduced through portal I and the arthroscope through portal J. The switching stick is then retracted back from the pectoralis major but still pushes the conjoint tendon laterally and

now also functions to elevate the subscapularis. Electrocautery creates the split in the subscapularis, medially and laterally, at the level of the switching stick. The split is made medially to expose the glenoid neck and laterally to the insertion of the subscapularis on lesser tuberosity (Fig. 19-14) while the stick still pushes the conjoint tendon.

4. Harvesting the Coracoid

1. The arthroscope is moved into portal I and a switching stick is introduced into portal D to lift the tissues above the coracoid and create a working space.

2. Electrocautery is used to define the space between the conjoint tendon and the pectoralis minor tendon, and then the pectoralis minor tendon is removed from the coracoid at the level of the bone (Fig. 19-15). Inferiorly, the pectoralis minor tendon is

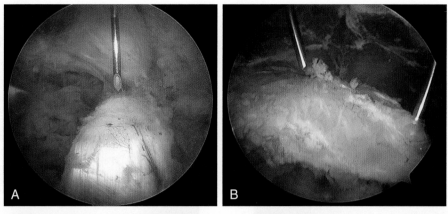

Figure 19-16. A and **B,** Needles being introduced from above the coracoid.

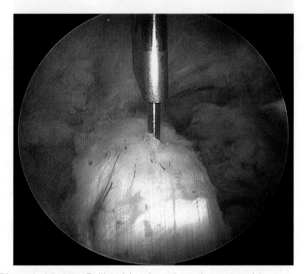

Figure 19-17. Drill guide placed on the coracoid.

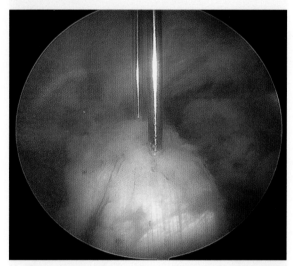

Figure 19-18. Position of K-wires on the coracoid.

bluntly dissected to free any adhesions and to protect the musculocutaneous nerve and brachial plexus. The inferior surface of the coracoid is then exposed with the help of electrocautery.

3. Portal H is created to allow superior access to the coracoid. Two needles are introduced from just above the coracoid to locate the tip and the midpoint of the coracoid (Fig. 19-16A and B). This ensures the proper position of the coracoid drill guide for the creation of portal H.

4. The drill guide is introduced from portal H. This drill guide is placed over the coracoid at the junction of the medial one third and lateral two thirds and 2 to 3 mm medial to the tip of coracoid (Fig. 19-17). The alpha hole of the guide is drilled with a Kirschner (K) wire. The drill guide is rotationally aligned to stay perpendicular to the superior surface, and then the beta hole is drilled with another K-wire. The drill guide is then removed, and the position of the K-wire is checked (Fig. 19-18). The two holes are then drilled over the K-wire with the help of the step drill.

5. The step drill and K-wires are removed, and the holes are tapped to prepare for introduction of top hat screws. The two top hat screws are then introduced over K-wires (Fig. 19-19). An optional step at this point is to pass a wire suture through the holes to secure the washers and to facilitate the next step of harvesting the coracoid by the cannula.

6. Stress risers are created on the superior, inferior, and lateral aspects of the coracoid proximal to the beta hole and with the help of a bur introduced from portals H, D, and M. At this stage the double cannula is introduced from portal M before advancement to the controlled osteotomy step (Fig. 19-20). The arthroscope is moved to portal J and the electrocautery to portal I. A curved osteotome is then introduced from portal H (Fig. 19-21), and a controlled osteotomy of the coracoid is performed (Fig. 19-22).

7. The double cannula with two long plastic bullets is now advanced to reach the coracoid graft. The two plastic bullets are removed and replaced with two long screws. The graft must then be reduced into the cannula. This is done to gain control of the graft and

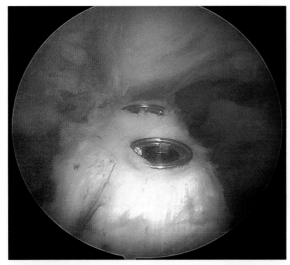

Figure 19-19. Top hats placed on the coracoid.

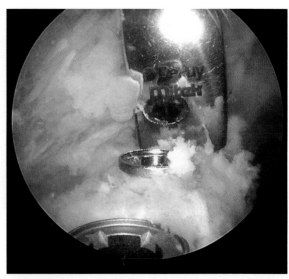

Figure 19-22. Osteotomy of the coracoid performed with a curved osteotome.

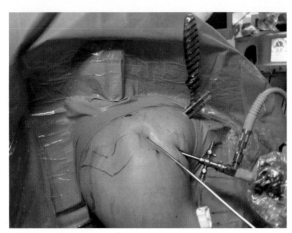

Figure 19-20. Plastic double cannula introduced from portal M just before the coracoid osteotomy.

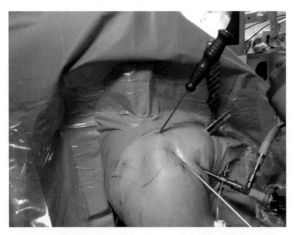

Figure 19-21. Curved osteotome introduced from the superior portal H.

is achieved by advancing the two long screws into the top hats of alpha and beta holes in the coracoid (Fig. 19-23A and B). The screws are advanced through the top hats and into the coracoid, where they engage the bone. This step can be secured by the use of the wire suture passed into the double-cannulated instrument before insertion of the long fixation screws. This step may help maintain control of the top hat in case it is loosely fixed to the coracoid.

8. The harvested graft is mobilized, and all adhesions are removed. This is achieved by a strong manipulation of the cannula to ensure total freedom of the coracoid process and upper part of the conjoint tendon, which will eventually cross above the inferior split portion of the subscapularis muscle. The mobilized coracoid usually has a medial spike arising from its base that must be trimmed to allow good bony contact with the glenoid (Fig. 19-23B). To achieve this, the assistant holds the scope, and the bur is held stationary while the coracoid is manipulated around the bur to allow accurate debridement of the graft and to minimize any risk to the plexus (Fig. 19-24).

5. Coracoid Transfer

The graft is then manipulated to reach the glenoid neck (Fig. 19-25). This is made possible by elevating the subscapularis split with the switching stick introduced from the posterior portal. A second switching stick, introduced under the deltoid through the lateral D portal, is used as a lever arm (Fig. 19-26) to angulate the scapula posteriorly, which helps facilitate the graft positioning on the glenoid neck while the arm is placed in discrete forward flexion and full internal

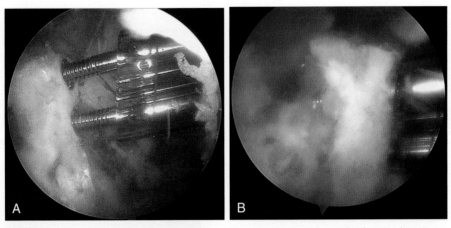

Figure 19-23. A and **B,** Gaining control of the coracoid by advancing long screws in the top hats.

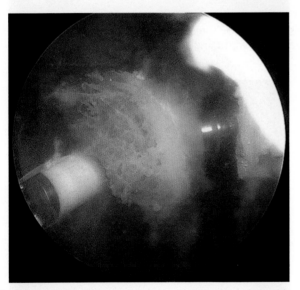

Figure 19-24. Removing bone spike on the bone with a bur while the coracoid is held stationary.

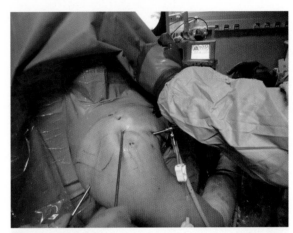

Figure 19-26. Switching sticks used to orient the glenoid more laterally.

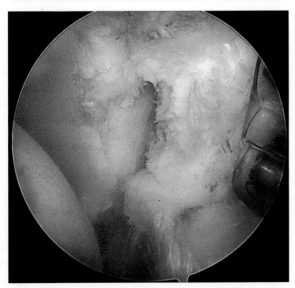

Figure 19-25. Placing the coracoid on the glenoid.

rotation at the shoulder to decrease the subscapularis tension.

6. Coracoid Fixation

While the arthroscope remains in portal J, the graft is positioned flush with the glenoid bone, medial to the cartilage in the predetermined position; two long K-wires are inserted through the coracoid positioning cannula, passing through the graft and the glenoid to achieve temporary fixation. The wires emerge posteriorly through the skin, and clips are placed on each (Fig. 19-27). At this step it is crucial to verify the position of the graft by moving the scope to different portals to verify the three-dimensional position of the coracoid. It is recommended to place the scope in portals I, D, and A to verify the exact position. If the position is not good, it is easy to remove the wires and to reposition the graft in a more adequate location. Once the position is controlled and validated, final fixation is performed. The long screw in the alpha hole is removed, and a 3.2 glenoid drill is passed over the K-wire. The length of the definitive screw can be read from the depth gauge on

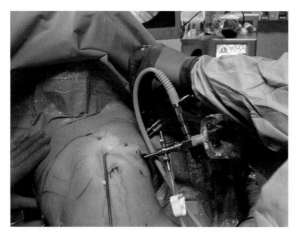

Figure 19-27. K-wires through the long screws in the double cannula and exiting posteriorly.

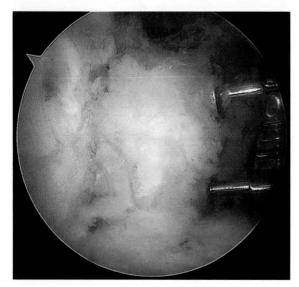

Figure 19-28. Screws placed in the alpha and beta holes through the double cannula.

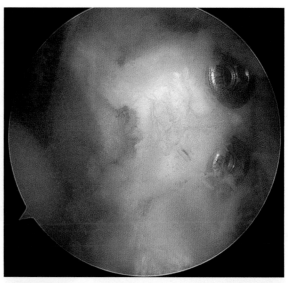

Figure 19-29. Checking the final position of the graft; graft flush with the glenoid.

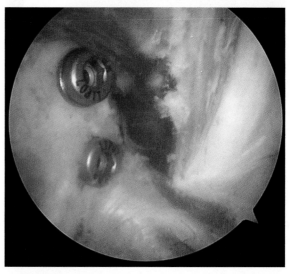

Figure 19-30. Final graft with the conjoint tendon acting as a sling crossing the subscapularis.

the drill. The drill is removed, and a definitive screw is placed in this hole. The same action is repeated for the beta hole, and a definitive screw is placed (Fig. 19-28). The K-wires are then removed, and the final position of the graft is checked through portals D, J, and A (Figs. 19-29 and 19-30).

RESULTS

To date we have performed more than 300 arthroscopic Latarjet procedures. We analyzed our first 100 consecutive procedures, performed from 2003 to May 2008. The study group included 98 patients whose average age was 27.5 years. Eventually we had 62 patients available for review at 18-month clinical follow-up.[10] We had 80% excellent results and 18% good results. All patients returned to work at a mean of 2 months.

We have also analyzed our results in our 200 available cases (presently unpublished). Our data show 197 cases with excellent stability and 185 patients having returned to full mobility.

POSTOPERATIVE CONSIDERATIONS

Rehabilitation

Postoperatively the patients require no immobilization and may begin full active range of movements immediately. They can return to work as soon as pain allows, and sports at 3 to 4 weeks. High-risk and contact sports are allowed only after 6 to 8 weeks.

Complications

In our published series of 100 cases, there were two perioperative hematomas, one intraoperative graft fracture, one transient musculocutaneous nerve palsy, three instances of partial osteolysis around the graft, and four nonunions of graft with the glenoid.[10]

Our unpublished analysis of 200 cases has shown eight cases of malunion of the graft and three cases with stiffness of the shoulder with return of normal function within 6 months. Screws were removed in 11 cases at a later date, and three cases were revised with use of an iliac crest bone graft (Eden-Hybinette procedure).

We also had early infection in three cases. These cases were subsequently treated with arthroscopic debridement and lavage. Infection resolved in all the cases after initial debridement and antibiotics. In our opinion, infection was probably related to inadequate asepsis caused by improper draping of the area around the M portal. As the M portal is quite medial in the chest, particular attention should be paid and care should be taken to keep it in the sterile aseptic surgical field.

CONCLUSION

The technique of arthroscopic Latarjet has evolved over last 8 years and now allows reproducible steps with use of a dedicated set of instruments. As the procedure is performed entirely under arthroscopic control, it provides excellent visibility of many important anatomic structures. The all-arthroscopic nature of the procedure also provides a powerful tool that allows the surgeon to visualize the coracoid graft in relation to the glenoid and thus control its final position. We believe this step is tremendously important and critical to the success of the Latarjet procedure regardless of whether the open or arthroscopic technique is used. We usually visualize the final graft position through three different portals and can place the graft in the desired position. However, an important requirement and caveat is that there should be a bloodless surgical field to have good visibility during the entire procedure. This requires a dedicated anesthesiologist to control hemodynamic variations and maintain low mean arterial pressure during the procedure. The critical steps in the procedure, such as making a good coracoid osteotomy with appropriate placement of top screws, an adequate subscapularis split, and visualization of placement of the graft in the desired location, all require excellent arthroscopic visualization. When executed appropriately, all these steps result in an excellent final result. The final outcome is therefore a coracoid bone block with sling effect in the exact desired location, allowing the patient to have good stability and to start active range-of-motion exercises soon after the surgery.

REFERENCES

1. Boileau P, Villalba M, Hery JY, et al. Risk factors for recurrence of shoulder instability after arthroscopic Bankart repair. *J Bone Joint Surg Am.* 2006;88: 1755-1763.
2. Tauber M, Resch H, Forstner R, et al. Reasons for failure after surgical repair of anterior shoulder instability. *J Shoulder Elbow Surg.* 2004;13:279-285.
3. Allain J, Goutallier D, Glorion C. Long-term results of the Latarjet procedure for the treatment of anterior instability of the shoulder. *J Bone Joint Surg Am.* 1998;80: 841-852.
4. Collin P, Rochcongar P, Thomazeau H. [Treatment of chronic anterior shoulder instability using a coracoid bone block (Latarjet procedure): 74 cases]. *Rev Chir Orthop Reparatrice Appar Mot.* 2007;93:126-132.
5. Hovelius L, Sandstrom B, Sundgren K, et al. One hundred eighteen Bristow-Latarjet repairs for recurrent anterior dislocation of the shoulder prospectively followed for fifteen years: study I—clinical results. *J Shoulder Elbow Surg.* 2004;13:509-516.
6. Hovelius LK, Sandstrom BC, Rosmark DL, et al. Long-term results with the Bankart and Bristow-Latarjet procedures: recurrent shoulder instability and arthropathy. *J Shoulder Elbow Surg.* 2001;10:445-452.
7. Hovelius L, Vikerfors O, Olofsson A, et al. Bristow-Latarjet and Bankart: a comparative study of shoulder stabilization in 185 shoulders during a seventeen-year follow-up. *J Shoulder Elbow Surg.* 2011;20:1095-1101.
8. Walch G. La luxation récidivante antérieure de l'épaule. *Rev Chir Orthop.* 1991;77(suppl 1):177-191.
9. Walch G, Boileau P. Latarjet-Bristow procedure for recurrent anterior instability. *Tech Shoulder Elbow Surg.* 2000;1:256-261.
10. Lafosse L, Lejeune E, Bouchard A, et al. The arthroscopic Latarjet procedure for the treatment of anterior shoulder instability. *Arthroscopy.* 2007;23(11):1242.e1-5.

Chapter **20**

Arthroscopic Rotator Cuff Repair: Single-Row Technique

L. Pearce McCarty III

Chapter Synopsis

- Arthroscopic repair of the rotator cuff with a single row of suture anchor fixation represents a well-established, well-reported technique with a high rate of success. Single-row arthroscopic rotator cuff repair can be executed consistently and effectively with relative ease. As with any technique—open or arthroscopic—proper tear pattern recognition and mobilization are essential elements to an appropriate repair. Advantages over more recent double-row techniques include reduced implant cost and in most cases decreased complexity and operative time.

Important Points

- Indicated for symptomatic patients with full-thickness tearing of the rotator cuff who have failed or are inappropriate candidates for nonoperative management
- Implemented arthroscopically with a single row of suture anchor fixation

Clinical and Surgical Pearls

- Accurate identification of the tear is essential to planning and executing an appropriate repair.

- Effective mobilization of the torn tendon(s) via a variety of releases and use of adjunct repair techniques such as margin convergence are vital to performing a repair with minimal tension.
- Methodic anchor insertion and suture passage in either a strict anterior-to-posterior or a posterior-to-anterior direction simplifies suture management, expediting the repair process.

Clinical and Surgical Pitfalls

- Inadequate lateral and posterior subacromial bursectomy can lead to compromised visualization secondary to swelling from arthroscopic fluid.
- Anchors that back out with a light tug on the suture limbs should be replaced with a larger-diameter anchor, without repunching or retapping of the pilot hole.
- Attempting to manage more than one suture through a given cannula during knot tying can lead to significant suture entanglement.

Although the use of arthroscopic techniques for operative repair of the rotator cuff has become increasingly common, controversy has emerged between advocates of single-row anchor fixation and those who advise use of two such rows (e.g., "double row," "dual row," "suture bridge," "transosseous equivalent"). Proponents of single-row fixation cite decreased cost and decreased operative time and point out the dearth of clinical outcome studies that justify use of double-row techniques. Proponents of double-row fixation, on the other hand, cite biomechanical advantages that include

superior repair strength[1] and footprint coverage,[2] decreased micromotion at the tendon-bone interface,[3] and increased, more homogenous pressure distribution across the repair site.[4] All of these factors, they suggest, may translate into improved healing potential at the tendon-bone interface. More recently, arthroscopic non–anchor-based transosseous techniques have been developed and may hold significant promise, but for the time being they remain out of mainstream practice.

Although investigations continue to pursue an answer to the question, "Is more better?" with respect to fixation, the use of single-row fixation remains an acceptable and in most cases less technically challenging arthroscopic repair technique for repair of the rotator cuff. Furthermore, given certain time-tested principles of rotator cuff repair, such as minimization of tension at the repair site, larger L-shaped, reverse-L–shaped, and U-shaped tears may be better suited to a single-row approach, particularly if they are chronic or acute-on-chronic with limited mobility, as efforts toward "anatomic" footprint coverage may result in excessive repair tension. Finally, regardless of the technique used for repair, the need for recognition of tear size and pattern, execution of necessary mobilization procedures including interval slides when indicated, appropriate footprint preparation, effective suture management, and appropriate rehabilitation remain essential elements of any properly performed arthroscopic rotator cuff repair.

PREOPERATIVE CONSIDERATIONS

History

- Distant or recent traumatic event, most commonly a fall from standing height with subsequent temporary inability to actively abduct the arm away from the side
- Nighttime pain
- Difficulty with overhead activity secondary to pain and/or "quick" fatigue
- Difficulty with outstretched activity secondary to pain and/or quick fatigue

Signs and Symptoms

- Anterolateral or direct lateral shoulder pain that may radiate down to, but rarely beyond, the elbow
- Dull ache at rest that may become sharp with overhead or outstretched use of the involved extremity

Physical Examination

- Observable atrophy in the supraspinatus and/or infraspinatus fossae (large or chronic tears)
- Tenderness to palpation over the anterolateral shoulder or greater tuberosity
- Reproducible anterolateral or lateral shoulder pain on manual motor testing of the rotator cuff
- Weakness with manual motor testing of the rotator cuff (large or chronic tears)
- Positive "hornblower's sign" with massive posterolateral tears (inability to actively externally rotate with the arm supported in 90 degrees of abduction)
- Positive lift-off test with massive anterosuperior tears

Imaging

- Plain radiographs consisting of Grashey, outlet, and axillary views for the following:
  - Evidence of greater tuberosity fracture when a history of trauma is present.
  - Acromial morphology including identification of enthesophyte on outlet view and os acromiale on axillary view.
  - Presence of static superior migration of the humeral head with respect to the glenoid. Note that the presence of such static changes together with a large or massive tear serves as a relative contraindication to operative repair. Superior static migration is the condition to look for on plain radiographs. Presence of a massive tear is inferred from the presence of observable static migration.
  - Presence of degenerative, chronic changes such as osteophyte formation along the inferior anatomic neck of the humeral head, acetabularization of the undersurface of the acromion, sclerosis and "rounding off" of the greater tuberosity, narrowing of the glenohumeral joint space, and loss of sphericity of the humeral head.
- Magnetic resonance imaging (MRI) for the following:
  - Identification of tear size, degree of retraction, tendon quality, and presence of intratendinous delamination and potentially recognition of tear pattern (Fig. 20-1).
  - Quantification of associated muscle belly atrophy and fatty infiltration. Note this is best performed on T1-weighted sagittal oblique views at the first cut in which the scapular spine becomes visible

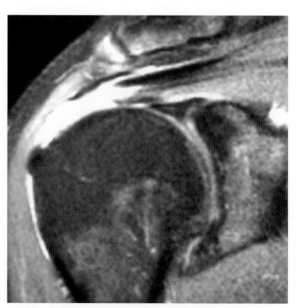

Figure 20-1. Proton density, fat-saturated coronal magnetic resonance image depicting full-thickness tearing of the supraspinatus with delamination and a moderate degree of tendon retraction.

and can be useful in determining the reparability of the tear.

- Identification of associated, potentially surgical pathology such as acromioclavicular arthritis or osteolysis, partial-thickness tearing or subluxation of the long head of the biceps tendon, articular cartilage defects, labral pathology, calcific tendonitis, intra-articular loose bodies, and subscapularis pathology.

- Ultrasonography
  - Inexpensive alternative to MRI for soft tissue evaluation
  - Highly dependent on technical skill of ultrasonographer
  - Offers ability to perform dynamic evaluation

Tear Size and Classification

Size (Anterior-to-Posterior Dimension)

- Small: Up to 1 cm
- Medium: 1-3 cm
- Large: 3-5 cm
- Massive: Greater than 5 cm or involving three or more tendons of the rotator cuff

Classification

- Partial-thickness
  - Bursal-sided
  - Articular-sided
  - Intrasubstance
- Full-thickness
  - Crescent
  - U-shaped
  - L-shaped
  - Reverse-L–shaped

Fatty Infiltration

- Goutallier classification[5]
  - Grade 0—No fatty deposits
  - Grade 1—Some fatty streaks
  - Grade 2—More muscle than fat
  - Grade 3—As much muscle as fat
  - Grade 4—Less muscle than fat

Indications and Contraindications

Indications

- Acute, traumatic full-thickness tear in an active, otherwise healthy individual capable of complying with postoperative protocol.
- Full-thickness tear with associated, appropriate pain recalcitrant to nonoperative treatment. Note that pain out of proportion to objective findings and/or pain in a distribution inconsistent with rotator cuff pathology should prompt further diagnostic

investigation and consideration of alternative diagnoses such as complex regional pain syndrome and cervical spine disease.

Contraindications

- Heavy smoking (relative)
- Concomitant adhesive capsulitis (relative)
- Complex regional pain syndrome
- Active infection
- Changes consistent with rotator cuff tear arthropathy (e.g., static proximal migration of the humeral head on plain radiography)
- Stage 4 fatty infiltration with significant muscle belly atrophy and significant tendon retraction (e.g., to glenoid rim) (relative)

SURGICAL TECHNIQUE
Anesthesia and Positioning

The surgeon should base anesthetic choice on consideration of patient preference, medical comorbidities (e.g., presence of morbid obesity or chronic obstructive pulmonary disease (COPD) may increase risk of respiratory compromise with interscalene regional block should the long thoracic nerve be affected), and skill of the anesthesiologist, but some combination of endotracheal, laryngeal mask airway, and regional anesthesia will typically be used.

Use of regional anesthesia such as an interscalene block with an indwelling catheter offers the patient effective pain control in the outpatient setting by extending the analgesic effects of the block for several days postoperatively. This can potentially reduce a patient's need for postoperative narcotic pain medication and thereby diminish the risk of associated side effects such as nausea, constipation, urinary retention, and narcosis.

Positioning may be either beach chair or lateral decubitus, depending on surgeon preference. However, beach chair positioning permits the surgeon to manipulate the humerus freely to improve arthroscopic access to the greater tuberosity, particularly during anchor placement.

Surgical Landmarks, Incisions, and Portals

Landmarks

- Coracoid process
- Clavicle
- Acromion
- Scapular spine

Portals

Portal placement determines to a great extent the ease with which one may execute the rotator cuff repair

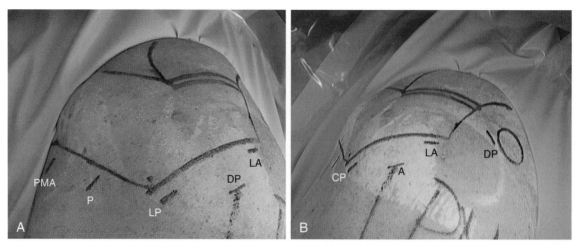

Figure 20-2. **A,** Surface landmarks of the shoulder, posterolateral view, depicting surface locations of the posteromedial accessory portal *(PMA)*, posterior portal *(P)*, lateral-posterior portal *(LP)*, direct lateral portal *(DP)*, and lateral-anterior portal *(LA)*. The acromial outline is drawn around its inferior palpable border. **B,** Surface landmarks of the shoulder, anterolateral view, depicting surface locations of the tip of the coracoid process *(CP)*, anterior portal *(A)*, LA, and DP.

(Fig. 20-2). Portal "crowding" should be avoided with the use of spinal needle localization of portal sites under direct arthroscopic visualization. The introduction of a spinal needle under direct arthroscopic visualization permits one to determine the precise proximity of one portal to another. In addition, one should not hesitate to establish additional viewing portals depending on the size and configuration of the tear pattern. Commonly used portals include the following:

- Anterior (lateral to the tip of the coracoid process and inferior to the acromioclavicular joint).
- Direct lateral (in line with posterior border of distal clavicle). This is a useful viewing and working portal, particularly for antegrade suture passing with a variety of commercially available antegrade, mechanical, penetrating suture passers.
- Posterior (in "soft spot" that defines posterior border of glenohumeral joint; standard initial intra-articular and bursal space viewing portal).
- Lateral-anterior (off the lateral border of the anterolateral corner of the acromion; this is a useful portal for anchor placement and suture management).
- Lateral-posterior (off the lateral border of the posterolateral corner of the acromion; this is a useful portal for viewing as well as anchor placement in cases of large and massive posterolateral tears).
- Posteromedial (approximately 3 cm medial to the standard posterior portal; this is a useful portal for suture passage with a penetrating suture grasper for large and massive posterolateral tears.
- Percutaneous (for anchor placement when necessary).

Examination Under Anesthesia and Diagnostic Arthroscopy

Examination under anesthesia should include careful documentation of passive range of motion as well as glenohumeral stability in the anterior, posterior, and inferior (sulcus) directions. Diagnostic arthroscopy of both the glenohumeral joint and bursal space should be performed according to the same meticulous sequence regardless of the ultimate arthroscopic procedure and should include evaluation of the following, at a minimum:

- Articular cartilage of the humeral head and glenoid
- Rotator cuff including particular evaluation of the subscapularis
- Long head of the biceps tendon and associated coracohumeral ligament (CHL)
- Glenoid labrum including the middle glenohumeral ligament and anterior and posterior bands of the inferior glenohumeral ligament
- Axillary pouch
- Subscapularis recess
- Subacromial space
- Subcoracoid space
- Acromioclavicular joint

Specific Steps

Specific steps for this procedure are outlined in Box 20-1.

1. Identification of Tear Size and Pattern

Accurate identification of tear size and pattern represents an essential initial step in arthroscopic repair of the rotator cuff, as it dictates which releases are needed, whether or not margin convergence will be necessary, and the proper location of anchor placement and suture passage for anatomic reduction of the torn rotator cuff tendon (Fig. 20-3). Often it is helpful to view the tear pattern from at least two portals and manipulate its free

margin with a tissue grasper before determining its classification.

Adhesions in the bursal space and bursal "leaders" (areas where the bursa has scarred to the leading edge of the free margin of the rotator cuff, giving a false impression of where the tear begins and ends) should be debrided to define the tear pattern accurately. In general, one must remember that tears of the supraspinatus and infraspinatus reduce to the tuberosity in a posteromedial-to-anterolateral direction, rather than directly medially to laterally. Specific tear patterns and considerations unique to each are as follows:

- *Crescent tears:* Most commonly found in cases of acute trauma, these are semilunar or crescent in shape with an apex that easily, *with minimal tension,* reduces to the tuberosity; no margin convergence or advanced releases are needed.
- *U-shaped tears:* Most commonly found in the acute-on-chronic or chronic setting, these have a shape

---

BOX 20-1 Surgical Steps

1. Identification of tear size and pattern
2. Associated procedures when indicated
3. Mobilization of rotator cuff and margin convergence
4. Preparation of tuberosity and tendon
5. Anchor placement
6. Suture passage
7. Knot tying
8. Inspection and evaluation of repair integrity

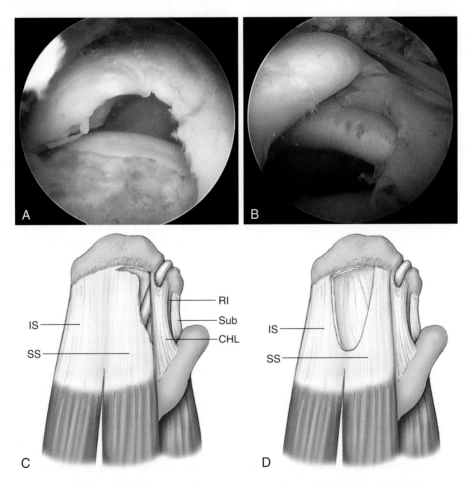

Figure 20-3. A, Arthroscopic image from a direct lateral portal of a left shoulder with a typical crescent tear pattern of the supraspinatus with minimal tendon retraction. **B,** Arthroscopic image from a direct lateral portal in a right shoulder of a typical reverse-L tear pattern of the supraspinatus. The long head of the biceps is visible anteriorly, deep to the long limb of the L. **C,** A typical L-shaped tear pattern of the supraspinatus. **D,** A typical U-shaped tear pattern of the supraspinatus. *CHL,* Coracohumeral ligament; *IS,* infraspinatus tendon; *RI,* rotator interval; *SS,* supraspinatus tendon; *Sub,* subscapularis tendon.

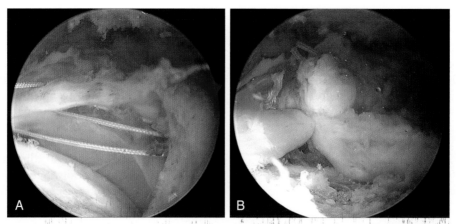

Figure 20-4. A, Arthroscopic image from a direct lateral portal in a left shoulder of a U-shaped tear. Multiple side-to-side sutures have been passed in preparation for a margin convergence. **B,** On completion of the margin convergence, the free margins of the anterior and posterior limbs of the U-shaped tear have been both approximated to each other and advanced significantly toward the prepared tuberosity.

similar to the crescent pattern but with a retracted apex that does not easily reduce to the tuberosity. Often, release techniques such as CHL release and anterior or posterior interval slides as well as side-to-side margin convergence must be executed to permit repair this type of tear to the tuberosity.

- *L-shaped and reverse-L–shaped tears:* These may be found in acute, traumatic, or chronic cases and involve a medial-to-lateral, longitudinal extension through the rotator interval (L-shaped, left shoulder) or supraspinatus-infraspinatus interval (reverse-L–shaped, left shoulder) as well as an anterior-to-posterior crescent component; these tears require side-to-side repair of the longitudinal component with subsequent repair of the anterior-posterior component to the tuberosity.

2. Associated Procedures When Indicated

Associated procedures may include, for example, subacromial decompression, distal clavicle resection, coracoid decompression, or biceps tenotomy or tenodesis.

Note that one should avoid release of the coracoacromial ligament and aggressive bony decompression in cases of large and massive tears to minimize risk of anterior-superior instability should the repair fail.

3. Mobilization of Rotator Cuff and Margin Convergence

Both posteromedial-to-anterolateral mobility and, in the case of U- and L-shaped tears, posterior-to-anterior mobility of the rotator cuff should be evaluated with use of a tendon grasper placed through either the direct lateral or lateral-anterior portal. Inability to reduce the tendon directly to bone with minimal tension indicates the need for one of potentially several in a series of

releases, particularly if direct tendon-to-tuberosity repair is planned. Properly performed releases can be highly effective in reducing tension at the repair site. Release, for example, of either the CHL or the superior glenohumeral ligament alone has been shown to reduce strain 25%, and release of both by up to 60%, depending on arm position.[6]

In performing a margin convergence for a chronic U- or L-shaped tear, the sutures are shuttled in side-to-side fashion; typically the posterior limb of the tear is advanced anterolaterally along the anterior limb, which is anchored along the CHL or, if intact, the anterior-most portion of the supraspinatus (Fig. 20-4). Sutures are passed through the most medial aspect of the tear first, progressing laterally. It is often helpful to view through a direct lateral or lateral posterior portal and work through a combination of anterior, posterior, and lateral-anterior portals. My preference is to use an antegrade NeedlePunch suture-passing device introduced through either the direct lateral or lateral-anterior portal and retrieve sutures through the anterior and posterior portals, respectively. Alternatively, penetrating graspers may be introduced simultaneously through the anterior and posterior portals and passed through the anterior and posterior limbs of the tendon, respectively. One of the penetrators is loaded with a free suture and "hands off" the suture to the other penetrator, which retrieves it.

Once the margin convergence portion of the repair has been completed, a standard single-row repair with a suture configuration of choice is executed. It can be helpful to "complete" the most lateral suture of the margin convergence with an anchor-based suture.

Common Releases

Common releases, in order from least to most aggressive, are described in the following paragraphs.

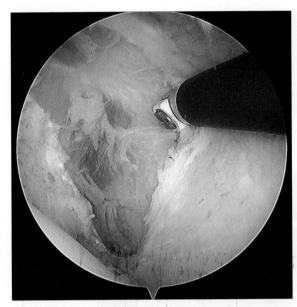

Figure 20-5. Posterior capsular release during mobilization of a large posterolateral tear. The muscle belly of the infraspinatus is visible through the aperture in the capsule.

Superior and Posterior Capsular Reflection

The glenohumeral capsular reflection onto the articular surface of the rotator cuff both superiorly and posteriorly may be thickened and may restrict mobilization of the tendon. Release is performed with a basket punch, radiofrequency, or hook-tip electrocautery type of device by viewing from a direct lateral portal and introducing the release device through the anterior portal for the superior capsular reflection or the lateral posterior portal for the posterior capsular reflection. Muscle fibers should be visible, particularly in the case of the posterior release, once the capsule has been divided (Fig. 20-5).

Coracohumeral Ligament from Base of Coracoid

The CHL is histologically a capsular element rather than a true ligament,[7] but nevertheless, particularly in the setting of a chronic retracted tear, it can serve to tether the anterior portion of the supraspinatus (as well as the superior aspect of the subscapularis). As has been demonstrated in the laboratory setting, it is possible to perform a safe, complete release of the CHL from an intra-articular approach by viewing from a posterior portal and working from an anterior portal.[8] A radiofrequency probe or hook-tipped cautery device is introduced through the anterior portal and used to peel the medial attachment of the CHL from the lateral aspect of the coracoid base until the coracoacromial ligament is visible. Visualization of the coracoacromial ligament confirms complete release of the CHL. Note that this technique also constitutes a variant of what has been described as an "anterior interval slide in continuity,"

which permits preservation of the medial aspect of the CHL for potential use in a margin convergence.[9]

Anterior Interval Slide (Traditional)

The "anterior interval" constitutes the division between the supraspinatus and subscapularis—that is, the rotator interval—and can be divided back to the base of the coracoid process to increase mobilization of the supraspinatus in a lateral direction. An increased lateral excursion of up to 2 cm has been described with this technique.[10] One must include the base of the coracoid process in this release to complete it. One or two side-to-side sutures can be used to advance the supraspinatus along the intact, anterior portion of the CHL to close the interval.

Posterior Interval Slide

For significantly retracted tears, particularly posterolateral tears involving both the supraspinatus and infraspinatus (Fig. 20-6A), a posterior interval slide allows significant mobilization of both tendons toward the greater tuberosity. The "posterior interval" constitutes the division between the supraspinatus and infraspinatus tendons. For this slide to be performed, the individual muscle bellies of the supraspinatus and infraspinatus are defined by skeletonization of the scapular spine (Fig. 20-6B). Note that although the two muscle bellies are well defined, there is crossover between the fibers of the two tendons more laterally. A traction suture is then placed in each tendon, and arthroscopic scissors are used to divide the supraspinatus and the infraspinatus back to the base of the scapular spine (Fig. 20-6C and D). The suprascapular nerve and artery run along the base of the scapular spine through the spinoglenoid notch, and care should be taken to avoid iatrogenic injury to these structures. Once the tendons have been divided, one can typically reduce the infraspinatus to its insertion on the greater tuberosity with ease and repair it in single-row fashion with one or two anchors (Fig. 20-6E). A series of side-to-side sutures can then be passed from the supraspinatus to the anterior margin of the repaired infraspinatus such that the latter is advanced laterally along the former. The supraspinatus is then repaired in standard single-row fashion directly to the tuberosity (Fig. 20-6F). Up to 4 cm of increased lateral excursion of the supraspinatus can be obtained with this technique.[10] In my experience, the lateral excursion of the infraspinatus is also significantly increased.

4. Preparation of Tuberosity and Tendon

A mechanical bur or shaver should be used to lightly abrade the bone of the greater tuberosity such that a smooth surface with punctate bleeding results (Fig. 20-7). One should avoid disruption of the cortex, as this may compromise the purchase of suture anchors used in the repair.

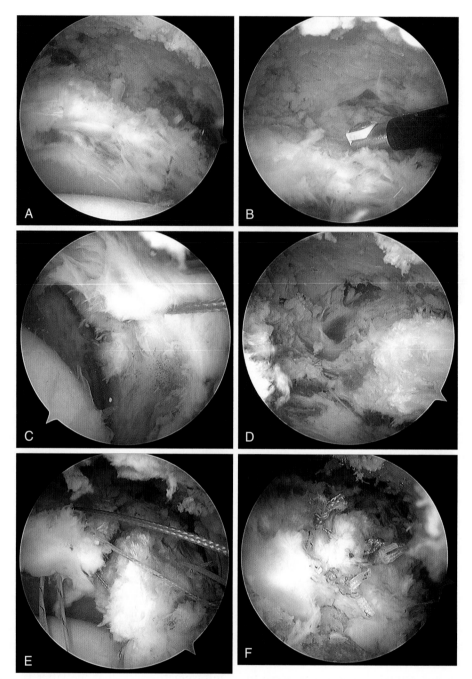

Figure 20-6. A, Arthroscopic image from a direct lateral portal in a left shoulder of a large, relatively immobile U-shaped posterolateral tear with retraction to the glenoid rim. **B,** Exposure of the scapular spine permits accurate identification of the supraspinatus (anterior) and infraspinatus (posterior) muscle bellies and subsequently their respective tendons. **C,** The tendons of the supraspinatus and infraspinatus are tagged with traction sutures in preparation for a posterior interval slide. **D,** The tendons and muscle bellies of the supraspinatus and infraspinatus have been split back to the scapular spine. Note that the suprascapular nerve and artery lie within the adipose tissue at the base of the spine. **E,** The infraspinatus has been advanced and repaired independently of the supraspinatus, and a series of side-to-side sutures has been passed to both reapproximate the two tendons and assist with advancement of the supraspinatus. **F,** Completed repair with direct tendon-to-bone fixation of both the supraspinatus and infraspinatus.

In a similar fashion, a mechanized shaver should be used to debride the free margin of the torn rotator cuff of devitalized tissue before repair. It is often helpful to run the shaver on forward and minimize suction to avoid iatrogenic injury to the healthy portion of the tendon.

5. Anchor Placement

The lateral-anterior portal (off the lateral edge of the anterolateral corner of the acromion) is often the most useful portal for anchor placement. Large or massive posterolateral tears may necessitate use of the

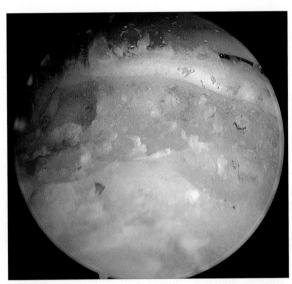

Figure 20-7. Preparation of greater tuberosity. Note punctate bleeding from prepared bony surface.

lateral-posterior portal as well. As a general rule of thumb, one should place anchors approximately 1 cm lateral to the articular margin, starting at or immediately posterior to the bicipital groove and spacing them approximately 1 cm apart across the anterior-to-posterior extent of the tear. Each anchor should be seated fully and "tug-tested" to ensure appropriate purchase, and sutures should be retrieved through a "waiting portal" until they are ready for passage through the rotator cuff.

6. Suture Passage

A systematic "same way every time" method of suture passage facilitates suture management and minimizes operative time. Sutures may be passed either immediately after each anchor has been placed or after all anchors have been placed. Either technique can be used effectively, but regardless, sutures should be stored in a waiting portal, retrieved through a working portal, and then stored in a waiting portal until ready to be tied. In addition, anchors should be placed and sutures passed sequentially in either an anterior-to-posterior or a posterior-to-anterior direction.

A number of different suture-passage devices can be used effectively, including penetrating graspers, antegrade needle punch devices (with or without auto–suture retrieval), and wire- or suture-based shuttle devices. I prefer use of an antegrade needle punch device that minimizes injury to tendon tissue during suture passage.

A variety of different suture patterns may also be used, and although certain configurations, such as the modified Mason-Allen and Mac[11] stitches, have demonstrated biomechanical superiority to simple sutures in

the laboratory setting, none has shown a clear advantage from a clinical outcome perspective. My preference when performing single-row repairs is to use triple-loaded anchors with a simple configuration when tendon quality is good, and a Mac stitch pattern when tendon quality is poor.

7. Knot Tying

Knot tying typically progresses from posterior to anterior, as suture limbs in the posterior aspect of the subacromial space may be more difficult to visualize than those in the anterior aspect, particularly after posterior bursal tissue has swollen and the rotator cuff has been reduced to the tuberosity. Any of a variety of different arthroscopic knots may be used, depending on surgeon preference. I prefer a nonsliding, nonlocking knot based on the Revo knot to minimize potential tissue laceration by the current generation of high–tensile strength sutures.

8. Inspection and Evaluation of Repair Integrity

The completed repair is inspected from both the subacromial and intra-articular spaces. In visualizing the repair within the subacromial space, it is important to internally and externally rotate the humerus to visualize the entire repair, particularly in cases of large and massive tears. An arthroscopic probe or Wissinger rod can be used to evaluate the integrity of the completed repair.

POSTOPERATIVE CONSIDERATIONS

Rehabilitation

Patients are placed in a sling with a small abduction pillow. Active hand, wrist, and elbow range-of-motion exercises are begun immediately, and pendulum exercises are begun 7 to 10 days postoperatively. Small- and medium-sized tears are sling-immobilized for 4 weeks, whereas large and massive tears are sling-immobilized for 6 weeks. After the period of sling immobilization has ended, an active-assisted, supine range-of-motion program is begun, consisting of scapular isometrics, ceiling punches, reverse pendulums, and forward elevation and external rotation in neutral abduction. Standing active range-of-motion is initiated 8 to 10 weeks postoperatively, along with gentle deltoid and rotator cuff isometrics. At 12 to 14 weeks postoperatively, rotator cuff strengthening is begun, progressing to strengthening as tolerated by 16 weeks. Modifications to these general guidelines are made with additional procedures, such as capsular release, subscapularis repair, and biceps tenodesis.

TABLE 20-1. Studies Comparing All-Arthroscopic Single-Row Rotator Cuff Repair with All-Arthroscopic Double-Row Rotator Cuff Repair

Study	Level of Evidence	Outcome
Lapner et al[12] (2011)	I	No clinical or radiographic difference
Burks et al[13] (2009)	I	No clinical or radiographic difference
Grasso et al[14] (2008)	I	No clinical difference (no imaging performed)
Franceschi et al[15] (2007)	I	No clinical or radiographic difference*

*Trend toward better restoration of footprint with double-row technique, but did not reach statistical significance.

Complications

- Infection
- Adhesive capsulitis
- Failure of the tendon to heal
- Complex regional pain syndrome
- Complications related to regional anesthesia (interscalene block)

RESULTS

The studies listed in Table 20-1 compared all-arthroscopic single-row rotator cuff repair with all-arthroscopic double-row rotator cuff repair.

REFERENCES

1. Lorbach O, Bachelier F, Vees J, et al. Cyclic loading of rotator cuff reconstructions: Single-row repair with modified suture configurations versus double-row repair. *Am J Sports Med.* 2008;36:1504-1510.
2. Apreleva M, Ozbaydar M, Fitzgibbons PG, et al. Rotator cuff tears: the effect of the reconstruction method on three-dimensional repair site area. *Arthroscopy.* 2002;18:519-526.
3. Ahmad CS, Stewart AM, Izquierdo R, et al. Tendon-bone interface motion in transosseous suture and suture anchor rotator cuff repair techniques. *Am J Sports Med.* 2005;33:1667-1671.
4. Park MC, Cadet ER, Levine WN, et al. Tendon-to-bone pressure distributions at a repaired rotator cuff footprint using transosseous suture and suture anchor fixation techniques. *Am J Sports Med.* 2005;33:1154-1159.
5. Goutallier D, Postel JM, Gleyze P, et al. Influence of cuff muscle fatty degeneration on anatomic and functional outcomes after simple suture of full-thickness tears. *J Should Elbow Surg.* 2003;12:550-554.
6. Hatakeyama Y, Itoi E, Urayama M, et al. Effect of superior capsule and coracohumeral ligament release on strain in the repaired rotator cuff tendon: a cadaveric study. *Am J Sports Med.* 2001;29:633-640.
7. Yang H, Tang K, Chen W, et al. An anatomic and histologic study of the coracohumeral ligament. *J Should Elbow Surg.* 2009;18:305-310.
8. Tetro AM, Bauer G, Hollstien SB, et al. Arthroscopic release of the rotator interval and coracohumeral ligament: an anatomic study in cadavers. *Arthroscopy.* 2002;18:145-150.
9. Lo IKY, Burkart SS. The interval slide in continuity: a method of mobilizing the anterosuperior rotator cuff without disrupting the tear margins. *Arthroscopy.* 2004;20(4):435-441.
10. Lo IKY, Burkhart SS. Arthroscopic repair of massive, contracted, immobile rotator cuff tears using single and double interval slides: technique and preliminary results. *Arthroscopy.* 2004;20:22-33.
11. Ma CB, MacGillivray JD, Clabeaux J, et al. Biomechanical evaluation of arthroscopic rotator cuff stitches. *J Bone Joint Surge Am.* 2004;86:1211-1216.
12. Lapner P, Bell K, Sabri E, et al. *A multicenter randomized control trial comparing single row with double row fixation in arthroscopic rotator cuff repair. presented AOSSM annual meeting.* San Diego, CA: 2011.
13. Burks RT, Crim J, Brown N, et al. A prospective randomized clinical trial comparing arthroscopic single- and double-row rotator cuff repair: Magnetic resonance imaging and early clinical evaluation. *Am J Sports Med* 2009;37:674-682.
14. Grasso A, Milano G, Salvatore M, et al. Single-row versus double-row arthroscopic rotator cuff repair: a prospective randomized clinical study. *Arthroscopy.* 2009;25:4-12.
15. Franceschi F, Ruzzini L, Longo UG, et al. Equivalent results of arthroscopic single-row and double-row suture anchor repair for rotator cuff tears: a randomized controlled trial. *Am J Sports Med.* 2007;35:1254-1260.

SUGGESTED READINGS

Goutallier D, Postel JM, Gleyze P, et al. Influence of cuff muscle fatty degeneration on anatomic and functional outcomes after simple suture of full-thickness tears. *J Should Elbow Surg.* 2003;12:550-554.
Lo IKY, Burkart SS. The interval slide in continuity: a method of mobilizing the anterosuperior rotator cuff without disrupting the tear margins. *Arthroscopy.* 2004;20(4):435-441.
Lo IKY, Burkhart SS. Arthroscopic repair of massive, contracted, immobile rotator cuff tears using single and double interval slides: technique and preliminary results. *Arthroscopy.* 2004;20:22-33.

Chapter 21

Arthroscopic Rotator Cuff Repair: Double-Row Techniques

Andrew Riff, Adam B. Yanke, Geoffrey S. Van Thiel, and Brian J. Cole

Chapter Synopsis
- Double-row and suture bridge repair techniques provide improved footprint coverage, pressurized contact area, reduced motion at the footprint tendon-bone interface, and greater load to failure. It is believed that improved contact characteristics will help maximize healing potential between repaired tendons and the greater tuberosity.

Important Points
- Double-row rotator cuff repair may improve healing biology and biomechanics.

Clinical and Surgical Pearls
- Properly prepare the subacromial space to ensure adequate access to the area where the lateral row will be located.
- Margin convergence should be performed for U-shaped tears to avoid tension overload of the central sutures.
- The lateral-row suture anchors must be placed as lateral as possible to avoid overcrowding of the tuberosity with implants and to maximize repair site contact.

- Suture bridge repair constructs create optimal footprint restoration and rotator cuff–to-tuberosity contact mechanics.

Clinical and Surgical Pitfalls
- The rotator cuff tear pattern must be recognized for an appropriate strategy to be designed for mobilization and repair of the tear.
- The medial-row suture anchors must be placed as medial as possible, adjacent to the articular cartilage, to maximize and reproduce contact at the repair site and to avoid overcrowding of the greater tuberosity with implants.

Videos
- Video 21-1: Scorpion
- Video 21-2: Four-Suture Bridge
- Video 21-3: Six-Suture Bridge for Massive Tears

Open rotator cuff repairs were commonly performed in a transosseous fashion. With the advent of arthroscopic rotator cuff repair, this method was abandoned for simpler configurations such as single-row repair. With improved surgical instrumentation and surgeon skill, the focus has returned to repair methods that attempt to recreate the biomechanics of original transosseous repairs. These repair constructs include double-row, transosseous equivalent, and transosseous techniques. The development of improved rotator cuff repair techniques has been motivated by the relatively high failure and retear rates, reaching 30% to 94%, with particularly high recurrence rates for massive tears or older patients.[1,2] Failure modes can include implant failure,

gap formation, or breakdown at the suture-tendon interface. Likely multiple factors contribute to failure of repair, which can be reduced by proper initial fixation, limitation of gap formation, and increase in the load sharing of the construct across the tendon unit. With an average footprint of 350 mm^2, a single-row repair does not reproduce the native supraspinatus footprint.[3,4] Biomechanical studies have demonstrated that double-row and suture bridge repair techniques provide improved footprint coverage,[5] a pressurized contact area and contact pressure at the footprint,[6,7] reduced motion at the footprint tendon-bone interface,[8] improved resistance to rotational forces,[9] and greater load to failure.[5,10,11,29] It is believed that improved contact characteristics will help maximize healing potential between repaired tendons and the greater tuberosity. Despite the numerous theoretical and biomechanical advantages, clinical data to corroborate biomechanical superiority had been lacking. Recent clinical trials comparing single-row and double-row arthroscopic repair in the treatment of rotator cuff tears have demonstrated improved postoperative cuff strength and decreased rate of retear with double-row repairs, particularly in tears larger than 30 mm.[12,13]

PREOPERATIVE CONSIDERATIONS

History

- Anterolateral shoulder pain frequently radiating toward the deltoid insertion.
- Usually insidious in onset, although patients may recall specific trauma.
- The pain is usually dull at rest.
- The pain is frequently exacerbated by overhead and reaching activities (combing hair, reaching into an overhead cabinet, and, in large multitendon tears, reaching into a back pocket).
- Night pain when sleeping on the affected side.
- Weakness with overhead activity.

Physical Examination

- Atrophy of the supraspinatus and infraspinatus.[14]
- Subacromial crepitation.
- Decreased active range of motion (ROM).
- Tenderness over greater tuberosity.
- Presence of impingement signs such as those revealed by the Neer test (sensitivity, 0.79; specificity, 0.53) and Hawkins-Kennedy test (sensitivity, 79%; specificity, 59%).[15]
- Supraspinatus tears may be evidenced by weakness to forward elevation, Jobe empty can test (sensitivity, 53%; specificity, 82%), and drop arm test (sensitivity, 35%; specificity, 88%).[16]
- Infraspinatus tears may be evidenced by weakness to external rotation or the external rotation lag sign (ERLS).
- Hornblower's sign may be indicative of severe degeneration or absence of the teres minor muscle (sensitivity, 95%; specificity, 92%).[17] To assess for the hornblower's sign, the examiner places the patient's shoulder in 90 degrees of abduction, the elbow in 90 degrees of flexion, and the shoulder in maximal external rotation. Inability to maintain external rotation is suggestive of significant teres minor degeneration.
- Subscapularis tears may be evidenced by limited internal rotation, lift-off test, belly press test

(Napoleon test), and bear hug test. The high specificity associated with the bear hug (92%) and belly press tests (98%) makes them valuable tests for ruling in subscapularis muscle tears.[18]
  - Lift-off test: The patient is instructed to place the hand of the same side as the affected shoulder against his or her lumbar spine and then to lift the hand off the back. Inability to lift off indicates a subscapularis tear.
  - Belly press test: The hand is used to press into the patient's abdomen, and the elbow is brought forward past the body midline. Inability to bring the elbow anteriorly past midline indicates a subscapularis tear.
  - Bear hug test: The patient is instructed to place the hand of the same side as the affected shoulder on the superior aspect of the contralateral shoulder. The patient tries to hold the starting position by means of resisted internal rotation while the examiner tries to pull the patient's hand superiorly off the shoulder with an external rotation force. Inability to maintain the starting position indicates a subscapularis tear.

Imaging

- Plain radiographs including a true anteroposterior (Grashey) view and an axillary view may demonstrate degenerative changes, calcific tendinitis, contributing acromial morphology and, most important, proximal humerus migration.
- Ultrasonography is a noninvasive, inexpensive test with good sensitivity (85%) and specificity (92%).[14] Drawbacks of ultrasonography are that it is operator dependent and less sensitive for partial-thickness tears (sensitivity, 66%; specificity, 94%).[14]
- Magnetic resonance imaging (MRI) is the standard imaging study (sensitivity, 86%; specificity, 90.4%).[14] It delineates which tendons are involved, degree of retraction, muscle atrophy, and fatty infiltration of the muscle bellies (degree of fatty degeneration can be graded according to the Goutallier classification).[19]
- Magnetic resonance arthrography is the most sensitive and specific technique for diagnosis of full-thickness rotator cuff tears (sensitivity, 95.4%; specificity, 98.9%) and partial-thickness rotator cuff tears (sensitivity, 85.9%; specificity, 96.0%).[14]

Indications and Contraindications

Indications

Full-thickness tears, young age (physiologic age below 60 years), high activity level, relative acuteness of the tendon tear, full passive ROM, and completion of 3 months of nonoperative treatment are features supporting early operative treatment.[24]

Contraindications

Partial-thickness tears, older age (physiologic age above 60 years), low demand, mild symptoms, and relative chronicity (increased Goutallier stage) of the tendon tear are features supporting nonoperative treatment.[20]

SURGICAL TECHNIQUE

Anesthesia and Positioning

The type of anesthesia to be administered should be determined by discussion among the surgeon, anesthesiologist, and patient regarding their preferences. The procedure may be performed with regional anesthesia with sedation or general anesthesia. The patient may be positioned in either the beach chair or the lateral decubitus position. The beach chair position is more familiar to many surgeons and is often easier for conversion to an open procedure. The lateral decubitus position allows better access to concomitant pathology and provides traction on the arm, which enhances visualization in the subacromial space.

Surgical Landmarks and Portals

Landmarks

- Clavicle
- Acromion
- Scapular spine
- Acromioclavicular joint
- Coracoid process

Portals

- Posterior portal
- Posterolateral portal
- Lateral portal
- Anterior portal

Examination Under Anesthesia and Diagnostic Arthroscopy

Examination under anesthesia confirms passive ROM. In the event of significant stiffness, capsular release or manipulation under anesthesia may be required. Diagnostic arthroscopy is performed in a stepwise fashion to evaluate the following:

- Anterior, posterior, and superior labrum
- Intra-articular biceps tendon
- Rotator cuff
- Humeral and glenoid cartilage

BOX 21-1 Surgical Steps

1. Tear pattern recognition
2. Tear mobilization
3. Greater tuberosity preparation
4. Margin convergence if necessary
5. Medial-row suture anchor placement
6. Medial suture passage
7. Lateral-row suture anchor placement

Specific Steps

Specific steps of the procedure are outlined in Box 21-1.

1. Tear Pattern Recognition

Diagnostic arthroscopy is performed through a standard posterior portal then the anterior rotator interval portal. Evaluation should include the following structures: glenohumeral articular surface, biceps tendon, labrum, supraspinatus, infraspinatus, and subscapularis. After completion of the intra-articular portion of the arthroscopy, the trocar and cannula for the arthroscope are passed through the posterior portal, aiming superior to the subacromial space. Entrance into the subacromial space is confirmed by ease of movement in the axial plane. This sweeping motion can also aid in improving visualization by freeing soft tissue adhesions. The anterolateral portion of the acromion should be easily identified by tactile feedback; this is where the surgeon should plan to enter the subacromial space. This trocar is then passed through the anterior portal, where a 6-mm cannula is placed over the trocar and advanced into the subacromial space. The blunt trocar is replaced with the arthroscope, and the subacromial space is visualized. An 18-gauge spinal needle is used to localize the lateral portal, made at the posterior border of the acromioclavicular joint, permitting in-line visualization of the supraspinatus. A 2-cm vertical incision is created, and the shaver can be introduced to perform the bursectomy, allowing for tear pattern recognition. Care is taken to extend the bursectomy laterally to ensure visualization of the planned lateral row. The arthroscope is then transitioned to the direct lateral portal for viewing. Most U-shaped, L-shaped, and crescent-shaped tears are amenable to double-row repair constructs as long as the lateral edge can be reduced to the lateral aspect of the greater tuberosity. Acromioplasty is performed when necessary. The anterolateral accessory portal is established just off the anterolateral edge of the acromion through spinal needle localization. One should ensure that the portal is allowing adequate access to the planned repair site before creation. An 8-mm cannula is inserted into this portal.

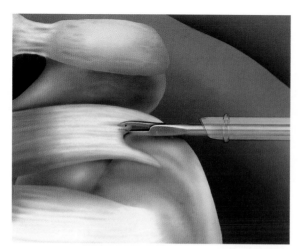

Figure 21-1. Assessment of the size and lateral mobility of the tear with use of a soft tissue grasper from the lateral portal.

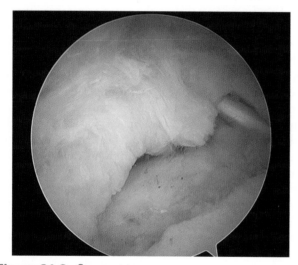

Figure 21-2. Crescent tear.

2. Tear Mobilization

The size and lateral mobility of the tear are assessed by grasping the tear edge with a tissue grasper and pulling laterally (Fig. 21-1). Crescent-shaped tears mobilize easily to the lateral aspect of the greater tuberosity footprint with minimal tension and do not require releases or mobilization techniques (Fig. 21-2). With the camera in the lateral portal, anterior and posterior tear mobility is assessed by pulling the anterior rotator cuff tear limb posterior and the posterior rotator cuff tear limb anterior. For U-shaped tears, the anterior and posterior tear limbs both have mobility. L-shaped tears have asymmetric limb mobility. Typically the posterior limb is more mobile than the anterior limb. A double-row repair requires adequate lateral mobilization of the tendon so that it may cover the entire footprint in the lateral direction (Fig. 21-3). Many chronic tears are immobile, and mobilization techniques may be required

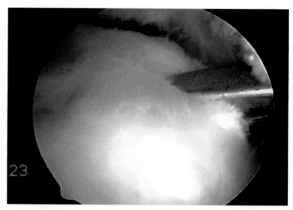

Figure 21-3. Crescent-shaped tear demonstrating full mobility to cover entire footprint in double-row repair.

to reduce the tendon to the greater tuberosity. When necessary, excursion can be increased with capsular release above the labrum, excision of superior fibrous adhesions, or release of the coracohumeral ligament and rotator interval.

3. Greater Tuberosity Preparation

The soft tissue on the greater tuberosity footprint is debrided and the cortical bone is abraded to stimulate healing. Care is taken to avoid complete decortication, which could compromise suture anchor fixation strength.

4. Margin Convergence

U- and L-shaped tears often have poor lateral mobility, and margin convergence sutures are necessary to reduce the tear volume and strain on the repair (Fig. 21-4). While viewing from the lateral portal, the surgeon passes free No. 2 sutures through the anterior limb of the rotator cuff and then the posterior limb to form a simple suture configuration (Fig. 21-5A). The suture-passing sequence is repeated for the necessary number of sutures to convert the U- or L-shaped component to a crescent-shaped tear. Two to four sutures are typically placed. Knot tying for these sutures is delayed until after the medial row of suture anchors has been placed to avoid restricting exposure to the medial tuberosity. Tying of the margin convergence sutures converts the U-shaped tear to a crescent-shaped tear, and the techniques for crescent-shaped tear repair are then carried out (Fig. 21-5B).

5. Medial-Row Suture Anchor Placement

The repair sequence involves placement of a medial row of suture anchors followed by suture passage through the tendon in a mattress fashion. The medial-row anchors are positioned as medial as possible adjacent to the articular surface of the humerus (Fig. 21-6). For a typical crescent-shaped supraspinatus tear, two anchors are placed, one in the anterior third and one in the

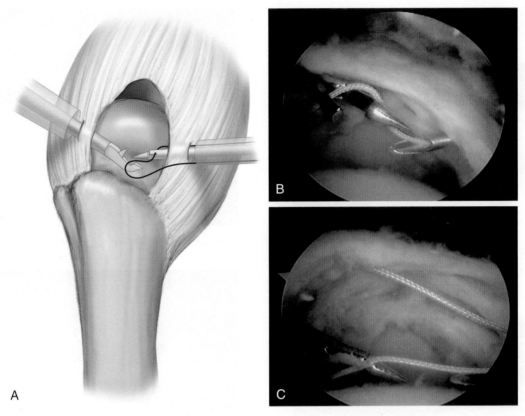

Figure 21-4. Technique of margin convergence with the suture introduced through the anterior cuff tear limb and retrieved through the posterior cuff tear limb. **A,** Position of suture-passing instruments. **B** and **C,** Suture placed with visualization from the lateral portal.

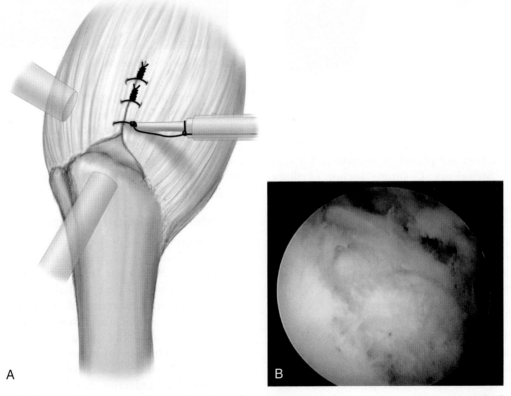

Figure 21-5. A, After margin convergence sutures have been tied, a crescent-shaped tear is obtained. **B,** Crescent-shaped tear as visualized from the posterior portal.

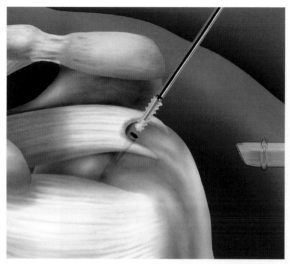

Figure 21-6. Medial-row anchor placement adjacent to the articular surface.

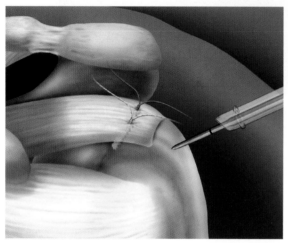

Figure 21-7. Punch placed at the lateral margin of the greater tuberosity.

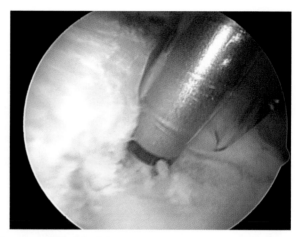

Figure 21-8. Medial row.

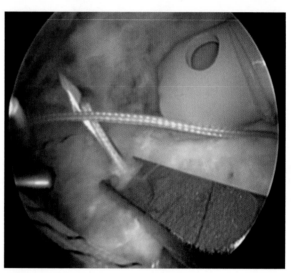

Figure 21-9. Scorpion suture passer.

posterior third of the footprint (Fig. 21-7). For larger tears, more anchors are placed as necessary. We typically use the SwiveLock C suture anchor (Arthrex, Naples, FL), which is double loaded with two sutures (a No. 2 FiberWire and 2-mm-wide FiberTape). Anchors are inserted at a 45-degree ("dead man's") angle to increase resistance to pull-out (Fig. 21-8). When anchors are being inserted, care should be taken to avoid overlapping tunnels. Anchors are typically placed from posterior to anterior.

6. Medial Suture Passing

If margin convergence sutures are placed, they are tied before medial anchor suture passage. Once the medial row of anchors is in place, sutures are passed through the cuff tissue with the use of suture-passing instruments 10 to 12 mm medial to the lateral edge of the rotator cuff tear. FiberWire sutures are typically passed with a pointed passing instrument such as the Penetrator (Arthrex) and tied in a horizontal mattress fashion. FiberTape sutures are passed with the Scorpion Suture Passer, which allows passage of an inverted mattress suture in one step (Fig. 21-9, Video 21-1). Once passed, the FiberTape sutures are left untied and parked outside the shoulder.

7. Lateral-Row Suture Anchor Placement

Through tying down of the FiberWire sutures medially, medial tension is established and the cuff tear is reduced into place at the greater tuberosity. At this point, one FiberTape limb from each medial anchor (anterior and posterior anchors) is retrieved through the accessory posterolateral cannula and threaded through the eyelet of a lateral anchor device such as the PushLock (Arthrex) (Fig. 21-10). Once both suture limbs are appropriately tensioned, the suture is secured in place with a hemostat. After tear reduction has been assessed, a hole is then punched at the intended site for the lateral implant, just lateral to the lateral edge of the tuberosity to

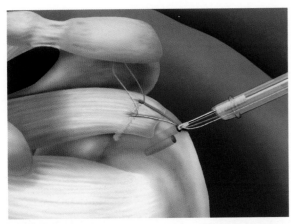

Figure 21-10. PushLock lateral anchor device.

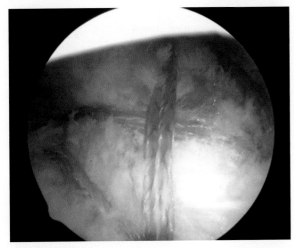

Figure 21-11. Four-suture bridge.

accommodate the posterior lateral anchor. Once the hole has been tapped, the anchor is introduced and secured into place while tension is maintained on each suture limb. The process is repeated for the anterior implant, and the final repair is evaluated. The anchors are placed lateral to the lateral edge of the footprint to fully maximize the tendon-to-footprint contact. Most commonly, for typical tears the end result is a four-suture bridge construct with cruciate suture configuration (Fig. 21-11, Video 21-2) or, less often, a six-suture bridge construct for massive tears (Video 21-3).

POSTOPERATIVE CONSIDERATIONS

Patients are placed in a sling with a small abduction pillow. The sling is worn continuously for 6 weeks except for bathing. During the first 6 weeks, active elbow, wrist, and hand exercises are performed. From 6 to 12 weeks, passive and active-assisted ROM is initiated. After 12 weeks, active motion and gentle strengthening are initiated. More aggressive strengthening is initiated at 4 months.

Complications

- Failure of tendon to heal
- Stiffness
- Missed pathologic changes: acromioclavicular joint arthritis, biceps tendinitis
- Infection

RESULTS

Several laboratory studies indicate improved strength of fixation to cyclic loading for double-row rotator cuff repairs compared with single-row rotator cuff repairs.[21,22] Other studies have demonstrated that traditional transosseous repair techniques have superior restoration of footprint coverage,[5] pressurized footprint contact area,[6,7] and decreased motion at the footprint tendon-bone interface.[8] Conventional double-row rotator cuff techniques have also been compared in the laboratory with newer suture bridge rotator cuff repair techniques.[23] For strength of fixation, the four-suture bridge technique had significantly higher ultimate load-to-failure values, with no difference in gap formation to cyclic loading. Furthermore, the suture bridge rotator cuff repair provided more pressurized contact area and mean pressure over the repaired rotator cuff tendon insertion compared with a double-row technique.

Whereas theoretical and biomechanical support for double-row repair is abundant, until recently there has been a paucity of clinical evidence supporting double-row techniques. In the last few years, a number of trials have been performed comparing single and double-row techniques with regard to subjective functionality questionnaires, cuff strength, and objective rates of cuff tear recurrence (Table 21-1).[12,13,24-32] Although these trials demonstrate a general trend toward improved subjective functionality with double-row repairs compared with single-row repairs with use of validated questionnaires such as those for the Constant score, American Shoulder and Elbow Surgeons (ASES) scale, University of California at Los Angeles (UCLA) shoulder rating scale, Single Assessment Numeric Evaluation (SANE), Western Ontario Rotator Cuff (WORC) index, or Disabilities of the Arm, Shoulder and Hand (DASH) measure, none of these trials demonstrates a statistically significant improvement in functionality. Nevertheless, double-row techniques appear to yield a statistically significant improvement in external rotation and abduction strength in the setting of tears greater than 3 cm in diameter.[13,26,30] More important, these trials demonstrate lower rates of cuff tear recurrence in patients undergoing double-row repair than those undergoing single-row repair.[12,29] These findings have been corroborated by a systematic review of 23 articles comparing retear rates for transosseous, single-row, double-row,

Text continued on p. 238

TABLE 21-1. Clinical Trials Comparing Single-Row Techniques with Double-Row Techniques

Study	N (SR/DR)	Follow-up	Age (Range)	Inclusion	Exclusion	Tear Size/Severity
Aydin et al[24] (2010)	68 (34/34)	Min, 2 y (mean, 36)	58 (36-69)	Full-thickness tear on MRI Tear of any RC tendon Amendable to SR/DR repair	Smoking Autoimune/rheumatologic disease Steroid use Traumatic tears Tears requiring side-to-side repair Large U-shaped tears No SLAP, Bankart, chondral lesions	<3 cm
Burks et al[25] (2009)	40 (20/20)	1 y	56 (43-74)	Full-thickness tear on MRI Ability to complete serial MRIs Ability to complete PT Amendable to SR/DR repair	Smoking Autoimmune/rheumatologic disease Steroid use Previous rotator cuff surgery on affected shoulder Irreparable tear Worker's compensation claims Subscapularis tear Tear requiring side-to-side repair	1-4.5 cm 1-3 cm in size–33 (SR, 18; DR, 15) >3 cm in size–7 (SR, 2; DR, 5)
Carbonel et al[26] (2012)	160 (80/80)	2 y	55.5	Full-thickness tear on MRI Tears >1 cm	GH osteoarthritis Other shoulder pathology (ipsilateral or contralateral) Tears >5 cm Retracted or immobile tears Fatty degeneration (Fuchs grade 4) Steroid use Inability to complete questionnaire	1-5 cm–160 (SR, 80; DR, 80) 1-3 cm in size–104 (SR, 51; DR, 53) 3-5 cm in size–56 (SR, 29; DR, 27)

Scoring Systems	Single Row	Double Row	*P* Value	Surgical Time (min)			Patient Satisfaction (Single/Double)	*P* Value
				Single Row	Double Row	*P* Value		
Constant	82.2 (range, 72-96)	78.8 (range, 68-94)		87 (58-137)	108 (70-181)			
Percent intact (MRI)	90%	80%	NR					
WORC	84.8 (18.4)	87.9 (20.0)	.24					
Constant	77.8 (9.0)	74.4 (18.4)	.98					
ASES	85.9 (14.0)	85.5 (20.0)	.67					
UCLA	28.6 (3.6)	29.5 (5.6)	.17					
SANE	90.9 (11.0)	89.9 (20.0)	.53					
Ext rot (N-m)	17.2 (7.7)	16.7 (7.5)	.86					
Int rot (N-m)	28.1 (13.8)	28.8 (14.4)	.69					
Percent intact (MRI)	81%	90%	>.05					
UCLA	28.9 ± 2.4	29.5 ± 1.6	.359					
Constant	79.8 ± 6.6	79.7 ± 3.2	.875					
ASES	84.6 ± 6.1	85.2 ± 3.2	.940					
External rotation	59.0 ± 6.7	58.6 ± 4.0	.774					
Internal rotation	55.7 ± 6.6	55.8 ± 4.3	.772					
Flexion	153.9 ± 10.2	159.2 ± 6.8	.003					
Abduction	154.3 ± 10.0	159.3 ± 6.8	.007					
Flexion SSI	0.75 ± 0.06	0.78 ± 0.04	.027					
Abduction SSI	0.76 ± 0.06	0.78 ± 0.04	.358					
Internal rotation SSI	0.79 ± 0.05	0.81 ± 0.04	.009					
External rotation SSI	0.80 ± 0.05	0.81 ± 0.03	<.001					
UCLA	27.1 ± 1.9	28.2 ± 1.4	.019					
Constant	75.2 ± 7.0	77.0 ± 2.4	.137					
ASES	80.3 ± 6.2	83.2 ± 3.1	.032					
External rotation	54.2 ± 6.6	56.3 ± 3.8	.002					
Internal rotation	51.0 ± 5.5	52.9 ± 3.7	.007					
Flexion	145.8 ± 9.8	153.1 ± 7.0	.002					
Abduction	146.3 ± 9.7	153.1 ± 7.0	.004					
Flexion SSI	0.70 ± 0.05	0.74 ± 0.03	.002					
Abduction SSI	0.72 ± 0.05	0.74 ± 0.03	.100					

Continued

TABLE 21-1. Clinical Trials Comparing Single-Row Techniques with Double-Row Techniques—cont'd

Study	N (SR/DR)	Follow-up	Age (Range)	Inclusion	Exclusion	Tear Size/Severity
Charousset et al[12] (2007)	66 (35/31)	Min, 2 y (mean, 28.7 mo)	59 (32-74)	Full-thickness supraspinatus tear	Previous surgery on affected shoulder Adhesive capsulitis Shoulder instability >1/3 of subscapularis or infraspinatus	Distal–54 (SR, 29; DR, 25) Intermediate–10 (SR, 5; DR, 5) Retracted–2 (SR, 1; DR, 1)
Franceschi et al[27] (2007)	60 (30/30)	Min 18 mo (mean, 22.5 mo)	61.7 (43-80)	Full-thickness tear on MRI Symptoms >3 mo Refractory to non-op therapy Sufficiently mobile tear	Fracture of glenoid, greater, or lesser tuberocity Inflammatory arthritis Retracted tendons not amenable to double-row repair Prior surgery on affected shoulder Inability to complete questionnaire	>3 cm 3-5 cm in size–39 (SR, 18; DR, 21) >5 cm in size–13 (SR, 8; DR, 5)
Koh et al[28] (2011)	62 (31/31)	Min, 2 y (mean, 31.9 mo)	61.3 (43-78)	Full-thickness tear on MRI	Irreparable tears Prior surgery on affected shoulder Fracture or dislocation Infection Inflammatory disease Open repair	2-4 cm
Ma et al[22] (2012)	53 (27/26)	Min, 2 y (mean, 33.4 mo)	61 (40-80)	Full-thickness tear >1 cm Amendable to SR/DR repair	Tear <1 cm Involvement of subscapularis Degenerative GH arthritis RC arthropathy Prior shoulder surgery Irreparable tears	>1 cm (all) 1-3 cm in size–36 (SR, 19; DR, 17) >3 cm in size–17 (SR, 9; DR, 9)
Mihata et al[29] (2011)	172 (65/107)	Min, 2 y (mean, 38.5 mo)	63 (18-82)	Full-thickness tear on MRI		All

Scoring Systems	Single Row	Double Row	P Value	Surgical Time (min)			Patient Satisfaction (Single/Double)	P Value
				Single Row	Double Row	P Value		
Internal rotation SSI	0.76 ± 0.04	0.78 ± 0.02	.026					
External rotation SSI	0.76 ± 0.05	0.78 ± 0.02	.019					
Percent intact (CT arthrography)	40%	60%	.03				Very satisfied: 21/25	0.91
Contrast	82.7	80.7	.4				Satisfied: 6/7	
Pain (max 15 pts)	13.9	13.2	.5				Disappointed: 1/1	
Activity (max 20 pts)	19.2	18.96	.51				Unsatisfied: 0/0	
Mobility (max 40 pts)	39.2	37.8	.1					
Strength (max 25 pts)	10.3	10.6	.78					
Percent intact (MRI)	54%	69%	>.05	42 ± 18.9	65 ± 23.4	0.005		
UCLA	32.9 (29-35)	33.3 (30-35)	>.05					
Forward flexion (deg)	159 (150-170)	156 (140-170)	>.05					
External rotation (deg)	132.4 (90-140)	131.3 (85-137)	>.05					
Internal rotation (deg)	37.3 (27-42)	40.3 (26-43)	>.05					
Percent intact (MRI)	38%	70%	.124	115.8 ± 25.0	214.5 ± 19.7	0.033	Excellent: 14/14	0.314
Pain (VAS)	1.5 ± 1.9	2.0 ± 2.4	.40				Good: 11/13	
Constant	85.4 ± 13.8	82.5 ± 21.9	.90				Fair: 5/1	
ASES	85.9 ± 15.2	83.4 ± 20.9	.76				Poor: 1/3	
UCLA	29.3 ± 5.2	29.8 ± 6.7	.39					
Percent intact (MR arthrography)	63%	77%	.63					
UCLA	31.4 ± 3.34	31.53 ± 3.4	.89					
ASES	91.25 ± 2.36	91.38 ± 2.36	.85					
Abduction strength (kg)	4.91 ± 0.8	5.01 ± 0.62	.63					
External rotation strength (kg)	6.86 ± 0.84	7.03 ± 0.78	.46					
UCLA	32.63 ± 2.83	32.06 ± 3.2	.95					
ASES	92.16 ± 2.19	92.12 ± 2.15	>.99					
Abduction strength (kg)	5.31 ± 0.57	5.18 ± 0.60	.85					
External rotation strength (kg)	7.52 ± 0.60	7.34 ± 0.58	.78					
UCLA	28.5 ± 2.67	30.56 ± 3.75	.53					
ASES	89.13 ± 0.99	90 ± 2.23	.82					
Abduction strength (kg)	3.99 ± 0.36	4.74 ± 0.60	.04					
External rotation strength (kg)	5.43 ± 0.59	6.47 ± 0.82	.03					
Percent intact (MRI)	89%	95%	>.05					
ASES	95.6 (11.1)	97.4 (9.1)	NR					
JOA	95.8 (9.5)	98.0 (5.3)						
UCLA	34.0 (3.9)	34.2 (3.5)						

Continued

TABLE 21-1. Clinical Trials Comparing Single-Row Techniques with Double-Row Techniques—cont'd

Study	N (SR/DR)	Follow-up	Age (Range)	Inclusion	Exclusion	Tear Size/Severity
						Small to medium–124 (SR, 57; suture bridge, 67)
						Large to massive–48 (SR, 8; suture bridge, 40)
Park et al[30] (2008)	78 (40/38)	25.1 mo (mean, 22-30 mo)	55.8 (28-78)	Full-thickness tear on MRI	Fracture or dislocation	All
						<3 cm in size–46 (SR, 25; DR, 21)
						>3 cm in size–32 (SR, 15; DR, 17)
Pennington et al[32] (2010)	132 (78/54)	2 y	54	Full-thickness tear on MRI	Tears <1.5 cm or >4.5 cm	1.5-4.5 cm
						2.5-3.5 cm
Sugaya et al[31] (2005)	80 (39/41)	Min, 2 y (mean, 35 mo)	57.9 (34-73)	Full-thickness tear on MRI	Glenoid fracture Bankart lesion Partial-thickness tear	<1 cm in size–16 (SR, 6; DR, 6) 1-3 cm in size–34 (SR, 17; DR, 17) 3-5 cm in size–25 (SR, 14; DR, 11) >5 cm in size–5 (SR, 2; DR, 3)
						<3 cm–50
						>3 cm–30

ASES, American Shoulder and Elbow Surgeons Index; CT, computed tomography; DR, double-row; ext, external; GH, glenohumeral; int, internal; JOA, Japanese Orthopaedic Association; MRI, magnetic resonance imaging; N-m, newton-meter; PT, physical therapy; RC, rotator cuff; rot, rotation; SANE, Single Assessment Numeric Evaluation; SLAP, superior labrum, anterior to posterior; SR, single-row; SSI, shoulder strength index; UCLA, University of California Los Angeles scale; VAS, visual analog scale; WORC, Western Ontario Rotator Cuff Index.

Scoring Systems	Single Row	Double Row	P Value	Surgical Time (min)			Patient Satisfaction (Single/Double)	P Value
				Single Row	Double Row	P Value		
Percent intact (MRI)	96.50%	97%	>.05					
Percent intact (MRI)	38%	93%	<.01					
ASES	91.6 ± 4.48	92.97 ± 2.27	.09					
Constant	76.68 ± 8.56	79.66 ± 4.52	.06					
SSI (abductor)	0.53 ± 0.22	0.79 ± 0.11	<.01					
SSI (int rot)	0.71 ± 0.16	0.81 ± 0.11	<.01					
SSI (ext rot)	0.66 ± 0.18	0.77 ± 0.15	<.01					
ASES	92.76 ± 4.16	92.76 ± 2.45	.99					
Constant	79.44 ± 8.11	79.52 ± 5.36	.97					
SSI (abductor)	0.78 ± 0.14	0.79 ± 0.11	.86					
SSI (int rot)	0.81 ± 0.13	0.82 ± 0.10	.92					
SSI (ext rot)	0.82 ± 0.12	0.74 ± 0.15	.07					
ASES	89.67 ± 4.45	93.24 ± 2.08	.01					
Constant	72.07 ± 7.4	79.82 ± 3.34	<.01					
SSI (abductor)	0.71 ± 0.15	0.82 ± 0.11	.04					
SSI (int rot)	0.73 ± 0.18	0.81 ± 0.12	.15					
SSI (ext rot)	0.74 ± 0.16	0.81 ± 0.14	.16					
Percent intact (MRI)	80%	68%	.017					
UCLA	29.6	29.3	.8					
ASES	86.9	91.6	<.8					
VAS	1.1	0.4	<.5					
Supraspinatus (lb)	13	16	<.02					
Infraspinatus (lb)	20	21	<.4					
Subscapularis (lb)	27	29	<.8					
Percent intact (MRI)	72%	76%	.03					
UCLA	32.4 (4.7)	33.1 (3.4)	.44					
ASES	92.9 (12.1)	94.6 (9.3)	.49					
Percent intact (MRI)	87%	100%	<.01					
Percent intact (MRI)	56%	71%	>.12					

and suture bridge repairs; this study demonstrated significantly lower retear rates in double-row repair methods when compared with single-row methods for tears greater than 1 cm.[33]

REFERENCES

1. Boileau P, Brassart N, Watkinson DJ, et al. Arthroscopic repair of full-thickness tears of the supraspinatus: does the tendon really heal? *J Bone Joint Surg Am.* 2005;87(6): 1229-1240.

2. Galatz LM, Ball CM, Teefey SA, et al. The outcome and repair integrity of completely arthroscopically repaired large and massive rotator cuff tears. *J Bone Joint Surg Am.* 2004;86(2):219-224.

3. Dugas JR, Campbell DA, Warren RF, et al. Anatomy and dimensions of rotator cuff insertions. *J Shoulder Elbow Surg.* 2002;11(5):498-503.

4. Ruotolo C, Fow JE, Nottage WM. The supraspinatus footprint: an anatomic study of the supraspinatus insertion. *Arthroscopy.* 2004;20(3):246-249.

5. Apreleva M, Ozbaydar M, Fitzgibbons PG, et al. Rotator cuff tears: the effect of the reconstruction method on three-dimensional repair site area. *Arthroscopy.* 2002;18 (5):519-526.

6. Bishop J, Klepps S, Lo IK, et al. Cuff integrity after arthroscopic versus open rotator cuff repair: a prospective study. *J Shoulder Elbow Surg.* 2006;15(3):290-299.

7. Maguire M, Goldberg J, Bokor D, et al. Biomechanical evaluation of four different transosseous-equivalent/suture bridge rotator cuff repairs. *Knee Surg Sports Traumatol Arthrosc.* 2011;19(9):1582-1587.

8. Ahmad CS, Stewart AM, Izquierdo R, et al. Tendon-bone interface motion in transosseous suture and suture anchor rotator cuff repair techniques. *Am J Sports Med.* 2005;33 (11):1667-1671.

9. Park MC, Idjadi JA, ElAttrache NS, et al. The effect of dynamic external rotation comparing 2 footprint-restoring rotator cuff repair techniques. *Am J Sports Med.* 2008; 36(5):893-900.

10. Baums MH, Buchhorn GH, Gilbert F, et al. Initial load-to-failure and failure analysis in single- and double-row repair techniques for rotator cuff repair. *Arch Orthop Trauma Surg.* 2010;130(9):1193-1199.

11. Pauly S, Fiebig D, Kieser B, et al. Biomechanical comparison of four double-row speed-bridging rotator cuff repair techniques with or without medial or lateral row enhancement. *Knee Surg Sports Traumatol Arthrosc.* 2011;19(12): 2090-2097.

12. Charousset C, Grimberg J, Duranthon LD, et al. Can a double-row anchorage technique improve tendon healing in arthroscopic rotator cuff repair? a prospective, nonrandomized, comparative study of double-row and single-row anchorage techniques with computed tomographic arthrography tendon healing assessment. *Am J Sports Med.* 2007;35(8):1247-1253.

13. Ma HL, Chiang ER, Wu HT, et al. Clinical outcome and imaging of arthroscopic single-row and double-row rotator cuff repair: a prospective randomized trial. *Arthroscopy.* 2011;28(1):16-24.

14. de Jesus JO, Parker L, Frangos AJ, et al. Accuracy of MRI, MR arthrography, and ultrasound in the diagnosis of rotator cuff tears: a meta-analysis. *AJR Am J Roentgenol.* 2009;192(6):1701-1707.

15. Hegedus EJ, Goode A, Campbell S, et al. Physical examination tests of the shoulder: a systematic review with meta-analysis of individual tests. *Br J Sports Med.* 2008;42(2):80-92.

16. Park HB, Yokota A, Gill HS, et al. Diagnostic accuracy of clinical tests for the different degrees of subacromial impingement syndrome. *J Bone Joint Surg Am.* 2005;87 (7):1446-1455.

17. Walch G, Boulahia A, Calderone S, et al. The 'dropping' and 'hornblower's' signs in evaluation of rotator-cuff tears. *J Bone Joint Surg Br.* 1998;80(4):624-628.

18. Barth JRH, Burkhart SS, Beer JFD. The bear-hug test: a new and sensitive test for diagnosing a subscapularis tear. *Arthroscopy.* 2006;22(10):1076-1084.

19. Goutallier D, Postel JM, Bernageau J, et al. Fatty muscle degeneration in cuff ruptures. Pre- and postoperative evaluation by CT scan. *Clin Orthop Relat Res.* 1994;(304): 78-83.

20. Oh LS, Wolf BR, Hall MP, et al. Indications for rotator cuff repair. *Clin Orthop Relat Res.* 2007;455:52-63.

21. Kim DH, Elattrache NS, Tibone JE, et al. Biomechanical comparison of a single-row versus double-row suture anchor technique for rotator cuff repair. *Am J Sports Med.* 2006;34(3):407-414.

22. Ma CB, Comerford L, Wilson J, et al. Biomechanical evaluation of arthroscopic rotator cuff repairs: double-row compared with single-row fixation. *J Bone Joint Surg Am.* 2006;88(2):403-410.

23. Park MC, Elattrache NS, Tibone JE, et al. Part I: Footprint contact characteristics for a transosseous-equivalent rotator cuff repair technique compared with a double-row repair technique. *J Shoulder Elbow Surg.* 2007;16(4): 461-468.

24. Aydin N, Kocaoglu B, Guven O. Single-row versus double-row arthroscopic rotator cuff repair in small- to medium-sized tears. *J Shoulder Elbow Surg.* 2010;19(5):722-725.

25. Burks RT, Crim J, Brown N, et al. A prospective randomized clinical trial comparing arthroscopic single- and double-row rotator cuff repair: magnetic resonance imaging and early clinical evaluation. *Am J Sports Med.* 2009;37(4):674-682.

26. Carbonel I, Martinez AA, Calvo A, et al. Single-row versus double-row arthroscopic repair in the treatment of rotator cuff tears: a prospective randomized clinical study. *Int Orthop.* 2012:1-7.

27. Franceschi F, Ruzzini L, Longo UG, et al. Equivalent clinical results of arthroscopic single-row and double-row suture anchor repair for rotator cuff tears. *Am J Sports Med.* 2007:1-7.

28. Koh KH, Kang KC, Lim TK, et al. Prospective randomized clinical trial of single- versus double-row suture anchor repair in 2- to 4-cm rotator cuff tears: clinical and magnetic resonance imaging results. *Arthroscopy.* 2011; 27(4):453-462.

29. Mihata T, Watanabe C, Fukunishi K, et al. Functional and structural outcomes of single-row versus double-row versus combined double-row and suture-bridge repair for

rotator cuff tears. *Am J Sports Med.* 2011;39(10): 2091-2098.

30. Park JY, Lhee SH, Choi JH, et al. Comparison of the clinical outcomes of single- and double-row repairs in rotator cuff tears. *Am J Sports Med.* 2008;36(7):1310-1316.

31. Sugaya H, Maeda K, Matsuki K, et al. Functional and structural outcome after arthroscopic full-thickness rotator cuff repair: single-row versus dual-row fixation. *Arthroscopy.* 2005;21(11):1307-1316.

32. Pennington WT, Gibbons DJ, Bartz BA, et al. Comparative analysis of single-row versus double-row repair of rotator cuff tears. *Arthroscopy.* 2010;26(11):1419-1426.

33. Duquin TR, Buyea C, Bisson LJ. Which method of rotator cuff repair leads to the highest rate of structural healing?: a systematic review. *Am J Sports Med.* 2010;38(4): 835-841.

34. Ma H-L, Chiang E-R, Wu H-TH, et al. Clinical outcome and image of arthroscopic single-row and double-row rotator cuff repair: a prospective randomized trial. *Arthroscopy.* 2012;28(1):16-24.

Chapter 22

Arthroscopic Subscapularis Repair

Lucas R. Wymore, Anthony A. Romeo, and R. Alexander Creighton

Chapter Synopsis
- Arthroscopic subscapularis repairs are becoming more common, and outcomes are similar to those of open repairs. Many times the tear is an upper border injury that can easily be addressed with arthroscopic techniques. This chapter outlines the preoperative assessment, technique, and outcomes of successful arthroscopic subscapularis repairs.

Important Points
- Patients often are seen after a traumatic event with internal rotation weakness and pain.
- Physical examination tests that isolate the subscapularis include the belly press, lift-off, and bear hug tests.
- The entire shoulder should be carefully examined to evaluate for other causes of pathology.
- It is paramount to have the repair be tension free and attached securely to the lesser tuberosity.

Clinical and Surgical Pearls
- An interscalene block or catheter can reduce the anesthetic required and help with postoperative pain.

- The comma sign can make identification of the tendon tear easier.
- Coracoidplasty can increase working space during the procedure and decreases impingement postoperatively.
- Place anchors inferiorly to superiorly, and tie knots superiorly to inferiorly.
- Use of a limb positioner can aid in anchor placement, allowing appropriate angle tension of repair while sutures are being tied.
- Check motion after repair to aid in the initial safe range of motion for postoperative rehabilitation.

Clinical and Surgical Pitfalls
- Straying medial to the coracoid places neurovascular structures at risk.
- Do not fail to address concomitant pathology.
- Do not overtension the repair.

As arthroscopic techniques in shoulder surgery have improved, recognition of subscapularis tendon injuries has increased. Although isolated subscapularis tears continue to be rare, estimated at 5% of rotator cuff tears,[1] they are increasingly being seen in association with other supraspinatus, infraspinatus, and teres minor tears, with an incidence estimated at 27% to 43%.[2] Because of this, there has been increased interest in arthroscopic subscapularis tendon repairs. The main advantages of an arthroscopic repair of the subscapularis tendon are smaller incisions, less postoperative pain, and the ability to better visualize and address coexisting pathologic processes, including labral tears,

long head biceps injury, and superior and posterior rotator cuff tears. This chapter addresses the preoperative considerations and the techniques involved in performing an arthroscopic subscapularis repair.

PREOPERATIVE CONSIDERATIONS

History

Often there is a history of trauma, which may include an abduction and external rotation moment, direct blow, heavy lifting, or traction injury.[3] For degenerative tears, the patient may report a gradual worsening of anterior shoulder pain without specific trauma. Patients may note difficulty with internal rotation—for example, in tucking in a shirttail. Consider a full differential diagnosis for anterior shoulder pain, including acromioclavicular joint arthrosis or dislocation, biceps tendon tears or inflammation, anterior capsulolabral damage, and fractures of the lesser tuberosity.

Physical Examination

A complete shoulder examination should begin with observation, range of motion, and strength testing. The most common physical examination findings associated with a subscapularis tear are weakness and pain with isolation of internal rotation. External rotation is evaluated with the arm at the side and compared with the contralateral extremity.

It is important to isolate the subscapularis muscle from other internal rotators during examination. Owing to the high association with biceps tendon pathology, careful examination with the Speed and O'Brien tests is also important. The belly press test is performed by asking the patient to press the ipsilateral hand on the abdomen, maintaining the elbow anterior to the body. The belly press test result is considered positive if the patient is not able to keep the elbow anterior to the trunk or if the wrist is flexed in attempting to press into the abdomen. The lift-off test requires the patient to be able to place the ipsilateral hand behind the back. The patient is asked to lift the hand off the back; if the patient is unable to do so, the test result is considered positive. The most sensitive test is the bear hug test.[4] The patient places his or her ipsilateral hand on the contralateral shoulder with the elbow elevated forward. The test result is positive if the surgeon is able to lift the patient's hand off the shoulder.

Imaging

A standard shoulder imaging series including an axillary view is obtained to assess for alternative pathologic changes, such as fractures and glenohumeral arthritis. Magnetic resonance imaging is the gold standard imaging modality for diagnosis of subscapularis tendon tears and evaluation of muscle belly quality, fatty infiltration, and displacement of the long head of the biceps tendon (Fig. 22-1). Magnetic resonance arthrography improves the sensitivity of diagnosis of partial tears and labral and biceps pathology. In addition, the coracohumeral distance is measured from the tip of the coracoid to the humerus on an axial cut with the smallest distance.[2] A distance of 6.5 mm is considered narrowed. The tendon should be assessed on both axial and sagittal images, with verification of its insertion on the lesser tuberosity.

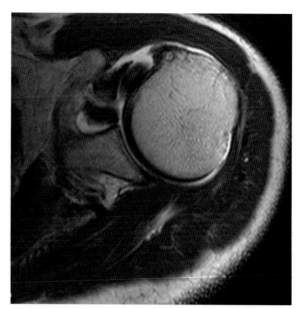

Figure 22-1. Magnetic resonance image of a torn subscapularis.

Indications and Contraindications

Indications for subscapularis repair are pain and weakness nonresponsive to conservative management. Important secondary indications are restoration of shoulder strength and function and treatment of recurrent shoulder instability.

Relative contraindications to arthroscopic repair include lack of pain, severe atrophy, retraction or significant fatty degeneration on magnetic resonance imaging, and rotator cuff tear arthropathy. For patients with massive tears, significant retraction, or atrophy, we recommend open surgery including pectoralis major tendon transfer and possible tissue augmentation. Absolute contraindications are severe medical illness that precludes anesthesia, and active infection. The decision to perform an arthroscopic or open procedure should be based on the surgeon's individual comfort level with the chosen technique.

SURGICAL TECHNIQUE
Anesthesia and Positioning

Most patients are placed under general anesthesia. We prefer to supplement every case with an interscalene block or nerve catheter depending on the skill and comfort of the anesthesiologist. This reduces the amount of anesthetic required during the case and improves postoperative pain control. If the patient's medical condition does not allow general anesthesia, regional anesthesia can be used along with sedation.

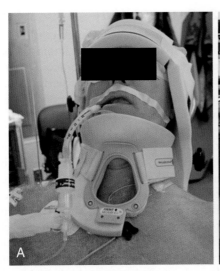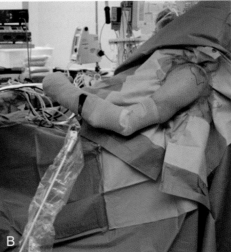

Figure 22-2. Positioning of the patient.

We prefer the beach chair position for arthroscopic repairs of the subscapularis (Fig. 22-2). The upper extremity can be easily moved and rotated to better visualize the subscapularis and its insertion. Furthermore, the beach chair position allows the surgeon to convert easily to an open procedure if necessary.

The patient is aligned on the edge of the table so that the affected shoulder and scapula are exposed. The head is secured to the operating table with a headrest, and a Philadelphia collar (Philadelphia Cervical Collar Company, Thorofare, NJ) is used to prevent excessive motion in the neck. We use the Spider Limb Positioner (Smith & Nephew, London) to aid in arm positioning during the case.

Surgical Landmarks, Incisions, and Portals

We begin every case by outlining the bony landmarks on the skin, including posterior and anterior corners of the acromion, and the soft spot between the posterior clavicle and anterior scapular spine. A line is drawn between the two corners of the acromion. The anterior and posterior edges of the clavicle and scapular spine are marked next. The acromioclavicular joint is palpated and marked. A circle is drawn over the prominence of the coracoid.

The posterior portal is the first portal to be established. With use of a three-finger shuck, the index finger of the same hand as the shoulder being operated on is placed in the soft spot between the clavicle and scapular spine. The middle finger is placed on the coracoid, and the thumb feels the interval between the infraspinatus and teres minor.

The anterior portal is generally placed just lateral to the coracoid and below the coracoacromial ligament.

This portal can easily be established with an outside-in technique localizing with a spinal needle or an inside-out technique over a Wissinger rod. An accessory anterolateral portal is made in all subscapularis repairs. This portal is located in the rotator interval anterior and medial to the anterolateral corner of the acromion. This places it about 1 to 2 cm superior and 2 cm lateral to the standard anterior portal. A spinal needle is used to localize this portal, with an intra-articular entrance site just posterior to the native biceps tendon. After the portal is made, it is enlarged to allow the placement of a threaded 8-mm clear cannula. It is important not to place the two anterior portals too close to each other. When there is also an associated superior rotator cuff tear, this portal may be placed through the defect.

Examination Under Anesthesia and Diagnostic Arthroscopy

Examination of both shoulders under anesthesia is performed on every patient after induction of anesthesia but before positioning, checking range of motion and instability. Any previous surgical scars are marked and reused if possible.

We start by performing diagnostic arthroscopy. Any intra-articular pathology is addressed. A dynamic examination of the subscapularis insertion is performed by advancing the arthroscope to the anterior aspect of the glenohumeral joint and moving the arm internally and externally with the aid of the arm positioner. If significant retraction has occurred, it is possible to see the conjoined tendons and note the medial displacement of the long head of the biceps. A probe or a grasper can be used to examine the extent of the tear. We also identify the comma sign—the torn superior glenohumeral ligament and coracohumeral ligament, which remain attached to and identify the superior and lateral margin of the subscapularis tendon[5] (Fig. 22-3).

Surgical Procedure

Specific steps for this procedure are outlined in Box 22-1.

1. Biceps Tendon

In many cases of significant subscapularis tear, the biceps tendon is subluxed medially. We prefer to release the biceps tendon intra-articularly at the superior labrum and to perform biceps tenodesis once the subscapularis repair has been completed. This approach improves intra-articular visualization and prevents postoperative pain related to the biceps tendon. We do consider a biceps tenotomy alone in select patients, but this is based on preoperative discussion with the patient.

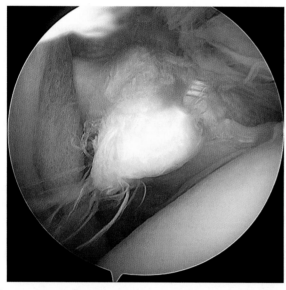

Figure 22-3. Subscapularis tear with comma sign.

2. Coracoidplasty

This step is somewhat analogous to performing a subacromial decompression. Removal of bone from the posterolateral tip of the coracoid creates extra space for subscapularis repair to be performed, and it decreases impingement by allowing more space for the repaired tendon.[6]

We start with debridement of the capsular tissue of the rotator interval at the superior edge of the subscapularis to expose the coracoid. We use the anterior portal and keep the shaver on the lateral edge of the coracoids to protect the neurovascular structures medially. Once the coracoid is reached, an electrothermal device is used to further remove the soft tissue attachment on the tip of the coracoid and expose the undersurface. A 4.0-mm bur is then used to remove about 5 mm of the posterolateral tip of the coracoid, again working through the anterior portal (Fig. 22-4). This area can be quite vascular, and prompt attention to any bleeding is required to maintain visualization.

3. Mobilization of Subscapularis

Through the anterior portal, the mobility of the torn subscapularis is assessed via grasper. If the tendon can be reduced to the lesser tuberosity without tension, one can proceed to the repair. If the tendon is not mobile, soft tissue dissection must be performed. First, the soft

---

BOX 22-1 Surgical Steps

1. Biceps tendon
2. Coracoidplasty
3. Mobilization of subscapularis
4. Preparation of the tendon edge and lesser tuberosity
5. Anchor placement
6. Suture management and passage
7. Additional anchor placement
8. Knot tying

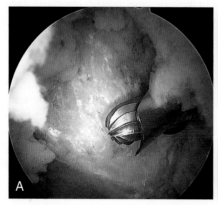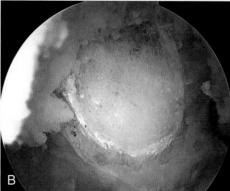

Figure 22-4. Coracoidplasty.

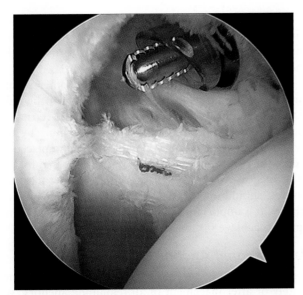

Figure 22-5. Mobilization of the subscapularis.

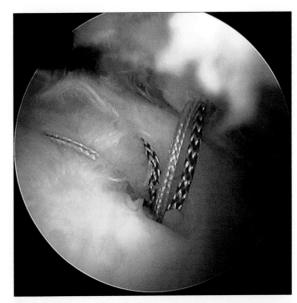

Figure 22-7. Anchor placement.

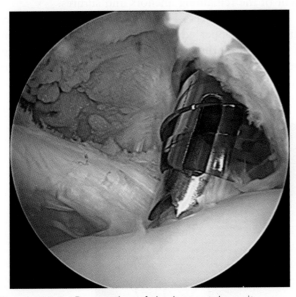

Figure 22-6. Preparation of the lesser tuberosity.

tissue attachments between the coracoid and subscapularis are released (Fig. 22-5). A release of the coracohumeral ligament and the anterior capsule is also helpful. Finally, a shaver, basket, or electrothermal device should release the middle glenohumeral ligament.

4. Preparation of the Tendon Edge and Lesser Tuberosity

A 4.5-mm shaver is inserted through the anterior portal and used to freshen up and remove the frayed edges of the torn subscapularis. The shoulder is then internally rotated and slightly abducted so the lesser tuberosity can be visualized (Fig. 22-6). A 4.0-mm bur is placed through the anterolateral portal and used to prepare the

bony bed for suture anchor placement. In most cases the tendon insertion is slightly medialized, and a small amount of the articular surface is included in the resection.

5. Anchor Placement

The suture anchors are placed through the anterior portal with the arm in external rotation (Fig. 22-7). We use double-loaded anchors for better stability for the repair. We place the anchors initially at the inferior edge of the subscapularis footprint and proceed superiorly, separating the anchors by 5 to 8 mm. In general, partial repairs can be accomplished with one or two anchors; typically three anchors are required for complete ruptures.

6. Suture Management and Passage

To aid in suture management, a switching stick is placed through the anterior cannula, and the cannula is removed. The sutures are then pulled out of the cannula, and a hemostat is placed on them. The cannula is placed back over the switching stick into the joint. This leaves the anterior cannula empty to facilitate the use of shuttling devices. To perform the repair, a combination of instruments may be used, including a curved Spectrum device (Linvatec, Utica, NY), a penetrator (Arthrex, Naples, FL), or a SixTer device (Mitek, Raynham, MA).

The suture limb that will be placed in the subscapularis is pulled from the anterior portal out through the anterolateral portal by a crochet hook. The one-step device or the Spectrum device is placed through the anterior portal and used to penetrate the tendon (Fig. 22-8). The suture should be passed at an angle from lateral to medial through the entire thickness of the tendon.

Once the passage device has penetrated through the tendon, its polydioxanone (PDS) suture is advanced and retrieved with the crochet hook through the anterolateral portal, or the permanent suture is grasped with the one-step device (Fig. 22-9).

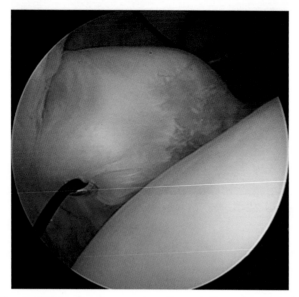

Figure 22-8. Passing a suture through the subscapularis with spectrum.

The anchor suture is then fixed to the PDS suture and shuttled through the tendon and back out the anterior portal. Care must be taken not to unload the anchor.

The same process is repeated for the other suture limb, resulting in a mattress configuration in the subscapularis tendon. Once both limbs have been retrieved, they are placed outside of the anterior cannula by the switching stick technique. A hemostat is again placed to secure the two limbs, and the process is repeated for the next anchor. At the end of this process, two mattress sutures should be passed through the subscapularis tendon. It is important to place the sutures at least 5 mm apart to achieve optimal fixation.

7. Additional Anchor Placement

It is up to the surgeon's preference to tie sutures immediately or after placement of all remaining anchors. We prefer to tie the sutures last because in our hands this allows better visualization and thus improved placement of the remaining anchors and sutures.

The same process is repeated to place the sutures through the upper edge of the tendon. Only one limb of the second suture on the last anchor is placed through the tendon. This will be the first suture to be tied and will allow restoration of the height of the tendon.

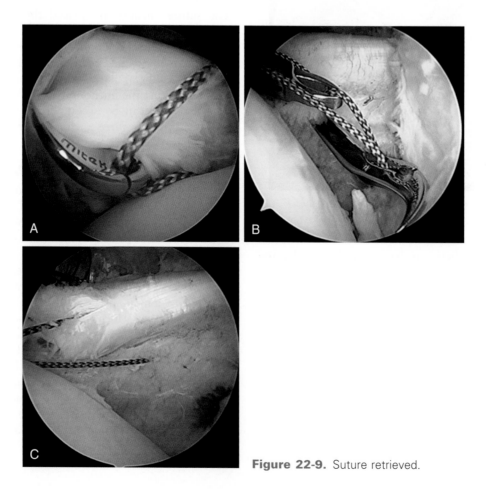

Figure 22-9. Suture retrieved.

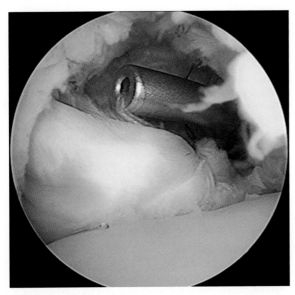

Figure 22-10. Suture tying.

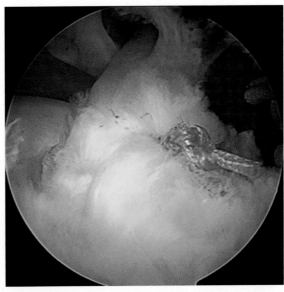

Figure 22-11. Final results with knot on tendon side of repair.

8. Knot Tying

The anterolateral portal is used for arthroscopic knot tying, as it allows the surgeon to pass-point the knots and provides a better angle of approach to the tendon. We start by tying the most superior suture to set the position of the remaining sutures.

A crochet hook is used to retrieve the two limbs of the most superior suture out of the anterolateral portal. Multiple alternating half hitches with alternating posts are placed, and the suture ends are cut (Fig. 22-10). The process is repeated for the second suture on the proximal anchor, followed by the inferior anchor. Ideally, the sutures are tied to place the knot on the tendon side of the repair, not the tuberosity (Fig. 22-11).

The arm is rotated to inspect the security of the repair and the tied knots. Motion is assessed to determine limits for the postoperative rehabilitation program. Subacromial pathology can be addressed at this time, and a biceps tenodesis can be performed if indicated. Wounds are closed in a standard fashion, and the arm is placed into an abduction pillow sling.

POSTOPERATIVE CONSIDERATIONS

Rehabilitation

For the first 2 weeks, we allow forward elevation to 90 degrees and internal rotation to the abdomen. We limit external rotation to what was determined to be secure

intra-operatively. From 2 to 6 weeks, we allow external rotation as tolerated without stretching or manipulation by a physical therapist. Forward elevation is increased to 140 degrees.

At 6 weeks, the sling is discontinued, and we begin active range of motion with progression to full motion as tolerated. We do not start strengthening until 12 weeks after surgery.

Sports-related rehabilitation is initiated at 5 months postoperatively. We allow return to collision sports at 9 months. Patients should expect maximal improvement to occur by about 12 months postoperatively.

Complications

Complications are those seen with arthroscopic shoulder surgery and rotator cuff repair. These include stiffness, repair failure, infection, and rarely nerve damage.

RESULTS

As the technique has become more common, more results have been published showing significant improvement compared with preoperative function and scores. The results of recent outcomes are summarized in Table 22-1. These studies suggest excellent early and midterm results with improvement in patient pain and function. We believe that a secure repair can be accomplished arthroscopically and that outcomes are similar to those reported to follow traditional open techniques.

TABLE 22-1. Clinical Results of Arthroscopic Subscapularis Repairs

Study	Follow-up	Outcome
Romeo (2005)	27 months	Forward elevation improved from 138 to 161 degrees External rotation improved from 70 to 86 degrees ASES score improved from 46 to 82 Simple shoulder test score improved from 7 to 10 of 12 79% good to excellent results
Bennett[7] (2003)	Minimum of 2 years	Constant score improved from 43 to 74 ASES score improved from 16 to 74 VAS for pain dropped from 9 to 2 of 10 Function improved from 25% to 82%
Burkhart and Tehrany[8] (2002)	10.7 months	Forward elevation improved from 96 to 146 degrees UCLA score improved from 10.7 to 30.5 92% good to excellent results
Adams et al[1] (2008)	Median 5 years	80% good to excellent 88% patient satisfaction ASES score improved from 40.5 to 91.2 UCLA score improved from 15.7 to 31.6
Lafosse et al[3] (2007)	Mean 29 months	Constant score improved from 58 to 96 UCLA score improved from 16 to 32 Forward elevation improved from 146 to 175 degrees External rotation improved from 50 to 60.3 degrees

ASES, American Shoulder and Elbow Surgeons scale; *UCLA,* University of California at Los Angeles shoulder rating scale; *VAS,* visual analogue scale.

REFERENCES

1. Adams CR, Schoolfield JD, Burhkart SS. The results of arthroscopic subscapularis tendon repairs. *Arthroscopy.* 2008;24:1381-1389.
2. Koo SS, Burkhart SS. Subscapularis tendon tears, identifying mid to distal footprint disruptions. *Arthroscopy.* 2010;26:1130-1134.
3. Lafosse L, Jost B, Reiland Y, Audebert S, et al. Structural integrity and clinical outcomes after arthroscopic repair of isolated subscapularis tears. *Journal of Bone and Joint Surgery Am.* 2007;89:1184-1193.
4. Burkhart SS, Brady PC. Arthroscopic subscapularis repair: surgical tips and pearls A to Z. *Arthroscopy.* 2006;22:1014-1027.
5. Lo IKY, Burkhart SS. The comma sign: an arthroscopic guide to the torn subscapularis tendon. *Arthroscopy.* 2003;19:334-337.
6. Bennett WF. Arthroscopic repair of isolated subscapularis tears: a prospective cohort with 2- to 4-year follow-up. *Arthroscopy.* 2003;19:131-143.
7. Burkhart SS, Tehrany AM. Arthroscopic subscapularis tendon repair: technique and preliminary results. *Arthroscopy.* 2002;18:454-463.
8. Richards DP, Burkhart SS, Campbell SE. Relation between narrowed coracohumeral distance and subscapularis tears. *Arthroscopy.* 2005;21:1223-1228.

SUGGESTED READING

Lo IK, Burkhart SS. The etiology and assessment of subscapularis tendon tears: a case for subcoracoid impingement, the roller-wringer effect, and TUFF lesions of the subscapularis. *Arthroscopy.* 2003;19: 1142-1150.

Chapter 23

Mini-Open Rotator Cuff Repair

Gregory P. Nicholson and James Hammond

Chapter Synopsis
- Mini-open rotator cuff repair techniques evolved to minimize morbidity from open techniques. This technique has been proven to provide reliable clinical improvements in patients with rotator cuff tears. Specific technical points will be given to aid the surgeon in obtaining reliable results.

Important Points
- Mini-open techniques can be used in most patients with rotator cuff tear.
- Detailed history and physical examination, appropriate imaging, and preoperative planning will help indicate patients for surgery.
- Treatment may differ in acute versus chronic tears.

Clinical and Surgical Pearls
- Performing expeditious arthroscopy is important to limit soft tissue fluid extravasation.
- Adequate bursectomy and limited acromioplasty will aid visualization.

- Rotation of the arm will help determine the extent of the tear.
- Tendon tear pattern, tendon quality, and tendon mobility are important factors to determine before proceeding with repair.
- Appropriate releases may be require to provide a tension-free repair.
- Double-row repair techniques may provide greater pull-out strength than single-row repair.

Clinical and Surgical Pitfalls
- Avoid excessive retraction on the deltoid.
- Monitor the distal end of the split, and use stay sutures to avoid axillary nerve injury.
- Massive cuff tears and subscapularis tears may be difficult to repair owing to visualization, rotation of the arm, and abduction.

 Video
- Video 23-1: Mini-Open Rotator Cuff Repair

Rotator cuff surgery is among the most commonly performed orthopedic procedures and is continually evolving. Large open procedures historically have had good clinical results but with the risk of significant morbidity. The increased morbidity related to the detachment of the deltoid from the acromion in open approaches could be functionally disabling. This has led to the advent of mini-open and all-arthroscopic techniques that bypass this portion of the procedure. These techniques have lessened the morbidity and have achieved success rates that approach those of open surgery in most studies. Pain relief and restoration of function are the primary goals of rotator cuff repair surgery. Structurally, cuff tendon healing with preservation of functional muscle with minimal atrophy and fatty infiltration is the goal.

This chapter will focus on the mini-open technique and outcomes.

PREOPERATIVE CONSIDERATIONS

History

Determining the pathologic origin of shoulder pain can be challenging for even the most astute diagnostician. Rotator cuff tears are commonly associated with impingement signs such as lateral deltoid pain, night pain, and pain with overhead activity. The symptoms can progress to pain at rest. Rotator cuff tears are often multifactorial in origin. There are extrinsic factors, such as patient anatomy with acromial morphology, patient activity levels, repetitive trauma, acute one-time trauma, and associated pathology, that contribute to tendon failure. There are intrinsic factors, such as patient age, tendon biology, and comorbid conditions such as diabetes and smoking, that are associated with cuff tears. A careful history can help sort out acute, acute on chronic, and chronic aspects of the condition.

Physical Examination

Examination of the shoulder girdle is important to observe for any muscular atrophy that might be visually perceptible in the supraspinatus and infraspinatus fossae. Palpation of the shoulder for areas of pain is important. Range of motion of the shoulder is critical to assess. Assess passive versus active range of motion in all planes. Compare the affected side with the unaffected side. Patients with tears can demonstrate good passive motion but can lack active reproduction of motion. This can be particularly evident with loss or weakness of external rotation or internal rotation. Manual muscle strength testing can identify areas of weakness or pain. Other specific maneuvers including impingement sign, response to a subacromial injection (the impingement test), pain at the AC joint, pain of the biceps groove, and the external rotation lag sign and Hornblower's signs can be helpful in the diagnosis of rotator cuff pathology. The cervical spine should be evaluated, and a neurologic examination should be performed also.

Imaging

Imaging should include plain radiography with three standard views of the shoulder: a true anteroposterior (AP) view of the glenohumeral joint (a Grashey view), an outlet view, and an axillary view. Acromial morphology on the outlet and AP views can reveal encroaching morphology, acromial bone spurs, and outlet narrowing resulting from shape and tilt of the bony anatomy. Arthritic changes may be apparent, as well as calcific tendinosis on plain radiographs. Cystic changes at the rotator cuff insertion should also be assessed. An os acromiale usually will be evident on the axillary lateral view. It will also be important to evaluate the acromioclavicular joint for changes. Measurement of the acromiohumeral interval is also important to determine if a rotator cuff defect is allowing superior migration of the humeral head. A measurement of less than 7 mm is indicative of significant superior migration of the humeral head.

Magnetic resonance imaging (MRI) without contrast is useful in working up rotator cuff tears. Tears are best assessed on the coronal T2-weighted images, but T1-images are also helpful. Important information to collect includes (1) whether tears are full or partial thickness, (2) amount of retraction, (3) whether muscle atrophy is present, and (4) presence of fatty infiltration. Associated pathology is also important to note, including biceps pathology.

Ultrasound has proved to be a useful modality to assess rotator cuff tears as well. Multiple studies have demonstrated its efficacy in not only diagnosing rotator cuff tears, but also evaluating the healing of tears postoperatively. More investigation will continue to define the usefulness in expanding the indications for its use.

Indications

Rotator cuff repair may be indicated for patients who have symptoms (pain and altered function) and in whom conservative management has failed. The symptoms are continuing to affect their occupation, recreation, sleep, and activities of daily living and have not resolved with appropriate therapy, medical management, time, and activity modification. Also, the rotator cuff tear is thought to be reparable on MRI evaluation. Indications for rotator cuff surgery have been challenged in recent literature. In December 2010 the American Academy of Orthopaedic Surgeons (AAOS) released its guidelines on optimizing the management of rotator cuff problems.[1] These guidelines were created by a panel of experts who performed a systematic review of the literature in an effort to delineate appropriate recommendations based on a review of articles. The guidelines state that there is weak evidence for repair of acute tears and that surgical intervention is an option for those with chronic, symptomatic, full-thickness repairs. These recommendations were the result of what was described as a paucity of high-level randomized controlled trials in the literature.

There are some generally accepted principles that have come from the literature. Acute tears, in which an event happens with a resultant decrease in function, are generally treated earlier than chronic tears. Chronic tears were found in 39% of cadavers by DePalma and colleagues[2] and on MRI in 54% of 60-year-old individuals.[3] Thus, asymptomatic tears are not to be addressed surgically. Tears thought to be ideal for clinical success are smaller tears with minimal retraction, no atrophy, and no fatty infiltration and heal postoperatively.

All-arthroscopic techniques have continued to improve, gain in popularity, and achieve results similar to those of other techniques. Nho and colleagues[4] performed a systematic review of the literature regarding all-arthroscopic techniques versus mini-open repair. Based on included studies they determined that results were equivalent between arthroscopic and mini-open techniques in terms of shoulder function and clinical outcome. There was a trend toward higher complication rates in the mini-open repair group. Their final statement was that both techniques are effective, and one should choose the technique that is most reproducible in his or her hands.

There are certain situations in which it has been argued that a mini-open procedure would be more advantageous than an all-arthroscopic surgery. These include retracted cuffs, larger tears, and tears involving the subscapularis and biceps dislocation as well as revision cuff surgery. However, these issues are difficult to address through any surgical technique.

SURGICAL TECHNIQUE

Anesthesia and Positioning

Anesthesia can be performed in a regional, general, or combined manner. Popular regional techniques include interscalene or supraclavicular blocks. The surgery can then be performed with sedation or general anesthesia. Rotator cuff repairs can be performed with the patient in a beach chair position or a lateral decubitus position. We prefer the beach chair position for rotator cuff surgery. The head is secured in a head holder, and the table is reclined to about a 60-degree angle. Rolled towels are placed behind the medial border of the scapula, and a padded bolster is attached to the table to allow the surgical arm to rest on and keep the arm from falling. All bone prominences are protected, as is the peroneal nerve distally. The arm is prepared and draped free in the normal sterile fashion.

Surgical Landmarks and Incisions

Surgical landmarks identified before incision include the acromion, clavicle, and coracoid process. Arthroscopic portals and the mini-open incision are based off of these landmarks. Typically, standard posterior, anterior, and anterolateral portals are used. The mini-open incision is made in an anterosuperior location to maximize exposure to the footprint of the supraspinatus. This incision can be made along Langer's lines, making it more cosmetic.

Specific Steps

Specific steps of this procedure are outlined in Box 23-1. Diagnostic arthroscopy of the glenohumeral joint is performed, and any operative issues are addressed. It is important to identify the long head of the biceps tendon, its exit from the glenohumeral joint, and any injury to the biceps sling or subscapularis complex. Bursoscopy and subacromial decompression with bursectomy and anteroinferior arthroscopic acromioplasty are performed (Fig. 23-1). Attempts are made to minimize the

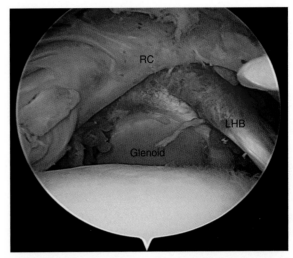

Figure 23-1. Large rotator cuff tear where the glenoid and biceps complex are viewed from the subacromial space. Note the retracted rotator cuff *(RC)* in the superior portion of the view.

BOX 23-1 Surgical Steps

1. Diagnostic arthroscopy
2. Arthroscopic debridement, bursectomy, and acromioplasty
3. Anterosuperior incision
4. Develop skin flaps
5. Split the deltoid
6. Complete bursectomy, lysis of adhesions for visualization
7. Expose cuff tear
8. Prepare footprint
9. Cuff repair via preferred suture technique
10. Evaluate repair
11. Wound irrigation
12. Closure

---

time spent performing arthroscopy to decrease the amount of fluid extravasation in the tissues.

Mini-open rotator cuff repair is then initiated. Dissection is taken down to the deltoid fascia, and skin and subcutaneous flaps are created to fashion a mobile window. The raphe between the anterior and lateral heads of the deltoid is identified, and the interval is opened. This is typically from the lateral border of the acromion to a distance of 3 to 4 cm laterally down the deltoid. Blunt dissection can free up any subdeltoid adhesions. A stay suture can be placed at the inferior portion of the split to prevent unintended extension and possible injury to the axillary nerve.

The subdeltoid and subacromial bursa is then exposed after placement of retractors under the deltoid edges. Any bursa still obscuring the rotator cuff is then

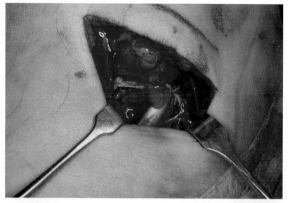

Figure 23-2. Exposure of the rotator cuff tear with bursal tissue in place. It is important to remove bursal tissue and delineate the true tear.

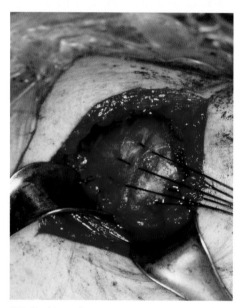

Figure 23-3. Use of sutures to ensure appropriate mobilization of the tendon to its footprint before tying.

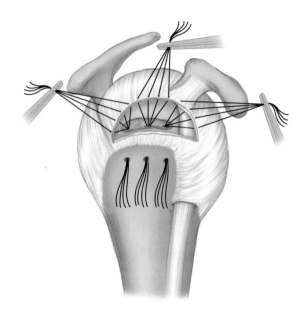

Figure 23-4. Simple suture configuration with transosseous bone tunnels used in lieu of suture anchors.

sharply excised, and the arm is rotated to expose the rotator cuff tear (Fig. 23-2). The supraspinatus tendon is the most frequently torn tendon, but internal rotation will assist in identifying any infraspinatus extension. It is also important to identify the biceps as it enters the rotator interval and determine if any extension or subscapularis involvement is present. Time should be taken to fully identify the rotator cuff, the tear pattern, the amount of retraction, tendon mobility, and the tendon quality. Placing a traction stitch with nonabsorbable suture (No. 2 Ethibond) into the tendon edge can help determine the best reduction maneuver (Fig. 23-3). Keep in mind that the reduction typically requires lateral and anterior movement to restore the footprint.

Releases are sometimes required to restore tendon mobility to the native footprint. Ensure that the tendon is sufficiently released from subacromial tissues. The rotator interval can be released to free up the anterior edge of the supraspinatus. Occasionally the supraspinatus can be retracted and adherent to the coracoid, requiring release from its bony base. Care should be taken to not dissect around the inferomedial portion of the coracoid, which puts the deep neurovascular structures at risk. Also ensure that the inferior border is free from glenohumeral joint adhesions, which are typically addressed during arthroscopy.

The footprint of the rotator cuff insertion can then be prepared, if this was not already completed during the arthroscopic portion of the procedure. A rasp or rongeur can be used to clear any soft tissue from the footprint and create a bleeding bony bed. Fealy and colleagues[5] reported that the lowest cuff vascularity is at the anchor site or cancellous trough, which supports this rationale.

There are several rotator cuff attachment options to choose from when the mini-open technique is used. Bone tunnels are the gold standard option, but suture anchors are another possibility (Fig. 23-4). Bone tunnels are completed by drilling into the footprint with a 2-mm drill bit and drilling a second hole that connects to the medial side from the lateral cortex. A sturdy free needle can facilitate this process. Drill holes are typically 1 cm apart across the entirety of the vacant footprint.

Suture anchors can be used in a similar fashion. They are usually placed along the articular margin, creating a medial row, and newer knotless anchors can then be added to create a lateral row, which completes the double-row technique. There has been much published about differing patterns of double-row suture constructs compared with single-row techniques. In general, studies are demonstrating greater pull-out strength with double-row versus single-row techniques, but a clinical difference has yet to be truly delineated.

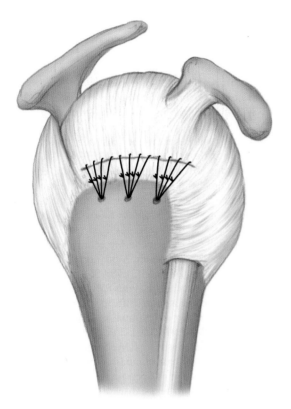

Figure 23-5. Completion of the repair. It is important to assess the repair under a range of motion to assess tension and reduction.

TABLE 23-1. Outcomes in the Literature

Study	Follow-up	Outcomes
Papadopoulos et al[8] (2011)	3.5 years	MOR, large or massive tears 93% good or excellent results
Osti et al[9] (2010)	2 years	No difference between AACR and MOR in tears smaller than 3 cm
Hanusch et al[10] (2009)	27 months	MOR, large or massive tears 87.5% satisfied
Mohtadi et al[11] (2008)	28 months	MOR significantly better than open at 3 months and equal at 28 months
Morse et al[12] (2008)	Meta-analysis	No difference between AACR and MOR
Nho et al[4] (2007)	Systematic review	No difference between AACR and MOR
Pearsall et al[13] (2007)	50 months	No difference between AACR and MOR small-to-medium tears

AACR, All-arthroscopic cuff repair; *MOR,* mini-open cuff repair.

Once the anchor and bone tunnel and suture construct of choice have been completed, the shoulder is taken through a range of motion to assess the repair (Fig. 23-5). Particular attention should be paid to evaluation of tension at the repair site. This provides a level of confidence in the ability to allow range of motion in the postoperative period. The wound is then copiously irrigated, the stay stitch and retractors are removed, and the deltoid fascia is approximated. The subcutaneous tissue is closed with an absorbable suture, followed by the skin. Sterile dressings are then placed, followed by a cryotherapy device and a sling. Depending on the quality of repair, an abduction pillow may be added.

POSTOPERATIVE CONSIDERATIONS

Rehabilitation

Sling use is continued for the first 4 to 6 weeks postoperatively. Early passive range of motion is initiated on day 1 with limitations given as needed based on intraoperative assessment of the repair. Supine passive forward flexion and supine external rotation begin on day 1 with the assistance of a therapist. The patient is taught to perform circular Codman exercises while bending over to 90 degrees at the waist. All exercises in

the immediate postoperative period must be done passively. At 6 weeks postoperatively, active exercises and light activity are permitted. Resistive exercises for the deltoid and rotator cuff are allowed after 3 months.

Complications

Several complications can accompany the mini-open rotator cuff repair.[6] Axillary nerve injury can occur if the deltoid split extends 4 to 5 cm distal to the lateral acromion. The stay suture can help prevent this extension. There have been reports of shoulder stiffness after mini-open rotator cuff repairs. It was felt that the smaller aperture in the deltoid for access to the tear may have been a function of significant pulling force from the retractors. The deltoid may have been injured locally, leading to significant stiffness.[7] As with any tendon repair technique, nonhealing or retearing can occur. Failure of the repair can be defined as clinical failure with persistence of pain and decreased function or as anatomic failure with nonhealing of the tendon to bone. Studies have shown that one does not necessarily lead to the other, but in general a tendon that heals to bone leads to better clinical results in both pain and function. Massive or large tears may have pain relief with nonhealing tears, but with persistent functional deficit.

RESULTS

Mini-open rotator cuff repair has been documented to produce significant clinical improvement in patients (Table 23-1). Since the previous edition was published, several studies have evaluated mini-open rotator cuff repairs. As previously mentioned, a systematic review of arthroscopic and mini-open repair was performed by Nho and colleagues[4] in 2007, with the previously stated results. In addition, a meta-analysis was performed by Morse and colleagues[12] in 2008. Their review of studies from 1966 to 2006 found five studies that met their criteria and found no difference between arthroscopic and mini-open repair groups.

Several other studies have documented comparison between mini-open and arthroscopic repair groups. Overall, no significant differences between groups have been identified. In addition, several studies have documented improvement in patients with large and massive tears after mini-open rotator cuff surgery.

REFERENCES

1. American Academy of Orthopaedic Surgeons. *Guideline on optimizing the management of rotator cuff problems.* Rosemont, IL: American Academy of Orthopaedic Surgeons; 2008.
2. DePalma A, Callery G, Bennett G. Variational anatomy and degenerative lesions of the shoulder joint. *Instr Course Lect.* 1949;6:255-281.
3. Sher JS, Uribe JW, Posada A, et al. Abnormal findings on magnetic resonance images of asymptomatic shoulders. *J Bone Joint Surg Am.* 1995;77(1):10-15.
4. Nho SJ, Shindle MK, Sherman SL, et al. Systematic review of arthroscopic rotator cuff repair and mini-open rotator cuff repair. *J Bone Joint Surg Am.* 2007;89(Suppl 3): 127-136.
5. Fealy S, Adler R, Drakos M, et al. Patterns of vascular and anatomical response after rotator cuff repair. *Am J Sports Med.* 2006;34:120-127.
6. Craig E. Mini-open and open techniques for full-thickness rotator cuff repairs. In: Craig E, ed. *The Shoulder. Master Techniques in Orthopaedic Surgery.* Philadelphia: Lippincott Williams & Wilkins; 2004:309-340.
7. Cohen BS, Nicholson GP, Romeo AA. Arthroscopic rotator cuff repair: is mini-open just of historical interest? *Curr Opin Orthop.* 2001;12331-12336.
8. Papadopoulos P, Karataqlis D, Boutsiadis A, et al. Functional outcome and structural integrity following mini-open repair of large and massive rotator cuff tears: a 3-5 year follow-up study. *J Shoulder Elbow Surg.* 2011;20(1): 131-137.
9. Osti L, Papalia R, Paganelli M, et al. Arthroscopic vs mini-open rotator cuff repair. A quality of life impairment study. *Int Orthop.* 2010;34(3):389-394.
10. Hanusch BC, Goodchild L, Finn P, Rangan A. Large and massive tears of the rotator cuff: functional outcome and integrity of the repair after a mini-open procedure. *J Bone Joint Surg Br.* 2009;91(2)201-205.
11. Mohtadi NG, Hollinshead RM, Sasyniuk TM, et al. A randomized clinical trial comparing open to arthroscopic acromioplasty with mini-open rotator cuff repair for full-thickness rotator cuff tears: disease-specific quality of life outcome at an average 2-year follow-up. *Am J Sports Med.* 2008;36(6):1043-1051.
12. Morse K, Davis AD, Afra R, et al. Arthroscopic versus mini-open rotator cuff repair: a comprehensive review and meta-analysis. *Am J Sports Med.* 2008;36(9):1824-1828.
13. Pearsall 4th AW, Ibrahim KA, Madanagopal SG. The results of arthroscopic versus mini-open repair for rotator cuff tears at mid-term follow-up. *J Orthop Surg Res.* 2007;2:24.

Chapter 24

Open Rotator Cuff Repair

John W. Sperling

Chapter Synopsis

- This chapter provides an overview of open rotator cuff repair. Preoperative considerations, surgical technique, postoperative rehabilitation, and published results are discussed.

Important Points

- It is very important to rule out other potential processes that can mimic shoulder pain, such as cervical radiculopathy.
- The surgeon needs to clearly understand the ability of the patient to comply with postoperative rehabilitation and restrictions.
- Advanced imaging studies such as magnetic resonance imaging and ultrasound provide important information about the size of the tear, amount of retraction, and muscle degeneration.

Clinical and Surgical Pearls and Pitfalls

- Systematic releases of the rotator cuff are essential to mobilize the tendon and reduce tension on the repair.
- A strong and meticulous repair of the deltoid is essential to avoid postoperative dehiscence.
- Careful identification of both the deep and superficial deltoid fascial layers is critical during the exposure and later repair.

Multiple facets need to be incorporated for a successful rotator cuff repair to be achieved. The process starts with a thorough understanding of the patient's symptoms, motivation, and ability to comply with postoperative restrictions. Careful examination together with appropriate imaging studies allows proper surgical planning.

PREOPERATIVE CONSIDERATIONS

History

Evaluation of the patient with a rotator cuff tear begins with a thorough history. It is critically important to understand the severity of the symptoms and the patient's ability to comply with postoperative restrictions. The surgeon also needs to elucidate the primary complaint, whether it is pain, weakness, or loss of motion, to better determine and guide the patient's expectations.

The history ascertains the patient's dominant extremity as well as occupation. The duration of pain and dysfunction is determined, as well as whether they started with a specific traumatic event. To understand the severity of pain and the degree to which it interferes with the quality of life, patients are asked to rate the pain on a scale of 1 to 10 at rest, with activities, and at night. The patient is also asked about specific alleviating and aggravating factors. Last, patients are asked to localize the pain—whether it occurs over the anterolateral aspect of the shoulder or radiates in a more radicular pattern down the entire arm, possibly consistent with a neurologic component of pain.

If possible, the results of prior studies are obtained, and prior treatment attempts and their results are reviewed. With a history of prior shoulder surgery, operative notes and images can help further delineate the pathologic process.

A focused review of systems is performed to rule out the possibility of other pathologic processes that frequently cause or mimic shoulder pain, such as inflammatory arthritis, cervical radiculopathy, and even thoracic neoplasias. A list of medications and associated medical problems should be recorded.

Physical Examination

Physical examination includes inspection and palpation of the entire shoulder, followed by specialized functional tests. Inspection assesses soft tissue swelling, deformity, or atrophy. Palpation comprises an examination of the cervical spine, acromioclavicular joint, and bicipital groove. The neurovascular examination of the extremities includes assessment of strength, sensation, and reflexes.

Subsequently, active and passive shoulder motion is recorded for forward flexion, abduction, internal rotation, and external rotation. Strength is graded on a scale of 1 to 5 for internal rotation, external rotation, flexion, extension, and abduction. Impingement tests have been found to be fairly nonspecific but can help elucidate a diagnosis of subacromial impingement; weakness is suggestive of a tear of the rotator cuff. More specialized tests include the lift-off and belly press tests for subscapularis function, as well as external rotation strength, and the lag sign for infraspinatus function; these allow more sensitive assessment of muscle strength.

Imaging

Radiography

Three radiographic views are routinely obtained: 40-degree posterior oblique views with internal and external rotation and an axillary view. One may observe superior subluxation of the humeral head and a decrease in the acromial-humeral distance with significant rotator cuff deficiency. One caveat is that with posterior subluxation, there can be the false appearance of superior humeral head subluxation. There may be sclerosis or rounding of the greater tuberosity with rotator cuff disease as well. The axillary view allows assessment of glenohumeral cartilage loss and subluxation. In addition, one may choose to obtain a Neer outlet view to evaluate acromial morphologic features.

Advanced Imaging Studies

Multiple options are available to further investigate the integrity of the rotator cuff, including arthrography, computed tomographic arthrography, magnetic resonance imaging, and ultrasonography. The decision of which test to perform is based on the individual surgeon's preference. Magnetic resonance imaging provides important additional information about tear size and configuration, degree of retraction, and muscle atrophy or degeneration.

Indications and Contraindications

After the information obtained from the history, physical examination, and imaging studies has been integrated, one determines the diagnosis and can present treatment options to the patient. It is critical to understand the patient's goals and expectations for surgery. Clearly, the primary indication for rotator cuff surgery is pain relief; recovery of strength and function is less predictable. Contraindications include active or recent infection, significant medical comorbidities, and an inability to follow the postoperative restrictions and rehabilitation regimen.

A detailed conversation with the patient then occurs concerning treatment options. The risk, benefits, and alternatives to surgical repair are discussed in detail. The decision to employ specific techniques, such as open versus arthroscopic repair, is based on the individual surgeon's preference and familiarity with each technique. I individualize this decision for each patient on the basis of the age of the patient, the physical demands on the shoulder, the size and configuration of the tear, and a primary or revision setting. My practice consists primarily of performing arthroscopic rotator cuff repair. However, the technique of open repair may be particularly useful in the revision setting when multiple anchors are already present within the humeral head. In addition, open repair may be considered in the young, active heavy laborer with a large rotator cuff tear.

SURGICAL TECHNIQUE

Anesthesia and Positioning

A combination of regional anesthesia and light sedation or general anesthesia is commonly used for rotator cuff repair, which increasingly is being performed on an outpatient basis. The patient is carefully padded and placed in the beach chair position. The waist should be in approximately 45 degrees of flexion, and the knees in 30 degrees of flexion. The table may be slightly rolled away from the surgical shoulder.

Surgical Landmarks

In nearly all patients, regardless of size, one can palpate the posterior scapular spine. The lateral border of the acromion, the anterior border of the acromion, and the anterior portion of the clavicle and coracoid are then marked with a sterile marker (Fig. 24-1). If one is performing arthroscopy before the open repair, one may wish to mark out the standard anterior incision and attempt to place the incision for the anterior portal in line with this future incision.

Specific Steps

Specific steps for this procedure are outlined in Box 24-1.

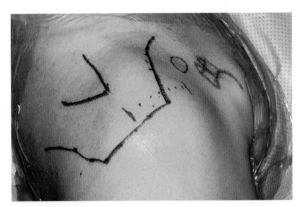

Figure 24-1. The landmarks on the shoulder are identified and marked. A 4- to 5-cm incision is made parallel to the lateral border of the acromion.

BOX 24-1 Surgical Steps

1. Incision
2. Deltoid split
3. Rotator cuff repair
4. Deltoid repair

There is significant variability in the skin incision used for open rotator cuff repair, including oblique incisions, horizontal incisions, and vertical incisions. The choice of which incision to use is based on the individual surgeon's preference.

1. Incision

An incision is made over the anterior superior aspect of the shoulder parallel with the lateral border of the acromion in line with the Langer lines. The length of the skin incision is typically 4 to 5 cm. The skin is incised, as well as the fat. The skin flaps are carefully developed and mobilized.

2. Deltoid Split

The deltoid muscle insertion into the acromion is clearly identified. There is significant variability among surgeons with regard to the technique with which they take down the deltoid (Fig. 24-2). In this example, the deltoid is taken down off the anterior aspect of the acromion with full-thickness sleeves (Fig. 24-3). One must take great care to ensure that this includes both the deep and superficial fascia of the deltoid. The surgeon then has the option either of splitting the deltoid in line with the fibers starting from the acromioclavicular joint anteriorly for approximately 3 cm or of extending the deltoid detachment posteriorly over the lateral border of the acromion. The extent of the deltoid detachment over the lateral acromion border can be modified on the basis of the size of the rotator cuff tear. One must be careful to avoid splitting the deltoid laterally in line with its fibers

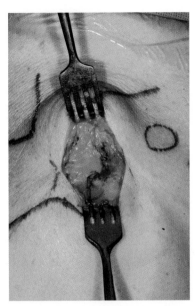

Figure 24-2. The area of deltoid to be taken off the acromion is carefully outlined.

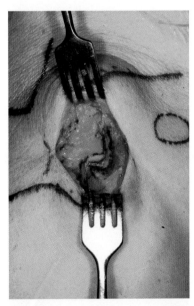

Figure 24-3. Full-thickness flaps of the deltoid including the superficial and deep layers of fascia are taken down.

more than 4 or 5 cm from the acromial border to protect the axillary nerve. However, in most cases, no more than a 2-cm split in line with the fibers of the deltoid is necessary. One can mark the area where the proximal deltoid split is made with a retention stitch (Fig. 24-4). An additional stitch is usually placed distally in the deltoid split to prevent propagation (Fig. 24-5).

3. Rotator Cuff Repair

On the basis of the surgeon's preference, an acromioplasty may then be performed (Fig. 24-6). The torn rotator cuff edges are identified, and retention stitches are placed (Fig. 24-7). Systematic releases are then

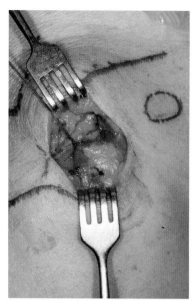

Figure 24-4. A marking stitch is placed in the corner of the deltoid to ensure proper alignment of the deltoid at the time of repair.

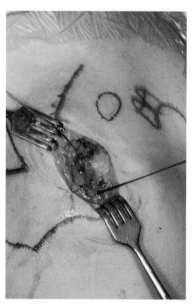

Figure 24-5. A stitch is placed in the distal deltoid split to prevent propagation.

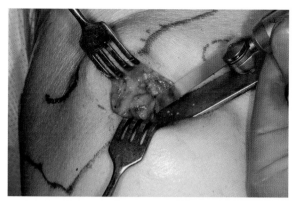

Figure 24-6. An acromioplasty may be performed on the basis of the surgeon's preference.

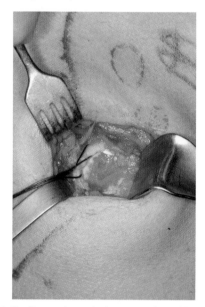

Figure 24-7. Retention stitches are placed in the rotator cuff tear.

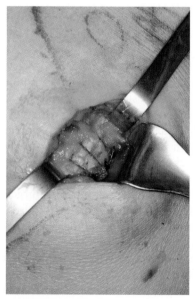

Figure 24-8. Rotator cuff repair is performed in this circumstance with tendon-to-bone stitches.

performed to mobilize the tendon. Specifically, one releases overlying bursal adhesions from the torn rotator cuff. Frequently there is scarring of the coracohumeral ligament to the rotator cuff that must be released. One may also perform intra-articular releases between the labrum and rotator cuff. Care must be taken not to injure the suprascapular nerve in performing medial releases.

The tendon edges are freshened. The rotator cuff repair can then be performed on the basis of the tear configuration (Fig. 24-8). It is my preference in performing a tendon-to-bone repair to use modified Mason-Allen stitches placed through bone tunnels.

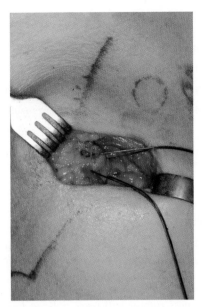

Figure 24-9. Drill holes are placed in the acromion for deltoid repair.

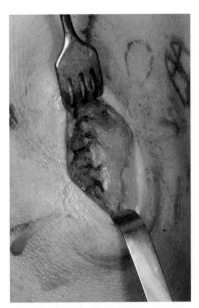

Figure 24-11. Final deltoid repair.

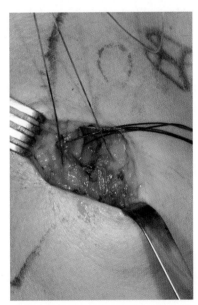

Figure 24-10. The corner of the deltoid is sutured back to its anatomic location.

4. Deltoid Repair

For closure, a meticulous repair of the deltoid is required. At the end of the procedure, the deltoid is repaired back in a tendon-to-tendon as well as a tendon-to-bone manner (Figs. 24-9 to 24-11). Drill holes are placed through the acromion with tendon-to-bone stitches. In addition, the split within the deltoid itself is repaired with multiple side-to-side stitches. Complications in this approach may be related to deltoid dehiscence postoperatively.

POSTOPERATIVE CONSIDERATIONS

Rehabilitation

The patient is placed in a shoulder immobilizer. Passive range-of-motion exercises are started with parameters determined at the time of surgery. Pulley and wand exercises are incorporated into the rehabilitation program from week 3 to week 6 on the basis of the individual patient. The patient then progresses to gentle isometric strengthening exercises.

RESULTS

Results of selected series of open rotator cuff repairs are listed in Table 24-1.

A study by Hawkins and colleagues[2] of 100 rotator cuff repairs at a mean follow-up of 4.2 years revealed that 86% had no or slight pain. All patients underwent acromioplasty in addition to the rotator cuff repair. The average abduction improved from 81 to 125 degrees postoperatively. Of 100 patients, 94 considered themselves improved with the surgery. Ellman and colleagues[3] reported the results of open rotator cuff repair in 50 patients with a mean follow-up of 3.5 years. The results were satisfactory in 84% and unsatisfactory in 16%.

Neer and colleagues[4] reviewed the results of 245 shoulders that underwent rotator cuff repair. Acromioplasty was also performed in 243 of 245 shoulders. Excellent or satisfactory results were obtained in 91% of the shoulders. Cofield and colleagues[1] reviewed the results of 105 shoulders with a chronic rotator cuff tear that underwent open surgical repair and acromioplasty

TABLE 24-1. Results of Open Rotator Cuff Repair

Study	No. of Patients	Mean Age	Mean Follow-up	Outcomes
Cofield et al[1] (2001)	105	58 years	13.4 years	80% satisfactory-excellent results
Hawkins et al[2] (1985)	100	51 years	4.2 years	94% subjective improvement
Ellman et al[3] (1986)	50	60 years	3.5 years	84% satisfactory results
Neer et al[4] (1988)	245	59 years	NA	91% satisfactory-excellent results
Millet et al[5] (2011)	233	58 years	6.3 years	94% survivorship at 5 years

and were observed for an average of 13.4 years. There was satisfactory pain relief in 96 of 105 shoulders. The most frequent complication was apparent failure of rotator cuff healing. Five patients underwent repeated repair. Tear size was found to be the most important determinant of outcome with regard to active motion, strength, rating of the result, satisfaction of the patient, and need for reoperation.

Millet and colleagues recently published the outcome of open rotator cuff repair in 233 patients at a mean follow-up of 6.3 years. In this cohort, 11% of patients underwent an additional surgical procedure. There was significant improvement in the American Shoulder and Elbow Surgeons scale (ASES) score from 56 preoperatively to 88 at the most recent follow-up. The survivorship was 94% at 5 years and 83% at 10 years.[5]

REFERENCES

1. Cofield RH, Parvizi J, Hoffmeyer PJ, et al. Surgical repair of chronic rotator cuff tears: a prospective long-term study. *J Bone Joint Surg Am.* 2001;83:71-77.
2. Hawkins RJ, Misamore GW, Hobeika PE. Surgery for full thickness rotator cuff tears. *J Bone Joint Surg Am.* 1985;67:1349-1355.
3. Ellman H, Hanker G, Bayer M. Repair of the rotator cuff: end-result study of factors influencing reconstruction. *J Bone Joint Surg Am.* 1986;68:1136-1144.
4. Neer CS, Flatow EL, Lech O. Tears of the rotator cuff—long term results of anterior acromioplasty and repair. *Orthop Trans.* 1988;12:735.
5. Millet PJ, Horan MP, Maland KE, et al. Long-term survivorship and outcomes after surgical repair of full thickness rotator cuff tears. *J Shoulder Elbow Surg.* 2011;2: 1-7.

Chapter 25

Tendon Transfers for Rotator Cuff Insufficiency

Jay Boughanem, Tyler Fox, and Laurence D. Higgins

Latissimus Dorsi Transfer

Chapter Synopsis

- The management of patients with unacceptable shoulder pain and weakness associated with chronic irreparable rotator cuff tears remains a challenging problem. In appropriately selected patients latissimus dorsi tendon transfer may be an appropriate salvage option for patients with irreparable posterosuperior rotator cuff tears.

Important Points

- Preoperative patient selection is key to achieving good outcomes.
- It has been suggested that improved tendon transfer healing rates with decreased rates of postoperative rupture can be obtained by harvest of the latissimus dorsi tendon from the humerus with a wafer of bone.

Clinical and Surgical Pearls

- Position the latissimus transfer laterally over the tuberosity to achieve greater external rotation moment
- A fascia lata graft may be added to augment tendon transfer length and/or strength of fixation

Clinical and Surgical Pitfalls

- Often overlooked contraindications to latissimus dorsi tendon transfer include preoperative shoulder pseudoparalysis and subscapularis insufficiency.

Pectoralis Major Transfer

Important Points

- Anterior stability of the glenohumeral joint is enhanced when the split pectoralis major tendon is routed in the retrocoracoid space underneath, rather than above, the conjoint tendon in line with the force vector of the deficient subscapularis.
- Retrocoracoid transfer provides superior restoration of rotational strength, and the posterior vector of the transfer is optimized in this position.

Clinical and Surgical Pearls

- Partial subscapularis repair, if possible, is helpful to improve results.

Clinical and Surgical Pitfalls

- Avoid far medial dissection to prevent nerve injury to the sternal head of the pectoralis major.

Direct primary repair achieves reliable pain relief and functional improvement in the majority of rotator cuff tears.[1-3] However, less commonly, very large musculotendinous defects, static superior subluxation of the humeral head, chronicity, and poor bone or tendon tissue quality may preclude successful primary repair.[2,4-7] In such cases, alternative reconstructive surgical techniques should be considered. Historically, the management of irreparable massive rotator cuff tears had encompassed a wide range of surgical procedures, including open or arthroscopic debridement, muscle or tendon transposition (upper subscapularis, teres minor, teres major, latissimus dorsi, pectoralis major, trapezius, deltoid, biceps, and triceps), tendon allografts, synthetic graft material, xenograft, and arthroplasty.[8-15]

Although debridement may allow pain relief in the low-demand patient,[16,17] function is not reliably restored.[2,18] Bridging of tendinous gaps with allografts and xenografts has not gained widespread acceptance because of variable functional results and inability to reestablish the length-tension relationship of the rotator cuff.[19] If the coracoacromial arch is intact, hemiarthroplasty may offer some relief in the setting of rotator cuff arthropathy,[20,21] but this treatment rarely addresses functional limitations.[22] Recently, reverse total shoulder arthroplasty has offered a promising solution for pain relief and concomitant functional improvement in older patients with irreparable tears; however, long-term data on the longevity of these prostheses are not available in the United States. Furthermore, a reverse prosthesis alone will not restore an external rotation deficit, which can be a persistent source of disability. For younger, high-demand patients, local or regional muscle and tendon transfers are viable treatment options that provide a vascularized, functional replacement of the affected musculotendinous unit when other repair methods are likely to fail.

When a musculotendinous unit has become torn and retracted from its insertion, the constituent muscle fibers undergo atrophy secondary to disuse. Concomitantly, fatty infiltration of the muscle interstitium results from macroarchitectural changes in the muscle fiber pennation angle.[23] Once these changes have occurred, the muscle may not generate the strength and excursion necessary for normal function, even after successful primary repair.[1,2,6,23,24] Even if excursion is sufficient to allow primary repair, fatty infiltration appears to be an irreversible event that may permanently compromise mechanical integrity of the musculotendinous unit.

Several donor muscles about the shoulder girdle have been shown to possess a suitable vector of pull, with adequate strength and amplitude to act as a surrogate rotator cuff tendon.[25-33,54] Empirically derived functional tendon transfers, of proven efficacy in foot and hand surgery, have been used to restore shoulder function after obstetric palsy in children.[29,34] The analogous situation in the adult can result from brachial plexopathy and iatrogenic, inherited, or degenerative injury to the neuromusculotendinous unit of the rotator cuff. Advancement or transposition of local and regional muscles has been described to treat commonly occurring massive degenerative rotator cuff tears.[6,11,13] The two patterns of massive, irreparable rotator cuff tears are posterior superior and anterior superior configurations. Posterior superior rotator cuff tears are the most common type and involve the supraspinatus and infraspinatus (and occasionally the teres minor) tendons. Anterior superior rotator cuff tears involve the

TABLE 25-1. Local and Regional Tendon Transfer Options for Muscle Deficits About the Shoulder

Deficit	Transfer Option
Infraspinatus (posteroinferior cuff)	Teres alone
Supraspinatus	Latissimus with or without teres major
Subscapularis (anterosuperior cuff)	Pectoralis major (split, clavicular head or sternal head)
Serratus anterior	Pectoralis major (split, sternal head)
Trapezius	Rhomboid, levator advancement (Eden-Lange procedure)

supraspinatus and the subscapularis. In this chapter, we review two reliable regional tendon transfers for treatment of the most commonly occurring deficits in the rotator cuff: the irreparable, massive posterior superior rotator cuff tear and the irreparable subscapularis tear (Table 25-1).

LATISSIMUS DORSI TRANSFER FOR POSTERIOR SUPERIOR ROTATOR CUFF TEARS

PREOPERATIVE CONSIDERATIONS

The latissimus dorsi transfer is primarily indicated for patients with unacceptable pain and functional deficits caused by a chronic, irreparable, massive tear of the posterosuperior rotator cuff. Because there is no strict preoperative definition of an irreparable tear, the clinician must use a constellation of findings on the history, physical examination, and radiographic workup to ascertain the feasibility of primary rotator cuff repair. Large chronic tears with associated poor tendon and bone quality may not be suitable for primary repair.

History

- Insidious onset of shoulder pain and loss of function during months to years
- Fatigue or pain with use of the arm in abduction
- External rotation weakness
- Prior failed surgery on the rotator cuff

Physical Examination

- Atrophy of the spinati may be noted, indicating a chronic, massive tear.
- Active forward flexion and external rotation are limited compared with the contralateral side. Motor testing of the supraspinatus and infraspinatus demonstrates weakness.
- Passive motion should be well maintained in the tendon transfer candidate.
- External rotation lag (a difference in passive and active external rotation arc) is indicative of a massive posterior cuff tear. An external rotation lag sign that persists in abduction, termed the *signe du clarion* ("hornblower's sign"), indicates extension of the tear into the teres minor[35] (Fig. 25-1).
- Subscapularis function is intact (Gerber lift-off test).
- It may be advantageous to perform an impingement test with a lidocaine injection into the subacromial space to test rotator cuff strength if the examination is limited by pain.

Imaging

- True anteroposterior (AP), scapular-Y, and axillary lateral views of the shoulder.
- Plain films may demonstrate static superior subluxation of the humeral head. An acromiohumeral distance of less than 7 mm (normal, 10.5 mm) suggests an irreparable tear of the infraspinatus (Fig. 25-2A).
- Magnetic resonance imaging (MRI) is performed to characterize the status of the rotator cuff tendons and to evaluate muscle atrophy and fatty infiltration.[50]

- A *massive tear*, defined as a tear encompassing two or more tendons, with grade 3 or 4 fatty infiltration of the rotator cuff musculature on MRI or computed tomography (CT) portends a poor prognosis for a successful primary repair and therefore is an indication for tendon transfer (Fig. 25-2B).[7]

Contraindications

Not all patients with massive, irreparable rotator cuff tears require surgery. Some patients with massive cuff

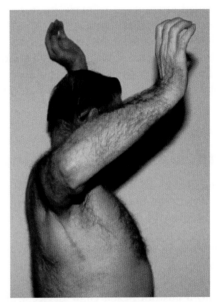

Figure 25-1. "Hornblower's sign": pathognomonic for massive posterior cuff tear.

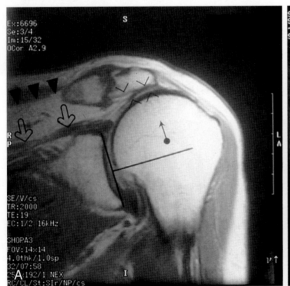
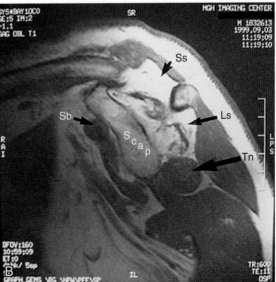

Figure 25-2. A, Magnetic resonance image demonstrating superior subluxation of the humeral head indicating massive rotator cuff tear. **B,** Grade 4 fatty infiltration of two rotator cuff muscles. *(From Warner JJP. Management of irreparable rotator cuff tears: The role of tendon transfer. In: Sim FH, ed. Instructional Course Lectures. Rosemont, IL: American Academy of Orthopaedic Surgeons; 2001.)*

tears experience minimal pain and maintain good overall shoulder function. Reconstructive efforts in such patients are unnecessary.

Patients with massive, irreparable rotator cuff tears often demonstrate pseudoparalysis, or the inability to initiate abduction. This finding is a contraindication to latissimus dorsi tendon transfer. Isolated loss of forward elevation alone is not reliably restored by this technique. In addition, patients with anterosuperior rotator cuff tears involving the subscapularis, such that the lift-off test result is positive, are not good candidates for latissimus transfer.

Prior failed attempts at primary rotator cuff repair are not necessarily contraindications to a latissimus transfer, but more limited gains in satisfaction and function should be expected.[36] Other relative contraindications include deltoid dysfunction, shoulder stiffness, severe rotator cuff tear arthropathy, and infection.

SURGICAL TECHNIQUE

Anesthesia and Positioning

The patient is assessed by the anesthesiologist preoperatively for the use of an interscalene block and catheter. However, because the interscalene block does not extend to the axilla, general anesthesia is necessary. We have had experience in positioning one of two ways—the beach chair or the lateral decubitus position.

If the beach chair position is selected, the patient is placed onto a custom beach chair device with retractable kidney rests, providing maximal exposure (T-Max Shoulder Positioner, Tenet Medical Engineering, Calgary, Canada). The beach chair position is relatively contraindicated in obese patients because of difficulty with surgical field exposure in the axilla. After induction, the patient is placed as far laterally on the table as possible to facilitate positioning of the surgeon during exposure. A first-generation cephalosporin is administered for prophylaxis. The operative limb and hemi-torso are

prepared and draped in the usual sterile fashion and then secured by means of a sterile pneumatic arm holder (Spider Limb Positioner, Tenet Medical Engineering, Calgary, Canada). With this position the surgeon may easily approach the superior shoulder and the axilla without the need of an assistant to hold the extremity (Fig. 25-3).

Alternatively, the lateral decubitus position may be used. After induction, the patient is placed into the lateral decubitus position on the far lateral side of a standard operating table. A full-length beanbag supports the patient's body, with an axillary roll in place on the contralateral side. The Tenet arm holder is positioned at the midportion of the bed on the ventral side of the patient. Preparation and draping proceed in the standard fashion, with care taken to provide adequate exposure superiorly and posteriorly (Fig. 25-4).

Surgical Landmarks and Incisions

Landmarks

- Anterosuperior exposure: acromion, acromioclavicular joint, clavicle, and coracoid process. The

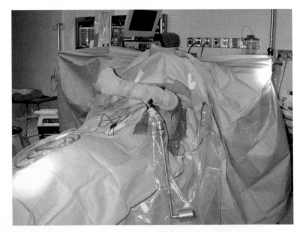

Figure 25-3. Beach chair position.

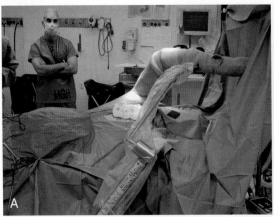
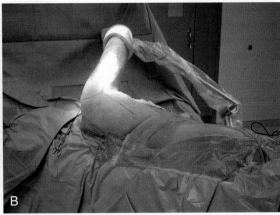

Figure 25-4. Lateral decubitus position.

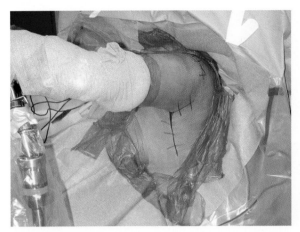

Figure 25-5. Posterior incision for latissimus dissection.

BOX 25-1 Surgical Steps: Latissimus Dorsi Transfer

1. Superior exposure, cuff assessment, mobilization
2. Greater tuberosity preparation (with anchor placement)
3. Posteroinferior exposure and mobilization of the latissimus tendon
4. Tendon transfer
5. Tendon fixation
6. Closure

---

incision is Langer's lines over the lateral third of the acromion, beginning at the posterior edge of the acromion and extending anteriorly 1 cm lateral to the coracoid process.

- Posteroinferior exposure: anterior border of the latissimus, triceps muscle belly, posterior deltoid. The posteroinferior incision of the latissimus dorsi is drawn parallel to the anterior border of the latissimus approximately 6 to 8 cm distal to the axillary fold. Proximally, the incision is curved superiorly parallel to the posterior axillary line to allow access to the posterior aspect of the deltoid (Fig. 25-5).

Structures at Risk

- Latissimus transfer: axillary nerve, radial nerve, brachial artery, thoracodorsal neurovascular pedicle

Specific Steps

Specific steps of this procedure are outlined in Box 25-1.

1. Superior Exposure, Cuff Assessment, and Mobilization

We approach the rotator cuff first during the procedure to allow assessment of cuff tissue and placement of anchors before harvesting of the latissimus. A No. 10 scalpel is used to incise skin and subcutaneous tissue to the level of the deltoid fascia. Sharp dissection with the

scalpel is used to develop skin flaps at this level adequate to allow visualization of the lateral acromion and interval between the anterior and middle deltoid. Electrocautery is used to secure hemostasis, and self-retaining retractors are placed.

Next, the electrocautery is used to split the deltoid in line with its fibers for a distance of 4 to 5 cm between the anterior and middle heads of the deltoid. The anterior deltoid may be reflected subperiosteally off the acromion by means of the electrocautery to provide visualization of the rotator cuff, if necessary. The interval between the anterior deltoid and coracoacromial arch is identified, and the coracoacromial ligament attachment to the acromion is preserved. The subacromial bursa is excised. Placement of Army-Navy retractors or a self-retaining subacromial spreader may be useful for exposure of the rotator cuff. The torn edges of the rotator cuff are then tagged with No. 3 Ethibond, and a systematic release of the rotator cuff is performed. A No. 15 scalpel is employed to release the coracohumeral ligament, extra-articular subacromial adhesions, and the superior capsule of the glenohumeral joint just deep to the rotator cuff. Care is taken not to release more than 1.8 cm medial to the glenoid to avoid iatrogenic injury to the suprascapular nerve. If the biceps tendon is present, it is released from the supraglenoid tubercle and tenodesed in the biceps groove. Once releases have been performed, the compliance and excursion of the cuff are assessed for the possibility of primary repair (Fig. 25-6).

2. Greater Tuberosity Preparation (with Anchor Placement)

If primary repair is deemed to be not feasible, the rotator cuff tendon edges are freshened with a scalpel and the greater tuberosity is prepared with a rongeur on its anterolateral surface. The footprint must be placed laterally enough to allow creation of an external rotation moment for the transferred tendon. Suture anchors are then placed to allow multiple fixation points and to reestablish the rotator cuff footprint, depending on the tear pattern. A moistened saline gauze is then packed into the wound, and attention is turned to the posteroinferior exposure (Fig. 25-7).

3. Posteroinferior Exposure and Mobilization of the Latissimus Tendon

With the arm holder in a position of abduction and maximal internal rotation, attention is turned to the posteroinferior incision. The skin is incised with a No. 10 scalpel, and skin flaps are developed above the level of the superficial fascia (Fig. 25-8A). By sharp dissection, the anterior border of the latissimus is defined. Posteriorly, the teres major, long head of the triceps, and posterior deltoid are identified. Careful dissection anteriorly will identify the neurovascular pedicle of the

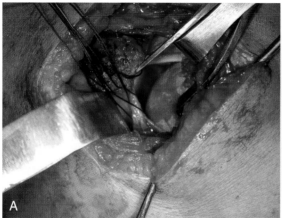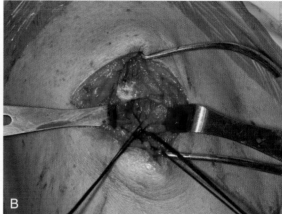

Figure 25-6. Mobilization and assessment of rotator cuff.

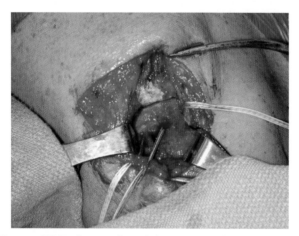

Figure 25-7. Preparation of the greater tuberosity for tendon insertion. Note lateral placement of anchors on tuberosity.

latissimus approximately 10 cm from the musculotendinous junction.[52] If the muscle portion of the teres major is distinct from the latissimus posteriorly, this interval may be developed distally to further isolate the latissimus. However, the bellies of these two muscles are often confluent. In this case, dissection is carried superiorly just off the anterior border of the latissimus to its insertion, which is identified by the long, flat tendon insertion on the anterior humerus. Exposure is facilitated by maximal internal rotation and abduction of the brachium. Once the insertion has been identified, the tendon is released under direct vision with a No. 15 scalpel, with care taken to avoid the radial and axillary nerves, which are close. The rest of the muscle belly may then be liberated of any adhesions to the chest wall in a retrograde fashion (Fig. 25-8B).

4. Tendon Transfer

After the latissimus has been identified and mobilized, a running locking stitch of No. 3 Ethibond is placed in the tendon, and final releases are performed distally (Fig. 25-9A). Adequate excursion of the tendon may be

tested by the ability to elevate the tendon superior to the level of the acromion (Fig. 25-10A). If this maneuver cannot be performed, further dissection of the thoracodorsal neurovascular pedicle may be performed as necessary, remembering that the average length of the pedicle is 8.4 cm. Alternatively, consideration may be given to augmentation of the graft with autogenous tissue (i.e., hamstring tendons) or soft tissue allografts to gain more length (Fig. 25-9B).

Once it has been determined that the tendon has enough length and excursion to reach the insertion site on the greater tuberosity, a subdeltoid tunnel is developed by a curved clamp inserted proximal to distal from the anterosuperior exposure to the posteroinferior exposure. The plane between the deltoid and teres minor is bluntly dissected, and the previously placed tagging sutures are drawn proximally through the soft tissue tunnel in an anterograde fashion. The axillary nerve is lateral to the passage of the tendon. Adequate excursion within the tunnel is confirmed by placing the tendon on the intended insertion site (Fig. 25-10B).

5. Tendon Fixation

Tendon fixation is performed to the insertion site with the arm in 45 degrees of abduction and 30 degrees of external rotation by means of horizontal mattress sutures from the suture anchors. Frequently, slight external rotation may be needed to secure the tendon without too much tension. If the mobilized remnant of the rotator cuff will reach the insertion site, it may be incorporated into the fixation of the latissimus tendon or secured with No. 5 FiberWire sutures in a Mason-Allen configuration through bone tunnels to the greater tuberosity (Fig. 25-11).

6. Closure

The deltoid is then repaired to the acromion through bone tunnels with No. 5 FiberWire (Fig. 25-12). All wounds are closed with 2-0 Vicryl sutures, followed by 3-0 Monocryl. Drains may be left in the wounds

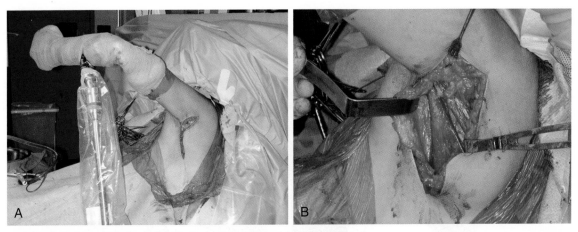

Figure 25-8. A, Posteroinferior incision. **B,** Mobilization of latissimus tendon.

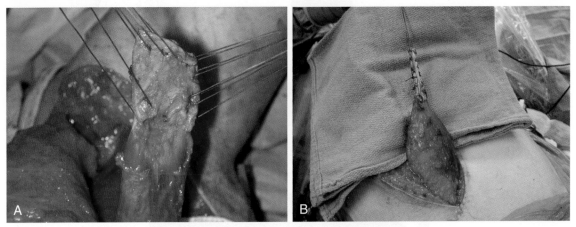

Figure 25-9. A, Preparation of latissimus tendon. **B,** Latissimus with the addition of fascia lata graft to reinforce tendon and attain length.

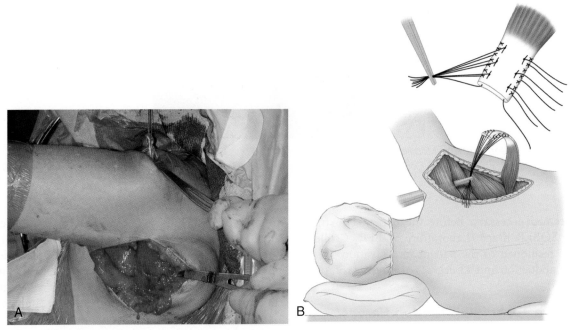

Figure 25-10. A, Testing adequate mobilization and excursion of the tendon transfer. **B,** Passage of tendon. *(From Warner JJP. Management of irreparable rotator cuff tears: The role of tendon transfer. In: Sim FH, ed.* Instructional Course Lectures. *Rosemont, IL: American Academy of Orthopaedic Surgeons; 2001.)*

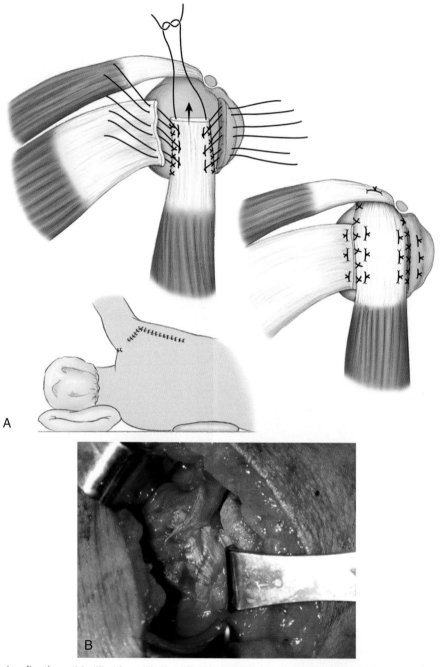

Figure 25-11. Tendon fixation. *(Modified from Higgins LD, Warner JJP. Massive tears of the posterosuperior rotator cuff. In: Warner JJP, Iannotto JP, Flatow EI, eds.* Complex and Revision Problems in Shoulder Surgery. *2nd ed. Philadelphia: Lippincott Williams & Wilkins; 2005.)*

if it is deemed necessary. Before the patient is extubated, the SOBER brace (Laboratoire SOBER, Crolles, France) is fashioned to the patient in a position of 45 degrees of abduction and 45 degrees of external rotation (Fig. 25-13).

Alternative Technique: Tendon Harvest with Bone

Citing high rates of postoperative rupture of the latissimus dorsi tendon transfer, Tauber et al have proposed an alternative technique of tendon harvest.[53] Instead of sharp removal of the latissimus tendon from the humerus, the tendon in harvested with a small piece of bone. The tendon and attached bone fragment can then be repaired through transosseous tunnels to the greater tuberosity with the potential for bone-to-bone healing. Using this technique, Moursy and colleagues[42] have reported improved clinical outcomes with a significant decrease in rates of postoperative rupture of the tendon transfer.

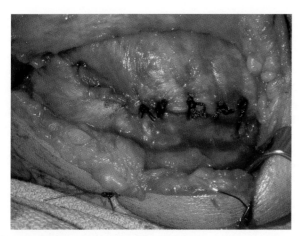

Figure 25-12. Deltoid repair.

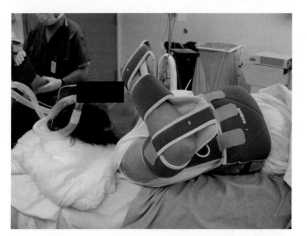

Figure 25-13. Application of SOBER brace in 45 degrees of abduction and external rotation before extubation. *(Modified from Higgins LD, Warner JJP. Massive tears of the posterosuperior rotator cuff. In: Warner JJP, Iannotto JP, Flatow EI, eds. Complex and Revision Problems in Shoulder Surgery. 2nd ed. Philadelphia: Lippincott Williams & Wilkins; 2005.)*

The rotator cuff and greater tuberosity are approached and prepared as described previously. The latissimus tendon, however, is approached through an axillary incision. With the arm held in an abducted position, an 8-cm incision is created in the posterior axillary fold perpendicular to the long axis of the arm. The posterior brachial cutaneous nerve is protected, and subcutaneous dissection proceeds until the latissimus dorsi and teres major tendons are exposed. The radial nerve is identified and carefully protected as it crosses the anterior border of the latissimus approximately 3 cm medial to the shaft of the humerus. A Hohmann retractor is then placed beneath the radial nerve and short head of the biceps and used to carefully retract them anteriorly away from the latissimus tendon insertion. Extreme care must be taken to avoid traction injury to the radial nerve from this retractor. The latissimus dorsi tendon is separated from the teres major, initially remote from the

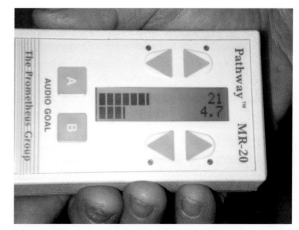

Figure 25-14. A biofeedback device is used to retrain the latissimus in its transferred location. (Pathway Biofeedback Device, Prometheus Group, Dover, NH.)

tendinous insertion. A sharp osteotome is then used to harvest the latissimus tendon with a small cortical fragment of bone approximately 3 mm in diameter. Tagging sutures are then placed, and the tendon passed as described previously. A bone trough corresponding to the dimensions of the harvested bone fragment is then created in the greater tuberosity. The transferred tendon and attached bone fragment are then secured into the trough with transosseous sutures.[37]

POSTOPERATIVE CONSIDERATIONS

Rehabilitation

The postoperative protocol is designed to protect tendon healing to bone while maintaining adequate excursion of the tendon through the submuscular tunnel and preventing glenohumeral stiffness and postsurgical adhesions. The patient is instructed to wear the SOBER brace continuously in abduction and external rotation for 6 weeks. During this time, passive abduction with external rotation above the plane of the brace (greater than 45 degrees) is instituted with physical therapy. Internal rotation and adduction are not permitted. At 6 weeks, the brace is removed and gentle activities of daily living are allowed with gentle mobilization of the extremity in physical therapy.

At the 3-month mark, active strengthening of the rotator cuff and tendon transfer is allowed. The normal vector of the latissimus is one of adduction, internal rotation, and extension. However, in its new position, the transfer must act out of phase as an external rotator. Therefore, muscle reeducation is performed with the aid of a biofeedback device (Fig. 25-14). An electrode is placed on the latissimus, which senses contraction and provides auditory and visual feedback to the patient. With the shoulder positioned in the midrange of

TABLE 25-2. Results of the Latissimus Dorsi Transfer

Author	No. of Patients	Follow-up	Outcomes
Aoki et al[9] (1996)	12	35 months	66% good-excellent UCLA score Forward flexion improved 36 degrees
Miniaci and MacLeod[37] (1999)	17 revision	51 months	82% satisfactory UCLA score Forward flexion improved 59 degrees External rotation improved 12 degrees
Warner and Parsons[3] (2001)	16 revision 6 primary	29 months 25 months	Postoperative score of 70% Forward flexion improved 60 degrees External rotation improved 37 degrees Postoperative score of 55% Forward flexion improved 43 degrees External rotation improved 29 degrees
Gerber et al[27] (1988)	4	14 months	75% good-excellent results Forward flexion improved 88 degrees Abduction improved 75 degrees External rotation improved 23 degrees
Gerber[6] (1992)	16	33 months	Postoperative normal age-adjusted Constant score of 73 Adequate pain relief in 94% of patients Forward flexion improved 52 degrees External rotation improved 13 degrees
Gerber et al[24] (2006)	69	53 months	Subjective shoulder value improved from 28% to 66% Age- and gender-matched Constant score improved from 55 to 73 Pain improved from 6 to 12 (of a possible 15 points) Forward flexion improved 19 degrees External rotation improved 7 degrees
Habermeyer et al[40] (2006)	14	32 months	Constant score improved from 46 to 74 Forward flexion improved 51 degrees External rotation improved 14 degrees
Moursy et al[42] (2009)	42 (Group A: 22 without bone; Group B: 20 with bone)	47 months	Group A: Four postoperative tendon ruptures, Constant score improved from 43 to 65 Group B: No postoperative tendon ruptures, Constant score improved from 40 to 74 Statistically significant improvement in outcome with harvest of tendon with bone

UCLA, University of California at Los Angeles shoulder rating scale.

abduction, the patient is instructed to adduct the arm, causing contraction of the latissimus. The therapist then assists the arm into forward flexion and external rotation during this maneuver, making a J shape in space. With time the patient learns how to contract the latissimus to execute abduction and external rotation. Full retraining of the muscle may take up to 12 months.

Complications

Complications of latissimus dorsi transfer include infection, scar tenderness (contraction of the axillary scar if it crosses perpendicular to the axilla), and pseudoparesis of the shoulder. As with any rotator cuff surgery, deltoid injury and axillary nerve injury may occur as well. If Resch's technique of latissimus tendon harvest with a bone fragment is used, then particular attention must be paid to limiting traction on the radial nerve to avoid injury to this structure. To prepare a more predictable

bony fragment, we now use a small oscillating saw rather than an osteotome to prepare this harvest. Late failure of the transfer has been variably reported, but if this is an intraoperative concern, the tendon may be augmented with autogenous fascia lata.[37]

RESULTS

Results of the latissimus dorsi transfer have been reported by Gerber and colleagues,[38] Aoki and colleagues,[9] Miniaci and MacLeod,[39] Warner and Parsons,[3] and Habermeyer and colleagues.[40] Good to excellent subjective results have been demonstrated in 13 of 16 patients[38] and 8 of 12 patients.[9] In Gerber's series, pain relief at rest was satisfactory in 94% of patients, and pain with exertion was 75% at 65 months postoperatively. Functionally, average improvement has ranged from 36 to 53 degrees in flexion and 14 degrees in external rotation. Habermeyer found an increased

Constant score from 46 to 76 at 32 months postoperatively with a single-incision technique.

More recent midterm results (53 months) by Gerber and Hersche[41] showed that patients maintained improvements in pain and function (subjective shoulder value increase from 28% to 66%; age- and gender-matched Constant score increase from 55 to 73).

Results in the setting of a failed prior attempt at rotator cuff repair have been less predictable. Warner and Parsons found that only 8 of 16 patients had adequate pain relief in the setting of a revision surgery, with an average gain in flexion of 44 degrees. In contrast, a satisfactory outcome was obtained in five of six patients who had the transfer as a primary procedure. Negative prognostic factors in the setting of a revision included prior deltoid injury, stiffness, and poor tendon quality of the remaining rotator cuff.

To improve the security of fixation of the transferred tendon and reduce postoperative rupture rates, Moursy and colleagues have advocated a modified technique of latissimus tendon harvest with a fragment of bone.[42] A group of 22 patients in whom the standard technique of tendon harvest was used were retrospectively compared with a group of 20 patients treated with a modified technique of tendon harvest with bone. The authors reported improvements in postoperative strength and range of motion with decreased pain in both groups, but with statistically superior results in the patients treated with the modified technique. At final follow-up, MRI revealed tendon transfer rupture and retraction in four patients treated with the standard technique but no patients in the modified technique group.

Irreparable rotator cuff tears continue to be a challenging problem for the reconstructive shoulder surgeon. For the appropriately chosen patient, latissimus dorsi transfer has been shown to provide reliable pain relief and improved function. Further study is necessary to delineate the future role of tendon transfers in the setting of prior arthroplasty or revision surgery, especially when patients have continued weakness of the external rotators (Table 25-2).

transfer has been described as a reasonable alternative in those instances to improve pain and function in shoulders in which the pain is attributed to the lack of a force couple with an intact posterior rotator cuff.[44] The patient's humeral head, however, must be centered in the preoperative axillary radiograph because this tendon transfer will not recenter the humeral head on the glenoid. Static anterior or anterosuperior subluxation of the humeral head is a contraindication to pectoralis major tendon transfer. In addition, the remainder of the rotator cuff should ideally be intact, including the supraspinatus. The pectoralis major transfer is therefore indicated for patients with unacceptable pain and functional deficits caused by a chronic, irreparable, tear of the subscapularis. Multiple techniques have been described for this transfer, including transfer of one or both heads of the tendon superficial or deep to the conjoined tendon to insert on the lesser tuberosity.[12,48,49] Our preferred method, transfer of the sternal head of the pectoralis, is described here.[36]

History

- Prior surgical injury to the subscapularis
- Prior instability surgery
- Shoulder arthritis status post–total shoulder replacement[51]
- Insidious onset of shoulder pain and loss of function
- Remote traumatic injury (external rotation)

Physical Examination

- Positive lift-off test result, positive belly press test result
- Internal rotation weakness
- Increased passive external rotation compared with the contralateral side (Fig. 25-15)

PECTORALIS MAJOR TRANSFER FOR SUBSCAPULARIS INSUFFICIENCY

PREOPERATIVE CONSIDERATIONS

Indications

Tendon retraction and fatty infiltration may preclude primary repair of the subscapularis.[43] Pectoralis major

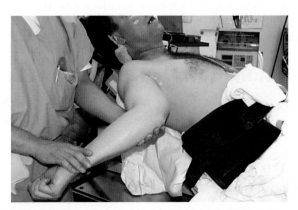

Figure 25-15. Increased passive external rotation as compared with the contralateral side.

Imaging

- Shoulder AP, axillary, and scapular-Y plain films
- MRI with T1 or equivalent sequences *or* CT scan to evaluate for fatty atrophy

Pertinent Positive Findings

- Tendon retraction on axial cuts
- Greater than grade 2 fatty infiltration of subscapularis on CT or MRI

Contraindications

Primary subscapularis tendon repair is preferable if possible. If the subscapularis insufficiency is a component of a massive irreparable anterosuperior rotator cuff tear, the patient may be best served by a reverse shoulder prosthesis if he or she meets the criteria for that salvage procedure. Combined latissimus and pectoralis major tendon transfers have not yielded satisfactory results in our experience.[8] Concurrent infection, stiffness, and medical comorbidities may preclude pectoralis major transfer. Anterior-superior escape or anterior subluxation of the humeral head relative to the glenoid on axillary views or on axial CT are contraindications to pectoralis major transfer.

SURGICAL TECHNIQUE

Anesthesia and Positioning

The patient is placed onto a custom beach chair device with retractable kidney rests, providing maximal exposure (T-Max Shoulder Positioner). After induction, the patient is placed as far laterally on the table as possible, to facilitate surgeon positioning during exposure. The operative limb and hemi-torso are prepared and draped in the usual sterile fashion and then secured by means of a sterile pneumatic arm holder (Spider Limb Positioner). With this position the surgeon may easily approach the superior shoulder and the axilla without the need of an assistant to hold the extremity (see Fig. 25-3).

Examination Under Anesthesia

Before draping, the passive external rotation of the affected and the unaffected contralateral arm is assessed (see Fig. 25-15).

Surgical Landmarks and Incisions

Deltopectoral approach: The lateral aspect of the coracoid and the deltoid insertion serve as the boundaries

---

> **BOX 25-2** Surgical Steps for Pectoralis Major Transfer
>
> 1. Deltopectoral approach
> 2. Evaluation and mobilization of the subscapularis tendon
> 3. Preparation of the lesser tuberosity
> 4. Preparation of the retrocoracoid space
> 5. Harvest of the sternal head of the pectoralis major tendon
> 6. Transfer under the clavicular head and through the retrocoracoid space
> 7. Fixation to the humeral head

of the deltopectoral incision with distal extension to visualize the pectoralis insertion.

Structures at Risk

- The axillary nerve courses over the belly of the subscapularis and is at risk throughout the mobilization of the subscapularis.
- The medial pectoral nerve is at risk during dissection and mobilization of the sternal head of the pectoralis if dissection is carried too medially. Injury to this nerve results in denervation of the transferred muscle.
- Axillary artery.
- Musculocutaneous nerve with retrocoracoid transfer.

Specific Steps

Specific steps of this procedure are outlined in Box 25-2.

1. Deltopectoral Approach

With the arm in slight forward flexion, abduction, and neutral rotation, a standard deltopectoral approach, extending from the lateral aspect of the coracoid toward the insertion of the deltoid, is employed for initial exposure. With the cephalic vein taken either laterally or medially (taking it medially avoids injury by the deltoid retractors), the interval between the pectoralis major and deltoid is exposed and maintained. The clavipectoral fascia is incised, and the conjoined tendon is retracted medially. Externally rotate the arm to expose the lesser tuberosity.

2. Evaluation and Mobilization of the Subscapularis Tendon

The subscapularis tendon deficiency may initially be difficult to appreciate, as the lesser tuberosity is often enveloped in scar tissue. After this scar has been excised and the bone of the lesser tuberosity is exposed, identification of the torn edge of the subscapularis tendon is attempted. The remnant tendon is tagged with 3.0 braided suture and mobilized from under the conjoint tendon with a combination of blunt and sharp dissection. Care is taken to protect the axillary nerve on the anterior inferior aspect of the subscapularis during dissection. If the subscapularis tendon is of poor quality or irreparable, the pectoralis major transfer is used. However, the tendon and scarred remnants of subscapularis were mobilized as far medially, superiorly, and inferiorly as possible, and an attempt can be made to attach the tendon and remnants to the lesser tuberosity.

3. Lesser Tuberosity Preparation

The lesser tuberosity is gently decorticated by using a shaver and a bur to obtain a bleeding bed. Suture anchors or transosseous sutures can be placed in preparation to receive the sternal head of pectoralis major.

4. Preparation of the Retrocoracoid Space

Anterior stability of the glenohumeral joint is enhanced when the split pectoralis major tendon is routed in the retrocoracoid space underneath, rather than above, the conjoint tendon in line with the force vector of the deficient subscapularis. Retrocoracoid transfer provides superior restoration of rotational strength, and the posterior vector of the transfer is optimized in this position. Passing the tendon in the retrocoracoid space also interposes muscle between the coracoid process and the humeral head and increases passive muscle tension.

The space between the pectoralis minor and the conjoined tendon is entered, and the area behind the conjoined tendon is exposed. The musculocutaneous nerve and its entrance into the muscle are located. This step is important for the assessment of the space for the transferred muscle when it passes between the nerve and the conjoined tendon. The interval between the pectoralis minor muscle and the conjoined tendon is opened so that the nerve can be identified visually; alternatively, the nerve can be palpated.

The interval between the nerve and the conjoined tendon dictates how much muscle needs to be harvested to be passed easily, so this stage is completed before the sternal head is harvested.

5. Harvest of Sternal Head of the Pectoralis Major Tendon

The pectoralis major harvest is accomplished after adequate estimation of the retrocoracoid space in the previous step. The interval between the sternal and clavicular heads of the pectoralis major tendon is best delineated at its humeral insertion. Placing the muscle under tension by abducting and externally rotating the shoulder facilitates the differentiation of the sternal and clavicular portions of the pectoralis major. Often a stripe of fatty tissue may be present in the plane between the two muscles (Fig. 25-16A). A Cobb elevator, No. 15 scalpel blade, or Metzenbaum scissors are used to isolate the tendon of the sternal head as it inserts inferior and deep to the clavicular head (Fig. 25-16B and C). The tendon is then detached sharply off the bone. After No. 2 braided nonabsorbable traction sutures have been placed into the tendon in a Mason-Allen fashion, blunt dissection between the muscle bellies of the sternal and clavicular heads proceeds medially. The medial and lateral pectoral nerves are safe as long as one stays lateral to the pectoralis minor and less than 8.5 cm from the humeral insertion of the pectoralis major.

6. Transfer Under the Clavicular Head and Through the Retrocoracoid Space

After the sternal head is sufficiently mobilized, a Kelly clamp is passed from superior to inferior, deep to the clavicular head of the pectoralis major and deep to the conjoint tendon. The traction sutures are grasped with this clamp to transfer the sternal head under the clavicular head (Fig. 25-17). Thus the muscle is advanced behind the conjoined tendon but anterior to the musculocutaneous nerve.

7. Fixation to the Humeral Head

The arm is then placed into the patient's physiologic amount of passive external rotation, as determined by the nonoperative arm during the examination under anesthesia. The transferred sternal head of the pectoralis major is then fixed to the lesser tuberosity with anchors or transosseous sutures.

POSTOPERATIVE CONSIDERATIONS

Rehabilitation

- Sling for 6 weeks with only passive range of motion to protect the transfer and limit scarring.
- Begin active-assisted range of motion after 6 weeks.
- Start active range of motion at 2 months.
- Strengthening may begin after 4 months.
- Return to sport or work after 6 months.

Complications

- Recurrent instability
- Avulsion of transferred pectoralis tendon
- Infection

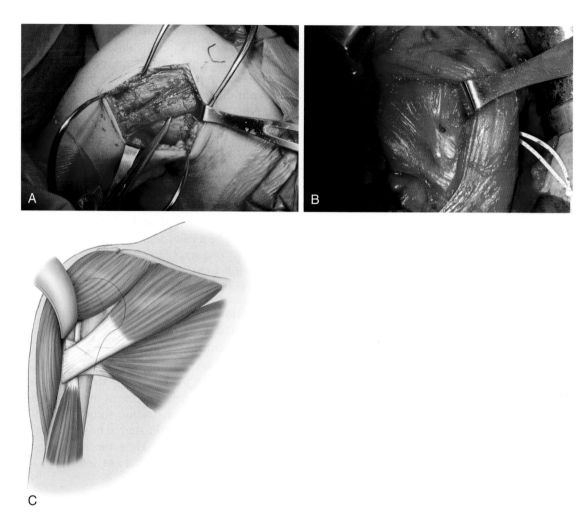

Figure 25-16. A, Identification of sternal and clavicular heads of pectoralis major. **B,** Sternal head of pectoralis major. **C,** Schematic of relationship of clavicular and pectoral head insertions.

- Deep vein thrombosis
- Coracohumeral impingement
- Nerve injury

RESULTS

The split tendon transfer has limited value in the management of patients with irreparable subscapularis insufficiency after shoulder replacement. In our experience, split tendon transfer in such patient populations has very limited success in improving pain or the Constant score. In patients with isolated subscapularis insufficiency after a failed stabilization procedure, improvement in pain and function can be expected in those who have a concentric glenohumeral joint preoperatively. However, if the shoulder joint is subluxed or not

concentric the transfer of pectoralis tendon is more likely to fail, an alternative treatment such as a bone block, transfer of the coracoid or capsular reconstruction using tendon allograft or autograft, or reverse arthroplasty in selected cases should be considered as a salvage procedure. In patients with irreparable subscapularis insufficiency in the setting of massive rotator cuff tear, significant improvement with the split pectoralis major transfer can be anticipated, in our opinion if (1) there is a concentric joint preoperatively and (2) no supraspinatus or infraspinatus atrophy is present. Grade 3 or 4 fatty infiltration of supraspinatus and infraspinatus is associated with failure of pectoralis major transfer. Better results are obtained if the subscapularis tendon can be partially or complete repaired concomitantly with the pectoralis major transfer (Table 25-3).

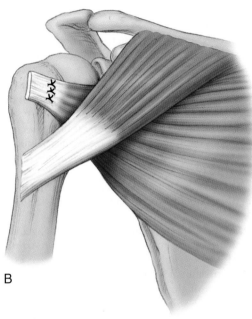

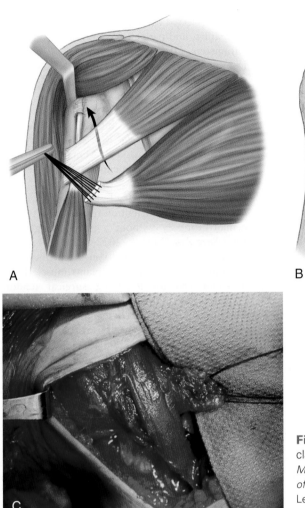

Figure 25-17. Transfer of tendon under clavicular head. *(Modified from Warner JJP. Management of irreparable rotator cuff tears: The role of tendon transfer. In: Sim FH, ed. Instructional Course Lectures. Rosemont, IL: American Academy of Orthopaedic Surgeons; 2001.)*

TABLE 25-3 Results of the Pectoralis Major Transfer

Author	No. of Patients	Follow-up (mo)	Outcomes
Gavrilidis et al[56] (2010)	15	37	Constant score improved from 52 to 68; 85% intact transferred pectoralis major on MRI evaluation
Elhassan et al[47] (2008)	30	24	
Group 1 (failed instability)	11	49	Pain 7.5 to 3.8 and Constant score 41 to 61
Group 2 (failed arthroplasty)	8	53	Pain 7.8 to 6.1 and Constant score 33 to 42
Group 3 (massive RCT)	11	57	Pain 7.9 to 4.2 and Constant score 23 to 52
Warner et al[55] (2004)	11	38	ASES score improved from 42 to 61 81% of patients satisfied
Aldridge et al[8] (2004)	11	31	Constant score improved from 21% to 36% 63% of patients satisfied
Gerber et al[57] (2003)	30	32	Constant score improved from 47% to 70% 82% good or excellent result
Galatz et al[12] (2003)	14	18	79% of patients satisfied
Resch et al[16] (2000)	12	28	Constant score improved from 27% to 67% 75% good or excellent result

ASES, American Shoulder and Elbow Surgeons scale; *RCT,* rotator cuff tear.

REFERENCES

1. Gazielly DF, Gleyze P, Montagnon C. Functional and anatomical results after rotator cuff repair. *Clin Orthop Relat Res.* 1994;304:43-53.
2. Harryman DT, Mack LA, Wang KY. Repairs of the rotator cuff: Correlation of functional results with integrity of the cuff. *J Bone Joint Surg Am.* 1991;73:982-989.
3. Warner JJP, Parsons M. Latissimus dorsi transfer: a comparative analysis of primary and salvage reconstruction of massive, irreparable rotator cuff tears. *J Shoulder Elbow Surg.* 2001;10:514-521.
4. Apoil A, Augereau B. Deltoid flap repair of large losses of substance of the shoulder rotator cuff. *Chirurgie.* 1985;11:287-290.
5. Arntz CT, Matsen III FA, Jackins S. Surgical management of complex irreparable rotator cuff deficiency. *J Arthroplasty.* 1991;6:363-370.
6. Gerber C. Latissimus dorsi transfer for the treatment of irreparable tears of the rotator cuff. *Clin Orthop Relat Res.* 1992;275:152-160.
7. Goutallier D, Postel JM, Bernageau J, et al. Fatty muscle degeneration in cuff ruptures: Pre- and postoperative evaluation by CT scan. *Clin Orthop Relat Res.* 1994;304:78-83.
8. Aldridge JM, Atkinson TS, Mallon WJ. Combined pectoralis major and latissimus dorsi tendon transfer for massive rotator cuff deficiency. *J Shoulder Elbow Surg.* 2004;13:621-629.
9. Aoki M, Okamura K, Fukushima S, et al. Transfer of latissimus dorsi for irreparable rotator cuff tears. *J Bone Joint Surg Br.* 1996;78:761-766.
10. Beauchamp M, Beaton DE, Barnhill TA, et al. Functional outcome after L'Episcopo procedure. *J Shoulder Elbow Surg.* 1998;7:90-96.
11. Cofield RH. Subscapularis muscle transposition for repair and chronic shoulder cuff tears. *Surg Gynecol Obstet.* 1982;154:667-672.
12. Galatz LM, Connor PM, Calfee RP, et al. Pectoralis major transfer for anterior-superior subluxation in massive rotator cuff insufficiency. *J Shoulder Elbow Surg.* 2003;12:1-5.
13. Neer CS, Flatow EL, Lech O. Tears of the rotator cuff: Long term results of anterior acromioplasty and repair. *Orthop Trans.* 1988;12:735.
14. Neviaser JS, Neviaser RJ, Neviaser TJ. The repair of chronic massive ruptures of the rotator cuff of the shoulder by use of a freeze-dried rotator cuff. *J Bone Joint Surg Am.* 1978;60:681-684.
15. Neviaser RJ, Neviaser TJ. Transfer of the subscapularis and teres minor for massive defects of the rotator cuff. In: Bayley IL, Kessel L, eds. *Shoulder Surgery.* Berlin: Springer; 1982:60-63.
16. Resch H, Povacz P, Ritter E, et al. Transfer of the pectoralis major muscle for the treatment of irreparable rupture of the subscapularis tendon. *J Bone Joint Surg Am.* 2000;82:372-382.
17. Rockwood CA, Burkhead WZ. Management of patients with massive rotator cuff debridement. *Orthop Trans.* 1988;12:12, 190.
18. Burkhart SS. Arthroscopic débridement and decompression for selected rotator cuff tears: Clinical results, pathomechanics, and patient selection based on biomechanical parameters. *Orthop Clin North Am.* 1993;24:111-123.
19. DeFranco MJ, Derwin K, Iannotti JP. New therapies in tendon reconstruction. *J Am Acad Orthop Surg.* 2004;12:298-304.
20. Hockman DE, Lucas GL, Roth CA. Role of the coracoacromial ligament as restraint after shoulder hemiarthroplasty. *Clin Orthop Relat Res.* 2004;419:80-82.
21. Laudicina L, D'Ambrosia R. Management of irreparable rotator cuff tears and glenohumeral arthritis. *Orthopedics.* 2005;28:382-388.
22. Hettrich CM, Weldon 3rd E, Boorman RS, et al. Optimizing the glenoid contribution to the stability of a humeral hemiarthroplasty without a prosthetic glenoid. *J Bone Joint Surg Am.* 2004;86:2022-2029.
23. Meyer DC, Hoppeler H, von Rechenberg B, et al. A pathomechanical concept explains muscle loss and fatty muscular changes following surgical tendon release. *J Orthop Res.* 2004;22:1004-1007.
24. Gerber C, Maquieira G, Espinosa N. Latissimus dorsi transfer for the treatment of irreparable rotator cuff tears. *J Bone Joint Surg Am.* 2006;88:113-120.
25. Cleeman E, Hazrati Y, Auerbach JD, et al. Latissimus dorsi tendon transfer for massive rotator cuff tears: a cadaveric study. *J Shoulder Elbow Surg.* 2003;12:539-543.
26. Comtet JJ, Herzberg G, Naasan IA. Biomechanical basis of transfers for shoulder paralysis. *Hand Clin.* 1989;5:1-14.
27. Gerber C, Vinh TS, Hertel R, et al. Latissimus dorsi transfer for treatment of massive tears of the rotator cuff: a preliminary report. *Clin Orthop Relat Res.* 1988;232:51-61.
28. Herzberg G, Urien JP, Dimnet J. Potential excursion and relative tension of muscles in the shoulder girdle: Relevance to tendon transfers. *J Shoulder Elbow Surg.* 1999;8:430-437.
29. Hoffer MM, Wickenden R, Roper B. Brachial plexus birth injuries: Results of tendon transfer of the rotator cuff. *J Bone Joint Surg Am.* 1978;60:691-695.
30. Jonsson B, Olofsson BM, Steffner LC. Function of the teres major, latissimus dorsi, and pectoralis major muscles: a preliminary study. *Acta Morphol Neerl Scand.* 1971;9:275.
31. L'Episcopo JB. Tendon transplantation in obstetrical paralysis. *Am J Surg.* 1934;25:122-125.
32. Rockwood Jr CA, Williams Jr GR, Burkhead Jr WZ. Debridement of degenerative, irreparable lesions of the rotator cuff. *J Bone Joint Surg Am.* 1995;77:857-866.
33. Wirth MA, Rockwood Jr CA. Operative treatment of irreparable rupture of the subscapularis. *J Bone Joint Surg Am.* 1997;79:722-731.
34. Covey DC, Riordan DC, Milstead ME, et al. Modification of the L'Episcopo procedure for brachial plexus birth palsies. *J Bone Joint Surg Br.* 1992;74:897-901.
35. Hertel R, Ballmer FT, Lombert SM, et al. Lag signs in the diagnosis of rotator cuff rupture. *J Shoulder Elbow Surg.* 1996;5:307-313.

36. Shiino K. Ueber die bewegungen im schultergelenk und die arbeitsleistung der schultermuskeln. *Arch Anat Phys Abtlg Anatomie.* 1913;(suppl):1-89.

37. Warner JJP, Gerber C. Treatment of massive rotator cuff tears: posterior-superior and antero-superior. In: Iannotti JP, ed. *The Rotator Cuff: Current Concepts and Complex Problems.* Rosemont, IL: American Academy of Orthopaedic Surgeons; 1998:59-94.

38. Gerber C, Meyer DC, Schneeberger AG, et al. Effect of tendon release and delayed repair on the structure of the muscles of the rotator cuff: an experimental study in sheep. *J Bone Joint Surg Am.* 2004;86:1973-1982.

39. Miniaci A, MacLeod M. Transfer of the latissimus dorsi muscle after failed repair of a massive tear of the rotator cuff. *J Bone Joint Surg Am.* 1999;81:1120-1127.

40. Habermeyer P, Magosch P, Rudolph T, et al. Transfer of the tendon of latissimus dorsi for the treatment of massive tears of the rotator cuff: a new single incision technique. *J Bone Joint Surg Br.* 2006;88:208-212.

41. Gerber C, Hersche O. Tendon transfers for the treatment of irreparable rotator cuff defects. *Orthop Clin North Am.* 1997;28:195-203.

42. Moursy M, Forstner R, Koller H, et al. Latissimus dorsi tendon transfer for irreparable rotator cuff tears: a modified technique to improve tendon transfer integrity. *J Bone Joint Surg Am.* 2009;91:1924-1931.

43. Warner JJP. Management of massive irreparable rotator cuff tears: The role of tendon transfer. AAOS *Instr Course Lect.* 2001;50:63-71.

44. Jost B, Puskas GJ, Lustenberger A, et al. Outcome of pectoralis major transfer for the treatment of irreparable subscapularis tears. *J Bone Joint Surg Am.* 2003;85:1944-1951.

45. Phipps GJ, Hoffer MM. Latissimus dorsi and teres major transfer to rotator cuff for Erb's palsy. *J Shoulder Elbow Surg.* 1995;4:124-129.

46. Watson M. Major ruptures of the rotator cuff: the results of surgical repair in 89 patients. *J Bone Joint Surg Br.* 1985;67:618.

47. Elhassan, B. Ozbaydar M. Transfer of pectoralis major for the treatment of irreparable tears of subscapularis. *J Bone Joint Surg Br.* 2008;90:1059-1065.

48. Gerber A, Clavert P, Millett PJ, et al. Split pectoralis major and teres major tendon transfers for reconstruction of irreparable tears of the subscapularis. *Tech Shoulder Elbow Surg.* 2004;5:5-12.

49. Konrad GG, Sudkamp NP, Kreuz PC, et al. Pectoralis major tendon transfers above or underneath the conjoint tendon in subscapularis-deficient shoulders an in vitro biomechanical analysis. *J Bone Joint Surg Am.* 2007;89:2477-2484.

50. Meyer DC, Pirkl C, Pfirrmann CW, et al. Asymmetric atrophy of the supraspinatus muscle following tendon tear. *J Orthop Res.* 2005;23:254-258.

51. Miller BS, Joseph TA, Noonan TJ, et al. Rupture of the subscapularis tendon after shoulder arthroplasty: diagnosis, treatment, and outcome. *J Shoulder Elbow Surg.* 2005;14:492-496.

52. Schoierer O, Herzberg G, Berthonnaud E, et al. Anatomical basis of latissimus dorsi and teres major transfers in rotator cuff tear surgery with particular reference to the neurovascular pedicles. *Surg Radiol Anat.* 2001;23:75-80.

53. Tauber M, Moursy M, Forstner R, et al. Latissimus dorsi tendon transfer for irreparable rotator cuff tears: a modified technique to improve tendon transfer integrity: surgical technique. *J Bone Joint Surg Am.* 2010;92:226-239.

54. Zachary RB. Transplantation of teres major and latissimus dorsi for loss of external rotation at shoulder. *Lancet.* 1947;2:757.

55. Gerber A, Calvert P, Millet P, et al. Split pectoralis major and teres major tendon transfers for reconstruction of irreparable tears of the subscapularis.. *Tech Shoulder Elbow Surg.* 2004;5(1):5-12.

56. Gavrilidis I, Kircher J, Magosch P, et al. Pectoralis major transfer for the treatment of irreparable anterosuperior rotator cuff tears. *Int Orthop.* 2010;34(5):689-694.

57. Jost B, Puskas GJ, Lustenberger A, et al. Outcome of pectoralis major transfer for the treatment of irreparable subscapularis tears. *J Bone Joint Surg Am.* 2003;85-A(10):1944-1951.

Chapter 26

Arthroscopic Repair of Superior Labral Anterior-Posterior Lesions by the Single-Anchor Double-Suture Technique

Joseph P. Burns, Max Tyorkin, and Stephen J. Snyder

Chapter Synopsis
- Diagnosis and management of symptomatic superior labral anterior-posterior (SLAP) lesions can be a difficult task, and the surgical technique has evolved considerably over the past 25 years. Arthroscopic suture anchor repair is now the standard of care and can be formed safely and quickly with only a few precise steps. For most lesions, a balanced, strong repair to the supraglenoid tubercle can provide reliable results with a single double-loaded anchor.

Important Points
- The most important consideration in the management of SLAP lesions is establishing the proper diagnosis. Symptomatic SLAP lesions are fairly rare and must be differentiated from degenerative tearing, normal anatomic variants, and biceps pathology.
- Agreement among history, physical examination findings, imaging, and arthroscopic findings is ideal
- Although a repair can be quick and easy, requiring only a few steps, the steps are very precise and must be performed with careful dexterity.

Clinical and Surgical Pearls
- If the history, examination findings, and magnetic resonance imaging (MRI) scans all do not agree, be sure to carefully rule out other shoulder pathology before tightening a superior labrum.

- Be sure to be comfortable identifying normal anatomic variants such as the Buford complex, sublabral foramen, and a degenerative labrum.
- Three surgical portals are recommended for a SLAP repair; however, a posterolateral accessory portal, also known as the *Wilmington portal,* can be necessary for placing suture anchors for tears extending posteriorly.
- The anterosuperior portal (ASP) is the most important portal and should be placed before the anterior midglenoid portal, using a spinal needle under direct visualization.
- Debridement of labrum and bone must remove all damaged tissue and create an optimal healing environment in a poorly vascularized area.

Clinical and Surgical Pitfalls
SLAP repair steps have been simplified, but they must be carried out with the utmost precision. Surgical pitfalls occur when anchors are improperly placed (e.g., too proud, too loose), cartilage is iatrogenically damaged (e.g., drill bit skiving, suturing devices), or stitching is careless (e.g., overtightening the biceps, multiple passes through labrum).

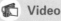 **Video**
- Video 26-1: Arthroscopic repair of a type II SLAP lesion

Tears of the superior labrum were first described by Andrews and colleagues in 1985[1] and later named and classified by Snyder and colleagues in 1990.[2] Since that time, the treatment of superior labral anterior-posterior (SLAP) lesions has evolved from debridement to repair using drill holes, tacks, and now suture anchors. With minor variations in technique only, most surgeons currently advocate the use of one or more suture anchors on the edge of the glenoid to stabilize and restore labral and biceps anchor anatomy. With only level III and IV evidence available in the literature, and a good deal of confusion regarding accurate diagnosis of a symptomatic SLAP lesion, there is still a great deal to be learned. Over the past 25 years, we have been working to develop a better understanding of SLAP lesions. This chapter represents our current management strategy.

PREOPERATIVE CONSIDERATIONS
History

A thorough history is essential in elucidating an injury to the superior labrum. Typically the patients are young male athletes who report shoulder pain exacerbated by overhead activity, or male or female patients who have sustained a traumatic traction or compression injury to the shoulder.[2,3] This is often associated with popping, snapping, catching, or locking, similar to mechanical symptoms that may be associated with a meniscal tear in the knee.[4,5] SLAP lesions must be differentiated from other pathologic processes of the shoulder, such as instability, impingement, rotator cuff tear, and acromioclavicular joint disease. Without a clear history of throwing overuse or trauma, the diagnosis must be questioned.

Physical Examination

Unfortunately, there is no single physical examination test that is specific and sensitive for a SLAP lesion, although several have been described. Both the comprehensive physical examination and the history are essential in raising the index of suspicion for a possible SLAP lesion. A complete examination is important but not accurate in predicting with certainty the existence of a SLAP lesion, although there are several tests that may prove useful. The biceps tension (Speed) test was the most accurate in several studies.[6-8] The Speed test result is positive when pain is elicited with resisted forward elevation of the fully supinated arm with the elbow extended and the arm flexed to 90 degrees. The compression-rotation sign described by Andrews and colleagues[9] is demonstrated with the patient supine, the shoulder elevated to 90 degrees, and the elbow flexed to 90 degrees. An axial load is then applied to the humerus to compress the glenohumeral joint while the arm is rotated. A positive test result is pain as well as mechanical symptoms elicited during this test. The O'Brien sign, or the active compression test, is elicited by first placing the arm in 90 degrees of forward flexion and 10 to 20 degrees of adduction. The arm is then fully internally rotated into the thumb-down position. The patient is then asked to resist downward pressure to the arm that is applied by the examiner. Pain is often produced when an unstable superior labrum is present. The test is then repeated but with the arm in full supination;

the pain should be decreased in this position compared with the initial position for the test result to be considered positive. We consider mechanical pain and one or more positive provocative tests to be consistent with a "suspicious physical examination."[10]

Imaging

As with most shoulder disease, standard radiographic evaluation includes four views of the shoulder (anteroposterior, axillary, outlet, and acromioclavicular joint views). Although plain radiographs are not specific for labral disease, they are important to rule out other, coexisting pathologic processes of the shoulder.

Although very high–quality magnetic resonance imaging (MRI) machines and very experienced evaluators may not need gadolinium-enhanced arthrograms to achieve similar sensitivity, MRI with arthrogram is still the most reliable imaging test of choice. Normal anatomic variations around the superior labrum can make MRI findings nonspecific, and the gold standard in diagnosing SLAP lesions is still arthroscopy itself, but the presence of paralabral cysts and coronal images with contrast extension under the superior labrum and extending laterally *into* the substance of the labrum are most commonly associated with true SLAP lesions (Fig. 26-1). MRI is also useful to evaluate for concomitant pathologic changes, such as rotator cuff tears, acromioclavicular joint disease, and biceps disease.

Indications and Contraindications

A combination of knowledge of anatomy (anatomic variants), patient history (traumatic event, overhead athlete), physical examination findings ("suspicious" provocative test results), MRI findings (contrast into labral tissue), and arthroscopy findings (detached unstable labrum and biceps anchor) with no other obvious explanation for the symptoms will give the best chance to correctly diagnose a SLAP lesion. Diagnostic arthroscopy is indicated when a SLAP tear is suspected in a symptomatic patient in whom a course of nonoperative treatment has failed but who otherwise has the corresponding history, physical examination, and MRI findings. Indications for repair are still being defined. We have developed and published an algorithm that can assist in the decision-making process (Fig. 26-2).[10]

SURGICAL TECHNIQUE
Anesthesia and Positioning

Once general endotracheal anesthesia has been achieved, with or without interscalene block, the patient is placed in the lateral decubitus position and supported with a

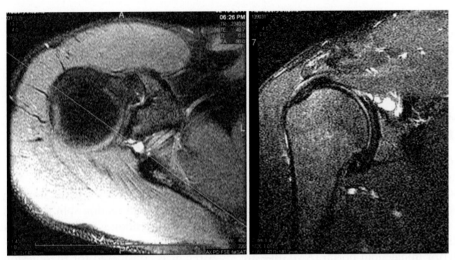

Figure 26-1. T2-weighted axial and coronal images of a type II superior labral anterior-posterior lesion with a paralabral cyst.

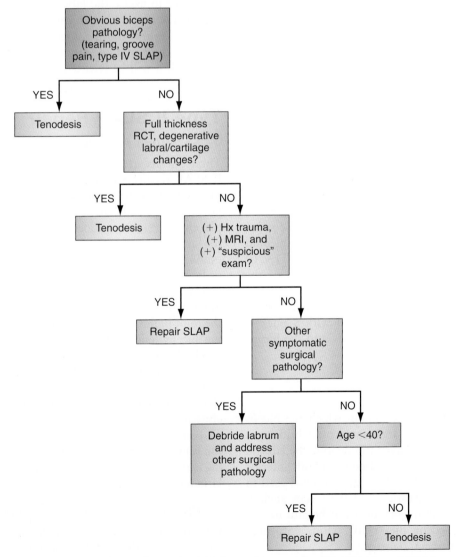

Figure 26-2. Algorithm for management of superior labral anterior-posterior (*SLAP*) lesion. *MRI,* Magnetic resonance imaging; *RCT,* rotator cuff tear.

beanbag. The shoulder is examined for stability and then prepared and draped. The arm is suspended in 10 pounds of balanced skeletal traction in a position of approximately 70 degrees of abduction and 10 degrees of forward flexion.

Surgical Landmarks, Incisions, and Portals

Bony landmarks of the acromion and clavicle are carefully and accurately outlined on the skin. A standard posterior arthroscopy portal is made, and the arthroscope is introduced into the joint. After diagnostic arthroscopy has confirmed the presence of the SLAP lesion, two anterior portals—an anterosuperior portal (ASP) and an anterior midglenoid portal (AMGP)—are created in the rotator interval using an outside-in technique as described later in the section on specific steps.

Examination Under Anesthesia and Arthroscopy

Examination under anesthesia is performed to evaluate the mobility and stability of the joint. This is followed by complete diagnostic arthroscopy from both anterior and posterior portals. The superior labrum is best visualized from the posterior portal and palpated with a probe from the anterior superior portal. When a SLAP lesion is present, the labrum may be frayed, torn, or completely detached or a combination of these. As categorized by Snyder and colleagues,[3] there are four basic types. A type I SLAP lesion has a frayed superior labrum, but the biceps anchor attachment to the superior glenoid is intact. Type II lesions have a separation of the superior labrum and biceps anchor from the superior glenoid with or without fraying of the superior labrum. Type III lesions appear similar to a bucket-handle tear of the meniscus; the superior labrum is torn, but it may or may not be displaced with an otherwise normal biceps anchor. Type IV is similar to type III with a bucket-handle labral tear, but the tear extends into the biceps tendon.

Specific Steps

Type I and type III SLAP lesions in which the biceps anchor is otherwise stable are treated by debridement alone. We use a 4.2-mm shaver and debride the labrum to a smooth edge. The shaver is used from both anterior and posterior portals. After shaving, a probe is used to evaluate the remaining labrum and the biceps anchor. Occasionally a radiofrequency device is helpful to stabilize the edges, used on the "cold" setting with high flow to minimize thermal damage.

Type II lesions are repaired by a single-anchor double-suture technique as outlined in Box 26-1.

Type IV lesions are treated similarly to type II lesions unless the biceps tendon split is severe. When more than 50% of the tendon is included with the displaced labral tear, one must consider performing a biceps tenodesis. A repair is considered for these lesions only in patients younger than 25 years, and they are counseled postoperatively regarding the possible need for biceps tenodesis in the future. In cases of mild biceps involvement, we prefer to excise the labral fragment along with the attached portion of torn biceps. If the remaining tendon appears healthy and the anchor is stable, then it is left alone. If the remaining tendon appears degenerative or damaged, it will be released and tenodesed.

Single-Anchor, Double-Suture Type II SLAP Repair

1. Establish Portals

Three portals are used for a standard single-anchor type II SLAP repair: posterior, anterosuperior and anterior midglenoid. (Percutaneous portals for the Wilmington portal area can be used for additional suture anchor placement for lesions extending far posteriorly.) With the arthroscope in the standard posterior portal, we establish the anterior superior portal with an outside-in technique. A spinal needle determines the ideal location. Insert the needle approximately 1 cm anterior to the anterolateral corner of the acromion such that it enters the joint in the superior edge of the rotator interval over the biceps tendon. Ensure that the needle can readily reach the 12-o'clock position on the glenoid passing posterior to the biceps (Fig. 26-3). After making an incision with a No. 11 blade in Langer's lines, insert a clear, smooth, plastic 6-mm operating cannula along the chosen path.

Next, establish an anterior midglenoid portal with the same outside-in technique as outlined before, entering through the rotator interval just above the subscapularis tendon, and place a cannula.

2. Prepare the Labrum and Glenoid

Debride any remaining soft tissue off the superior glenoid below the detached labrum-biceps anchor. Trim all fraying of the labrum until all fragments have been removed. The posterior portion of the lesion and glenoid

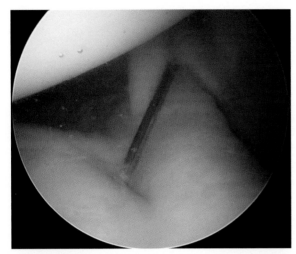

Figure 26-3. Viewed from the posterior portal, a spinal needle locates the ideal position for anterosuperior portal creation.

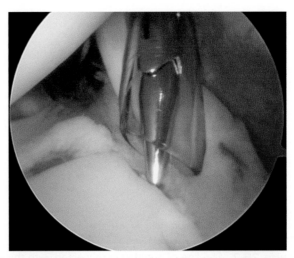

Figure 26-5. The suture anchor drill with inserter guide is ideally placed through the anterosuperior portal, posterior to the biceps tendon, at the anatomic origin of the biceps.

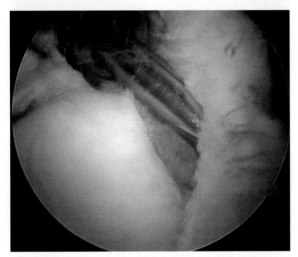

Figure 26-4. A 4.2-mm shaver is used to completely debride all damaged labrum and prepare a bleeding bony bed for repair.

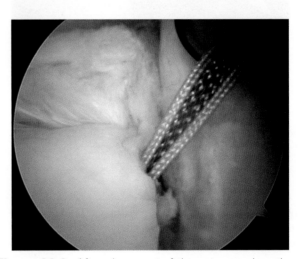

Figure 26-6. After placement of the suture anchor, the two suture limbs are identified as anterior and posterior.

are best trimmed with the shaver in the posterior portal and the arthroscope anteriorly. The superior glenoid rim and neck are only slightly decorticated down to a bleeding surface, with care taken not to remove excessive bone (Fig. 26-4). The bone here is often relatively soft, and use of a bur is seldom necessary.

3. Anchor Placement

Through the ASP, insert a small, double-loaded anchor into the 12-o'clock position in the glenoid, posterior to the biceps tendon. Coming behind the biceps tendon helps to stabilize the inserter and avoid skiving (Fig. 26-5). Anchor insertion is performed in the center of the biceps origin on the glenoid tubercle (Fig. 26-6). If possible, align the anchor eyelet such that an anterior and a posterior suture are present.

4. Suture Identification, Separation, and Passage

With a crochet hook, identify all four suture limbs, which suture is more posterior and which is more anterior, and then which of each suture's limbs is on the labral side of the eyelet and which is on the glenoid side of the eyelet. Retrieve the two limbs on the glenoid side of the anchor islet (one limb from each suture), taking them into the AMGP. Store them outside the cannula with a switching stick. Next, retrieve the two remaining labral-side limbs into the AMGP, where they are saved for shuttling through the labrum.

Using a medium-sized Spectrum crescent suture hook (Linvatec, Largo, FL) loaded with a No. 1 polydioxanone (PDS) suture (monofilament suture), enter the joint through the ASP. Rehearse the motion posterior to the

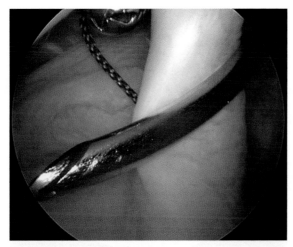

Figure 26-7. The line of suturing is rehearsed with the stitcher before labral penetration.

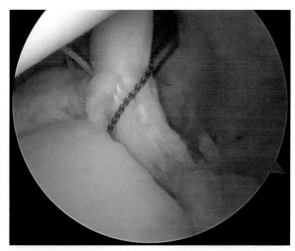

Figure 26-9. After the passage of the two suture limbs, anterior and posterior sutures are ready for tying.

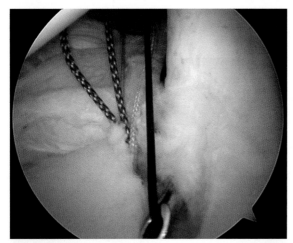

Figure 26-8. The stitcher is passed one time, directly through the center of the biceps origin, and a shuttle is passed out the anterior midglenoid.

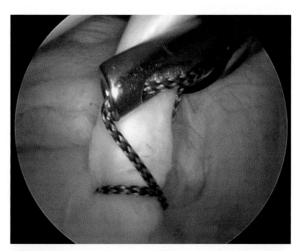

Figure 26-10. Tying takes place through the anterosuperior portal—posterior suture then anterior suture. Posts and knots are placed away from the glenoid surface.

biceps to gain muscle memory (Fig. 26-7). (Unsuccessful pass attempts cause iatrogenic damage to the labrum.) Puncture the superior labrum and biceps tendon with the suture hook placed directly on the superior side of the middle of the biceps anchor. Aim the needle to exit just below the avulsed labrum, adjacent to the prepared bone of the biceps footprint. (Avoid penetrating the biceps too far from the base, as this will lead to shortening of the tendon when the sutures are tied.) Grasp the PDS through the AMGP (Fig. 26-8). At once, load and shuttle *both* labrum limbs back through the superior labrum and out the ASP.

5. Tie Sutures—Posterior and Anterior

Using a crochet hook from behind the biceps, pull the two limbs of the posterior suture into the ASP (Fig. 26-9). From the ASP, the posterior suture and then the anterior suture can be tied sequentially (Fig. 26-10), one

on each side of the biceps, keeping the knots away from the glenoid. The final construct should be a balanced repair of the entire biceps anchor, stable to probing but not so tight as to strangulate the tissue (Fig. 26-11). In cases of posterior or anterior extension, additional anchors are placed as needed. Portals are closed in standard fashion with buried 4-0 monofilament absorbable suture and Steri-Strips.

POSTOPERATIVE CONSIDERATIONS

Rehabilitation

The shoulder is protected in a 15-degree UltraSling (DJO Global, Inc., Vista, CA). The patient should begin elbow, wrist, and hand exercises immediately, with gentle pendulum exercises after 1 week. The shoulder

TABLE 26-1. Published Literature Regarding the Outcomes of Superior Labral Anterior-Posterior Repair with Suture Anchors

Study	Follow-up	Outcome	Return to Prior Athletic Level	Level of Evidence
Morgan et al[11] (1998)	Mean 12 months	84% excellent	84%	IV
O'Brien et al[12] (2002)	Mean 3.7 years (2-7.4 years)	71% good-excellent (patient satisfaction)	52%	IV
Kim et al[13] (2002)	Mean 33 months	94% satisfactory (UCLA)	22%	IV
Rhee et al[14] (2005)	Mean 33 months	86% good-excellent (UCLA)	76%	IV
Cohen et al[4] (2006)	Mean 44 months	69% good-excellent (patient satisfaction)	48%	IV
Ide et al[15] (2005)	Mean 41 months	90% good-excellent (Rowe)	75%	IV
Enad et al[16] (2007)	Mean 31 months	80% good-excellent (UCLA)	77%	IV
Yung et al[17] (2008)	28 months	87% good-excellent (UCLA)	92%	IV
Boileau et al[18] (2009)	Mean 35 months	40% satisfied	20%	III
Brockmeier et al[6] (2009)	Mean 32 months	87% good-excellent (patient satisfaction)	71%	IV
Alpert et al[9] (2010)	2 years minimum	88% satisfied		III
Friel et al[19] (2010)	Mean 3.4 years	80% good-excellent (UCLA)	62%	IV

UCLA, University of California at Los Angeles shoulder rating scale.

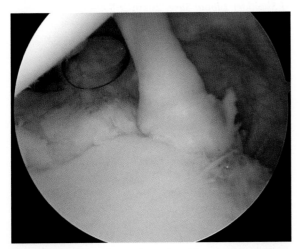

Figure 26-11. A balanced repair with one suture tied on either side of the tendon, without excessive tension.

should be protected from excess stress on the biceps tendon for 12 weeks. Progressive resistance exercises are allowed at 6 weeks. For pitchers, if there are no limitations on motion and the patient is asymptomatic, interval throwing is allowed after 4 months, throwing from the mound at 6 months, and full velocity throwing at 7 months.

Complications

- Missed coexisting shoulder disease.
- Failure to insert anchor properly. Anchors left too proud can cause serious damage to the humeral

chondral surface. Anchors that are too loose will pull out, and the procedure will be difficult to revise.
- Failure to recognize anatomic variants (e.g., Buford complex, sublabral hole).
- Stiffness with loss of external rotation.

RESULTS

In patients who have been selected for repair carefully, results are reliably good; 80% or more good to excellent results are reported in most published literature. Overhead throwing athletes tend to have fewer excellent results in most literature. There is still significant debate over SLAP repair versus biceps tenodesis and the ideal age for SLAP repair. The published results using modern suture anchor technique are referenced in Table 26-1.

REFERENCES

1. Andrews JR, Carson WG Jr, McLeod WD. Glenoid labrum tears related to the long head of the biceps. *Am J Sports Med.* 1985;13:337-341.
2. Snyder SJ, Banas MP, Karzel RP. An analysis of 140 injuries to the superior glenoid labrum. *J Shoulder Elbow Surg.* 1995;4:243-248.
3. Snyder SJ, Karzel RP, Del Pizzo W, et al. SLAP lesions of the shoulder. *Arthroscopy.* 1990;6:274-279.
4. Cohen DB, Coleman S, Drakos MC, et al. Outcomes of isolated type II SLAP lesions treated with arthroscopic fixation using a bioabsorbable tack. *Arthroscopy.* 2006; 22:136-142.

5. Glousman R, Jobe F, Tibone J, et al. Dynamic electromyographic analysis of the throwing shoulder with glenohumeral instability. *J Bone Joint Surg Am.* 1988;70:220-226.

6. Brockmeier SF, Voos JE, Williams RJ III, et al. Outcomes after arthroscopic repair of type-II SLAP lesions. *J Bone Joint Surg Am.* 2009;91:1595-1603.

7. Franceschi F, Longo UG, Ruzzini L, et al. No advantages in repairing a type II superior labrum anterior and posterior (SLAP) lesion when associated with rotator cuff repair in patients over age 50: a randomized controlled trial. *Am J Sports Med.* 2008;36:247-253.

8. Gorantla K, Gill C, Wright RW. The outcome of type II SLAP repair: a systematic review. *Arthroscopy.* 2010;26:537-545.

9. Alpert JM, Wuerz TH, O'Donnell TF, et al. The effect of age on the outcomes of arthroscopic repair of type II superior labral anterior and posterior lesions. *Am J Sports Med.* 2010;Aug 25.

10. Burns JP, Bahk M, Snyder SJ. Superior labral tears: repair versus biceps tenodesis. *J Shoulder Elbow Surg.* 2011;20 (2 Suppl):S2-S8.

11. Morgan CD, Burkhart SS, Palmeri M, et al. Type II SLAP lesions: three subtypes and their relationships to superior instability and rotator cuff tears. *Arthroscopy.* 1998;14:553-565.

12. O'Brien SJ, Allen AA, Coleman SH, et al. The transrotator cuff approach to SLAP lesions: technical aspects for repair and a clinical follow-up of 31 patients at a minimum of 2 years. *Arthroscopy.* 2002;18:372-377.

13. Kim SH, Ha KI, Kim SH, et al. Results of arthroscopic treatment of superior labral lesions. *J Bone Joint Surg Am.* 2002;84:981-985.

14. Rhee YG, Lee DH, Lim CT. Unstable isolated SLAP lesion: Clinical presentation and outcome of arthroscopic fixation. *Arthroscopy.* 2005;21:1099.

15. Ide J, Maeda S, Takagi K. Sports activity after arthroscopic superior labral repair using suture anchors in overhead throwing athletes. *Am J Sports Med.* 2005;33:507-514.

16. Enad JG, Kurtz CA. Isolated and combined Type II SLAP repairs in a military population. *Knee Surg Sports Traumatol Arthrosc.* 2007;15:1382-1389.

17. Yung PS, Fong DT, Kong MF, et al. Arthroscopic repair of isolated type II superior labrum anterior-posterior lesion. *Knee Surg Sports Traumatol Arthrosc.* 2008;16:1151-1157.

18. Boileau P, Parratte S, Chuinard C, et al. Arthroscopic treatment of isolated type II SLAP lesions: Biceps tenodesis as an alternative to reinsertion. *Am J Sports Med.* 2009;37:929-936.

19. Friel NA, Karas V, Slabaugh MA, et al. Outcomes of type II superior labrum, anterior to posterior (SLAP) repair: prospective evaluation at a minimum two-year follow-up. *J Shoulder Elbow Surg.* 2010;19:859-867.

Chapter 27

Arthroscopic and Open Decompression of the Suprascapular Nerve

Umasuthan Srikumaran, Lewis L. Shi, Jeffrey D. Tompson, Laurence D. Higgins, and Jon J.P. Warner

Chapter Synopsis
- Suprascapular nerve compression at the suprascapular notch can cause significant shoulder pathology. This condition can be surgically managed with arthroscopic or open release of the suprascapular transverse ligament.

Important Points
- Superior and posterolateral shoulder pain is common.
- Space-occupying lesions or dynamic conditions can cause suprascapular neuropathy.
- Carefully rule out other, more common causes of shoulder pathology.
- Electromyography can support diagnosis, but if negative, fluoroscopically guided anesthetic and cortisone injection can be used to confirm diagnosis.

Clinical and Surgical Pearls
- Achieve good visualization in the subacromial space before exposing the suprascapular notch.

- Use the anterior border of the supraspinatus and the coracoclavicular ligaments as landmarks to guide dissection.
- Protect the suprascapular nerve during resection of the transverse suprascapular ligament.

Clinical and Surgical Pitfalls
- Inadequate visualization:
    - Perform a thorough subacromial bursectomy.
    - Use arthroscopic instrumentation to retract during dissection and suprascapular nerve release.
- Difficulty identifying transverse suprascapular ligament:
    - Mark out surface anatomy; use landmarks (anterior border of supraspinatus, coracoclavicular ligaments, coracoid base) starting laterally and follow medially. Localize with spinal needles as needed.

Suprascapular neuropathy is thought to result from compression or tethering of the nerve as it courses under the suprascapular notch (Fig. 27-1). Compression of the suprascapular nerve (SSN) can result from a variety of causes that narrow the notch: supraglenoid cysts, fracture of the scapular notch with resultant callus formation,[1] an enlarged or thickened transverse scapular ligament, hardware from prior surgical interventions, or any space-occupying lesion in the region of the notch.[1-4] Tethering of the nerve results from more dynamic mechanisms: retraction as the result of massive rotator cuff tears, repetitive traction injuries in overhead athletes such as volleyball players and pitchers, and traumatic stretch injuries associated with glenohumeral dislocations or proximal humerus fractures.[5-10] Injuries to the nerve can result in inflammation and swelling of the nerve, causing further compression at the suprascapular notch.

PREOPERATIVE CONSIDERATIONS

The diagnosis of suprascapular neuropathy can be challenging, as the presenting symptoms are generally nonspecific. Patients most often describe a deep or dull aching pain in the posterolateral aspect of the dominant

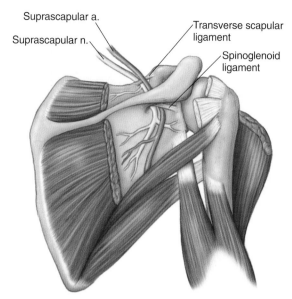

Suprascapular a.

Suprascapular n.

Transverse scapular ligament

Spinoglenoid ligament

Figure 27-1. Anatomic course of suprascapular nerve under the transverse scapular ligament and spinoglenoid notch. *a*, artery; *n*, nerve.

shoulder or directly above the supraspinatus fossa.[11] Patients may also report weakness, particularly in abduction and external rotation. Symptoms may start immediately after a traumatic injury or may develop slowly over time.[11,12] Chronic conditions may be more common in individuals with substantial overhead demands, whether athletic or work related.

Owing to the nonspecific nature of the patient's complaints, it is important to perform a complete examination of the neck and shoulder to determine if other conditions (rotator cuff pathology, stiffness, arthritis, acromioclavicular disease, cervical radiculopathy, fractures) are responsible for the patient's symptoms or are associated with SSN pathology. Accordingly, the surgeon should thoroughly assess (and compare with the uninvolved side) the appearance of the shoulder, range of motion (actively and passively), strength, and distal neurologic function, in addition to performing typical provocative maneuvers.

On physical examination it is important to completely visualize the shoulders from posteriorly to detect associated atrophy of the supraspinatus and infraspinatus fossa. Isolated infraspinatus fossa atrophy suggests that the nerve injury is at the level of the spinoglenoid notch. Weakness in abduction and external rotation may also be evident. Maneuvers attempting to place the SSN under tension may reproduce the patient's symptoms. Lafosse and colleagues suggest a stretch test that laterally rotates the head away from the involved shoulder while also retracting the shoulder posteriorly.[13] Cross-body adduction and internal rotation may also reproduce pain by tensioning the spinoglenoid ligament and further tethering the shoulder nerve.[14]

Imaging is used primarily to assess for the commonly associated conditions mentioned previously, but also to evaluate for space-occupying lesions near the suprascapular or spinoglenoid notch. The degree of atrophy of the supraspinatus and infraspinatus muscles can also be determined with computed tomography (CT) or magnetic resonance imaging (MRI). Additional diagnostic studies include electromyography and nerve conduction velocity tests.[9,15] The reliability of these tests is unclear. If the surgeon has a high degree of suspicion for SSN pathology, a fluoroscopically guided injection of anesthetic and cortisone into the suprascapular notch can be performed.

Indications

- Patients with a space-occupying lesion at the suprascapular notch with pain and weakness
- Patients with electromyographic evidence of suprascapular neuropathy
- Patients with a negative electromyogram (EMG) who experience substantial relief of their symptoms with fluoroscopically guided injection of anesthetic and cortisone
- Patients with massive rotator cuff tears with either a positive EMG or relief of their symptoms with fluoroscopically guided injection of anesthetic and cortisone

Contraindications

- Patients with cervical radiculopathy (address underlying spine pathology first)
- Patients with brachial plexitis (follow conservatively until resolution of general inflammation)
- Patients who do not experience any relief of symptoms after fluoroscopically guided injection of anesthetic and cortisone, in the absence of a space-occupying lesion

SURGICAL TECHNIQUE

SSN release can be approached arthroscopically or by open technique. We prefer an arthroscopic approach in most cases, as it is minimally invasive, provides excellent visualization, allows for assessment of the subacromial space and glenohumeral joint, and limits associated surgical morbidity. An open approach may be required in settings where visualization is poor arthroscopically owing to scarring or in situations where partial hardware removal is required (e.g., tip of a previously placed glenoid screw).

In either approach, the surgery can be performed with the patient under regional or general anesthesia with or without an interscalene nerve block. The patient is placed in the beach chair position with the involved extremity in an adjustable arm holder.

Open Suprascapular Nerve Release

Specific steps of this procedure are outlined in Box 27-1.

When an open approach is used, a trapezius-splitting exposure allows for access to the suprascapular notch.[16] Bony surface landmarks include the scapular spine, lateral acromion, clavicle, and coracoid. The SSN runs 4.5 cm medial to the posterior edge of the acromion. A longitudinal incision is made beginning anteriorly over the trapezius and continuing posteriorly over the spine of the scapula (Fig. 27-2). The trapezius is then elevated off the spine of the scapula and off the medial acromion and split longitudinally, with the incision curved somewhat anteriorly relative to the acromioclavicular joint.

The supraspinatus muscle belly is identified and carefully retracted posteriorly (Fig. 27-3). The coracoid base can be found by locating the coracoclavicular ligaments and following them inferiorly and medially. The transverse scapular ligament runs perpendicularly to the coracoclavicular ligaments and over the suprascapular notch. Immediately above the ligament are the suprascapular vessels, and below is the SSN. Gentle retraction of these structures will allow resection of the ligament, sharply or with a Kerrison rongeur (Fig. 27-4). On rare occasions the ligament may be ossified and require removal with the use of small osteotomes. Ligament release may not completely free the nerve, necessitating additional bony resection around the notch. As part of the closure, the trapezius is reattached to the scapular spine with sutures through bur holes.

BOX 27-1 Surgical Steps: Open Suprascapular Nerve Release

1. Trapezius-splitting exposure to allow for access to the suprascapular notch.
2. Identify bony surface landmarks: scapular spine, lateral acromion, clavicle, coracoid.
3. Locate the suprascapular nerve 4.5 cm medial to the posterior edge of the acromion.
4. Make a longitudinal incision beginning anteriorly over the trapezius and continuing posteriorly over the spine of the scapula.
5. Elevate the trapezius off of the spine of the scapula and off the medial acromion and split longitudinally, curving the incision somewhat anteriorly relative to the acromioclavicular joint.
6. Identify the supraspinatus muscle belly and carefully retract posteriorly. Locate the coracoid base and transverse scapular ligament.
7. Resect the ligament, sharply or with a Kerrison rongeur. On rare occasions the ligament may be ossified and require removal with the use of small osteotomes. Ligament release may not completely free the nerve, necessitating additional bony resection around the notch.
8. Reattach the trapezius to the scapular spine with sutures through bur holes.

Arthroscopic Suprascapular Nerve Release

Specific steps of this procedure are outlined in Box 27-2.

Standard portal placement is used as for routine shoulder arthroscopy. Additional portals for SSN release include an anterolateral portal for visualization and superior portals for instrumentation (Fig. 27-5). Diagnostic arthroscopy and completion of other surgical procedures, such as rotator cuff repair, are performed before SSN release.

The arthroscopic posterior approach for SSN release has been described by Bhatia and colleagues[17] and Lafosse colleagues.[18,19] The first step is to prepare the subacromial space by removing the subacromial bursa. Visualization can then occur from laterally or anterolaterally. Identification of the anterior border of the supraspinatus can help guide medial dissection. The coracoclavicular ligaments serve as an anterior landmark and further guide dissection medially and inferiorly along the coracoid base.

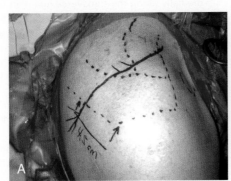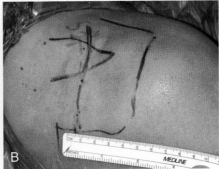

Figure 27-2. Saber saw incision over the suprascapular nerve during an open release. Suprascapular nerve is 4.5 cm medial to the posterolateral edge of the acromion.

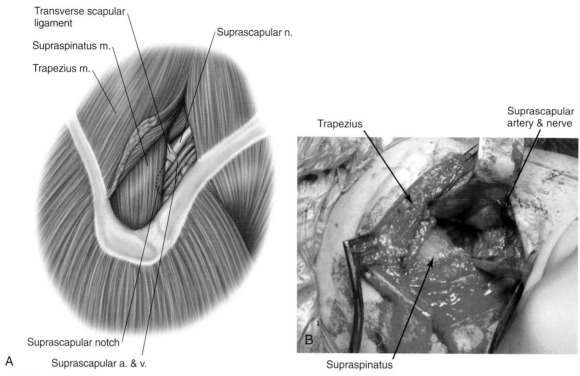

Transverse scapular ligament

Suprascapular n.

Supraspinatus m.

Trapezius m.

Trapezius

Suprascapular artery & nerve

Suprascapular notch

A

Suprascapular a. & v.

Supraspinatus

B

Figure 27-3. After the trapezius is split, the supraspinatus muscle is exposed. This is then retracted posteriorly. *a,* artery; *m,* muscle; *n,* nerve.

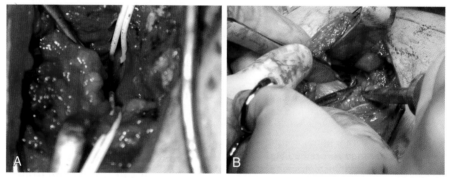

A

B

Figure 27-4. A, Suprascapular nerve is tagged with a vessel loop and protected. **B,** The transverse scapular ligament is then resected.

BOX 27-2 Surgical Steps: Arthroscopic Suprascapular Nerve Release

1. Use standard portal placement as for routine shoulder arthroscopy. Additional portals include an anterolateral portal for visualization and superior portals for instrumentation.

2. Perform diagnostic arthroscopy and complete other surgical procedures, such as rotator cuff repair, before suprascapular nerve release.

3. Prepare the subacromial space by removing the subacromial bursa.

4. Identify the anterior border of the supraspinatus. The coracoclavicular ligaments serve as an anterior landmark and further guide dissection medially and inferiorly along the coracoid base.

5. Create an accessory superior portal with the assistance of a spinal needle.

6. Use a blunt trocar through this portal to retract tissue medially along the transverse ligament to identify the suprascapular vessels and the suprascapular nerve.

7. A second superior portal can be made next to the first superior portal to allow for additional instrumentation to release the nerve. Visualize the transverse ligament, and introduce arthroscopic scissors through the second superior portal.

8. The blunt trocar can be positioned inferior to the ligament to protect the nerve while it is released with the arthroscopic scissors or biter.

9. Probe the nerve to ensure that the decompression is adequate and that scar tissue is removed.

An accessory superior portal can then be made with the assistance of a spinal needle. This portal is generally 1 to 2 cm medial to the acromioclavicular joint on the skin. The spinal needle should be directed anterior to the supraspinatus muscle toward the coracoid base,

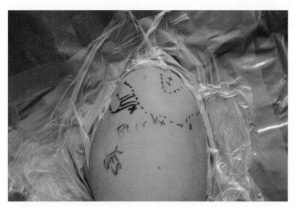

Figure 27-5. Arthroscopic portals for a left shoulder suprascapular nerve release. Lateral is the viewing portal, and working portals are superior medial—one for retraction and another for arthroscopic scissors.

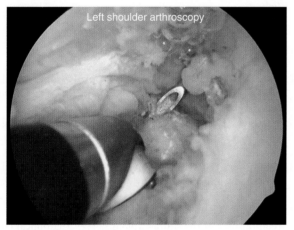

Figure 27-6. Viewed from the lateral portal, a spinal needle is placed from the superior medial portal toward the base of the coracoid. The transverse scapular ligament is further medial than this.

adjacent to the transverse suprascapular ligament (Fig. 27-6). A blunt trocar can then be used through this portal to retract tissue medially along the transverse ligament to identify the suprascapular vessels and the SSN (Fig. 27-7).

A second superior portal can be made next to the first superior portal to allow for additional instrumentation to release the nerve (Fig. 27-8). With the blunt trocar providing gentle retraction, the transverse ligament is adequately visualized, and arthroscopic scissors can be introduced through the second superior portal.

The blunt trocar can be positioned inferior to the ligament to protect the nerve while it is released with the arthroscopic scissors or biter. We use a small biter with a blunt tip so that it may retract the nerve away while the ligament is being cut. On occasion the suprascapular transverse ligament may be partially or completely ossified. In these cases, small osteotomes can be introduced arthroscopically to release the nerve. Alternatively, a Kerrison rongeur may be used to remove bone above the nerve. Use of a motorized bur in this region is not recommended. After the release, the nerve is probed to ensure that the decompression is adequate and that scar tissue is removed (Fig. 27-9).

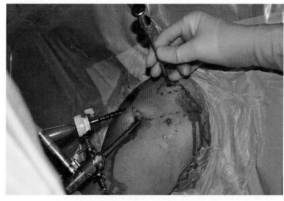

Figure 27-7. A blunt trocar is then placed in this portal to retract the suprascapular artery medially.

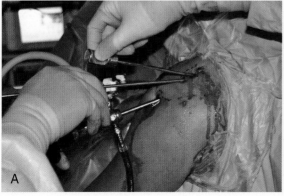
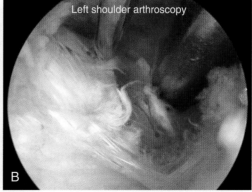

Figure 27-8. The second superior medial portal is made to insert cutting instrument.

TABLE 27-1. Clinical Results After Suprascapular Nerve Release

Study	No. of Patients	Average Follow-up (mo)	Clinical Outcome
Shah et al[20] (2011), level IV case series	24 (no rotator cuff disease)	22.5	17/24 (71%) would have surgery again
			18/24 (75%) had improved ASES scores (from 36.6 to 70.6)
			17/24 (71%) had improved SSV scores (from 37.7 to 64.8)
Lafosse et al[19] (2007), level IV case series	10	15	9/10 (90%) rated result as excellent
			Of 8 postoperative electromyograms, 7 demonstrated complete normalization of motor fiber latency and motor action potentials
			Constant scores improved from 60.3 to 83.4
			Abduction and external rotation strength improved
Kim et al[21] (2005), level IV case series	39	18	28/31 (90%) improved to grade 4 supraspinatus strength; 3/31 (10%) to grade 3
			Of 31 patients with preoperative pain, 100% had improvement postoperatively

ASES, American Shoulder and Elbow Surgeons scale; *SSV,* subjective shoulder value.

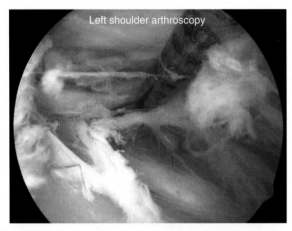
Left shoulder arthroscopy

Figure 27-9. A probe freeing up the suprascapular nerve after the ligament has been released.

POSTOPERATIVE CONSIDERATIONS

Postoperative rehabilitation is generally limited by other procedures that were concurrently performed, such as rotator cuff repair. If SSN release is preformed in isolation, a postoperative sling is used only for comfort for the first 24 to 48 hours. Passive and active range of motion can begin in the first week. Strengthening can commence when full active and passive range of motion is achieved.

RESULTS

Clinical results after release of the SSN are likely to vary based on the cause of neuropathy and whether rotator cuff pathology was present. The scientific literature is presently limited to several case series and is summarized in Table 27-1. In general, patients can expect pain

relief as well as improved function and strength. The procedure carries minimal risk, as no surgical complications are reported in the few series that have been published.

REFERENCES

1. Solheim LF, Roaas A. Compression of the suprascapular nerve after fracture of the scapular notch. *Acta Orthop Scand.* 1978;49:338-340.
2. Maquieira GJ, Gerber C, Schneeberger AG. Suprascapular nerve palsy after the Latarjet procedure. *J Shoulder Elbow Surg.* 2007;16:e13-15.
3. Moore TP, Fritts HM, Quick DC, et al. Suprascapular nerve entrapment caused by supraglenoid cyst compression. *J Shoulder Elbow Surg.* 1997;6:455-462.
4. Warner JP, Krushell RJ, Masquelet A, et al. Anatomy and relationships of the suprascapular nerve: Anatomical constraints to mobilization of the supraspinatus and infraspinatus muscles in the management of massive rotator-cuff tears. *J Bone Joint Surg Am.* 1992;74:36-45.
5. Albritton MJ, Graham RD, Richards RS, 2nd, et al. An anatomic study of the effects on the suprascapular nerve due to retraction of the supraspinatus muscle after a rotator cuff tear. *J Shoulder Elbow Surg.* 2003;12:497-500.
6. Asami A, Sonohata M, Morisawa K. Bilateral suprascapular nerve entrapment syndrome associated with rotator cuff tear. *J Shoulder Elbow Surg.* 2000;9:70-72.
7. de Laat EA, Visser CP, Coene LN, et al. Nerve lesions in primary shoulder dislocations and humeral neck fractures. A prospective clinical and EMG study. *J Bone Joint Surg Br.* 1994;76:381-383.
8. Ferretti A, Cerullo G, Russo G. Suprascapular neuropathy in volleyball players. *J Bone Joint Surg Am.* 1987;69:260-263.
9. Mallon WJ, Wilson RJ, Basamania CJ. The association of suprascapular neuropathy with massive rotator cuff tears:

A preliminary report. *J Shoulder Elbow Surg.* 2006;15: 395-398.

10. Ringel SP, Treihaft M, Carry M, et al. Suprascapular neuropathy in pitchers. *Am J Sports Med.* 1990;18:80-86.

11. Cummins CA, Messer TM, Nuber GW. Suprascapular nerve entrapment. *J Bone Joint Surg Am.* 2000;82: 415-424.

12. Martin SD, Warren RF, Martin TL, et al. Suprascapular neuropathy. Results of non-operative treatment. *J Bone Joint Surg Am.* 1997;79:1159-1165.

13. Lafosse L, Piper K, Lanz U. Arthroscopic suprascapular nerve release: Indications and technique. *J Shoulder Elbow Surg.* 2011;20:S9-13.

14. Plancher KD, Luke TA, Peterson RK, et al. Posterior shoulder pain: A dynamic study of the spinoglenoid ligament and treatment with arthroscopic release of the scapular tunnel. *Arthroscopy.* 2007;23:991-998.

15. Vad VB, Southern D, Warren RF, et al. Prevalence of peripheral neurologic injuries in rotator cuff tears with atrophy. *J Shoulder Elbow Surg.* 2003;12:333-336.

16. Post M. Diagnosis and treatment of suprascapular nerve entrapment. *Clin Orthop Relat Res.* 1999;92-100.

17. Bhatia DN, de Beer JF, van Rooyen KS, et al. Arthroscopic suprascapular nerve decompression at the suprascapular notch. *Arthroscopy.* 2006;22:1009-1013.

18. Lafosse L, Tomasi A. Technique for endoscopic release of suprascapular nerve entrapment at the suprascapular notch. *Tech Shoulder Elbow Surg.* 2006;7:1-6.

19. Lafosse L, Tomasi A, Corbett S, et al. Arthroscopic release of suprascapular nerve entrapment at the suprascapular notch: Technique and preliminary results. *Arthroscopy.* 2007;23:34-42.

20. Shah AA, et al. Clinical outcomes of suprascapular nerve decompression. *J Shoulder Elbow Surg.* 2011;20: 975-982.

21. Kim DH, et al. Management and outcomes of 42 surgical suprascapular nerve injuries and entrapments. *Neurosurgery.* 2005;57:120-127.

SUGGESTED READINGS

Boykin RE, Friedman DJ, Higgins LD, et al. Suprascapular neuropathy. *J Bone Joint Surg Am.* 2010;92:2348-2364.

Piasecki DP, Romeo AA, Bach BR, Jr, et al. Suprascapular neuropathy. *J Am Acad Orthop Surg.* 2009;17:665-676.

Chapter 28

Arthroscopic Subacromial Decompression and Distal Clavicle Excision

Eric J. Strauss and Michael G. Hannon

Chapter Synopsis

- Arthroscopic subacromial decompression is one of the most commonly performed procedures about the shoulder. Distal clavicle excision may be performed as part of the same procedure via the indirect approach. The history and physical examination in addition to targeted diagnostic imaging are essential to confirm the diagnosis of shoulder impingement and/or acromioclavicular joint degeneration. Good to excellent clinical results can be expected in approximately 80% of patients.

Important Points

- All patients should undergo a minimum of 3 to 6 months of nonoperative treatment for shoulder impingement syndrome and acromioclavicular joint pain, including activity modification, physiotherapy, nonsteroidal anti-inflammatory drugs (NSAIDs), and corticosteroid injections.
- Absolute contraindications to subacromial decompression include the presence of rotator cuff arthropathy or a massive irreparable rotator cuff tear.
- Absolute contraindications to a distal clavicle excision include preexisting acromioclavicular joint instability.

Clinical and Surgical Pearls

- Subacromial decompression may be performed via the classic or cutting block technique.
- The acromioplasty should be visualized in two planes to ensure a smooth, even resection.
- Distal clavicle excision may be performed via the direct or indirect approach based on the pathology being treated.
- Adequate bony resection is needed, with care taken to ensure that no superior bone is left in situ while preserving the superior joint capsule to avoid destabilizing the acromioclavicular joint.

Clinical and Surgical Pitfalls

- Pitfalls in subacromial decompression include inadequate resection, over-resection leading to fracture, and poor portal placement leading to technical difficulties.
- Pitfalls in distal clavicle excision include over-resection leading to acromioclavicular joint instability, retained superior bone, and inadequate resection leading to residual symptoms.

The concept of shoulder impingement was first described by Meyer in 1937. Later, Neer expanded on Meyer's work, describing the successive stages of impingement (Box 28-1). Shoulder impingement syndrome is characterized by anterior shoulder pain worsened with overhead activity. Shoulder impingement syndrome is thought to be caused by an anatomic narrowing of the subacromial space by the structures forming the coracoacromial arch leading to progressive bursitis, tendinitis, and rotator cuff tearing. Arthroscopic subacromial decompression has become one of the most common surgical procedures involving the shoulder, both as primary treatment for shoulder impingement syndrome and as a routine practice in arthroscopic rotator cuff repair to create an adequate working space and protect the repair construct.

Acromioclavicular (AC) joint degeneration and pain may exist alone or in combination with shoulder impingement. Arthroscopic subacromial decompression and distal clavicle excision are naturally paired procedures, as the two can be performed simultaneously via the indirect distal clavicle excision technique. In the less common situation in which AC joint arthritis exists in isolation, the direct distal clavicle excision technique may be used.

PREOPERATIVE CONSIDERATIONS

History

The patient's history coupled with a thorough physical examination will establish the diagnosis of subacromial impingement or AC joint degeneration. The importance of this evaluation cannot be overstated, as failure of both subacromial decompression and distal clavicle excision often relates to initial diagnostic errors and missed associated pathology.

As part of the patient's initial history, his or her hand dominance and occupation should be noted. A thorough review of the patient's pain symptoms, including duration, palliative and provoking activities, pain radiation, severity, and the character of the pain must be elicited. Any previous treatments for shoulder pain including courses of physiotherapy, corticosteroid injections, or pain medications are important aspects of the history. Operative reports should be obtained for any previous surgical procedures involving the shoulder.

Classically, patients with symptoms related to impingement have anterolateral shoulder pain, exacerbated by overhead activities. They may report difficulty with activities of daily living that require overhead motion, such as combing hair or reaching into cabinets. These patients often have night pain, especially when they lie on the affected side. One should be aware that young, overhead throwing athletes may develop secondary outlet impingement after chronic internal impingement owing to anterior capsular laxity and posterior capsular contracture.

A small subset of patients with AC joint pathology may be the prototypical heavy laborer or weightlifter with localized pain and tenderness to palpation over the AC joint. Unfortunately, most patients with AC joint pathology have much vaguer, more poorly localized symptoms.

Physical Examination

On physical examination of the shoulder, patients with impingement syndrome are said to have positive Neer and Hawkins signs. They may have tenderness to palpation at the greater tuberosity and demonstrate a painful arc syndrome, defined as pain between 60 and 120 degrees of forward elevation in the scapular plane. The infraspinatus test is performed with the patient's elbows flexed to 90 degrees and the arms adducted to the side. A positive test result is defined as pain and/or weakness when the patient attempts to resist an internal rotation force applied by the examiner. A Neer test may be performed, whereby a diagnostic subacromial injection of 10 mL of lidocaine is provided to assess for relief of symptoms with provocative testing. Park and colleagues reported that the combination of three positive test results—specifically the Hawkins sign, the painful arc sign, and the infraspinatus test result—had a 95% posttest probability for *any* degree of impingement.[1]

Multiple physical examination maneuvers to identify AC joint pathology have been described, including direct tenderness to palpation of the AC joint, the cross-arm adduction test, the O'Brien test, and the Paxinos test. An intra-articular diagnostic lidocaine injection remains the gold standard for diagnosis of AC joint pathology, although Partington and Broome demonstrated in a cadaveric study that nearly one third of attempted AC joint injections may be extra-articular.[2]

In addition to impingement and AC joint arthritis, the differential diagnosis of shoulder pain is broad and includes glenohumeral arthritis, adhesive capsulitis, multidirectional instability, symptomatic os acromiale, biceps tendon pathology, and cervical radiculopathy. One should also be aware that failure to recognize AC joint degeneration and pain concomitant with impingement may lead to a failed subacromial decompression.[3]

Imaging

After an initial impression is formed from the history and physical examination, imaging modalities may be used to confirm the diagnosis of impingement or AC joint arthritis or both and to rule out some of the more common causes of shoulder pain often mistaken for these two entities. Radiographs of the involved shoulder should include a true anteroposterior (AP) view of the shoulder (Fig. 28-1), a scapular-Y view (Fig. 28-2), an axillary view, and a Zanca view of the distal clavicle. Magnetic resonance imaging may assist in identifying

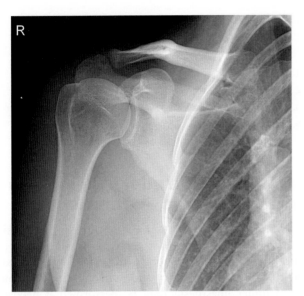

Figure 28-1. Preoperative anteroposterior radiograph of the right shoulder.

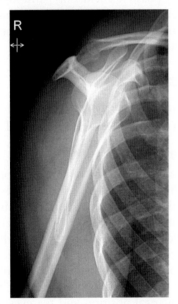

Figure 28-2. Preoperative scapular-Y radiograph of the right shoulder demonstrating a subacromial spur.

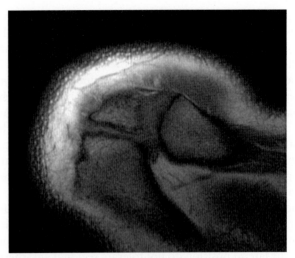

Figure 28-3. Magnetic resonance image shows widening at site of an unstable os acromiale.

rotator cuff or labral pathology, AC joint edema, or biceps tendon pathology, as well as an unstable os acromiale (Fig. 28-3).

Indications and Contraindications

All patients with impingement should undergo a minimum of 3 to 6 months of nonoperative treatment including nonsteroidal anti-inflammatory drugs (NSAIDs), a subacromial corticosteroid injection, physiotherapy, and modalities. A prospective series by Cummins and colleagues has demonstrated that nearly 80% of patients

with symptoms of impingement will have symptomatic resolution without the need for surgery at 2 years of follow-up.[4] Nonoperative treatment for AC joint pathology is similar. In addition, activity modification should be encouraged, including cessation of all aggravating activities. Physical therapy may be beneficial in those cases in which impingement and AC joint pain coexist, but it is typically not beneficial in isolated cases of AC joint pathology. For patients with persistent symptoms and functional limitation despite an adequate trial of nonoperative care, shoulder arthroscopy is indicated for management of the pathology.

Contraindications to arthroscopic subacromial decompression and distal clavicle excision are few. If a patient has rotator cuff arthropathy or a massive irreparable rotator cuff tear, the coracoacromial ligament should be preserved to prevent the development of anterosuperior escape; thus subacromial decompression is contraindicated. In cases of preexisting AC joint instability resulting from grade III or higher AC joint injury, distal clavicle excision is contraindicated without a concomitant stabilization procedure.

SURGICAL TECHNIQUE

Anesthesia and Positioning

Subacromial decompression and distal clavicle excision can be performed with the patient under regional anesthesia with an interscalene nerve block; with general anesthesia; or with a combined approach. Regional anesthesia can provide enhanced efficiency perioperatively (i.e., block room) as well as improved postoperative pain control, with small associated risks of complications such as intraneural injection, pneumothorax, and cardiac toxicity. Traditionally, hypotensive anesthesia with systolic blood pressure below 100 mm

Hg has been advocated to enhance visualization and ease of subacromial decompression. A case series by Pohl and Cullen reported several serious medical complications associated with hypotension, specifically in the upright beach chair position, including stroke and death.[5] The practice of deliberate hypotension in the beach chair position should be approached with caution.

It is possible to perform each procedure with the patient in either the beach chair or the lateral decubitus position. There are various advantages and disadvantages typically associated with each patient position. One may argue that the lateral decubitus position is more advantageous for a subacromial decompression, as traction on the upper extremity opens up the glenohumeral joint and subacromial space. However, patients in the lateral position do not tolerate regional anesthesia well; thus general anesthesia is required. It is the senior author's preference to use the beach chair position for both subacromial decompression and distal clavicle excision. This position provides a familiar anatomic orientation, provides for improved access to anterior portal sites, allows easy conversion to an open procedure if required, and lends itself to a regional anesthetic technique.[6]

Surgical Landmarks, Incisions, and Portals

Landmarks

- Acromion
- Scapular spine
- AC joint
- Clavicle
- Coracoid

Portals and Approaches

- Subacromial decompression and indirect acromioclavicular resection
  - Anterior working portal
  - Posterior scope portal
  - Lateral working portal
- Direct acromioclavicular resection
  - Anterior portal
  - Posterior portal

Structures at Risk

- Subacromial decompression and indirect acromioclavicular resection
  - Anterior portal: brachial plexus, axillary artery
  - Posterior portal: axillary nerve, posterior circumflex humeral artery
  - Lateral portal: axillary nerve
- Direct acromioclavicular resection
  - Anterior portal: brachial plexus, axillary artery

BOX 28-2 Surgical Steps: Subacromial Decompression

1. Set-up and equipment
2. Glenohumeral arthroscopy
3. Acromial exposure
4. Acromioplasty

Examination Under Anesthesia and Diagnostic Arthroscopy

A complete shoulder examination under anesthesia allows for assessment of symmetry in all planes of motion with the contralateral arm, as well as an assessment of ligamentous laxity and joint stability. Manipulation under anesthesia may be performed if needed. Diagnostic arthroscopy should proceed systematically as in all arthroscopic cases. Particular attention should be paid to any possible coexisting pathology found that had been previously undiagnosed, including subtle glenohumeral arthritic changes, biceps pathology, labral tears, and intra-articular loose bodies.

Specific Steps

Subacromial Decompression

Specific steps of this procedure are outlined in Box 28-2.

1. Set-up and Equipment

The patient is positioned on a standard operating table with a beach chair extension placed at the head. The back of the table is elevated to approximately 70 degrees, the table is placed in 15 degrees of Trendelenburg, and the table is flexed at the patient's knees, which are supported with pillows. Foot pumps are applied bilaterally to serve as intraoperative deep vein thrombosis (DVT) prophylaxis. Care is taken to ensure that the patient's neck is in a neutral position and the eyes and ears are appropriately protected while the head positioner is secured. The contralateral arm is placed in a well-padded arm holder affixed to the table. The surgeon's initials, which were marked in the holding area, are once again identified on the operative arm and circled as confirmation by the surgical assistant. The patient is then prepared and draped in the usual sterile fashion, with an arthroscopic extremity drape. The operative extremity is held with a pneumatic limb positioner (Fig. 28-4). The surgeon confirms that prophylactic antibiotics have been given before incision. At this point the formal time out is called.

2. Glenohumeral Arthroscopy

All bony landmarks are then identified with a sterile marking pen (Fig. 28-5). The portals are marked before

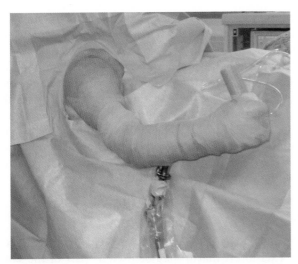

Figure 28-4. A patient is placed in the upright beach chair position with a pneumatic arm positioner.

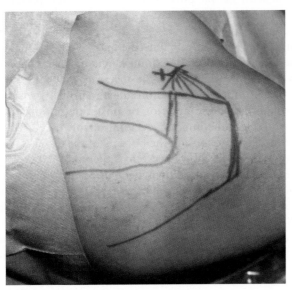

Figure 28-5. Overhead view of the patient's right shoulder demonstrating the marking of all relevant bony landmarks: acromion, scapular spine, acromioclavicular joint, clavicle, and coracoid.

the start of the procedures, as landmarks may become more difficult to appreciate as the shoulder becomes swollen intraoperatively. The posterior portal incision is marked out as a 1-cm vertical line at the soft spot approximately 2 cm posterior and 1 cm medial to the posterolateral corner of the acromion. The anterior portal is marked just lateral to the tip of the coracoid. The glenohumeral joint is insufflated with approximately 20 mL of normal saline. Starting with the posterior incision, a No. 11 blade is used to incise through skin only. The blunt trocar is used to insert the arthroscopic sheath through the posterior deltoid. The step-off between the posterior glenoid and the capsule can be palpated with the tip of the trocar. The trocar is

then advanced through the capsule and into the glenohumeral joint. The anterior portal is created through the rotator interval with spinal needle localization under direct visualization, and a 7-mm cannula is placed. Diagnostic arthroscopy commences in a systematic fashion. The arthroscopic pump pressure is generally set at 50 mm Hg and modified as needed to maintain adequate visualization. Any additional intra-articular pathology identified at this time may be addressed before subacromial decompression.

3. Acromial Exposure

After glenohumeral arthroscopy has been completed and any intra-articular pathology has been identified and treated, the joint is suctioned of all fluid and attention is turned to the subacromial space. The blunt trocar and arthroscopic sheath are redirected into the subacromial space. The trocar and sheath should be placed just deep to the posterolateral corner of the acromion, aiming toward the center of the acromion. The thumb of the nondominant hand may be placed on the posterolateral corner of the acromion as a mechanical block to prevent inadvertent passing of the trocar into the subcutaneous tissue above the acromion in an obese patient. The tip of the blunt trocar can be used to palpate the bony undersurface of the acromion to confirm positioning. Several sweeping motions medially and laterally can break up subacromial adhesions and create a potential space in which to work.

The lateral working portal is localized with the help of an 18-gauge spinal needle. This portal is made no more than 3 to 4 cm off of the lateral aspect of the acromion to protect the axillary nerve. The portal must be placed sufficiently anteriorly to allow access to the anterior acromion for acromioplasty. Once needle localization has verified that the instruments will be able to access the anteromedial acromion and the AC joint, a 1-cm vertical incision through skin is made. In general an arthroscopic cannula is not needed for this portal unless a rotator cuff repair is planned. A motorized shaving instrument with teeth is used to perform the initial bursectomy and improve the subacromial working space (Fig. 28-6). In general, the bursectomy should start anterolaterally and proceed medially and posteriorly. Care is taken during the bursectomy to avoid debridement of the deltoid muscles fibers or the intact rotator cuff.

Next the anterolateral corner of the undersurface of the acromion can be palpated and identified with the radiofrequency probe. Soft tissue is removed from the undersurface of the acromion with the radiofrequency probe, including the coracoacromial ligament, clearly outlining the borders of the acromion. When the coracoacromial ligament is fully released, the subdeltoid fascia can be identified. The acromial branch of the thoracoacromial artery may be encountered during coracoacromial ligament resection and should be cauterized.

4. Acromioplasty

A motorized oval bur or bone cutting shaver is inserted through the lateral working portal to begin the acromioplasty. The resection begins at the anterolateral corner of the acromion and proceeds medially (Fig. 28-7A). The level of resection may be set with an initial pass from anterior to posterior. The width of the bur itself can be used as a gauge of the resection level. Small strokes with intermittent bursts of suction lead to efficient acromioplasty while maintaining adequate visualization. One should verify that the acromion has been burred to a flat surface by confirming the resection with the camera in the posterior as well as the lateral portal (Fig. 28-7B). The reverse cutting feature may be used to "polish" the resection. After the resection has been completed, the

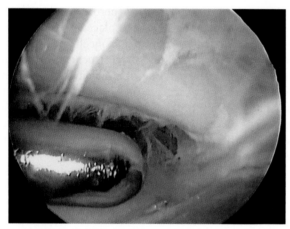

Figure 28-6. Subacromial view demonstrating the bursectomy.

arthroscopic shaver is reinserted and run in the subacromial space to clear the space of any free bony fragments and debris.

Some surgeons prefer to perform the acromioplasty via a cutting block technique as described by Sampson.[7] Again, the level of the resection is initially set with the bur from the lateral working portal. Then the arthroscope and bur are exchanged. Resection proceeds from posterior to anterior, with the posterior acromion used as a level or cutting block to ensure an evenly resected acromioplasty.

Distal Clavicle Excision via the Indirect Approach

The advantage of the indirect approach for distal clavicle excision is that it may be used as part of the same surgical procedure in patients who have concomitant impingement and AC joint pathology, with use of the same arthroscopic portals. The senior author prefers to perform distal clavicle excisions with the arthroscope in the lateral portal providing a head-on view of the AC joint. An 18-gauge spinal needle may be used to localize the orientation of the AC joint percutaneously. Alternatively, direct pressure on the distal clavicle can aid in its visualization. The radiofrequency probe is inserted through either the anterior or posterior portal and is used to clear the inferior AC joint of soft tissue attachments, clearly exposing the borders of the distal clavicle (Fig. 28-8). The motorized bur is then inserted through the anterior portal, allowing for direct working access to the AC joint. Resection of the AC joint begins anteriorly on the lateral aspect of the distal clavicle (Fig. 28-9). Approximately 5 to 10 mm of distal clavicle is excised, with care taken to ensure that no superior bone is left in situ while protecting the superior and posterior

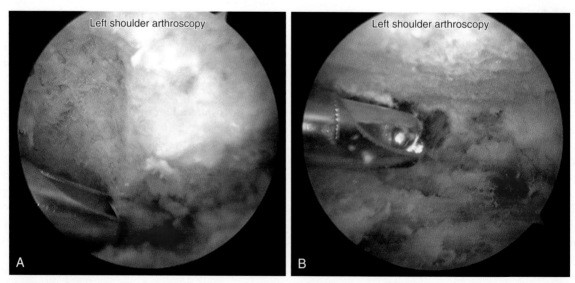

Figure 28-7. **A,** Subacromial view demonstrating initial lateral resection of the acromion. **B,** Similar view demonstrating completed acromioplasty with even resection.

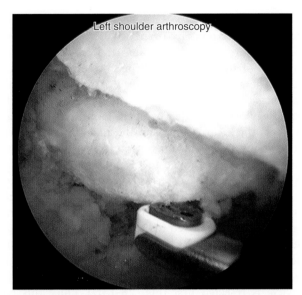

Figure 28-8. Subacromial view with arthroscope in the lateral portal demonstrating soft tissue clearance of the distal clavicle with the radiofrequency probe coming in from the anterior portal.

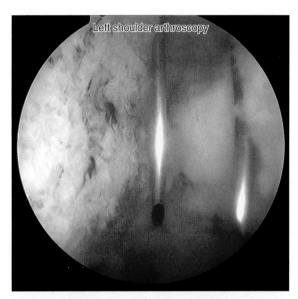

Figure 28-10. Subacromial view with the arthroscope through the anterior portal demonstrating two parallel spinal needles outlining the extent of resection of the distal clavicle.

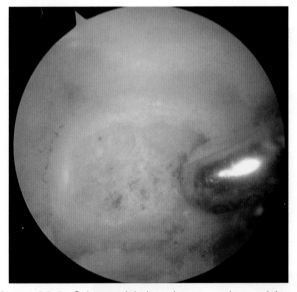

Figure 28-9. Subacromial view demonstrating excision of the anterior half of the distal clavicle.

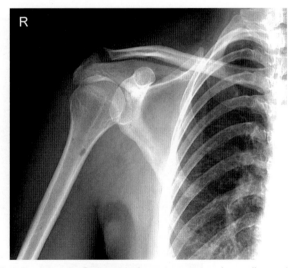

Figure 28-11. Postoperative anteroposterior radiograph of the right shoulder of the patient in Figure 28-1 demonstrating a distal clavicle excision.

aspects of the joint capsule so as not to destabilize the AC joint. Resection depth can be judged by using the bur (typically 5.5 mm) as a measuring device against the intact posterior aspect of the distal clavicle. Last, the arthroscope may be brought through the anterior portal to assess the final distal clavicle resection. We routinely place two parallel spinal needles at the resection edges to assess and document the adequacy of distal clavicle excision (Fig. 28-10). The arthroscopic shaver is then run in the subacromial space to ensure that all bony debris has been removed. A postoperative shoulder series is typically obtained to document the AC joint

resection (Fig. 28-11) and subacromial decompression (Fig. 28-12).

Distal Clavicle Excision via the Direct Approach

In patients with isolated AC joint pathology, the direct approach may be used. Two portals, the anterosuperior and posterosuperior, are used (Fig. 28-13A). First, a-22 gauge needle is used to determine the orientation of the AC joint (Fig. 28-13B). The joint is insufflated with 5 to 10 mL of normal saline. Next, the positions of the anterior and posterior portals are localized with use of

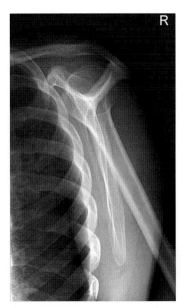

Figure 28-12. Postoperative scapular-Y view of the right shoulder of the patient in Figure 28-2 after subacromial decompression.

two additional 22-gauge needles. The portals should each be approximately 1 cm off of the anterior and posterior border of the AC joint, respectively. Free fluid flow out of the needles confirms intra-articular placement. The anterior viewing portal is made first with a stab incision with a No. 11 blade along the path of the previously placed needle. After the trocar has been used to insert the arthroscopic sheath, a small joint arthroscope is inserted. Instruments should pass at approximately a 30-degree angle to the horizontal plane (Fig. 28-13C). Next, the posterior working portal is made under direct visualization. A 3-mm shaver is brought into the joint from posterior to anterior. The fibrocartilaginous disk is removed to create some working space. Next, an electrocautery device is used to lift the capsule off the distal clavicle. A 5.5-mm round bur is used to resect the distal clavicle. The posterior half of the distal clavicle is resected first (Fig. 28-13D). Once this has been completed, the instruments are switched and the anterior resection is performed from the anterior working portal, using the posterior resection as a guide.

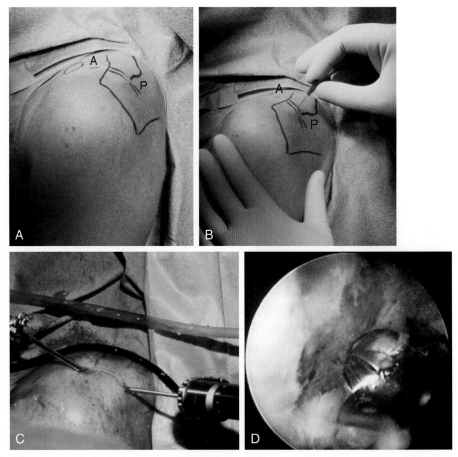

Figure 28-13. A, Direct acromioclavicular resection portal sites for a left shoulder, which include the anterior *(A)* and posterior *(P)* portals. **B,** A 22-gauge spinal needle is used to localize the precise position of the acromioclavicular joint. **C,** The outside view showing the arthroscope entering the anterior portal and the motorized bur in the posterior portal. **D,** Intra-articular view with the arthroscope in the anterior portal and the bur seen in the posterior portal.

TABLE 28-1. Outcomes After Arthroscopic Subacromial Decompression and Distal Clavicle Excision

Study	Follow-up	No. of Patients	Outcome
Clinical Results After Subacromial Decompression			
Ellman[8] (1987)	17 months (12-36 months)	49	88% good-excellent
Roye et al[9] (1995)	41 months (2-7 years)	88	89% good-excellent 68% throwing athletes
Stephens et al[10] (1998)	8 years 5 months (6-10 years)	82	81% good-excellent 67% throwing athletes
Clinical Results After Subacromial Decompression and Distal Clavicle Excision			
Kay et al[11] (2003)	6 years (3.9-9 years)	20	100% good-excellent
Lozman et al[12] (1995)	32 months (minimum 2 years)	18	89% good-excellent
Martin et al[13] (2001)	4 years 10 months (3-8 years)	31	100% good-excellent
Clinical Results After Direct Distal Clavicle Excision			
Auge and Fischer[14] (1998)	18.7 months (12-25 months)	10	100% good-excellent 100% osteolysis
Flatow et al[15] (1995)	31 months (24-49 months)	41	93% osteoarthritis or osteolysis 58% acromioclavicular hypermobility

Again the arthroscopic shaver is run in the joint to clear any residual bony debris.

POSTOPERATIVE CONSIDERATIONS

Rehabilitation

Patients are discharged home with enteric-coated aspirin 325 mg daily for DVT prophylaxis as well as oxycodone for pain control. They are instructed to remain in a sling postoperatively for approximately 48 hours and then to remove the sling daily for pendulum-type exercises. They are encouraged to ice the shoulder to reduce postoperative pain and swelling. If desired, a cryotherapy pack may be used. The patients are weaned from the sling as they continue to recover. Formal physical therapy begins after the initial postoperative visit at 7 to 10 days. Passive and active range of motion is allowed in all planes. Strengthening exercises may be initiated once the patient's pain is well controlled and the range of motion is nearly symmetrical with that on the contralateral side.

Complications

Complications from subacromial decompression include inadequate decompression, regrowth of previous spurs, excessive acromial resection with fracture, infection, continued pain, neurovascular injury, and medical complications. In general, infection and neurovascular complications are rare. Failure to diagnose and treat other causes of shoulder pain is a common reason for residual postoperative pain. Additional complications specific to distal clavicle excision include AC joint instability caused by over-resection and residual pain from inadequate AC joint resection.

RESULTS

After arthroscopic subacromial decompression, good to excellent results can be expected in approximately 80% of patients. In patients with coexisting subacromial impingement syndrome and AC degenerative joint disease, concomitant subacromial decompression and distal clavicle excision yields good to excellent results in nearly 90% of patients. For isolated AC joint disease, direct distal clavicle excision yields good to excellent results in more than 90% of patients (Table 28-1).

REFERENCES

1. Park HB, Yokota A, Gill HS, et al. Diagnostic accuracy of clinical tests for the different degrees of subacromial impingement syndrome. *J Bone Joint Surg.* 2005;87(7): 1446-1455.
2. Partington PF, Broome GH. Diagnostic injection around the shoulder: hit and miss? A cadaveric study of injection accuracy. *J Shoulder Elbow Surg.* 1998;7(2):147-150.
3. Dopirak R, Ryu RK. Management of the failed arthroscopic subacromial decompression: causation and treatment. *Sports Med Arthrosc.* 2010;18(3):207-212.
4. Cummins CA, Sass LM, Nicholson D. Impingement syndrome: temporal outcomes of nonoperative treatment. *J Shoulder Elbow Surg.* 2009;18(2):172-177.

5. Pohl A, Cullen DJ. Cerebral ischemia during shoulder surgery in the upright position: a case series. *J Clin Anesth*. 2005;17(6):463-469.

6. Peruto CM, Ciccotti MG, Cohen SB. Shoulder arthroscopy positioning: lateral decubitus versus beach chair. *Arthroscopy*. 2009;25(8):891-896.

7. Sampson TG, Nisber JK, Glick JM. Precision acromioplasty in arthroscopic subacromial decompression of the shoulder. *Arthroscopy*. 1991;7(3):301-307.

8. Ellman H. Arthroscopic subacromial decompression: analysis of one- to three-year results. *Arthroscopy*. 1987; 3:173-181.

9. Roye R, Grana W, Yates C. Arthroscopic subacromial decompression: two to seven-year follow-up. *Arthroscopy*. 1995;11:301-306.

10. Stephens S, Warren R, Payne L, et al. Arthroscopic acromioplasty: a 6- to 10-year follow-up. *Arthroscopy*. 1998;14:382-388.

11. Kay S, Dragoo J, Lee R. Long-term results of arthroscopic resection of the distal clavicle with concomitant subacromial decompression. *Arthroscopy*. 2003;19: 805-809.

12. Lozman P, Hechtman K, Uribe J. Combined arthroscopic management of impingement syndrome and acromioclavicular arthritis. *J South Orthop Assoc*. 1995;4: 177-181.

13. Martin S, Baumgarten T, Andrews J. Arthroscopic resection of the distal aspect of the clavicle with concomitant subacromial decompression. *J Bone Joint Surg Am*. 2001;83:328-335.

14. Auge W, Fischer R. Arthroscopic distal clavicle resection for isolated atraumatic osteolysis in weight lifters. *Am J Sports Med*. 1998;26:189-192.

15. Flatow EL, Duralde XA, Nicholson GP, et al. Arthroscopic resection of the distal clavicle with a superior approach. *J Shoulder Elbow Surg*. 1995;4:41-50.

Chapter 29

Arthroscopic Management of Glenohumeral Arthritis

Rachel M. Frank, Geoffrey S. Van Thiel, and Nikhil N. Verma

Chapter Synopsis

- Glenohumeral degenerative disease is a growing problem in the active patient population. Patient discomfort may be related to isolated articular cartilage disease, but may also result from other glenohumeral abnormalities, including labral, rotator cuff, and/or long head of the biceps tendon pathology. Although shoulder arthroplasty remains the gold standard for reducing pain in patients with advanced shoulder arthritis, it is typically not the most appropriate option for the relatively young patient who wishes to remain active without postoperative activity limitations. Therefore shoulder arthroscopy has become an increasingly popular treatment option for this challenging patient population, with a growing body of literature supporting its ability to improve pain and function while potentially delaying the need for arthroplasty.

Important Points

- Surgery may be indicated after failure of nonoperative management, including activity modification, physical therapy, nonsteroidal anti-inflammatory drugs, and/or injections.
- Examination may reveal crepitus, locking, or clicking.
- Decreased range of motion with pain at the extremes can often be addressed arthroscopically.

Clinical and Surgical Pearls

- Arthroscopic techniques include debridement, synovectomy, chondroplasty, capsular release, and subacromial decompression.
- For isolated lesions, microfracture can be considered.
- A complete capsular release will often provide good relief and improved range of motion.
- The lateral position allows for better access to the inferior aspect of the glenoid for a complete capsular release.
- The best surgical candidates include those with preserved joint space with a concentric glenoid and an absence of large osteophytes.
- Patients who respond to glenohumeral injections are more likely to respond to arthroscopic treatment.

Clinical and Surgical Pitfalls

- Patients with grade 4 bipolar disease, narrowed joint space (<2 mm), biconcave glenoid, and large osteophytes are at an increased risk of failure.
- When considering an isolated chondral lesion found at arthroscopy, it is crucial to determine if the lesion is truly responsible for the patient's symptoms, or if it is simply incidental in nature.
- Care must be taken during an inferior capsular release, given the proximity of the axillary nerve.

Glenohumeral degenerative disease is a growing problem in the relatively young, active patient population. Patients with shoulder arthritis have increased pain and decreased function compared with patients with normal shoulder joints,[1] and such symptoms can certainly have a significant impact on quality of life, particularly at a younger age. However, given the complexity of the shoulder joint, it can be difficult to determine the exact pain generator (Fig. 29-1). Articular cartilage degradation can contribute to the patient's symptoms, as can other shoulder pathologies including synovitis and capsulitis, labral tears, rotator cuff pathology, and long head of the biceps (LHB) tenosynovitis. Thus a comprehensive diagnostic and therapeutic approach is necessary.

Nonoperative treatment techniques including activity modification, physical therapy, nonsteroidal anti-inflammatory drugs (NSAIDs), and intra-articular

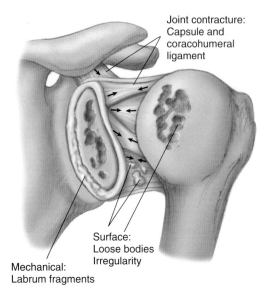

Joint contracture:
Capsule and
coracohumeral
ligament

Surface:
Loose bodies
Irregularity

Mechanical:
Labrum fragments

Figure 29-1. Sources of pain in an arthritic glenohumeral joint. *(Modified from Gartsman GM: Shoulder Arthroscopy. 2nd ed. Philadelphia: Elsevier; 2008.)*

injections of corticosteroids and/or hyaluronic acid solutions (off-label use) are typically effective as first-line options; however, their effects are often temporary.[2,3] Surgical options are varied and range from simple arthroscopic debridement to total shoulder arthroplasty. Arthroplasty has certainly shown favorable outcomes with regard to pain relief; however, postoperative limitations and risks can be significant in an active patient.

Nonarthroplasty alternatives, including arthroscopic debridement, are increasingly attractive options in contemporary orthopedics.[4-7] Shoulder arthroscopy and debridement is a commonly used initial surgical technique in the approach to treating patients with early glenohumeral degeneration, and several authors have demonstrated its potential for decreasing pain, improving function, and potentially delaying the need for eventual arthroplasty.[8-15] These debridement and arthroscopic procedures often include a combination of debridement, chondroplasty, synovectomy, capsular release, and subacromial decompression (SAD). However, it is important to keep in mind that the goal of arthroscopy at this stage is not to cure the underlying disease process (arthritis) but rather to provide symptomatic improvement and maintenance of function for as long as possible.

PREOPERATIVE CONSIDERATIONS

History

Classically, patients with shoulder arthritis will have decreased range of motion (ROM) and global pain associated with activities or motion, most commonly in the older patient. A history of trauma or weightlifting should be solicited in a younger patient. As with most shoulder conditions, night pain may be a prominent component of the patient's complaints. The onset is usually insidious and has been progressively affecting the patient's activity level. A history of prior treatments such as injections and NSAIDs should be solicited. Such conservative measures may provide temporary relief and improved function, but with time the pain may be refractory to these modalities. However, the key in the history is not diagnosing the "degenerative condition," but rather determining associated and contributing pathologies and developing a treatment algorithm.

The activity level of the patient should be determined, as well as the postoperative goals. Is the patient a sedentary household ambulator who wants to be able to reach things without pain, or is he or she an avid tennis player who hopes to return to some level of sport? This initial fact will guide decision making as to whether the patient is a good candidate for arthroplasty, or whether a less invasive technique such as arthroscopy should be tried first. The onset of pain is also important, as are the characteristics of the discomfort. An acute onset suggests an exacerbation of a concomitant pathology. Pain at the extremes of motion may be the result of decreased motion and capsulitis rather than the underlying degeneration, which may also cause pain in mid-ROM. A sensation of "popping" or "clicking" can be attributed to loose bodies or chondral irregularity, and pain isolated to the anterior aspect of the shoulder may occur secondary to biceps tendonitis. Nonetheless, a complete history related to the shoulder joint should be completed, and the recognition of concomitant pathologies is essential.

Furthermore, it is imperative for the orthopedic surgeon to ask about previous shoulder injuries and procedure(s), as certain implants and techniques have well-documented correlations with the development of arthritis. For example:

- Instrumentation leading to chondrolysis[16]
- Labral repair with anchors or tacks
- Techniques involving thermal capsulorrhaphy leading to chondrolysis[17]
- Use of postoperative intra-articular pain pump[18,19]
- History of a proximal humerus fracture
- History of recurrent instability

Physical Examination

A complete physical examination of both shoulders should be performed for every patient with possible glenohumeral arthritis. After visualization of the shoulder, standard range-of-motion, strength, sensation, and stability tests should be performed, followed by any special tests deemed appropriate. The physical examination should be completed with the mindset that the patient has an underlying degenerative condition and that accompanying pathology can be treated to improve the symptomatology. The cervical spine examination must also be performed to rule out referred pain. All examination findings must be compared with the contralateral shoulder to determine what is abnormal versus a normal variant for that patient. Typical physical examination findings include the following:

- Decreased ROM—specific documentation with preoperative ROM is essential
- Sensation of crepitus, clicking, catching, or locking
  - *Note:* Some patients may have painless crepitus, and although this may signal articular cartilage disease, this is likely not the source of the patient's symptoms (incidental finding).
- Limited ROM compared with normal shoulder
  - Decreased forward flexion in patients with large inferior humeral head bone spur
  - Decreased external rotation in patients with flattened humeral head
  - Pain at extremes of motion
- Possible point tenderness
  - Especially if a component of bursitis is present
  - Evaluation for tenderness over the LHB
  - Evaluation for tenderness over the acromioclavicular (AC) joint
- Provocative testing such as LHB tension signs
- Normal strength, though examination can be limited by pain
- Neurovascular examination to document normal status

Imaging

Imaging is useful in the evaluation of the patient with glenohumeral degenerative joint disease (DJD), and the typical modalities include radiographs, magnetic resonance imaging (MRI), and computed tomography (CT).

- Plain radiographs
  - Standard: anteroposterior (AP), axillary lateral, and scapular-Y views
    - Evaluation of glenohumeral joint space, inferior humeral osteophytes, proximal humeral migration
  - West Point axillary view:
    - Helpful for evaluating glenoid bone loss ("bony Bankart")
  - Stryker notch view:
    - Helpful for evaluating humeral head bone loss (Hill-Sachs lesions)
  - Axillary view:
    - Necessary for the evaluation of glenoid morphology (biconcave glenoid, posterior erosion, anterior bone loss)
    - Evaluation of remaining joint space (millimeters)
- MRI (without contrast) can show the following:
  - Status of articular cartilage and subchondral bone
  - Loose bodies
  - Joint effusions
  - Soft-tissue pathologies (labrum, rotator cuff, biceps tendon)
- CT (with three-dimensional reconstruction) can show the following:
  - Postoperative hardware from previous surgeries
  - Bony defects of the humeral head and glenoid
  - Glenoid version or erosion

Indications and Contraindications

Indications

Once the requisite nonoperative management has failed, the first step in indicating a patient for arthroscopic management of glenohumeral DJD is determining whether he or she will substantially benefit from the procedure in comparison to an index arthroplasty. Consideration for arthroscopic management includes young patients with high activity goals, early degenerative disease with some remaining joint space, and a concentric glenoid. As the results of arthroscopic intervention are variable, primary arthroplasty should be considered in older patients, those with sedentary activity goals, and patients with end-stage arthritis with no remaining joint space or significant glenoid biconcavity or erosion. Once this decision point has been passed, an evaluation for concomitant pathology as a contributing source of pain should be performed. Some patients have significant chondral lesions that are relatively asymptomatic with other pathology being the inciting factor. Thus it is essential to specifically determine the possible pain generators to be addressed at the time of surgery. It is imperative that the surgeon not "treat" the image or arthroscopic findings; instead, he or she should identify pathology that correlates with clinical symptoms.

Contraindications

Relative contraindications include no remaining joint space with large osteophytes or nonconcentric glenoid with posterior erosion. In addition, elderly patients with a low level of function who wish to undergo one procedure and return to their activities would be better served by an arthroplasty.

Pearls

- Preoperative diagnostic injections performed under sterile conditions can help locate the specific site of pain (e.g., subacromial, biceps, intra-articular source, AC joint).

- It can be difficult to differentiate the symptoms and physical examination findings caused by impingement from those caused by diffuse osteoarthritis.
  - For this reason, the diagnosis of arthritis is sometimes not made until the time of arthroscopy.
- Understand the patient's goals for after surgery.
  - Unrealistic patient expectations must be addressed, and ultimately the patient may be deemed not appropriate for surgery.
- Understand the patient's anatomy and the severity of disease before performing arthroscopy.
  - Patients with residual joint space and no osteophytes will likely benefit.
  - Patients with severe, grade 4 bipolar disease, decreased joint space of less than 2 mm, and/or large osteophytes may not benefit and may need a more definitive procedure.
  - Arthroscopic debridement is contraindicated in patients with severe posterior glenoid erosion or glenoid biconcavity.
  - Pain at extremes of motion (likely because of osteophytes and/or inflamed synovium) and pain at rest (likely a result of synovitis) are commonly relieved with arthroscopy.[20]
  - Pain during mid-ROM (likely caused by extensive articular surface damage) is likely too advanced to be relieved with arthroscopy.[20]
  - Increased ROM achieved by arthroscopic debridement and capsule release can provide significant relief.

SURGICAL TECHNIQUE

Anesthesia and Positioning

Arthroscopic management of glenohumeral arthritis is typically performed with the patient under general anesthesia with an interscalene block or interscalene block with sedation. The nerve block is useful especially in the postoperative period for pain control. Most arthroscopic techniques used for shoulder arthritis can be performed with both the beach chair and the lateral decubitus position. Surgeon experience, preference, and comfort should determine which positioning is appropriate for any given patient, as neither position has been shown to be superior with regard to easier setup or better surgical access.[21] After appropriate setup, skin preparation and draping can occur according to the surgeon's preference. The senior surgeon (N.N.V.) prefers to use the lateral position for this procedure, as it allows improved access to the inferior aspect of the glenohumeral joint for capsular release and osteophyte debridement.

In the beach chair position, the patient is placed supine on the operating room table, with the head, neck, and torso supported in a neutral position. A variety of table attachments and/or straps can be used to position the head appropriately. The hips are flexed at 45 to 60 degrees, the knees are flexed to 30 degrees, and the patient is placed in 10 to 15 degrees of Trendelenburg. All bony prominences must be padded. The patient should be moved to the edge of the table so that the operative shoulder is essentially free and not supported by the table. The operative extremity can also be supported by an optional arm-positioning device that can aid in traction and distraction.

In the lateral position the patient should be placed on a bean bag or supported with another device and all bony prominences completely padded. The patient's torso can then be rolled approximately 25 degrees posterior to position the glenoid parallel to the floor. An axillary roll is placed under the chest distal to the axilla. The arm is then suspended, prepared, and placed in a traction sleeve with neutral rotation. The traction device is placed in 45 degrees of abduction and 15 degrees of forward flexion. Ten pounds of weight are then used for both distraction and abduction traction (20 pounds total).

Examination Under Anesthesia

Every shoulder should undergo an examination under anesthesia (EUA) before the arthroscopy is begun. The EUA is extremely helpful in determining ROM and stability of the affected shoulder, which can sometimes be obscured during a clinical examination owing to patient guarding and pain. The ROM should be compared with that of the contralateral shoulder, in particular forward flexion, abduction, external rotation at the side, external rotation in abduction, internal rotation, and external rotation. Stability should also be compared with that of the contralateral shoulder, although instability is generally not encountered in patients with glenohumeral arthritis.

Surgical Landmarks, Incisions, and Portals

Standard shoulder arthroscopy portals are used for most arthroscopic procedures for treatment of glenohumeral arthritis. Accurate portal placement is essential, especially for the posterior portal, which is the main visualization used for diagnostic arthroscopy. Surgical landmarks are key for making accurate portal placements. The anterior, posterior, and lateral borders of the acromion can be palpated easily and drawn with a sterile marking pen. The coracoid process (typically found 2 to 3 cm inferior to the AC joint), clavicle, and spine of the scapula can also be easily palpated and drawn. The posterior portal is placed through the "soft spot," which can be appreciated by palpation approximately 2 cm inferior and 1 cm medial to the posterolateral acromion. With the lateral decubitus position, the posterior portal should be shifted to a position 1 cm distal and 1 cm medial to the posterolateral corner of the acromion. The anterior portal is the working portal for most arthroscopic shoulder procedures and can be placed under direct visualization with a spinal needle. This portal is placed 2 to 3 cm inferior to the antero-lateral edge of the acromion, lateral to the coracoid, and runs through the rotator interval.

Specific Steps

Specific steps of this procedure are outlined in Box 29-1.

Diagnostic Arthroscopy

Diagnostic arthroscopy should always be performed to identify normal anatomic and pathoanatomy. A step-wise approach is helpful with this portion of the proce-dure and allows the surgeon to consistently evaluate all relevant structures, including the labrum, rotator cuff, capsule, glenohumeral ligaments, and biceps tendon. Surgical findings should be correlated with preoperative history and physical examination findings to determine pathology related to patient symptoms. Common find-ings of glenohumeral arthritis found during diagnostic arthroscopy include the following:

- Synovitis
- Labrum fraying
- Articular cartilage degenerative changes (Fig. 29-2)
- Capsular tightness
- Loose bodies (Fig. 29-3)

Debridement, Synovectomy, and Chondroplasty

For the symptomatic patient with diffuse glenohumeral arthritis, debridement, capsular release, and chondro-plasty are often the first-line arthroscopic procedures used. Although the natural history of these procedures is largely unknown, favorable short-term outcomes have been reported in the literature (Table 29-1). During debridement, loose and redundant tissue is removed, including inflamed synovium (synovectomy) and loose

cartilage flaps (chondroplasty). Both thermal and mechanical debridement techniques have been described. A thermal device is often used for the initial synovec-tomy and is helpful in maintaining hemostasis. The labrum, loose chondral flaps, and loose bodies can be addressed with a full-radius arthroscopic shaver, typi-cally 4.0 mm. Maintaining the shaver on suction is helpful, as it increases the flow of saline through the joint and therefore the flow of the debrided tissue out of the joint. Although labral fraying or detachment is commonly encountered, labral repair is generally not indicated, as it would result in further tightening of a stiff shoulder and likely worsening of symptoms.

Osteophytes are removed with either a mechanical bur or an osteotome, and loose bodies are removed with a grasper. Large osteophytes located on the anterior and posterior aspects of the glenoid can also be removed; this technique, referred to as *recontouring* of the glenoid, changes the shape and concavity of the glenoid to restore

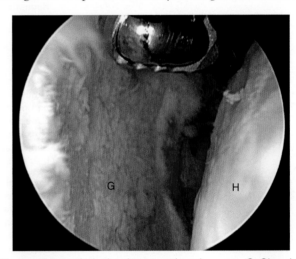

Figure 29-2. Articular degenerative changes. *G,* Glenoid; *H,* humerus.

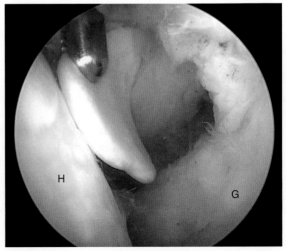

Figure 29-3. Loose bodies in the glenohumeral joint removed through an anterior portals. *G,* Glenoid; *H,* humerus.

BOX 29-1 Surgical Steps
1. Examination under anesthesia
2. Diagnostic arthroscopy
3. Debridement
4. Synovectomy
5. Chondroplasty
6. Capsular release
7. Subacromial decompression
8. Microfracture (if deemed appropriate by specific pathology)

TABLE 29-1. Selected Outcomes

Study	No. of Shoulders	Average Follow-up (mo)	Outcome	Notes
Van Thiel et al[14] (2010)	71	27	Significant improvements (*P* < .05) in ASES, SST, VAS scores and range of motion Postoperative SANE score 71.1 Postoperative Constant score 78.5 Postoperative UCLA score 28.3	Sixteen patients progressed to arthroplasty at 10.1 months after debridement Risks included grade 4 bipolar changes, joint space <2 mm, and/or large osteophytes
Kerr et al[11] (2008)	20	20 (minimum 12)	Patients with unipolar lesions had better outcomes than those with bipolar lesions All but three patients had SANE scores of ≥60	Patients <55 years All with grade 2-4 articular cartilage changes Three patients went on to arthroplasty
Richards and Burkhart[13] (2007)	9	14	Preoperative FF 132, ER 43, IR 17 Postoperative FF 153, ER 59, IR 48	Preliminary results only as part of a technique paper
Cameron et al[8] (2002)	61	minimum 24 (45 patients)	Significant improvement (*P* < .0001) in pain and motion in 88% Repeat surgery in 87%	All with grade 4 articular cartilage lesions With and without capsular release Concomitant procedures (acromioplasty, DCR, labral debridement or repair) did not have negative effect
Guyette et al[10] (2002)	36	60	Patients with grade 1, 2, or 3 changes had mean follow-up L'Insalata score of 90 Patients with grade 4 had mean follow-up L'Insalata score of 50 Radiographic arthrosis correlated but was less reliable	All patients received SAD (all patients had subacromial impingement in addition to glenohumeral arthritis)
Weinstein et al[15] (2000)	25	34 (minimum 12)	Excellent results: 2 patients (8%) Good results: 19 patients (72%) Unsatisfactory results: 5 patients (20%) Of 12 patients with marked preoperative stiffness, 83% had improved range of motion postoperatively	Of note, 52% of patients had grade 2 arthritic changes or lower

ASES, American Shoulder and Elbow Surgeons scale; *DCR*, distal clavicle resection; *ER*, external rotation; *FF*, forward flexion; *IR*, internal rotation; *SAD*, subacromial decompression; *SANE*, Single Assessment Numeric Evaluation; *SST*, Simple Shoulder Test; *UCLA*, University of California at Los Angeles shoulder rating scale; *VAS*, visual analogue scale.

its normal axis of curvature to redistribute contact area and pressure.

Capsular Release

Capsular release is an essential component to the procedure in any patient with a moderate loss of motion, as many of these patients are functionally symptomatic from decreased ROM. In general, a shoulder is a good candidate for capsular release when there is a loss of 15 to 20 degrees in any plane. A complete circumferential capsular release is often performed, including the rotator interval, but a limited release can be completed if there is a significant deficit in one plane. The procedure is typically performed with either a thermal coagulation device or an arthroscopic cutter (i.e., "biter") (Fig. 29-4). The anterior capsule must be dissected free from the underlying subscapularis tendon; it should be noted that the thermal device is not recommended for release of the inferior capsule given the proximity of the axillary nerve (Fig. 29-5). Furthermore, the surgeon must be cognizant of the nerve in this location with either device. If needed, the accessory posterior-inferior portal can be helpful for safely addressing this region, especially during capsular release and osteophyte resection. Richards and Burkhart[13] have described their technique for performing a release of the rotator interval, anterior capsule, posterior capsule, and axillary recess in addition to debridement, using the arthroscopic shaver as well as electrocautery probes, and have described preliminary data with improvements in ROM.

Subacromial Decompression

Patients with glenohumeral osteoarthritis may also have impingement, and SAD is often performed concomitantly with arthroscopic debridement. SAD in these settings is typically limited to bursectomy only, unless there is an exceptionally large bone spur. The indication for acromioplasty should be carefully considered, as it may lead to increased bleeding and eventual scarring and fibrosis, leading to a new source of pain and stiffness for the patient. The diagnosis of impingement can be difficult, as many symptoms overlap with findings of early to moderate glenohumeral arthritis. Furthermore, reported clinical outcome data often include frequent concomitant procedures, and it can be extremely difficult, if not impossible, to determine if the symptomatic relief provided by surgery was related to the debridement, to the SAD, or to both.

Microfracture

We have described the use of microfracture in a small patient population with good outcomes.[22] In the majority of patients with diffuse DJD of the shoulder, microfracture is not an option. However, in the younger patient with a focal defect, microfracture may be beneficial. Portal placement is important; the anterior portal can be placed more laterally when performed on the anterosuperior glenoid, and a lower portal just above the subscapularis is used when the defect is located more inferiorly. Posterior glenoid lesions can be accessed with a posterior 7-o'clock position (right shoulder) portal, and most lesions on the humerus are reached through the standard anterior portal facilitated by internal and external rotation of the arm. Once localized, standard microfracture technique is used as described for the knee (Fig. 29-6).

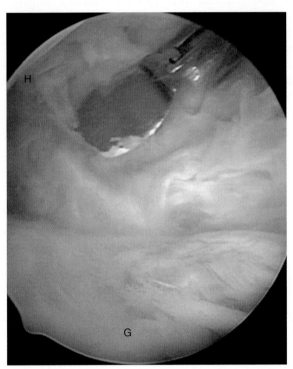

Figure 29-4. Capsular release around the inferior aspect of the glenoid viewed from an anterior portal. *G,* Glenoid; *H,* humerus.

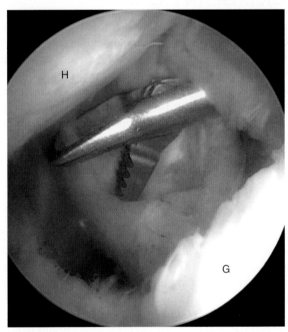

Figure 29-5. Release of the capsule overlying the subscapularis viewed from the posterior portals. *G,* Glenoid; *H,* humerus.

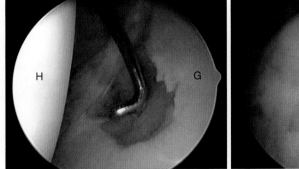 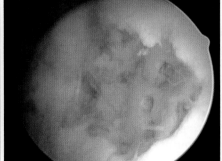

Figure 29-6. A, Full-thickness chondral defect of the glenoid viewed from the posterior portal. **B,** Microfracture holes created via standard microfracture technique throughout the prepared glenoid defect.

Other Possible Concomitant Procedures

Several other procedures can be performed at the time of arthroscopic debridement for glenohumeral arthritis. Each of these procedures should be performed only in properly indicated patients with explicit preoperative informed consent documented. Specific discussion of each of these techniques is beyond the focus of this chapter, but they are discussed throughout other chapters within the text:

- Biceps tenotomy or tenodesis
- Distal clavicle excision
- Rotator cuff repair

POSTOPERATIVE CONSIDERATIONS

Unrestricted, active ROM is permitted and should be encouraged as soon as the first postoperative day. All patients, and especially those who underwent capsular release, can experience a considerable amount of pain postoperatively, and although intra-articular pain catheters were used in the past, recent reports suggest an association with the development of glenohumeral chondrolysis. The preoperative regional block should aid in postoperative pain control in addition to adequate oral analgesics.

Rehabilitation

As mentioned in the previous section, unrestricted ROM is allowed immediately after surgery. A sling may be worn for comfort but should be discontinued as soon as possible. Patients should begin working on regaining full ROM as soon as possible under the guidance of a physical therapist, especially those who underwent capsular release. Rotator cuff strengthening should begin 3 to 4 weeks after surgery. Patients can return to work and activities as soon as they are comfortable.

Complications

The complication rate for shoulder arthroscopy is low. With more involved procedures, including inferior capsular release and glenoid osteophyte resection, the risk of bleeding increases, though it is still low. One must be aware of pertinent shoulder neurovascular anatomy to avoid damaging nerves and vessels, in particular the axillary nerve when working inferiorly, and the musculocutaneous nerve during the placement of the anterior portal. The most frequent negative outcome after arthroscopic debridement is persistent pain that is unresponsive to arthroscopic intervention, with subsequent need for shoulder arthroplasty.

RESULTS

Currently there is a paucity of studies available describing clinical outcomes following arthroscopic management of glenohumeral arthritis. The few studies that do exist have provided evidence that arthroscopic techniques may improve shoulder pain and function for patients with arthritic changes. More specifically, based on the work of Van Thiel and colleagues,[14] patients with unipolar lesions and limitations in ROM can expect good pain relief and significant improvements in shoulder function and ROM. However, patients with bipolar changes, significant radiographic joint space narrowing, or large osteophytes will not do as well with a debridement procedure. The authors listed in Table 29-1 have also demonstrated these predictive factors; in general, patients with significant bipolar changes will not do as well. Furthermore, a large percentage of patients can expect a significant increase in ROM postoperatively. Nevertheless, longer-term studies are needed to determine if the results stand over time. A summary of recent studies[8,10,11,13-15] is presented in Table 29-1.

REFERENCES

1. Matsen 3rd FA, Ziegler DW, DeBartolo SE. Patient self-assessment of health status and function in glenohumeral degenerative joint disease. *J Shoulder Elbow Surg.* 1995; 4(5):345-351.
2. Silverstein E, Leger R, Shea KP. The use of intra-articular hylan G-F 20 in the treatment of symptomatic osteoarthritis of the shoulder: a preliminary study. *Am J Sports Med.* 2007;35(6):979-985.
3. Sinha I, Lee M, Cobiella C. Management of osteoarthritis of the glenohumeral joint. *Br J Hosp Med (Lond).* 2008; 69(5):264-268.
4. Chong PY, Srikumaran U, Kuye IO, et al. Glenohumeral arthritis in the young patient. *J Shoulder Elbow Surg.* 2011;20(2 Suppl):S30-S40.
5. Cole BJ, Yanke A, Provencher MT. Nonarthroplasty alternatives for the treatment of glenohumeral arthritis. *J Shoulder Elbow Surg.* 2007;16(5 Suppl):S231-S240.
6. Denard PJ, Wirth MA, Orfaly RM. Management of glenohumeral arthritis in the young adult. *J Bone Joint Surg Am.* 2011;93(9):885-892.
7. Elser F, Braun S, Dewing CB, et al. Glenohumeral joint preservation: current options for managing articular cartilage lesions in young, active patients. *Arthroscopy.* 2010;26(5):685-696.
8. Cameron BD, Galatz LM, Ramsey ML, et al. Nonprosthetic management of grade IV osteochondral lesions of the glenohumeral joint. *J Shoulder Elbow Surg.* 2002;11(1):25-32.
9. Ellman H, Harris E, Kay SP. Early degenerative joint disease simulating impingement syndrome: arthroscopic findings. *Arthroscopy.* 1992;8(4):482-487.
10. Guyette TM, Bae H, Warren RF, et al. Results of arthroscopic subacromial decompression in patients with subacromial impingement and glenohumeral degenerative

joint disease. *J Shoulder Elbow Surg.* 2002;11(4): 299-304.

11. Kerr BJ, McCarty EC. Outcome of arthroscopic débridement is worse for patients with glenohumeral arthritis of both sides of the joint. *Clin Orthop Relat Res.* 2008; 466(3):634-638.

12. Ogilvie-Harris DJ, Wiley AM. Arthroscopic surgery of the shoulder. A general appraisal. *J Bone Joint Surg Br.* 1986;68(2):201-207.

13. Richards DP, Burkhart SS. Arthroscopic débridement and capsular release for glenohumeral osteoarthritis. *Arthroscopy.* 2007;23(9):1019-1022.

14. Van Thiel GS, Sheehan S, Frank RM, et al. Retrospective analysis of arthroscopic management of glenohumeral degenerative disease. *Arthroscopy.* 2010;26(11):1451-1455.

15. Weinstein DM, Bucchieri JS, Pollock RG, et al. Arthroscopic débridement of the shoulder for osteoarthritis. *Arthroscopy.* 2000;16(5):471-476.

16. McNickle AG, L'Heureux DR, Provencher MT, et al. Post-surgical glenohumeral arthritis in young adults. *Am J Sports Med.* 2009;37(9):1784-1791.

17. Lubowitz JH, Poehling GG. Glenohumeral thermal capsulorrhaphy is not recommended—shoulder chondrolysis requires additional research. *Arthroscopy.* 2007;23(7): 687.

18. Anakwenze OA, Hosalkar H, Huffman GR. Case reports: two cases of glenohumeral chondrolysis after intraarticular pain pumps. *Clin Orthop Relat Res.* 2010;468(9): 2545-2549.

19. Solomon DJ, Navaie M, Stedje-Larsen ET, et al. Glenohumeral chondrolysis after arthroscopy: a systematic review of potential contributors and causal pathways. *Arthroscopy.* 2009;25(11):1329-1342.

20. Steinmann SP, Carroll RM, Levine WN. Arthroscopic Management of Glenoid Arthritis. In: Miller MD, Cole BJ, eds. *Textbook of Arthroscopy.* Philadelphia: Saunders; 2004:259-265.

21. Peruto CM, Ciccotti MG, Cohen SB. Shoulder arthroscopy positioning: lateral decubitus versus beach chair. *Arthroscopy.* 2009;25(8):891-896.

22. Frank RM, Van Thiel GS, Slabaugh MA, et al. Clinical outcomes after microfracture of the glenohumeral joint. *Am J Sports Med.* 2010;38(4):772-781.

Chapter 30

Arthroscopic Capsular Release for the Treatment of Stiff Shoulder Pathology

Gregory P. Nicholson

Chapter Synopsis
- The arthroscopic management of stiff shoulder pathology is detailed. The diagnosis, imaging, indications for operative treatment, and specific technique of arthroscopic capsular release, along with aftercare, are detailed.

Important Points
- Shoulders that have not responded to appropriate conservative treatment and have had symptoms for over 4 months are candidates for arthroscopic capsular release.
- An existing shoulder arthroplasty implant may be more effectively treated by open release technique.
- Shoulder stiffness can be caused or maintained by involvement of the glenohumeral capsule, the rotator interval, or the subacromial space. All areas can and should be evaluated and released if involved.
- All causes of shoulder stiffness can be addressed by arthroscopic technique.

Clinical and Surgical Pearls
- Technically challenging procedure because of limited space. Be patient!
- Know your chosen pump and fluid flow characteristics.
- I prefer the 3.5-mm ArthroWand bipolar cautery device to perform the release. It provides a bloodless release of the capsule and is stiff enough to access tight areas, and the right angle can cut through the thickened capsule.
- The goal is a balanced release. Proceed from superior to inferior to access the contracted capsule. Anterior, posterior, and inferior areas should be addressed if involved.

Clinical and Surgical Pitfalls
- Approximately 20% of postrelease patients experience increasing stiffness 3 to 5 weeks postoperatively. This is an inflammatory flare-up and can be treated appropriately.
- Manipulation before release should be avoided. It can cause soft tissue and bone injury. It also creates bleeding that makes visualization difficult during arthroscopy.

The diagnosis of shoulder stiffness, also termed *frozen shoulder* or *adhesive capsulitis*, is one of exclusion. It is a clinical syndrome characterized by painful restricted passive and active range of motion. It is associated with night pain and pain with activities.[1-5] This clinical entity has been difficult to classify and follows an unpredictable clinical course.[1,3,6,7] Etiologic factors in the pathophysiology of the disease include idiopathic causes, posttraumatic conditions, diabetes, and postsurgical factors; the condition can arise even as a consequence of prolonged impingement syndrome.[4,5,8-11] It appears that susceptible shoulders respond to an insult in a common pathway of expression. This is a glenohumeral synovitis. If this process continues unabated, the capsule will become thickened and disorganized in its collagen structure and actually become contracted.[12,13] The time course of the process and recovery is unpredictable. The true cause, diagnostic criteria, pathophysiology, treatment methods, and natural history of this condition are under debate and investigation.[1,4-8,14-16] There are patients who do not respond to time, proper therapy, injections, or anti-inflammatory medications and who are profoundly affected by the shoulder stiffness. These patients can be offered an arthroscopic capsular release.

PREOPERATIVE CONSIDERATIONS

History

The majority of adhesive capsulitis patients with an idiopathic cause are women between the ages of 35 and 60 years. A history should be taken for other contributing factors, especially endocrine abnormalities such as diabetes or hypothyroidism. A history of trauma or surgery is important to note. A neurologic history is important to note for possible involvement of cervical disease. The type of a prior surgical procedure on or around the shoulder is important to know, and a previous operative note can be helpful.

Physical Examination

Adhesive capsulitis, or frozen shoulder, is a limitation of motion without an obvious clinical reason for the loss of motion such as arthritis or previous fracture of the shoulder. Thus a comprehensive examination of the shoulder and cervical spine needs to be performed. The examiner should evaluate passive motion and active motion in forward elevation in the plane of the scapula, external rotation at the side, and internal rotation. In a painful shoulder, internal rotation behind the back can be painful. It is helpful to evaluate internal rotation with the arm abducted in the scapular plane approximately 40 degrees and then let the forearm drop toward the floor. The rotation can be seen and measured, and the early movement of the scapula can easily be seen in patients with posterior capsular involvement. The affected side should always be compared with the unaffected side. Inspection for atrophy around the shoulder girdle should be done. Evaluation for acromioclavicular (AC) joint pain, impingement-type pain, and cervical radicular symptoms must be done. In this step-wise fashion the examiner can determine the motion planes that are involved, and any contributing factors to the loss of motion and pain patterns. It can be helpful to do differential injections around the shoulder to determine pathologic locations and contributions. A subacromial injection of anesthetic can eliminate subacromial pain and allow the examiner to evaluate the shoulder with that area temporarily "eliminated" as a pain generator. An injection in the glenohumeral joint itself can eliminate glenohumeral pain. This can allow the examiner to evaluate shoulder motion again with pain eliminated. If the motion is remarkably improved, it may not be a true shoulder stiffness problem. However, most of the time the injections help the pain aspect but the

range of motion is not improved, confirming a diagnosis of stiffness.

Imaging

Plain radiographs will evaluate conditions such as arthritis of the glenohumeral joint, calcific tendonitis, and subacromial impingement. A true anteroposterior (AP) view of the glenohumeral joint, an axillary view, and an outlet view should be performed. Magnetic resonance imaging (MRI) can evaluate for rotator cuff pathology, but in a true adhesive capsulitis picture, MRI will exclude other pathology. Bone scan, computed tomography (CT), and electromyography are rarely necessary for the evaluation of frozen shoulder. Arthrography with limited joint volume was at one time felt to be a gold standard–type test,[3] but it is not necessary for the diagnosis of shoulder stiffness if a proper history is obtained and a proper physical examination is performed. Another diagnostic test can be physical therapy. A patient who does not respond to or who actually gets worse with a therapy program designed specifically for shoulder stiffness can be a candidate for arthroscopic capsular release.

Conservative Treatment

Conservative treatment should always be attempted. As mentioned previously, injections can relieve pain and facilitate therapy. The pathophysiology is that of glenohumeral inflammation. Corticosteroid injections into the glenohumeral joint can decrease the inflammatory response, relieve pain, and allow better motion. An oral steroid medication can also be used. Gentle range of motion and stretching are instituted. Nonsteroidal anti-inflammatory drugs (NSAIDs) can be used after or in conjunction with steroids. If the pain is relieved, most patients can accept the limitations of motion.[6,7] This allows more time to restore motion and function.

Indications for Surgical Intervention

Some patients do not respond to conservative management. A recalcitrant frozen shoulder is one that has had symptoms for over 4 months and has not responded to a surgeon-directed therapy program directed toward the diagnosis of shoulder stiffness. This program should be given at least 6 weeks to show progress. If patients still have sleep disturbance, pain, and limitation of motion that affects their occupation, recreation, and sleep, then it is time to consider an arthroscopic capsular release.[4,17,18] The cause of the stiffness has been found to not have a significant effect on the outcome of arthroscopic capsular release; thus the procedure is equally effective across causes.[4]

Contraindications to Arthroscopic Capsular Release

If the patient has motion loss and a shoulder prosthesis in place, an open approach may be preferred. If motion loss is present along with a history of an open instability repair that used a subscapularis shortening procedure, again, an open approach may be preferred.

SURGICAL TECHNIQUE

Anesthesia and Positioning

By definition there is restricted range of motion of the shoulder; thus there is small joint volume, and small movements can help intra-articular exposure. For this reason the preference is for the beach chair position with the arm free. The lateral position with the arm in traction will restrict ability to rotate the shoulder during the procedure, and traction will not open up the stiff joint. A combined anesthetic technique is preferred. A scalene regional block for intraoperative and postoperative pain relief is preferred. A general anesthetic can then be used. If the patient is going to be admitted for therapy, an in-dwelling scalene catheter can be used for prolonged pain control. The surgeon should choose the option based on the patient, the anesthesia experience, and surgeon experience.

The patient is placed in the beach chair position with a small towel roll under the medial border of the scapula. The landmarks of the scapular spine, acromion, and coracoid are marked out after standard preparation and draping. An assessment of motion is made with the patient under anesthesia (Fig. 30-1). No manipulation is performed at this time. It would create bleeding within the glenohumeral joint and make for a more difficult procedure.

Equipment and Instruments

Surgeon knowledge of the chosen pump is underrated but important. Proper fluid management during the case facilitates a clear field and prevents unnecessary swelling. It is helpful to use a 1:300,000 dilution of epinephrine in the fluid. This helps prevent nuisance bleeding. My preference for the release instrument is the ArthroWand bipolar cautery device (ArthroCare, Sunnyvale, CA). The 3.5-mm, 90-degree (non-TurboVac) model allows a 3.5-mm swathe of tissue to be cut without bleeding. It is a stiff instrument that allows the surgeon to cut the tissue both by pushing away and by pulling back toward the portal. The right angle at the tip allows the surgeon to cut into tissue and around corners. Other devices have been used to perform the capsular release including monopolar devices, basket cutters, and shavers.[4,5,8,10,14,15,17-19] A combination of release tools can be used depending on surgeon preference.

Specific Steps

Specific steps of this procedure are outlined in Box 30-1.

After motion assessment, the glenohumeral joint in insufflated with saline with an 18-gauge spinal needle from the posterior portal. The posterior portal is made

---

BOX 30-1 Surgical Steps: Arthroscopic Capsular Release

1. Limited synovectomy
2. Rotator cuff interval and anterosuperior release
3. Inferior release
4. Portal change and posterior superior release
5. Gentle manipulation

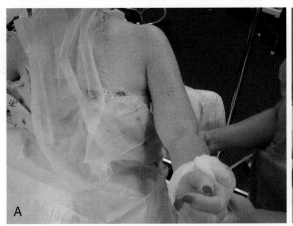 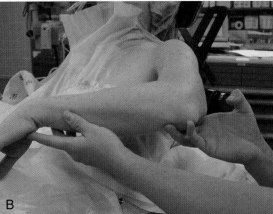

Figure 30-1. Preoperative range of motion assessment in a left shoulder with the patient in the beach chair position under anesthesia. **A,** External rotation is markedly limited at the side to only approximately 10 degrees. **B,** Internal rotation with the arm in 40 degrees of abduction in the scapular plane reveals that the forearm falls only to parallel to the floor. This represents approximately 20 degrees of internal rotation motion.

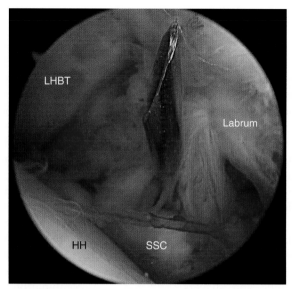

Figure 30-2. The initial arthroscopic view of the contracted arthroscopic triangle in a left shoulder. A spinal needle is in the middle of the interval. Note the gelatinous synovitis over the biceps and anterior capsule. *HH,* Humeral head; *SSC,* subscapularis tendon; *LHBT,* long head of the biceps tendon.

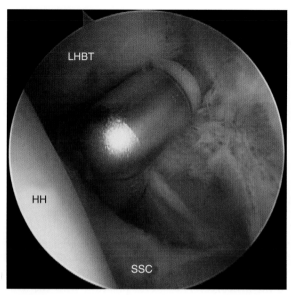

Figure 30-3. The ArthroWand device (ArthroCare, Sunnyvale, CA) begins the release at the biceps root. The tip is turned into the tissue. The release will be carried down the glenoid rim in an extra-labral fashion. *HH,* Humeral head; *LHBT,* long head of the biceps tendon; *SSC,* subscapularis tendon.

approximately 2 cm medial and inferior to the postero-lateral corner of the acromion. A stab wound is made at this spot, and the blunt obturator for the arthroscopic sheath is introduced into the joint. The joint is con-tracted and the capsule is thickened. The tip of the scope sheath is aimed at the superior aspect of the glenoid toward the long head of biceps origin. This will allow the arthroscopic sheath to enter a more open area of the joint and avoid articular cartilage damage.

The arthroscope is connected, and visualization of the arthroscopic triangle is achieved. The arthroscopic triangle formed by the long head of the biceps tendon, the glenoid, and the top of the subscapularis tendon is typically contracted and involved with a red, gelatinous synovitis (Fig. 30-2). The spinal needle is inserted ante-riorly just lateral to the tip of the coracoid and into the arthroscopic triangle. A stab wound is made anteriorly, and a smooth cannula is placed into the joint through the arthroscopic triangle. Fluid flow will allow visualiza-tion. The shaver is brought in to debride the accessible synovitis. This gelatinous synovium is easily debrided without significant bleeding. At this point the smooth cannula is removed and the ArthroWand is brought in anteriorly down the track exited by the cannula. There is no need to attempt to bring the device through the cannula. The cannula will restrict mobility.

The arthroscopic capsular release must begin supe-riorly and proceed inferiorly. The shoulder must be "unzipped." The cautery device begins the release just below the biceps tendon in the rotator interval (Fig. 30-3). The "base" of the triangle is released and then

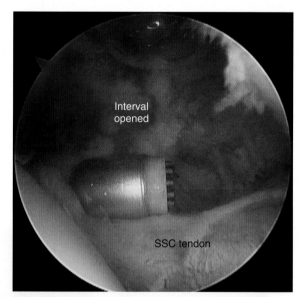

Figure 30-4. The left shoulder viewed from the posterior portal after release of the rotator interval. The subscapularis tendon is clearly visible, and the triangle size is larger. The release of the interval allows improved external rotation and the ability to continue the release inferiorly. *SSC,* subscapularis.

carried across the top of the subscapularis tendon (Fig. 30-4). This provides mobility to proceed inferiorly. An extralabral capsular release is performed (Fig. 30-5). The thickened capsule is cut or released by the cautery device. Mobility and visualization in the inferior aspect of the joint improves as the release continues from

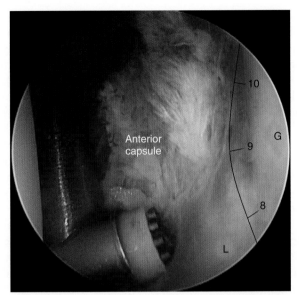

Figure 30-5. In this left shoulder, the arthroscope is moved inferiorly and the ArthroWand (ArthroCare, Sunnyvale, CA) begins to release the anterior capsule. The tip of the cautery device is turned into the tissue. An advantage of the ArthroWand is its flexible stiffness. The surgeon can cut the tissue by either pulling back toward or pushing away from the portal entry site. *G*, Glenoid; *L*, labrum.

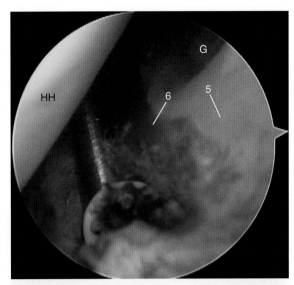

Figure 30-7. The cautery has stayed along the glenoid and released the capsule down around and beyond the 6-o'clock position. *G*, Glenoid; *HH*, humeral head.

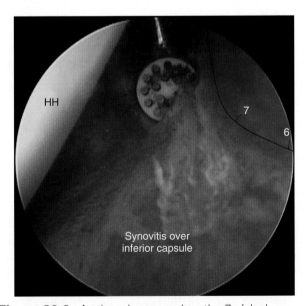

Figure 30-6. As the release reaches the 7-o'clock position (5-o'clock position in a right shoulder), the cautery tip is turned up away from the axillary nerve. The bipolar device can still cut the capsule or debulk it in this method. Note the extensive red synovitis on the inferior capsule. *HH*, Humeral head.

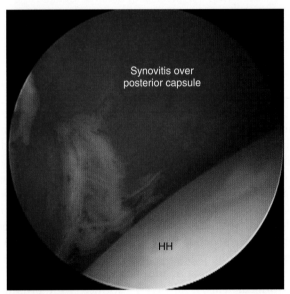

Figure 30-8. The arthroscope is now in the anterior portal looking posteriorly in this left shoulder. The posterior capsule is thickened and covered with the typical synovitis material seen in adhesive capsulitis pathology. The posterior capsule will be released in a similar fashion as the anterior capsule. *HH*, Humeral head.

superior to inferior down the anterior capsule (Fig. 30-6). As the ArthroWand cautery device gets down inferiorly (from the 5- to 7-o'clock position), the device is turned facing superiorly to cut the capsule (Fig. 30-7). This prevents injury to the axillary nerve. The device is

also kept along the rim of the glenoid. Drifting away from the glenoid rim can endanger the axillary nerve.

Once the 5- or 6-o'clock position has been reached, then the arthroscope is switched to the anterior portal and the cautery device to the posterior portal. The capsular release is now repeated from superior to inferior and extralabral, but along the posterior capsule (Fig. 30-8). The region above the biceps origin, the postero-superior recess, should be addressed and released if

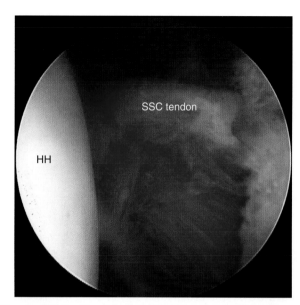

Figure 30-9. The left shoulder viewed anteriorly after complete release and placement of the shoulder through a full range of motion. The subscapularis muscle belly is now seen with the shoulder in external rotation. The contracted capsule is no longer seen. *HH,* Humeral head; *SSC,* subscapularis.

found to be contracted. This capsular area can restrict the excursion of the supraspinatus tendon unit.

After the capsule has been circumferentially released, the subacromial space should be evaluated. In patients with previous surgery or impingement pathology, the subacromial space can be involved.[4,5,11,17,18] The necessary debridement of adhesions and possible acromioplasty should be performed. If the patient has developed AC joint pain during the stiffness process, it should be addressed at this time. Then the shoulder should be put through a range of motion. A sequence of forward elevation in the plane of the scapula, external rotation at the side, abduction, and internal rotation should be performed. This is always performed with proximal pressure on the humerus. It should not be a forceful manipulation. A few soft releases may be felt, representing the last few contractures being lysed. This is not a true manipulation. The capsular release provides for a controlled, bloodless, atraumatic manipulation with this range of motion at the end of the procedure (Fig. 30-9).

POSTOPERATIVE CONSIDERATIONS

Patients can be admitted for a 24-hour stay to allow for physical therapy while the scalene regional block is in effect. This provides an opportunity for pain-free motion exercises. It also shows the patients that motion has

been restored and can be achieved without pain. This is a big psychological step for many patients who have battled pain, poor motion, and dysfunction for a prolonged time period. If the surgeon elects to treat in the hospital in this fashion after arthroscopic capsular release, it is recommended to try to do the case early in the morning so that the therapist can see the patient while the block is still in effect. Analgesics and NSAIDs are routinely used to control pain and inflammation. We have used a derotation sling and wedge (Apex sling, EBI, Parsippany, NJ) to place the shoulder in a neutral position and avoid the internally rotated position that a traditional sling would achieve.

Outpatient therapy emphasizing motion for forward elevation, external rotation, and internal rotation is performed 3 days a week for 3 weeks, and then 2 days a week for 3 more weeks. Patients are instructed to do range-of-motion exercises everyday at home for 20 to 30 minutes, three times a day. Isometric strength and resistive strength exercises are not prescribed until motion is pain-free, flexible, and consistent. The time to achieve this and progress to strengthening is approximately 6 to 8 weeks. The time to final pain-free range of motion is approximately 6 to 10 weeks.[4,10,15,16] The need for home continuous passive motion therapy is rare. It should be considered for patients who may be at higher risk for slow progress, such as diabetics with profound motion loss (external rotation at side less than 0 degrees), or those in whom a previous stiffness procedure (manipulation or release procedure) has failed.

Complications

The goal is a balanced capsular release. This cannot be accomplished with manipulation alone. One of the pitfalls is to not accomplish the balanced release and to leave one of the previously mentioned areas not addressed. Thus the surgeon should always assess and address the anterior, inferior, and posterior capsular regions. The interval should always be released and the subacromial space evaluated. Even with good technique I have found that approximately 20% of patients will develop a transient decrease in motion 3 to 5 weeks after the procedure. The shoulder motion becomes less flexible and can actually become very "rubbery" and painful. This is an inflammatory flare-up and has been describe by other authors.[4,16] It should be recognized and the patient reassured and treated with patience, anti-inflammatory medication, and, if not contraindicated, either a Medrol Dosepak or intra-articular steroid injection. The issue should resolve in 3 to 6 weeks.

Other potential complications include injury to the axillary nerve, fracture of the humerus, damage to the joint surface, and recurrent stiffness. There is also the risk of complications from the scalene block. In my experience the complication rate has been very low, and

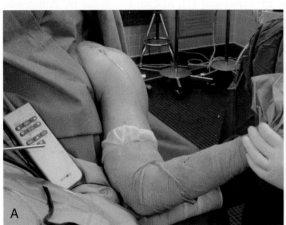
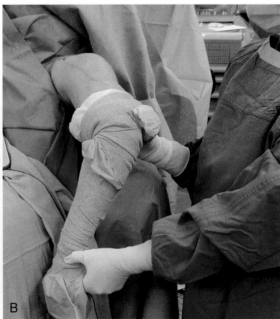

Figure 30-10. The left shoulder after release. **A,** External rotation at the side is now 65 degrees. **B,** Internal rotation reveals that the forearm can rotate and point almost directly at the floor. Significant gain in rotational arc has been achieved.

no patient has developed recurrent stiffness after arthroscopic capsular release.

RESULTS

Arthroscopic capsular release has shown the ability to consistently restore range of motion, improve shoulder function, and relieve pain for shoulder stiffness from a variety of causes (Fig. 30-10).[4,5,8-11,14-16,19] It has possibly shortened the natural history of this not fully understood clinical entity. Reports on outcomes have shown a time to achieve final pain-free range of motion of 6 to 10 weeks. The time in formal therapy has averaged 2.5 months. The recurrence of stiffness has not been seen. The average improvement in range of motion has been 73 degrees for forward elevation, 44 degrees in external rotation, and eight spinal segments in internal rotation. The cause of the stiffness has been shown to not have an effect on motion, pain, or patient satisfaction. Diabetic frozen shoulder has shown a trend toward a longer time to achieve final range of motion, but significant improvements in motion, pain, and function have been reported.[4]

REFERENCES

1. Grey RG. The natural history of "idiopathic" frozen shoulder. *J Bone Joint Surg Am.* 1978;60:564.
2. Murnaghan JP. Frozen shoulder. In: Rockwood CA Jr, Matsen FA III, eds. *The Shoulder.* Vol. 2. Philadelphia, 1993, Saunders, 837-861.
3. Nevaiser RJ, Nevaiser TJ. Frozen shoulder: diagnosis and management. *Clin Orthop Relat Res.* 1987;223: 59-64.
4. Nicholson GP. Arthroscopic capsular release for stiff shoulders. effect of etiology on outcomes. *Arthroscopy.* 2003;19(1):40-49.
5. Ozaki J, Nakagawa Y, Sukurai G, et al. Recalcitrant chronic adhesive capsulitis of the shoulder. *J Bone Joint Surg Am.* 1989;71:1511-1515.
6. Griggs SM, Ahn A, Green A. Idiopathic "Adhesive capsulitis": a prospective functional outcome study of non-operative treatment. *J Bone Joint Surg Am.* 2000;82: 1398-1407.
7. Shaffer B, Tibone JE, Kerlan RK. Frozen shoulder: a long term follow-up. *J Bone Joint Surg Am.* 1992;74: 738-746.
8. Ogilivie-Harris DJ, Myerthall S. The diabetic frozen shoulder: arthroscopic release. *Arthroscopy.* 1997;13: 1-18.
9. Ticker JB, Beim GM, Warner JJP. Recognition and treatment of refractory posterior capsular contracture of the shoulder. *Arthroscopy.* 2000;16:27-34.
10. Warner JJP, Allen A, Marks P, et al. Arthroscopic release of chronic refractory capsular contracture of the shoulder. *J Bone Joint Surg Am.* 1996;78:1808-1816.
11. Warner JJP, Allen A, Marks PH, et al. Arthroscopic release of post-operative capsular contracture of the shoulder. *J Bone Joint Surg Am.* 1997;79:1151-1158.
12. Hannafin JA, DiCarlo EF, Wickiewicz TL. Adhesive capsulitis: capsular fibroplasia of the glenohumeral joint. *J Shoulder Elbow Surg.* 1994;3:S5.
13. Rodeo SA, Hannafin JA, Tom J, et al. Immunolocalization of cytokines in adhesive capsulitis of the shoulder. *J Orthop Res.* 1997;15(3):427-436.

14. Pearsall AW, Osbahr DC, Speer KP. An arthroscopic technique for treating patients with frozen shoulder. *Arthroscopy*. 1999;15:2-11.

15. Segmuller HE, Taylor DE, Hogan CS, et al. Arthroscopic treatment of adhesive capsulitis. *J Shoulder Elbow Surg*. 1995;4:403-408.

16. Watson L, Dalziel R, Story I. Frozen shoulder: a 12-month clinical outcome trial. *J Shoulder Elbow Surg*. 2000;9:16-22.

17. Nicholson GP. Adhesive Capsulitis. Manipulation or arthroscopic capsular division. In: Barber FA, Fischer SP, eds. *Surgical Techniques for the Shoulder and Elbow*. New York, NY: Thieme Medical Publishers; 2003:127-130.

18. Nicholson GP, Ticker JB. Arthroscopic capsular release. In: Imhoff AB, Ticker JB, Fu F, eds. *Atlas of Shoulder Arthroscopy*. London: Martin Dunitz; 2003:343-351.

19. Harryman DT, Matsen FA, Sidles JA. Arthroscopic management of refractory shoulder stiffness. *Arthroscopy*. 1997;13:133-147.

Chapter 31

Arthroscopic and Open Management of Scapulothoracic Disorders

Kevin M. Doulens and John E. Kuhn

Chapter Synopsis

- Scapulothoracic bursitis, crepitus, dyskinesis, and winging are related conditions of the shoulder that are frequently seen together. Crepitus, or snapping scapula, may be asymptomatic or may be seen with bursitis. Nonoperative treatment is often effective and includes corticosteroid injections in the scapulothoracic bursae and physical therapy. Surgery to resect inflamed bursae and/or bony prominences may be performed arthroscopically or via an open procedure. When long thoracic nerve palsies do not recover, a transfer of the sternal head of the pectoralis major muscle is recommended.

Important Points

- Scapulothoracic bursitis, crepitus, dyskinesis, and winging are often seen together.
- Crepitus may be asymptomatic or a finding in patients with "hidden agendas."
- Physical therapy and injections of corticosteroids are often successful for the treatment of bursitis and dyskinesis.
- Surgery to resect the bursa or remove bony prominences can be performed via an open procedure or arthroscopically with predictably good results.
- Long thoracic nerve palsies may take over a year to recover; surgery should be reserved for patients who have no clinical or electromyographic improvement after a lengthy period of nonoperative treatment.

Clinical and Surgical Pearls

- Imaging of the scapulothoracic articulation is important to identify bony or soft tissue tumors as a source of symptoms.
- Arthroscopy of the scapulothoracic articulation is facilitated by putting the patient's arm behind the back in a "chicken wing" position.
- Open resection of the superomedial angle of the scapula requires meticulous repair of the periscapular muscles.
- When a pectoralis transfer is performed for a long thoracic nerve palsy, the end of the tendon should meet the scapula with the graft used for augmentation.

Clinical and Surgical Pitfalls

- Scapulothoracic crepitus and voluntary scapular winging may be used by patients to achieve secondary gain.
- Pneumothorax is a risk for injections of the scapulothoracic articulation. This may be reduced by placing the arm behind the back in a chicken wing position and by use of imaging.
- Portals placed too far from the medial border of the scapula during scapulothoracic arthroscopy may put the dorsal scapular nerve at risk.
- The suprascapular nerve and artery are at risk for medial dissection during open resection of the superomedial angle of the scapula.

Knowledge about the interplay of structures and biomechanics surrounding the scapula and its role in shoulder motion is evolving steadily. The result is that our understanding of shoulder disease is also increasing. It is becoming clear that processes affecting the scapula in turn greatly influence the function of the shoulder.[1]

Conditions of the scapulothoracic articulation can be broadly divided into four main disease processes: bursitis, crepitus, dyskinesis, and winging. Each of these is a unique entity, but they are often seen in combination.

Scapulothoracic bursitis manifests as posterior shoulder pain with range of motion. The patient can often

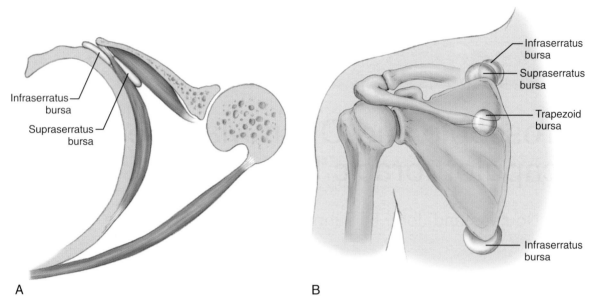

Figure 31-1. Bursae about the scapula. A number of bursae have been described about the scapula, including the two major bursae (infraserratus and supraserratus) and the four minor or adventitial bursae. (*Modified from Kuhn JE, Hawkins RJ. Evaluation and treatment of scapular disorders. In: Warner JJP, Iannotti JP, Gerber C, eds:* Complex and Revision Problems in Shoulder Surgery. *Philadelphia: Lippincott-Raven; 1997.*)

localize the pain under the scapula. Two major bursae are consistently identified: the infraserratus bursa between the serratus and the chest wall and the supraserratus bursa between the subscapularis and the serratus (Fig. 31-1). In addition, four minor adventitial bursae have been described.[2] Clinically significant bursitis tends to affect two areas most commonly: the superior medial angle and the inferior angle. The bursae at these locations are minor adventitious bursae that may become apparent only when they are inflamed. Through a process that is similar to subacromial bursitis, repetitive motion of the scapula over the rib cage causes inflammation and edema in the bursae. As with other types of bursitis, this process can be initially treated with rehabilitation and judicious corticosteroid injections.[3] This is often sufficient to quiet the process and relieve the patient's symptoms. On occasion the bursitis is refractory to medical management, and surgical intervention in the form of a bursectomy is required.

Scapular crepitus is a process whereby palpable and often audible noises are generated under the scapula. Of significance in this process is that not all crepitus is painful or pathologic, and the volume of the noise does not correlate with the severity of the pain. Crepitus ranges from mild, painless subscapular crunching to painless but loud snapping and from minimal discomfort to disabling pain. In most patients, symptomatic scapulothoracic crepitus is associated with bursitis.

Winging of the scapula is a finding that may result from many causes. In athletes, winging is typically seen as an isolated palsy of the serratus caused by a long thoracic nerve neurapraxic injury. Winging may also be seen with profound scapular bursitis or may manifest as part of scapular dyskinesis. Scapular dyskinesis is defined as abnormal motion of the scapula characterized by medial border or inferior angle prominence, early excessive scapular elevation and shrugging, or rapid downward rotation during lowering of the arm.[1] A static abnormality of scapular position, called the *SICK scapula* (*s*capular malposition, *i*nferior medial border prominence, *c*oracoid pain and malposition, and dys*k*inesis of scapular movement), probably represents a more severe state of this condition.[4] Whereas dyskinesis is likely to be the most common finding in the athlete with shoulder pain, it is best treated with appropriate rehabilitation and will not be explored in detail in this chapter. Winging caused by bursitis typically resolves with treatment of the bursitis. Winging caused by long thoracic nerve injury resolves spontaneously in most athletes; when it persists, surgical intervention can be considered.

PREOPERATIVE CONSIDERATIONS

History

Many scapulothoracic conditions in athletes are related to other pathologic processes in the shoulder, and therefore the history should include a thorough orthopedic review of systems. A typical history of the patient with a scapulothoracic disorder includes the following:

- Pain with activity greater than pain at rest
- Painful crepitus
- Increased pain on carrying or lifting objects away from the body
- Pain at the superior angle of the scapula
- Pain near other scapulothoracic muscles

Physical Examination

The physical examination for scapulothoracic disorders requires the physician to stand behind the patient, who is disrobed or wearing a sports bra. The scapular position at rest should be noted. A scapula that is depressed, anteriorly tilted, and internally rotated suggests a SICK scapula and typically has tenderness at the pectoralis minor insertion on the coracoid.[4] The patient is asked to elevate and then lower the arms while the physician looks for dyskinesis. Crepitus can be heard, and the location of crepitus (superomedial angle or inferior angle) frequently can be determined by careful palpation. Provocative testing to elicit winging can be performed by having the patient push off from the wall or elevate the arms against resistance (Fig. 31-2).

Imaging

Radiography

Radiographs are helpful to find subscapular bone prominences (Fig. 31-3) and include the following views:

- True anteroposterior view
- Axillary view
- Scapular-Y view (Fig. 31-3A)

Other Modalities

Magnetic resonance imaging and computed tomographic scans are usually not necessary but can be helpful in identifying soft tissue and bone lesions (Fig. 31-3B).

Electromyography

If winging of the scapula is thought to be of neurologic origin, electromyography will assist in the diagnosis. Serial studies every 3 to 4 months can document recovery of an injured long thoracic nerve.

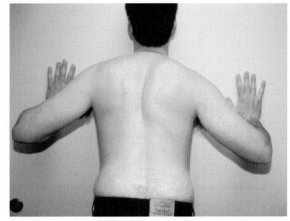

Figure 31-2. Winging of the scapula. Winging can be accentuated by pushing off from a wall or by resisting forward elevation.

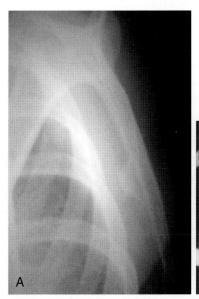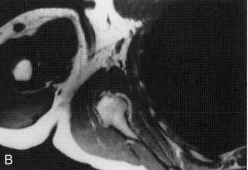

Figure 31-3. Subscapular bone prominences associated with scapulothoracic disorders. The osteochondroma **(A)** is the most common tumor of the scapula. The corresponding magnetic resonance image demonstrates reactive bursal tissue with high signal around the osteochondroma **(B)**.

Indications and Contraindications

Most scapulothoracic problems in athletes are not treated surgically. Rehabilitation focused on pectoralis minor stretching, serratus and lower trapezius strengthening, posterior capsule stretching, and core strengthening will treat the SICK scapula and scapular dyskinesis.[4] Patients with scapular bursitis and milder forms of crepitus will often respond to similar rehabilitation and the judicious use of corticosteroid injections. With the mixing of steroid and local anesthetic, injections can be therapeutic and diagnostic, perhaps giving an indication of potential postsurgical results. Athletes with long thoracic nerve injury can be monitored for many months with serial electromyography as the nerve typically recovers spontaneously, occasionally taking up to 2 years. Bracing may help with symptom relief while the nerve recovers. When nonoperative approaches fail, surgery may be considered for these conditions.

There are no absolute contraindications to surgery of the scapula; however, physicians must be cautious of the patient with less-than-obvious pathologic changes, the patient with questionable responses to therapy and injection, and the patient who may have a voluntary component to the complaint. Scapulothoracic crepitus often exists without symptoms. In addition, some patients who have secondary gain develop voluntary scapular winging. Patients with secondary gain, unrecognized scapular dyskinesis, and voluntary winging will have predictably poor postsurgical outcomes.

SURGICAL TECHNIQUE: BURSECTOMY AND PARTIAL SCAPULECTOMY

Anesthesia and Positioning

Positioning of the patient is similar for both bursectomy and partial scapulectomy. The prone position is used, often with a bolster under the lateral chest to cause the rib cage to rise and the shoulder to fall forward, thereby making the scapula more prominent. The surgical preparation should extend from C5 to L1 and include the entire back and the arm of the involved side.

Specific Steps

Bursectomy

Specific steps of this procedure are outlined in Box 31-1.

Scapulothoracic bursectomy can be performed in an open or an endoscopic fashion. The open procedure has a distinct advantage in that it allows direct visualization of adventitial bursae whose position and plane of dissection might be anatomically variable.

BOX 31-1 Surgical Steps: Bursectomy, Open or Arthroscopic

1. Skin incision medial to scapula
2. Levator and rhomboids dissected subperiosteally off medial scapula (open only)
3. Plane between subscapularis and chest wall developed and bursae resected
4. Muscles reapproximated to scapula and skin closed

In the open procedure for a superior medial bursectomy, the incision is placed medial to the superior vertebral border of the scapula. The trapezius is split in line with its fibers, and the levator scapulae and rhomboids are exposed. The levator and rhomboids are then incised off of the medial border of the scapula in a subperiosteal fashion. A plane is then developed between the serratus anterior under the scapula and the chest wall. The thickened bursa can be dissected from this space. The levator, rhomboids, and trapezius are then reapproximated to the scapula, and the skin is closed. Postoperatively, the patient uses a sling for comfort and begins passive physical therapy immediately. Once the periscapular muscles have healed adequately at approximately 3 to 4 weeks, active motion is initiated. Strengthening can begin at 12 weeks. For symptomatic inferior angle bursae, the incision can be made along the inferior medial border just distal to the angle. The trapezius and then the latissimus dorsi are split in line with their fibers, allowing direct access to the inferior angle and the bursa. After the bursa has been excised, the muscles are reapproximated and skin is closed. Postoperative care and rehabilitation are the same.

The endoscopic approach to scapulothoracic bursitis involves the use of two or three portals to access the subscapular space.[5] The patient may be positioned in either the prone or the lateral position. All portals must be kept at least 2 cm medial to the medial border of the scapula to prevent injury to the dorsal scapular nerve (Fig. 31-4). Elevation of the scapula can be achieved by putting the arm behind the back in a "chicken wing" position or using a hook retractor.[6]

The first portal is inserted medial to the scapula and midway between the scapular spine and the inferior angle. Insufflation of the infraspinatus bursa with injection will help identify the plane of surgery. The blunt obturator and endoscope can then be inserted into the bursa. The second portal can be either superior or inferior, depending on the location of the pathologic process. The superior portal is made, once again at least 2 cm medial to the medial border of the scapula at the level of the scapular spine. This will allow access to the superior medial angle. If required, a third portal can be made at the inferior angle of the scapula in a similar fashion

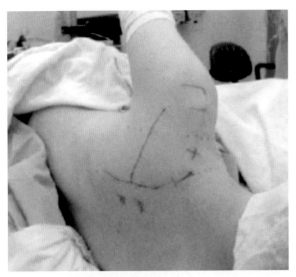

Figure 31-4. Endoscopic portals for scapulothoracic bursectomy. *(From Pavlik A, Ang K, Coghlan J, Bell S. Arthroscopic treatment of painful snapping of the scapula by using a new superior portal. Arthroscopy. 2003;19:608-612.)*

BOX 31-2 Surgical Steps: Scapulectomy

1. The skin is incised.
2. The trapezius is split and dissected from the spine of the scapula.
3. The superomedial angle is dissected free.
4. The superomedial angle is resected with a saw.
5. The medial border of the supraspinatus is repaired to the rhomboid-serratus-subscapularis flap, and the inferior border and trapezius are repaired to bone.

---

to access the inferior portion.[7] In all these portals, landmarks are few, and hemostasis is critical to allow adequate visualization. Once the bursectomy has been performed, the portals are closed and the patient is placed into a sling. Activity is performed as tolerated.

Partial Scapulectomy

Specific steps of this procedure are outlined in Box 31-2.

Painful scapulothoracic crepitus and its most dramatic presentation, the snapping scapula, are both treated with a partial scapulectomy when conservative measures fail. The pathologic lesion is generally at the superior medial angle, and so excision of this corner of the scapula is often successful at relieving symptoms. As in the bursitis procedures, the patient is placed prone.

The incision is placed along the medial border of the scapula from the level of the scapular spine inferiorly to the superomedial angle (Fig. 31-5). The skin is elevated in a subcutaneous plane, exposing the spine of the scapula laterally. The trapezius is split in line with its fibers and elevated from the spine of the scapula, and the plane between the undersurface of the trapezius and

the supraspinatus is developed. Starting along the spine, the supraspinatus is then dissected free from medial to lateral in a subperiosteal fashion until the edge of the scapular notch can be palpated. It is important to not extend farther lateral as damage to the suprascapular nerve and artery can occur. Starting once again along the medial border, the levator and rhomboids are elevated off subperiosteally. With the superior medial border exposed, the dissection is carried subperiosteally around the border and under the scapula to peel the serratus and subscapularis off the bone. This is most easily done with a Cobb elevator. Once both sides of the scapula have been exposed, the superior corner can be resected. This cut is made with an oscillating saw and runs from the base of the scapular spine to approximately 4 or 5 cm lateral along the superior edge of the scapula. Once again, care must be taken to not disturb the contents of the scapular notch. With the superior medial angle resected, the plane between the supraspinatus and the combined muscle flap are sutured together with No. 2 permanent suture. The trapezius is secured to the spine of the scapula. The skin is closed, and the patient is placed into a sling.

Passive range of motion can begin immediately. Active exercises start at 6 weeks, and strengthening begins at 12 weeks.

Scapular Winging

Operative treatment of scapular winging for patients whose therapy fails and who remain symptomatic is an attempt to restore stability in the face of a known deficiency. Because restoration of normal anatomy is not possible, these surgeries will have varying degrees of success and probably will not be able to return athletes to high levels of function.

Transfer of the sternal head of the pectoralis major muscle is the most popular therapy for permanent serratus anterior palsy (Fig. 31-6). For this procedure, the patient is placed in the lateral decubitus position. Either one or two incisions can be used. For a single incision, it is made across the axilla from the border of the pectoralis major anteriorly to the inferior angle of the scapula. The sternocostal head lies under the clavicular head at the insertion into the humerus. The sternocostal head is released and redirected back toward the inferior tip of the scapula. Because this muscle alone is generally not long enough to reach without excessive tensioning, an autologous fascia lata or hamstring tendon graft from the ipsilateral leg is harvested. The fascia lata graft is tubularized and sewn into the end of the pectoralis major tendon. The distal tip of the scapula is then cleared of soft tissues, and a small hole is made in the tip. The graft is then passed through the hole and sutured back onto itself. Enough tension is applied so that the end of the pectoralis tendon is in contact with the scapula.

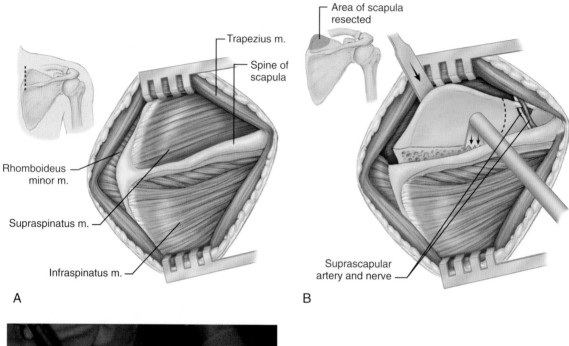

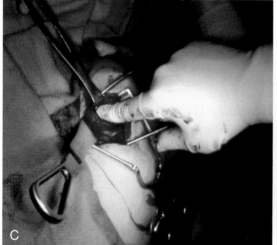

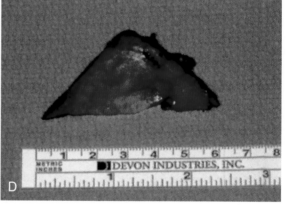

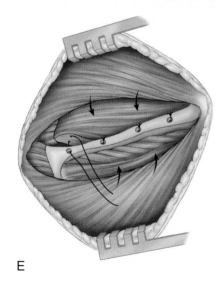

Figure 31-5. Partial scapulectomy. **A,** The skin incision is made in Langer's lines, and the trapezius is dissected from the spine of the scapula. **B,** The superomedial angle is resected after it has been dissected in a subperiosteal fashion in the plane between supraspinatus and the rest of the scapular muscles. **C,** An acromial retractor is placed between the subscapularis and the scapula, and the superomedial angle is cut with a saw. **D,** The resected superomedial angle is triangular with a base of about 5 cm. **E,** The medial border of the supraspinatus is repaired to the rhomboid-serratus-subscapularis flap, and the inferior border and trapezius are repaired to bone. *m,* Muscle. *(A, B, and E, Modified from Kuhn JE, Hawkins RJ. Evaluation and treatment of scapular disorders. In: Warner JJP, Iannotti JP, Gerber C, eds.* Complex and Revision Problems in Shoulder Surgery. *Philadelphia: Lippincott-Raven; 1997.)*

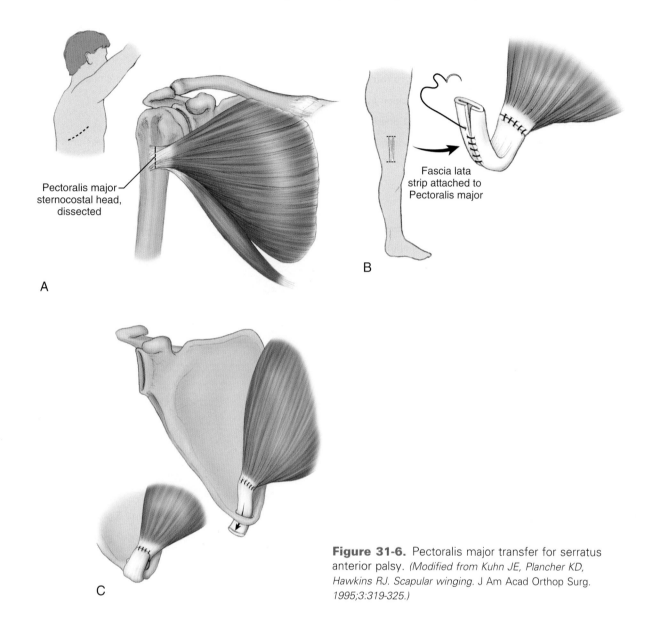

Figure 31-6. Pectoralis major transfer for serratus anterior palsy. *(Modified from Kuhn JE, Plancher KD, Hawkins RJ. Scapular winging.* J Am Acad Orthop Surg. *1995;3:319-325.)*

The patient is placed into a sling, and postoperative passive range of motion is begun immediately. Active motion is begun at 6 weeks, and strengthening begins at 12 weeks.

POSTOPERATIVE CONSIDERATIONS

Rehabilitation

The patient is kept in immobilization for up to 6 weeks after muscle transfer. Passive therapy is begun immediately to avoid stiffness, and active motion is allowed at week 6. After these procedures, strengthening rehabilitation is begun at around 12 weeks.

Complications

Any surgery that involves dissection under the scapula has the potential for chest wall complications, most notably pneumothorax. Postoperative radiographs will help identify any involvement of the lungs. Incisions and portals made midline to the medial border of the scapula can lead to dorsal scapular nerve injury. Splitting of the trapezius does not interfere with its innervation. If the superomedial angle of the scapula is resected too far laterally, the suprascapular nerve and artery are at risk.

RESULTS

The results of these different procedures vary (Tables 31-1 to 31-3). Bursectomy and partial scapulectomy are

TABLE 31-1. Results of Scapulothoracic Bursectomy*

Study	Number and Technique	Outcome
Ciullo and Jones[8] (1993)	13 arthroscopic bursectomies	100% return to preinjury activity
McCluskey and Bigliani[9] (1991)	9 open bursectomies	89% good-excellent
Nicholson and Duckworth[10] (2002)	17 open bursectomies	100% relief of pain
Sisto and Jobe[11] (1986)	4 open bursectomies	4/4 returned to professional pitching

*All are level IV case series.

TABLE 31-2. Results of Partial Scapulectomy for Scapulothoracic Crepitus*

Study	Number and Technique	Outcome
Arntz and Matsen[12] (1990)	12 patients, 14 shoulders	86% complete relief
Harper et al[13] (1999)	7 arthroscopic resections	6 successful, 1 failure
Lehtinen et al[5] (2004)	6 open, 6 combined open and scope, 2 scope, 2 bursectomies	13/16 (81%) satisfied
Pavlik et al[7] (2003)	10 arthroscopic resections	4 excellent, 5 good, 1 fair
Richards and McKee[14] (1989)	3 open resections	100% success in pain relief

*All reports are level IV case series.

TABLE 31-3. Results of Pectoralis Major Transfers for Serratus Anterior Palsy*

Study	No. Transfers	Outcome
Connor et al[15] (1997)	11 pectoralis	10/11 satisfactory
Gozna and Harris[16] (1979)	3 pectoralis	3/3 successful
Iceton and Harris[17] (1987)	15 pectoralis	9 satisfactory, 2 fair, 4 failures
Noerdlinger et al[18] (2002)	15 pectoralis	2 excellent, 5 good, 4 fair, 4 poor
Steinmann and Wood[19] (2003)	9 pectoralis	4 excellent, 2 good, 3 poor

*All reports are level IV case series.

surgeries with high success rates and satisfaction of patients. Muscle transfers and sling procedures have lower and less predictable results but may still be beneficial to the patient in terms of pain relief and improved function.

REFERENCES

1. Kibler WB, McMullen J. Scapular dyskinesis and its relation to shoulder pain. *J Am Acad Orthop Surg.* 2003;11: 142-151.
2. Kuhn JE, Plancher KD, Hawkins RJ. Symptomatic scapulothoracic crepitus and bursitis. *J Am Acad Orthop Surg.* 1998;6:267-273.
3. Chang WH, Im SH, Ryu JA, et al. The effects of scapulothoracic bursa injections in patients with scapular pain: a pilot study. *Arch Phys Med Rehabil.* 2009;90:279-284.
4. Burkhart SS, Morgan CD, Kibler WB. The disabled throwing shoulder: spectrum of pathology. Part III: the SICK scapula, scapular dyskinesis, the kinetic chain, and rehabilitation. *Arthroscopy.* 2003;19:641-661.
5. Lehtinen JT, Macy JC, Cassinelli E, et al. The painful scapulothoracic articulation. *Clin Orthop Relat Res.* 2004;423:99-105.
6. Thomas DM, Hansen U, Owens BD. Hook retraction for scapulothoracic arthroscopy. *Am J Orthop.* 2011;40: 372-373.
7. Pavlik A, Ang K, Coghlan J, et al. Arthroscopic treatment of painful snapping of the scapula by using a new superior portal. *Arthroscopy.* 2003;19:608-612.
8. Ciullo JV, Jones E. Subscapular bursitis: conservative and endoscopic treatment of "snapping scapula" or "washboard syndrome." *Orthop Trans.* 1993;16:740.
9. McCluskey III GM, Bigliani LU. Surgical management of refractory scapulothoracic bursitis. *Orthop Trans.* 1991;15:801.
10. Nicholson GP, Duckworth MA. Scapulothoracic bursectomy for snapping scapula syndrome. *J Shoulder Elbow Surg.* 2002;11:80-85.

11. Sisto DJ, Jobe FW. The operative treatment of scapulothoracic bursitis in professional pitchers. *Am J Sports Med*. 1986;14:192-194.
12. Arntz CT, Matsen III FA. Partial scapulectomy for disabling scapulothoracic snapping. *Orthop Trans*. 1990;14: 252-253.
13. Harper GD, McIlroy S, Bayley JI, et al. Arthroscopic partial resection of the scapula for snapping scapula: a new technique. *J Shoulder Elbow Surg*. 1999;8:53-57.
14. Richards RR, McKee MD. Treatment of painful scapulothoracic crepitus by resection of the superomedial angle of the scapula: a report of three cases. *Clin Orthop Relat Res*. 1989;247:111-116.
15. Connor PM, Yamaguchi K, Manifold SG, et al. Split pectoralis major transfer for serratus anterior palsy. *Clin Orthop Relat Res*. 1997;341:134-142.
16. Gozna ER, Harris WR. Traumatic winging of the scapula. *J Bone Joint Surg Am*. 1979;61:1230-1233.
17. Iceton J, Harris WR. Treatment of winged scapula by pectoralis major transfer. *J Bone Joint Surg Br*. 1987;69: 108-110.
18. Noerdlinger MA, Cole BJ, Stewart M, et al. Results of pectoralis major transfer with fascia lata autograft augmentation for scapula winging. *J Shoulder Elbow Surg*. 2002;11:345-350.
19. Steinmann SP, Wood MB. Pectoralis major transfer for serratus anterior paralysis. *J Shoulder Elbow Surg*. 2003;12:555-560.

SUGGESTED READINGS

Kuhn JE, Plancher KD, Hawkins RJ. Scapular winging. *J Am Acad Orthop Surg*. 1995;3:319-325.
Kuhn JE, Plancher KD, Hawkins RJ. Symptomatic scapulothoracic crepitus and bursitis. *J Am Acad Orthop Surg*. 1998;6:267-273.
Lazar MA, Kwon YW, Rokito AS. Snapping scapula syndrome. *J Bone Joint Surg Am*. 2009;91:2251-2261.
Manske RC, Reiman MP, Stovak ML. Nonoperative and operative management of snapping scapula. *Am J Sports Med*. 2004;32:1554-1565.

Chapter 32

Scapulothoracic Fusion

James Hammond, Geoffrey S. Van Thiel, Nathan Mall, and Anthony A. Romeo

Chapter Synopsis
- Scapulothoracic arthrodesis is a complex procedure that is used in salvage situations. Conditions for which this procedure is indicated are typically facioscapulohumeral dystrophy or conditions that lead to periscapular muscle or nerve injury that causes significant winging. Pain and loss of motion are the persistent symptoms. Results can be good when the procedure is used in the right patient population.

Important Points
- Scapulothoracic arthrodesis is a salvage procedure.
- Adequate understanding of the anatomy is key to a successful procedure.
- Detailed history and physical examination, appropriate imaging, and preoperative planning will help determine whether surgery is indicated.

Clinical and Surgical Pearls
- Use of adequate positioning and draping aids in adequate exposure and surgery.
- Take time to release the rhomboids and ensure you are in the space between the serratus anterior and the ribcage.
- Remove interposing tissue and achieve adequate bony contact between the ribs and the scapula for optimal fusion mass.
- Care should be taken to protect the pleura and avoid pulmonary injury.
- Apply enough tension on the wires to provide adequate compression, but without overtensioning.
- Use appropriate postoperative protocols to allow time to achieve sufficient fusion.

Clinical and Surgical Pitfalls
- Appropriate patient selection is paramount.
- Failure to remove sufficient soft tissue can compromise fusion.
- Aggressive decortication can result in scapular perforation or fracture.

The scapulothoracic articulation is one of four joints that work in concert to allow the shoulder to have the greatest range of motion of any joint in the body. Scapulothoracic motion is a significant contributor because it helps account for one third of shoulder elevation. Causes of dysfunction of the scapulothoracic joint can essentially be broken into two categories: dystrophic and nondystrophic. The primary dystrophic cause is facioscapulohumeral dystrophy (FSHD). Nondystrophic causes include peripheral nerve injury, failed tendon transfers for nerve injury, brachial plexus injuries, and stroke. These conditions ultimately alter the stability of the scapular platform and affect glenohumeral motion. Commonly this manifests as scapular winging and loss of shoulder motion that lead to pain. Scapulothoracic arthrodesis has been described as a viable salvage operation.[1,2] The goal of this procedure is to create a solid union between the anterior surface of the scapula and the posterior thorax to stabilize this articulation, restore some level of function, and alleviate pain.[3]

PREOPERATIVE CONSIDERATIONS

History

At presentation, patients may have FSHD—a genetic disorder that leads to progressive muscular weakness and muscle loss and primarily affects face, shoulder, and upper arm muscles. This condition affects about 5 per 100,000 people. Genetic studies often demonstrate a deletion in the long arm of chromosome 4. Facial symptoms often accompany this condition and can vary from ptosis to speech problems.[4] Brachial plexus injuries from birth or recent trauma may be noted. Trauma or other conditions may be elucidated that have lead to muscle injury or peripheral nerve injury.

Physical Examination

Primarily patients have pain combined with loss of forward elevation and abduction. Depending on the cause, various forms of scapular winging may be present. Medial winging of the scapula caused by serratus anterior or long thoracic nerve injury typically occurs with superior migration and medial rotation of the inferior border of the scapula. Lateral winging of the scapula caused by trapezius or spinal accessory nerve injury is associated with inferior migration and lateral rotation of the inferior border of the scapula. More subtle winging resulting from rhomboid or dorsal scapular nerve injury will manifest similarly to lateral winging with inferior migration and lateral rotation of the inferior border. In most patients the deltoid and rotator cuff function is preserved. Range of motion is usually less than 90 degrees of forward elevation and abduction. Atrophy of the shoulder girdle should also be noted. These visual cues will help lead the examiner to determine if any nerve injury is present and which nerves are involved. Another test that is helpful is to stabilize the scapula with one's hand and determine if the patient's range of motion improves. This will provide insight to the possible motion to be gained from the procedure by providing a stable platform for function.

Imaging

No imaging modalities will provide significant insight into this particular diagnosis. The pathology is a dynamic phenomenon and is not structural. Plain radiographs may demonstrate abnormal scapular positioning with significant elevation of the superomedial border or lateral translation depending on the underlying pathology. Nerve injury patterns might be identified on magnetic resonance imaging (MRI) but again are not diagnostic. Electromyography can be useful in determining nerve injury and the extent of injury. It is important to identify whether transient neurapraxic changes are present versus a more permanent injury. Neurapraxic injuries resulting from trauma often will spontaneously recover within 1 year. These patients often can be followed and conservative measures used to maintain range of motion and muscle strength in functioning groups.

Indications

Indications for scapulothoracic fusion include pain and persistent loss of function. These basic complaints can be related to nerve injury with persistent electromyographic changes for longer than 1 year with no recovery, FSHD, or other neuromuscular disease. In these patients, extensive physical therapy and other conservative measures have typically failed. Some patients have undergone muscle transfers for scapular winging caused by nerve injury, yet have persistent symptoms. Patients with FSHD are not candidates for muscle transfers owing to the global nature of the disease process, and fusion is indicated. Scapulothoracic arthrodesis is essentially a salvage procedure for these patients.

Contraindications

Axillary nerve injury and poor deltoid function are contraindications for scapulothoracic arthrodesis. The deltoid becomes one of the prime movers for shoulder function and range of motion with fusion and must be working properly. Relative contraindications include poor bone quality, smoking, and significant pulmonary compromise. Fusion does alter rib cage excursion, which can affect respiratory function.

SURGICAL PROCEDURE

Anesthesia and Positioning

The patient is brought to the operating room and given preoperative antibiotics. After induction of general anesthesia and intubation, the patient is moved to a prone position. Care must be taken to ensure that the patient's abdomen is free to maximize ventilation and minimize intra-abdominal pressure. Bony prominences should be padded and the arms should be in a position to avoid awkward shoulder positioning and nerve compression. The operative arm is placed in 90 degrees of abduction and external rotation with 30 degrees of horizontal adduction. The upper arm, neck, and spine all the way to the posterior superior iliac spine should be prepped into the surgical field. This allows for some movement of the extremity and harvesting of bone graft during the procedure.

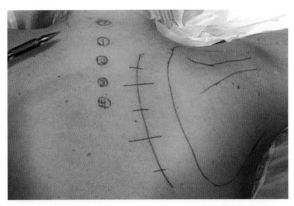

Figure 32-1. Patient position with anatomic landmarks drawn and planned incision.

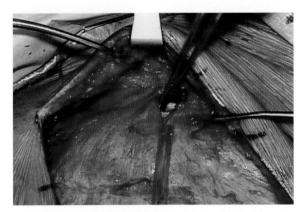

Figure 32-2. Split made in the trapezius to expose the medial border of the scapula.

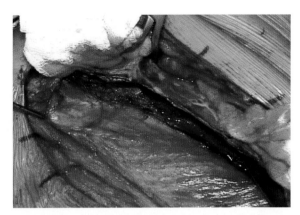

Figure 32-3. Use of the towel clip and tension allows exposure of the medial scapular border and release of rhomboids.

Surgical Landmarks

Surgical landmarks that should be marked before the procedure include the spinous processes of C7 to T4, the associated thoracic ribs, and the superior, medial, and lateral borders of the scapula (Fig. 32-1). Typically with the arm positioned as described earlier, the spine of the scapula overlies the fourth rib and the scapula is rotated approximately 30 degrees in relation to the spinous processes.

Specific Steps

Box 32-1 outlines the specific steps of this procedure.

After surgical timeout an incision is made along the medial border of the scapula, and subcutaneous flaps are raised to expose the trapezius over the entire dimension of the scapula. A split is then made in the trapezius to identify the medial border of the scapula (Fig. 32-2). The supraspinatus and infraspinatus are then subperiosteally elevated to expose the medial scapula for about 3 cm. A towel clip is then used to pull on the scapula, which puts tension on the rhomboids and levator scapulae muscles (Fig. 32-3). These muscles are raised from

BOX 32-1 Surgical Steps

1. Position prone with 90 degrees of abduction and 30 degrees of horizontal adduction.
2. Identify appropriate landmarks and incision orientation.
3. Create skin flaps to expose the entire scapula.
4. Incise the trapezius to expose the medial border of the scapula.
5. Raise flaps of supraspinatus, infraspinatus, and teres minor.
6. Elevate the medial border of the scapula to tension the rhomboid major and minor and elevate them.
7. Mobilize serratus and subscapularis ventrally about 3 cm laterally.
8. Remove scapulothoracic bursa and expose the third through sixth ribs.
9. Circumferentially expose these ribs while protecting the neurovascular structures off the inferior border.
10. Decorticate the posterior ribs and the ventral scapular body.
11. Pass Luque wires under each rib.
12. Obtain bone graft from posterior superior iliac spine and place around ribs and scapula.
13. Fashion 4.5-mm plate to dorsal scapula and drill holes, protecting the pleura underneath.
14. Pass wires and tension through plate.
15. Place final bone graft medial to border.
16. Reattach muscle layers to scapula.
17. Perform final subcutaneous and skin closure.

the medial border of the scapula and tagged (Fig. 32-4). Care is taken at this point to enter the scapulothoracic space between the serratus and the ribcage and to not enter the interval between the serratus and the subscapularis. Visualization or palpation of the rib helps to ensure that the correct space has been entered.

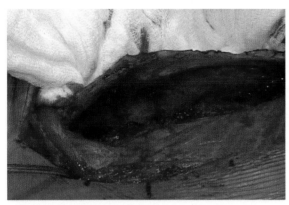

Figure 32-4. Medial scapular border exposed after mobilization of the musculature.

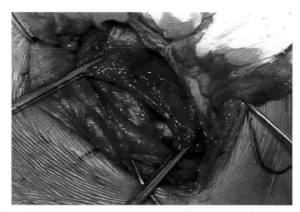

Figure 32-6. Removal of bursal tissue from between the ribs and the scapula.

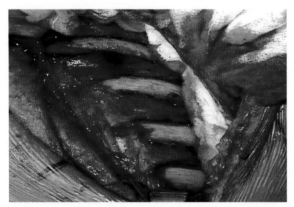

Figure 32-5. Exposure of the posterior ribs. Care must be taken to avoid the inferior neurovascular structures during dissection.

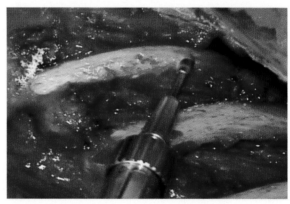

Figure 32-7. Gentle decortication of the posterior ribs with a high-speed bur assists in achieving fusion.

Attention is then turned to identification of the seventh cervical spinous process, which then allows identification of the third through sixth ribs. These ribs are then circumferentially exposed (Fig. 32-5). Care must be taken inferior on each rib to separate out the intercostal neurovascular bundle and minimize injury to these structures. Attention must also be paid in dissecting the parietal pleura from the rib surface, allowing passage of wires and minimizing injury to these structures.

At this point there should be excellent bony apposition between the anterior surface of the scapula and the posterior rib surface. Any intervening soft tissues should be removed at this time (Fig. 32-6). These bony surfaces are then lightly decorticated with a high-speed bur. A malleable retractor can be placed under each rib to protect the lung tissue from the bur (Fig. 32-7). The scapula is also decorticated on the ventral surface to allow adequate bleeding bone surface for fusion. The scapular body becomes quite thin away from the medial border, and bone perforation can occur with decortication.

A four- or five-hole 4.5-mm reconstruction plate is selected and contoured, and the wires are passed under the ribs and through the scapula/plate (Fig. 32-8). Drill holes are then placed through the scapula and centered over the fourth, fifth, and sixth ribs. Again the malleable retractor is used to protect the underlying pleural tissue. The spine of the scapula is reassessed to ensure it lies over the fourth rib with the desired 30 degrees of rotation. A looped 18-gauge Luque wire is positioned under each rib and then the loop is cut, which creates two wires under each rib (Fig. 32-9). The fourth rib wires are passed first and lightly tensioned over the plate. The fifth and sixth rib wires are tensioned. The wires under the third rib are passed through a drill or bur hole and tensioned, as well.

To ensure that no pleural injury has occurred, sterile saline is next poured into the wound. A deep breath is then provided by the anesthesia staff, and the surgeon should observe for any bubbles that may appear. Bubbles are indicative of a pleural injury and if present may necessitate the use of a chest tube postoperatively.

Bone graft is then obtained from the posterior superior iliac spine and placed between the scapula and each rib (Fig. 32-10). Allograft bone can be added to provide enough graft between the scapula and ribs. Once the graft is in place, one final check should be made to

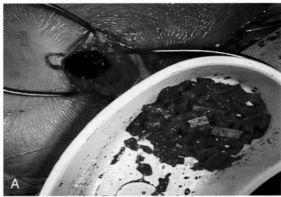

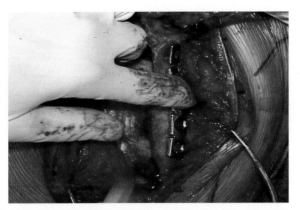

Figure 32-8. Contour the plate to fit the dorsal scapular surface inferior to the spine of the scapula.

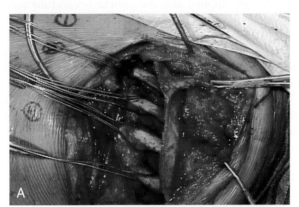

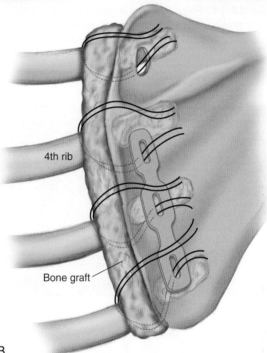

Figure 32-10. A, Obtain bone graft from posterior superior iliac crest. **B,** Bone graft is passed under the scapula for 3 to 5 cm over each rib. The wires are then tensioned and the remainder of the bone graft is placed at the medial border of the scapula.

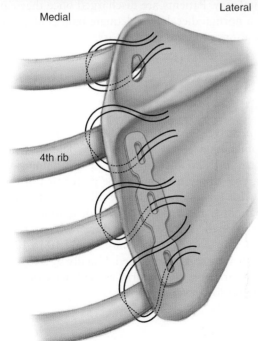

Figure 32-9. A, Passage of Luque wires under each rib. **B,** Wire setup. Two wired passed under each rib with one limb through the hole in the scapula and plate and the other limb over the construct. These are tied and tensioned individually.

ensure that the appropriate position has been maintained. In addition to the 30-degree rotation, the medial border should be about 5 to 7 cm lateral to the spinous processes. The wires then undergo sequential tightening to compress the scapula to the ribs (Fig. 32-11). The plate aids in dispersing forces and avoiding cutout of the thin bone of the scapula. Remaining bone graft is then placed along the medial border of the scapula and the exposed ribs (Fig. 32-12).

The surrounding musculature is then repaired back to the scapula. The supraspinatus and infraspinatus are allowed to fall naturally back into their respective fossae and sutured medially into place. The rhomboids are then reattached to the medial border of the scapula and the wound is closed in layers (Fig. 32-13). Sterile

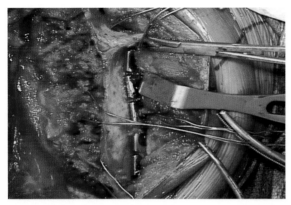

Figure 32-11. Place final bone graft adjacent to medial scapular border after passage of Luque wires through drill holes and plate before sequential tightening.

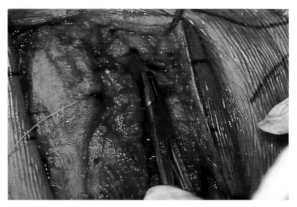

Figure 32-13. Reattach rhomboids to medial scapular border.

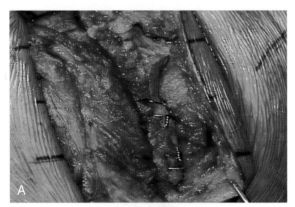

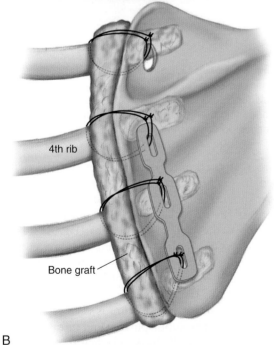

4th rib

Bone graft

B

Figure 32-12. A, Final construct before closure. **B,** Final bone graft, plate, and tensioned wires. Spine of the scapula positioned at the fourth rib.

dressings are applied and the patient is carefully rolled to a supine position. Care is taken to minimize scapular motion during this process. The arm is immobilized in 10 degrees of external rotation, 15 degrees of abduction, and neutral flexion and extension of the shoulder.

The patient is typically kept in the hospital for 72 to 96 hours to monitor for pulmonary complications, pain control, and initiation of physical therapy. A chest radiograph is taken in the recovery room and repeated on postoperative day 1 to evaluate for pneumothorax and/or pulmonary effusion. Findings of careful neurovascular examination are also monitored during the hospital stay. Patients are discharged once they can tolerate a normal diet, have adequate pain control on oral medications, and are ambulatory.

POSTOPERATIVE CONSIDERATIONS

Postoperative rehabilitation begins with strict sling immobilization for 4 to 6 weeks. The patient is to perform no shoulder motion or pendulums. Hand, wrist, and elbow motion can be performed in the sling only with no significant lifting allowed. After 6 weeks the patient is allowed to perform pendulums and begin active-assisted range of motion, which is slowly advanced to active range of motion. At 10 to 12 weeks, strengthening can be advanced. Usually by 3 to 4 months patients are able to perform typical activities of daily living and low-level activities.

RESULTS

Scapulothoracic fusion is a rare procedure, and therefore the literature on results and outcomes is limited to level IV case series (Table 32-1). Glenn and Romeo reported on 25 patients who underwent 32 scapulothoracic fusions. Eighteen of these patients had FSHD, and

TABLE 32-1. Summary of the Literature on Scapulothoracic Fusions

Author	No. of Patients (Extremities)	Age (y) (Range)	Diagnosis	Technique	Follow-up (mo) (Range)	Flexion Preop	Flexion Postop	Abduction Preop	Abduction Postop	FEV1	Satisfied (%)	Complications (%)	Type
Ketenjian[14] (1978)	3 (5)	24 (24-27)	FSH	Mersilene tape or fascia lata	34 (20-60)			56	87.6			None reported	
Letournel et al[8] (1990)	9 (16)	23 (17-35)	FSH	Plates, wires, overlying rib	69 (24-133)	75	108	77	102	NS			PTx—3 PEff—1 Fx—1 NU—1 SFx—2
Twyman et al[12] (1996)	6 (12)	30 (17-44)	FSH	Wires, ICBG	49 (12-80)	56	96	63	91	NS			SFx—1 BW—3 NU—1 NP—1 HTx—1
Andrews et al[9] (1998)	6 (10)	23 (17-33)	FSH	Wires, ICBG	73 (28-120)	52.5	111	56.5	112	NS			PTx—1 PEff—1 BW—6
Berne et al[7] (2003)	33 (49)	28 (16-56)	FSH	Plates, wires, overlying rib	102 (12-257)	69	81	70	81		93%		NU—1 BW—2 PTx—5 PEff—4 Fx—2 SFx—2 NP—2 PHW—2
Bizot et al[15] (2003)	10 (10)	39 (22-57)	SAP	Wires, ICBG	76 (12-180)	83	101	72	93		75%	38%	NU—1 FS—1
Diab et al[5] (2005)	8 (11)	17 (11-21)	FSH	Wires, washers, plates, ICBG	72 (24-120)	75	102.7	75	105.5			18%	PHW—2
Jeon et al[6] (2005)	6 (6)	30 (22-39)	ND	Wire, rush rod, ICBG	49 (28-89)			80	98		100%		
Rhee and Ha[10] (2006)	6 (9)	25 (15-37)	FSH	Vertical plate and wires, ICBG	102 (56-118)	71	109	76	108	NS			PEff—1
Ziaee et al[13] (2006)	6 (8)	25.4	FSH	Plates, wires	32.5 (14-55)	64	104	67.5	112.5			25%	HTx—2
Demirhan et al[11] (2009)	13 (18)	29 (20-50)	FSH	Wires, ICBG	36 (24-87)	47.2	102.2	55.6	126.1	NS		11%	NU—2 BW—1 PHW—1

All studies were level IV evidence.

BW, Broken wire; FEV1, forced expiratory volume in 1 second; FS, frozen shoulder; FSH, facioscapulohumeral dystrophy; Fx, fracture; HTx, hemothorax; ICBG, iliac crest bone graft; ND, nondystrophic disorders; NP, nerve palsy; NS, not significant; NU, nonunion; PEff, pulmonary effusion; PHW, painful hardware; PTx, pneumothorax; SAP, serratus anterior palsy; SFx, stress fracture.

seven were secondary to posttraumatic injuries. The average gain in forward flexion was 38 degrees, and external rotation improved 6 degrees. Improvements were noted in the Simple Shoulder Test and American Shoulder and Elbow Surgeons scores.[3] FSHD patients make up the majority of those who undergo scapulothoracic fusion. Several case series have reported results of this procedure for other diagnoses, which reveal similar outcomes to those with FSHD.[4,5] Another study by Berne and colleagues[6] reviewed 49 shoulders in 33 patients with FSHD and was a continuation of the study by Letournel and colleagues.[7] The authors in these studies used a technique similar to that described in this chapter, in which wires are passed through the scapula and a plate. Results yielded an average increase in forward flexion of 12 degrees and an average increase in abduction of 11 degrees at a mean follow-up of 102 months. Several authors noted a significant decrease in motion as the length of follow-up increased, as a result of progressive weakness in the deltoid as the patients aged; however, several other studies demonstrated nearly 30-degree improvements in flexion and abduction despite average follow-up of about 6 years.[5,8-10] Pain relief was cited in all articles; however, only two studies reported validated outcome scores or pain scales.[10,11] Patients can also be expected to have preserved lung function, with several studies demonstrating no significant change in forced expiratory volume in 1 second (FEV_1) from preoperative status to final follow-up.[5,8-10,12,13] Complications were quite common, and patients and parents should be warned of a complication rate of 5% to 25%, with pneumothorax, hardware complications and fractures being the most common. Scapulothoracic fusion is a salvage procedure that is a useful and predictable procedure in a specific population. Excellent pain relief and improved function can be achieved in patients with scapular winging from multiple causes, but in particular in those with FSHD.

REFERENCES

1. DeFranco MJ, Nho S, Romeo AA. Scapulothoracic fusion. *J Am Acad Orthop Surg.* 2010;18:236-242.

2. Krishnan SG, Hawkins RJ, Michelotti JD, et al. Scapulothoracic arthrodesis: indications, technique, and results. *Clin Orthop Relat Res.* 2005;435:126-133.

3. Glenn RE, Romeo AA. Scapulothoracic arthrodesis: indications and surgical technique. *Tech Shoulder Elbow Surg.* 2005;6(3):178-187.

4. Fascioscapulohumeral dystrophy. PubMed Health. www.ncbi.nlm.nih.gov/pubmedhealth/PMH0001726/. Obtained Sept 7, 2011.

5. Diab M, Darras BT, Shapiro F. Scapulothoracic fusion for facioscapulohumeral muscular dystrophy. *J Bone Joint Surg Am.* 2005;87:2267-2275.

6. Jeon IH, Neumann L, Wallace WA. Scapulothoracic fusion for painful winging of the scapula in nondystrophic patients. *J Shoulder Elbow Surg.* 2005;14:400-406.

7. Berne D, Laude F, Laporte C, et al. Scapulothoracic arthrodesis in facioscapulohumeral muscular dystrophy. *Clin Orthop Relat Res.* 2003:106-113.

8. Letournel E, Fardeau M, Lytle JO, et al. Scapulothoracic arthrodesis for patients who have facioscapulohumeral muscular dystrophy. *J Bone Joint Surg Am.* 1990;72:78-84.

9. Andrews CT, Taylor TC, Patterson VH. Scapulothoracic arthrodesis for patients with facioscapulohumeral muscular dystrophy. *Neuromuscul Disord.* 1998;8:580-584.

10. Rhee YG, Ha JH. Long-term results of scapulothoracic arthrodesis of facioscapulohumeral muscular dystrophy. *J Shoulder Elbow Surg.* 2006;15:445-450.

11. Demirhan M, Uysal O, Atalar AC, et al. Scapulothoracic arthrodesis in facioscapulohumeral dystrophy with multifilament cable. *Clin Orthop Relat Res.* 2009;467:2090-2097.

12. Twyman RS, Harper GD, Edgar MA. Thoracoscapular fusion in facioscapulohumeral dystrophy: clinical review of a new surgical method. *J Shoulder Elbow Surg.* 1996;5:201-205.

13. Ziaee MA, Abolghasemian M, Majd ME. Scapulothoracic arthrodesis for winged scapula due to facioscapulohumeral dystrophy (a new technique). *Am J Orthop (Belle Mead NJ).* 2006;35:311-315.

14. Ketenjian AY. Scapulocostal stabilization for scapular winging in facioscapulohumeral muscular dystrophy. *J Bone Joint Surg Am.* 1978;60:476-480.

15. Bizot P, Teboul F, Nizard R, et al. Scapulothoracic fusion for serratus anterior paralysis. *J Shoulder Elbow Surg.* 2003;12:561-565.

Chapter 33

Biceps Tenodesis: Arthroscopic and Open Techniques

Shane Hanzlik and Michael J. Salata

Chapter Synopsis
- Biceps tenodesis is an effective treatment for pathology of the long head of the biceps tendon. This chapter discusses both open and arthroscopic methods for performing tenodesis, explaining the procedures in a stepwise manner. Common pitfalls and clinical pearls are also discussed.

Important Points
- Be sure that concomitant problems such as rotator cuff pathology are diagnosed and addressed.
- Thoroughly evaluate the biceps tendon arthroscopically by pulling the extra-articular portion into the joint. Arthroscopic findings should correlate with the clinical examination.
- Meticulous tunnel preparation is the key to the min-open subpectoral tenodesis technique.

Clinical and Surgical Pearls
- Make the skin incision more inferior than might seem appropriate. There is no reason for the incision to extend above the inferior border of the pectoralis major.
- Placing the lateral retractor through the pectoralis tendon one third above the inferior border allows for excellent exposure of the tunnel entry site.
- Careful placement of the medial retractor is mandatory. The structures at risk include the brachial artery and musculocutaneous nerve.

- Center the guide pin medially to laterally 1 cm above the inferior border of the pectoralis tendon. Be sure the reamer enters perpendicular to the humerus, and *do not* violate the posterior cortex.
- Use of the tap allows for easier screw placement. Be sure to remove all soft tissue at the tunnel entry (a bovie is helpful) to minimize difficulty in starting the screw.
- It is better to err on the side of too short than too long; it is very difficult to overtighten the repair.

Clinical and Surgical Pitfalls
- It is not uncommon to begin the dissection either too proximal or too lateral. If the anatomy described in the chapter is not easily identified, consider reorienting before further dissection.
- Leaving tendon in the intertubercular groove may be a source of persistent discomfort or "groove pain." This can be a pitfall of arthroscopic techniques.
- Avoid retractor misplacement or overzealous medial retraction; this can damage the musculocutaneous nerve.
- Violation of the posterior humeral cortex with interference screw fixation can lead to humerus fracture and should be avoided.

Pathology of the long head of the biceps tendon (LHBT) has long been recognized as a significant cause of anterior shoulder pain that can affect the scope and quality of a patient's activity level.[1-3] The diagnosis of this particular disease process can be challenging because there are many sources that can produce anterior shoulder pain.

While debate exists about whether pathology of the LHBT is a primary disease process[2] or is secondary to concurrent disease processes such as impingement or subscapularis dysfunction,[1,3] the end result is a painful shoulder that can be a persistent cause of disability for patients who are often young and active. Treatment methods devised for the surgical management of biceps pathology and include tenotomy,[4-6] tenodesis,[7-9] and tendon relocation with reconstruction of the biceps pulley.[10]

Multiple surgical procedures have been described to address the pathology associated with the LHBT. Although the pathologic tendon was commonly debrided or treated with tenotomy in the past, tenodesis has become a more common method of treatment. Currently, there is no clear consensus as to whether tenotomy or tenodesis is superior[4]; biomechanical[2,3,5,11,12] and clinical[8,13,14] studies have shown both procedures to be effective. Tenodesis is more commonly being performed over tenotomy for several reasons, including improved cosmetic appearance, maintenance of elbow flexion and supination strength, and maintenance of the biceps muscle length-tension relationship.[9]

The course of the LHBT is unique, and the path taken by the tendon can contribute to pathologic conditions that result in a painful shoulder. The tendon is intra-articular, but transitions to an extrasynovial portion that averages 9 cm in length and 5 to 6 cm in diameter. The tendon originates from the superior glenoid tubercle and the superior labrum,[12] which is known as the biceps anchor. From this starting position the tendon exits the glenohumeral joint by passing through the rotator interval descending into the intertubercular groove. The "bicipital groove" has been reported to be variable in its dimensions, with an average depth of 4.3 mm.[15] This variation has been reported to be a factor in biceps instability and other pathologic conditions including tendinopathy of the LHBT.[15,16] The LHBT is contained between the greater and lesser tuberosities by a sling of tissue composed of fibers from the anterior rotator cuff (supraspinatus and subscapularis), the coracohumeral ligament, and the superior glenohumeral ligament (SGHL).[11] The SGHL, which arises from the supraglenoid and the base of the coracoid, travels within the rotator interval, forming a semicircular sling anteriorly for the lateral part of the intra-articular LHBT before attaching at the lesser tuberosity of the proximal humerus.[17] Pain localized to the bicipital groove can be a cause of failure for those patients undergoing a proximal biceps tenodesis or tenotomy when adhesions are present.

Both arthroscopic and open techniques can be used for tenodesis. Fixation methods include interference screws, suture anchors, fixation to the coracoid process, or suture fixation to the rotator interval. Interference screw fixation has been shown to be a superior method in terms of biomechanical load to failure compared with suture anchor or soft tissue fixation. Some surgeons believe that failure to remove diseased tendon from the bicipital groove and retention of pain-generating synovial tissue in this confined space may be a cause of failure for some forms of tenodesis. Although both arthroscopic and open techniques will be discussed in this chapter, a mini-open subpectoral biceps tenodesis with a soft tissue interference screw is our preference.

PREOPERATIVE CONSIDERATIONS

History

- Pain is localized to the anterior aspect of the shoulder (in or near the location of the bicipital groove). This pain may or may not radiate to the biceps muscle belly distally
- Associated shoulder pathology may include rotator cuff disease, glenohumeral arthritis, subscapularis pathology, previous fracture, and superior labral pathology (superior labral anterior-posterior [SLAP] tears)
- Pain occurs with functions that require use of the biceps: forward shoulder elevation, active forearm supination, active elbow flexion.

Physical Examination

- Tenderness over the bicipital groove, which lies 7 cm distal to the acromion, is the most common finding in this patient population[14] and is seen to migrate laterally with external rotation and medially with internal rotation of the shoulder.
- Pain is elicited by tests specific for biceps pathology:
  - Speed test: Pain elicited by resisted forward flexion.
  - Yergason test: Result is considered positive if anterior shoulder pain is experienced with resisted forearm supination.[13]
- The biceps tendinosis test (BTT) described by Mazzocca and colleagues[9] is a test to diagnose pain from biceps pathology located in the subpectoral triangle. A two-part test, the BTT begins with examiner placing his or her index finger into the axilla underneath the pectoralis major tendon, allowing palpation of the biceps in this region. If the patient's discomfort is reproduced and is asymmetrical to the contralateral (normal) side, a combination of local anesthetic and steroid is injected into the glenohumeral joint. The patient is then allowed to rest for 3 to 5 minutes, and the first part of the test is repeated. If a significant portion of the patient's pain is relieved, the test result is considered positive; this is indicative of biceps pathology.

Imaging

- Standard shoulder plain radiographs may include true anteroposterior (AP), scapular oblique, and axillary views.
- Magnetic resonance imaging (MRI) or magnetic resonance arthrography is performed as indicated for associated pathology such as rotator cuff disease or superior labral pathology.

- Musculoskeletal ultrasound can include dynamic testing when the differential diagnosis includes a subluxing biceps tendon.

Indications and Contraindications

The decision to treat biceps pathology should be predicated on the fact that conservative management, including a period of rest from aggravating activities, a course of physical therapy that may include active release therapy, and corticosteroid injections, has failed. When nonoperative management has been shown to be unsuccessful and the patient's clinical history and physical examination findings are consistent with the diagnosis of biceps pathology, surgical management can be selected. A careful screen for associated pathology is mandatory to rule out other concomitant shoulder conditions that may be mimicking or contributing to the patient's anterior shoulder complaints. Although these conditions should be screened for and corrected when present, they are by no means contraindications to biceps surgery.

Inability to tolerate the anesthetic that is necessary for shoulder surgery is the only true contraindication to this procedure. In patients with osteopenia or osteoporosis, interference screw fixation should be weighed against the possible risk of fracture.

SURGICAL TECHNIQUE

Anesthesia and Positioning

- The beach chair or lateral position may be used. We prefer to use a standard beach chair position (table back to 90 degrees) for the arthroscopic portion of the procedure and then to recline the back of the table to 30 to 45 degrees for the exposure and tenodesis portion of the procedure.
- For exposure and visualization the senior author (M.S.) finds it easier to use a pneumatic arm-positioning device to hold the arm in 80 to 90 degrees of forward elevation, 45 degrees of abduction, and neutral to slight external rotation.
- Anesthesia is typically general anesthesia with an interscalene block placed preoperatively. Adequate local anesthesia is required at the site of the exposure because this area is covered variably by the nerve block.

Surgical Landmarks, Incisions, and Portals

Landmarks
- Acromion
- Clavicle and acromioclavicular (AC) joint

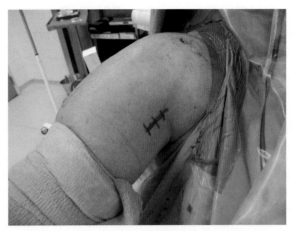

Figure 33-1. A 1-to 1.5-cm incision is made just distal to the inferior border of the pectoralis major tendon at the medial aspect of the axillary fold.

- Coracoid
- Pectoralis major tendon

Portals
- Standard posterior viewing portal
- Standard anterior working portal through the rotator interval
- Other portals as necessary for concomitant procedures

Incisions
- A 1- to 1.5-cm incision is made just distal to the inferior border of the pectoralis major tendon at the medial aspect of the axillary fold (Fig. 33-1).
- Structures at risk with this approach include the cephalic vein, musculocutaneous nerve, and pectoralis major tendon.

Examination under Anesthesia and Diagnostic Arthroscopy

- Examination under anesthesia should be performed on all patients undergoing shoulder arthroscopy. Assessment of glenohumeral range of motion (ROM) should be performed, and the necessity of a capsular release determined at this point of the procedure. Glenohumeral stability should also be assessed and documented.
- Diagnostic arthroscopy should include a systematic assessment of the glenohumeral joint including the biceps tendon, the articular cartilage of the glenoid and humerus, the subscapularis tendon, the intra-articular appearance of the posterior rotator cuff tendons, and the appearance of the superior labrum as well as the labrum in its entirety.

Specific Steps for Mini-Open Subpectoral Tenodesis with Interference Screw

Box 33-1 lists the specific steps for this procedure.

1. Arthroscopic Preparation

The arthroscope is placed in the standard posterior portal and introduced atraumatically into the glenohumeral joint. A systematic review of the glenohumeral joint is then performed. The biceps is inspected, and the extra-articular portion is pulled into the joint with the use of a probe. Injection of the tendon or fraying is consistent with bicipital disease and is documented. More than 30% to 50% of biceps fraying is considered by most authors to be the threshold for definitive treatment with tenotomy or tenodesis.

2. Biceps Tenotomy

Although there are multiple ways to perform tenotomy of the biceps, it is the senior author's preferred technique to use a basket forceps inserted through the anterior portal, which is cannulated. The biceps tendon is transected at the superior labral junction.

3. Exposure

The arm is forward flexed to about 90 degrees, abducted to 45 degrees, and placed in neutral to slight external rotation. The inferior border of the pectoralis major tendon is then palpated and marked with a skin marker. A 2- to 4-cm incision is then made in line with the axillary fold and carried through the skin and subcutaneous tissues to the level of the fascia overlying the pectoralis major and the short head of the biceps. The interval between the pectoralis and short head of the biceps muscle is then identified and the fascia is incised in line with the incision. Blunt dissection with a finger is then performed, and the undersurface of the pectoralis tendon is freed of adhesions. The bicipital groove should be easily palpated at this point with the LHBT residing within it on the back of the pectoralis major. If the anatomy is not easily identified, the dissection is likely too lateral or proximal. A large pointed Hohmann retractor is placed through the pectoralis tendon at the junction of the superior two thirds and distal one third over the lateral cortex of the humerus. A second blunt Chandler retractor is placed medially, with great care taken to hug the humerus and avoid interposing soft tissue because overzealous retraction medially or failure to stay next to bone can injure the musculocutaneous nerve (Fig. 33-2). The LHBT at the musculotendinous junction is visualized and retrieved with a right angle clamp or with the surgeon's finger and delivered into the wound (Fig. 33-3).

4. Tunnel Preparation

Many methods exist for the remainder of the operation. It is the senior author's preference to use a commercially available tenodesis system called the Biceptor system (Smith & Nephew, Andover, MA) (Fig. 33-4). The area 1 cm proximal to the inferior border of the pectoralis major tendon in the bicipital groove is identified. A 2.4-mm guide pin is advanced through the near cortex to the far cortex but should not engage the far cortex because this could lead to a stress riser (Fig. 33-5). The placement of the guide pin should be perpendicular to the humerus and should be central from medial to lateral. An 8-mm acorn reamer is then used to over-ream the guide pin through the near cortex (Fig. 33-6). Again, great care should be taken to avoid any violation of the posterior cortex. The reamer is then backed out, the wound is copiously irrigated, and all bony debris is removed (Fig. 33-7). The tunnel is then tapped to a depth of 15 mm with the tap provided on the instrument set.

5. Tenodesis

The appropriate biceps fork is then selected (8 mm) and used to push the biceps tendon into the prepared tunnel. The fork is placed 1 cm proximal to the

---

BOX 33-1 Surgical Steps for Mini-Open Subpectoral Tenodesis with Interference Screw

1. Arthroscopic preparation
2. Biceps tenotomy
3. Exposure
4. Tunnel preparation
5. Tenodesis
6. Closure

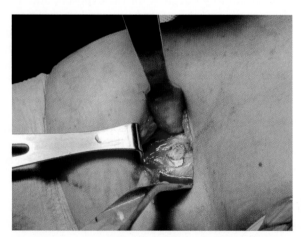

Figure 33-2. A blunt Chandler retractor is placed medially to hug the humerus without interposing soft tissue, because overzealous retraction medially or failure to stay next to bone can injure the musculocutaneous nerve.

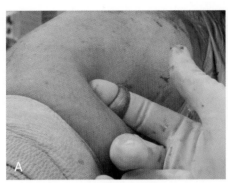
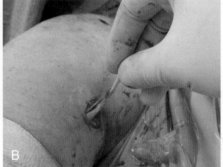

Figure 33-3. The long head of the biceps tendon at the musculotendinous junction is visualized and retrieved with the surgeon's finger and delivered into the wound.

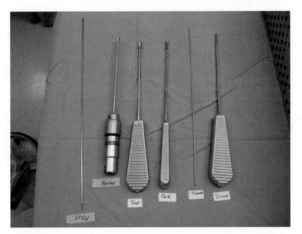

Figure 33-4. The Biceptor system (Smith & Nephew, Andover, MA).

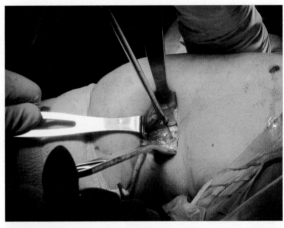

Figure 33-6. An 8-mm acorn reamer is used to over-ream the guide pin through the near cortex.

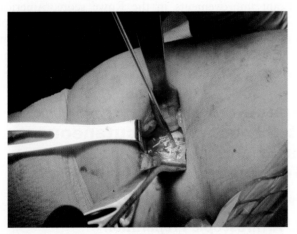

Figure 33-5. A 2.4-mm guide pin is advanced through the near cortex to the far cortex but should not engage the far cortex because this may lead to a stress riser.

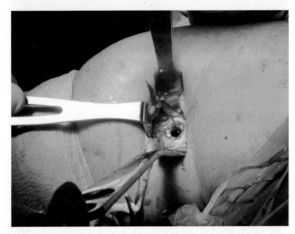

Figure 33-7. The reamer is backed out, the wound is copiously irrigated, and all bony debris is removed.

musculotendinous junction. On the back table the 1.5-mm tendon pin is secured to the bi-grip pin puller, and this construct is then inserted through the tendon fork and hammered to just engage the posterior cortex. This will secure the tendon in the tunnel (Fig. 33-8). The bi-grip pin puller is then removed and the tendon fork

withdrawn. Excess tendon is trimmed and residual tendon is pushed deep into the tunnel with forceps. An 8 × 15 mm polyetheretherketone (PEEK) interference screw (Biceptor Screw, Smith & Nephew) is then placed on the cannulated screwdriver, and this is introduced over the 1.5-mm guidewire. The screw is then advanced

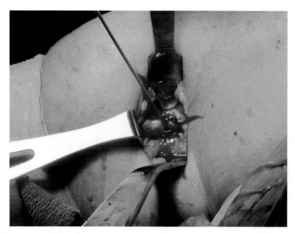

Figure 33-8. A 1.5-mm tendon pin is secured to the bi-grip pin puller, and this construct is then inserted through the tendon fork and hammered to just engage the posterior cortex. This will secure the tendon in the tunnel.

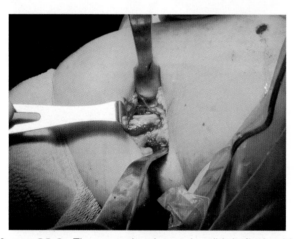

Figure 33-9. The screw is advanced until it is flush with the near cortex.

until it is flush with the near cortex (Fig. 33-9). Care should be taken to be sure the screw is not advanced too far or left proud. Tension is assessed; the wound is again copiously irrigated, and hemostasis is ensured.

6. Closure

If the fascia can be easily identified, No. 0 Vicryl is used for fascial closure. The deep dermal layer is closed with a 2-0 Vicryl suture, and a running subcutaneous closure of the skin is performed with a 3-0 Monocryl stitch. Dermabond is then used to seal the wound, given its proximity to the axilla.

Postoperative Considerations

Follow-up

The patient is seen in the office 7 to 10 days postoperatively; the suture ends are clipped and the wound is assessed. The standard three radiographic views are repeated to assess for tunnel location.

BOX 33-2 Surgical Steps for the Arthroscopic Percutaneous Intra-articular Transtendon Technique

1. Arthroscopic preparation
2. Suture passage
3. Biceps tenotomy
4. Suture retrieval and knot tying

Rehabilitation

Rehabilitation is often dictated by any concomitant procedures performed (e.g., rotator cuff repair). For tenodesis performed in isolation:

- Motion: Progress from passive to active and active-assisted ROM
- Strengthening: Begins at 12 weeks postoperatively
- Full activity: Unrestricted at 4 to 6 months postoperatively

Complications

- Infection
- Construct failure
- Persistent pain
- Musculocutaneous nerve injury
- Humerus fracture
- Hematoma or seroma

Results

Published data on this technique show statistically significant improvements in the Rowe score, American Shoulder and Elbow Surgeons scale (ASES) score, simple shoulder test score, and Constant-Murley score and a significant decrease in the visual analogue pain scale result.

Specific Steps for the Arthroscopic Percutaneous Intra-articular Transtendon Technique[18]

Box 33-2 lists the specific steps of this procedure.

1. Arthroscopic Preparation

The patient is placed in either the beach chair or the lateral position. For placement of the arthroscope, a standard posterior portal is created with the arm at the side. This allows for visualization of the glenohumeral joint. After visualization has been achieved, an anterior portal is established in the rotator interval. The biceps tendon is then examined with use of a probe through the anterior portal and by pulling the extra-articular portion of the biceps tendon into the joint. For maximal excursion, the arm is forward flexed with the elbow flexed.

2. Suture Passage

The bicipital groove is then palpated, and the correct site for spinal needle placement is confirmed with the arthroscope. A spinal needle is inserted from the anterior aspect of the shoulder through the transverse humeral ligament and into the bicipital groove, piercing the biceps tendon (Fig. 33-10). A No. 1 polydioxanone (PDS) bioabsorbable suture is then threaded through the spinal needle and pulled through the anterior portal with a grasper. Under arthroscopic visualization a second spinal needle is inserted from the anterior shoulder to pierce the transverse humeral ligament and biceps tendon near the first suture (Fig. 33-11). A second No.

1 PDS bioabsorbable suture is passed through the needle and pulled out through the anterior portal with a grasper. These two bioabsorbable sutures are then used to pull a No. 2 braided, nonabsorbable suture through the biceps tendon. This is done by tying one end of the No. 2 suture to one strand of PDS and pulling from the anterior shoulder puncture site through the biceps tendon and then out through the anterior cannula. The end that was pulled through the anterior cannula is then tied to the free end of the other PDS suture and pulled back through the anterior cannula, through the biceps tendon, and then out through the anterior shoulder puncture wound. These steps are then repeated for a second mattress suture, securing the biceps tendon (Fig. 33-12).

3. Biceps Tenotomy

After the two mattress sutures have secured the biceps tendon, arthroscopic scissors or a biter can be used to cut the biceps tendon proximal to the sutures. Any remaining stump of biceps anchor should be debrided to form a smooth and stable rim on the superior labrum (Fig. 33-13).

4. Suture Retrieval and Knot Tying

For retrieval of the sutures, a lateral portal is created in the shoulder and the suture ends are located in the subacromial space. Each suture end is pulled out through the lateral portal with a grasper. They are then tied with use of standard arthroscopic knot-tying techniques. This will create a mattress-type suture in the biceps

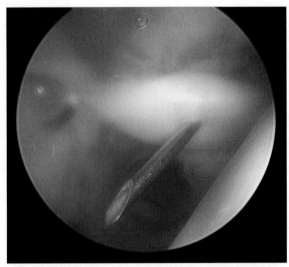

Figure 33-10. A spinal needle is inserted from the anterior aspect of the shoulder through the transverse humeral ligament and into the bicipital groove, piercing the biceps tendon.

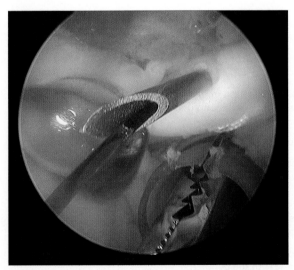

Figure 33-11. Under arthroscopic visualization a second spinal needle is inserted from the anterior shoulder to pierce the transverse humeral ligament and biceps tendon near the first suture.

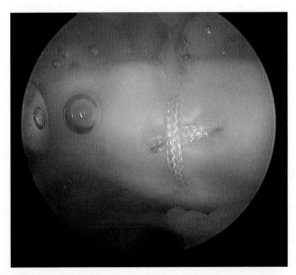

Figure 33-12. The end that was pulled through the anterior cannula is tied to the free end of the other polydioxanone (PDS) suture and pulled back through the anterior cannula, through the biceps tendon, and then out through the anterior shoulder puncture wound. These steps are then repeated for a second mattress suture, securing the biceps tendon.

tendon, securing it to the transverse humeral ligament in the bicipital groove.

RESULTS

Table 33-1 presents results of these procedures.

Tenotomy

Biceps tenotomy has been shown to be effective in pain relief in numerous studies. Kelly and colleagues[5] reported on 40 patients who underwent arthroscopic release of

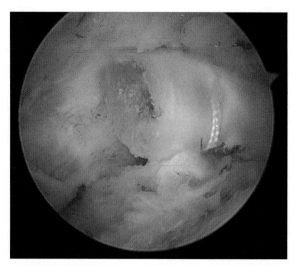

Figure 33-13. After the two mattress sutures have secured the biceps tendon, arthroscopic scissors or a biter can be used to cut the biceps tendon proximal to the sutures. Any remaining stump of biceps anchor should be debrided to form a smooth and stable rim on the superior labrum.

LHBT. Ninety-six percent of patients were relieved of the tenderness to palpation in the intertubercular groove. However, 70% of patients had a "Popeye" sign, and 38% of patients had fatigue discomfort symptoms. The authors advocated tenotomy for individuals over the age of 60 who were not manual laborers. Similarly, Kempf and colleagues[19] advocated LHBT tenotomy in elderly patients with significant biceps pathology. They reported on 210 patients with arthroscopically treated rotator cuff tears of whom 18% underwent tenotomy of LHBT. When compared with the nontenotomized group, the tenotomized group had statistically significant improvements in the level of physical activity, active mobility, and pain parameters. Gill and colleagues[4] demonstrated that arthroscopic biceps tendon release for treatment of bicipital tenosynovitis, dislocation, or partial rupture can yield favorable results. The average ASES score was 81.8. More than 96% of patients did not require any pain medication at follow-up.

Mini-Open Subpectoral Tenodesis

The mini-open subpectoral tenodesis has been proven effective in pain relief as well as having low rates of complications. Nho and colleagues[20] reported that the incidence of complications after subpectoral biceps tenodesis with interference screw fixation in a population of 353 patients over the course of 3 years was 2.0%. Also, they reported a 0.57% incidence of failure of fixation and a 0.57% incidence of persistent bicipital pain. Millett and colleagues[21] reviewed 34 patients who underwent open biceps tenodesis with interference screw fixation technique and reported no failures of

TABLE 33-1. Results of Studies of Tenotomy and Mini-Open Subpectoral Tenodesis

Author	No. of Patients	Results
Tenotomy		
Kelly et al[5] (2005)	40	96% relieved of tenderness to palpation in the intertubercular groove; 70% had a "Popeye" sign; 38% fatigue discomfort symptoms
Kempf et al[19] (1999)	210	Tenotomized group (18%) had statistically significant improvements in the level of physical activity, active mobility, and pain parameters
Gill et al[4] (2001)	30	Average ASES score 81.8; more than 96% did not require any pain medication at follow-up
Mini-Open Subpectoral Tenodesis		
Nho et al[20] (2010)	353	Incidence of complications after interference screw fixation 2.0%; incidence of failure of fixation 0.57%; incidence of persistent bicipital pain 0.57%
Millet et al[21] (2008)	34	No failures of fixation at average follow-up of 13 months; one patient with persistent bicipital groove tenderness (3% of the cohort)
Mazzocca et al[9] (2008)	41	Pain in the subpectoral triangle in 7% at follow-up (mean of 1.1 on 10-point pain-scale); one failure (2%) resulting from rerupture of the tendon

ASES, American Shoulder and Elbow Surgeons scale.

fixation at an average of 13 months after surgery. Millett and colleagues also reported one patient with persistent bicipital groove tenderness, which represented 3% of the cohort. Mazzocca and colleagues[9] studied 41 patients at approximately 1 year after open subpectoral biceps tenodesis with use of interference screw fixation. Seven percent of patients reported pain in the subpectoral triangle at follow-up, with a mean of 1.1 on a 10-point pain-scale. There was one failure (2%) caused by reruption of the tendon. Nevertheless, all patients, including the patient with the failed tenodesis, reported statistically significant improvement in ASES, Rowe, Simple Shoulder Test (SST), Constant-Murley, and Single Assessment Numeric Evaluation (SANE) scores from baseline to final follow-up, and the open subpectoral biceps tenodesis was able to restore biceps symmetry in 35 of 41 patients.

REFERENCES

1. Hitchcock HH, Bechtol CO. Painful shoulder: observations on the role of the tendon of the long head of the biceps brachii in its causation. *J Bone Joint Surg Am.* 1948;30(2):263-273.
2. Post M, Benca P. Primary tendinitis of the long head of the biceps. *Clin Orthop Relat Res.* 1989;(246): 117-125.
3. Walch G, Nové-Josserand L, Boileau P, et al. Subluxations and dislocations of the tendon of the long head of the biceps. *J Shoulder Elbow Surg.* 1998;7(2):100-108.
4. Gill TJ, McIrvin E, Mair SD, et al. Results of biceps tenotomy for treatment of pathology of the long head of the biceps brachii. *J Shoulder Elbow Surg.* 2001;10(3): 247-249.
5. Kelly AM, Drakos MC, Fealy S, et al. Arthroscopic release of the long head of the biceps tendon: functional outcome and clinical results. *Am J Sports Med.* 2005;33(2): 208-213.
6. Walch G, Edwards TB, Boulahia A, et al. Arthroscopic tenotomy of the long head of the biceps in the treatment of rotator cuff tears: clinical and radiographic results of 307 cases. *J Shoulder Elbow Surg.* 2005;14(3):238-246.
7. Berlemann U, Bayley I. Tenodesis of the long head of biceps brachii in the painful shoulder: improving results in the long term. *J Shoulder Elbow Surg.* 1995;4(6): 429-435.
8. Boileau P, Krishnan SG, Coste JS, et al. Arthroscopic biceps tenodesis: a new technique using bioabsorbable interference screw fixation. *Arthroscopy.* 2002;18(9): 1002-1012.
9. Mazzocca AD, Cote MP, Arciero CL, et al. Clinical outcomes after subpectoral biceps tenodesis with an interference screw. *Am J Sports Med.* 2008;36(10):1922-1929.
10. McClelland D, Bell SN, O'Leary S. Relocation of a dislocated long head of biceps tendon is no better than biceps tenodesis. *Acta Orthop Belg.* 2009;75(5):595-598.
11. Habermeyer P, Magosch P, Pritsch M, et al. Anterosuperior impingement of the shoulder as a result of pulley lesions: a prospective arthroscopic study. *J Shoulder Elbow Surg.* 2004;13(1):5-12.
12. Vangsness Jr CT, Jorgenson SS, Watson T, et al. The origin of the long head of the biceps from the scapula and glenoid labrum. An anatomical study of 100 shoulders. *J Bone Joint Surg Br.* 1994;76(6):951-954.
13. Yergason RM. Supination sign. *J Bone Joint Surg.* 1931;13:160.
14. Sethi N, Wright R, Yamaguchi K. Disorders of the long head of the biceps tendon. *J Shoulder Elbow Surg.* 1999;8(6):644-654.
15. Cone RO, Danzig L, Resnick D, et al. The bicipital groove: radiographic, anatomic, and pathologic study. *AJR Am J Roentgenol.* 1983;141(4):781-788.
16. Ward AD, Hamarneh G, Schweitzer ME. 3D bicipital groove shape analysis and relationship to tendopathy. *J Digit Imaging.* 2008;21(2):219-234.
17. Werner A, Mueller T, Boehm D, et al. The stabilizing sling for the long head of the biceps tendon in the rotator cuff interval. A histoanatomic study. *Am J Sports Med.* 2000;28(1):28-31.
18. Sekiya JK, Elkousy HA, Rodosky MW. Arthroscopic biceps tenodesis using the percutaneous intra-articular transtendon technique. *Arthroscopy.* 2003;19(10): 1137-1141.
19. Kempf JF, Gleyze P, Bonnomet F, et al. A multicenter study of 210 rotator cuff tears treated by arthroscopic acromioplasty. *Arthroscopy.* 1999;15:56-66.
20. Nho SJ, Reiff SN, Verma NN, et al. Complications associated with subpectoral biceps tenodesis: low rates of incidence following surgery. *Shoulder Elbow Surg.* 2010; 19(5):764-768.
21. Millett PJ, Sanders B, Gobezie R, et al. Interference screw vs. suture anchor fixation for open subpectoral biceps tenodesis: does it matter? *BMC Musculoskelet Disord.* 2008;9:121.

Chapter 34

Anatomic Acromioclavicular Joint Reconstruction

Knut Beitzel, Simone Cerciello, and Augustus D. Mazzocca

Chapter Synopsis

- Acromioclavicular joint injuries are among the most common shoulder injuries. Classification and indication for surgical or nonsurgical treatment are based on clinical and radiologic findings. Recent surgical techniques allow for anatomic reconstruction of the instable joint.

Important Points

- Classification is based on both clinical and radiologic examination findings.
- High-grade injuries—typically types IV, V, and VI, with greater than 100% displacement in either a posterior or inferior direction—are typically treated surgically.
- Surgical techniques should aim toward anatomic reconstruction of the acromioclavicular and coracoclavicular ligaments.

Clinical and Surgical Pearls

- Include the sternoclavicular joint in the operative field to allow wide exposure.
- Place a small towel bump under the medial scapular edge.
- Perform glenohumeral arthroscopy to evaluate for possible associated glenohumeral lesions.
- Instead of repositioning of the head, the clavicle can be displaced anteriorly with a towel clip to allow access for conoid tunnel drilling.

- The skin incision is over the coracoid process, more medial than usual (not over the acromioclavicular joint).
- The medial skin incision allows direct visualization of the coracoclavicular ligament and coracoid.
- Tag the deltoid and trapezial fascia for good repair.
- If sutures are passed laterally to medially, make sure the medial coracoid base is exposed and position a Darrach retractor on the medial base to "catch" the passing device.
- Do not power-spin the reamer out to avoid tunnel widening.
- The 5.5 × 8 mm polyetheretherketone (PEEK) screws are inserted into a 5.5-mm bone tunnel (line to line).
- Insert the screw anterior to the graft to adequately recreate the posteriorly positioned coracoclavicular ligaments.
- A postoperative platform brace (Lehrman) is prescribed for 6 weeks.

Clinical and Surgical Pitfalls

- Nonanatomic tunnel placement resulting from improper patient positioning and surgical exposure
- Difficult graft passage because of improper graft preparation
- Insufficient repositioning of the joint in chronic cases because of soft tissue or scar tissue interposition

Acromioclavicular (AC) joint separation represents one of the most common shoulder injuries in general orthopedic practice. The most common mechanism of this injury is a fall with a direct force to the lateral aspect of the shoulder and with the arm in an abducted position.

Depending on the magnitude of injury to the AC joint capsule and ligaments as well as to the coracoclavicular (CC) ligaments, these injuries can be classified by increasing severity as type I through type VI. Typically, the first- and second-degree sprains of the AC joint, otherwise known as type I and type II injuries, are treated conservatively; most affected patients return to preinjury status.

No overall consensus exists on treatment for type III dislocations according to Rockwood's classification, although a trend toward initial nonoperative treatment is presently favored in most cases. Some of these conservatively treated patients will have persistent pain and an inability to return to their sport or job. Subsequent surgical stabilization, albeit delayed, has still allowed return to sport or work in such cases. However, consideration of other factors, such as type of sport, timing of injury relative to athletic season, position in which the athlete competes, or throwing demands, may alter the procedure. In light of the controversy and clear lack of evidence supporting acute surgical management of grade III AC separations, we recommend that all patients be treated initially with 3 to 4 weeks of nonoperative management. A patient with a grade III AC separation qualifies for surgical reconstruction after a failed short course of nonoperative management as defined by persistent symptoms.

High-grade injuries—typically types IV, V, and VI—with greater than 100% displacement in either a posterior or inferior direction are typically treated surgically.

Currently a wide range of procedures aimed at a permanent reduction of AC joint dislocations exists. However, none of these has been shown to be the overall gold standard. Most of the current techniques focus on reconstruction of the CC ligaments in reference to anatomic studies emphasizing the biomechanical importance of the CC ligaments for vertical stability of repairs of the AC joint. From a biomechanical perspective, the importance of the CC ligaments and AC ligaments in controlling superior and horizontal translation of the distal clavicle has been elucidated. Open and arthroscopically assisted procedures are currently known. Of these, anatomic techniques focus on reconstruction of both the conoid and trapezoid ligaments. However, improved horizontal stability may further be facilitated by a reconstruction of the CC ligaments in an early stage after injury with an approach of clavicle and acromion, allowing subsequent healing of the torn AC and CC ligaments. Alternatively, an additional reconstruction of the AC ligaments could be performed, which is seen as advantageous especially in chronic instabilities with decreased healing potential of the AC ligaments.

We advocate use of a separate, more robust graft source, semitendinosus tendon rather than the coracoacromial ligament, and an anatomic procedure to achieve optimal postoperative results. The anatomic coracoclavicular reconstruction (ACCR) enables simultaneous reconstruction of the CC ligaments (trapezoid and conoid) and the AC ligaments for optimized restoration of biomechanical function. This technique restores function of both the CC ligaments and the AC ligaments in an anatomic procedure with the use of an allogenic or autologous tendon graft (semitendinosus).

PREOPERATIVE CONSIDERATIONS

The pain associated with AC joint injury may be difficult to localize because of the complex sensory innervation of the joint. An acute injury as described earlier is an important indicator in the diagnosis. Conversely, the lack of a discrete injury with AC joint pain and joint separation is more consistent with a degenerative condition. Given an acute injury, it is important to determine the level of perceived pain, its location, and any history of previous shoulder injuries. During examination, the patient should be upright so that the weight of the arm helps exaggerate any deformities. If a patient has more pain than is expected for a simple AC joint injury, then there should be high suspicion for a coronoid fracture or a type IV injury with displacement of the clavicle through the trapezial fascia. An examination for neural injuries, vascular injuries, or additional injuries of the adjoining joints should always be completed.

History

- Acute traumatic event versus chronic instability
- Current pain, physical limitations, and disability
- Failure of at least 3 months of conservative treatment
- Age of the patient (physeal fractures)
- Prior surgical procedures (distal clavicle resection)
- Status post–distal clavicular fracture (not always obvious)
- Posterior headache (nuchae)

Physical Examination

- AC joint examination
  - Inspection (Fig. 34-1)
  - Tenderness to palpation
  - Anterior-posterior translation or mobility
  - Superior-inferior translation or mobility
  - Reduction of the distal clavicle with shoulder shrug differentiates type III from type V (distal clavicle buttonhole through deltotrapezial fascia)
- Range of motion
  - Arm positioning limitation
  - Inability to lift arm
  - Pain with forward elevation and wing out
- Strength testing

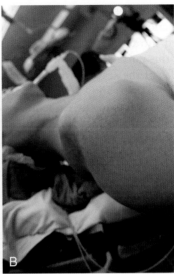
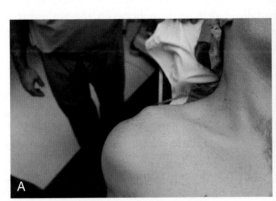

Figure 34-1. High-grade (type V) acromioclavicular separation. **A,** Anteroposterior view. **B,** Lateral view.

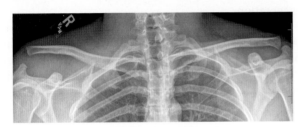

Figure 34-2. Preoperative radiograph.

Differential Diagnosis

Other causes of pain must be ruled out:

- Cervical spine disease: trapezial spasm
- Thoracic outlet syndrome
- Scapular dyskinesis
- Hyperlaxity
- Coracoid fracture

Factors Affecting Surgical Planning

- Traumatic skin lesions, prior surgeries, incisions

Imaging

- Standard imaging
  - Bilateral Zanca view: 10- to 15-degree cephalad tilt (Fig. 34-2)
  - Axillary, outlet, and anteroposterior views of the shoulder in the scapular plane
- Additional imaging
  - Cross-arm adduction view: anteroposterior shoulder—measure clavicle override

  - Magnetic resonance imaging: labral injury masquerading as AC joint pain
  - Computed tomographic scan: nondisplaced lateral clavicle or acromion fracture

Indications

- No absolute indications exist.
- Type I and II lesions are generally treated conservatively.
- Instability after distal clavicle excision.
- Treat type III lesions initially with 3 to 4 weeks of nonoperative management. Reconstruction is advocated even for symptomatic type III injuries in laborers, throwers, and overhead athletes.
- Operative treatment is generally the accepted method for complete AC joint injuries (types IV, V, and VI).

Contraindications

- Asymptomatic and painless functional grade I, II, and III separations

SURGICAL PLANNING

- Reasonable expectations of the patient and compliance with postoperative regimen
- Graft choice: semitendinosus allograft or autograft
- Postoperative sling immobilization for 6 weeks

SURGICAL TECHNIQUE

Anesthesia and Positioning

The patient is positioned in a beach chair position with a special emphasis on good access to the clavicle for placement of the bone tunnels. Turning the head slightly in the opposite direction and making sure that the head can be repositioned intraoperatively have been shown to be beneficial for this purpose. A small bump is placed at the medial border of the scapula to stabilize the AC joint for reduction. This also allows the shoulder to fall posteriorly, improving access to the coracoid. The sternoclavicular joint is included in the surgical field, and access to the posterior aspect of the clavicle should be possible.

Examination under Anesthesia

- Evaluate anterior-posterior translation as well as superior-inferior translation of the distal clavicle.
- Evaluate glenohumeral range of motion and stability.

Surgical Landmarks and Portals

Landmarks

- Clavicle
- Acromion
- Coracoid process

Portals

- Scope first to evaluate and address possible concomitant glenohumeral lesions
- Standard posterior arthroscopy port
- Anterior rotator interval port

Specific Surgical Steps for Anatomic Coracoclavicular Reconstruction

Specific steps of the procedure are outlined in Box 34-1.

Exposure

A No. 10 blade scalpel is used to make a 6-cm longitudinal incision, centered over or slightly medial to the coracoid. Medial and lateral skin flaps are elevated with a needle-tipped bovie. Gelpi retractors assist with exposure. The deltotrapezial fascia is dissected, and generous skin flaps are raised above the fascia to improve visualization. The fascia is incised in line with the natural demarcation between the trapezius insertion onto the posterior aspect of the clavicle and the deltoid origin on the anterior clavicle. This incision extends medially beyond the conoid ligament insertion. Maintaining full-thickness flaps and detaching the complete anterior deltoid insertion at this point are critical to obtaining a good closure. In addition, tagging stitches are placed in the flaps at the medial extent of the exposure to facilitate accurate reapproximation. Freeing the clavicle and AC joint of soft tissues that are preventing joint reduction completes the exposure (Fig. 34-3). The distal clavicle should be preserved in general, and a careful distal resection of 5 mm of the distal clavicle should be performed only in advanced and symptomatic degeneration.

The medial and lateral coracoid base is exposed with a Cobb elevator. A headlight may be useful for this portion of the procedure. Care is taken to avoid excessive medial dissection to prevent musculocutaneous nerve injury.

Passage of the Shuttle Suture Under the Coracoid

A specially designed cannulated passing device (Arthrex, Naples, FL) is passed medially to laterally around the coracoid. A FiberWire or FiberStick (Arthrex) is then shuttled through the cannulated handle and retrieved laterally at the tip. This passing stitch is later used for graft passage around the coracoid (Fig. 34-4).

An alternative means of coracoid graft fixation is biotenodesis screw fixation of the looped end of the semitendinosus graft in a coracoid base bone tunnel. This is best achieved by positioning the 7-mm offset anterior cruciate ligament guide on the medial coracoid base and reaming an 8- or 9-mm bone tunnel.

BOX 34-1 Surgical Steps

1. Exposure
2. Passage of the shuttle suture under the coracoid
3. Clavicular tunnels
4. Graft preparation
5. Graft passage
6. Clavicle reduction
7. Graft fixation
8. Acromioclavicular joint capsular ligament repair
9. Closure

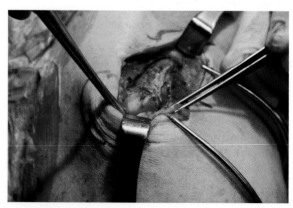

Figure 34-3. Initial exposure.

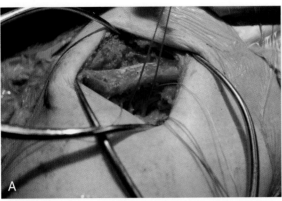
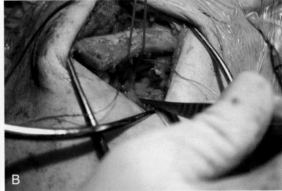

Figure 34-4. A, FiberWire around the coracoid. **B,** Close-up view.

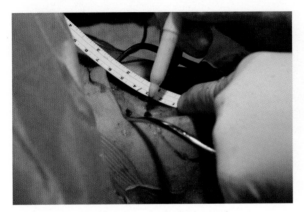

Figure 34-5. Marking the clavicular tunnels.

Clavicular Tunnels

The conoid ligament tunnel is established with a guide pin drilled 4.5 cm medial from the intact lateral distal clavicle edge and positioned along the posterior superior cortex. The pin is directed at 30 degrees anterior, aiming toward the coracoid. A second guide pin is drilled central on the clavicle's anteroposterior dimension and 1.5 cm lateral to the medial pin. This tunnel will be used to reconstruct the trapezoid ligament and is again directed 30 degrees anteriorly toward the coracoid (Figs. 34-5 and 34-6). A 5.5-mm reamer is used to ream both tunnels (Fig. 34-7). The reamer is removed by hand twisting after penetration of the far cortex to avoid tunnel widening with subsequent taping.

Graft Preparation

An allograft semitendinosus graft is contoured to fit through a 5.5-mm tunnel. No. 2 FiberWire is used to place baseball stitches at each end of the graft (Fig. 34-8).

Graft Passage

The initially passed FiberWire or FiberStick is used to shuttle the prepared semitendinosus graft along with an additional No. 2 FiberWire around the coracoid process. The accessory FiberWire will provide secondary fixation. The free ends of the semitendinosus graft along with the free No. 2 FiberWire are shuttled into the respective clavicular bone tunnels by use of a suture-passing device (Fig. 34-9).

Clavicle Reduction

Pushing up on the elbow to elevate the scapulohumeral complex reduces the AC joint. At this step, a possible posterior displacement must be considered and if necessary prevented, and all soft tissue restraints must be debrided within the AC joint. Before fixation, the quality of reduction is examined visually and radiographically ("mini C-arm"). Anatomic reduction of the AC joint is critical. We recommend fixing the AC joint in a slightly over-reduced position (2 to 3 mm) to compensate for the anticipated loss of reduction, which generally occurs in the postoperative period.

Graft Fixation

The graft exiting the posteromedial (conoid ligament) tunnels is secured first. A 5.5- × 8-mm polyetheretherketone (PEEK) tenodesis screw (Arthrex) is then used for graft fixation. With countertension on the opposite graft end, the PEEK screw is inserted flush to the cortical surface into the conoid tunnel.

It is placed in the anterior aspect of the tunnel, and tension is maintained on the graft during fixation. The other limb of the graft exiting the trapezoid tunnel is again cyclically tensioned to remove any slack before being secured with a second interference screw. The nonresorbable suture is then tied on the superior aspect of the clavicle for additional security after the suture has been passed through the cannulated portion of the screw.

Acromioclavicular Joint Capsular Ligament Repair

The shorter limb of graft exiting the conoid tunnel is sewn into the longer limb, which is then looped over the top of the AC joint to reinforce this repair. High-strength nonabsorbable suture is used to take the lateral

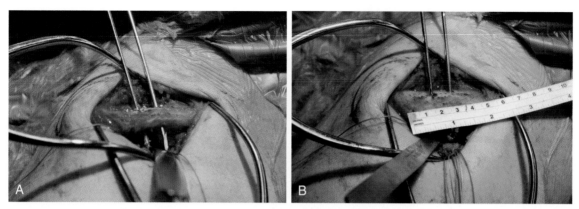

Figure 34-6. A, Guide pins in the tunnels. **B,** Measuring the distance between guide pins.

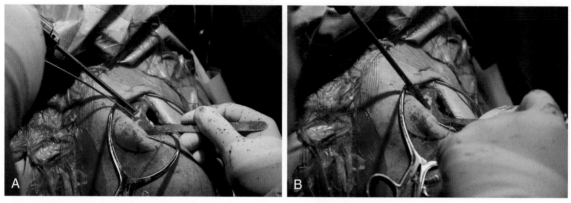

Figure 34-7. A, Reaming the coracoid tunnel. **B,** Reaming the trapezoid tunnel.

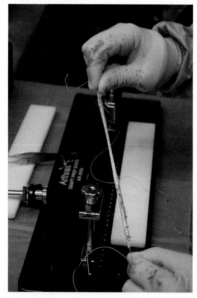

Figure 34-8. Graft preparation.

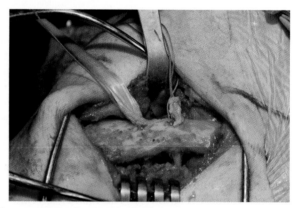

Figure 34-9. Passage of the graft.

limb (trapezoid) and suture it into the most posterior tissue on the acromial side of the joint. The remaining graft is then taken posteriorly and sutured to the trapezial fascia, creating the posterior AC ligament. No. 2 FiberWire stitches are used to imbricate the superior AC joint capsular ligaments in a pants-over-vest

configuration. This will offer additional anteroposterior stability to the reconstruction. The deltotrapezial fascia is also repaired in this step if full-thickness flaps of fascia and AC joint capsular ligament were elevated in a single layer.

Closure

After copious wound irrigation, the subcutaneous tissues are closed with 2-0 Vicryl sutures. A 3-0 Monocryl is used to perform a subcutaneous skin closure. The wound is injected with bupivacaine.

TABLE 34-1. Results of Studies of Acromioclavicular Joint Reconstruction

Study	Type	Native Coracoclavicular Ligament	Anatomic Coracoclavicular Ligament Reconstruction	Coracoacromial Transfer
Lee et al[1] (2003)	Cadaver	650 N (load to failure)	700 N (load to failure) Semitendinosus	150 N (load to failure)
Costic et al[2] (2004)	Cadaver	60.8 ± 5.2 N/mm (stiffness) 560 ± 206 N (load to failure)	23.4 ± 5.2 N/mm (stiffness) 406 ± 60 N (load to failure) Semitendinosus	
Grutter and Petersen[3] (2005)	Cadaver	815 N	774 N Flexor carpi radialis	483 N
Mazzocca et al[4] (2006)	Cadaver		396.4 ± 136.42 N	354.3 ± 100.26 N

N, Newton.

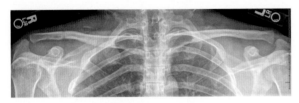

Figure 34-10. Postoperative radiograph.

POSTOPERATIVE CONSIDERATIONS

Follow-up

- Sutures are removed at 1 week.
- Patients are seen at 1, 2, 3, and 6 months and then annually.
- Postoperative radiographs include bilateral Zanca views to measure coracoid-clavicular distance (Fig. 34-10).

Rehabilitation

- A platform brace (Lehrman) is worn for 6 weeks.
- Immediate pendulum exercises are begun, with limitation of passive external rotation to 30 degrees and passive forward flexion to 90 degrees.
- Active range of motion is started at 8 weeks.
- Strengthening is started at 12 to 16 weeks.
- Sports-specific activities and return to full athletics are allowed at 16 to 24 weeks.
- Return to heavy labor is allowed at 6 months.

Complications

- Infection
- Construct failure
- Sterile abscess from FiberWire or PEEK screw reaction
- Potential clavicle fracture from stress riser effect on bone tunnels

- Potential musculocutaneous nerve injury
- Persistent pain

RESULTS

Results of studies of AC joint reconstruction are shown in Table 34-1.

REFERENCES

1. Lee SJ, Nicholas SJ, Akizuki KH, et al. Reconstruction of the coracoclavicular ligaments with tendon grafts. *Am J Sports Med.* 2003;31:648-654.
2. Costic RS, Labriola JE, Rodosky ME, et al. Biomechanical rationale for development of anatomical reconstruction of coracoclavicular ligaments after complete acromioclavicular joint dislocations. *Am J Sports Med.* 2004;32:1929-1936.
3. Grutter PW, Petersen SA. Anatomical acromioclavicular ligament reconstruction. *Am J Sports Med.* 2005;31:1-6.
4. Mazzocca AD, Santangelo SA, Johnson ST, et al. A biomechanical evaluation of an anatomical coracoclavicular ligament reconstruction. *Am J Sports Med.* 2006;34:236-246.

SUGGESTED READINGS

Beitzel K, Cote MP, Apostolakos J, Solovyova O, et al. Current concepts in the treatment of acromioclavicular joint dislocations. *Arthroscopy.* 2013;29(2):387-397.

Debski RE, Parson IM, Woo S, et al. Effect of capsular injury on acromioclavicular joint mechanics. *J Bone Joint Surg Am.* 2001;83:1344-1351.

Geaney LE, Miller MD, Ticker JB, et al. Management of failed AC joint reconstruction: causation and treatment. *Sports Med Arthrosc.* 2010;18:167-172.

Jari R, Costic RS, Rodosky MW, et al. Biomechanical function of surgical procedures for acromioclavicular joint dislocations. *J Arthroscopy.* 2004;20:237-245.

Jones HP, Lemos MJ, Schepsis AA. Salvage of failed acromioclavicular joint reconstruction using autogenous semitendinosus tendon from the knee. *Am J Sports Med.* 2001;29:234-237.

Chapter 35

Management of Pectoralis Major Muscle Injuries

Robert M. Coale and Jon K. Sekiya

Chapter Synopsis

- Pectoralis major muscle tears are being increasingly reported. The mechanism of injury and physical examination are key components to diagnosis of this injury. Full-thickness tears in patients wishing to return to preinjury levels are best treated with surgical repair.

Important Points

- Full-thickness tears are commonly diagnosed on physical examination findings alone.
- Return to full function of patients with full-thickness tears can be achieved with surgical repair.
- Chronic neglected tears have improved results with surgical care compared with those treated nonoperatively.
- Elderly patients, patients with muscle belly tears, and patients with partial-thickness tears are generally best treated with nonsurgical management.
- Partial-thickness tears can be confirmed with advanced imaging if necessary.

Clinical and Surgical Pearls

- The fixation technique should be based on the individual's anatomy with regard to the ability to retract the deltoid and/or remaining clavicular head when the choice of suture anchors or transcortical window-based fixation is made.
- Identification of both heads of the pectoralis major as well as its footprint is necessary for anatomic repair.
- Secure traction suture fixation to the retracted tendon stump with gentle lysis of adhesions facilitates low tension repair.
- Use of the intact muscle heads may facilitate repair technically and biologically.

Clinical and Surgical Pitfalls

- Avoid iatrogenic injury to the long head of the biceps tendon when preparing the cortical bed and footprint. Obtain a plain radiograph series to rule out concomitant injuries.
- If obtaining a magnetic resonance imaging scan, ensure that axial images of the entire insertion site, including its distal-most extent, are collected.

Since the first described report of a pectoralis major muscle rupture in 1822, our understanding of the injury has evolved. Previously, pectoralis major tears were recognized as rare injuries incurred by manual laborers who could tolerate functionally negligible strength losses. Before the year 2000, the number of cases reported in the literature was below 150; however, since the year 2000, over 220 additional cases have been reported. This coincides with the increase in the number of individuals pursuing athletic endeavors, as well as those pushing the limits of human performance in training for such sports.[1-3] These athletes cannot continue their sport at the same level without maximal clinical outcome, which is most reliably obtained by surgical repair. Pectoralis major muscle injuries have been, are, and will remain a traditional topic of orthopedics in which our understanding of anatomy lays the groundwork for a thorough history coupled with a complete physical examination to reach the diagnosis. We are able to apply advancing surgical methods to provide our patients with the best possible outcome based on the needs of the individual.

PREOPERATIVE CONSIDERATIONS

History

Men in the third and fourth decades of life are those primarily affected by pectoralis major muscle injuries.[1,4] Most commonly, tears occur as complete distal tears at or near the insertion on the humerus but can also occur at the musculotendinous junction.[1,4-6] Tears generally involve the sternal head but can also involve both heads or the clavicular head alone.[3]

The pectoralis major muscle is responsible for adduction and internal rotation and contributes to forward flexion. It originates broadly from the clavicle, the sternum, the ribs (first through sixth), and the aponeurosis of the external oblique muscle; however, it inserts in a more focal manner on the anterior aspect of the proximal humerus.[7,8] The pectoralis major is a unique muscle capable of maximal power production over a broad range of velocities of muscle shortening. It is composed of a larger sternal head and a smaller clavicular head; the sternal head has a bilaminar insertion of three segments anteriorly and three segments posteriorly.[7] Within the anterior layer, each successive segment insertion and origin is more inferior and deep. Within the posterior layer, each successive segment remains more inferior and deep in origin, but its insertion is more superior.[7]

Mechanisms include indirect injury such as from weightlifting and gymnastics and less often direct trauma such as shotgun-firing and seatbelt injuries. Indirect injury most commonly occurs during near-maximal eccentric contraction in a mechanically unfavorable extended, abducted, and externally rotated position. This is classically represented at the end of the eccentric portion of a bench-press repetition. Nearly 50% of all cases reported since 1972 have occurred during bench-press.[1,3,5,6,8-14] Fiber bundle lengths are relatively shorter and have greater lateral pennation angles in the more inferior segments.[7,8] The inferior fibers are lengthened 30% to 45% of their resting fiber length when stretched and receive maximal load with minimal overlap, placing them at a mechanical disadvantage. This combination of fiber bundle length and pennation angle is the prime reason that most tears involve this region of the muscle.[7,8]

Physical Examination

Often, clinical suspicion based on the mechanism of injury combined with the focal physical examination findings leads to the correct diagnosis. The hallmark finding is the asymmetrical contour of the axillary fold when the shoulder is positioned in 90 degrees of abduction, slight extension, and external rotation. Asymmetry can also be seen within the muscle belly with resisted adduction and internal rotation of the shoulder. Palpation of a defect within the axillary fold confirms the suspicion. Often a subcutaneous band passing from the fascia over the pectoralis major into the upper arm remains intact and palpable. Impressive amounts of ecchymosis to the shoulder girdle are commonly present. Although development of a large hematoma is not typical, it should be recognized. Potential complications including life-threatening infections have been reported secondarily; thus the clinician should have an index of suspicion.[15-17]

Imaging

Imaging modalities can be used as adjuncts in diagnosis and surgical planning. A standard shoulder radiographic series should be obtained to identify the presence of a bony avulsion, which may alter surgical planning, and also to identify rare concurrent injuries including proximal humeral fractures and shoulder dislocation.[18-20] Advanced imaging is best used, to confirm the clinician's suspicion of a partial-thickness tear that would generally be treated nonoperatively.

Indications and Contraindications

Muscle belly tears, partial-thickness tears, and tears in the elderly are in most cases best treated nonoperatively, whereas full-thickness distal tears are best treated operatively depending on individual patient factors including age, cosmetic concerns, and activity goals.

SURGICAL TECHNIQUE

Anesthesia and Positioning

General anesthesia, with accompanying paralytics or with an effective regional nerve block, is optimal to achieve full muscle relaxation to assist in mobilization of the retracted tendon stump. The modified beach chair position with a flexion angle of approximately 45 degrees is used. A small roll of sheets may be placed under the patient's scapula to allow greater motion of the shoulder during repair. The operative arm may be held by an assistant or with the use of a hydraulic positioning device to optimize the operative window.

Surgical Landmarks

Manual palpation or cupping of the hand over the deltoid permits accurate determination of the deltopectoral interval. An incision of approximately 6 to 10 cm based on the inferior half of a standard deltopectoral incision is used. Care is taken to avoid unnecessary dissection into the axilla to prevent potential infection from opportunistic bacterial flora.

Examination Under Anesthesia

Visual examination for asymmetry of the axillary fold compared with the contralateral limb should be performed. This can be optimally viewed with the shoulder held in 90 degrees of abduction with external rotation (Fig. 35-1). Manual palpation of the defect in the same position easily identifies the tear.

Specific Steps

Box 35-1 outlines the specific steps of this procedure.

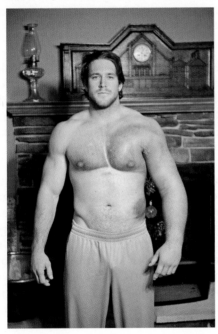

Figure 35-1. Physical examination of a patient with a left pectoralis major muscle rupture with development of significant ecchymosis.

1. Exposure

Preinjecting the skin with bupivacaine (Marcaine) or ropivacaine and epinephrine (prepackaged standard) (1:1000) or epinephrine and normal saline (with or without Marcaine) can be used to improve hemostasis. Initial sharp dissection is performed with the shoulder in a position of neutral rotation, slight flexion, and slight abduction for optimal identification of the delto-pectoral interval. Care is taken to protect the cephalic vein throughout the procedure. When possible, we prefer to dissect the cephalic vein laterally with the deltoid, particularly in tears involving the clavicular head. It is intimately associated with the clavicular head of the pectoralis major and may make the already difficult process of mobilization of the pectoralis major more technically demanding. The cephalic vein has multiple deltoid branches that supply it, and protecting this association may be advantageous to the upper extremity.

Once the interval has been dissected, the deltoid is retracted and the pectoralis major defect is identified. If the defect is repaired within the first 7 to 10 days, a hematoma is often encountered early during the exposure. With a later repair, a pseudomembrane is formed about the pectoralis major stump containing serosanguineous fluid. With manual palpation the retracted tendon stump is usually easily identified (Fig. 35-2). In most cases a small amount of tendon remains attached to the proximal retracted muscle. Thorough dissection to determine the extent of head involvement is

---

BOX 35-1 Surgical Steps

1. Exposure
2. Tendon-muscle mobilization
3. Tendon reattachment
4. Closure

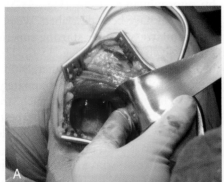
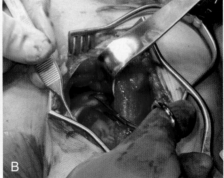

Figure 35-2. Rupture identification. **A,** Clavicular head is identified and retracted superiorly to find the space previously occupied by the ruptured sternal head. **B,** Stump of the retracted ruptured sternal head is identified with intact clavicular head retracted superiorly.

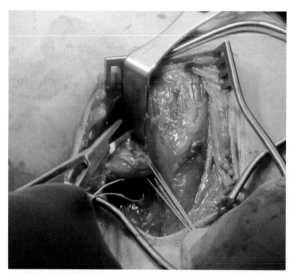

Figure 35-3. Placement of traction sutures in a modified Mason-Allen configuration.

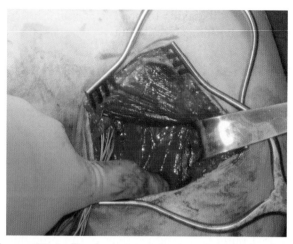

Figure 35-4. The footprint of the insertion site has been exposed just lateral to the long head of the biceps tendon, deep to the clavicular head. The cortex has been denuded approximately 3 mm in width and 4 cm in length.

paramount. More commonly the sternal head is involved, or portions thereof. Given the complex anatomic insertion on the humerus, each head should be identified so that anatomic repair can be achieved. Care should be taken to stay within the appropriate layer and to avoid dissecting too deeply and into the chest wall.

2. Tendon-Muscle Mobilization

The tendon stump should be carefully tagged with approximately four No. 2 nonabsorbable braided sutures in a modified Mason-Allen configuration (Fig. 35-3). With gentle traction, the adhesions preventing normal excursion of the muscle can be identified and carefully released. Slow constant tension can also result in significant gains in muscle excursion. It is usually best to perform adhesion releases by spreading with scissors, because forceful blunt dissection can often cause further damage to the remaining musculotendinous interface, thus compromising repair.

3. Tendon Reattachment

Once the anatomy has been defined and the excursion is that of low tension for repair, the footprint of the humeral insertion site can be prepared. The deltoid is retracted laterally and the intertubercular groove is identified by palpation. Identification of the groove and protection of the biceps tendon should be performed throughout the procedure to avoid iatrogenic injury to the long head of the biceps tendon. The biceps tendon sheath can be gently retracted medially and will assist in preventing inadvertent injury. The insertion site is visualized. In the rare case that a sufficient tendinous portion is remaining on the humerus, primary tendon-to-tendon repair can be undertaken. More commonly, diminutive soft tissue is left and it is debrided without

compromising the repair. When the clavicular head remains intact, it should be retracted superiorly and laterally because the insertion site of the sternal head is deep and slightly distal to that of the clavicular head.

The insertion site is then debrided of soft tissue, and an area of cortical bone 3 mm in width by 4 cm in length is denuded to a bleeding bed (Fig. 35-4). This can be performed with a combination of a curette and a motorized bur. The cortex should not be aggressively compromised, because fixation methods include anchors or transcortical bridges that rely on its integrity.

Often the size of the patient determines the best method of fixation. Because these injuries more often occur in more muscularly developed patients, visualization of the insertion site becomes difficult. Given this set of conditions, suture anchors may be the best method of fixation because creation of a bony bridge requires more extensive visualization. When using suture anchors, we prefer to use four single-loaded anchors with No. 2 nonabsorbable braided suture. Anchors are placed within the preprepared footprint, evenly spaced by approximately 1 cm (Fig. 35-5). Multiple suture techniques have been described. We prefer to place horizontal mattress sutures starting superiorly and working progressively inferiorly (Fig. 35-6). The shoulder should be in a position of approximately 15 to 30 degrees of internal rotation and approximately 15 degrees of forward flexion to remove as much stress as possible for ease of opposition to ensure the best repair. Once all sutures have been passed, they should sequentially be tied from superior to inferior (Fig. 35-7). After the horizontal mattresses have been tied with use of a free needle, each limb of the previously place modified Mason-Allen sutures is passed through any remaining uninjured head and tied successively (Fig. 35-8). This restores the anatomic bilaminar tendon, further enhances

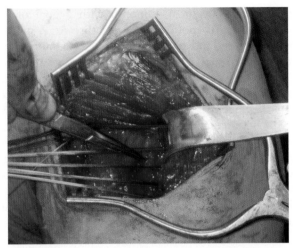

Figure 35-5. Anchors have been placed in the preprepared footprint. The biceps is noted with the snap to be just medial to the footprint and uninjured.

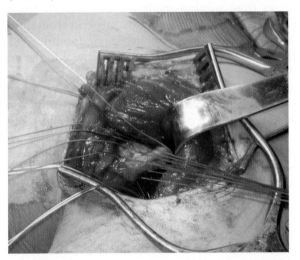

Figure 35-6. Anchor sutures have been passed medial to previously placed modified Mason-Allen sutures in a horizontal mattress fashion.

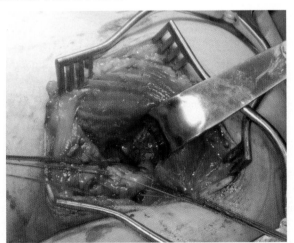

Figure 35-7. The horizontal mattress sutures are tied sequentially from superior to inferior with traction applied to modified Mason-Allen sutures and the arm held in slight forward flexion and internal rotation.

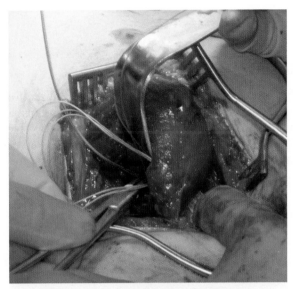

Figure 35-8. Both limbs of the previously placed modified Mason-Allen sutures are placed through the intact clavicular head.

healing to intact tissue, and shares load from the previously placed horizontal mattress sutures.

In patients with chronic retracted ruptures in which the surgeon is unable to obtain sufficient excursion for repair despite adequate relaxation and releases, augmentation may be appropriate. A tibialis anterior allograft is prepared on the back table with a No. 2 nonabsorbable suture in a running fashion to both ends. A 6-mm graft is the goal size. A 7-mm unicortical tunnel is drilled in the cortex at the middle of the pectoralis major footprint just lateral to the biceps groove. The graft is then secured within the tunnel, and a 5.5-mm bioabsorbable screw is used as fixation. The graft is then passed from deep to superficial through the inferior aspect of the pectoralis major stump sequentially with use of a Pulvertaft technique from inferior to superior (Fig. 35-9). Once the graft has been passed through the length of the stump, it is secured to itself with multiple figure-of-eight sutures with No. 2 nonabsorbable suture. It is important to place appropriate tension on the repair to restore an adequate length-tension relationship as well as provide optimal cosmesis.

4. Closure

Once repair is completed, the wound is irrigated and meticulous hemostasis is maintained. The retractors are removed and the cephalic vein is inspected for trauma. The interval is then closed with gently approximated No. 2 nonabsorbable sutures. Final wound closure is completed with a 3-0 absorbable deep dermal stitch followed by a running 4-0 absorbable subcuticular stitch. A sterile dressing is applied, and the patient is placed in a shoulder immobilizer sling with the hand at the abdomen to prevent abduction and external rotation that may stress the repair.

POSTOPERATIVE CONSIDERATIONS

Rehabilitation

The patient remains in a shoulder immobilizer for a period of at least 6 weeks. Passive pendulums and passive forward elevation to 130 degrees may begin 1 week postoperatively. A strong emphasis on periscapular strengthening should continue with scapular protraction, retraction, and elevation throughout rehabilitation. Passive range of motion in all planes to pain

tolerance may begin at 1 month with a goal of full normal range of motion at 2 months. At 2 months postoperatively and once normal range of motion has been achieved, active and active-assisted range of motion is initiated. Rotator cuff strengthening exercises may begin once active range of motion is full. Advanced strengthening programs with the use of free weights may be initiated at 6 months postoperatively, beginning with low weights and high repetitions. At this time, gradual return to sport and work duties may begin under controlled conditions. Full return is permitted when the patient is pain free, has full strength, and has full range of motion. Heavy bench-pressing is discouraged indefinitely.

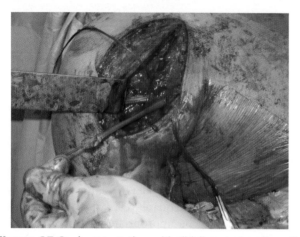

Figure 35-9. Augmentation with tibialis anterior allograft via a Pulvertaft technique in a patient with a chronic retracted pectoralis major stump.

Complications

Although rare, complications from the injury itself as well as from surgical treatment can occur. Iatrogenic long head biceps tendon rupture can occur from surgical trauma, because the pectoralis major footprint is less than 3 mm in thickness and directly lateral to the intertubercular groove. In preparing the bony bed for reattachment, violation of the long head of the biceps tendon can occur if meticulous technique is not used.[21] Wound infection remains a concern with operative intervention, given the incision's proximity to the axilla. Other, rare complications that have been reported include the development of heterotopic ossification, compartment syndrome, and infected hematomas.[15,22-26]

TABLE 35-1. Outcomes of Pectoralis Major Muscle Rupture

Author	Study	Results
Aarimaa et al[28] (2004)	33 repairs	33 repairs: 13 excellent, 17 good, 3 fair
	Meta-analysis of 73 cases	*Meta-analysis of 73 cases:* 32 acute repairs (<3 weeks): 18 excellent, 12 good, 2 fair 19 delayed (>3 weeks): 8 excellent, 11 good 22 nonoperative: 1 excellent, 16 good, 5 fair
Antosh et al[9] (2009)	14 ruptures	8 repaired (<6 weeks): 4 very satisfied, 4 satisfied, 3 excellent function, 4 good function, 1 average function 6 repaired (>6 weeks): 3 very satisfied, 2 satisfied, 1 unsatisfied, 2 excellent function, 1 good function, 2 average function, 1 poor function
Bak et al[4] (2000)	Meta-analysis of 72 cases	Surgical repair: 88% excellent-good (statistically better if repaired within 8 weeks of injury) Nonoperative: 27% excellent-good
Hanna et al[11] (2001)	22 ruptures	10 repaired: peak torque 99% of uninjured side 12 nonoperative: peak torque 56% of uninjured side
Ponchini et al[14] (2010)	20 ruptures	10 repaired: 7 excellent, 2 good, 1 bad, peak torque deficit 13.7% 10 nonoperative: 2 good, 5 fair, 3 bad, peak torque deficit 41.2%
Schepsis et al[3] (2000)	17 ruptures	6 acute repairs (<2 weeks from injury): 96% subjective, 102% isokinetic strength 7 chronic repairs (>2 weeks from injury): 93% subjective, 94% strength 4 nonoperative: 51% subjective, 71% strength
Wolfe et al[8] (1992)	8 ruptures	4 repaired: peak torque 105.8% compared with normal side 4 nonoperative: peak torque deficit 29.9% compared with normal side

RESULTS

It is well established that full-thickness distal pectoralis major tears are best treated by surgical repair. Numerous studies have reported that acute surgical intervention, generally less than 8 weeks from injury, achieves optimal and near normal outcomes Table 35-1. Surgical treatment of delayed or neglected full-thickness tears also results in outcomes superior to those treated nonoperatively, though acute treatment is preferred. Repairs have been described in patients up to 13 years after the injury with near-normal outcomes.[27] Surgical treatment outcomes are superior to outcomes of nonoperative treatment in subjective scoring, functional assessments including isokinetic testing, and cosmesis.[3,4,11,14,28] A recent prospective study revealed a 41.2% deficit in peak torque in horizontal adduction in the nonoperative group compared with 13.7% in the operative group. Numerous studies have shown no significant change in operatively treated isokinetic strength when compared with the contralateral limb.[3,8,11] Case reports have demonstrated that after surgical repair even the most elite athletes are able to return to sport and achieve the highest goals. One case report reveals a patient winning the national powerlifting championship in bench-press after repair.[29] Another reports an individual earning a gold medal in Olympic wrestling after having undergone repair.[30] No case reports exist of patients with full-thickness tears treated nonoperatively returning to this level of competition.

REFERENCES

1. Kretzler HH, Richardson AB. Rupture of the pectoralis major muscle. *Am J Sports Med.* 1989;17:453-458.
2. McEntire JE, Hess WE, Coleman SS. Rupture of the pectoralis major muscle: a report of eleven injuries and review of fifty-six. *J Bone Joint Surg Am.* 1972;54:1040-1045.
3. Schepsis AA, Grafe MW, Jones HP, et al. Rupture of the pectoralis major muscle: outcome after repair of acute and chronic injuries. *Am J Sports Med.* 2000;28:9-15.
4. Bak K, Cameron EA, Henderson IJP. Rupture of the pectoralis major muscle: a meta-analysis of 122 cases. *Knee Surg Sports Traumatol Arthrosc.* 2000;8:113-199.
5. Connell DA, Potter HG, Sherman MF, et al. Injuries of the pectoralis major muscle: evaluation with MR imaging. *Radiology.* 1999;210:785-791.
6. Zvijac JE, Schurhoff MR, Hechtman KS, et al. Pectoralis major tears: correlation of magnetic resonance imaging and treatment strategies. *Am J Sports Med.* 2006;34;289-294.
7. Fung L, Wong B, Ravichandiran K, et al. Three-dimensional study of pectoralis major muscle and tendon architecture. *Clin Anat.* 2009;22:500-508.
8. Wolfe SW, Wickiewicz TL, Cavanaugh JT. Ruptures of the pectoralis major muscle: an anatomic and clinical analysis. *Am J Sports Med.* 1992;20:587-593.
9. Antosh IJ, Grassbaugh JA, Parada SA, et al. Pectoralis major tendon repairs active-duty population. *Am J Orthop.* 2009;38:26-30.
10. Carrino JA, Chandnanni VP, Mitchell DB, et al. Pectoralis major muscle and tendon tears: diagnosis and grading using magnetic resonance imaging. *Skeletal Radiol.* 2000;29:205-313.
11. Hanna CM, Glenny AB, Stanley SN, et al. Pectoralis major tears: comparison of surgical and conservative treatment. *Br J Sports Med.* 2001;35:202-206.
12. He ZM, AO YF, Wang JQ, et al. Twelve cases of the pectoralis major muscle tendon rupture with surgical treatment—an average of 6.7-year follow-up. *Chin Med J (Engl).* 2010;123:57-60.
13. Kakwani RG, Matthews JJ, Kumar KM, et al. Rupture of the pectorals major muscle: surgical treatment in athletes. *Int Orthop.* 2007;31:159-163.
14. de Castro Pochini A, Ejnisman B, Andreoli CV, et al. Pectoralis major muscle rupture in athletes: a prospective study. *Am J Sports Med.* 2010;38:92-98.
15. Patissier P. Traite des maladies des artisans. Paris: 163,1822.
16. Chapple K, Kelty C, Irwin LR, et al. Traumatic abscess of pectoralis major. *Arch Orthop Trauma Surg.* 2000;120: 479-481.
17. Beloosesky Y, Hendel D, Weiss A, et al. Rupture of the pectoralis major muscle in nursing home residents. *Am J Med.* 2001;111:233-235.
18. Verfaillie SM, Claes T. Bony avulsion of the pectoralis major muscle. *J Shoulder Elbow Surg.* 1996;5:327-329.
19. Kono M, Johnson EE. Pectoralis major tendon avulsion in association with a proximal humerus fracture. *J Orthop Trauma.* 1996;10:508-510.
20. Arciero RA, Cruser DL. Pectoralis major rupture with simultaneous anterior dislocation of the shoulder. *J Shoulder Elbow Surg.* 1997;6:318-320.
21. Provencher MT, Handfield K, Boniquit NT, et al. Injuries to the pectoralis major muscle. *Am J Sports Med.* 2010;38: 1693-1705.
22. Purnell R. Rupture of the pectoralis major muscle: a complication. *Injury.* 1988;19:284.
23. Pitts RT, Garner HW, Ortiguera CJ. Pectoralis major avulsion in a skeletally immature wrestler: a case report. *Am J Sports Med.* 2010;38:1034-1037.
24. Simionian PT, Morris ME. Pectoralis tendon avulsions in skeletally immature. *Am J Orthop.* 1996;25:563-564.
25. Rehman A, Robinson P. Sonographic evaluation of injuries of the pectoralis muscles. *Am J Roent.* 2005;184: 1205-1211.
26. Letenneur M. Rupture sous cutanie du muscle grand pectoral. *Inf Section Med J.* 1861;52:202-205.
27. Anbari A, Kelly 4th JD, Moyer RA. Delayed repair of a ruptured pectoralis major muscle: a case report. *Am J Sports Med.* 2000;28:254-256.
28. Aarimaa V, Rantanen J, Heikkila J, et al. Rupture of the pectoralis major muscle. *Am J Sports Med.* 2004;32: 1256-1262.
29. Urs ND, Jani DM. Surgical repair of rupture of the pectoralis major muscle: a case report. *J Trauma.* 1976;16: 749-750.
30. Pavlik A, Csepai D, Berkes I. Surgical treatment of pectoralis major rupture in athletes. *Knee Surg Sports Traumatol Arthrosc.* 1998;6:129-133.

Chapter 36

Nonarthroplasty Options for Glenohumeral Arthritis and Chondrolysis

Rachel M. Frank, Lucas S. McDonald, and Matthew T. Provencher*

Chapter Synopsis

- Glenohumeral arthritis and chondrolysis remain problematic for the active patient population. Total shoulder arthroplasty is successful at relieving pain and restoring function; however, concerns regarding component loosening, ability to perform high-level athletic activity, and the potential need for revision surgery make this option less attractive, especially in a younger patient population. With recent advances in diagnostic modalities, surgical techniques, and biologic implants, the treatment algorithm for these difficult patients continues to evolve. When nonoperative treatment fails, there are several nonarthroplasty surgical options for these patients, including palliative, reparative, restorative, and reconstructive techniques.

Important Points

- Patient age and desired activity level are important preoperative considerations.
- Global location of the defect (glenoid surface, humeral head, or bipolar "kissing" lesions), local location of the defect (central, peripheral), and size, depth, and containment of the defect must be thoroughly assessed for optimal management.
- A true anteroposterior (AP) and axillary views should be used to assess for subtle glenohumeral joint space changes.
- Bony version should be assessed. Nonarthroplasty options have limited success if extensive posterior or posteroinferior glenoid bone loss is present.
- Assess posterior humeral translation on the glenoid. If posterior subluxation is present, this may indicate worse outcomes with nonarthroplasty options.
- Advanced (bipolar) glenohumeral disease can be initially treated with nonarthroplasty options, including capsular release and synovectomy, with less predictable results for interpositional arthroplasty and biologic options.

Clinical and Surgical Pearls

- Isolated chondral lesions of the glenohumeral joint are rare, but can be debilitating. It is crucial to identify which lesions are incidental and which are truly symptomatic.
- Range-of-motion deficits may exist as a manifestation of cartilage damage, arthritis, and resultant capsular synovitis, thickening, and contracture.
- Nonarthroplasty techniques include palliative, reparative, restorative, and reconstructive surgical techniques.
- Arthroscopic debridement including synovectomy and tailored capsular release (capsulectomy) can help treat range-of-motion deficits.
- When performing microfracture long-handled curettes and awls are used to create clean lesion edges and adequate marrow stimulation.
- Autologous chondrocyte implantation has been described for isolated humeral head defects.
- Osteochondral autografts and allografts can be used to treat lesions with combined cartilage and bone loss.
- Interpositional arthroplasty uses a variety of allograft materials including lateral meniscus, Achilles tendon, and fascia lata.

Clinical and Surgical Pitfalls

- Contraindications: infection, extensive bipolar lesions, bone loss (especially posterior bone erosion)
- Surgical pitfalls: not obtaining clean or vertical walls during microfracture, incomplete debridement, incomplete capsular release, axillary nerve injury (closest between the 5- and 7-o'clock positions inferiorly), incomplete pain relief because of extensive disease

---

*The views expressed in this article are those of the authors and do not reflect the official policy or position of the Department of the Navy, Department of Defense, or the United States Government.

Glenohumeral arthritis and chondrolysis in the young, active patient population represent difficult clinical scenarios for even the most experienced of orthopedic surgeons. Even the diagnosis of symptomatic cartilage lesions can be challenging, as these patients often have multiple injuries and varying pain complaints making it difficult to determine which pathology is the primary generator of symptoms. A thorough understanding of shoulder pathoanatomy is critical for appropriate clinical decision making to provide effective treatment. Overall, the diagnosis of a symptomatic chondral injury is one of exclusion.[1] Whereas isolated articular cartilage lesions of the glenohumeral joint are rare, these lesions can become extremely painful and functionally limiting. Nonoperative treatment includes activity modification, physical therapy, nonsteroidal anti-inflammatory drugs (NSAIDs), and intra-articular injections of corticosteroids and/or hyaluronic acid solutions (off-label usage). Unfortunately, their effects are usually temporary at best. Surgical options range from simple arthroscopic treatment to arthroplasty. Total shoulder arthroplasty remains the gold standard for glenohumeral arthritis treatment and is successful at relieving pain and restoring function. Concerns regarding component loosening, ability to perform high-level athletic activity, and the potential need for early revision surgery make this a less attractive option in a younger patient population. Other surgical treatment options range from palliative arthroscopic debridement and capsular release (capsulectomy) to reparative (microfracture), restorative (osteochondral autograft or allograft and autologous chondrocyte implantation [ACI]), and reconstructive surgical techniques (biologic resurfacing). With recent advances in diagnostic modalities, surgical techniques, and biologic implants, the treatment algorithm for these difficult patients is evolving, and no single nonarthroplasty option has been identified as the gold standard. The purposes of this chapter are to provide an overview of the typical patient with glenohumeral arthritis or chondrolysis, to discuss patient evaluation and appropriate clinical decision making, and finally to describe the various nonarthroplasty surgical treatment options for these challenging clinical situations.

PREOPERATIVE CONSIDERATIONS

History

As previously described, articular cartilage lesions of the shoulder are often incidental findings discovered during preoperative imaging studies or during diagnostic arthroscopy. Treating asymptomatic lesions can be detrimental because the true cause of symptoms may be ignored or missed, and the treatment itself may cause further damage to the chondral surface. It is critical to determine if glenoid or humeral head articular cartilage lesions are truly symptomatic, and the diagnostic approach begins with a thorough patient history. In patients with multiple shoulder pathologies and those who have undergone prior operations, it is even more challenging to determine if current articular defects were actually responsible for their previous, preoperative symptoms. In addition, patients with previous shoulder surgery and intra-articular pain pump placement are at risk for the development of postsurgical glenohumeral chondrolysis.[2-7] During the initial office visit, the clinician should inquire about the following:

- Mechanism of injury (traumatic versus insidious onset)
- Current symptoms (may point to alternative diagnosis)
  - Locking
  - Clicking
  - Crepitus
  - Pain (e.g., rest pain, activity-related pain, night pain)
  - Stiffness
  - Inability to use arm above head
  - Instability
  - Numbness or tingling
- Previous nonsurgical and surgical treatment of the shoulder
- Response to prior treatment
- Patient's activity level
- Post-treatment goals
  - Allows the surgeon to address patient expectations, ensuring these are aligned with treatment options and outcomes

Signs and Symptoms

Patients with glenohumeral chondrolysis typically have vague shoulder complaints including activity pain and motion loss. Night pain is a common complaint, though nonspecific in nature. Popping or clicking sensations are often associated with articular cartilage defects. Shoulder swelling often points to articular pathology; however, this can also result from soft-tissue injuries including rotator cuff lesions. Numbness and tingling of the involved extremity are typically not seen in these patients and should direct the clinician to an alternative diagnosis. Patients may also report sudden pain and locking in specific shoulder positions associated with engagement of articular lesions.

Physical Examination

A complete physical examination of both shoulders should be performed for every patient being evaluated for symptomatic chondral defects. Range of motion

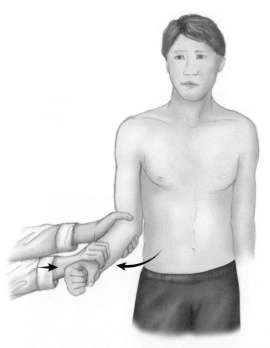

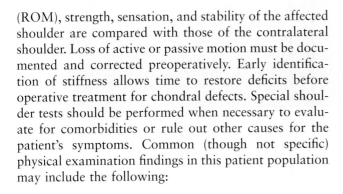

Figure 36-1. Examination of external rotation at the side that is contracted, with tight external rotation at the side.

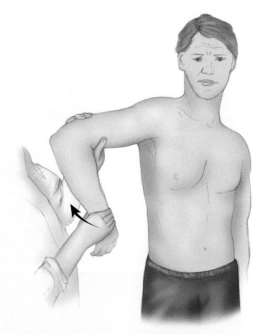

Figure 36-2. Examination of abduction internal rotation contracture of patient, showing contracture and facial pain in internal rotation (abducted internal rotation).

(ROM), strength, sensation, and stability of the affected shoulder are compared with those of the contralateral shoulder. Loss of active or passive motion must be documented and corrected preoperatively. Early identification of stiffness allows time to restore deficits before operative treatment for chondral defects. Special shoulder tests should be performed when necessary to evaluate for comorbidities or rule out other causes for the patient's symptoms. Common (though not specific) physical examination findings in this patient population may include the following:

- Tenderness to palpation—rule out subacromial bursitis
- Decreased ROM
  - Decreased forward flexion caused by an inferior humeral head spur.
  - Decreased external rotation caused by a flattened humeral head.
  - Decreased external rotation at the side (ERs) can indicate anterior capsular contracture, including the rotator interval, the superior and middle glenohumeral ligament, and the coracohumeral ligament (Fig. 36-1).
  - Decreased abduction and external rotation (ABER) can indicate anterior and anteroinferior capsule contracture.
  - Decreased abduction and internal rotation (ABIR) can indicate posterior and posteroinferior capsule contracture (Fig. 36-2).

  - Decreased abduction (ABD) can indicate inferior capsule contracture and possible involvement of the superior capsule or superior labral anterior-posterior (SLAP) region.
- Crepitus with ROM—painless versus painful
- Clicking, catching, or locking with ROM
- Normal strength and sensation

Imaging

Imaging studies are routinely used in the evaluation of glenohumeral chondral lesions and typically include radiographs, magnetic resonance imaging (MRI), magnetic resonance arthrography (MRA), and computed tomography (CT). Despite advances in imaging techniques, glenohumeral articular surface defects may not be easily seen on plain radiographs or with other advanced imaging modalities, and glenohumeral arthroscopy remains the gold standard for diagnosis. Imaging is, however, extremely helpful not only for diagnosis, but especially for preoperative planning. Specific planning considerations include the chondral anatomy of the shoulder joint. Normally the humeral head cartilage is thickest in the center (1.2 to 1.3 mm thick) and thinner at the periphery (less than 1.0 mm thick).[8] In contrast, the glenoid cartilage is thickest along the periphery, tapering centrally to the bare area where it is completely devoid of cartilage. Knowledge of normal anatomy in conjunction with information supplied by imaging studies helps determine the

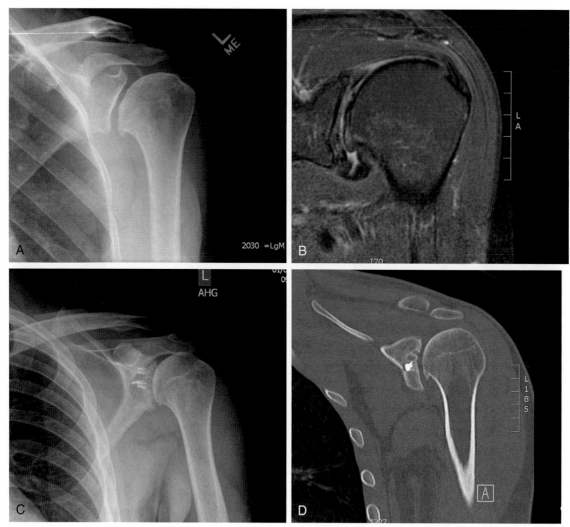

Figure 36-3. A, True anteroposterior (AP) Grashey view of a 36-year-old man with early degenerative glenohumeral joint and bipolar cartilage. **B,** Coronal magnetic resonance arthrogram of the shoulder shown in **A** better demonstrates the bipolar cartilage and early bony changes. **C,** AP view of a shoulder with anchors in the superior quadrant of the glenoid. One of the anchors had eroded through the glenoid and was in contact with the humeral head. **D,** Coronal computed tomography scan of the shoulder shown in **C** demonstrating glenoid cystic changes and small humeral head osteophyte.

significance of lesions based on their location along the humeral head and/or glenoid surface.

Radiographs

Every patient should undergo a standard radiographic series of the shoulder including an anteroposterior (AP) view, a true AP view (especially important to assess subtle joint space changes), a scapular-Y view, and an axillary lateral view. These views evaluate the joint space for glenohumeral arthritis and may show overt bony abnormalities. Other specific radiographs include the Stryker notch view to evaluate Hill-Sachs lesions and the Garth (apical oblique) view to evaluate glenoid bone loss[4] (Fig. 36-3). The earliest signs of

glenohumeral wear are usually in the posteroinferior quadrant of the shoulder and may demonstrate joint space narrowing or subtle posterior joint subluxation (Fig. 36-4).

Magnetic Resonance Imaging and Magnetic Resonance Arthrography

MRI and MRA are the imaging modalities of choice for the evaluation of glenohumeral chondral surface lesions. In addition to evaluating the articular surface, MRI and MRA can detect subchondral bone changes and concomitant soft tissue ligamentous, labral, and rotator cuff pathology.[9,10] All sequences should be analyzed, though the T2-weighted image (with and without fat

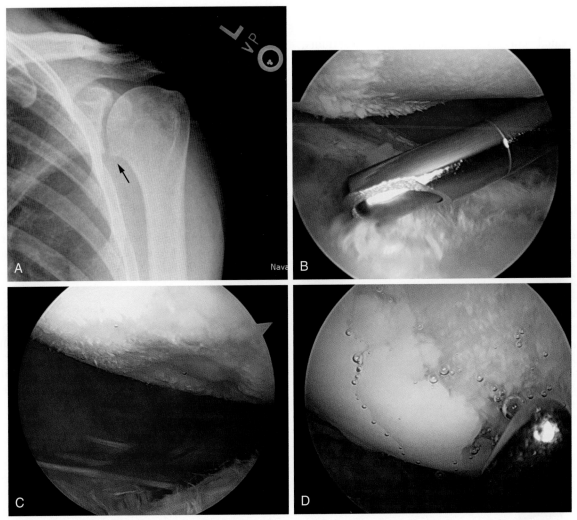

Figure 36-4. A, True anteroposterior (AP; Grashey) radiograph of a 27-year-old man 6 months after an arthroscopic Bankart repair with an inert plastic (polyetheretherketone [PEEK]) anchor. There is a small osteophyte that is evident only on the true AP view. **B,** The anchor eroded through the glenoid, causing linear stripe wear and full-thickness cartilage loss on the humeral head, demonstrated in this arthroscopic image with the arthroscope inserted from the posterior portal. Additional examples of focal humeral head defects demonstrate a concentric humeral head defect **(C)** and stripe wear **(D)**.

suppression) and the T1-weighted fat-suppressed three-dimensional spoiled gradient-echo technique are most helpful.

Computed Tomography

CT images provide a global evaluation of the glenohumeral joint, which is enhanced with three-dimensional reconstructions of images. Although not routinely obtained as part of a workup for suspected glenohumeral arthritis or chondrolysis, CT scans are useful for operative planning in patients requiring more invasive osteochondral reconstruction for full-thickness cartilage defects that include subchondral bone.

Indications and Contraindications

Relative Indications

- Younger than 50 years
- Active
- Symptomatic
- Failed nonoperative treatment
- Realistic postoperative goals
- No other causal pathology

Relative Contraindications

- Significant joint space narrowing
- Infection

- Significant glenoid version or structural abnormalities
- Untreated concomitant injuries (e.g., instability, rotator cuff)
- Unrealistic postoperative goals
- Unwillingness to comply with postoperative rehabilitation regimen

SURGICAL TECHNIQUE

Specific steps of the procedure are outlined in Box 36-1.

Anesthesia and Positioning

Depending on surgeon and anesthesiologist preference, the majority of procedures for glenohumeral arthritis

---

BOX 36-1 Surgical Techniques

Palliative: debridement, capsular release and capsulectomy, synovectomy

Reparative: microfracture

Restorative: osteochondral autograft, osteochondral allograft, autologous chondrocyte implantation (ACI)

Reconstructive: biologic resurfacing of glenoid with or without biologic resurfacing or nonbiologic resurfacing of humeral head

---

and chondrolysis are performed with the patient under general anesthesia with an interscalene block. Alternatively, sedation with an interscalene block can also be used. The interscalene block not only helps minimize the amount of intraoperative anesthetic needed but also helps with immediate postoperative pain management. Positioning is in the beach chair or lateral decubitus position and depends on the procedure being performed and surgeon preference. For arthroscopic procedures we prefer the lateral decubitus position with the arm placed in balanced suspension as this offers ease of access to all quadrants of the shoulder, facilitating capsular and synovial exposure for capsulectomy, debridement, and any concomitant arthroscopic procedures. If an open procedure is performed, such as allograft or interpositional arthroplasty, we prefer the beach chair position.

Beach Chair Setup

- The patient is placed supine at the lateral edge of the table so the operative shoulder is unimpaired (Fig. 36-5).
  - The medial border of the scapula is bolstered with two towels, facilitating scapular protraction against the chest wall.
  - A commercially available arm-positioning device can assist with traction and distraction.

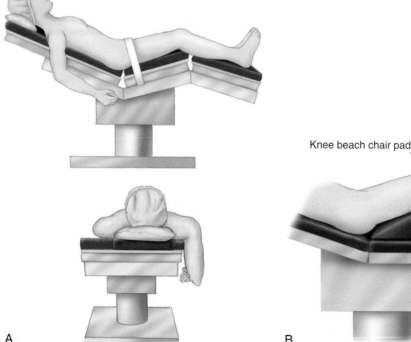

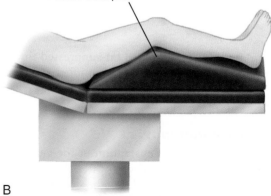

Knee beach chair pad

A   B

Figure 36-5. The beach chair setup. **A,** Supine, with the patient at the lateral edge of the table so the operative shoulder is unimpaired. All bony prominences are well padded. Head, neck, and torso are supported in a neutral position. Hips are flexed 45 to 60 degrees while the knees are flexed to 30 degrees. **B,** A knee beach chair pad may be used to assist with positioning.

- All bony prominences are well padded.
  - Protect the nonoperative olecranon.
  - Protect the peroneal nerves at the knee.
  - Protect bilateral calcanei.
- Head, neck, and torso are supported in a neutral position.
- Hips are flexed 45 to 60 degrees while the knees are flexed to 30 degrees.
  - Use a knee beach chair pad to assist with positioning.

Lateral Decubitus Setup

- Patient is positioned with the operative side up, supported with a bean bag or alternative support.
- All bony prominences are well padded.
  - The torso is rolled 25 degrees posterior, which positions the glenoid parallel to the floor and opens the shoulder joint.
- An axillary roll is placed under the chest four fingerbreadths distal to the axilla.
- The arm is prepared for surgery and placed in a suspension sleeve with neutral rotation before attachment to a suspension device.
- The arm is balanced in suspension at 45 degrees of ABD and 15 degrees of forward flexion.

Surgical Landmarks, Incisions, and Portals

- Landmarks include the coracoid process, the acromion, the deltoid insertion, and the axillary crease.
- Use standard arthroscopy portals for arthroscopic techniques.
- Use the deltopectoral approach for open techniques.
  - Identify and preserve the cephalic vein (generally retract laterally).
- At-risk structures include the musculocutaneous nerve, the axillary nerve, and the anterior humeral circumflex artery (blood supply to the humeral head) (Fig. 36-6).

Examination Under Anesthesia

An examination under anesthesia (EUA) should be performed before the beginning of arthroscopy and helps evaluate the following:

- ROM including flexion, ABD, ERs, ABER, ABIR
  - This provides information to plan tailored capsular releases.
- Stability
- Areas of mechanical click or "engagement" of the humeral head on the glenoid

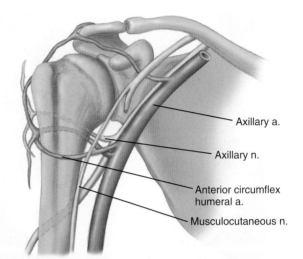

Axillary a.

Axillary n.

Anterior circumflex humeral a.

Musculocutaneous n.

Figure 36-6. The at-risk neurovascular structures of the shoulder with the deltopectoral approach include the axillary nerve, the musculocutaneous nerve, and the anterior circumflex humeral artery (blood supply to a large portion of the humeral head). *a,* Artery; *n,* nerve.

Specific Surgical Techniques and Steps

Palliative Arthroscopic Procedures

- Debridement (please see previous chapter for complete description of surgical technique).
- Capsulectomy: This is the first-line treatment for nonarthroplasty treatment of glenohumeral arthritis and associated motion loss. Tailored capsular release is based on ROM deficits in specific planes and can greatly improve ROM and provide pain relief (Fig. 36-7).
1. Position the patient in the lateral decubitus position.
2. Use standard posterior and midglenoid arthroscopic portals.
3. With the arthroscope inserted from posterior, a capsular release is performed with an arthroscopic basket cutter. The release is started superiorly at the rotator interval, and the capsule is released from anterosuperior to anteroinferior at the labral-capsular junction.
4. Care is taken not to release deeper than 2 to 3 mm to protect the axillary nerve, which is closest at the 5- to 7-o'clock position.
5. The arthroscope is switched to the anterior portal, and the basket cutter is inserted percutaneously (without a cannula) through the posterior portal. The release is completed posteroinferiorly to posterosuperiorly.
6. A radiofrequency device use is described for capsular releases. We prefer to limit use to synovial debridement and hemostasis after release, to avoid potential iatrogenic injury to the axillary

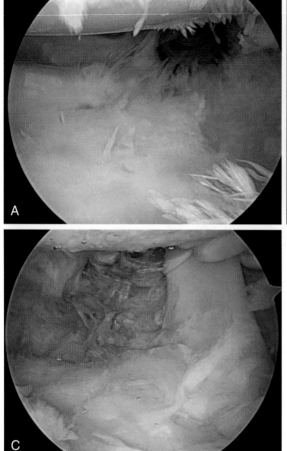

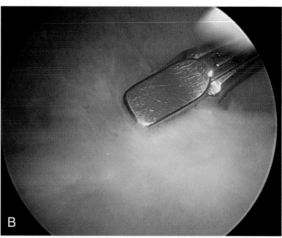

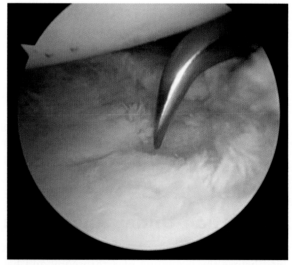

Figure 36-7. A, An example of extensive cartilage loss on the humeral head in a 29-year-old man. **B,** The patient underwent an initial capsular release arthroscopically; the arthroscopic biter is inserted from the anterior portal with the arthroscope posteriorly. **C,** The rotator interval tissue is usually scarred and inflamed, shown here with arthroscope from posteriorly, and should also be extensively debrided. This patient was eventually treated with a bulk fresh osteochondral allograft (two 18-mm plugs) to the humeral head.

nerve or other structures around the glenohumeral joint.

7. Once arthroscopy is completed, a gentle manipulation under anesthesia in all planes of motion is performed with the patient remaining in the lateral decubitus position.

Reparative Arthroscopic Procedures

Microfracture (Fig. 36-8) may be performed with or without a capsulectomy. Microfracture is best performed on isolated glenoid and/or humeral head lesions. (Please see previous chapters for a complete description of surgical technique.) Surgical pearls are as follows:

- Long-handled arthroscopic curettes and awls help achieve arthroscopic access to all areas of the glenohumeral joint.
- It is important to gently remove the layer of calcified cartilage from the injured area with a curette, small bone-cutting shaver, or burr.
- Microfracture holes are placed at approximately 5- to 7-mm intervals and 3 to 4 mm deep.
- Arthroscopic pump pressure is decreased to ensure marrow bleeding from the microfracture sites.

Figure 36-8. An example of microfracture to the posteroinferior glenoid.

Restorative Techniques

Restorative surgical techniques for glenohumeral cartilage defects aim to *restore* the damaged articular surface and include the use of osteochondral autografts, osteochondral allografts, and ACI as an off-label indication.

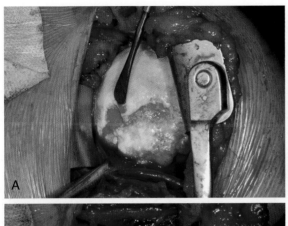
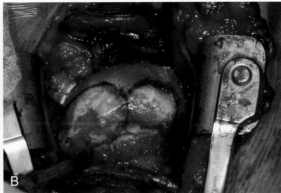
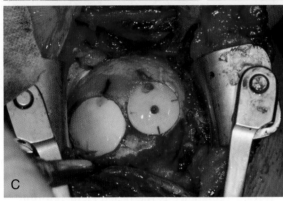

Figure 36-9. An example of a 25-year-old male patient with isolated humeral head cartilage damage (grade IV) treated with a fresh osteochondral allograft, two plugs (one 18 mm, one 20 mm), in the inferior aspect of the humeral head.

These techniques can be used as the primary procedure (especially in patients with large isolated defects); however, more often these are used in patients in whom debridement and/or microfracture procedures have already failed. These techniques are more invasive than palliative and reparative techniques and typically require a shoulder arthrotomy with a subscapularis and a capsular takedown.

Osteochondral Autograft

1. Use the standard deltopectoral approach (Fig. 36-9).
2. Perform a subscapularis takedown and a capsular takedown. If the lesion is superior and anterior in the humeral head, a limited (superior half only) subscapularis takedown may be sufficient.
3. The area to be grafted (typically on the humeral head) is identified and sized.
4. Obtain osteochondral autograft bone from the contralateral or ipsilateral knee. This can be performed in an arthroscopically assisted manner using commercially available autograft plug harvesters and implanters. Typically, a 6- to 10-mm bone plug is used. One should consider the curvature of the injured area to ensure optimal plug fit.
5. The knee donor autograft plug is obtained in a size-matched manner, including about 8 mm.
6. The recipient area to be grafted is cored to the same depth after the donor core has been confirmed for proper depth and orientation.

7. The donor graft is gently tamped into position flush with the native articular cartilage.
8. The shoulder capsule is closed in a typical fashion. Avoid overtensioning the capsule, and perform a meticulous subscapularis repair.
9. The deltopectoral approach is closed in a layered fashion, and the patient is placed in a padded ABD sling.

Osteochondral Allograft

1. Similar to the procedure noted previously, except that the allograft is a fresh donor allograft.
2. Fresh humeral head, glenoid, and distal tibia (for the glenoid) have all been described for allograft treatment of isolated large osteochondral lesions. These also have the advantage of providing bony augmentation for areas of bone loss, injury, or necrosis.
3. The fresh donor bone is sized using commercially available allograft donor and recipient systems to match the recipient.
4. Typically these donor cores are 15 to 25 mm for the humeral head and smaller for the glenoid.
5. Contrary to the autograft procedure, with this procedure the recipient is prepared first to get the diameter and depth of the area to be grafted. A typical depth (to minimize the burden of bone and potential allograft marrow elements) is 4 to 6 mm of subchondral bone.

6. Care is taken to keep the recipient preparation drill flush to the articular margins, and if possible to include the entire lesion. Copious irrigation is used to cool the bone.

7. Once sized, the donor graft is harvested on the back table. The core is sized appropriately and pulse-lavaged with 2 to 3 L of lactated Ringer's solution.

8. The donor graft is gently tamped into position, flush with the native articular cartilage.

9. The shoulder capsule is closed in a typical fashion. Avoid overtensioning the capsule, and perform a meticulous subscapularis repair.

10. The deltopectoral approach is closed in a layered fashion, and the patient is placed in a padded ABD sling.

Autologous Chondrocyte Implantation (U.S. Food and Drug Administration Off-Label Use in the Shoulder)

1. Before implantation, the cartilage cells must be harvested and cultured, which takes approximately 4 to 6 weeks. An initial surgery is performed to confirm the glenohumeral lesion, usually in conjunction with knee arthroscopy to harvest the cartilage for ACI.

2. Use the standard deltopectoral approach.

3. Perform a subscapularis and a capsular takedown.

4. The contralateral (or ipsilateral) proximal tibia is prepared and draped for harvesting of the periosteal flap that will be sutured around the defect to contain the ACI cells.

5. The lesion is prepared with standard ACI technique using small curettes, smoothing the bone, and ensuring near-vertical walls.

6. The periosteal patch is smoothed over the lesion and gently stretched thin.

7. A 6-0 colored Vicryl suture is used to repair the patch with multiple interrupted sutures. A small entry area under the flap is left for implantation of the cultured chondrocytes.

8. Before injection of the cells, fibrin glue is used to seal the edges of the periosteal patch to ensure a watertight repair.

9. Cultured chondrocyte cells are then injected underneath the flap and sutured in place, with fibrin glue used to complete the watertight repair.

10. The shoulder capsule is closed in a typical fashion. Avoid overtensioning the capsule, and perform a meticulous subscapularis repair.

11. The deltopectoral approach is closed in a layered fashion, and the patient is placed in a padded ABD sling.

Reconstructive Techniques

Reconstructive surgical techniques aim to *reconstruct* the more severely damaged glenohumeral joint. These techniques are often used in patients with advanced unipolar or bipolar disease and are considered the last resort before total shoulder arthroplasty. Patients with bipolar disease have much poorer surgical outcomes and should be approached with caution. Surgical options include biologic resurfacing of the glenoid combined with either a biologic or nonbiologic resurfacing of the humeral head. Currently, biologic resurfacing of the humeral head remains investigational, and the only cases reported involve the use of osteochondral allograft or ACI. More commonly, nonbiologic reconstruction of the humeral head with implant resurfacing or hemiarthroplasty is performed with a concomitant biologic resurfacing of the glenoid. Biologic glenoid resurfacing options include allograft interposition with lateral meniscus, Achilles tendon or tensor fascia lata, and/or processed tissue graft interposition with dermal patch regenerative tissue matrix or porcine small intestine submucosa. The dermal patch is available in the form of 4×4 cm^2 sheets that are 1 to 2 mm thick, which can be customized to the desired shape and size of the patient's glenoid.

Open Lateral Meniscus Allograft or Dermal Patch Resurfacing Technique

1. Our preference is the beach chair position.

2. Use a standard deltopectoral approach.

3. Prepare the humeral head and any necessary soft tissue or capsular releases.

4. The glenoid labrum is left in situ to serve as an anchor for fixation of the graft.

5. Remove the remaining glenoid articular cartilage with a curette.

6. Perform concentric reaming of the glenoid, starting with a small reamer.

    a. Starting small avoids damage to the native labral tissue.

7. Place nonabsorbable sutures through the labrum, in positions that allow for six to eight points of circumferential fixation to the glenoid.

    a. Lateral meniscus fixation (Fig. 36-10):

        i. Sutures from the labrum are passed through the lateral meniscal allograft.

        ii. Orient the graft so that the anterior and posterior horns face anteriorly and the thickest portion of the graft covers the posterior portion of the glenoid.

        iii. Suture the horns together to provide stability during peripheral fixation.

        iv. Tie each circumferential suture, leaving fixation of the horns to the anterior aspect of the glenoid for last.

        v. Glenoid anchors may be used for posterior or other hard to reach areas.

        vi. Once the allograft is in place, carefully anteriorly dislocate the humerus, allowing for humeral head hemiarthroplasty insertion.

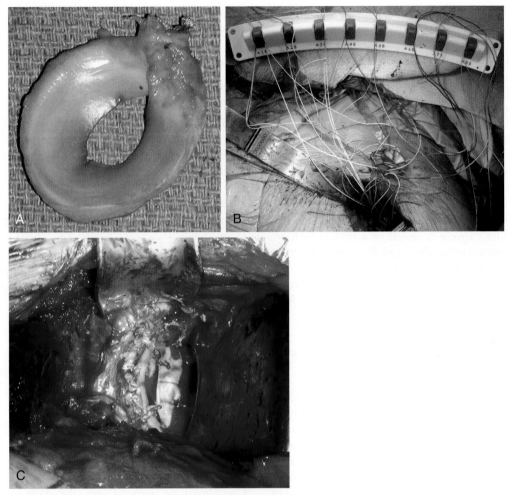

Figure 36-10. A lateral meniscus interpositional arthroplasty in a 23-year-old female patient with focal glenoid loss and nearly normal humeral head cartilage. The lateral meniscus is inserted after meticulous glenoid preparation (cartilage debridement, gentle reaming, and suture tying to an intact labrum or anchor usage) through an open approach and sutured into position.

    vii. Perform the humeral head hemiarthroplasty or humeral head resurfacing (humeral head focal defect cap, or large head cap) per surgeon preference.

    viii. Reduce the shoulder.

       a) Assess conformity of the implanted component and graft.

       b) Assess the glenohumeral ROM and stability.

b. Dermal patch resurfacing (Fig. 36-11):

    i. Allow the graft to thaw and hydrate per manufacturer's protocol.

    ii. Perform the humeral head hemiarthroplasty first.

    iii. Reduce the shoulder, and assess conformity of the implant with the native articular surface.

    iv. Insert retractors to displace the implanted humeral head posteriorly.

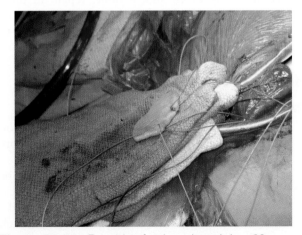

Figure 36-11. Example of a dermal patch in a 28-year-old man with near-complete glenoid cartilage loss and grade I to II diffuse humeral head changes.

v. Cut the thawed graft to the appropriate size and shape.

vi. Secure the graft to the glenoid by individually passing sutures from the labrum through the edges of the graft material.

vii. Glenoid anchors may be used for posterior or other hard to reach areas.

viii. Use of sequential suture passage and tying allows for tensioning of the dermal patch over the glenoid surface.

ix. Reduce the shoulder.
   a) Assess conformity of the implanted component and graft.
   b) Assess glenohumeral ROM and stability.

8. The shoulder capsule is closed in a typical fashion. Avoid overtensioning the capsule, and perform a meticulous subscapularis repair.

9. The deltopectoral approach is closed in a layered fashion, and the patient is placed in a padded ABD sling.

POSTOPERATIVE CONSIDERATIONS

Most patients can be discharged from the hospital on the day of surgery. Some patients may stay overnight for additional pain control or if a postoperative drain is placed. Patients return to the clinic 7 to 10 days postoperatively for a wound check and for radiographs including a true AP view. The early and late restrictions on activity depend on the procedure performed. For arthroscopic procedures, unrestricted passive and active ROM is encouraged as early as the first postoperative day, especially for those with capsular release and/or microfracture. For open procedures a sling is used for protection and comfort, and activity is dictated by the subscapularis takedown and, if done, repair. In these cases external rotation is protected and limited to 20 to 30 degrees with no active internal rotation for 5 to 6 weeks while the patient is in a sling.

Rehabilitation

Arthroscopic Procedures

- Unrestricted passive to active ROM is allowed on the first postoperative day. Rehabilitation is more restricted if microfracture is performed.
  - A sling is provided for comfort only and can be removed per patient tolerance.
  - Early scapular stabilization exercises are started.
- Light strengthening is started at 4 to 6 weeks, though generally dictated by subscapularis repair.
- Unrestricted strengthening is started at 12 weeks.
- Unrestricted activities are allowed at 16 weeks.
- Performance of overhead competitive athletics is allowed at 6 months.

- All stages are begun earlier if debridement alone is performed.

Open Procedures

Phase 1: 0 to 6 Weeks

- Pendulum exercises up to 800 per day
- Sling use for 4 to 6 weeks
- Active use of the hand, the wrist, and the elbow
- Active-assisted ROM to 120 degrees of flexion and to 75 degrees of ABD

Phase 2: 7 to 12 Weeks

- Progress from active-assisted to active ROM.
- Begin and progress with deltoid and rotator cuff isometric strengthening.
  - Exceptions: Internal rotation is limited.
- Begin and progress with periscapular muscular strengthening.

Phase 3: 13 Weeks to 6 Months

- Start internal rotation strengthening.
- Progress with the remainder of strengthening.

Phase 4: 6 Months and Beyond

- Consider return to competitive overhead athletics.

Complications

Complications depend on the type of procedure performed. With arthroscopic procedures, the overall complication rate is low. The most reported major complications include damage to the neurovascular structures, including the axillary nerve in working inferiorly and the musculocutaneous nerve in placing the anterior portal. With open procedures the complication rate is also low, comparable to that of total shoulder arthroplasty. Complications include damage to the axillary and musculocutaneous nerves, infection, and failure of repair. In working with allograft tissue, there is a low but serious risk of disease transmission, including human immunodeficiency virus (HIV) and hepatitis.

RESULTS

Reports of outcomes after palliative, reparative, restorative, and reconstructive surgical techniques for glenohumeral articular defects are limited. These procedures are relatively new, and techniques are constantly evolving, making it difficult to perform long-term, prospective, randomized clinical trials. Currently the majority of studies available are case reports, case series, and retrospective cohort studies. A summary of selected studies representing all procedures is available in Table 36-1.

TABLE 36-1. Selected Outcomes

	Procedure	No. of Shoulders	Average Follow-up	Outcomes	Notes
Van Thiel et al[11] (2010)	Arthroscopic debridement	71	27 months	Significant improvements (*P* < .05) in ASES, SST, VAS scores, ROM Postoperative SANE score 71.1 Postoperative Constant score 78.5 Postoperative UCLA score 28.3	16 patients progressed to arthroplasty at 10.1 mo
Frank et al[12] (2010)	Arthroscopic microfracture	17	28 months	Significant improvements (*P* < .05) in VAS, ASES, and SST scores	Procedure best if isolated, unipolar glenoid or HH lesion
Millett et al[13] (2010)	Arthroscopic microfracture	31	47 months	Significant improvements (*P* < .05) in ability to work, ADLs, sports activity, and ASES score	Procedure best if isolated, small, HH lesion
Scheibel et al[14] (2004)	Osteochondral autograft to HH	8	33 months	6 pain free 2 reduced pain MRI scan with graft incorporation and congruent articular surfaces in 7 of 8	Patients with traumatic grade IV chondral lesions of HH
Yagishita and Thomas[15] (2002)	Femoral head allograft to HH	1	24 months	Pain free with no recurrent instability	
Chapovsky and Kelly[9] (2005)	Osteochondral allograft plugs to HH engaging Hill-Sachs lesion	1	12 months	Full return to athletics Pain free	
Gerber and Lambert[16] (1996)	Osteochondral allograft plugs to HH reverse Hill-Sachs lesions	4	68 months	Good to excellent outcomes in 3 AVN development in 1	All HH defects with >40% articular surface involvement
McCarty and Cole[17] (2007)	Osteochondral allograft to HH, lateral meniscal allograft to glenoid	1	24 months	ASES score 83, SST score 8 FF 90 to 160 degrees ER 40 to 50 degrees	Patient with bipolar GH chondrolysis after arthroscopic thermal capsulorrhaphy
McNickle et al[5] (2009)	Osteochondral allograft to HH, lateral meniscus allograft to glenoid (1 patient with HH treatment only)	8	37 months	Improvements in SST, ASES, and VAS scores	All patients with extensive postsurgical glenohumeral arthritis
Romeo et al[18] (2002)	ACI to focal defect of HH	1	12 months	Full painless ROM	Patient with focal defect s/p arthroscopic capsulorrhaphy with radiofrequency device
Burkhead and Hutton[19] (1995)	HH hemiarthroplasty with biologic resurfacing to glenoid (TFL or anterior capsule)	6 (14 in series, 6 with follow-up)	28 months	Reduction in pain in all cases Improvement in FF, ER, and IR 5 of 6 with excellent outcomes 1 of 6 satisfactory outcome	
Lee et al[20] (2009)	HH hemiarthroplasty with biologic resurfacing to glenoid (anterior capsule)	18	4.8 years	ASES score 74.4 Constant score 71.4 FF 130 degrees, ABD 122 degrees, ER 39 degrees 83% satisfied	56% with moderate to severe glenoid erosion on postoperative radiographs

Continued

TABLE 36-1. Selected Outcomes—cont'd

	Procedure	No. of Shoulders	Average Follow-up	Outcomes	Notes
Krishnan et al[21] (2008)	Biologic resurfacing to glenoid with TFL (n = 11), anterior capsule (n = 7), Achilles tendon (n = 18)	36	7 years	ASES score 39 to 91 Good to excellent in 86%	Radiographs with mean 7.2 mm glenoid erosion, which appeared to stabilize at 5 years postoperatively
Elhassan et al[22] (2009)	HH hemiarthroplasty with biologic resurfacing to glenoid (Achilles tendon, TFL, or anterior capsule)	13	14 months	10 of 13 converted to TSA at mean 14 months postoperatively 2 of 13 with postoperative infection Overall 92.3% failure rate	Authors reported technique as unreliable
Nicholson et al[23] (2007)	HH implant resurfacing with lateral meniscus allograft to glenoid	30	18 months	ASES score 38 to 69 SST score 3.3 to 7.8 VAS score 6.4 to 2.3 (pain) FF 96 to 139 degrees ER 26 to 53 degrees 94% satisfied	Revision surgery for complications in 5 patients within first year
Wirth[24] (2009)	HH hemiarthroplasty with lateral meniscus allograft to glenoid	30 (90% follow-up)	35 months	Significant improvements in ASES, SST, and VAS scores in all patients	16% reoperation rate (half because of failure of meniscal construct)
Huijsmans et al[25] (2004)	Dermal patch to glenoid	6	6 months	Preliminary improvements	
Savoie et al[26] (2009)	Arthroscopic glenoid resurfacing with biologic patch	23	3-6 years	75% satisfied ASES score 22 to 78* UCLA score 15 to 29* Rowe score 55 to 81* Constant score 26 to 79*	5 patients converted to TSA, but 4 of 5 underwent resurfacing again

*$P < .05$.

ABD, abduction; *ACI,* autologous chondrocyte implantation; *ADLs,* activities of daily living; *ASES,* American Shoulder and Elbow Surgeons scale; *AVN,* avascular necrosis; *ER,* external rotation; *FF,* forward flexion; *HH,* humeral head; *IR,* internal rotation; *TFL,* tensor fascia lata; *MRI,* magnetic resonance imaging; *ROM,* range of motion; *SANE,* Single Assessment Numeric Evaluation; *s/p,* status post; *SST,* simple shoulder test; *TSA,* total shoulder arthroplasty; *UCLA,* University of California at Los Angeles shoulder rating scale; *VAS,* visual analogue scale.

REFERENCES

1. Cole BJ, Yanke A, Provencher MT. Nonarthroplasty alternatives for the treatment of glenohumeral arthritis. *J Shoulder Elbow Surg.* 2007;16:S231-S240.
2. Bailie DS, Ellenbecker TS. Severe chondrolysis after shoulder arthroscopy: a case series. *J Shoulder Elbow Surg.* 2009;18:742-747.
3. Busfield BT, Romero DM. Pain pump use after shoulder arthroscopy as a cause of glenohumeral chondrolysis. *Arthroscopy.* 2009;25:647-652.
4. Kang RW, Frank RM, Nho SJ, et al. Complications associated with anterior shoulder instability repair. *Arthroscopy.* 2009;25:909-920.
5. McNickle AG, L'Heureux DR, Provencher MT, et al. Postsurgical glenohumeral arthritis in young adults. *Am J Sports Med.* 2009;37:1784-1791.
6. Saltzman M, Mercer D, Bertelsen A, et al. Postsurgical chondrolysis of the shoulder. *Orthopedics.* 2009;32: 215.
7. Solomon DJ, Navaie M, Stedje-Larsen ET, et al. Glenohumeral chondrolysis after arthroscopy: a systematic review of potential contributors and causal pathways. *Arthroscopy.* 2009;25:1329-1342.
8. Fox JA, Cole BJ, Romeo AA, et al. Articular cartilage thickness of the humeral head: an anatomic study. *Orthopedics.* 2008;31.
9. Chapovsky F, Kelly JD 4th. Osteochondral allograft transplantation for treatment of glenohumeral instability. *Arthroscopy.* 2005;21:1007.
10. Gold GE, Reeder SB, Beaulieu CF. Advanced MR imaging of the shoulder: dedicated cartilage techniques. *Magn Reson Imaging Clin N Am.* 2004;12:143-159, vii.
11. Van Thiel GS, et al. Retrospective analysis of arthroscopic management of glenohumeral degenerative disease. *Arthroscopy.* 2010;26(11):1451-1455.
12. Frank RM, et al. Clinical outcomes after microfracture of the glenohumeral joint. *Am J Sports Med.* 2010;38(4): 772-781.

13. Millett PJ, et al. Outcomes of full-thickness articular cartilage injuries of the shoulder treated with microfracture. *Arthroscopy.* 2009;25(8):856-863.

14. Scheibel M, et al. Osteochondral autologous transplantation for the treatment of full-thickness articular cartilage defects of the shoulder. *J Bone Joint Surg Br.* 2004; 86(7):991-997.

15. Yagishita K, Thomas BJ. Use of allograft for large Hill-Sachs lesion associated with anterior glenohumeral dislocation. A case report. *Injury.* 2002;3(9):791-794.

16. Gerber C, Lambert SM. Allograft reconstruction of segmental defects of the humeral head for the treatment of chronic locked posterior dislocation of the shoulder. *J Bone Joint Surg Am.* 1996;78(3):376-382.

17. McCarty LP III, Cole BJ. Reconstruction of the glenohumeral joint using a lateral meniscal allograft to the glenoid and osteoarticular humeral head allograft after bipolar chondrolysis. *J Shoulder Elbow Surg.* 2007;16(6): e20-e24.

18. Romeo AA, et al. Autologous chondrocyte repair of an articular defect in the humeral head. *Arthroscopy.* 2002; 18(8):925-929.

19. Burkhead WZ Jr, Hutton KS. Biologic resurfacing of the glenoid with hemiarthroplasty of the shoulder. *J Shoulder Elbow Surg.* 1995;4(4):263-270.

20. Lee KT, Bell S, Salmon J. Cementless surface replacement arthroplasty of the shoulder with biologic resurfacing of the glenoid. *J Shoulder Elbow Surg.* 2009;18(6): 915-919.

21. Krishnan SG, et al. Humeral hemiarthroplasty with biologic resurfacing of the glenoid for glenohumeral arthritis. Surgical technique. *J Bone Joint Surg Am.* 2008;90 (Suppl 2 Pt 1):9-19.

22. Elhassan B, et al. Soft-tissue resurfacing of the glenoid in the treatment of glenohumeral arthritis in active patients less than fifty years old. *J Bone Joint Surg Am.* 2009; 91(2):419-424.

23. Nicholson GP, et al. Lateral meniscus allograft biologic glenoid arthroplasty in total shoulder arthroplasty for young shoulders with degenerative joint disease. *J Shoulder Elbow Surg.* 2007;16(5 Suppl):S261-S266.

24. Wirth MA. Humeral head arthroplasty and meniscal allograft resurfacing of the glenoid. *J Bone Joint Surg Am.* 2009;91(5):1109-1119.

25. Huijsmans PE, et al. The treatment of glenohumeral OA in the young and active patient with the Graft Jacket: preliminary results. *J Bone Joint Surg Br.* 2005;87-B (Suppl III):275.

26. Savoie FH III, Brislin KJ, Argo D. Arthroscopic glenoid resurfacing as a surgical treatment for glenohumeral arthritis in the young patient: midterm results. *Arthroscopy.* 2009;25(8):864-871.

SUGGESTED READINGS

Cole BJ, Yanke AMT. Provencher Nonarthroplasty alternatives for the treatment of glenohumeral arthritis. *J Shoulder Elbow Surg.* 2007;16:S231-S240.

McCarty LP 3rd, Cole BJ. Nonarthroplasty treatment of glenohumeral cartilage lesions. *Arthroscopy.* 2005;21: 1131-1142.

Provencher MT, Navaie M, Solomon DJ, et al. Joint chondrolysis. *J Bone Joint Surg Am.* 2011;93:2033-2044.

Solomon DJ, Navaie M, Stedje-Larsen ET, et al. Glenohumeral chondrolysis after arthroscopy: a systematic review of potential contributors and causal pathways. *Arthroscopy.* 2009;25:1329-1342.

Chapter 37

Biologics in Rotator Cuff Repair

Salma Chaudhury and Scott A. Rodeo

Chapter Synopsis

- High failure rates after rotator cuff repairs have encouraged the search for biologics that may stimulate improved healing. This chapter will consider a number of different biologic approaches to augmenting rotator cuff repairs. Key cytokine and growth factors that play important roles are identified as potential targets for biologic therapies. The efficacy and limitations of a number of commercially available biologic treatments are considered, including drug therapies, platelet-rich plasma, structural support with scaffolds, and more novel cellular therapies. Techniques to indirectly modulate the biologic milieu of rotator cuff tendons are also considered, such as encouragement of neovascularization and mechanical loading.

Important Points

- Modulation of cytokines and growth factors in the biologic milieu surrounding rotator cuff tendons may enhance healing.
- A number of drugs have been identified that potentially impair tendon healing, such as cyclooxygenase 2 inhibitors and fluoroquinolones; their judicious use after rotator cuff surgeries is advised.
- The role of platelet-rich plasma in rotator cuff repairs remains unproven and requires further investigation.
- Concerns persist about the efficacy of a number of synthetic and biologic scaffolds for augmenting rotator cuff repairs.
- Stem cell therapies alone have failed to result in improved rotator cuff healing. Enhanced stem cell function and tendon healing may occur through modulation of cell cytokine expression.

Rotator cuff pathologies are among the most common causes of shoulder pain. The incidence of rotator cuff tears is known to increase with age, particularly over the age of 50 years. Torn rotator cuff tendons are associated with increased pain and poorer shoulder function. A significant proportion of torn rotator cuff tendons retear after surgical repairs, and failure rates of 30% to 70% are frequently reported. The biologic milieu that precedes and follows rotator cuff tears has been shown to contribute to rotator cuff tear pathogenesis. The increasing health burden of rotator cuff tears has encouraged investigation into biologic adjuncts that may be used to augment surgical repairs of rotator cuff tendons with the aim of ultimately reducing high failure rates. It is hoped that biologic adjuncts will encourage regeneration of functional tendon tissue rather than mechanically inferior scar tissue that usually forms at the healing rotator cuff enthesis (Fig. 37-1).[1]

This chapter explores a number of biologic approaches used to treat rotator cuff tears in addition to surgical repairs, such as drug, scaffold, and cellular therapies, as well as mechanical modulation of the healing environment. Drugs and systemic factors that impair tendon-bone healing also are considered.

DRUG TREATMENTS THAT IMPROVE HEALING

Modulating Cytokines and Growth Factors

The biologic milieu surrounding healing rotator cuff tears is complex and affected by a number of factors that can be both helpful and detrimental to tendon regeneration. Manipulation of this biologic environment

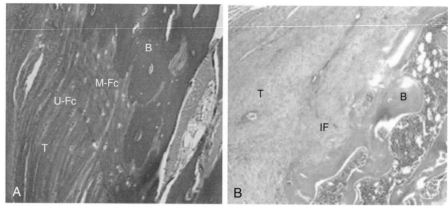

Figure 37-1. A, Histologic sections of a normal supraspinatus tendon insertion site demonstrates the four zones of a direct insertion: tendon *(T)*, unmineralized fibrocartilage *(U-Fc)*, mineralized fibrocartilage *(M-Fc)*, and bone *(B)*. **B,** This histologic section of the tendon-bone attachment site 4 weeks after supraspinatus tendon repair in a rat model shows the site is characterized by a fibrovascular scar tissue interface *(IF)* without formation of an intermediate zone of fibrocartilage between tendon *(T)* and bone *(B)*. *(From Kovacevic D, Rodeo SA. Biological augmentation of rotator cuff tendon repair. Clin Orthop Relat Res. 2008;466:622-633.)*

may tip the balance to favor tendon healing rather than tendon breakdown. A number of growth factors and cytokines related to extracellular matrix (ECM) regulation and turnover have been shown to play a role in rotator cuff tear pathogenesis. Modulation of these growth factors is proposed to enhance tendon healing, and a number of biologic moieties have been delivered to rotator cuff repair sites in an attempt to augment the rotator cuff tendon-bone interface.

Increasing cell numbers and their proliferation is proposed to increase tendon healing. One such cytokine that stimulates tendon regeneration is transforming growth factor β_1 (TGF-β_1), through its effects on cell replication and hyperplasia. However, a number of cytokines affect multiple pathways and can result in negative as well as positive effects on tendon healing. TGF-β_1 also increases smooth muscle actin (SMA) levels, which are thought to contribute to tendon retraction after tears.

Matrix metalloproteinases (MMPs) and their inhibitors (tissue inhibitors of matrix metalloproteinases [TIMPs]) control the balance between synthesis and degradation of the ECM. The most important regulators of the ECM include MMPs 1, 2, 3, 9, and 10 as well as TIMPs 2, 3, and 4. Manipulation of MMP-related pathways are proposed to encourage tendon regeneration. Tetracyclines inhibit collagenase via an interleukin (IL)-1β–mediated release of MMP-3. One such example, doxycycline, was reported to improve the histology and mechanics of rotator cuff tendon healing in a rat model.[2]

Recapitulating embryonic tendon differentiation may help to replicate the scarless healing process that is seen in the embryo. TGF-β_3 plays a role in wound healing and embryonic tendon development, and therefore a number of studies have investigated the effects of localized TGF-β_3 delivery to healing tendon sites.[3,4] TGF-β_3 delivery resulted in improved collagen I expression, vascularity, cellularity and cell proliferation. Improvements in histology and mechanical properties were also noted (Fig. 37-2).

Effects of some growth factors may be temporally mediated and depend on the phase of healing during which they are delivered. For example, fibroblast growth factor 2 (FGF-2) delivered both with and without scaffolds was found to improve the histology and biomechanical properties of healing supraspinatus tears in rats at early rather than later time points.[5,6] Another cytokine that is thought to be detrimental to rotator cuff healing is the proinflammatory mediator tumor necrosis factor α (TNF-α), and its effects appear to be affected by timing. A study of the effects of TNF-α blockade found an early improvement in mechanical properties only at 2 and 4 weeks, but the improvement was no longer present at 8 weeks.[7]

Ultimately, the effectiveness of cytokine- or growth factor–mediated enhancement of rotator cuff healing may be determined by a number of factors related to delivery, such as concentration, timing of delivery, and delivery modality. One interesting approach taken was to coat sutures with platelet-derived growth factor (PDGF-BB), and although it improved the histology of the rotator cuff, there was no effect on mechanical properties.[8] Biologic and synthetic scaffolds are increasingly used as a delivery vehicle for growth factors, to ensure localized delivery and retention. Targeted delivery can be achieved by seeding transduced cells that express desired factors to the site of the rotator cuff repair.

Another approach to ensure higher levels of growth factor and cytokine delivery is to use concentrated autologous platelets as a delivery vehicle in the form of

FIBROCARTILAGE FORMATION

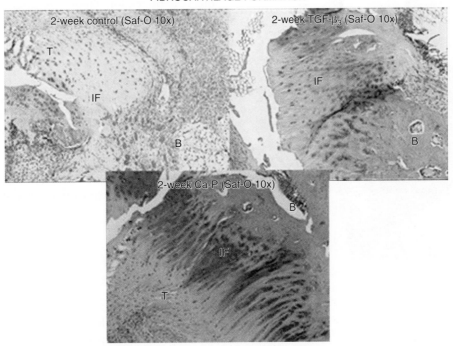

Figure 37-2. Representative safranin O–stained tissue sections of the healing enthesis at 2 weeks after surgery. There is more fibrocartilage present in the experimental groups compared with the control group. *T*, Tendon; *IF*, interface; *B*, bone. *(From Kovacevic D, Fox AJ, Bedi A, et al. Calcium-phosphate matrix with or without TGF-β3 improves tendon-bone healing after rotator cuff repair. Am J Sports Med. 2011;39:811-819.)*

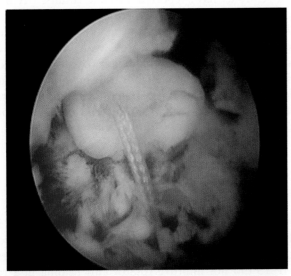

Figure 37-3. Arthroscopic image of platelet-rich fibrin matrix augmentation during rotator cuff repair, fixed with sutures.

platelet-rich plasma (PRP), which is classified as an autologous blood product rather than a drug (Fig. 37-3). Few randomized controlled trials have studied PRP application to rotator cuff repairs, and these studies have failed to demonstrate an improvement in healing after PRP treatment, which calls into question the efficacy of PRP use for rotator cuff tears. Two randomized controlled trials looking at the effects of platelet-rich fibrin matrix in 88 and 79 patients found there was no significant difference in clinical outcomes or healing rates compared with primary closures alone.[9,10] However, a smaller randomized controlled trial in 20 patients reported a significant increase in blood flow in the PRP group, but this did not translate to improved clinical scores.[11] Questions remain about the ideal concentration system, cellular content, platelet count, and timing of delivery.

Enhancing Bony Healing at the Enthesis

In addition to targeting tendon healing, a number of osteoinductive strategies have focused on bone healing at the rotator cuff enthesis. Bone morphogenetic protein (BMP) plays a role in both fibrocartilage and tendon formation. When recombinant BMP-12 was applied to torn rotator cuff tendons in sheep with use of different carriers, the fibrocartilage and tendon strength was significantly improved at 9 weeks (Fig. 37-4).[12] A cocktail of osteoinductive factors, including BMP-2, BMP-7, FGF, and TGF-β$_1$ and TGF-β$_2$ was found to improve fibrocartilage formation and mechanical properties in a sheep rotator cuff repair model, although the regenerated tissue consisted of scar tissue.[13] Cartilage-derived morphogenetic protein 2 (CDMP-2) was delivered to a rat rotator cuff tear model and significantly improved the histologic and morphologic appearance of the

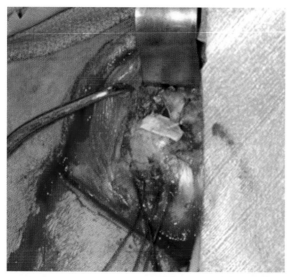

Figure 37-4. Image of application of collagen sponge containing BMP-12 at the tendon-bone interface during a rotator cuff repair. *(From Seeherman HJ, Archambault JM, Rodeo SA, et al. rhBMP-12 accelerates healing of rotator cuff repairs in a sheep model. J Bone Joint Surg Am. 2008;90:2206-2219.)*

healing enthesis.[14] A novel approach to encouraging enthesis healing is to use parathyroid hormone, which modulates osteoclastic resorption and osteoblastic bone formation. A different approach may be to prevent excessive loading of the repaired tendon by temporarily paralyzing the muscle. Botulinum toxin A–mediated paralysis has been investigated and was found to delay the formation of fibrocartilage and mineralized bone at days 21, 28, and 56.[15]

DRUGS THAT POTENTIALLY IMPAIR HEALING

Analgesics

Analgesics such as nonsteroidal anti-inflammatory drugs (NSAIDs) and corticosteroids are the among the most common drugs used to reduce pain and impaired function associated with rotator cuff tears. Although these drugs often reduce symptoms, there is increasing evidence that they may actually impair tendon healing through a number of adverse effects on cellular behavior such as cell apoptosis as well as inhibition of cell proliferation and migration. Cyclooxygenase-2 (COX-2) inhibitors indomethacin and celecoxib have been shown to inhibit key mediators that stimulate tendon healing, such as prostaglandin E_2 (PGE$_2$).[16] Corticosteroids have been shown to impair tendon ultrastructure by impairing collagen organization (Fig. 37-5). The resulting weakening of collagen fibers may reduce the tendon fiber's ability to transmit loads and increase

the risk of tendon failure. Anabolic steroids such as nandrolone have also been shown to induce inflammation and reduce tendon strength.

Antibiotics

Fluoroquinolone antibiotics have been reported to induce tendinopathies and tendon ruptures in a number of published cases.[17] Fluoroquinolones are thought to exert their effect through MMPs and other ECM constituents, resulting in collagen disruption and reduced mechanical properties. Therefore fluoroquinolone prescription after rotator cuff repairs should be avoided when possible.

STRUCTURAL SUPPORT FOR HEALING

Mechanical reinforcement of the healing rotator cuff enthesis with scaffolds is proposed to help reduce high failure rates after repairs (Fig. 37-6). A number of scaffolds composed of different animal- and human-derived tissue as well as synthetic materials are commercially available.[18] Several thousand scaffolds are reportedly used annually. Clinical studies of augmenting repairs with scaffolds have reported variable results.[19] A biologic scaffold composed of dermis of small intestinal submucosa was used clinically in the past. However, these scaffolds were associated with a number of disadvantages, such as induction of foreign body responses, risk of zoonotic DNA transmission, cost, and additional operating time. Demonstration of greater clinical efficacy and safety profiles is required before more widespread usage can be recommended.

CELL-MEDIATED TENDON HEALING

Attempts to enhance stem cell function have resulted in cell modulation to express different cytokines and cell signals. Genetic modification of stem cells to express BMP-13 did not improve rotator cuff healing in a rat model.[20] However, stem cell transfection with genes to express factors that play a role in tendon embryogenesis, such as membrane type 1 metalloprotease (MT1-MMP) and scleraxis, resulted in improved histologic and mechanical properties of rotator cuff tendons (Fig. 37-7).[21,22]

Alternative cell sources have been studied to determine if they are able to stimulate improved tendon regeneration, as this would avoid ethical and regulatory issues linked to stem cells. Tendon fibroblasts that expressed insulinlike growth factor (IGF-I) or PDGF-β have been shown to improve the histology of healing

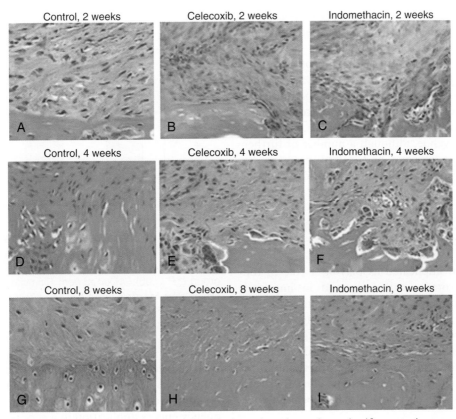

Figure 37-5. Photomicrograph demonstrating tendon-bone insertion site at 2 weeks (**A,** control group; **B,** celecoxib group; **C,** indomethacin group), 4 weeks (**D,** control group; **E,** celecoxib group; **F,** indomethacin group), and 8 weeks (**G,** control group; **H,** celecoxib group; **I,** indomethacin group) after surgery (hematoxylin and eosin, ×320). *(From Cohen DB, Kawamura S, Ehteshami JR, Rodeo SA. Indomethacin and celecoxib impair rotator cuff tendon-to-bone healing. Am J Sports Med. 2006;34:362-369.)*

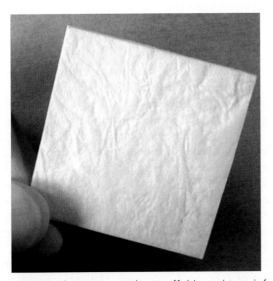

Figure 37-6. An augmentation scaffold used to reinforce a rotator cuff repair.

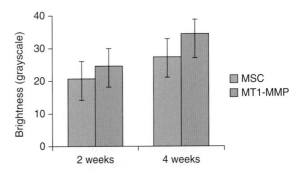

Figure 37-7. Collagen fiber organization as determined by the level of birefringence of picrosirius-stained slides under polarized light microscopy. There were no differences found between groups at either time point. Bar graphs represent the mean for each group, and error bars represent ±1 standard deviation. *MSC,* Mesenchymal stem cell; *MT1-MMP,* membrane type 1 matrix metalloproteinase. *(Modified from Gulotta LV, Kovacevic D, Montgomery S, et al. Stem cells genetically modified with the developmental gene MT1-MMP improve regeneration of the supraspinatus tendon-to-bone insertion site. Am J Sports Med. 2010;38:1429-1437.)*

tendons. In addition to localized delivery of tenocytes, fibroblasts and endothelial cells are other potential candidates for cell-mediated tendon healing. Cells have been seeded onto scaffolds, with the aim of achieving more targeted and sustained delivery, and a few animal studies have reported improved histologic and mechanical properties. Cellular augmentation of rotator cuff repairs, particularly with modified stem cells, is a promising therapeutic avenue, although a number of further issues surrounding efficacy and safety need to be addressed before potential clinical application.

SYSTEMIC FACTORS THAT IMPAIR HEALING

Smoking has been implicated as playing a role in the pathogenesis of rotator cuff tears and in impaired healing. Using a rat supraspinatus model, nicotine was found to impair cell proliferation and collagen formation, as well as reduce mechanical properties at early time points.[23] Diabetes results in increased advanced glycation end products (AGEs) that are thought to impair collagen material properties. The clinical effects of smoking on rotator cuff healing have not been well described.

A rat model of diabetes with sustained hyperglycemia resulted in a disorganized histologic appearance and inferior mechanical properties of rotator cuff tendon. A clinical study of patients with diabetes did not report any effect on clinical scores or range of movement, although diabetic patients did have increased complications from rotator cuff surgeries.[24]

INDIRECT MODULATION OF BIOLOGY

Impaired vascular supply to the rotator cuff is proposed to predispose to rotator cuff tears, and the relatively avascular "critical zone," which is 1 cm away from the supraspinatus insertion, has been identified as an area that is prone to tendon failure. A number of approaches that aim to enhance the vasculature of healing rotator cuffs have been investigated. Topical glyceryl trinitrate patches were applied to patients with chronic supraspinatus tendinopathy as part of a double-blind randomized controlled trial. An improvement was noted in pain, function, and tendon forces.

Manipulation of the vasculature of rotator cuff tendons is proposed to be achievable through sound waves and radiation, such as extracorporeal shock wave therapies (ESWT), bipolar radiofrequency energy, or low-intensity pulsed ultrasound (LIPUS) therapy. Clinical studies, however, have not reported positive effects,

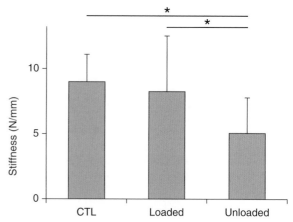

Figure 37-8. The loaded group had a significantly higher stiffness than the unloaded group. Stiffness in the unloaded group was significantly lower than the control group (*$P < .05$). *(Modified from Thomopoulos S, Zampiakis E, Das R, Silva MJ, Gelberman RH. The effect of muscle loading on flexor tendon-to-bone healing in a canine model. J Orthop Res. 2008;26:1611-1617.)*

with reduced tissue perfusion reported after a clinical study of ESWT for rotator cuff tendinopathy. Similarly, no improvement was reported after bipolar radiofrequency energy application in a supraspinatus rat model.

The biologic environment surrounding rotator cuff repairs may be indirectly modulated through mechanical stimulation. Loading is known to encourage improved organization of the tendon ECM. A canine study of the effects of postoperative loading on healing reported that loading across the repair site resulted in improved mechanical properties.[25] The ideal amount and timing of loads during the rehabilitation period remains undefined (Fig. 37-8).

CONCLUSION

High failure rates after rotator cuff repairs have encouraged the investigation of biologic therapies that may enhance rotator cuff repairs. Modulation of cytokines and growth factors in the surrounding biologic milieu may encourage regeneration of native functioning tendon tissue rather than poor-quality scar tissue. Ensuring localized delivery of growth factors and cytokines can be challenging and may be a key determinant of successful outcomes. PRP is one approach to delivering factors in concentrated platelets; however, its efficacy for enhancing rotator cuff repairs remains unproven. A number of options are available for mechanical augmentation of repairs using scaffolds, with varying reports of successful outcomes. Delivery of cells to the site of the repair may provide appropriate cellular signals during healing, and transduced stem cells are a promising avenue for future research.

REFERENCES

1. Kovacevic D, Rodeo SA. Biological augmentation of rotator cuff tendon repair. *Clin Orthop Relat Res.* 2008;466(3):622-633.
2. Bedi A, Fox AJS, Kovacevic D, et al. Doxycycline-mediated inhibition of matrix metalloproteinases improves healing after rotator cuff repair. *Am J Sports Med.* 2010;38(2):308-317.
3. Kovacevic D, Fox AJ, Bedi A, et al. Calcium-phosphate matrix with or without TGF-β3 improves tendon-bone healing after rotator cuff repair. *Am J Sports Med.* 2011;39(4):811-819.
4. Manning CN, Kim HM, Sakiyama-Elbert S, et al. Sustained delivery of transforming growth factor beta three enhances tendon-to-bone healing in a rat model. *J Orthop Res.* 2011;29(7):1099-1105.
5. Ide J, Kikukawa K, Hirose J, et al. The effect of a local application of fibroblast growth factor–2 on tendon-to-bone remodeling in rats with acute injury and repair of the supraspinatus tendon. *J Shoulder Elbow Surg.* 2009;18(3):391-398.
6. Ide J, Kikukawa K, Hirose J, et al. The effects of fibroblast growth factor–2 on rotator cuff reconstruction with acellular dermal matrix grafts. *Arthroscopy.* 2009;25(6):608-616.
7. Gulotta LV, Kovacevic D, Cordasco F, et al. Evaluation of tumor necrosis factor β blockade on early tendon-to-bone healing in a rat rotator cuff repair model. *Arthroscopy.* 2011;27(10):1351-1357.
8. Uggen C, Dines J, McGarry M, et al. The effect of recombinant human platelet-derived growth factor BB-coated sutures on rotator cuff healing in a sheep model. *Arthroscopy.* 2010;26(11):1456-1462.
9. Castricini R, Longo UG, De Benedetto M, et al. Platelet-rich plasma augmentation for arthroscopic rotator cuff repair. *Am J Sports Med.* 2011;39(2):258-265.
10. Rodeo SA, Delos D, Williams RJ, et al. The effect of platelet-rich fibrin matrix on rotator cuff tendon healing: A prospective randomized clinical study. *Am J Sports Med.* 2012;40(6):1234-1241.
11. Zummstein MA, Lesbats V, Trojani C, et al. A new technique of biologic augmentation in repair of chronic rotator cuff tears using autologous platelet rich fibrin (PRF): vascularization response and tendon healing in a prospective randomized trial. Presented at the Open Meeting of the Americal Shoulder and Elbow Surgeons, New Orleans, LA,2010.
12. Seeherman HJ, Archambault JM, Rodeo SA, et al. rhBMP-12 accelerates healing of rotator cuff repairs in a sheep model. *J Bone Joint Surg Am.* 2008;90(10):2206-2219.
13. Rodeo SA, Potter HG, Kawamura S, et al. Biologic augmentation of rotator cuff tendon-healing with use of a mixture of osteoinductive growth factors. *J Bone Joint Surg Am.* 2007;89(11):2485-2497.
14. Murray DH, Kubiak EN, Jazrawi LM, et al. The effect of cartilage-derived morphogenetic protein 2 on initial healing of a rotator cuff defect in a rat model. *J Shoulder Elbow Surg.* 2007;16(2):251-254.
15. Thomopoulos S, Kim HM, Rothermich SY, et al. Decreased muscle loading delays maturation of the tendon enthesis during postnatal development. *J Orthop Res.* 2007;25(9):1154-1163.
16. Cohen DB, Kawamura S, Ehteshami JR, et al. Indomethacin and celecoxib impair rotator cuff tendon-to-bone healing. *Am J Sports Med.* 2006;34(3):362-369.
17. Stinner DJ, Orr JD, Hsu JR. Fluoroquinolone-associated bilateral patellar tendon rupture: A case report and review of the literature. *Mil Med.* 2010;175(6):457-459.
18. Derwin KA, Badylak SF, Steinmann SP, et al. Extracellular matrix scaffold devices for rotator cuff repair. *J Shoulder Elbow Surg.* 2010;19(3):467-476.
19. Longo UG, Lamberti A, Maffulli N, et al. Tendon augmentation grafts: a systematic review. *Br Med Bull.* 2010;94:165-188.
20. Gulotta LV, Kovacevic D, Packer JD, et al. Adenoviral-mediated gene transfer of human bone morphogenetic protein-13 does not improve rotator cuff healing in a rat model. *Am J Sports Med.* 2011;39(1):180-187.
21. Gulotta LV, Kovacevic D, Montgomery S, et al. Stem cells genetically modified with the developmental gene MT1-MMP improve regeneration of the supraspinatus tendon-to-bone insertion site. *Am J Sports Med.* 2010;38(7):1429-1437.
22. Gulotta LV, Rodeo SA. Emerging ideas: evaluation of stem cells genetically modified with scleraxis to improve rotator cuff healing. *Clin Orthop Relat Res.* 2011;469(10):2977-2980.
23. Bedi A, Fox AJ, Harris PE, et al. Diabetes mellitus impairs tendon-bone healing after rotator cuff repair. *J Shoulder Elbow Surg.* 2010;19:978-988.
24. Chen AL, Shapiro JA, Ahn AK, et al. Rotator cuff repair in patients with type I diabetes mellitus. *J Shoulder Elbow Surg.* 2003;12(5):416-421.
25. Thomopoulos S, Zampiakis E, Das R, et al. The effect of muscle loading on flexor tendon-to-bone healing in a canine model. *J Orthop Res.* 2008;26(12):1611-1617.

Chapter 38

Tendon Augmentation Devices in Rotator Cuff Repair

Stephen J. Snyder and Joseph P. Burns

Chapter Synopsis
- Massive degenerative rotator cuff tears are a difficult problem for all shoulder surgeons to reconstruct. In select patients it is now reasonable to arthroscopically reconstruct the cuff with a biologic matrix. Our experience has proven that good pain relief and improvement in strength and motion can be expected with a properly performed allograft cuff replacement. This chapter reviews the steps of the operation as performed at the Southern California Orthopedic Institute (SCOI).

Important Points
- The patient should have good passive and active-assisted motion of the shoulder and minimal arthritis.
- All graft materials are not the same. The graft must be chosen with care, avoiding materials that are weak or likely to incite inflammatory reactions, especially those with cross-linked collagen that are likely to retard cellular in-growth.
- The operation should be rehearsed in the model laboratory until the steps are second nature for the surgeon and the staff.
- The patient should understand that this operation, even when completely successful, will never result in a "normal" shoulder. There will always be weakness, especially in external rotation.

Clinical and Surgical Pearls
- Be comfortable with use of the scope in all three subacromial portals.

- Never cross a suture over another; keep each successive suture anterior and parallel to all others.
- Use a reverse cutting needle to pass the short-tail interference knot (STIK) sutures through the graft.
- Do not allow slack in the sutures when pulling the STIK sutures into the shoulder; pull the medial sutures first, and take up slack in all others.
- Create numerous bone marrow vents in the tuberosity to allow a rich "crimson duvet" to form over the graft.

Clinical and Surgical Pitfalls
- It is important to monitor surgical time. If the operation takes more than 2½ hours, remove the traction sleeve for 15 minutes to guard against ischemia or nerve damage.
- Never put the graft in too much tension. The most important goal is that the graft heal. The natural elasticity of the graft will help protect it from suture cutout. As the graft is repopulated with host cells, it will attain a more tendon-like tone.
- Be very careful when positioning the patient for surgery. The prolonged surgical time will increase the risk of pressure points on the nerves and skin.

Video
- Video 38-1: Reconstruction of a massive rotator cuff tear using acellular human dermal matrix allograft

With the advent of magnetic resonance imaging (MRI) and our better understanding of the clinical evaluation and natural history of rotator cuff problems, orthopedic surgeons now have the tools to reduce the number of misdiagnosed and thus mismanaged rotator cuff tears. In addition, with modern shoulder arthroscopy techniques we have the ability to repair serious rotator cuff tears and thereby reduce the incidence and severity of the common sequela of chronic disability that often follows the failure to perform such repairs.

Unfortunately, there are still numerous patients in whom the initial injury is missed or in whom the pathology is so severe, with advanced tendon disease, that even an appropriate repair fails. In these situations the patient has a weak painful shoulder and very few acceptable surgical options. Current reports indicate failure rates of 41% to 94% for treatment of massive cuff tears.[1-4]

When the pain and disability from severe, nonrepairable rotator cuff disease are unacceptable, the only available choices for treatment include radical open surgery for a latissimus dorsi muscle transfer to replace the cuff, or some type of constrained total shoulder joint replacement, such as a reverse total shoulder. Both of these options offer some benefit but are considered, at best, unpredictable, especially in younger patients without arthritis.

The obvious solution to this serious quandary is to replace or reinforce the severely damaged cuff tendon with a substitute grafting material. In the past, grafts such as Teflon, fascia lata, biceps tendon, and freeze-dried cuff tendon have been tested, but none of these materials has been consistently successful. Although new materials are now available, orthopedists are understandably cautious when presented with any sort of graft material to replace this important tendon.

Currently there is resurgence in interest in biologically assisting the healing of the damaged rotator cuff either by augmentation of a weak tendon after direct repair or, in very difficult situations, by replacement of the deficient tendon with biologic materials. These new biologic materials are called *extracellular matrix* (ECM) grafts. Numerous classes of biologic matrices are available, including dermal allografts, dermal xenografts, resorbable and nonresorbable fabrics, and many other collagen and man-made products. Each material has unique properties that must be understood before its use in a patient is considered.[2,5-11]

With the advent of modern tissue banks offering safe, reliable, and readily available allograft tissue with proven success in reconstructing multiple other areas of the body, surgeons are now comfortable investigating the potential for replacing damaged rotator cuff tissue with a regenerative biologic matrix. Numerous animal laboratory studies support the concept that certain acellular dermal graft materials are successful for restoring deficient rotator cuff tendons.[12,13] Short-term to midterm results in humans are promising and have shown reliable improvement in shoulder function and pain scores. Rotator cuff reconstruction with a biologic matrix can now readily be performed arthroscopically in the outpatient surgical center with minimal morbidity to surrounding tissue.[14-16]

Characteristics of the ideal rotator cuff graft are presented in Box 38-1.

Our graft choice for this group of patients with chronic massive nonrepairable rotator cuff damage over

---

BOX 38-1 Characteristics of the Ideal Rotator Cuff Graft

- Negligible risk of disease transfer or inflammatory rejection
- Robust initial strength for preventing suture cutout
- Moderate elastic nature (stress shielding)
- Favorable handling characteristics (suitable for arthroscopic use)
- Rapidly repopulated with appropriate host cells (vascular channels)
- No or minimal cross-linked collagen
- Natural growth factors within the graft
- Readily available as a cryopreserved or ready-to-use product
- Reasonably priced
- Favorable clinical history of material (multiple previous human applications)
- Encouraging animal laboratory data
- U.S. Food and Drug Administration (FDA) approval for rotator cuff application

---

BOX 38-2 Surgical Steps

1. Complete initial preparation of the STIK sutures.
2. Perform shoulder evaluation, debridement, decompression, and preparation.
3. Insert the first suture anchor.
4. Measure the defect in the rotator cuff.
5. Prepare the graft.
6. Insert the anterior anchor and perform biceps tenodesis with an "Italian loop" stitch.
7. Attach the graft to the posterior and medial cuff.
8. Attach the graft to the anterior cuff and biceps tendon.
9. Deliver the graft into the shoulder.
10. Tie the STIK sutures.
11. Tie the anchored sutures.
12. Suture the lateral graft to bone.
13. Insert the third and fourth anchors.
14. Tie the anchored sutures.
15. Evaluate the repair.

STIK, Short-tail interference knot.

---

the past 6.5 years has been a human acellular dermal matrix allograft, GraftJacket (Wright Medical Technology, Arlington, VA).[14,16,17]

Use of an acellular human dermal allograft material as a "patch" graft is considered an off-label use by the U.S. Food and Drug Administration (FDA). When GraftJacket is used to augment a deficient tendon or bridge a cuff defect less than 1 cm, its use is considered "on label."

SURGICAL TECHNIQUE FOR COMPLETE REPLACEMENT OF A MASSIVE NONREPAIRABLE ROTATOR CUFF TENDON DEFECT

The specific steps of the procedure are outlined in Box 38-2.

Preparing the Graft

On the back table, tie 12 short-tail interference knots (STIK) sutures with three different-colored No. 2 braided polyester suture material. Form the STIK sutures by looping a suture around a 2-mm metal rod and tying a loop with a bulky knot below it. Test the strength of the knot by pulling firmly on the free end of the STIK suture while the loop is still on the post.

Make a knotted suture measuring device by tying a loop on one end of a No. 0 braided suture and forming simple half-hitch knots along the suture at 1-cm intervals for 5 cm, beginning 1 cm from the loop end. Load the nonloop end of the suture onto a single-eye knot pusher and pull it up to the loop knot. The loop end of the suture will be passed into the shoulder with the knot pusher so that it can be grasped with a small clamp via another portal, and the knotted suture can thus be laid along the edges of the cuff defect and measured by counting the knots.

Hydrate or otherwise prepare the graft in room temperature sterile saline if needed.

Shoulder Evaluation, Debridement, Decompression, and Preparation

The scope is positioned in any appropriate portal.

Begin by creating standard posterior midglenoid (PMG) and anterior midglenoid (AMG) portals, and place a 7-mm operating cannula in each one. Create the midlateral subacromial (MLSA) portal carefully. Use a spinal needle to select a location 4 cm lateral to the midpoint of the cuff defect. Insert an 8-mm docking cannula in this portal. All three cannulas are left in these portals for the entire procedure, and all stitching and knot-tying tools and the scope can be moved among these portals without need to remove the cannula.

Perform a 15-point evaluation of the shoulder, and document the condition of the cartilage surface, labrum, biceps subscapularis, synovium, and rotator cuff.

Prepare the shoulder joint by debriding the degenerative cuff edges and bursal scar. Repair any significant subscapularis or labral tissues as needed. Mobilize the medial stump of the rotator cuff by carefully releasing the scar and capsule just above the glenoid.

Prepare the bursa by smoothing the underside of the acromion and acromioclavicular joint if needed. Remove any suture anchors that are blocking the area of graft attachment in the area 3 cm lateral to the articular cartilage edge. Debride all soft tissue and lightly decorticate the greater tuberosity to expose the cancellous bone, including the area of the biceps groove. This will create a better surface for healing the biceps tenodesis.

Inserting the First Suture Anchor

The scope is placed in the MLSA portal at the "50-yard line" of the tear, or, if desired, the scope may be placed in a posterior lateral portal without use of an operating cannula.

Choose a spot for the first suture anchor with use of a spinal needle as a guide. The ideal position is a few millimeters anterior to the posterior edge of the cuff stump and 4 mm lateral to the edge of the articular cartilage.

Before inserting each anchor, use a small 1.2-mm bone punch to create a starter hole for each anchor. Also create four or five bone marrow vents by puncturing the exposed bone of the lateral tuberosity (away from the anchor sites). Always direct the punch vertically down the humerus and thus away from the subchondral bone area.

Insert the first triple-loaded suture anchor into the posterior pilot hole in a medial direction, passing approximately 45 degrees to the subchondral bone. The eyelet of the anchor is seated 1 mm below the bone surface and is always aligned in a medial-to-lateral direction so that it opens toward the edge of the cartilage and the medial cuff stump.

Perform a "partial cuff repair" by fixing the posterior edge of the remaining cuff to the tuberosity. Pass the medial limb of the most posterior suture from the posterior anchor through a healthy bite of posterior cuff near the attachment site on the bone. If a "suture shuttle" technique is used, first retrieve the index suture into the anterior mid-glenoid portal. Pass the shuttle device through the cuff stump with a crescent-shaped needle via the PMG cannula. Retrieve the shuttle into the AMG cannula, load the suture, and carry it back through the cuff and out the back. Tie the sutures with a sliding-locking knot. Clamp the remaining sutures next to the skin to hold them snugly.

Measuring the Defect in the Rotator Cuff

Insert the knotted suture measuring device with the single-eye knot pusher via the PMG cannula. Grasp the loop end of the suture with a small clamp inserted through the AMG cannula. Measure all four sides of the cuff defect, allowing 5 mm of overlap in each dimension. On the lateral edge measure from 5 mm posterior

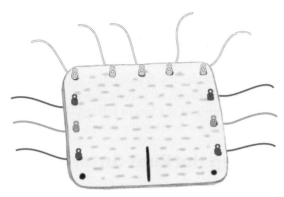

Figure 38-1. The graft is prepared for implantation by placement of short-tail interference knot sutures around the perimeter 5 mm from the edge.

to the posterior lateral anchor to the area of the biceps tendon or biceps groove. The measurement of the medial edge should likewise allow 5 mm of overlap on each side. A surgical technician records the measurements and creates a pattern on a surgical towel with a surgical marking pen. Mark a dot to indicate the locations for the STIK sutures 5 mm from the edge of the graft every 8 mm on the posterior, medial, and anterior borders. Also, place a dot at the anterior and posterior lateral corners to guide insertion of the middle anchor suture.

Inserting STIK Sutures in the Graft

On the back table, a surgical assistant (if available) prepares the graft at the same time as the surgeon inserts the second (anterior) anchor. Place the graft on the pattern that was created on the towel, and press it carefully to transfer the pattern to the graft. Cut the graft along the edge of the pattern and replace the remaining portion in the saline bath. Insert a STIK suture into each dot along the posterior, medial, and anterior edge, leaving the loop knot on the upper side (Fig. 38-1). Always use the smallest possible reverse cutting needle when passing sutures through the graft, and orient the bevel away from the edge to minimize creation of a stress riser. *Do not* insert a STIK suture in the most lateral of the anterior and posterior target spots. Return the graft to the saline until it is needed. Color the unknotted ends of the medial sutures with the skin marker to identify them during graft passage.

Inserting the Anterior Anchor and Performing Biceps Tenodesis with an "Italian Loop" Stitch

The scope is positioned in the lateral mid-glenoid (LMG) cannula or posterior lateral portal (Fig. 38-2).

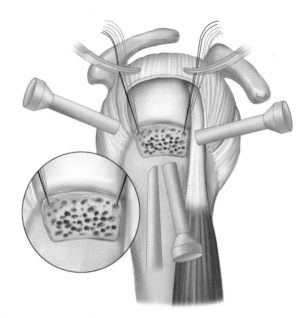

Figure 38-2. The three cannulas are in place and the bone has been prepared. Two anchors have been inserted and multiple bone marrow vents have been punched in the tuberosity.

Use the spinal needle as a guide for the anterior anchor. Insert it just posterior to the biceps tendon, 5 mm lateral to the articular cartilage. Retrieve the most anterior medial suture into the PMG cannula. Pass an appropriately curved suture needle via the AMG cannula through any rotator interval tissue and through the biceps tendon at the level of the anchor. Send the shuttle and retrieve it with a grasping clamp into the PMG cannula. Load the shuttle and carry the suture back through the biceps and into the AMG cannula. Retrieve the same suture again into the PMG cannula. Pass the shuttle again through the rotator interval and biceps tissue a few millimeters away from the initial pass. Send the shuttle again, retrieve it, and load the suture. Pull the shuttle out the AMG cannula to complete the Italian loop stitch. Tie the suture with a nonsliding "revo" knot. Clamp the remaining sutures snugly outside the skin.

Attaching the Graft to the Posterior and Medial Cuff

The scope is positioned in the AMG cannula.

Wrap a surgical towel around the arm 5 cm lateral to the LMG cannula and secure it with two clamps. Place the graft on the moistened towel and turn it so that the posterior edge is toward the cannula. Secure the STIK sutures by clamping them with an Alice clamp.

It is imperative to ensure that all sutures pass between and medial to the two suture anchors and their sutures and never pass between the sutures or lateral to them.

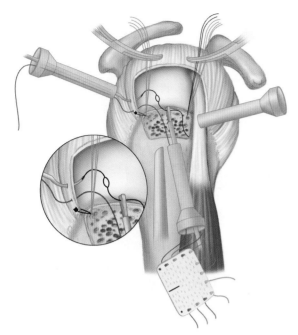

Figure 38-3. The short-tail interference knot sutures from the graft are passed through the cuff remnant with a crescent-shaped suture hook and a shuttle.

Each successive suture must pass parallel to the previous one and *anterior* to it. If the sutures do cross or are not parallel, they will twist when they are pulled to seat the graft.

Retrieve the medial limb of the center suture of the posterior anchor into the MLSA cannula. Be certain that the suture passes *medial* to the other suture and between the remaining sutures in the anchors. Pass the suture through the graft at the target spot on the posterior lateral corner. Tie a STIK suture on the topside of the suture and pull the other end to take up the slack so that the edge of the graft is 10 cm away from the lateral subacromial portal cannula. Hold the suture to the moist towel with a posterior Alice clamp. Clamp the remaining sutures with a rubber-tipped clamp outside the skin to hold them taut.

Choose the free end of the most lateral-posterior STIK suture and clamp it in the posterior Alice clamp in preparation for passing.

Pass a shuttle through the posterior cuff remnant 8 mm medial to the posterior suture anchor with a crescent hook and retrieve it *anterior* to the previous suture, between the anchored sutures and into the MLSA cannula (Fig. 38-3). Load the shuttle and carry it back through the cuff and into the PMG cannula.

Continue passing the remaining STIK sutures along the posterior edge of the cuff defect, placing each stitch 8 mm more medial than the previous one. Usually the crescent-shaped suture hook is best for all posterior sutures.

Alternative Stitching Method: Direct Suture Passage

The scope is positioned in the appropriate portal for best viewing.

Some surgeons prefer suturing with the direct pass method via the lateral portal. This method works well as long as the sutures are passed sequentially from posterior to anterior and great care is taken to avoid crossing the sutures. Load the needle with the free end of the STIK suture outside the MLSA cannula and pass it into the joint with the suturing device. Drive the needle through the cuff remnant and retrieve it from the top with a grasper in the PMG cannula.

Continue suturing along the medial edge of the cuff stump with use of the appropriate suture hook. Usually four or five sutures are used for the medial side. The free ends of the STIK sutures are left in the PMG cannula.

Attaching the Graft to the Anterior Cuff and Biceps Tendon

The scope is positioned in the PMG portal.

Stitch the anterior edge of the defect, following the same steps as previously but progressing from medial to lateral. Use the appropriate suture hook to pass the first STIK suture through the rotator interval tissue 8 mm from the anterior medial STIK suture. Do not pass the first anterior suture through the biceps because there is usually adequate tissue available.

Continue down the anterior defect, incorporating the rotator interval and biceps tissue in the remaining stitches. Leave the free ends of the STIK sutures in the AMG cannula.

Retrieve the medial end of the middle suture from the anterior anchor into the MLSA cannula. Be certain it passes medial to the other sutures in that anchor. Pass the suture from bottom to top through the graft, through the anterior-lateral target spot, and tie a STIK suture on the top. Pull up the slack and clamp the ends outside the skin (Fig. 38-4).

Delivering the Graft into the Shoulder

The scope is positioned outside the shoulder.

Orient the graft so that the medial edge is directed toward the cannula. A problem can occur if some of the sutures are slack and others tight when the graft is pulled into the MLSA cannula. Avoid this by locating the ends of the medial STIK sutures (colored purple) and taking up all slack by pulling on them outside the AMG and PMG cannulas. Pull on the free ends of the other STIK sutures and the two anchored sutures just enough to take up any slack. Roll the graft so that the knots are

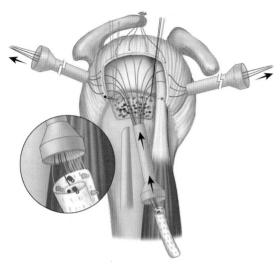

Figure 38-4. The graft is rolled and advanced into the cannula by pulling on the free end of the short-tail interference knot sutures.

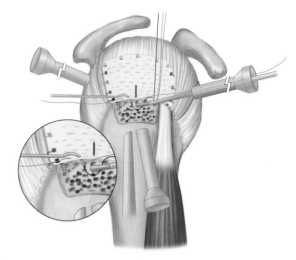

Figure 38-6. The sutures from the anchors are passed through the graft using curved suture hooks and suture shuttle relays.

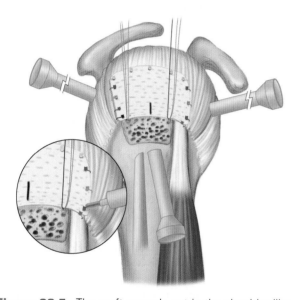

Figure 38-5. The graft spreads out in the shoulder like a parachute. The short-tail interference knot sutures are retrieved and tied around the perimeter.

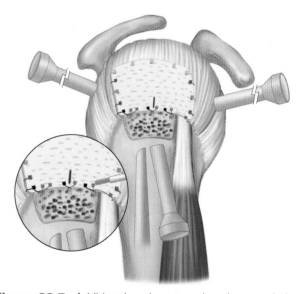

Figure 38-7. Additional anchors are placed as needed to complete the fixation of the lateral end of the graft to bone.

outside, and snug all sutures so that the graft is in the end of the cannula. Pull the medial (purple-colored) suture tails to lead the graft into the cannula (Fig. 38-5). Alternate pulling on the medial STIK sutures, and take up any slack of the other sutures. This stepwise method will prevent formation of any suture loops that can catch on the STIK sutures and cause the graft to seat improperly.

Tying the STIK Sutures

The scope is positioned in the MLSA cannula.

Retrieve all sutures from the PMG cannula into the AMG cannula except the most lateral STIK suture. Retrieve the knotted end of the posterior lateral-most STIK suture into the PMG cannula. Tie the sutures with a sliding-locking knot; use the unknotted end of the STIK suture and the post (Fig. 38-6).

Continue to retrieve the STIK sutures along the anterior edge from lateral to medial by first removing the free end and then the knotted end into the PMG cannula and tying them together (Fig. 38-7). All STIK sutures can be readily tied through the PMG cannula with the scope viewing from the MLSA cannula.

Tying the Anchored Sutures

Retrieve both ends of the anterior anchored suture that passes through the anterior-lateral graft into the AMG cannula. Cut off the knot and tie the sutures with a sliding-locking knot. Repeat the process for the posterior anchor suture.

Suturing the Lateral Graft to Bone

The scope usually is kept in the MLSA portal but can be changed as needed for best visualization.

Retrieve the medial end of the remaining suture from the posterior anchor into the AMG cannula. Pass a curved suture hook through the graft from top to bottom 5 mm anterior to the previous suture. Retrieve the shuttle and carry it into the AMG cannula. Load the shuttle and carry the suture through the graft and into the PMG cannula. Retrieve the other end of the suture and store both sutures tails in colored plastic suture protectors outside the PMG cannula. Repeat the stitching for the anterior anchored suture, and store it outside the AMG cannula in a colored plastic suture protector.

Inserting the Third and Fourth Anchors

Locate the centerline on the lateral edge of the graft. Determine how much space remains between the anterior and posterior sutures. If there is more than 1 cm on each side of the centerline, two double-loaded anchors are needed. Most often only one additional double-loaded anchor is required. If only one anchor is needed, seat it directly lateral to the resting position of the midlateral mark on the graft. Before inserting the anchor (or anchors), create additional bone marrow vents as needed. Pass the sutures from posterior to anterior, and store each in a colored suture protector outside the PMG cannula.

Tying the Anchored Sutures

Retrieve the sutures from the suture protectors in an anterior-to-posterior direction. Tie the sutures with the medial limb used for the post so that the knot sits on top of the graft. Tie all remaining sutures.

Evaluating the Repair

Carefully evaluate and document the entire repair. If there are any gaps along the edges, pass additional sutures. Seldom is this necessary. Turn off the fluid pump and observe while the bone marrow bubbles from the bone vents. This will form a "crimson duvet"

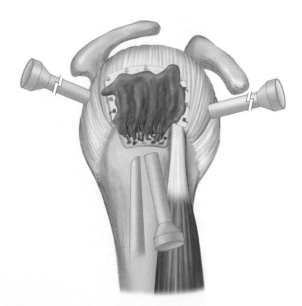

Figure 38-8. The arthroscopic pump is turned off; the bone marrow vents allow a rich clot, called a "crimson duvet," to form. It is the source of healing fibrin matrix rich in stem cells, platelets, and growth factors and new vascular access channels.

(Fig. 38-8) over the tuberosity, suture line, and graft, bringing new blood supply and forming a rich matrix clot replete with platelets and their growth factors and mesenchymal stem cells.

POSTOPERATIVE CONSIDERATIONS

Support the arm in 15 degrees of abduction in a pillow immobilizer. Begin elbow, wrist, and hand exercises the evening of surgery, with gentle pendulum circles at 1 week.

Delay formal physical therapy for 8 weeks and follow a slow progressive program similar to that for a massive cuff tear. Water therapy is very helpful at 6 to 8 weeks to allow passive motion without stress on the healing graft. Progress activities slowly; active-assisted lifting is allowed at 3 months. A gadolinium contrast MRI scan at 3 months will help in determining whether the graft has survived and in electing the progressive exercises and activities (Fig. 38-9).

DISCUSSION

Several questions concerning rotator cuff augmentation grafts remain to be answered.

- What is the optimal form of the ACM allograft— that is, what is the best graft material, how thick should it be, and what should be its configuration and source?

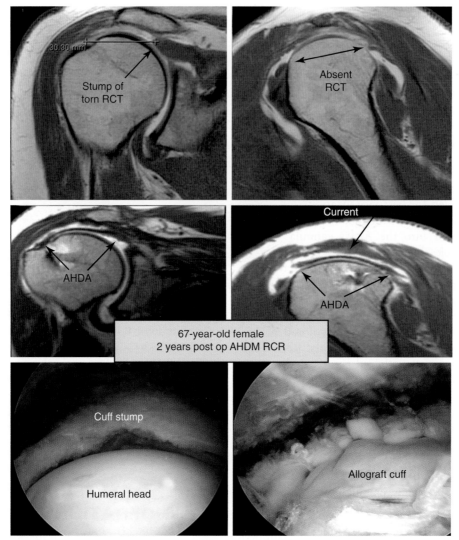

Figure 38-9. This sequence documents a massive nonrepairable rotator cuff tear that has been replaced by an allograft extracellular matrix. The gadolinium magnetic resonance imaging scan reveals the healed graft 1 year postoperatively. *AHDA,* acellular human dermal allograft; *RCT,* rotator cuff tendon.

- Is there an upper age cutoff that will limit the potential for successful healing of the graft?
- What is the ideal form of fixation? What is the ideal anchor and suture configuration?
- Are there potential benefits from use of additional growth factors or other biologic enhancements?
- Should the graft be preloaded with stem cells?
- Is it necessary to proceed slowly with rehabilitation?

Why Does this Form of Graft Often Work?

It is obvious that replacing a nonrepairable rotator cuff defect with an allograft matrix will never create a normal rotator cuff tendon. There will always be persistent weakness resulting from muscle atrophy and scarring and capsular tightness. The most noticeable

deficiency is often in strength of external rotation because there is less contribution from other muscles to aid the weakened infraspinatus.

The healed rotator cuff allograft does greatly improve shoulder pain and often helps with strength of elevation. The theoretical bases for these improvements, though not proven, are illustrated by the following scenarios:

- The living graft may improve function by reattaching any remaining rotator cuff muscle fibers from the supraspinatus and infraspinatus tendon stump to bone, allowing them once again function to assist in shoulder elevation and external rotation. In addition, if the fibers are viable they may be able to be strengthened by postoperative exercise.
- The healed graft that bridges between the cuff stump on three sides and the tuberosity may serve as a stabilizing unit, helping to hold the head in a more

natural position in the socket by reducing the proximal subluxation. This stabilizing function will assist the biomechanical force couple, improving the strength of the deltoid. This action is akin to closing the extensor hood in a boutonnière deformity of the finger.

- Having a smooth living soft tissue graft situated between the humerus and the acromion may be helpful by reducing contact pressure between the bones during elevation and rotation.
- Resealing the joint may improve the intra-articular milieu by reestablishing the capsule and joint fluid pressures and aiding in joint nutrition and physiologic balance.

CONCLUSION

We believe we have now documented that some types of acellular matrix graft are a viable solution, at least in the short term, for surgical salvage in selected patients with massive nonrepairable rotator cuff pathology. Of course, long-term follow-up is mandatory to determine the longevity and viability of the graft as well as patient satisfaction. Arthroscopic techniques permit us to treat the entire joint (e.g., biceps, subscapularis, labrum, synovium) without damage to the deltoid or large skin incisions in an outpatient setting. As more patients become available for longer follow-up, we will arrive at answers to the remaining questions and will have additional data to better address the lingering uncertainties.

REFERENCES

1. Cofield RH, Parvizi J, Hoffmeyer PJ, et al. Surgical repair of chronic rotator cuff tears. A prospective long-term study. *J Bone Joint Surg Am.* 2001;83:71-77.
2. Galatz LM, Ball CM, Teefey SA, et al. The outcome and repair integrity of completely arthroscopically repaired large and massive rotator cuff tears. *J Bone Joint Surg Am.* 2004;86:219-224.
3. Harryman DT, Mack LA, Wang KY, et al. Repairs of the rotator cuff. Correlation of functional results with integrity of the cuff. *J Bone Joint Surg Am.* 1991;73: 982-989.
4. Romeo AA, Hang DW, Bach Jr BR, et al. Repair of full thickness rotator cuff tears. Gender, age, and other factors affecting outcome. *Clin Orthop Relat Res.* 1999: 243-255.
5. Aurora A, McCarron J, Iannotti JP, et al. Commercially available extracellular matrix materials for rotator cuff repairs: state of the art and future trends. *J Shoulder Elbow Surg.* 2007;16(suppl):S171-S178.
6. Badylak SF, Freytes DO, Gilbert TW. Extracellular matrix as a biological scaffold material: structure and function. *Acta Biomater.* 2009;5:1-13.
7. Derwin KA, Badylak AD, Steinmann SP, et al. Extracellular matrix scaffold devices for rotator cuff repair. *J Shoulder Elbow Surg.* 2010;19:467-476.
8. MacGillivray JD, Romeo AA, Warren RF, et al. Biomechanical and biologic augmentation for the treatment of massive rotator cuff tears. *Am J Sports Med.* 2010;38: 619.
9. Derwin KA, Codsi MJ, Milks RA, et al. Rotator cuff repair augmentation in a canine model with use of a woven poly-L-lactide device. *J Bone Joint Surg Am.* 2009;91:1159-1171.
10. Iannotti JP, Codsi MJ, Kwon YW, et al. Porcine small intestine submucosa augmentation of surgical repair of chronic two-tendon rotator cuff tears. A randomized, controlled trial. *J Bone Joint Surg Am.* 2006;88:1238-1244.
11. Valentin JE, Badylak JS, McCabe GP, et al. Extracellular matrix bioscaffolds for orthopaedic applications. A comparative histologic study. *J Bone Joint Surg Am.* 2006; 88:2673-2686.
12. Adams JE, Zobitz ME, Reach Jr JS, et al. Rotator cuff repair using an acellular dermal matrix graft: an in vivo study in a canine model. *Arthroscopy.* 2006;22: 700-709.
13. Xu H, Wan H, Sandor M, et al. Host response to human acellular dermal matrix transplantation in a primate model of abdominal wall repair. *Tissue Eng Part A.* 2009;14:2009-2019.
14. Bond JL, Dopirak RM, Higgins J, et al. Arthroscopic replacement of massive, irreparable rotator cuff tears using a Graft-Jacket allograft: technique and preliminary results. *Arthroscopy.* 2008;24:403-409.
15. Burkhead WZ, Schiffern SC, Krishnan SG. Use of Graft Jacket as an augmentation for massive rotator cuff tears. *Semin Arthroplasty.* 2007;18:11-18.
16. Snyder SJ, Arnoczky SP, Bond JL, et al. Histologic evaluation of a biopsy specimen obtained 3 months after rotator cuff augmentation with GraftJacket Matrix. *Arthroscopy.* 2009;25:329-333.
17. Dopirak R, Bond JL, Snyder SJ. Arthroscopic total rotator cuff replacement with an acellular human dermal allograft matrix. *Int J Shoulder Surg.* 2007;1:7-15.

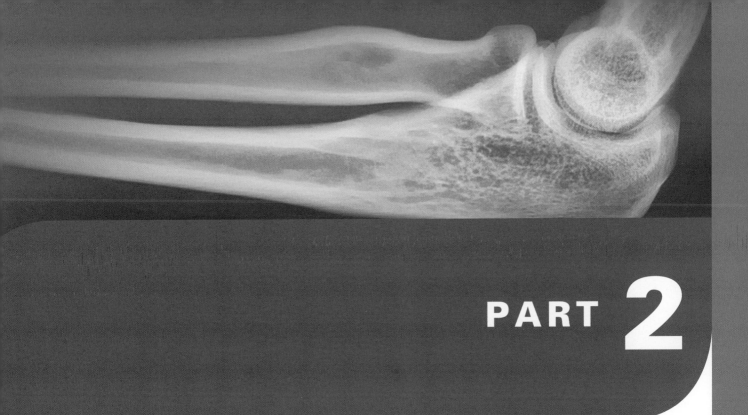

The Elbow

Chapter 39

Patient Positioning and Portal Placement

Frederick M. Azar and Richard Rainey

Chapter Synopsis

- A thorough understanding of the indications for elbow arthroscopy and the anatomic structures about the elbow allows safe and effective arthroscopic treatment of a number of elbow disorders. Appropriate patient positioning and correct portal placement are essential.

Important Points

- Thorough physical and imaging examinations are necessary for accurate diagnosis.
- A complete patient history is essential for identifying differential diagnoses.
- The most common contraindications to elbow arthroscopy are previous severe trauma and active infection.

Clinical and Surgical Pearls

- Before any portals are established, important anatomic structures should be marked on the extremity with indelible ink.
- Once the initial portal has been made, all subsequent portals should be made under direct visualization.
- Stab incisions should not be used to establish portals because they may damage neurovascular structures.
- Gravity or pump flow with pressures of 35 to 45 mm Hg will keep fluid from extravasating into soft tissues and causing compartment syndrome.

Clinical and Surgical Pitfalls

- The most common complication related to portal placement is nerve damage, which occurs in about 3% of procedures. Vulnerable nerves (ulnar, radial, posterior interosseous) should be identified and protected.

Elbow arthroscopy continues to evolve as a tool for diagnostic and therapeutic treatment of common and complex elbow problems. A thorough understanding of the anatomic structures and the surgical technique will allow safe and efficient treatment of these conditions.

PREOPERATIVE CONSIDERATIONS

Patient History

A thorough history of the patient's symptoms will help to elucidate a cause and allow the generation of a differential diagnosis that will aid in treatment.

A typical history should include information about the following:

- Acuity versus chronicity
- Location
- Type of symptoms (pain vs. mechanical)
- When the symptoms occur (with activity vs. at rest)
- Instability
- Swelling
- Neurovascular symptoms
- History of previous injury
- Previous treatment(s) and their effectiveness

Physical Examination

The physical examination of the patient goes beyond just the symptomatic elbow. An effort should be made to assess both upper extremities for evaluation of side-to-side asymmetry at the elbow and shoulder; the cervical spine should be examined when a patient gives a history of neurovascular complaints. Following these steps will aid in making a comprehensive decision

403

about the diagnosis instead of an isolated decision based on examination of only the affected elbow.

The examination should proceed in a sequential manner, beginning with inspection for and notation of any previous incisions or scars, swelling or fullness, and notable erythema. After the elbow has been inspected, palpation, again in a sequential fashion, will help to localize any areas of tenderness or pain. The elbow should be delineated into four regions for assessment: lateral, posterior, medial, and anterior. Because each region has anatomic structures that may account for the patient's symptoms, positive findings at a specific region or regions should aid in generating a differential diagnosis.

- Stability of the elbow should be tested in standard fashion with the appropriate tests based on the patient's history.
- Range of motion, including flexion-extension and pronation-supination, should be evaluated to identify any side-to-side differences and to ensure that functional motion has been preserved. The findings should be documented.
- Mechanical symptoms and their relative locations should be noted during active and passive motion of the elbow.
- The neurovascular status of the upper extremities should always be determined and documented.

Physical Examination Maneuvers

Medial Compartment

- Check for valgus instability. With the elbow flexed to 30 degrees to relax the anterior capsule and to free the olecranon from its bony articulation in the olecranon fossa, apply valgus stress with the arm in full supination.
- Discomfort along the medial aspect of the elbow may indicate ulnar collateral ligament (UCL) injury.
- Palpate the proximal flexor-pronator mass and medial epicondyle.
- Test resisted wrist flexion and forearm pronation; pain with these maneuvers may indicate medial epicondylitis or flexor-pronator tendon disease.
- Palpate the ulnar nerve in the cubital tunnel; flex and extend the elbow as the nerve is palpated to detect nerve subluxation.
- Assess the Tinel sign over the ulnar nerve in all three zones.

Posterior Compartment

- Palpate the triceps muscle insertion and the posterolateral and posteromedial joint to check for bone spurs or impingement.
- Perform the "clunk" test for posterior olecranon impingement: Grasp the patient's upper arm to stabilize the arm as the elbow is brought into full

extension. Pain with this maneuver may indicate compression of the olecranon into the fossa (valgus extension overload).

Lateral Compartment

- Palpate the lateral epicondyle and extensor origin to identify lateral epicondylitis or tendon disease.
- Pain with resisted wrist dorsiflexion and forearm supination is indicative of lateral epicondylitis.
- Palpate the radiocapitellar joint while the forearm is pronated and supinated to check for crepitus or catching, which may indicate chondromalacia.
- Inspect the "soft spot" to check for synovitis or effusion.

Stability

- The O'Driscoll posterolateral instability test can be performed to evaluate posterolateral rotatory instability. However, because of the patient's apprehension, the test result is usually negative. This test is best done with the patient under general anesthesia.

Range of Motion

- Flexion, extension, pronation, and supination are determined and compared with those of the opposite extremity.

Differential Diagnosis

The differential diagnosis can be based on the patient's subjective complaints or objective findings or both.

Lateral

- Radial head or neck fracture
- Lateral epicondylitis
- Extensor mechanism strain or avulsion
- Capitellar osteochondritis dissecans (OCD)
- Chondromalacia of the radial head or the capitellum
- Loose bodies
- Synovitis

Posterior

- Triceps tendinitis
- Triceps tendon avulsion
- Olecranon bursitis
- Olecranon stress fracture
- Posterior or posteromedial impingement
- Loose body
- Triceps enthesopathy

Medial

- Medial epicondyle fracture or avulsion
- Medial epicondylitis
- Flexor-pronator strain or avulsion

- Ulnar collateral ligament (UCL) sprain or rupture
- Ulnar neuritis
- Ulnar nerve subluxation

Anterior

- Distal biceps tendinitis
- Distal biceps tendon rupture
- Brachialis muscle strain
- Anterior capsular sprain
- Coronoid process fracture

Imaging

Radiography

Radiography may or may not help in confirming the diagnosis. All elbows should be imaged for assessment of bony pathology including fractures, subluxation, dislocation, or presence of loose bodies.

Views should include the following:

- Anteroposterior view: performed with the elbow in full extension
- Lateral view: performed with the elbow in 90 degrees of flexion
- Oblique view: rarely performed but may be useful in assessing for avulsions, fractures, or shear injuries
- Axial view: used to assess for signs of posteromedial impingement (posteromedial osteophytes)
- Gravity stress test view: special test used to assess for valgus laxity

Magnetic Resonance Imaging

Magnetic resonance imaging (MRI) is useful for assessing and confirming musculotendinous injuries of the extension and flexor origins, chondral lesions including radiocapitellar OCD, and ligamentous injuries including lateral ulnar collateral ligament (LUCL) and UCL injuries (best assessed by arthrography with injection of saline or gadolinium) and for detecting loose bodies.

Elbow Arthroscopy

Indications

- Synovectomy (partial or complete)
- Evaluation and treatment of OCD lesions of the capitellum
- Removal of posterior or posteromedial osteophytes
- Evaluation and removal of loose bodies
- Debridement of the joint of chondral lesions
- Capsular release
- Lysis of adhesions
- Pain with inconclusive examination and imaging

Contraindications

- Bony ankylosis
- Soft tissue contracture

- Local soft tissue infection
- Any alteration of the normal bony or soft tissue anatomy that would not allow safe entry of the arthroscope into the joint

SURGICAL TECHNIQUE

Anesthesia

Anesthesia options for this procedure include general or regional anesthesia, each of which has advantages and disadvantages. Advantages of general anesthesia include the ability to position the patient in any necessary position and the ability to achieve muscular relaxation. Disadvantages of general anesthesia include the need for increased postanesthesia recovery time, as well as the possibility of decreased pain relief postoperatively compared with regional anesthesia. Advantages of regional anesthesia include the ability to achieve excellent postoperative pain control and a decreased need for a long recovery time postoperatively. The disadvantages include inability to place the patient in any position, especially prone, and the inability to perform a reliable neurologic examination postoperatively.

Patient Positioning

Several patient positions can be used to safely perform elbow arthroscopy:

- Supine with the arm suspended from a suspension device
- Lateral decubitus position with or without the arm positioned over a post
- Prone with an arm board in place and the hand in the dependent position with the shoulder in neutral

Supine Position

Arthroscopy of the elbow with the patient supine can be done two ways: the standard supine position or the suspended supine position (Fig. 39-1). Both are useful, but the suspended supine position is used most often. With the use of either, the patient is placed supine on the operative table with the scapula at the edge of the table. The shoulder and elbow are abducted and flexed to 90 degrees. The upper extremity is held by a suspension or traction device (suspended position) or by operative personnel (standard position). We prefer the suspension setup. A well-padded, pneumatic tourniquet is placed high on the arm before the arm is prepared and draped. The hand and a portion of the forearm are placed into a sterile stockinette or impervious stockinette with a strap for suspension from the suspension or traction device. Usually 5 to 10 pounds of traction are used to maintain the elbow in the desired position.

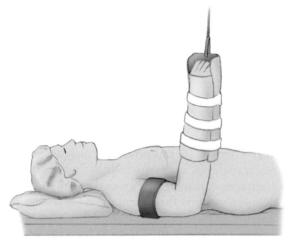

Figure 39-1. Supine position for elbow arthroscopy. *(Modified from Baker CL Jr, Jones GL. Current concepts. Arthroscopy of the elbow. Am J Sports Med. 1999;27:251-264.)*

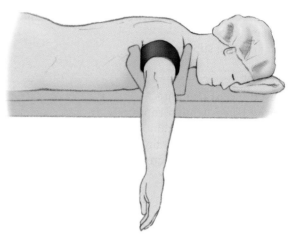

Figure 39-2. Prone position for elbow arthroscopy. *(Modified from Baker CL Jr, Jones GL. Current concepts. Arthroscopy of the elbow. Am J Sports Med. 1999;27:251-264.)*

The amount of weight necessary is based on the age and size of the patient. Use of the traction setup allows access to the medial and lateral portions of the elbow and eliminates the need for an assistant to hold the extremity. Flexion of the elbow to 90 degrees relaxes the neurovascular structures, allowing safe portal placement and access to the elbow joint. The forearm is easily supinated and pronated in this position as well.

If a suspension device is not available, then one or two arm boards can be used to support the operative extremity. This requires an assistant to hold the upper extremity with the elbow flexed to 90 degrees at all times. This setup is more stable but requires more operative personnel.

Prone Position

After secure intubation, the patient is repositioned prone, with care taken to place chest protectors to protect the torso and the airway (Fig. 39-2). The patient is then positioned close to the edge of the table on the operative side. The shoulder is abducted to 90 degrees, the elbow flexed to 90 degrees over a bolster, and the hand pointed toward the floor. A well-padded pneumatic tourniquet is then applied to the upper arm, and the upper extremity is moved through a full range of motion including flexion and extension. This is to ensure that the elbow can be placed in the position(s) necessary during surgery and to avoid shoulder hyperextension. Then the upper extremity is prepared and draped in normal sterile fashion.

Prone positioning has several advantages. First, no traction is needed because gravity assists with distending the joint as it hangs over the bolster. Second, the arm is more stable in this position, unlike in the supine position, in which the arm may swing medially or laterally when instruments are placed. Third, gravity and

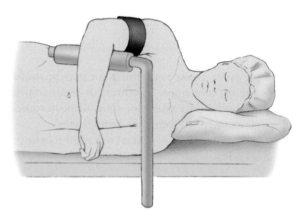

Figure 39-3. Lateral decubitus position for elbow arthroscopy. *(Modified from Baker CL Jr, Jones GL. Current concepts. Arthroscopy of the elbow. Am J Sports Med. 1999;27:251-264.)*

joint distention cause the neurovascular structures to fall away from the joint, decreasing the likelihood of neurovascular injury. Last, this position allows easy conversion to an open procedure if necessary.

Lateral Decubitus Position

After secure intubation, the patient is repositioned in the lateral position with the surgical side up (Fig. 39-3). A beanbag with suction or hip positioners will help maintain this position. All bony prominences are well padded distally, and the axilla is protected as needed with an axillary roll. A well-padded pneumatic tourniquet is placed high on the arm, and the arm is placed over a bolster after normal sterile preparation and draping.

This position allows easy access to the posterior compartment, as well as access to the medial and lateral aspects of the elbow.

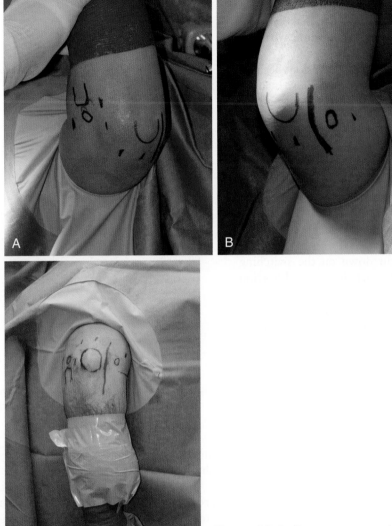

Figure 39-4. Bone anatomy and landmarks outlined before distention of the joint: radial head, medial and lateral epicondyles, olecranon, and course of the ulnar nerve.

Surgical Landmarks, Incisions, and Portals

General Principles

- Before making any incisions, mark important anatomic structures on the operative extremity with indelible ink (Fig. 39-4).
  - Mark all bony landmarks (radial head, olecranon tip, medial and lateral epicondyles, and capitellum).
  - Mark out the course of the ulnar nerve. Move the elbow through a range of motion to ensure that it does not subluxate from the cubital tunnel.
  - Identify and mark the course of all superficial nerves, and use a retractor to avoid the nerve when necessary.
  - Mark all portal sites.
- Distend the joint by placing an 18-gauge needle through the direct lateral portal site (soft spot) and injecting 20 to 40 mL of saline or lactated Ringer's solution into the joint.
- Initiate an anterolateral (our preference) or anteromedial portal after placing a second 18-gauge needle in the anticipated portal site.
- Use a blunt or conical trocar and cannula to trap the capsule over the radial head for anterolateral portal placement.

- Leave the 18-gauge needle in place in the soft spot to act as an outflow.
- Once the initial portal has been made, make all subsequent portals under direct visualization with use of an 18-gauge needle.
- When making portals, avoid "stab" incisions because these may injure neurovascular structures. Instead, lay the tip of the blade against the skin and pull the skin across the blade; this allows subcutaneous tissue and sensory nerves to fall away to a safe distance and reduces the risk of nerve injury. Spread the subcutaneous tissues with a mosquito hemostat to prevent damage to the superficial cutaneous nerves.
- A switching stick is useful when trying to establish the anteromedial portal from the anterolateral portal or vice versa. Pass the switching stick carefully across the joint and use it to tent the skin on the opposite side. Use the blade to cut down on the switching stick, and place a cannula over the exposed portion of the switching stick.
- Gravity flow or pump flow with pressures of 35 to 45 mm Hg will keep the fluid from extravasating into the soft tissues and causing a compartment syndrome.

Specific Portal Placement

Lateral Portals

The direct lateral portal lies in the center of a triangle formed by the lateral epicondyle, radial head, and olecranon (Fig. 39-5). This soft spot is easily palpated before distention. This approach passes through the anconeus muscle; it is used for initial joint distention and for lateral portal viewing. Watch for the posterior antebrachial cutaneous nerve, which passes within 7 mm.

The anterolateral portal lies 2 to 3 cm distal and 1 to 2 cm anterior to the lateral humeral epicondyle, within the sulcus between the radial head and capitellum anteriorly. These measurements may vary depending on the size of the patient, and portal placement depends on locating the radiocapitellar articulation. The anterolateral portal passes through the extensor carpi radialis brevis and the supinator muscle before reaching the capsule. This portal provides an excellent view of the medial capsule, medial plica, coronoid process, trochlea, and coronoid fossa. Watch for the posterior antebrachial cutaneous nerve, an average of 2 mm from the sheath; the radial nerve, which is usually 7 to 11 mm anteromedial to the portal, but may be as close as 2 or 3 mm; and the posterior interosseous nerve, 1 to 13 mm from the portal, depending on the degree of forearm pronation.

The middle anterolateral portal, located 1 cm directly anterior to the lateral epicondyle, provides access to the radiocapitellar joint and lateral compartment and is a good working portal for instrumentation. It also

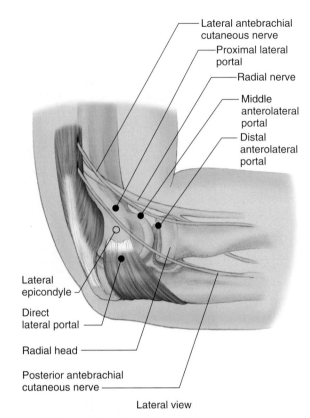

Figure 39-5. Lateral portals. *(Modified from Baker CL Jr, Jones GL. Current concepts. Arthroscopy of the elbow. Am J Sports Med. 1999;27:251-264.)*

functions as a good viewing portal for the anterior ulnohumeral joint.

The proximal anterolateral portal is made 1 to 2 cm proximal and 1 cm anterior to the lateral epicondyle. Stothers and colleagues described this portal as being safer than the middle anterolateral portal, which is safer than the standard distal anterolateral portal.

Medial Portals

The anteromedial portal is placed 2 cm anterior and 2 cm distal to the medial epicondyle (Fig. 39-6). It usually is placed under direct visualization with the use of an 18-gauge needle. The anteromedial portal passes between the radial aspect of the flexor digitorum sublimis and the tendinous portion of the pronator teres before entering the joint capsule. It allows examination of the radiocapitellar and humeroulnar joints, the coronoid fossa, the capitellum, and the superior capsule. Watch for the medial antebrachial cutaneous nerve, which is an average of 6 mm from the portal but may be as close as 1 mm; the median nerve, which is 19 mm anterolateral to the portal with the joint distended and 12 mm without distention; and the ulnar nerve, located an average of 21 mm from the portal. The portal is 17 mm posteromedial to the brachial artery.

The proximal medial (superomedial) portal is placed 1 cm anterior and 1 to 2 cm proximal to the medial

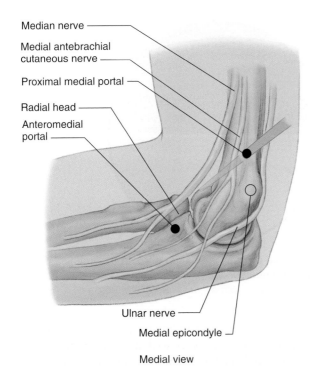

Figure 39-6. Medial portals. *(Modified from Baker CL Jr, Jones GL. Current concepts. Arthroscopy of the elbow.* Am J Sports Med. *1999;27:251-264.)*

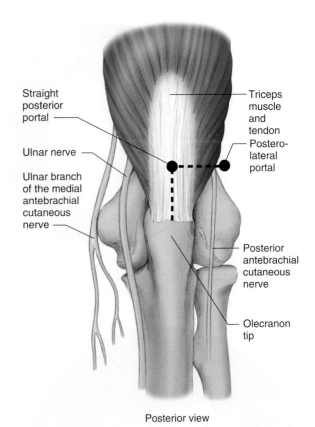

Figure 39-7. Posterior portals. *(Modified from Baker CL Jr, Jones GL. Current concepts. Arthroscopy of the elbow.* Am J Sports Med. *1999;27:251-264.)*

epicondyle and passes through a tendinous portion of the flexor-pronator group. This portal provides excellent viewing of the anterior compartment of the elbow, particularly the radiocapitellar joint. Watch for the median nerve, which is 22.3 mm from the portal.

Posterior Portals

The posterolateral portal is placed 2 to 3 cm proximal to the olecranon tip and just lateral to the lateral border of the triceps muscle (Fig. 39-7). This portal allows examination of the olecranon tip, olecranon fossa, and posterior trochlea.

The straight posterior portal is located over the center of the triceps tendon, 2 cm medial to the posterolateral portal and 3 cm proximal to the tip of the olecranon. This portal is helpful for removal of impinging olecranon osteophytes and loose bodies from the posterior elbow joint. Watch for the posterior and medial antebrachial cutaneous nerves, which lie on the lateral and medial aspects of the upper arm 23 to 25 mm medial to the straight posterior portal, and the ulnar nerve, located within 25 mm of the straight posterior portal.

Normal Arthroscopic Anatomy

Anterior Compartment

Through the anterolateral portal (Fig. 39-8), the coronoid and its articulation with the trochlea can be viewed.

Flexion and extension of the elbow bring the anterior trochlea into view. The brachialis tendon insertion can be evaluated on the coronoid process. The coronoid fossa can be seen proximal in the compartment. With the arthroscope directed medially, the medial portion of the capsule can be examined, including the anterior third of the anterior bundle of the ulnar collateral ligament. With proper orientation of the scope, the proximal ulna and medial gutter can be viewed. The sublime tubercle, with the intersection of the anteromedial capsule and the proximal medial ulna, can be evaluated.

Through the anteromedial portal (Fig. 39-9), the radial head and the radiocapitellar articulation can be identified. Supination and pronation of the forearm allow viewing of 75% of the surface of the radial head. The annular ligament can be noted crossing the radial neck, and the radial fossa can be evaluated with proximal viewing of the scope. The attachment of the capsule to the humerus can be seen superiorly. The scope can then be advanced to examine the lateral gutter, the undersurface of the capsule, and the origin of the extensor muscles to the lateral epicondyle. The articulations of the radius, ulna, and distal humerus can be viewed by placing the scope between the trochlear and capitellar ridges up to the medial border of the radial head.

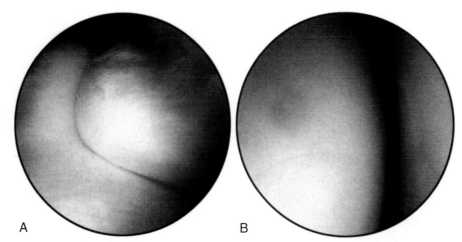

Figure 39-8. Anterolateral portal. **A,** Medial side of elbow; the coronoid process is on the right and the trochlea is on the left. **B,** Radiocapitellar joint with varus stress applied to expose the undersurface of the radial head. *(From Phillips BB: Arthroscopy of upper extremity. In: Canale ST, ed. Campbell's Operative Orthopaedics. 10th ed. St Louis: Mosby; 2003.)*

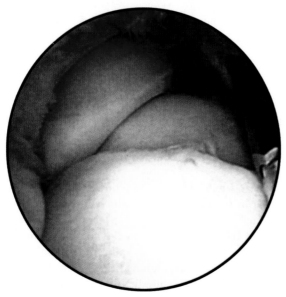

Figure 39-9. Anteromedial portal, anterior aspect of elbow. The coronoid and trochlea are in the foreground and the radiocapitellar joint is in the background, with the shaver just proximal to the radiocapitellar joint. The annular ligament is clearly seen. *(From Phillips BB: Arthroscopy of upper extremity. In: Canale ST, ed. Campbell's Operative Orthopaedics. 10th ed. St Louis: Mosby; 2003.)*

Lateral Compartment

Through the direct lateral portal (Fig. 39-10), the articulation of the olecranon, radial head, and capitellum can be seen. Again, supination and pronation of the forearm allow viewing of 75% of the radial head articular surface. The capitellum can be seen, and most of the smooth convex surface can be examined through this portal. The olecranon fossa can also be evaluated at this position. The scope can then be positioned posteriorly into the groove formed by the olecranon and trochlea.

The entire olecranon can be seen from this vantage. The apophyseal scar can be viewed at the midpoint as a bare area of roughened articular cartilage. The undersurface of the trochlea should be visible when the scope is turned anteriorly. The posterolateral corner and capsule are viewed by looking posteriorly from the olecranon-trochlear groove. The posterior compartment can then be viewed for establishment of the posterior portals. If the 4-mm arthroscope is too large for this portal, a 2.7-mm arthroscope can be used.

Posterior Compartment

The olecranon tip will be the first landmark seen through the posterolateral portal (Fig. 39-11). The triceps tendon insertion will be seen at the olecranon tip, where osteophyte formation may be noted posteromedially in patients with posterior impingement caused by valgus extension overload. The olecranon fossa and posterior trochlear surface also can be seen from this position. Normally 50% to 60% of the ulnar collateral ligament can be seen when the scope is pushed medially and the posteromedial corner of the elbow is seen. The ulnar nerve is superficial to this area of the elbow and must be identified and protected.

POSTOPERATIVE CONSIDERATIONS

Complications

- Neurovascular injury
- Arthrofibrosis
- Infection
- Articular cartilage injury
- Compartment syndrome secondary to excessive fluid extravasation

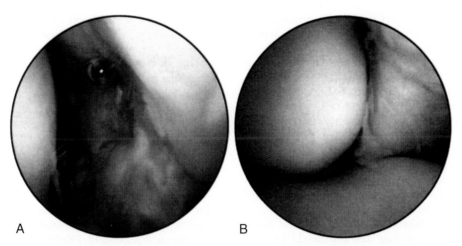

Figure 39-10. Direct lateral portal. **A,** Bare area of olecranon is right inside with trochlea on left. **B,** With the elbow flexed 90 degrees (patient supine), the articular surface of three bones can be seen. Radial head is superior left, ulna is superior right, and capitellum is inferior. *(From Phillips BB: Arthroscopy of upper extremity. In: Canale ST, ed. Campbell's Operative Orthopaedics. 10th ed. St Louis: Mosby; 2003.)*

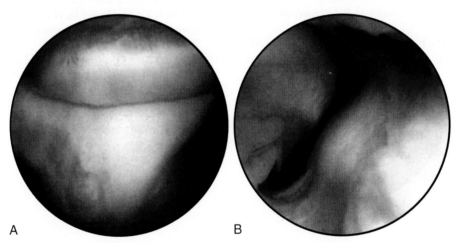

Figure 39-11. Posterolateral portal. **A,** Posterior compartment; tip of olecranon is superior, trochlea is inferior, and olecranon fossa is in foreground. **B,** Medial gutter with posterior aspect of ulnar collateral ligament on the right and distal humerus on the left. *(From Phillips BB: Arthroscopy of upper extremity. In: Canale ST, ed. Campbell's Operative Orthopaedics. 10th ed. St Louis: Mosby; 2003.)*

- Synovial-cutaneous fistula
- Complex regional pain syndrome

The most common complication related to portal placement is nerve damage, which occurs in about 3% of procedures. Most of these injuries are to cutaneous nerves and are transient, although there have been isolated reports of major neurovascular injuries. These include irreparable damage to the ulnar nerve; transection of the ulnar, radial, and posterior interosseous nerves; and compression neuropathy of the radial nerve.

Drainage from a portal site occurs in approximately 2.5% of patients, but deep infection is less frequent (approximately 1%).

SUGGESTED READINGS

Abboud JA, Ricchetti ET, Tjoumakaris F, et al. Elbow arthroscopy: basic setup and portal placement. *J Am Acad Orthop Surg.* 2006;14:312-318.

Ahmad CS, Vitale MS. Elbow arthroscopy: setup, portal placement, and simple procedures. *Instr Cours Lect.* 2011;60:171-180.

Andrews JR, Baumgarten TE. Arthroscopic anatomy of the elbow. *Orthop Clin North Am.* 1995;26:671-677.

Baker CL Jr. Normal arthroscopic anatomy of the elbow: prone technique. In: McGinty JB, Burkhart SS, Jackson RW, et al, eds. *Operative Arthroscopy.* 3rd ed. Philadelphia: Lippincott Williams & Wilkins; 2003.

Baker CL Jr, Shalvoy RM. The prone position for elbow arthroscopy. *Clin Sports Med.* 1991;10:623-628.

Bedi A, Dines J, Dines DM, et al. Use of the 70-degree arthroscope for improved visualization with common arthroscopic procedures. *Arthroscopy*. 2010;26:1684-1696.

Brach P, Goitz FJ. Elbow arthroscopy: surgical techniques and rehabilitation. *J Hand Ther*. 2006;19:228-236.

Dodson CC, Nho SJ, Williams RJ 3rd, et al. Elbow arthroscopy. *J Am Acad Orthop Surg*. 2008;16:574-585.

Field LD, Altchek DW, Warren RF, et al. Arthroscopic anatomy of the lateral elbow: a comparison of three portals. *Arthroscopy*. 1994;10:602-607.

Geib TM, Savoie FH 3rd. Elbow arthroscopy for posttraumatic arthrosis. *Instr Course Lect*. 2009;58:473-480.

Keener JD, Galatz LM. Arthroscopic management of the stiff elbow. *J Am Acad Orthop Surg*. 2011;19:265-274.

Kelly EW, Morrey BF, O'Driscoll SW. Complications of elbow arthroscopy. *J Bone Joint Surg Am*. 2001;83:25-34.

Kim SJ, Jeong JH. Technical note. Transarticular approach for elbow arthroscopy. *Arthroscopy*. 2003;19:E27.

Kim SJ, Jeong JH. Transarticular approach for elbow arthroscopy. *Arthroscopy*. 2003;19:E37.

Kim SJ, Moon HK, Chun YM, et al. Arthroscopic treatment for limitation of motion of the elbow: the learning curve. *Knee Surg Sports Traumatol Arthrosc*. 2011;19:1013-1018.

Meyers JF, Carson WG Jr. Elbow arthroscopy: supine technique. In: McGinty JB, Burkhart SS, Jackson RW, et al, eds. *Operative Arthroscopy*. 3rd ed. Philadelphia: Lippincott Williams & Wilkins; 2003.

Micheli LJ, Luke AC, Mintzer CM, et al. Elbow arthroscopy in the pediatric and adolescent population. *Arthroscopy*. 2001;17:694-699.

Miller CD, Jobe CM, Wright MH. Neuroanatomy in elbow arthroscopy. *J Shoulder Elbow Surg*. 1995;4:168-174.

Morrey BF. Complications of elbow arthroscopy. *Instr Course Lect*. 2000;49:255-258.

Noonberg GE, Baker CL Jr. Elbow arthroscopy. *Instr Course Lect*. 2006;55:87-93.

Rosenberg BM, Loebenberg MI. Elbow arthroscopy. *Bull NYU Hosp Jt Dis*. 2007;65:43-50.

Savoie FH 3rd. Guidelines to becoming an expert elbow arthroscopist. *Arthroscopy*. 2007;23:1237-1240.

Savoie FH III, Field LD. Arthrofibrosis and complications in arthroscopy of the elbow. *Clin Sports Med*. 2001;20:123-129.

Selby RM, O'Brien SJ, Kelly AM, et al. The joint jack: report of a new technique essential for elbow arthroscopy. *Arthroscopy*. 2002;18:440-445.

Steinmann SP, King GJW, Savoie FH III. Arthroscopic treatment of the arthritic elbow. *J Bone Joint Surg Am*. 2005;87:2114-2121.

Stothers K, Day B, Regan WR. Arthroscopy of the elbow: anatomy, portal sites, and a description of the proximal lateral portal. *Arthroscopy*. 1995;11:449-457.

Takahashi T, Iai H, Hirose D, et al. Distraction in the lateral position in elbow arthroscopy. *Arthroscopy*. 2000;16:221-225.

Tucker SA, Savoie FH 3rd, O'Brien MJ. Arthroscopic management of the post-traumatic stiff elbow. *J Elbow Shoulder Surg*. 2011;20(2 Suppl):S83-S89.

Zonno A, Manuel J, Merrell G, et al. Arthroscopic technique for medial epicondylitis: technique and safety analysis. *Arthroscopy*. 2010;26:610-616.

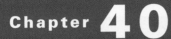

Chapter 40

Arthroscopic and Open Management of Osteochondritis Dissecans of the Elbow

Nicholas D. Iagulli, Larry D. Field, and Felix H. Savoie III

Chapter Synopsis

- Osteochondritis dissecans is a localized condition involving the articular surface resulting in separation of the articular cartilage and subchondral bone. The most common site of osteochondritis dissecans of the elbow is the capitellum, and it generally occurs in young athletes who report a history of overuse. Pain is the most common complaint, and radiographs are the initial diagnostic test of choice. Treatment decisions are based primarily on the integrity of the articular cartilage and whether the involved segment is stable, unstable but attached, or detached and loose. Stable lesions can be treated nonoperatively, whereas unstable or detached lesions often require surgery. Arthroscopic abrasion arthroplasty is the standard procedure of choice, except when the lesion involves over 50% of the articular surface or disrupts the lateral buttress. In this case, osteochondral autograft transplantation may have better results.

Important Points

- Stable lesions should be treated conservatively.
- Unstable lesions can be treated arthroscopically in the following circumstances:
  - Lesion involves less than 50% articular surface.
  - Lateral buttress is intact.

- Osteochondral autograft transplantation may be considered in large lesions involving the lateral buttress with engagement of radial head.

Clinical and Surgical Pearls

- Mark surface landmarks before arthroscopy.
- Insufflate elbow joint with saline before making portals.
- Anteromedial portal is made first anterior to muscular septum.
- Anterolateral portal is made under direct visualization.
- Lesion is best visualized with a 70-degree scope from posterior or lateral portal.
- Debride lesion through the soft-spot portal.

Clinical and Surgical Pitfalls

- Mechanical symptoms likely indicate an unstable lesion.
- Poor results after arthroscopic treatment have been reported in lesions that involve the lateral buttress.

Osteochondritis dissecans is a localized condition that involves the articular surface with separation of a segment of articular cartilage and subchondral bone. The most common site of osteochondritis dissecans of the elbow is the capitellum, although lesions have been reported in the trochlea, on the radial head, and on the olecranon and in the olecranon fossa.[1] Osteochondritis dissecans most often occurs in athletes ages 11 to 21 years who report a history of overuse.[2,3] The lesion generally involves only a segment of capitellum and is primarily located in a central or anterolateral position.[4,5] Appropriate treatment of this disorder remains controversial. Often treated with benign neglect, osteochondritis is a potentially sport-ending injury for an athlete and in the long term can lead to degenerative arthritis.[5,6]

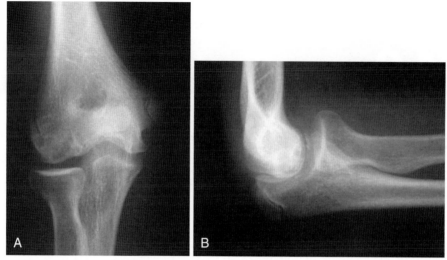

Figure 40-1. Anteroposterior (**A**) and lateral (**B**) radiographs demonstrating radiolucency and rarefaction typical of osteochondritis dissecans of the elbow.

PREOPERATIVE CONSIDERATIONS

History

Osteochondritis dissecans is primarily a disorder of the young athlete and rarely occurs in adults. The typical patient is age 11 to 21 years, with the majority being age 12 to 14 years.[2,3,7] Males are affected more than females; however, this disorder is prevalent among female gymnasts. The dominant arm is almost always involved, and bilateral involvement has been reported in 5% to 20% of cases.[8] A history of elbow overuse is often described in association with common sporting activities such as baseball, gymnastics, weightlifting, racquet sports, and cheerleading.[36]

Physical Examination

Most patients report pain, and it is usually insidious and progressive in nature. The pain is often localized over the lateral aspect of the elbow and is exacerbated by activities and relieved by rest. For some patients the location of pain may be poorly defined.[8]

On clinical examination, palpation laterally over the radiocapitellar joint reproduces tenderness. Elbow range of motion is limited, particularly in extension, and it is not uncommon to observe flexion contractures of 5 to 23 degrees.[2,10-13] A loss of elbow flexion is less common, whereas supination and pronation are rarely altered. Any complaints of clicking, catching, grinding, or locking suggest fragment instability or loose bodies. Crepitus and swelling may be present, as well.[2,3,8,9] Provocative tests such as the active radiocapitellar compression test may aid in making the diagnosis.[14] This test is performed by having the patient actively pronate and supinate the forearm with the elbow in full extension, allowing the dynamic muscle forces to compress across the radiocapitellar joint, thus reproducing symptoms.

Imaging

Plain radiographs are the initial diagnostic test of choice. Standard anteroposterior (AP) and lateral views of the elbow will usually show the classic findings of a radiolucency and rarefaction of the capitellum with flattening or irregularity of the articular surface. A rim of sclerotic bone often surrounds the radiolucent crater, which is typically located in the central or anterolateral aspect of the capitellum (Fig. 40-1). Loose bodies may be present if the necrotic segment becomes detached.

Additional studies may be indicated to further evaluate osteochondritis dissecans. Computed tomography (CT) is useful in determining the extent of the osseous lesion as well as the presence and location of loose bodies. CT arthrography more accurately defines the integrity of the articular surface.[15]

Magnetic resonance imaging (MRI) has become the standard modality for further evaluation.[2,16] MRI allows assessment of the articular surface and definition of the size and extent of the lesion (Fig. 40-2). Whereas early, stable lesions show signal changes on T1-weighted images, T2-weighted images remain normal. On the other hand, advanced lesions show signal changes on both T1- and T2-weighted images.[2,17] Loose in situ lesions often demonstrate a cyst under the lesion. Magnetic resonance arthrography (MRA) can improve the diagnosis of osteochondral lesions owing to penetration of contrast beneath the disrupted cartilage surface.[16,17]

Progress and healing can be monitored over time with plain radiographs. If the fragment remains stable,

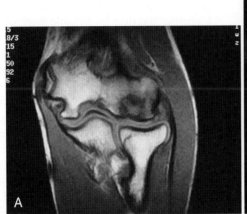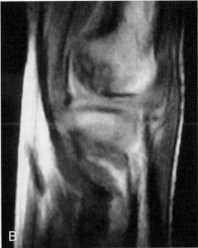

Figure 40-2. Coronal (**A**) and sagittal (**B**) magnetic resonance images of the same lesion shown in Figure 40-1. Increased signal of the T2 image indicates disruption of the articular surface.

the central sclerotic fragment gradually becomes less distinct and the surrounding area of radiolucency slowly ossifies. A nonhealing lesion in a patient who remains symptomatic despite conservative treatment should prompt the clinician to consider operative treatments.[2,5]

Indications and Contraindications

The proper treatment of osteochondritis dissecans lesions is a highly debated topic. Treatment options include nonoperative modalities, usually rest and avoidance of any aggravating activities, versus surgical management, which includes fragment excision, fragment fixation, and osteochondral autograft reconstruction of the lesion. Management decisions are based primarily on the integrity of the articular cartilage and status of the involved segment—that is, whether it is stable, unstable but attached, or detached and loose.

Stable lesions with intact cartilage and in situ subchondral fragments are managed conservatively.[2,8,16] Sports and other aggravating activities are stopped until symptoms have subsided, usually after a period of approximately 3 to 6 weeks. During this time we recommend protecting the elbow in a hinged elbow brace without limitations to motion. Athletes can usually return to sports without restrictions 3 to 6 months after initiation of treatment.[9] Patients with intact lesions that are identified early and treated conservatively have the best prognosis. However, it is prudent for the clinician to inform the family of possible long-term sequelae.[5,6,8,13,16,18,19]

Indications for surgical treatment include persistent or worsening symptoms despite prolonged conservative care, the presence of loose bodies, and evidence of lesion instability including violation of intact cartilage or detachment.[2,8,20,21] Multiple surgical techniques have been described and are discussed in the following sections.

NONOPERATIVE TREATMENT

Nonsurgical treatment is typically selected for patients with early-grade, stable lesions and involves activity modification with cessation of sports participation.[22-24] The duration of activity modification is dictated by symptomatology, with a typical regimen consisting of 3 to 6 weeks of rest followed by a return to sport in 3 to 6 months.[23,25] Recent studies have reported significantly improved rates of radiographic healing and subjective outcomes in terms of pain and return to sport in patients with open capitellar physes.[22,24] Nonoperative treatment is recommended for all stable lesions in patients with open capitellar physes.[24]

OPERATIVE TREATMENT

Operative intervention is indicated for lesions that do not improve with appropriate nonoperative treatment, the presence of loose bodies with mechanical symptoms, or the presence of an unstable lesion.[25,26] Multiple operative procedures have been described for treating these lesions, including drilling of the defect,[26] fragment removal with or without curettage or drilling of the residual defect,[5,6,13,18,26-28] fragment fixation by a variety of methods,[26,29-32] reconstruction with osteochondral autograft,[26,31,33-36] autologous chondrocyte implantation,[26,37] and closing-wedge osteotomy of the lateral condyle.[26,38] Making comparisons between the reported results of these various operative techniques is difficult because of their largely retrospective nature, the use of different outcome measurements, and the relative infrequency of osteochondritis dissecans.[26]

Open Surgical Approaches

Open procedures to remove fragments (Table 40-1) have demonstrated improved results with respect to pain and radiographic parameters when performed in patients with lesions measuring less than 50% of the capitellar articular width.[5,23,24] Other studies have shown that removal of loose bodies or excision of the fragment with or without drilling or curettage was not sufficient to regain full function and allow patients to return to their previous level of sport.[30,32,39] Kuwahata and Inoue[30] performed fragment fixation using a Herbert screw, whereas Takeda and colleagues[32] used pullout wiring for fixation (Table 40-2). Both studies performed cancellous bone grafting to fill the crater and possibly to enhance

fragment union. All patients showed complete reossification at follow-up, and most returned to their previous sporting activities. Nobuta and colleagues[40] found that fragment fixation by flexible wire or thread and revascularization by drilling was effective in patients whose lesion thickness was less than 9 mm (see Table 40-2). Takahara and colleagues[24] found significantly improved outcome in terms of pain in patients treated with fragment fixation with bone pegs (see Table 40-2).[41]

Osteochondral autograft transplantation (Fig. 40-3) was recently introduced as another treatment option for capitellar osteochondritis dissecans.[26,31,33-36] Indications for this procedure include lesions that involve more than 50% of the articular surface area, those with disruption of the lateral buttress (Fig. 40-4), and lesions that cause engagement of the radial head.[23,24,42] Cylindric osteochondral grafts are harvested from a donor site, typically the lateral femoral condyle, and the graft plug is

TABLE 40-1. Results of Open Fragment Excision of Osteochondritis Dissecans of the Elbow

Study	Follow-up	No. of Patients	Return to Sport	Comments
Bauer et al[6] (1992)	23 years	31	Unknown	40% recurrence of symptoms
Takahara et al[24] (2007)	9.6 years	55	27 (49%)	Results dependent on size of capitellar defect Better results with lesions measuring <50% of capitellar articular width

TABLE 40-2. Results of Open Fragment Fixation of Osteochondritis Dissecans of the Elbow

Study	Follow-up	No. of Patients	Return to Sport	Technique	Comments
Harada et al[29] (2002)	7.5 years	4	3 (75%)	Dynamic staples and bone graft	100% union rate
Kuwahata and Inoue[30] (1998)	32 months	7	7 (100%)	Herbert screw and bone graft	100% union rate
Nobuta et al[40] (2008)	17 months	28	19 (68%)	Flexible wire or thread with drilling	82% union rate
Takeda et al[32] (2002)	57 months	11	10 (91%)	Pullout wires and bone graft	100% union rate

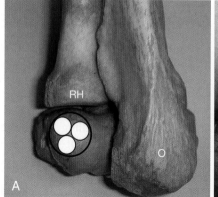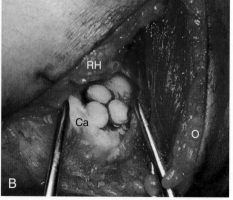

Figure 40-3. Osteochondral autograft reconstruction of osteochondritis dissecans lesion of the capitellum: schematic drawing (**A**) and intraoperative view (**B**). *Ca*, Capitellum; *O*, olecranon; *RH*, radial head. (*From Takahara M, Mura N, Sasaki J, et al. Classification, treatment, and outcome of osteochondritis dissecans of the humeral capitellum: Surgical technique. J Bone Joint Surg Am. 2008;90[Suppl 2 Pt 1]:47-62.*)

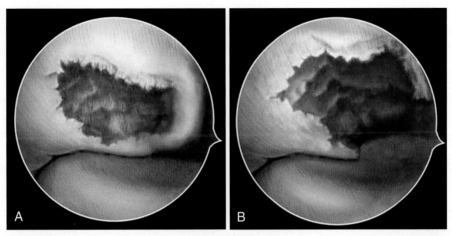

Figure 40-4. View of osteochondritis dissecans lesion of capitellum in a right elbow with patient in the prone position as viewed from the lateral portal. Contained osteochondritis dissecans lesion (**A**) with circumferential healthy cartilage present. Similar lesion with loss of lateral column support (**B**). *(From Baker CL 3rd, Romeo AA, Baker CL Jr. Osteochondritis dissecans of the capitellum. Am J Sports Med. 2010;38:1917-1928.)*

TABLE 40-3. Results of Osteochondral Autograft Reconstruction for Osteochondritis Dissecans of the Elbow

Study	Follow-up	No. of Patients	Return to Sport	Technique	Comments
Iwasaki et al[33] (2009)	45 months	19	17 (90%)	Autologous osteochondral mosaicplasty	No loose bodies or degenerative changes
Shimada et al[43] (2005)	25.5 months	10	8 (80%)	OATS	100% graft incorporation Increase in radiocapitellar joint congruency
Takahara et al[24] (2007)	2.9 years	15	11 (73%)	Fragment fixation with bone pegs or reconstruction with osteochondral plug grafts	Recommendations Fixation with bone graft for ICRS II and III OCA for ICRS IV
Yamamoto et al[36] (2006)	3.5 years	18	16 (89%)	OATS	All patients with good or excellent results

ICRS, International Cartilage Repair Society; *OATS,* Osteochondral Autograft Transplantation System; *OCA,* osteochondral autograft.

inserted perpendicular to the subchondral bone.[34,41] These authors[34,41] have suggested that this procedure may reduce the progression to osteoarthritis and lead to better long-term results.[39] Several reports have described success with osteochondral mosaicplasty with regard to clinical and radiographic findings at short-term follow-up (Table 40-3).[26,33,36,43]

A closing wedge osteotomy for the management of capitellar osteochondritis dissecans has been used by Kiyoshige and colleagues[38] to unload the radiocapitellar joint. This results in widening of the radiohumeral joint space, reduction of compression, and stimulation of revascularization and remodeling of the lesion.[38,39] This technique is reserved for early-grade lesions and is technically demanding.[23,38] Although almost all patients returned to full athletic activity in this series, minimal osteoarthritic changes and enlargement of the radial head occurred in all patients postoperatively.[38,39]

Arthroscopic Approaches

Arthroscopic surgery is becoming the standard procedure for treatment of capitellar osteochondritis dissecans.[39,44] Advantages of an arthroscopic approach include the minimally invasive nature of the procedure with the potential for early rehabilitation, excellent access to the lesion and the entire elbow joint, and the ability to identify and treat concomitant lesions including the removal of loose bodies.[26] Studies on arthroscopic debridement and abrasion arthroplasty (Table 40-4) have shown encouraging short-term and midterm results.[5,10,12,24,27,39,45-47] Long-term results are mixed, however, with variable return to sport and recurrence of loose bodies.[23,39]

Most surgeons use a variation of a six-portal approach (Fig. 40-5).[10,26,48,44] These portals include standard anteromedial, anterolateral, direct posterior,

TABLE 40-4. Results of Arthroscopic Treatment of Osteochondritis Dissecans of the Elbow

Study	Follow-up	No. of Patients	Return to Sport	Comments
Baumgarten et al[10] (1998)	4 years	16	13 (81%)	Slight capitellar flattening in eight patients
Bojanic et al[45] (2006)	1 year	3	3 (100%)	Microfractured lesion; postoperative MRI scan showed defects filled with hyaline-like tissue
Brownlow et al[46] (2006)	6.4 years	29	23 (79%)	At follow-up, 38% demonstrated DJD and loose bodies at follow-up
Byrd and Jones[27] (2002)	3.9 years	10	4 (40%)	No correlation between grade of lesion and postoperative outcomes or return to sport Potential poor prognosis with lesion extension into lateral border of capitellum
Rahusen et al[47] (2006)	3.8 years	15	12 (80%)	Significant improvement in pain No improvement in range of motion
Ruch et al[12] (1998)	3.2 years	12	3 (25%)	No functional limitation in 92% Improved extension seen postoperatively All demonstrated capitellar remodeling Lateral capsular fragment was associated with worse outcomes

DJD, degenerative joint disease; *MRI,* magnetic resonance imaging.

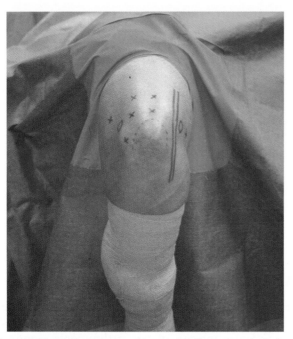

Figure 40-5. Common arthroscopic elbow portals (left elbow in the prone position with ulnar nerve marked).

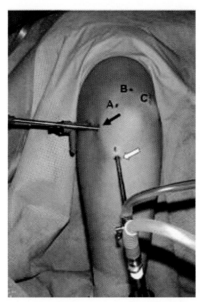

Figure 40-6. The distal ulnar portal *(white arrow)* approximately 3 to 4 cm distal to radiocapitellar joint and just lateral to the palpable posterior edge of the ulna. The black arrow indicates the soft-spot portal used as a working portal. *A,* Posterolateral portal for viewing of the olecranon fossa; *B,* direct posterior portal for working portal; and *C,* ulnar nerve. *(From Van Den Ende KI, McIntosh A, Adams J, et al. Osteochondritis dissecans of the capitellum: A review of the literature and a distal ulnar portal. Arthroscopy. 2011;27:122-128.)*

posterolateral, and dual direct-lateral portals.[26,48] Baumgarten and colleagues[10] identified the use of two direct lateral portals as the key to effective arthroscopic treatment of osteochondritis dissecans of the capitellum. Davis and colleagues[48] performed a cadaveric study evaluating the dual direct-lateral portals and found that 78% of the entire capitellar surface area was accessible through these portals. In addition, the portals remain safely proximal and posterior to the lateral ligamentous complex.[48] A distal ulnar portal (Fig. 40-6) has

recently been described and is placed approximately 3 to 4 cm distal to the posterior aspect of the radiocapitellar joint and just lateral to the palpable posterior edge of the ulna.[39] This portal is typically used as a viewing portal, whereas the standard soft-spot portal is used as a working portal.[39] Some authors have described an arthroscopic-assisted drilling method involving use of a hole drilled through the radius shaft.[49] The osteochondritis dissecans lesion can be completely reached by changing the flexion angle in both pronation and supination.[49] The angle of approach can be close to the posterior interosseous nerve, and the procedure requires drilling across the normal cartilage surface to the radius.[39,49]

Poor results after arthroscopic treatment have been noted in lesions that extend through the lateral margin of the capitellum resulting in the absence of a complete circumferential border of healthy articular cartilage and subchondral bone[12,26,27] (see Fig. 40-4). Byrd and Jones[27] postulated that the lateral fragment noted in the study by Ruch and colleagues[12] is similarly associated with loss of the lateral border of the capitellum and portends a possible poor prognosis.[26]

Our Preferred Technique: Arthroscopic Excision and Drilling

We use general anesthesia and the prone position for arthroscopic evaluation of the elbow. The patient is placed prone on the operating table over chest rolls to ensure adequate ventilation. The shoulder is abducted to 90 degrees, and the arm is supported by an arm positioner or an arm board (Fig. 40-7). The arm board is placed parallel to the operating table, centered at the shoulder. A sandbag, foam support, or rolled blankets are placed under the upper arm to elevate the shoulder and allow the elbow to rest in 90 degrees of flexion.

Surface landmarks are marked on the skin before creation of portals. Important landmarks to outline include the radial head, olecranon, lateral epicondyle, medial epicondyle, and ulnar nerve (see Fig. 40-5). Before the portals are made, the joint must be distended with 20 to 30 mL of sterile saline. This can be done by placing an 18-gauge spinal needle in either the olecranon fossa or the soft spot bounded by the lateral epicondyle, olecranon, and radial head. Neurovascular structures are displaced away from the joint with distention of the joint, which gives an additional margin of safety.[11,50]

The arthroscope is introduced through the proximal anteromedial portal. This portal is located 2 cm proximal to the medial epicondyle and just anterior to the medial intermuscular septum (Fig. 40-8). The medial intermuscular septum is identified by palpation, and the portal is made anterior to the septum so that the ulnar nerve is not injured. The blunt trocar is introduced into the portal, anterior to the septum, and aimed toward the radial head while maintaining contact with the anterior surface of the humerus. This allows the brachialis muscle to remain anterior and protect the median nerve and brachial artery. The trocar enters the elbow through the tendinous origin of the flexor-pronator group and medial capsule.[1] Once entrance into the joint has been confirmed, the anterolateral portal is established under direct visualization. The proximal anterolateral portal is positioned 2 cm proximal and 1 to 2 cm anterior to the lateral epicondyle (Fig. 40-9), and in some cases may be used as the initial portal in elbow arthroscopy. The blunt trocar is aimed toward the center of the joint while maintaining contact with the anterior humerus,

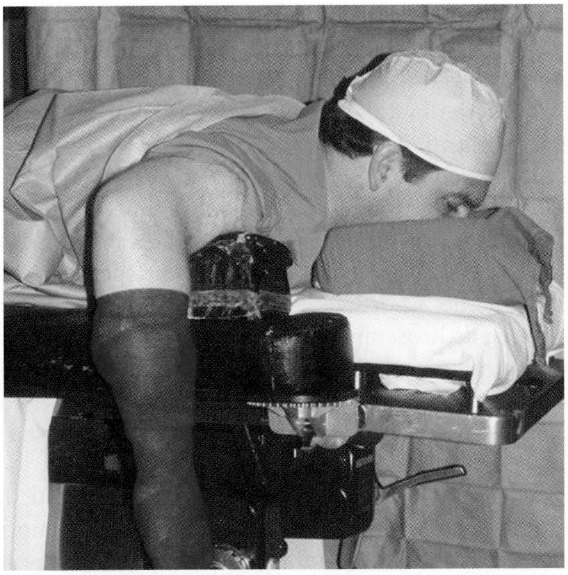

Figure 40-7. Prone position for arthroscopic treatment of the elbow pathology.

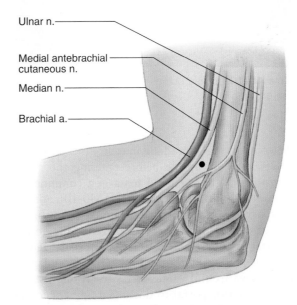

Ulnar n.

Medial antebrachial cutaneous n.

Median n.

Brachial a.

Figure 40-8. Illustration demonstrating anatomic positioning of the proximal anteromedial portal. *a*, artery; *n*, nerve.

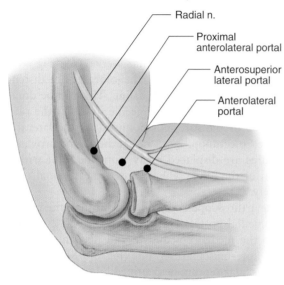

Figure 40-9. Illustration demonstrating anatomic positioning of common lateral arthroscopic portals. *n*, nerve.

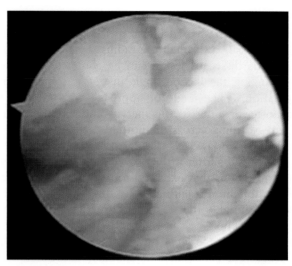

Figure 40-11. Posterolateral gutter of a patient with osteochondritis dissecans demonstrating synovitis and an inflamed posterolateral plica.

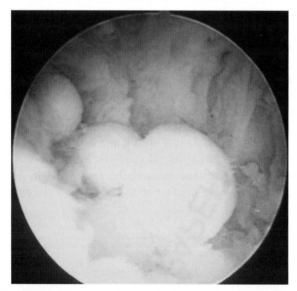

Figure 40-10. Loose bodies in the anterior compartment of the elbow.

and pierces the brachioradialis muscle, brachialis muscle, and lateral joint capsule before entering the anterior compartment. The coronoid fossa is a common place for loose bodies to be localized (Fig. 40-10). Although the osteochondritic lesion may be noted on the anterior aspect of the capitellum, it is most commonly noted on the posterior aspect and can be barely visualized with the scope in the anterior portal. One should always perform a varus and valgus stress test while the scope is in the anterior portal to document any concomitant instability of the elbow. Once a complete diagnostic arthroscopy of the anterior compartment of the elbow has been performed and any associated loose bodies

have been removed, the inflow cannula is left in the proximal anteromedial portal and the scope is transferred to a straight posterior portal. The straight posterior or transtriceps portal is located 3 cm proximal to the tip of the olecranon in the midline posteriorly (see Fig. 40-5).[27,51] This portal allows visualization of the entire posterior compartment as well as the medial and lateral gutters.[1] The blunt trocar is advanced toward the olecranon fossa through the triceps tendon and posterior joint capsule. The medial gutter is evaluated initially along with the olecranon fossa, and any loose bodies noted in either of these are removed. The arthroscope is then continued into the lateral compartment, and a soft-spot portal is established. In most cases of osteochondritis dissecans, a relatively large posterolateral plica will be noted, along with a significant amount of synovitis in the lateral compartment (Fig. 40-11). The soft-spot portal is located in the center of the triangular area bordered by the olecranon, lateral epicondyle, and the radial head. This portal is also known as the *direct lateral* or *midlateral portal* (see Fig. 40-5). The blunt trocar passes through the anconeus muscle and the posterior capsule and into the joint. This inflammatory tissue is excised through a posterior soft-spot portal. At this point the 30-degree arthroscope is removed and a 70-degree arthroscope is substituted through the posterior central portal. Use of the 70-degree arthroscope allows complete evaluation of the osteochondritis dissecans lesion of the capitellum (Fig. 40-12). The shaver is placed through the soft-spot portal, and any loose fragments of the osteochondritic area are debrided. The necrotic bone is then removed and, in an attempt to stimulate blood flow, multiple drill holes are placed into the main body of the capitellum with either a drill or an awl (Fig. 40-13).

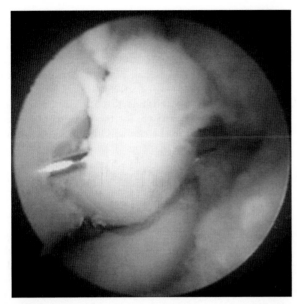

Figure 40-12. Arthroscopic management of a detached osteochondritic lesion of the capitellum as viewed from the anteromedial portal. The loose fragment is temporarily stabilized with a spinal needle before removal with a grasper from the anterolateral portal.

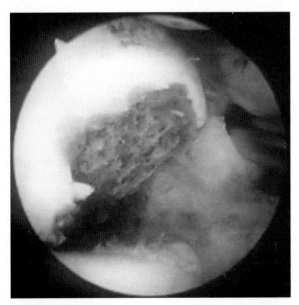

Figure 40-13. The subchondral base after excision of the fragment and debridement with a motorized shaver.

POSTOPERATIVE CONSIDERATIONS

Rehabilitation

Rehabilitation after surgery starts with the patient being placed into a double-hinged elbow brace with initiation of early motion. As the swelling and pain subside, the patient is allowed to resume athletic activities in the brace. The patient is gradually weaned from the brace 8 to 12 weeks postoperatively, as long as he or she remains free of significant pain or any mechanical symptoms.

Complications

Very few complications associated with the treatment of osteochondritis dissecans have been documented. One patient in our series developed severe arthritic changes in the radial head that required an additional surgery. To date, we have had no neurologic complications associated with the treatment of osteochondritis of the capitellum.

REFERENCES

1. Mitsunaga MM, Adishian DA, Bianco AJ Jr. Osteochondritis dissecans of the capitellum. *J Trauma*. 1982;22: 53-55.
2. Bradley J, Petrie R. Osteochondritis dissecans of the humeral capitellum: Diagnosis and treatment. *Clin Sports Med*. 2001;20:565-590.
3. Schenck RC Jr, Goodnight JM. Osteochondritis dissecans. *J Bone Joint Surg Am*. 1996;78:439-456.
4. Konig F. Ueber freie Korper in den Gelenken. *Deutsche Zeitschr Chir*. 1887;27:90-109.
5. Takahara M, Ogino T, Sasaki I, et al. Long term outcome of osteochondritis dissecans of the humeral capitellum. *Clin Orthop Relat Res*. 1999;363:108-115.
6. Bauer M, Jonsson K, Josefsson PO, et al. Osteochondritis dissecans of the elbow: A long-term follow up study. *Clin Orthop Relat Res*. 1992;284:156-160.
7. Pappas AM. Osteochondritis dissecans. *Clin Orthop Relat Res*. 1981;158:59-69.
8. Shaughnessy WJ. Osteochondritis dissecans. In: Morrey BF, ed. *The Elbow and Its Disorders*. 3rd ed. Philadelphia: WB Saunders; 2000, pp 255-260.
9. Peterson RK, Savoie FH III, Field LD. Osteochondritis dissecans of the elbow. *Instr Course Lect*. 1998;48: 393-398.
10. Baumgarten T, Andrews J, Satterwhite Y. The arthroscopic classification and treatment of osteochondritis dissecans of the capitellum. *Am J Sports Med*. 1998;26:520-523.
11. McManama GB Jr, Micheli LJ, Berry MV, et al. The surgical treatment of osteochondritis of the capitellum. *Am J Sports Med*. 1985;13:11-21.
12. Ruch D, Cory J, Poehling G. The arthroscopic management of osteochondritis dissecans of the adolescent elbow. *Arthroscopy*. 1998;14:797-803.
13. Woodward AH, Bianco AJ Jr. Osteochondritis dissecans of the elbow. *Clin Orthop Relat Res*. 1975;110:35-41.
14. Baumgarten TE. Osteochondritis dissecans of the capitellum. *Sports Med Arthrosc*. 1995;3:219-223.
15. Holland P, Davies AM, Cassar-Pullicino VN. Computed tomographic arthrography in the assessment of osteochondritis dissecans of the elbow. *Clin Radiol*. 1994;49: 231-235.
16. Takahara M, Shundo M, Kondo M, et al. Early detection of osteochondritis dissecans of the capitellum in young baseball players: report of three cases. *J Bone Joint Surg Am*. 1998;80:892-897.

17. Fritz RC, Stoller DW. The elbow. In: Stoller DW, ed. *Magnetic Resonance Imaging in Orthopaedics & Sports Medicine.* 2nd ed. Philadelphia: Lippincott-Raven; 1997, pp 743-849.
18. Jackson DW, Silvino N, Reiman P. Osteochondritis in the female gymnast's elbow. *Arthroscopy.* 1989;5:129-136.
19. Singer KM, Roy SP. Osteochondrosis of the humeral capitellum. *Am J Sports Med.* 1984;12:351-360.
20. Chess D. Osteochondritis. In: Savoie FH III, Field LD, eds. *Arthroscopy of the Elbow.* New York: Churchill Livingstone; 1996:77-86.
21. Nagura S. The so-called osteochondritis dissecans of Konig. *Clin Orthop Relat Res.* 1960;18:100-122.
22. Mihara K, Suzuki K, Makiuchi D, et al. Surgical treatment for osteochondritis dissecans of the humeral capitellum. *J Shoulder Elbow Surg.* 2010;19:31-37.
23. Ruchelsman DE, Hall MP, Youm T. Osteochondritis dissecans of the capitellum: Current concepts. *J Am Acad Orthop Surg.* 2010;18:557-567.
24. Takahara M, Mura N, Sasaki J, et al. Classification, treatment, and outcome of osteochondritis dissecans of the humeral capitellum. *J Bone Joint Surg Am.* 2007;89:1205-1214.
25. Yadao MA, Field LD, Savoie FH III. Osteochondritis dissecans of the elbow. *Instr Course Lect.* 2004;53:599-606.
26. Baker CL 3rd, Romeo AA, Baker CL Jr. Osteochondritis dissecans of the capitellum. *Am J Sports Med.* 2010;38(9):1917-1928.
27. Byrd T, Jones K. Arthroscopic surgery for isolated capitellar osteochondritis dissecans in adolescent baseball players: Minimum three-year follow-up. *Am J Sports Med.* 2002;30:474-478.
28. Tivnon MC, Anzel SH, Waugh TR. Surgical management of osteochondritis dissecans of the capitellum. *Am J Sports Med.* 1976;4:121-128.
29. Harada M, Ogino T, Takahara M, et al. Fragment fixation with a bone graft and dynamic staples for osteochondritis dissecans of the humeral capitellum. *J Shoulder Elbow Surg.* 2002;11:368-372.
30. Kuwahata Y, Inoue G. Osteochondritis dissecans of the elbow managed by Herbert screw fixation. *Orthopedics.* 1998;21:449-451.
31. Oka Y, Ikeda M. Treatment of severe osteochondritis dissecans of the elbow using osteochondral grafts from a rib. *J Bone Joint Surg Br.* 2001;83:838-839.
32. Takeda H, Watarai K, Matsushita T, et al. A surgical treatment for unstable osteochondritis dissecans lesions of the humeral capitellum in adolescent baseball players. *Am J Sports Med.* 2002;30:713-717.
33. Iwasaki N, Kato H, Ishikawa J, et al. Autologous osteochondral mosaicplasty for osteochondritis dissecans of the elbow in teenage athletes. *J Bone Joint Surg Am.* 2009;91(10):2359-2366.
34. Iwasaki N, Kato H, Ishikawa J, et al. Autologous osteochondral mosaicplasty for osteochondritis dissecans of the elbow in teenage athlete: Surgical technique. *J Bone Joint Surg Am.* 2010;92 Suppl 1 (Part 2):208-216.
35. Nakagawa Y, Matsusue Y, Ikeda N, et al. Osteochondral grafting and arthroplasty for end-stage osteochondritis dissecans of the capitellum: A case report and review of the literature. *Am J Sports Med.* 2001;29:650-655.
36. Yamamoto Y, Ishibashi Y, Tsuda E, et al. Osteochondral autograft transplantation for osteochondritis dissecans of the elbow in juvenile baseball players: Minimum 2-year follow-up. *Am J Sports Med.* 2006;34(5):714-720.
37. Iwasaki N, Yamane S, Nishida K, et al. Transplantation of tissue-engineered cartilage for the treatment of osteochondritis dissecans in the elbow: Outcomes over a four-year follow-up in two patients. *J Shoulder Elbow Surg.* 2010;19:e1-e6.
38. Kiyoshige Y, Takagi M, Yuasa K, et al. Closed-wedge osteotomy for osteochondritis dissecans of the capitellum: a 7- to 12-year follow-up. *Am J Sports Med.* 2000;28(4):534-537.
39. Van Den Ende KI, McIntosh A, Adams J, et al. Osteochondritis dissecans of the capitellum: A review of the literature and a distal ulnar portal. *Arthroscopy.* 2011;27(1):122-128.
40. Nobuta S, Ogawa K, Sato K, et al. Clinical outcome of fragment fixation for osteochondritis dissecans of the elbow. *Ups J Med Sci.* 2008;113(2):201-208.
41. Takahara M, Mura N, Sasaki J, et al. Classification, treatment, and outcome of osteochondritis dissecans of the humeral capitellum: Surgical technique. *J Bone Joint Surg Am.* 2008;90 Suppl 2 (Part 1):47-62.
42. Ahmad C, El Attrache N. Treatment of capitellar osteochondritis dissecans. *Tech Shoulder Elbow Surg.* 2006;7(4):169-174.
43. Shimada K, Yoshida T, Nakata K, et al. Reconstruction with an osteochondral autograft for advanced osteochondritis dissecans of the elbow. *Clin Orthop Relat Res.* 2005;435:140-147.
44. Savoie FH. Guidelines to becoming an expert elbow arthroscopist. *Arthroscopy.* 2007;23:1237-1240.
45. Bojanic I, Ivkovic A, Boric I. Arthroscopy and microfracture technique in the treatment of osteochondritis dissecans of the humeral capitellum: Report of three adolescent gymnasts. *Knee Surg Sports Traumatol Arthrosc.* 2006;14(5):491-496.
46. Brownlow HC, O'Connor-Read LM, Perko M. Arthroscopic treatment of osteochondritis dissecans of the capitellum. *Knee Surg Sports Traumatol Arthrosc.* 2006;14(2):198-202.
47. Rahusen FT, Brinkman JM, Eygendaal D. Results of arthroscopic débridement for osteochondritis dissecans of the elbow. *Br J Sports Med.* 2006;40(12):966-969.
48. Davis JT, Idjadi JA, Siskosky MJ, et al. Dual direct lateral portals for treatment of osteochondritis dissecans of the capitellum: An anatomic study. *Arthroscopy.* 2007;23:723-728.
49. Aria Y, Hara K, Fujiwara H, et al. A new arthroscopic-assisted drilling method through the radius in a distal-to-proximal direction for osteochondritis dissecans of the elbow. *Arthroscopy.* 2008;24:237e1-237e4.
50. Brown R, Blazina ME, Kerlan RK, et al. Osteochondritis of the capitellum. *J Sports Med.* 1974;2:27-46.
51. Menche DS, Vangsness CT Jr, Pitman M, et al. The treatment of isolated articular cartilage lesions in the young individual. *Instr Course Lect.* 1998;47:505-515.

Chapter 41

Arthroscopy for the Thrower's Elbow

Michael J. O'Brien and Felix H. Savoie III

The throwing motion in overhead athletes, particularly pitchers, places a tremendous amount of force across the medial ulnar collateral ligament (MUCL) on the medial side of the elbow. The anterior band of the MUCL is the primary restraint to valgus stress, especially at 20 to 120 degrees of flexion, where most athletic activity occurs (Fig. 41-1). The stress of the throwing motion can lead to developmental anatomic changes in the young thrower and places the overhead athlete at risk for specific injury patterns. Continued insult can lead to significant ligament and tendon injuries in the experienced athlete, valgus instability and attenuation of the MUCL, and posterior osteophyte formation.

During the pitching cycle the valgus stress applied to the extending elbow causes a wedging effect of the medial olecranon into the olecranon fossa (Fig. 41-2). The valgus stress on the elbow joint created by the humeral torque generated during pitching causes near-failure tensile stresses on the anterior band of the MUCL during the early acceleration phase of the throwing cycle. This repetitive microtrauma can lead to progressive valgus instability, with attenuation of the MUCL and subsequent posteromedial impingement of the elbow joint, and increased compressive forces across the radiocapitellar joint. This results in reactive osteophyte production on the posteromedial aspect of the olecranon (Fig. 41-3). The posteromedial osteophyte abuts the medial aspect of the olecranon fossa, causing pain, loose bodies, and a painful area of chondromalacia. Compressive and rotatory forces are increased across the radiocapitellar articulation, leading to the development of synovitis and osteochondral lesions (osteochondritis dissecans and osteochondral fractures) that can fragment and become loose bodies. This continuum of instability and impingement has been referred to as *valgus extension overload* (VEO).[1,2] It is associated

Ulnar collateral ligaments

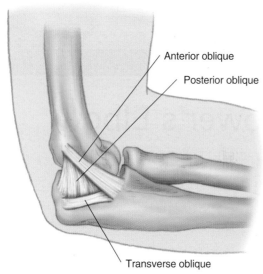

Anterior oblique

Posterior oblique

Transverse oblique

Figure 41-1. The medial ulnar collateral ligament is composed of the anterior band, posterior band, and transverse band.

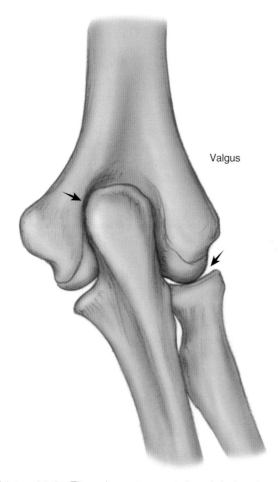

Valgus

Figure 41-2. The valgus stress produced during the throwing motion produces medial compartment distraction, lateral compartment compression, and posterior compartment impingement. *Arrows* indicate areas of impingement.

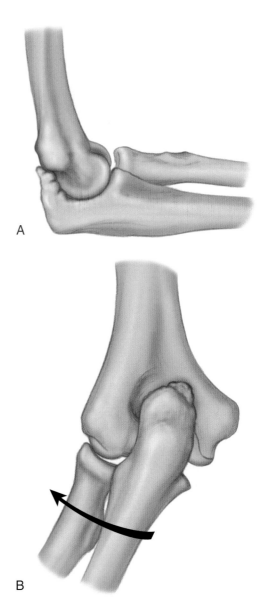

A

B

Figure 41-3. Valgus extension overload osteophyte formation on the posteromedial olecranon, and medial instability with insufficiency of the medial ulnar collateral ligament. *Arrows* show direction of force in valgus extension overload.

with medial compartment distraction, lateral compartment compression, and posterior compartment impingement.

Arthroscopic resection of the posteromedial osteophyte complex and removal of loose bodies can alleviate these painful symptoms experienced by overhead athletes. Kamineni and colleagues[3] found that the function of the anterior band of the MUCL is compromised by resection of the posteromedial olecranon of more than 3 mm. This must be taken into consideration before performance of debridement procedures for posteromedial impingement because excessive resection of bone may further destabilize the elbow and expose a compromised MUCL to further stress and failure.[4]

Identifying and preventing overuse injuries is the key, especially in the young pitcher. Joint injuries in the shoulder and elbow occur when motion segments of the kinetic chain are not properly coordinated during the throwing cycle. This can lead to poor pitching mechanics, overuse injuries, and structural damage. Injury prevention and rehabilitation should center on proper pitching mechanics, core and hip abductor strengthening, scapular control, internal rotation stretching, and joint range of motion.

PREOPERATIVE CONSIDERATIONS

History

When obtaining the history from the athlete, it is always important to elucidate the timing of the injury, chronicity of symptoms, and any previous injuries to the elbow, shoulder, or trunk. For the overhead athlete, it is imperative to also discuss features that relate to training and performance. The treating physician should inquire about any changes in training regimens, pitch counts, and types of pitches thrown; about any recent changes in performance such as changes in throwing velocity, loss of control, or loss of stamina; and whether the pain consistently occurs at a specific phase of the throwing cycle.

Athletes will have a chief complaint of posterior or posteromedial elbow pain in the dominant throwing arm. A loss of full extension may also be reported. Baseball players are by far the most commonly affected; the athlete will most often be a pitcher, although infielders and outfielders can also sustain these injuries. Athletes describe pain between the acceleration phase and the follow-through phase of the pitching motion[2] (Fig. 41-4). Whereas tears to the ulnar collateral ligament (UCL) usually occur suddenly, with a memorable "pop" and immediate searing pain felt during a single pitch, VEO more commonly develops slowly over time. Pitchers gradually become ineffective and may be able

to pitch for two or three innings, followed by a gradual loss of control that becomes evident. An early release because of posteromedial elbow pain will cause the ball to sail high. Chronic impingement and VEO can cause ulnar nerve irritation, loss of elbow extension, and posterior compartment arthritis. Athletes may report symptoms of catching or locking when loose bodies develop.

Physical Examination

A throwing athlete's arm undergoes bony as well as muscular hypertrophy.[5] One area of bony hypertrophy includes the medial aspect of the olecranon. The patient may experience tenderness over the tip of the olecranon or the medial aspect of the olecranon. A flexion contracture may be present. King and colleagues[6] reported that 50% of all pitchers have flexion contractures, and about 30% of these pitchers have cubitus valgus deformities.

Range of motion of the elbow should be tested and compared with the contralateral extremity. Flexion contracture may result from posterior osteophyte impingement or anterior capsular contracture, and crepitus may be associated with loose bodies. The ulnar nerve must be evaluated for anterior subluxation out of the groove.

- Tenderness at the posteromedial tip of the olecranon is pathognomonic.
- VEO test: extending the elbow while applying a valgus stress reproduces the pain.
- Posterior olecranon impingement or extension impingement test: pain elicited with forced terminal extension.
- Valgus stress test: increased medial joint space opening, loss of end point, or pain elicited is significant for UCL insufficiency.
- Milking maneuver and gliding valgus stress test: maneuver eliciting pain, instability, or apprehension signifies insufficiency of UCL.
- Examination of the elbow should also evaluate for other causes of medial-sided elbow pain, such as

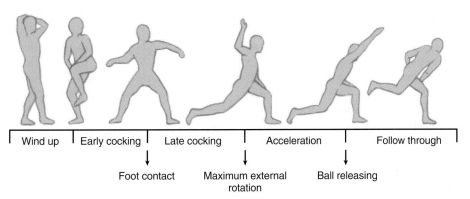

| Wind up | Early cocking | Late cocking | Acceleration | Follow through |

Foot contact   Maximum external rotation   Ball releasing

Figure 41-4. Pain associated with valgus extension overload occurs in the acceleration and follow-through phases of the pitching cycle.

isolated UCL insufficiency, ulnar neuropathy, medial epicondylitis, and flexor-pronator rupture.

Imaging

Routine radiographs should be obtained, including AP, lateral, and oblique images. A posterior osteophyte on the tip of the olecranon can usually be visualized on the lateral radiograph and on the anteroposterior view. Wilson and colleagues[2] described two oblique olecranon axial radiographs with the upper arm flat on the cassette and the elbow flexed 110 degrees. This visualizes the posteromedial aspect of the olecranon on profile, demonstrating posteromedial olecranon osteophytes and traction injuries to the medial epicondyle. Magnetic resonance imaging (MRI) and computed tomography (CT) can be helpful to further define the osteophytosis. MRI can also identify chondral lesions, loose bodies, and injury to the UCL.

Indications

Indications for surgery include continued pain, lack of function, and the inability of overhead throwing athletes to throw at a previous level, despite extensive nonoperative rehabilitation. Imaging studies must reveal osteophytes on the posteromedial aspect of the olecranon.

Contraindications

UCL insufficiency is a contraindication to isolated arthroscopic resection of the posterior osteophytes, as the athlete's problem will not be addressed and ultimately may worsen. Relative contraindications to elbow arthroscopy include severe bony or fibrous ankylosis, ulnar nerve subluxation, or previous surgery that has distorted the native anatomy, such as ulnar nerve transposition.

SURGICAL TECHNIQUE
Anesthesia and Positioning

Elbow arthroscopy is usually performed with the patient under general anesthesia. Performing the procedure with use of regional anesthesia is possible, although it makes postoperative neurologic examination difficult. Patient positioning can be supine with an arm-supporting device or in the prone or lateral decubitus position with the arm hanging over a bolster or arm holder. We prefer the prone position, as this stabilizes the elbow and upper arm and provides improved access to the posterior compartment. A pneumatic tourniquet is routinely applied, and the elbow is flexed over an arm holder. The elbow should be positioned and draped so

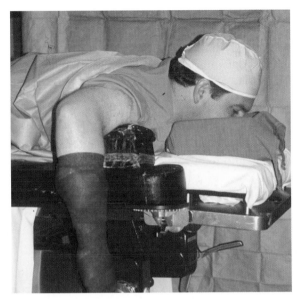

Figure 41-5. The prone position stabilizes the patient's upper arm and offers excellent access to the posterior compartment.

the proximal upper arm rests on the arm holder with the elbow flexed to 90 degrees and the antecubital fossa hanging free (Fig. 41-5).

Surgical Landmarks and Incisions

The olecranon is outlined, as well as the medial epicondyle, lateral epicondyle, and radial head. The ulnar nerve is drawn along its course. All anticipated portals are marked before beginning (Fig. 41-6).

Examination Under Anesthesia

Examination under anesthesia is crucial to evaluate for varus or valgus instability and to assess range of motion. A block to terminal extension may be hard (caused by posterior osteophyte impingement) or soft (caused by anterior capsular contracture). The ulnar nerve must be palpated and confirmed to lie in its groove. It must be confirmed that the ulnar nerve does not subluxate anteriorly with elbow flexion. If subluxation of the nerve occurs, the nerve must be identified and dissected free through an open medial incision before any medial arthroscopic portals are established.

Specific Steps

Specific steps of this procedure are outlined in Box 41-1.

Arthroscopy offers a complete diagnostic view of the entire elbow joint with limited morbidity. Pathology in both the anterior and posterior compartments of the elbow joint can be identified and treated. The standard

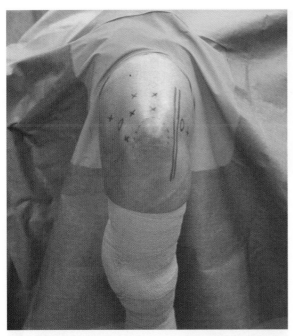

Figure 41-6. The standard portals for arthroscopy of the thrower's elbow include the proximal anteromedial portal, proximal anterolateral portal, direct posterior portal, posterolateral portal, and soft-spot portal.

BOX 41-1 Surgical Steps

1. Insufflate the elbow with 20 to 30 mL of normal saline.

2. Establish a proximal anterior medial portal for the arthroscope.

3. Establish a proximal anterior lateral portal using an outside-in technique with a spinal needle.

4. Perform diagnostic arthroscopy.

5. Address any osteochondral defects.

6. Perform an arthroscopic valgus stress test to evaluate for the presence of MUCL insufficiency.

7. Evaluate the posterior compartment.

8. Evaluate the olecranon for asymmetry.

9. Address any posteromedial spurs.

10. Inspect the humeral chondral surface opposite the spur.

11. Address any cartilage lesions.

12. Repeat assessment of valgus instability with an arthroscopic valgus stress test.

13. Perform MUCL reconstruction if insufficiency of the MUCL is present.

14. Evacuate arthroscopic fluid, close, and apply compressive bandage.

MUCL, Medial ulnar collateral ligament.

---

proximal anteromedial and proximal anterolateral portals are the workhorse portals for the anterior compartment. Direct posterior (transtriceps) and posterolateral portals provide safe access to the posterior compartment of the elbow.

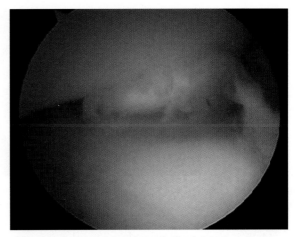

Figure 41-7. View of radiocapitellar joint showing osteochondral lesion on capitellum.

First, the elbow joint is insufflated with 20 to 30 mL of normal saline. This can be injected into the joint either through a direct posterior portal into the olecranon fossa or through the lateral soft-spot portal (between the lateral epicondyle, radial head, and olecranon). We begin by establishing a proximal anterior medial portal for the arthroscope. This portal is placed 2 cm anterior and 2 to 3 cm proximal to the medial epicondyle of the humerus. A 1-cm incision is made just through the skin in this location. A hemostat can be used to spread the subcutaneous fat until the medial intramuscular septum is palpated. A blunt-tipped trocar is then placed through the proximal medial portal, passing anterior to the medial intramuscular septum to avoid iatrogenic injury to the ulnar nerve, and advanced directly on bone along the anterior medial aspect of the distal humerus. The trocar is advanced toward the radiocapitellar joint and can be felt to pop through the anterior medial capsule of the elbow joint. This results in access to the joint. Next, a proximal anterior lateral portal is established through use of an outside-in technique with a spinal needle. This portal is located 1 cm anterior and 2 to 3 cm proximal to the lateral epicondyle of the humerus.

Diagnostic arthroscopy can then be performed in the anterior compartment to evaluate the synovium and articular cartilage. Loose bodies, often located in the coronoid fossa, may be identified and removed. The coronoid is inspected for the presence of a spur, and the anterior trochlea and coronoid fossa are evaluated for cartilage lesions. The anterior radiocapitellar joint can be inspected, and anterior cartilage defects on the radial head or capitellum can be identified (Fig. 41-7). If an osteochondral defect is identified on preoperative imaging studies, it can be addressed at this time through internal fixation, debridement, abrasion chondroplasty, or microfracture.

The arthroscope is then placed in the proximal anterior lateral portal, and an arthroscopic valgus stress test

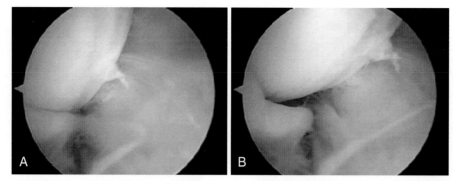

Figure 41-8. The arthroscopic valgus stress test. Gapping of more than 3 mm between the coronoid and medial trochlea signifies insufficiency of the medial ulnar collateral ligament.

(Fig. 41-8) is performed to evaluate for the presence of MUCL insufficiency.[1] While the medial compartment of the elbow is visualized, a valgus stress is applied manually to the elbow. A gap of 3 mm or more between the coronoid process and medial trochlea signifies incompetence of the MUCL.

After completion of evaluation of the anterior compartment, the posterior compartment is evaluated. The proximal anterior lateral portal is retained, and the inflow fluid is attached to this cannula to maintain distention of the joint. In evaluating the posterior compartment, the posterolateral portal is the viewing portal and the direct posterior portal, or transtriceps portal, is the working portal. The posterolateral portal is established for the arthroscope 3 cm proximal to the tip of the olecranon, and just lateral to the triceps tendon. The direct posterior portal can then be established as the working portal by splitting the triceps tendon in its midline 3 cm proximal to the tip of the olecranon.

Diagnostic arthroscopy of the posterior compartment allows inspection of the osteophyte complex on the posteromedial aspect of the olecranon, as well as the chondromalacia on the medial aspect of the olecranon fossa. Loose bodies can be identified and removed with a small grasper. The lateral gutter should always be evaluated, and the posterior radiocapitellar joint can be inspected for cartilage lesions. Loose bodies often reside in the lateral gutter, and a plica in the posterolateral aspect of the radiocapitellar joint may also be identified (Fig. 41-9); both can be resected through the lateral soft-spot portal. Excess soft tissue, including synovial reflections, can be removed from the tip of the olecranon and olecranon fossa.

The medial, lateral, and central olecranon are compared for asymmetry. A fragmented spur on the posteromedial olecranon is commonly encountered (Fig. 41-10). A probe or motorized shaver in the direct posterior portal can be used to measure the dimensions and extent of the spur. A ¼-inch osteotome, or a motorized bur with a gentle medial-to-lateral movement, can be used to remove the osteophytes from the posteromedial aspect of the olecranon.[7] As an added safety factor, a

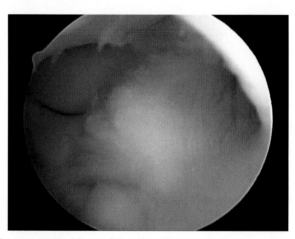

Figure 41-9. View of the lateral gutter from the posterolateral portal showing a plica posterior to the radiocapitellar joint.

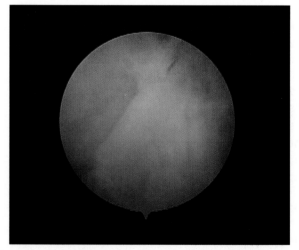

Figure 41-10. View of the posterior compartment showing an osteophyte complex on the posteromedial aspect of the olecranon.

retractor (often just a switching stick or freer) may be placed through an accessory portal 1 cm proximal to the standard posterior central portal and into the medial gutter. The use of this retractor holds the medial capsule and the overlying ulnar nerve away from the shaver or osteotome during posteromedial spur resection. Intra-operative fluoroscopy may be performed or a postero-anterior and lateral radiograph may be taken to ensure that all bony debris has been resected from the posterior compartment of the elbow. Once the osteophyte has been removed, the humeral chondral surface opposite the spur can be inspected more completely. If a cartilage lesion is present, it can be managed at this time at the surgeon's discretion. Loose chondral flaps should be debrided, and if necessary, microfracture can be performed.

Great care should be taken to avoid iatrogenic injury to the ulnar nerve. The ulnar nerve lies just superficial to the capsule in the posteromedial gutter. If a retractor is not used while working medially, limited suction should be employed, and a hooded bur can help protect the ulnar nerve from the bur. Care should also be taken to remove only the osteophyte and to leave the native olecranon bone. Kamineni and colleagues recommend limiting resection to the osteophyte alone and preserving as much normal olecranon bone as possible, to limit the potential for instability in the throwing athlete.[3,8] Resection of more than 3 mm of the normal posteromedial olecranon may place excess stress on an already compromised anterior band of the UCL.[3]

After resection of the posteromedial osteophyte, the arthroscope should be placed back into the proximal anterior lateral portal, and repeat assessment of valgus instability with an *arthroscopic valgus stress test* can again be performed. If removal of the posteromedialosteophyte causes an increase in the diastasis of the medial ulnohumeral joint, insufficiency of the MUCL is present, and MUCL reconstruction should be performed.

At the completion of the procedure, all arthroscopic fluid is evacuated from the joint through the anterior portal. Each portal is closed with a simple nylon suture, and a compressive dressing is applied to the elbow for the first 48 hours.

POSTOPERATIVE CONSIDERATIONS

Rehabilitation

Postoperative rehabilitation is started early and progressed rapidly for VEO and isolated spur resection. We often splint the elbow in full extension for 1 to 2 days before beginning rehabilitation. A sling is discouraged, as its use may cause a loss of extension. A cryocompression sleeve can be very helpful to help manage postoperative pain and swelling. Physical therapy and home exercises are begun early, usually on postoperative day 2 to 7, with the fundamental goal of restoration of full range of motion and joint flexibility. Establishment of full terminal extension is a primary goal of the early

phase of rehab, as a flexion contracture can develop and be devastating to the overhead athlete. Forearm terminal stretching of the flexor and extensor musculature is performed with the elbow in full extension and stretching the wrist in flexion and extension. An isotonic regimen of light weights and high repetitions is initiated. Wrist curls are initiated with a 1-pound weight and elbow curls with a 5-pound weight, and a rope curl-up bar can be used for the forearm flexors and extensors. Flexor-pronator mass strengthening can improve dynamic valgus stability. Therapeutic putty should be used throughout the day. Moist heat, ultrasound, iontophoresis, and deep tissue massage may be beneficial.

At approximately 4 to 6 weeks an interval throwing program can be initiated. This begins with a gentle long toss and progresses every week in length and velocity of throws. It is important that the patient be completely pain free at each level before progression (Fig. 41-11). Throwing time should be limited by the athlete's symptoms and should not exceed 30 to 45 minutes per day. Once throwing from the mound has been resumed, the athlete can increase throwing speed over several weeks until at full strength.

Complications

Complications after arthroscopic osteophyte resection for VEO are rare. Iatrogenic ulnar nerve injury can occur; therefore great care must be taken in working along the posteromedial gutter. Over-resection of the posteromedial olecranon can lead to further valgus instability and MUCL insufficiency. Checking for valgus instability arthroscopically after the resection is key.

RESULTS

Arthroscopy for the treatment of intra-articular pathology in the overhead athlete has become a safe and reliable technique (Table 41-1). Andrews and Carson[9] reported in 1985 on a preliminary study of 12 patients treated with elbow arthroscopy. These researchers noted an improvement from 50% preoperatively to 83% postoperatively in four objective criteria, and an improvement from 17% preoperatively to 58% postoperatively in four subjective criteria. Removal of loose bodies produced the best results.

Andrews and Timmerman[10] reviewed their results of arthroscopic and open elbow surgery in 72 professional baseball players. The most common diagnoses were posteromedial olecranon osteophytes (65%), intra-articular loose bodies (39%), UCL injury (25%), and ulnar neuritis (15%). The patients with posteromedial olecranon osteophytes had the highest rate of reoperation, and those who underwent MUCL reconstruction had a higher rate of return to play. The authors caution the treating clinician that procedures aimed at treating

RE-ENTRY THROWING PROGRAM
Phase I: Long Toss

- All baseball players must begin re-entry with long toss
- All throwing must be pain free
- Emphasize a "crow-hop" throw with follow-through
- Emphasize a high arc on the ball; no hard, ground-level throwing
- Always warm up first: jog, stretch, light toss (30-60 feet)
- Soreness is expected; rest and use ice or heat between throwing days
- Continue a maintenance strengthening program; perform after throwing
- Once able to complete 75 throws at 180 feet, begin gradual return to position

Step	Distance	Routine	Step	Distance	Routine
1	45 feet	Warm-up throws 25 throws Rest 15 minutes Warm-up throws 25 throws	7	120 feet	Warm-up throws 25 throws Rest 15 minutes Warm-up throws 25 throws
2	45 feet	Warm-up throws 25 throws Rest 10 minutes Warm-up throws 25 throws Rest 10 minutes 25 throws	8	120 feet	Warm-up throws 25 throws Rest 10 minutes Warm-up throws 25 throws Rest 10 minutes 25 throws
3	60 feet	Warm-up throws 25 throws Rest 15 minutes Warm-up throws 25 throws	9	150 feet	Warm-up throws 25 throws Rest 15 minutes Warm-up throws 25 throws
4	60 feet	Warm-up throws 25 throws Rest 10 minutes Warm-up throws 25 throws Rest 10 minutes 25 throws	10	150 feet	Warm-up throws 25 throws Rest 10 minutes Warm-up throws 25 throws Rest 10 minutes 25 throws
5	90 feet	Warm-up throws 25 throws Rest 15 minutes Warm-up throws 25 throws	11	180 feet	Warm-up throws 25 throws Rest 15 minutes Warm-up throws 25 throws
6	90 feet	Warm-up throws 25 throws Rest 10 minutes Warm-up throws 25 throws Rest 10 minutes 25 throws	12	180 feet	Warm-up throws 25 throws Rest 10 minutes Warm-up throws 25 throws Rest 10 minutes 25 throws

PITCHERS: progress to re-entry program from mound
POSITIONAL PLAYERS: progress to re-entry program from position
BATTING: with physician approval, progress to re-entry program for hitters

Phase II: Re-Entry for Pitchers

- Pitchers must be able to throw 75 times at 180 feet pain free
- All pitchers must follow this progression from the mound under supervision
- All throwing must be pain free
- Emphasize proper body mechanics and follow-through
- Throw from the mound under the supervision of a coach
  Always warm up first: jog, stretch, light toss (30-60 feet)
- Soreness is expected; rest and use ice or heat between throwing days
- Continue a maintenance strengthening program; perform after throwing

Step	Routine	Step	Routine
1	Long toss (90-120' × 50 throws) 15 fastballs at 50%	8	60 fastballs at 75%
2	Long toss (90-120' × 50 throws) 30 fastballs at 50%	9	45 fastballs at 75% 15 fastballs at BP
3	Long toss (90-120' × 25 throws) 45 fastballs at 50%	10	45 fastballs at 75% 30 fastballs at BP
4	Long toss (90-120' × 25 throws) 60 fastballs at 50%	11	30 fastballs at 75% 15 curveballs at 50% 45-60 fastballs at BP
5	Long toss (120-150' × 25 throws) 30 fastballs at 75%	12	30 fastballs at 75% 30 curveballs at 75% 30 fastballs at BP
6	30 fastballs at 75% 45 fastballs at 50%	13	30 fastballs at 75% 60-90 pitches in BP (25% curve)
7	45 fastballs at 75% 15 fastballs at 50%	14	Simulated game; progress by 15 throws per workout

Simulated Game Progression
1. 15 minute warm-up consisting of 50-80 pitches with gradually increasing velocity
2. 5-8 innings
3. 12-18 pitches per inning, including 6-10 fastballs
4. 9 minutes rest between innings

Phase II: Re-Entry for Infielders

- Infielders must be able to throw 75 times at 180 feet pain free before entering this phase
- All infield players (except catchers) must follow this progression
- All throwing must be pain free
- Emphasize proper body mechanics and follow-through
- Always warm up first: jog, stretch, light toss (30-60 feet)
- Soreness is expected; rest and use ice or heat between throwing days
- Continue a maintenance strengthening program; perform after throwing

Step	Routine
1	Warm up to 150 feet 20 throws from position Rest 10 minutes 20 throws from position 20 long tosses at 150 feet
2	Warm up to 150 feet 20 throws from position (10 backhand, 10 glove-side) Rest 10 minutes 20 throws from position (as above) 20 long tosses at 150 feet
3	Warm up to 150 feet 20 throws with feet planted (backhand side) Rest 5 minutes 20 throws with feet planted (backhand side) 20 long tosses at 150 feet
4	Warm up to 150 feet Fielding and batting practice 20 long tosses at 180 feet
5	Simulated game

Figure 41-11. An example of an interval throwing program—the Tulane Institute of Sports Medicine Re-entry Throwing Program.

Phase II: Re-Entry for Catchers

- Catchers must be able to throw 75 times at 180 feet pain free before entering this phase
- All throwing must be pain free
- Emphasize proper body mechanics and follow-through
- Always warm up first: jog, stretch, light toss (30-60 feet)
- Soreness is expected; rest and use ice or heat between throwing days
- Continue a maintenance strengthening program; perform after throwing

Step	Routine
1	Warm up to 150 feet 20 throws from 60 feet 20 throws from 90 feet 20 throws from 120 feet Rest 10 minutes 20 throws from squat at 60 feet 10 throws from squat at 90 feet 10 throws from squat at 120 feet 10 long tosses at 120 feet
2	Warm up to 150 feet 20 throws to mound from squat after pitch 10 throws to each base from squat after pitch Rest 10 minutes 30 throws to mound from squat after pitch 10 throws to each base from squat after pitch 20 long tosses at 150 feet
2	Warm up to 150 feet 20 throws to mound from squat after pitch 10 throws to each base from squat after pitch Rest 5 minutes 10 throws to each base after bunt 30 throws to mound standing 20 long tosses at 150 feet
4	Simulated game

LITTLE LEAGUE
RE-ENTRY THROWING PROGRAM
Phase I: Long Toss

- All baseball players must begin re-entry with long toss
- All throwing must be pain free
- Emphasize a "crow-hop" throw with follow-through
- Emphasize a high arc on the ball; no hard, ground-level throwing
- Always warm up first: jog, stretch, light toss (15-30 feet)
- Soreness is expected; rest and use ice or heat between throwing days
- Continue a maintenance strengthening program; perform after throwing
- Once able to complete 75 throws at 90 feet, begin gradual return to position

Step	Distance	Routine	Step	Distance	Routine
1	30 feet	Warm-up throws 25 throws Rest 15 minutes Warm-up throws 25 throws	5	60 feet	Warm-up throws 25 throws Rest 15 minutes Warm-up throws 25 throws
2	30 feet	Warm-up throws 25 throws Rest 10 minutes Warm-up throws 25 throws Rest 10 minutes 25 throws	6	60 feet	Warm-up throws 25 throws Rest 10 minutes Warm-up throws 25 throws Rest 10 minutes 25 throws
3	45 feet	Warm-up throws 25 throws Rest 15 minutes Warm-up throws 25 throws	7	90 feet	Warm-up throws 25 throws Rest 15 minutes Warm-up throws 25 throws
4	45 feet	Warm-up throws 25 throws Rest 10 minutes Warm-up throws 25 throws Rest 10 minutes 25 throws	8	90 feet	Warm-up throws 25 throws Rest 10 minutes Warm-up throws 25 throws Rest 10 minutes 25 throws

Phase II: Re-Entry for Outfielders

- Outfielders must be able to throw 75 times at 180 feet pain free before this phase
- All throwing must be pain free
- Emphasize proper body mechanics and follow-through
- Always warm up first: jog, stretch, light toss (60-90 feet)
- Soreness is expected; rest and use ice or heat between throwing days
- Continue a maintenance strengthening program; perform after throwing

Step	Routine
1	Warm up to 180 feet 15 throws from 120 feet Rest 10 minutes 20 throws from 120 feet 20 long tosses from 180 feet
2	Warm up to 200 feet 15 throws from 150 feet Rest 10 minutes 20 throws from 150 feet 20 long tosses from 200 feet
3	Warm up to 225 feet 15 throws from 180 feet Rest 10 minutes 20 throws from 180 feet 20 long tosses from 225 feet
4	Warm up to 250 feet 15 throws from 200 feet Rest 10 minutes 20 throws from 200 feet 20 long tosses from 250 feet
5	Warm up to 250 feet 5 throws to each cutoff (2nd, 3rd, home) Rest 5 minutes 6 throws to each cutoff 20 long tosses from 250 feet
6	Warm up to 250 feet 5 throws to each cutoff 5 throws to each base (2nd, 3rd, home) Rest 5 minutes 2 throws to each cutoff 3 throws to each base 20 long tosses from 250 feet
7	Warm up to 250 feet 5 throws to each cutoff 5 throws to each base Rest 5 minutes 5 throws to each cutoff 5 throws to each base 20 long tosses from 250 feet
8	Warm up to 250 feet Fielding practice (grounders, fly balls) 5 throws to each cutoff 5 throws to each base 20 long tosses from 250 feet
9	Simulated game

Figure 41-11, cont'd.

TABLE 41-1. Results of Arthroscopy for the Treatment of Intra-articular Pathology in the Overhead Athlete

Study	No. of Patients	Outcome
Andrews and Carson[9] (1985)	12	Improvement from 50% preoperatively to 83% postoperatively in four objective criteria Improvement from 17% preoperatively to 58% postoperatively in four subjective criteria
Andrews and Timmerman[10] (1995)	72	Patients with posteromedial olecranon osteophytes had the highest rate of reoperation Those who underwent MUCL reconstruction had a higher rate of return to play
Reddy et al[11] (2000)	187	Average Figgie score improved from 27.7 to 45.4 points, with the largest increase occurring in the pain score 51% achieved an excellent result, 36% a good result, 11% a fair result, and 4% a poor result Of baseball players, 47 (85%) of 55 were able to return to the same level of competition
Wilson et al[2] (1983)	5	Reoperation was required in one patient with severe chondromalacia of the olecranon articular surface
Bartz et al[12] (2001)	24	In 19 of 24, complete relief was obtained and patients were able to equal or exceed their preoperative throwing velocity 2 of 24 required reoperation for MUCL reconstruction
Fideler et al[13] (1997)	113	Excellent results in 113 professional baseball players treated arthroscopically for posterior impingement and loose bodies 74% returned to their preoperative level of sports
Bradley[14] (1995)	6	Good to excellent results were achieved in 6 patients

MUCL, Medial ulnar collateral ligament.

the secondary effects of MUCL insufficiency (such as posteromedial impingement) without addressing the underlying MUCL often produced an unsatisfactory outcome.

Reddy and colleagues[11] reviewed 187 elbow arthroscopies performed over a 7-year period. The most common diagnoses were posterior impingement (51%), loose bodies (31%), and degenerative joint disease (22%). The average Figgie score improved from 27.7 points to 45.4 points, with the largest increase occurring in the pain score. Fifty-one percent of patients achieved an excellent result, 36% a good result, 11% a fair result, and 4% a poor result. Of 55 baseball players, 47 (85%) were able to return to the same level of competition.

There are few published studies on the treatment of VEO in the throwing athlete. Wilson and colleagues[2] reported on five patients treated with open biplanar spur excision. Reoperation was required in one patient with severe chondromalacia of the olecranon articular surface. Bartz and colleagues[12] reported on 24 baseball pitchers treated with a mini-open technique. Of the 24 pitchers, 19 obtained complete relief and were able to equal or exceed their preoperative throwing velocity. Two patients required reoperation for MUCL reconstruction. In 1997, Fideler and colleagues[13] showed excellent results in 113 professional baseball players treated arthroscopically for posterior impingement and loose bodies; 74% returned to their preoperative level of sports. Bradley[14] showed that after 2 years,

six National Football League (NFL) linemen with posterior impingement treated arthroscopically had either an excellent or a good result.

REFERENCES

1. Miller CD, Savoie FH III. Valgus extension injuries of the elbow in the throwing athlete. *J Am Acad Orthop Surg.* 1994;2:261-269.
2. Wilson FD, Andrews JR, Blackburn TA, et al. Valgus extension overload in the pitching elbow. *Am J Sports Med.* 1983;11(2):83-88.
3. Kamineni S, ElAttrache NS, O'Driscoll SW, et al. Medial collateral ligament strain with partial posteromedial olecranon resection: A biomechanical study. *J Bone Joint Surg Am.* 2004;86:2424-2430.
4. Ahmad CS, Park MC, ElAttrache NS. Elbow medial ulnar collateral ligament insufficiency alters posteromedial olecranon contact. *Am J Sports Med.* 2004;32:1607-1612.
5. Jones HH, Priest JD, Hayes WC, et al. Humeral hypertrophy in response to exercise. *J Bone Joint Surg Am.* 1977;59:204-208.
6. King JW, Brelsford HJ, Tullos HS. Analysis of the pitching arm of the professional baseball pitcher. *Clin Orthop Relat Res.* 1969;67:116-123.
7. O'Holleran JD, Altchek DW. The thrower's elbow: arthroscopic treatment of valgus extension overload syndrome. *HSS J.* 2006;2(1):83-93.
8. Kamineni S, Hirohara H, Pomianowski S, et al. Partial posteromedial olecranon resection: a kinematic study. *J Bone Joint Surg Am.* 2003;85:1005-1011.

9. Andrews JR, Carson WG. Arthroscopy of the elbow. *Arthroscopy*. 1985;1(2):97-107.

10. Andrews JR, Timmerman LA. Outcome of elbow surgery in professional baseball players. *Am J Sports Med*. 1995; 23(4):407-413.

11. Reddy AS, Kvitne RS, Yocum LA, et al. Arthroscopy of the elbow: a long-term clinical review. *Arthroscopy*. 2000; 16(6):588-594.

12. Bartz RL, Lowe WR, Bryan WJ. Posterior elbow impingement. *Oper Tech Sports Med*. 2001;9:245-252.

13. Fideler BM, Kvitne RS, Jordan S. Posterior impingement of the elbow in professional baseball players. *J Shoulder Elbow Surg*. 1997;6:169-170.

14. Bradley JP. Arthroscopic treatment of posterior impingement of the elbow in NFL linemen. *J Shoulder Elbow Surg*. 1995;2:119-120.

Chapter 42

Arthroscopic Management of Elbow Stiffness

Debdut Biswas, Robert W. Wysocki, and Mark S. Cohen

Chapter Synopsis

- Contracture of the elbow is a common postinjury sequela of elbow trauma. Initial treatments are typically nonoperative and include static bracing and structured rehabilitation. For patients who experience suboptimal motion that severely limits their activities of daily living, surgical intervention is typically indicated. Arthroscopic techniques have recently emerged as an operative alternative to traditional open contracture release.

Important Points

- Arthroscopic release of a posttraumatic elbow is a technically demanding procedure that requires intimate knowledge of intracapsular elbow anatomy as well as skills in elbow arthroscopy.
- A thorough evaluation of the entire extremity should be performed preoperatively, including meticulous neurovascular evaluation of the ulnar nerve.
- A congruent ulnohumeral joint is necessary before pursuit of arthroscopic release; accordingly, severe contractures may be more reliably treated with an open surgical technique.
- Compliance with postoperative rehabilitation protocols is essential in ensuring recovery of elbow motion after surgical contracture release.

Clinical and Surgical Pearls

- The liberal use of retractors is highly recommended, especially after capsulectomy when fluid distention is difficult.
- The anterior release consists of debridement of the radial and coronoid fossae to remove impingement during elbow flexion.

- Anterior capsulectomy is technically easier from a medial-to-lateral direction and is performed more safely proximal to the trochlea to avoid injury to the radial nerve.
- Posterior release consists of debridement of the olecranon fossa as well as removal of osteophytes from the tip of the olecranon to allow for unimpeded elbow extension.
- We recommend ulnar nerve decompression in patients who demonstrate provocative ulnar neuropathic symptoms and in patients who experience a significant loss of flexion preoperatively.

Clinical and Surgical Pitfalls

- If visualization is compromised or if concern exists intraoperatively regarding the ability to safely perform an adequate release arthroscopically, the surgeon should be prepared to convert the procedure to an open approach.
- Anterior capsulectomy should be performed with extreme diligence, as the radial nerve lies directly anterior to the radiocapitellar joint; capsulectomy is most safely initiated proximal to the trochlea.
- Posteromedial capsulectomy places the ulnar nerve at risk of injury; we recommend identifying and decompressing the ulnar nerve through a limited open approach before proceeding with posteromedial capsulectomy.
- Risk to the ulnar nerve can be minimized by avoiding the use of suction or a bur in proximity to the nerve.

Loss of mobility represents the most common complication of elbow trauma. The predisposition of the elbow to develop posttraumatic contracture has been attributed to several factors, including the intrinsic congruity of the ulnohumeral articulation, the presence of three articulations within a synovium-lined cavity, and the intimate relationship of the capsule to the intracapsular ligaments and extracapsular muscles.[1-3]

Several authors have evaluated the elbow motion necessary to complete daily activities; these studies have reported that a majority of activities could be reasonably performed within a functional arc of 100 degrees (30 to 130 degrees) of flexion and extension of the elbow and 100 degrees of rotation of the forearm (50 degrees each for pronation and supination).[4] The inability of the elbow to achieve this motion after the occurrence of trauma may result in substantial impairment of upper extremity function, especially with the loss of elbow flexion and forearm supination, which are difficult to accommodate for.

Nonoperative management remains the initial modality of treatment and typically includes static splinting as well as structured rehabilitation and physical therapy dedicated toward regaining functional range of motion. These modalities are particularly useful for the first 6 to 12 months postinjury but become less successful in cases of more remote trauma. For patients whose elbow contracture is refractory to conservative measures, surgical debridement and release of the elbow are offered in an effort to restore functional motion of the joint. Although open approaches have been classically described for the surgical treatment of the posttraumatic elbow contracture, arthroscopic techniques have recently emerged as a less invasive alternative for the treatment of elbow stiffness and demonstrate similar efficacy within the literature.

PREOPERATIVE CONSIDERATIONS

History

It is imperative for the practitioner to determine the extent to which the loss of elbow motion compromises a patient's functional capabilities. The magnitude of functional impairment, rather than absolute loss of motion, ultimately directs management decisions when treating the patient with posttraumatic contracture of the elbow.

The details surrounding the initial injury as well as mechanism of trauma are important aspects of the history. Many of these patients will have undergone previous surgical treatment, and it is critical to obtain and review previous operative documentation, especially when arthroscopic treatment is being considered.

Complications related to initial treatments, including infection, neurologic deficits, or other ipsilateral limb injuries, all potentially influence future management. In addition, details regarding the patient's progress or, more important, lack of progress with structured rehabilitation should be elicited during the history taking.

Physical Examination

Physical examination begins with inspection of the entire upper extremity, specifically evaluating for deformity, swelling, and muscle atrophy while noting the location of any previous surgical incisions that would influence further surgical planning. Range-of-motion evaluation should include the hand, wrist, forearm, and elbow and should be compared with the contralateral, unaffected extremity. In the posttraumatic setting, loss of extension is more common than loss of flexion.

A careful neurovascular examination is essential, especially during the evaluation of ulnar nerve function. Residing in the cubital tunnel and adjacent to the medial joint capsule, the ulnar nerve may become entrapped in scar tissue along the medial elbow after trauma, which may result in posttraumatic ulnar neuropathy. Traction ulnar neuritis of the elbow may manifest as medial elbow pain, and patients may report sensory changes in an ulnar nerve distribution, particularly with elbow flexion. Patients with posttraumatic ulnar neuropathy may simply have loss of flexion and medial elbow pain in the absence of overt symptoms of ulnar neuropathy; thus a meticulous neurovascular evaluation, including assessment of two-point discrimination, pinch strength, and intrinsic muscle function, are essential to document the preoperative function of the ulnar nerve. Elbow stability must also be assessed, in particular to rule out subtle posterolateral rotatory instability as a cause of the patient's complaints of stiffness.

Imaging

Standard plain radiographs of the elbow are typically obtained and include anteroposterior, lateral, and oblique projections. Stress radiographs should be considered if elbow instability is suspected. Computed tomography (CT) is frequently performed, especially when the presence of heterotopic ossification (HO) or intra-articular loose bodies is suspected or if bony deformity or malunion is suspected in the setting of previous fracture. Three-dimensional CT reconstruction is typically helpful in further delineating bony and articular anatomy. Advanced imaging is important in documenting ulnohumeral joint congruency as well as any osseous impingement secondary to overgrowth in the olecranon or coronoid fossae that would directly limit motion. We have found magnetic resonance imaging (MRI) to have a limited role.

Indications and Contraindications

Nonoperative management is routinely initiated after the initial evaluation of the patient with a posttraumatic elbow contracture and typically includes a course of structured rehabilitation and the use of preadjusted static braces for passive progressive stretch of the soft tissues. Supervised therapy helps ensure compliance and can also be used to document progress with therapy.

Surgical management is indicated for patients who continue to experience significant loss of mobility with resultant impairment of upper extremity function and limitation with daily activities. Although a flexion contracture of at least 25 to 30 degrees and/or less than 110 to 115 degrees of active flexion was historically reported as an indication for surgical contracture release, surgical management may still be offered to certain patients who may require full or nearly full motion for specific lifestyle and employment demands. Patients typically must be at least 3 to 4 months removed from injury to allow them to achieve "tissue equilibrium," with maximal resolution of posttraumatic swelling and inflammation. Most important, patients must be willing to comply with the required extensive program of postoperative therapy, as operative outcomes depend on diligent participation in a structured rehabilitation program. This is especially true for adolescents, who may not be dedicated to improving their elbow motion.

Relative contraindications to arthroscopic elbow release include severe elbow contractures with minimal joint motion, prior ulnar nerve transposition surgery, and the presence of significant heterotopic bone; these patients are more reliably treated with extensive open debridement of the elbow to restore motion and protect the ulnar nerve. If there has been previous medial elbow surgery or ulnar nerve transposition and one is considering arthroscopic release, the ulnar nerve should be isolated and protected through a medial exposure before arthroscopy. If the ulnohumeral joint shows marked degenerative changes, a simple release of the joint may not lead to improved motion and may exacerbate pain in an arthritic joint. If advanced posttraumatic arthritis is observed in the ulnohumeral articulation, salvage-type procedures are often required if surgery is undertaken.[5]

Subtle elbow instability commonly manifests as loss of motion after elbow fracture or dislocation; accordingly, special attention should be devoted toward evaluating elbow stability either with stability testing on physical examination or with stress radiographs. If instability is present, then treatment typically would include ligament reconstruction with or without capsular release. The stiff and unstable elbow is a particularly challenging condition to treat. The priority is to achieve stability and to later restore motion, typically in a staged procedure.

SURGICAL TECHNIQUE

Arthroscopic release of a posttraumatic elbow is a technically demanding procedure that requires intimate knowledge of intracapsular elbow anatomy as well as advanced skills in elbow arthroscopy. Multiple portals are required, and diligent fluid management is essential, especially after capsulectomy when joint distention is more difficult. The use of joint retractors is typically required to achieve adequate visualization and facilitate appropriate surgical debridement.[6-10]

From a purely mechanical standpoint, to improve elbow extension, posterior impingement must be removed between the olecranon tip and the olecranon fossa. Anteriorly, tethering soft tissues such as the anterior joint capsule and any adhesions between the brachialis and the humerus must be released. Similarly, to improve elbow flexion, the surgeon must release any soft tissue structures posteriorly that may be tethering the joint. They include the posterior joint capsule and the triceps muscle, which can become adherent to the humerus. The surgeon must remove any bony or soft tissue impingement anteriorly, including any soft tissue overgrowth in the coronoid and radial fossae. There must be a concavity above the humeral trochlea and capitellum to accept the coronoid centrally and the radial head laterally for full flexion to occur (Fig. 42-1).

Anesthesia and Positioning

We typically favor a regional block, although general anesthesia may also be considered. We then position the patient in the lateral decubitus or prone position with the affected extremity facing up and all bony prominences well padded. A rolled blanket or elbow stirrup attachment for the operative table is positioned underneath the arm, allowing the elbow to move from 90 degrees of flexion to full extension. The video monitor, shaver system, camera control unit, and light source are positioned such that the surgeon has a clear view of the monitor. After the extremity has been sterilely prepared and draped up to the axilla, the hand and forearm are wrapped with an elastic bandage to limit fluid extravasation and a sterile pneumatic tourniquet is placed as proximally as possible around the arm (Fig. 42-2).

The major external landmarks and portal sites are then marked, including the olecranon and medial and lateral epicondyles, and the postulated path of the ulnar nerve is marked along the medial aspect of the elbow as a reminder of its position throughout the procedure (Fig. 42-2B). The extremity is exsanguinated with a compressive elastic bandage, and the tourniquet is inflated.

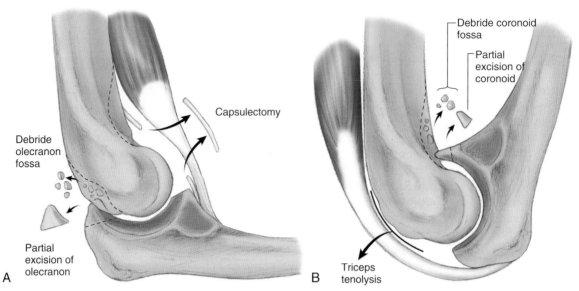

Figure 42-1. A, Improving elbow extension requires removal of posterior bony impingement and release of the anterior joint capsule. **B,** Improvement of flexion requires posterior soft tissue release and removal of any soft tissue or bony impingement anteriorly.

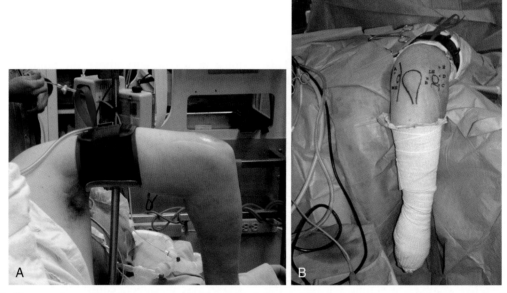

Figure 42-2. The arm is positioned over a padded lateral bolster, and the forearm is wrapped with an elastic bandage to limit fluid extravasation. Anatomic landmarks are marked: lateral epicondyle, medial epicondyle, proximal anteromedial portal, soft-spot portal, standard anterolateral portal, modified anterolateral portal, and proximal anterolateral portal. The expected path of the ulnar nerve is also depicted.

Surgical Landmarks, Incisions, and Portals

The elbow joint is insufflated with 30 mL of normal sterile saline solution through the soft spot outlined by the lateral epicondyle, radial head, and olecranon to facilitate entry into the intra-articular space with the arthroscope (Fig. 42-3).

Anteromedial Portal

The proximal anteromedial portal is created through a small stab incision, only through skin, 2 cm proximal and 2 cm anterior to the medial epicondyle, which on palpation should place this incision well anterior to the palpable medial intermuscular septum. Subcutaneous tissue is spread with a hemostat clamp (Fig. 42-4A), with great care taken to slide along the anterior humerus. The surgeon should have a sense of the trocar flipping back and forth from posterior to anterior along the septum, ensuring that the trajectory is anterior to the septum to protect the ulnar nerve. It should be noted that entry into the joint may be difficult, particularly in cases involving posttraumatic stiffness with a contracted capsule. Care must be taken to hug the anterior humeral cortex because the capsule can be quite adherent, pushing the instrument into an extra-articular plane. Beneath the capsule and in the joint, the trocar or switching stick can be used to lever anteriorly to help strip the brachialis from the capsule and develop a space in which to work.

The anterior joint compartment is then penetrated with a blunt trocar and cannula (Fig. 42-4B), with the tip of the trocar directed laterally toward the radial head. The trocar is then advanced gently through the capsule and exchanged for a long 2.7-mm (or standard 4.0-mm) 30-degree arthroscope. Gravity inflow of sterile saline is established to allow for distention of the

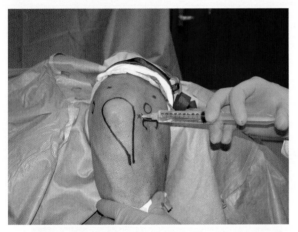

Figure 42-3. The elbow joint is insufflated with sterile saline through the lateral soft spot.

elbow capsule. Specialized cannulas that do not have any holes near the tip (Fig. 42-5) may be helpful. Use of standard cannulas can lead to the inadvertent entrance of fluid into the soft tissues while the joint is being visualized.

This medial portal allows excellent inspection of the lateral joint including the radial head, capitellum, and lateral capsule. An examination of the anterior elbow joint compartment is performed, evaluating for loose bodies, synovitis, and cartilage injury. The arthroscope is then directed laterally, and the camera is rotated to visualize the radiocapitellar joint in the horizontal plane.

If visualization is difficult, a retractor can be introduced through a proximal anterolateral portal (see later). With tensioning of the capsule anteriorly, improved visualization of the lateral capsule and soft tissues can be achieved; a Freer elevator is useful for this purpose.

Anterolateral Portal

After diagnostic arthroscopy of the anterior elbow through the medial portal, a modified anterolateral "working" portal is created either with an inside-out technique with a switching stick or with direct needle localization while viewing from the medial side.

The portal is typically 1 cm proximal and 1 cm anterior to the superior aspect of the capitellum. Through this portal (Fig. 42-6) any lateral synovitis may be debrided with a resector. It is of utmost importance to understand the position of the posterior interosseus nerve just anterior to the midline of the radiocapitellar joint to avoid inadvertent injury when advancing cutting or thermal instruments in the working portals.

Specific Steps

The specific steps of this procedure are outlined in Box 42-1.

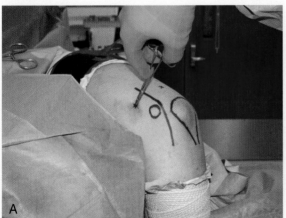
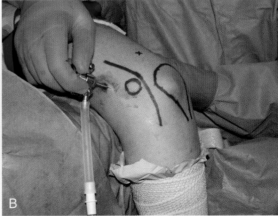

Figure 42-4. A, Subcutaneous tissue is first spread with a hemostat clamp when the anteromedial portal is being placed. **B,** The trocar is then introduced and directed inferiorly toward the anterior elbow capsule.

Anterior Release

After placement of anteromedial and anterolateral portals, the anterior joint is cleared of any synovitis or adhesions that are present. Typically the arthroscope is introduced through the anteromedial portal while instruments to be used for debridement are initially placed through the anterolateral portal. Mechanical instruments (e.g., shaver) are commonly used for debridement, although thermal devices may more easily facilitate the removal of soft tissue. If a surgeon elects

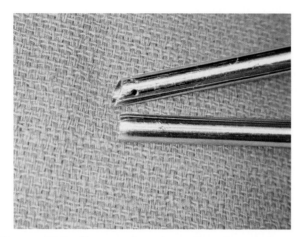

Figure 42-5. Close-up view shows the arthroscopic cannulas used for the elbow. Traditional cannulas *(top)* for larger joints commonly have an oblique end with holes near the tip to facilitate flow. Specialized cannulas *(bottom)* for the elbow do not have outflow holes. This is important because the distance between the cannula tip and the joint capsule can be quite small in the elbow, allowing fluid to extravasate inadvertently into the soft tissues. Fluid management is important in performing an elbow release arthroscopically.

to use thermal instruments, inflow should be gradually increased to avoid heat generation within the joint. The coronoid and radial fossae are debrided of any fibrous tissue down to the bony floor to allow articulation of the coronoid and radial head, respectively, during elbow flexion. The arthroscope and the working instruments must be alternated rapidly, efficiently, and effectively from medial to lateral positions during debridement (Figs. 42-7 and 42-8).

Following debridement of the coronoid and radial fossae, attention is next turned toward the anterior capsule. Special care is devoted to the radial nerve, which lies directly anterior to the capsule near the midline of the radiocapitellar joint. Accordingly, debridement of the anterior capsule directly off the humerus proximal to the trochlea is much safer than distal resection. The capsulotomy is usually initiated with a wide-mouthed duckling punch in a medial-to-lateral direction, viewing through the anterolateral portal; dissection in

---

BOX 42-1 Surgical Steps

1. Anterior release
   - Coronoid and radial fossa debrided above the articular surface, creating a concavity
   - Capsulectomy
2. Posterior release
   - Establishment of view by debridement of the olecranon fossa
   - Synovectomy
3. Ulnar nerve decompression and posteromedial capsulectomy
4. Closure

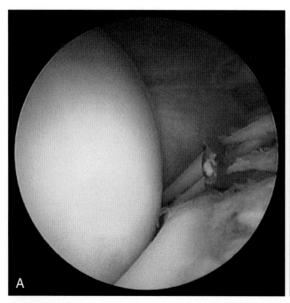
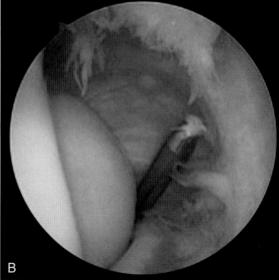

Figure 42-6. Arthroscopic view of elbow joint as viewed from medial portal with localization of anterolateral portal with 18-gauge spinal needle followed by placement of a blunt trocar through the joint.

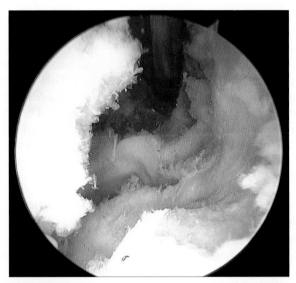

Figure 42-7. The coronoid and radial fossa have been debrided above the articular surface, creating a concavity and removal of any tissue that would cause impingement in flexion.

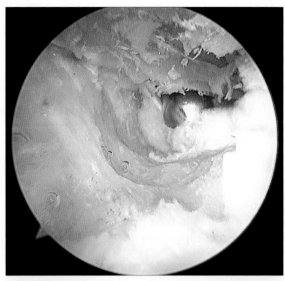

Figure 42-9. Capsulectomy has been performed anteriorly, revealing the undersurface of the brachialis. The capsular resection is performed proximal to the joint line; capsular debridement distal to the radiocapitellar joint would place the radial nerve, which lies directly anterior to the capsule at the joint line, at risk.

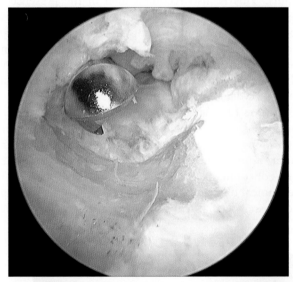

Figure 42-8. The concavity proximal to the trochlea is viewed from the lateral portal.

this direction is technically easier, as the interval between the capsule and the brachialis is more defined on the medial side. Use of a knife to extend the capsulotomy down to the level of the collateral ligaments on each side completes the capsulotomy. The capsular attachments should be resected off the humerus as far as the supracondylar ridges both medially and laterally.

Capsulectomy is then performed. Debridement performed near the level of the joint must be done with extreme diligence to avoid iatrogenic injury to the radial nerve. The capsulectomy should be performed on the medial side, extending from a proximal-to-distal direction. The lateral capsule should then be excised proximally and distally. This is the most dangerous aspect of the anterior release because the radial nerve is not protected behind the capsule but is located just anterior to the radial head, between the brachialis and the extensor carpi radialis brevis. If there is significant doubt regarding the tissue planes intraoperatively, simple capsulotomy off the humerus will often suffice for motion restoration if working toward complete capsulectomy is placing the radial nerve at risk (Fig. 42-9).

The use of retractors during anterior capsulectomy is heavily advocated, as their use greatly aids in visualization, can obviate the need for increased fluid pressure, and can aid in fluid management. This is especially true after the capsulectomy has begun, because fluid distention is less effective and extravasation into the periarticular soft tissues occurs more frequently. This must be limited, because it is much more difficult to work within the elbow after a significant amount of fluid has extravasated.

Posterior Release

After anterior release, we recommend maintaining a cannula in the anterior joint during the posterior release to establish outflow for the remainder of the procedure. With the elbow extended maximally to protect the posterior trochlea, a blunt elevator is used to blindly strip and clear the olecranon fossa and elevate the posterior joint capsule via tactile feedback. The posterior portals may then be placed. The posterolateral portal is started approximately 1 cm proximal to the midpoint between a line drawn from the olecranon tip to the lateral epicondyle. The posterior portal is established 3 to 4 cm above the olecranon tip in the midline.

With the arthroscope in the posterolateral portal and the shaver in the posterior portal, a view is first established by debridement of the olecranon fossa (Fig. 42-10). The camera is then turned to look in a distal direction. A radiofrequency ablation device can be used to debride dense scar tissue. The posterior capsule is freed from the humerus proximally, and it can be partially resected. Typically, this capsule is less hypertrophic than the anterior capsule. The capsule can then be elevated from the distal humerus with a shaver or periosteal elevator to further increase working space. A retractor placed in a proximal posterolateral portal is useful to maintain that space.

A synovectomy is then performed, with care taken to preserve the capsule to more easily perform the

capsulotomy later. Resection of osteophytes and removal of loose bodies are then carried out, particularly near the tip of the olecranon and the medial and lateral corners (Fig. 42-11). After bony and soft tissue debridement, the posterior capsule is resected. This is most easily performed with a shaver or radiofrequency ablation device through the posterolateral portal. The posterolateral capsule is initially resected, and the posteromedial capsule is release in cases in which there is a significant loss of flexion (flexion limited to below 90 to 110 degrees).

Posteromedial Capsulectomy and Ulnar Nerve Decompression

The ulnar nerve lies along the medial joint capsule in the cubital tunnel and may become enveloped in scar tissue and develop adhesions to the local soft tissues after trauma. We recommend that the ulnar nerve be released in all cases when preoperative symptoms exist or when provocative ulnar neuropathic symptoms exist (e.g., positive Tinel sign or positive elbow flexion test result). This is also recommended in the presence of significant preoperative loss of flexion, for which postoperative restoration in joint flexion may precipitate ulnar nerve symptoms. It has generally been recommended that ulnar nerve decompression be considered when preoperative elbow flexion is limited to less than 90 to 110 degrees.[11]

In cases in which posteromedial capsulectomy is considered, any mechanical or thermal instruments used along the medial ulnohumeral joint and medial gutter render the ulnar nerve susceptible to injury. The concomitant use of suction makes the use of mechanical burs and shavers more dangerous. Although the posteromedial capsulectomy may be performed

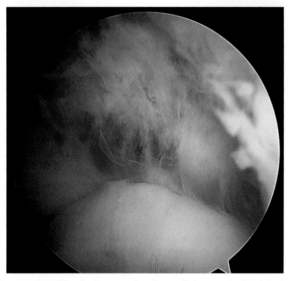

Figure 42-10. Arthroscopic view of the posterior joint, including fibrous tissue within the olecranon fossa.

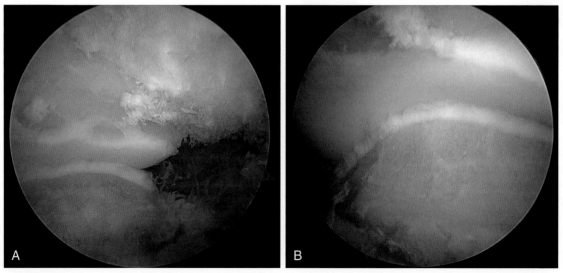

Figure 42-11. Lateral (**A**) and medial (**B**) views of the olecranon, demonstrating that the olecranon fossa and olecranon tip have been debrided of scar and osteophytes, removing any structures that impinged and prevented extension.

arthroscopically, our preference is to first identify and decompress the ulnar nerve through a limited open approach before arthroscopic procedures, particularly those in which a posteromedial release is anticipated. If a limited open approach is chosen for the nerve, it is much easier to perform before the arthroscopic joint release, as fluid extravasation and resultant swelling of the soft tissues can obscure tissue planes and local anatomy, rendering nerve dissection more difficult.

After ulnar nerve decompression, the posteromedial capsulectomy may be more safely performed. During the posteromedial release it is important to understand that the ulnar nerve is closer to the epicondyle than the tip of the olecranon, so release of the capsule is safer along the olecranon. A retractor placed in the proximal posterolateral portal or even in a proximal posterior portal (sometimes with two retractors used) is invaluable at this stage.

After anterior and posterior release, it is particularly important to document recovery of elbow motion intraoperatively. It is especially important to achieve terminal flexion and extension, in spite of soft tissue swelling, before leaving the operating room. If the ulnar nerve was decompressed, it can be left in the cubital tunnel (i.e., in situ decompression) or formally transposed anteriorly, depending on the surgeon's preference.

Closure

Two drains may be placed at the surgeon's discretion—one through the proximal anterolateral portal and one posteriorly, which is brought out through a separate exit wound. Portal sites and the ulnar nerve incision if used are closed with horizontal mattress sutures. The elbow is wrapped in a soft, compressive dressing; in our practice we prefer to cut out some of the dressing anteriorly (in the antecubital fossa) to allow more flexion postoperatively, as we start continuous passive motion (CPM) immediately.

POSTOPERATIVE CONSIDERATIONS

Follow-up

It is imperative that the surgeon follow these patients diligently in the postoperative period. Patients are typically seen in the office 10 to 14 days postoperatively for suture removal. Although most ultimate elbow motion is recovered during the first 6 to 8 weeks, patients can continue to make gains in terminal flexion and extension for several months postoperatively.

Rehabilitation

We typically prefer CPM that is begun immediately in the recovery room and continues throughout the patient's hospital stay. Formal therapy is commonly begun on postoperative day 1, when the dressing is removed, and edema-control modalities (e.g., edema sleeve, Ace wrap) are used to limit swelling. Active and gentle passive elbow motion is combined with intermittent CPM. Static progressive elbow bracing is begun early in the postoperative period. Flexion and extension are alternated based on the preoperative deficit and the early progress of the elbow. CPM should then be continued at home for 3 to 4 weeks along with a formal supervised rehabilitation program.

A nonsteroidal anti-inflammatory agent (e.g., indomethacin) is commonly prescribed as prophylaxis against HO for several weeks postoperatively. This also helps to limit inflammation of the periarticular soft tissues during rehabilitation.

With proper patient selection, results can be gratifying, with predictable recovery of a functional arc of elbow motion and pain relief.

Complications

Pathologic HO after contracture release has become rare, especially with the development of structured, supervised rehabilitation protocols in the immediate postoperative period. The use of pharmacologic prophylaxis has also limited the development of HO. Diligent radiographic follow-up of these patients, however, is the best way to monitor for the development of this complication.

In a retrospective review of elbow arthroscopies performed for varied orthopedic conditions, Kelly and colleagues reported four cases of deep infection, 33 cases of prolonged drainage from or superficial infection at a portal site, and 12 transient nerve palsies (five ulnar nerve, four superficial radial nerve, one posterior interosseous nerve, one medial antebrachial cutaneous nerve, and one anterior interosseous nerve).[8,9] Several other cadaveric studies have carefully described the relationship of neurovascular structures to portal sites and cannula positions; the work of these authors has improved the understanding of anatomy around the elbow and the importance of judicious portal placement.[12,13]

Several authors have suggested that the risk of nerve injury may be higher with arthroscopic versus open contracture release. This may be attributed to several factors, including surgeon experience and complexity of the surgery. The majority of iatrogenic nerve injuries occurred early during the initial reports of arthroscopic contracture release.[6,14-16] From our experience, we believe that the majority of intraoperative nerve injuries may be avoided by the diligent use of retractors, the avoidance of suction near a nerve, the use of a shaver instead of a bur near a nerve to avoid the "power-takeoff" effect in which the bur wraps tissue and pulls

TABLE 42-1. Studies of Efficacy of Arthroscopic and Open Elbow Contracture Release Procedures

Study	Methodology	Results
Savoie et al[17] (1999)	24 patients; arthroscopic debridement of coronoid and olecranon processes, olecranon fossa 18 patients underwent radial head resection	Average arc of motion 131 degrees, improvement of 81 degrees Significant decrease in VAS pain score (preoperative 8.2; postoperative 2.2)
Ball et al[18] (2002)	14 patients, arthroscopic contracture release	Average VAS satisfaction 8.4 of 10, VAS pain score 4.6 of 10 Mean flexion increased from 117.5 to 133 degrees, extension improved from 35.4 to 9.3 degrees Mean self-reported functional ability score 28.3 of 30
Nguyen et al[19] (2006)	22 patients, arthroscopic contracture release	Mean flexion improved from 122 degrees to 141 degrees ($P < .001$) Extension improved from 38 degrees to 19 degrees ($P < .001$) Mean arc improvement was 38 degrees ($P < .001$) Mean ASES-e score 31 of 36
Kelly et al[8] (2007)	25 elbows, arthroscopic debridement	24 were "better" or "much better" postoperatively 21 patients reported minimal or no pain Average flexion-extension arc improved by 21 degrees

ASES-e, American Shoulder and Elbow Surgeons Elbow form; *VAS,* visual analogue scale.

the nerve into it, and a thorough knowledge and understanding of where the nerves are and/or actually visualizing and retracting them. Most important, however, is that the surgeon may avoid a majority of these complications by recognizing the limits of arthroscopic technique and converting to an open approach in situations where contracture release is difficult or cannot be safely performed.

RESULTS

Several studies have reported the efficacy of both arthroscopic and open elbow contracture release procedures (Table 42-1). It is widely reported that after either treatment patients regain about 50% of lost motion. A meta-analysis of the literature suggests that 90% to 95% of patients regain lost motion (defined as at least a 10-degree increase in the arc of motion) and about 80% achieve a functional arc of motion (defined as ranging from 30 to 130 degrees); another 5% to 10% get to within 5 to 10 degrees of each end of this functional range.

REFERENCES

1. Akeson WH. An experimental study of joint stiffness. *J Bone Joint Surg Am.* 1961;43:1022-1034.
2. Akeson WH, Amiel D, Woo SL. Immobility effects on synovial joints the pathomechanics of joint contracture. *Biorheology.* 1980;17(1-2):95-110.
3. Cohen MS, Schimmel DR, Masuda K, et al. Structural and biochemical evaluation of the elbow capsule after trauma. *J Shoulder Elbow Surg.* 2007;16(4):484-490.
4. Morrey BF, Askew LJ, Chao EY. A biomechanical study of normal functional elbow motion. *J Bone Joint Surg Am.* 1981;63(6):872-877.
5. Jupiter JB, O'Driscoll SW, Cohen MS. The assessment and management of the stiff elbow. *Instr Course Lect.* 2003; 52:93-111.
6. Haapaniemi T, Berggren M, Adolfsson L. Complete transection of the median and radial nerves during arthroscopic release of post-traumatic elbow contracture. *Arthroscopy.* 1999;15(7):784-787.
7. Kelberine F, Landreau P, Cazal J. Arthroscopic management of the stiff elbow. *Chir Main.* 2006;25(Suppl 1): S108-S113.
8. Kelly EW, Bryce R, Coghlan J, et al. Arthroscopic debridement without radial head excision of the osteoarthritic elbow. *Arthroscopy.* 2007;23(2):151-156.
9. Kelly EW, Morrey BF, O'Driscoll SW. Complications of elbow arthroscopy. *J Bone Joint Surg Am.* 2001; 83(1):25-34.
10. Lynch GJ, Meyers JF, Whipple TL, et al. Neurovascular anatomy and elbow arthroscopy: inherent risks. *Arthroscopy.* 1986;2(3):190-197.
11. Antuna SA, Morrey BF, Adams RA, et al. Ulnohumeral arthroplasty for primary degenerative arthritis of the elbow: long-term outcome and complications. *J Bone Joint Surg Am.* 2002;84(12):2168-2173.
12. Kuklo TR, Taylor KF, Murphy KP, et al. Arthroscopic release for lateral epicondylitis: a cadaveric model. *Arthroscopy.* 1999;15(3):259-264.
13. MacAvoy MC, Rust SS, Green DP. Anatomy of the posterior antebrachial cutaneous nerve: practical information for the surgeon operating on the lateral aspect of the elbow. *J Hand Surg Am.* 2006;31(6):908-911.
14. Cohen AP, Redden JF, Stanley D. Treatment of osteoarthritis of the elbow: a comparison of open and arthroscopic debridement. *Arthroscopy.* 2000;16(7):701-706.
15. Marshall PD, Fairclough JA, Johnson SR, et al. Avoiding nerve damage during elbow arthroscopy. *J Bone Joint Surg Br.* 1993;75(1):129-131.
16. Papilion JD, Neff RS, Shall LM. Compression neuropathy of the radial nerve as a complication of elbow

arthroscopy: a case report and review of the literature. *Arthroscopy*. 1988;4(4):284-286.

17. Savoie FH, 3rd, Nunley PD, et al. Arthroscopic management of the arthritic elbow: indications, technique, and results. *J Shoulder Elbow Surg*. 1999;8(3): 214-219.

18. Ball CM, Meunier M, Galatz LM, et al. Arthroscopic treatment of post-traumatic elbow contracture. *J Shoulder Elbow Surg*. 2002;11(6):624-629.

19. Nguyen D, Proper SI, MacDermid JC, et al. Functional outcomes of arthroscopic capsular release of the elbow. *Arthroscopy*. 2006;22(8):842-849.

Chapter 43

Elbow Synovitis, Loose Bodies, and Posteromedial Impingement

Jamie L. Lynch, Matthew A. Kippe, and Kyle Anderson

Chapter Synopsis

- The most common indication for elbow arthroscopy in an athletic population is the presence of loose bodies. However, this diagnostic and therapeutic intervention can also be used for posteromedial impingement and synovial conditions that do not respond to nonoperative management. A thorough history and physical examination can guide the surgeon to proper diagnoses and subsequent use of elbow arthroscopy. Understanding the anatomy around the elbow is imperative to avoid described complications. Overall, if athletes have no associated elbow instability, most are able to return to the same level of their sport after arthroscopic elbow surgery.

Important Points

- Indications: Loose bodies and synovial conditions leading to mechanical symptom.
- Contraindications: Overlying cellulitis or altered elbow anatomy secondary to surgical or traumatic causes.
- Symptoms: Catching or locking of the elbow, limitations in range of motion, pain, and/or an effusion.
- Surgical technique: An examination under anesthesia should be used to evaluate the patient for instability. Typically, two anterior portals and two or three posterior portals are employed based on surgeon preference.

Clinical and Surgical Pearls

- Keep the elbow flexed at 90 degrees and distended with saline before initial portal placement to help protect neurovascular structures.
- Fluid inflow can be achieved through an 18-gauge needle in the midlateral portal, which may improve distention for joint entry.
- A spinal needle can help stabilize loose fragments and prevent migration during removal.
- Loose bodies can be brought toward the cannula by allowing fluid outflow from a side port.
- Large loose bodies can be removed in one motion along with the cannula.

Clinical and Surgical Pitfalls

- Maintain low suction on the shaver while working in the proximity of the capsule.
- The posterolateral cannula can be advanced into the radial gutter to facilitate placement of a midlateral portal.
- Minimize joint entry without the use of a cannula.
- Do not rely on the brachialis muscle for neurovascular protection.
- Consider the use of arthroscopic retractors for protection and visualization.

Athletic activities can lead to elbow inflammation and synovitis, joint degeneration, and formation of spurs and loose bodies. In fact, loose body removal represents the most common indication for elbow arthroscopy in this population.[1] Several of the conditions listed are specifically caused by the stress an athlete places on the elbow. Secondary to the high demands on an overhead athlete's elbow, a relatively small but acute deficit in range of motion (ROM) can be extremely disabling. With chronic motion loss, however, the athlete can adapt with greater ease. The necessary ROM varies with each sport, position, and the individual mechanics required to remain competitive.

Posteromedial impingement results from forces at the elbow that begin during late cocking and continue through acceleration and deceleration.[2] Valgus extension overload results in shear forces in the posterior elbow, whereas the anterior compartment experiences a tension force medially, with a compression force laterally.[3,4] Subsequent chondral changes to the olecranon and distal humerus are observed. With continuation of the offending activity, osteophyte formation typically occurs in the posteromedial elbow. Persistent throwing can cause osteophyte fracture and loose body formation.[4,5] Clinically, the athlete has pain and decreased ROM.

Similar to acute and chronic elbow injuries, synovial disorders may secondarily result in pain and mechanical symptoms that can hinder an athlete's performance. Diseases such as synovial chondromatosis, pigmented villonodular synovitis, and inflamed synovial plica can produce mechanical symptoms that alter normal elbow motion.[6-8] These conditions must not be overlooked, and the clinician should maintain a broad differential diagnosis because the athlete's symptoms may not be secondary to the activity, but rather intensified by the activity.

In the athletic population, elbow arthroscopy can be an effective tool for the removal of inflamed synovial tissue, osteophytes, and loose bodies. Regardless of cause, the procedure aims to resolve the clinical presentation resulting from acute and chronic injuries and synovial disorders, with the goal of returning an athlete to the previous level of competition.

PREOPERATIVE CONSIDERATIONS

History

A carefully obtained history provides the most important information. Symptoms are usually activity related. Patients may describe mechanical symptoms, such as catching, locking, and popping. The specific activity or timing within the activity can be important in determining the type of pathologic changes present. Take note of previous surgeries to the affected elbow, specifically ulnar nerve transpositions.

Typical History

- Insidious and progressive posterior elbow pain and limited elbow extension result from impinging posterior osteophytes; popping, locking, or catching suggests loose bodies.
- Symptoms are usually most prominent during the involved activity; the patient is often asymptomatic at rest.
- Specific timing of pain exacerbation during the activity can be revealing. Pain in late innings during pitching can indicate ligamentous disease often unmasked after forearm muscles fatigue, whereas arthrosis manifests more frequently with pain

and stiffness early in the morning or early in the activity.
- Specific timing of pain during the throwing motion itself can help differentiate between ligamentous injury (often most symptomatic during early acceleration) and impingement (which typically produces pain at ball release or follow-through).[1,9]
- The patient may report intermittent swelling after activity.
- Paresthesias may result from ulnar nerve irritation from either impinging spurs or traction during throwing.

Physical Examination

Any physical examination of a joint must consist of observation including resting position of the joint and evaluation of any skin breakdown, incisions, erythema, edema or effusion, and both passive and active ROM. Palpation of the elbow should be precise, and the examiner must focus on the underlying anatomy. For instance, medial epicondylitis can be distinguished from an ulnar collateral ligament (UCL) injury with purposeful and directed palpation, taking advantage of a thorough understanding of the local anatomy. Assessment of stability is also necessary. Furthermore, a full motor and sensory examination should be documented.

Brief examinations of the cervical spine, ipsilateral shoulder, wrist, and contralateral elbow are performed before the physical examination focuses on the elbow. Several conditions of the cervical spine and shoulder may cause elbow pain.

- ROM, loss of extension: Posterior olecranon spur, posterior compartment loose bodies, bridging osteophyte across olecranon fossa, anterior capsule contracture, collateral ligament contracture with or without ossification.
- ROM, loss of flexion: Coronoid spur, anterior compartment loose bodies, coronoid fossa spur, posterior capsule contracture or triceps adhesions, collateral ligament contracture.
- Palpation, with or without joint effusion, warmth, or crepitation: Medial, lateral or posterior tenderness can be associated with medial or lateral epicondylitis, triceps tendonitis, or an olecranon stress fracture; posteromedial tenderness with valgus hyperextension and posteromedial impingement[4]; or posterolateral tenderness with lateral synovial plicae.[6,7]
- Ligamentous stability: Medial collateral ligament insufficiency can lead to posteromedial impingement followed by spur formation, then fragmentation and loose bodies or loss of extension; valgus testing is performed with the elbow in pronation at 60 to 75 degrees of elbow flexion.[4,5,10]

- O'Driscoll's moving valgus test: Constant valgus torque is applied to a flexed elbow, and then the elbow is quickly extended. The result is positive if medial elbow pain is reproduced at the medial collateral ligament and is greatest between 120 degrees and 70 degrees.[11]
- Valgus extension overload test: Combined valgus and gentle terminal extension.[4]
- Neurovascular: Palpate the ulnar nerve during flexion and extension to determine if it subluxates, and assess a Tinel sign. Complete a distal examination for motor and sensory deficits.
- Intra-articular injections of a local anesthetic may be helpful in assessing an intra-articular versus an extra-articular pathologic process.

Imaging

Radiography

- Standard anteroposterior and lateral views are obtained (Fig. 43-1).

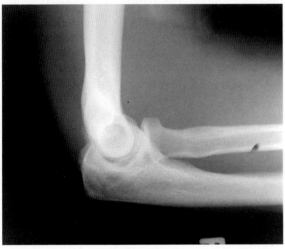

Figure 43-1. Lateral radiograph of a professional baseball player with pain and limited extension.

- The hyperflexion and external rotation view can increase visualization of the posteromedial olecranon out of its fossa (Fig. 43-2).
- When radiocapitellar disease is suspected, the external rotation view is obtained with the anterior elbow surface oriented at 40 degrees oblique relative to the cassette.

Other Modalities

- Computed tomographic scanning and magnetic resonance imaging without contrast enhancement can provide additional information and details about synovial disease, particularly loose bodies, osteophytes filling the olecranon and coronoid fossa, capsular thickening, and chondral thinning, as well as useful information about the integrity of the collateral ligaments (Fig. 43-3).
- Ultrasonography is an inexpensive modality that can provide additional information, especially in assessing collateral ligaments both statically and dynamically.
- Dynamic ultrasonography is performed for functional assessment. The performance of dynamic ultrasonography requires education and skill of the radiologist in applying a valgus stress to the elbow.
- The contralateral elbow can be evaluated to determine if gap formation is pathologic.
- We prefer magnetic resonance imaging to assess the structural integrity of the UCL and to evaluate for intra-articular disease.

Indications and Contraindications

In general, there are few absolute indications for surgery in dealing with an athlete. The primary indication is failure to return to competition after nonsurgical management. The most common indications for elbow arthroscopy in this population are removal of a loose

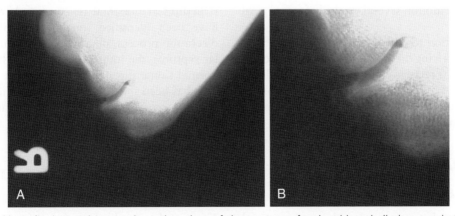

Figure 43-2. A, Hyperflexion and external rotation view of the same professional baseball player as in Figure 43-1 demonstrating posteromedial spur. **B,** Close-up view of the posteromedial fragment.

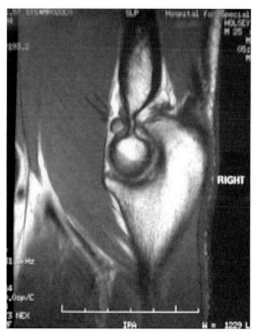

Figure 43-3. Magnetic resonance image demonstrating the position of a loose body within the elbow capsule at the coronoid fossa.

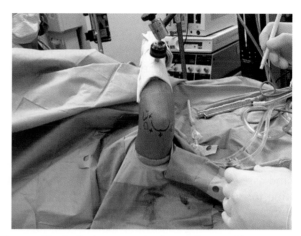

Figure 43-4. Arthroscopy in the supine position facilitates conversion to open procedures, such as a ligament reconstruction.

body that is closely correlated with mechanical symptoms and loss of motion. The simple appearance of a loose body on radiographs may not necessarily produce symptoms. Most patients report locking, catching, decreased ROM, or pain toward the extremes of motion.

In addition to osteophyte and loose body removal, arthroscopy is indicated for the treatment of synovial diseases, such as pigmented villonodular synovitis, synovial chondromatosis, and synovial plicae, which often produce debilitating pain, mechanical symptoms, and effusion.

For patients with synovitis, optimizing motion after elbow surgery including arthroscopic debridement is multifactorial. Both timing of surgery and preoperative ROM are important variables. In these patients, consideration can be given to the use of intra-articular corticosteroids to reduce synovial inflammation and maximize motion several weeks before surgical intervention.

A contraindication to elbow arthroscopy is any soft tissue infection overlying the joint without intra-articular infection. There is a relative contraindication for elbow arthroscopy in the setting of an alteration to the normal anatomy around the elbow, including but not limited to an ulnar nerve transposition or previous trauma.

SURGICAL TECHNIQUE

Anesthesia

The procedure can be performed with use of general anesthesia, regional anesthesia, or a combination

thereof, depending on the preferences of the surgeon, anesthesiologist, and patient. Most surgeons prefer a general anesthetic because it provides total muscle relaxation as well as allowing immediate postoperative neurologic assessment. The patient is positioned supine if arthroscopy is planned in combination with a reconstructive procedure.

Examination Under Anesthesia and Positioning

Before the patient is positioned for arthroscopy, an examination under anesthesia is performed to evaluate ROM as well as ligamentous stability. The supine position (Fig. 43-4) permits a smoother transition to an open procedure, such as collateral ligament reconstruction. Alternatively, arthroscopy can be performed in the prone position or the lateral decubitus position if a padded arm holder is available. Both of these positions can provide excellent arthroscopic exposure, but conversion to an open procedure can be more difficult.

The patient is properly positioned with the elbow flexed to 90 degrees, placing the anterior neurovascular structures at maximal relaxation. After the landmarks have been identified (medial and lateral epicondyle, olecranon process, ulnar nerve, and medial intermuscular septum), the joint is distended with 20 to 40 mL of normal saline through the lateral soft spot (Fig. 43-5). This has been shown in cadaveric studies to help protect neurovascular structures by increasing the distance between neurovascular structures and the portals by up to 1 cm.[12]

Surgical Landmarks, Incisions, and Portals

The number and placement of portals may differ, depending on the condition being treated. Most surgeons use two anterior portals and two or three posterior portals. Several studies have suggested different initial portal sites, and there continues to be considerable controversy about the safest initial portal.[12-18] We prefer proximal anterolateral portals. The most commonly used portals are described in Table 43-1.

Diagnostic Arthroscopy

Once the patient is positioned properly, the diagnostic arthroscopy is performed. The capsule and synovium may be thickened and inflamed, making introduction of the initial cannula difficult. In addition to a thorough inspection of both the anterior and posterior compartments, assessment of ligament integrity can be accomplished with provocative testing under direct intra-articular visualization.[5,20] It is important to understand that the entire medial collateral ligament (MCL) cannot be visualized intra-articularly.[20] Notably, a

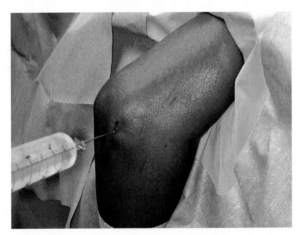

Figure 43-5. Before the surgeon establishes the first portal, the joint is distended with a saline injection through the midlateral soft spot.

negative valgus stress does not exclude significant partial tears of the ligament.[21]

Specific Steps

Box 43-1 outlines the specific steps of this procedure.

1. Establishment of Portals

Whether a lateral or medial portal is established first is a matter of the surgeon's preference. It is more important that the surgeon develop a routine that is thorough and can be performed consistently. In creating a portal, the use of a No. 15 blade to incise only epidermis and dermis followed by use of a hemostat for blunt dissection as opposed to plunging with a No. 11 blade can reduce injury to cutaneous and deep nerves.[7] A secondary portal can be established under direct visualization with spinal needle localization. Surgeons who advocate establishing a medial portal first and then a lateral portal under direct visualization argue that this is safer because the average distance between the medial portals and the median nerve is greater than the distance between the lateral portals and the radial or posterior interosseous nerve.[15] We begin by visualizing the anterior compartment first, allowing for adequate and maximal distention while creating anterior portals and treating anterior pathology. We prefer to establish a proximal lateral portal as described by Field and colleagues,[17] which is on average 13.7 mm from the radial

BOX 43-1 Surgical Steps
1. Establishment of portals
2. Anterior compartment assessment and debridement
3. Posterior compartment assessment and debridement
4. Closure

TABLE 43-1. Commonly Used Portals		
Portal	**Description**	**Nearest Neurovascular Structure**
Midlateral	"Soft spot"—center of triangle in olecranon, 7 mm	Posterior antebrachial radial head, capitellum cutaneous nerve
Proximal lateral[13]	2 cm proximal, 1 cm anterior to lateral epicondyle 7.9 mm extended, 13.7 mm flexed	Radial nerve
Anterolateral[14]	3 cm distal, 1 cm anterior to lateral epicondyle 1.4 mm extended, 4.9 mm flexed	Radial nerve
Proximal medial[2]	2 cm proximal medial epicondyle, anterior to intermuscular septum 12-23 mm	Median nerve
Anteromedial[14]	2 cm distal, 2 cm anterior to medial epicondyle 2 mm extended, 7 mm flexed	Median nerve
Posterolateral[19]	Proximal to olecranon, lateral edge of triceps ~15-20 mm	Radial nerve
Posterocentral[14]	Proximal to olecranon, through triceps tendon ~15-20 mm	Ulnar nerve, transtriceps

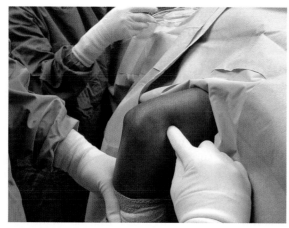

Figure 43-6. Proximal lateral portal. The portal is placed just anterior to the humerus where the supracondylar ridge meets the lateral epicondyle.

nerve in a flexed elbow (Fig. 43-6). This portal allows broad visualization of the anterior compartment.

2. Anterior Compartment Assessment and Debridement

When the procedure is started from a lateral portal, examination of the medial gutter is performed first, followed by a search for loose bodies across the entire anterior compartment from medial to lateral. All fragments should be removed when they are encountered, because visualization can change and loose bodies can move to a less accessible area during the procedure. An arthroscopic grasper or shaver is used for smaller fragments or fragments adherent to the capsule. A spinal needle can also be used to stabilize the fragment and prevent it from migrating into a recess. Fluid flow should be well controlled, especially once a loose body has been localized. Allowing outflow at the cannula can help bring the loose body toward the arthroscopic grasper. Very large loose bodies may need to be broken into smaller pieces to be removed through the cannula. This can also be accomplished by removal of the fragment and the cannula in one maneuver after the portal skin incision has been extended and the portal carefully dilated with a spreading clamp (Fig. 43-7). Grasping the loose body on end may improve ease of removal. The camera can also assist in pushing the fragment out through the portal while the loose body is gently and consistently being pulled by the grasper. At times a plica may be more easily resected by getting a rough edge started with either an arthroscopic bipolar or a retractable hook blade. It may be necessary to switch portals and view from the medial side to resect all pathologic tissue completely from the lateral compartment. In addition, a 70-degree scope can be used so the articular surfaces of the distal humerus, radius, and ulna can be clearly visualized.[19]

An arthroscopic valgus instability test can be performed during viewing from the proximal lateral or anterolateral portal. The medial aspect of the ulnohumeral joint is observed for any gap formation (Fig. 43-8). Any gap greater than 1 to 2 mm is considered abnormal.[5]

3. Posterior Compartment Assessment and Debridement

After evaluation and debridement of the anterior compartment, a cannula is left in place to maintain joint distention while the transition is made to the posterior compartment. Next, a posterolateral portal is established, which is located just radial to the triceps tendon and 2 to 3 mm proximal to the tip of the olecranon. This is the primary viewing portal for work to be done in the posterior compartment. Careful inspection will reveal loose bodies, spurs, chondromalacia, and fibrous debris. Debridement and loose body removal can be accomplished through a posterocentral (transtriceps) portal (Fig. 43-9). The olecranon should be probed because fibrous tissue can often hide fragmentation that may be a source of persistent pain. Extreme caution must be used in operating the motorized shaver, especially while suction is used, because of the proximity of the ulnar nerve along the posteromedial olecranon. The scope can be advanced into the midlateral viewing area to assess the radial gutter and to remove any remaining pathologic tissue along the posterior aspect of the radial head and capitellum. This can also be accomplished by use of a midlateral portal or a 70-degree scope to improve visualization of this small compartment. Most plicae are posterolateral and are best removed by viewing from posterolateral and working from the midlateral portal (Fig. 43-10). The plicae can be resected with a motorized shaver, with suction carefully controlled.

4. Closure

Portal incisions are closed with 4-0 nylon sutures in a simple interrupted fashion. Sterile dressings are applied, and the arm is placed in a sling for comfort.

POSTOPERATIVE CONSIDERATIONS

Rehabilitation

- Reduce inflammation in the immediate postoperative period with ice, elevation, and anti-inflammatory medication.
- Phase 1 (3 to 6 weeks): Passive ROM is started in the early postoperative period.
- Phase 2 (6 to 10 weeks): ROM exercises are continued with the addition of strengthening.

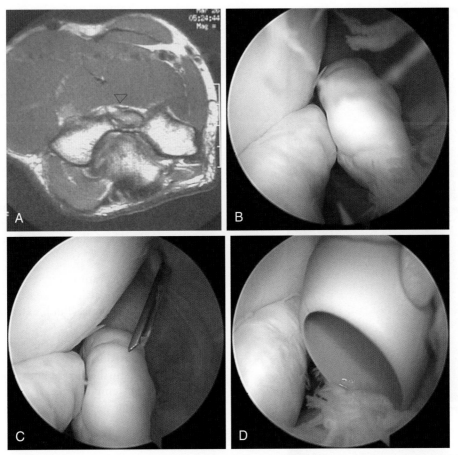

Figure 43-7. Loose body removal. **A,** Axial magnetic resonance image of a loose body in the coronoid fossa of the humerus causing mechanical symptoms. **B,** During arthroscopy, the loose body is visualized through the proximal lateral portal. **C,** A spinal needle is used to make an anteromedial portal under direct visualization as well as to prevent movement of the loose body. **D,** A cannula is placed in a proximal medial portal, through which the loose body was removed from the elbow joint.

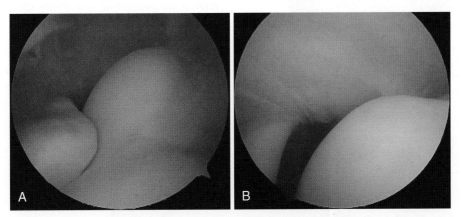

Figure 43-8. During diagnostic arthroscopy, ligamentous stability is assessed under direct visualization. **A,** Arthroscopic image of ulnohumeral joint without valgus stress applied. **B,** Arthroscopic image of medial opening of ulnohumeral joint with valgus stress.

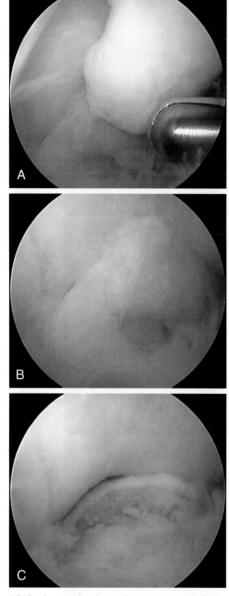

Figure 43-9. Loose body and spur removal from olecranon fossa. **A,** Large loose body in posterior compartment. **B,** After loose body has been removed, a large olecranon spur is revealed. **C,** Olecranon after spur removal, now with no mechanical blocks to extension.

- Phase 3: The focus is on advanced strengthening, resistive exercises, and sport-specific training, such as a graduated throwing program.
- General overall conditioning is emphasized throughout rehabilitation, including strengthening of adjacent joints, core strengthening, and cardiovascular training.

Complications

Elbow arthroscopy for the removal of loose bodies, debridement, and synovectomy is generally a safe procedure. Complications are uncommon and usually minor. The major concern is for the potential of neurovascular injury. The following complications have been reported[22-25]:

- Direct nerve laceration
- Transient nerve palsies caused by compression from levering instruments, fluid extravasation, or local anesthetic usage
- Postoperative stiffness
- Heterotopic ossification
- Potential for further loose body formation
- Subcutaneous emphysema
- Portal drainage
- Infection

RESULTS

Arthroscopy for the treatment of elbow joint synovitis and posteromedial impingement and for loose body removal in athletes can reduce pain and improve function. Most athletes are able to return to the same level of their sport after arthroscopic elbow surgery, particularly if no associated instability exists.[1,7,26-31] However, in certain athletes, depending on the type of sport and position played, reoperation rates are high, and return to the previous level of competition is less reliable.[26] Table 43-2 summarizes clinical results after elbow arthroscopy for posteromedial impingement, loose body removal, and treatment of common synovial diseases.

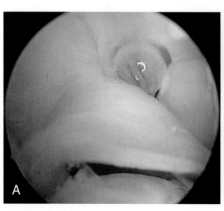

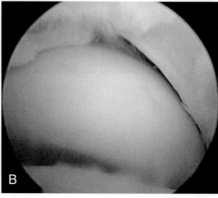

Figure 43-10. Lateral synovial plicae in a golfer causing pain and mechanical symptoms. **A,** Symptomatic lateral synovial plicae viewed from posterolateral portal. **B,** Radiocapitellar joint after removal of the lateral synovial plicae.

TABLE 43-2. Clinical Results of Elbow Arthroscopy for Loose Body, Synovial Plicae, and Osteophyte Removal

Author	Follow-up (mo)	Outcome
Wilson et al[4] (1983)	12	5/5 pitchers returned for at least one full season of maximum effectiveness
Andrews and Timmerman[26] (1995)	mean, 42 (minimum, 24)	47/59 professional baseball players returned for at least one season (however, 33% reoperation rate, and 25% required ulnar collateral ligament reconstruction)
Bradley[27] (1995)	24	6/6 excellent and good objective and subjective results
Reddy et al[31] (2000)	mean, 42.3 (range, 7-115)	47/55 baseball players returned to competition
Kim et al[7] (2006)	33.8 (range, 24-65.5)	11/12 athletes reported excellent outcome and returned to competition
Raushen et al[30] (2009)	38	16/16 elbows had good to excellent outcome; all but 2 athletes returned to activity at preoperative level (inclusion criteria: isolated posteromedial impingement)

REFERENCES

1. Ward WG, Anderson TE. Elbow arthroscopy in a mostly athletic population. *J Hand Surg Am.* 1993;18:220-224.
2. Maloney MD, Mohr KJ, el Attrache NS. Elbow injuries in the throwing athlete: Difficult diagnoses and surgical complications. *Clin Sports Med.* 1999;18:795-809.
3. Cain Jr EL, Dugas JR, Wolf RS, et al. Elbow injuries in throwing athletes: a current concepts review. *Am J Sports Med.* 2003;31:621-635.
4. Wilson FD, Andrews JR, Blackburn TA, et al. Valgus extension overload in the pitching elbow. *Am J Sports Med.* 1983;11:83-88.
5. Field LD, Altchek DW. Evaluation of the arthroscopic valgus instability test of the elbow. *Am J Sports Med.* 1996;24:177-183.
6. Clarke RP. Symptomatic, lateral synovial fringe (plica) of the elbow joint. *Arthroscopy.* 1988;4:112-116.
7. Kim DH, Gambardella RA, Elattrache NS, et al. Arthroscopic treatment of posterolateral elbow impingement from lateral synovial plicae in throwing athletes and golfers. *Am J Sports Med.* 2006;34:1-7.
8. Ofluoglu O. Pigmented villonodular synovitis. *Orthop Clin North Am.* 2006;37:23-33.
9. King JW, Brelsford HJ, Tullos HS. Analysis of the pitching arm of the professional baseball pitcher. *Clin Orthop Relat Res.* 1969;67:116-123.
10. Callaway GH, Field LD, Deng XH, et al. Biomechanical evaluation of the medial collateral ligament of the elbow. *J Bone Joint Surg Am.* 1997;79:1223-1230.
11. O'Driscoll SW, Lawton RL, Smith AM. The "moving valgus stress test" for medial collateral ligament tears of the elbow. *Am J Sports Med.* 2005;33(2):231-239.
12. Lynch GJ, Meyers JF, Whipple TL, et al. Neurovascular anatomy and elbow arthroscopy: inherent risks. *Arthroscopy.* 1986;2:191-197.
13. Adolfsson L. Arthroscopy of the elbow joint: a cadaveric study of portal placement. *J Shoulder Elbow Surg.* 1994;3:53-61.
14. Andrews JR, Carson WG. Arthroscopy of the elbow. *Arthroscopy.* 1985;1:97-107.
15. Baker CL, Jones GL. Arthroscopy of the elbow. *Am J Sports Med.* 1999;27:251-264.
16. Burman MS. Arthroscopy of the elbow joint: a cadaveric. *J Bone Joint Surg.* 1932;14:349-350.
17. Field LD, Altchek DW, Warren RF, et al. Arthroscopic anatomy of the lateral elbow: a comparison of three portals. *Arthroscopy.* 1994;10:602-607.
18. Poehling GG, Whipple TL, Sisco L, et al. Elbow arthroscopy. A new technique. *Arthroscopy.* 1989;5:222-224.
19. Bedi A, Dines J, Dines DM, et al. Use of the 70° arthroscope for improved visualization with common arthroscopic procedures. *Arthroscopy.* 2010;26(12):1684-1696.
20. Field LD, Callaway GH, O'Brien SJ, et al. Arthroscopic assessment of the medial collateral ligament complex of the elbow. *Am J Sports Med.* 1995;23:396-400.
21. Kooima CL, Anderson K, Craig JV, et al. Evidence of subclinical medial collateral ligament injury and posteromedial impingement in professional baseball players. *Am J Sports Med.* 2004;32:1602-1606.
22. Dexel J, Schneiders W, Kasten P. Subcutaneous emphysema of the upper extremity after elbow arthroscopy. *Arthroscopy.* 2011;27(7):1014-1017.
23. Kelly EW, Morrey BF, O'Driscoll SW. Complications of elbow arthroscopy. *J Bone Joint Surg Am.* 2001;83:25-34.
24. Marshall PD, Fairclough JA, Johnson SR, et al. Avoiding nerve damage during elbow arthroscopy. *J Bone Joint Surg Am.* 1993;74:129-131.
25. Sodha S, Nagda SH, Sennett BJ. Heterotopic ossification in a throwing athlete after elbow arthroscopy. *Arthroscopy.* 2006;22(7):802.e1-e3.
26. Andrews JR, Timmerman LA. Outcome of elbow surgery in professional baseball players. *Am J Sports Med.* 1995;23:407-413.
27. Bradley JP. Arthroscopic treatment of posterior impingement of the elbow in NFL lineman [abstract]. *J Shoulder Elbow Surg.* 1995;2:S119.

28. Fideler BM, Kvitne RS, Jordan S, et al. Posterior impingement of the elbow in professional baseball players: results of arthroscopic treatment [abstract]. *J Shoulder Elbow Surg.* 1997;6:169-170.

29. Ogilvie-Harris DJ, Schemitsch E. Arthroscopy of the elbow for removal of loose bodies. *Arthroscopy.* 1993;9: 5-8.

30. Rahusen FT, Brinkman JM, Eygendaal D. Arthroscopic treatment of posterior impingement of the elbow in athletes: a medium-term follow-up in sixteen cases. *J Shoulder Elbow Surg.* 2009;18(2):279-282.

31. Reddy AS, Kvitne RS, Yocum LA, et al. Arthroscopy of the elbow: a long term clinical review. *Arthroscopy.* 2000;16:588-594.

Chapter 44

Arthroscopic Management of the Arthritic Elbow

Julie E. Adams, Justin P. Strickland, and Scott P. Steinmann

Chapter Synopsis

- Arthroscopy of the elbow can be useful for diagnostic and therapeutic reasons. This chapter highlights the indications, techniques, outcomes, and complications of this procedure.

Important Points

- Although plain radiographs may be adequate for preoperative planning, three-dimensional computed tomographic scanning is helpful.
- Pain at the end arcs of motion or presence of a discrete lesion (osteochondral defect, loose body) are good indications for this procedure. Patients with pain throughout the arc of motion may not benefit as much from this procedure.
- Elbow arthroscopy is a technically difficult procedure with a real potential for complications.

Clinical and Surgical Pearls

- An arm holder made specifically for elbow arthroscopy may make positioning easier.
- If the lateral decubitus position is used, the elbow should be positioned high in the operative field. This helps eliminate impingement of the arthroscope and instruments against the patient's body or surgical drapes.
- The patient is tilted slightly toward the surgeon to prevent the arm holder from impinging on the antecubital fossa.
- Elevation of the patient's arm overhead in a fully extended Statue of Liberty position overnight can help quickly remove postoperative swelling to allow early active motion.

Clinical and Surgical Pitfalls

- Any portal can be used as an initial starting portal. However, the anterolateral portal is closest to a major nerve (radial nerve), and care should be taken to establish this portal in the correct position.
- Avoid suction on the shaver in the anterior aspect of the joint under usual circumstances, as the suction may inadvertently pull structures into the shaver or bur.
- Attempt to do all bone work first in the elbow joint before removing capsule. This helps limit edema and potentially protects vital structures.
- Heterotopic bone can form even after an arthroscopic procedure. To potentially limit this process, remove as many bone fragments as possible.

Arthroscopy of the elbow is indicated for diagnostic therapeutic purposes in the setting of elbow arthritis and may be useful to treat many of the pathologic changes encountered with osteoarthritis, inflammatory arthritis, and posttraumatic conditions.[1,2]

Because of the complex articular and neurovascular anatomy about the elbow joint, elbow arthroscopy is technically challenging. Potential advantages of an arthroscopic approach over an open surgery include improved articular visualization, decreased postoperative pain, and the potential for faster postoperative recovery. To date, however, conclusive evidence of improved outcomes over open procedures are lacking.

This chapter provides an overview of arthritic conditions about the elbow and tips and techniques for safer and effective arthroscopy of the elbow joint.

PREOPERATIVE CONSIDERATIONS

History

Posttraumatic arthritis, osteoarthritis, hemophilic arthritis, and inflammatory arthritis may affect the elbow joint. Pain is a common complaint; however, patients may also report stiffness, weakness, instability, mechanical symptoms, or cosmetic deformity.[3] A description of the degree and direction of motion loss and presence and occurrence of pain is an important part of the history.

A history of trauma may be elicited from patients. The most common injury that may cause posttraumatic arthritis is a comminuted intra-articular fracture resulting in articular incongruity.[3] Posttraumatic contractures caused solely by capsular fibrosis may be secondary to hemarthrosis from various traumatic causes. The patient should be asked whether he or she had physical therapy, whether it was painful or relatively benign, and whether splints had been used for short- or long-term sessions.

Osteoarthritis involving the elbow is most commonly seen in the dominant arm of men with a history of heavy labor, weightlifters, and throwing athletes.[3] Crutch ambulators may also be more prone to this condition. These patients are commonly in the third to eighth decades. Patients typically report pain at extremes of motion with loss of terminal extension more than loss of flexion. Patients with osteoarthritis who may benefit from arthroscopic debridement typically lack significant pain in the mid-arc of motion; rather, pain will be noted more at the end arc of flexion and/or extension owing to impinging terminal osteophytes. The presence of mid-arc of motion discomfort or pain throughout the arc of motion may be indicative of more widespread joint changes that may not respond as well to arthroscopic debridement.

Symptomatic rheumatoid arthritis of the elbow fortunately is becoming less common with the advent of disease-modifying agents but can be quite debilitating when it does occur. Both elbows are commonly involved, and patients initially have pain and swelling from synovitis and effusion. More severe involvement with loss of bone and failure of the soft tissues around the elbow joint may cause instability, which may accelerate articular destruction as a result of subluxation or malalignment.[4,5]

Patients with hemophilia commonly develop arthropathy of the elbow. This appears to be related to some threshold of clinical or subclinical intra-articular bleeding, which seems to result in potentiation of an inflammatory cascade leading to worsening synovial proliferation and hemarthroses, with subsequent arthritis. Patients may report recurrent intra-articular bleeds caused by proliferative synovitis, or the secondary arthritic changes that ensue.[6]

Physical Examination

On examination, patients with osteoarthritis will commonly have pain at the endpoints of motion and/or mechanical symptoms. Lack of terminal extension is common, along with loss of terminal flexion. Likewise, patients with inflammatory or hemophilic arthritis will commonly have synovitis about the joint. In all types of arthritis, crepitus may also be present. It is important to record the passive and active ranges of motion. This aids in quantifying the functional deficits while determining the success of treatment. Although difficult, it may be useful to differentiate between a "soft" and "hard" endpoint, as this may lead the examiner to determine the cause of stiffness. A complete neurovascular examination should always be performed. The physical examination findings are then correlated with the radiographic findings.

Imaging

Anteroposterior, lateral, and oblique plain film views of the elbow are obtained. On radiographic examination of the typical osteoarthritic or posttraumatic elbow, osteophytes may be seen on the olecranon and coronoid processes and also in the olecranon and coronoid fossae. Many patients have loose bodies, and presence of a loose body on an elbow radiograph is in most instances a sign of an underlying and more substantial degenerative process.

Computed tomography with three-dimensional reformatting may be especially helpful for visualizing osseous anatomy and aiding in the development of the preoperative plan.

Indications

Surgery on an arthritic elbow may be indicated for patients with functional loss of motion, mechanical symptoms caused by loose bodies, and/or pain. Those with synovitis or hemophilic bleeds recalcitrant to medical management may also be candidates for surgical management.

SURGICAL TECHNIQUE

Anesthesia and Positioning

We prefer to use general anesthesia. This permits the patient to be placed in either a prone or a lateral decubitus position, which might not be tolerated by an awake patient managed with a regional block. In addition, lack of paralysis allows the nerve to respond if dissection is too close; furthermore, the status of the major peripheral nerves may be established immediately after surgery.

Placement of the patient in the lateral decubitus position allows excellent access to the elbow joint (Fig. 44-1). The arm is placed in a padded arm holder that is attached to the side of the table. A low-profile elbow arm holder specifically designed for this purpose may be used.

A nonsterile tourniquet is then placed on the arm at the level of the arm holder, and the arm is firmly secured to the arm holder. This facilitates arthroscopy by keeping the arm stable, just as a knee holder maintains stability during knee arthroscopy. The elbow should be positioned slightly higher than the shoulder. This allows 360-degree exposure of the elbow joint, eliminating the potential for impingement of the arthroscope or other instruments against the side of the body (Fig. 44-2).

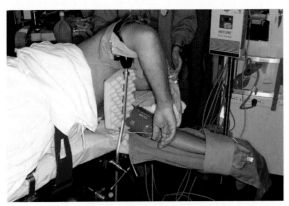

Figure 44-1. The lateral decubitus position for elbow arthroscopy. The arm is placed into a specially designed elbow arm holder with a nonsterile tourniquet. The arm is strapped into the arm holder to secure it during arthroscopic manipulation. The opposite arm is draped out on an arm board.

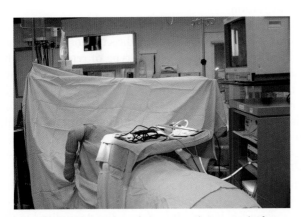

Figure 44-2. Overview of the operating room before elbow arthroscopy is begun. The patient is in lateral decubitus position. The monitor is placed opposite the surgeon for ease of viewing.

Surgical Landmarks, Incisions, and Portals

All portal sites are marked before surgery or insufflation of the joint, when the elbow is not distended or edematous and palpation of osseous landmarks is more precise (Fig. 44-3). Surface landmarks that should be marked include the lateral epicondyle, medial epicondyle, radial head, capitellum, ulnar nerve, and olecranon. The ulnar nerve is palpated to determine its location and to ensure that it does not subluxate from the cubital tunnel.

An 18-gauge needle is placed through the planned anterolateral portal. The elbow is then distended with 20 to 30 mL of saline. When the joint is distended, entry into the joint is easier and potentially safer. Attempting to enter a nondistended elbow joint accurately with a trocar is considerably difficult.

Initial portal entry can be performed safely from either the medial or the lateral side, depending on the preference of the operating surgeon. All portals are made with a knife blade, which is drawn across the skin to ensure that only the skin, and not the underlying soft tissue, is divided. The neurovascular structure that is at greatest risk of injury from a lateral portal is the radial nerve. There are two techniques commonly used to reduce the risk of injury to that nerve. One option is to establish an anterolateral portal as soon as the joint is distended, before fluid extravasation makes it difficult to see and to feel the anatomic landmarks. The anterolateral portal is established just anterior to the sulcus between the capitellum and the radial head. A second option is to establish an anteromedial portal first, and then make the anterolateral portal with an inside-out approach under direct visualization. The anteromedial portal is a safe distance away from the median and ulnar nerves; once it is established, under direct visualization with the arthroscope inside the joint, an anterolateral portal is established by placing a spinal needle into the joint and next placing a trocar and cannula. This can

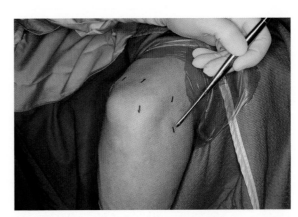

Figure 44-3. Intraoperative view of portal placement. The retractor is demonstrating the standard anterolateral portal.

be a safe technique in experienced hands, but simply observing from inside of the joint, as is done with this technique, does not guarantee that the spinal needle and trocar are not being passed through the radial nerve.

Once the arthroscope (4-mm, 30-degree) has been placed into the joint, visualization is maintained by pressure distention of the capsule or mechanical retraction. Both methods work, but excessively high fluid pressures may lead to fluid extravasation during the course of a long arthroscopic procedure. The retractors can be simple lever retractors such as a Howarth elevator or large Steinmann pins. They are placed into the elbow joint through an accessory portal, which is typically 2 to 3 cm proximal to the arthroscopic viewing portal. With the capsule and overlying soft tissue held away from the bone with the retractors, adequate visualization can be achieved with a high-flow, low-pressure system.

Direct Lateral or Midlateral Portal

The direct lateral or midlateral ("soft spot") portal is located at the center of the triangle bounded by the olecranon, lateral epicondyle, and radial head. It is difficult to visualize the anterior aspect of the joint from this portal; however, it provides a good view of the posterior aspect of the capitellum, radial head, and radioulnar articulation. This is helpful, especially when one is examining a patient with osteochondritis dissecans of the capitellum. Because of the shallow nature of this portal and the limited space in which to work, it can be helpful to use a 2.7-mm arthroscope.

Anteromedial Portal

The anteromedial portal is placed 2 cm distal and 2 cm anterior to the medial epicondyle (Fig. 44-4). Instruments placed through this portal tend to penetrate the common flexor origin and the brachialis before entering the joint. Before any medial portals are placed, the ulnar nerve should be palpated and checked for any tendency

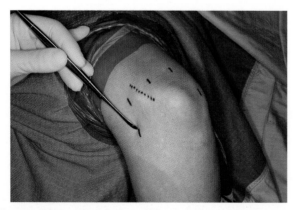

Figure 44-4. Medial view of intraoperative portal placement demonstrating the anteromedial portal with the retractor. The dotted line represents the ulnar nerve.

to subluxate from the cubital tunnel. The medial antebrachial cutaneous nerve is most at risk with this portal. The median nerve is farther away, an average of 7 mm from the portal.

Posterior Portals

Two portals are necessary to visualize the posterior aspect of the elbow joint. The fat pad normally occupies a large portion of the potential space. A second portal is usually established simultaneously with the first because debridement with an arthroscopic shaver will be needed immediately to obtain a visible working space. The location of the ulnar nerve is confirmed before the first portal is established. Unlike the anterior portals, in which palpation of the median or radial nerve is not possible, posterior portals can typically be established safely once the ulnar nerve has been identified.

The posterolateral portal is excellent for initial viewing of the posterior aspect of the elbow. It is made level with the tip of the olecranon, with the elbow flexed 90 degrees, at the lateral joint line. The trocar should be aimed at the center of the olecranon fossa. The direct posterior portal is established 3 cm proximal to the tip of the olecranon, at the proximal margin of the olecranon fossa. The triceps is thick at this point, and a knife blade is used to incise directly into the posterior joint. After this portal has been made, a shaver or radiofrequency probe can be placed into the joint and debridement can be performed. Loose bodies and osteophytes on the olecranon fossa can be removed through this portal while the surgeon views through the posterolateral portal. The arthroscope and the shaver can be switched back and forth to complete the debridement. Because of the frequent switching between portals and the relative safety of the portal location, it is not necessary to use a cannula in the posterior aspect of the elbow joint. However, an outflow cannula can be maintained in the anterior aspect of the elbow joint to limit fluid extravasation.

A good location for an initial posterior retractor portal is 2 cm proximal to the directly posterior portal. A Howarth elevator or similar type of retractor can be used to elevate the joint capsule out of view while not interfering with the working instruments. This can help with visualization of the medial and lateral gutters and also the release of a tight posterior aspect of the capsule in a stiff elbow.

Distal Ulnar Portal

The distal ulnar portal is particularly useful for visualizing the posterior capitellum, especially in the setting of osteochondral lesions. It is placed 3 to 4 cm distal to the posterior portion of the radiocapitellar joint, just radial to the palpable dorsal crest of the ulna. After incision of the skin, a straight hemostat is passed along the radial border of the ulna directed proximally toward the radio-capitellar joint, and the intended portal site is expanded. This may then be replaced by the trocar and then the arthroscope. Progressive visualization of the capitellum is facilitated by additional flexion of the elbow. It is useful to visualize through this portal while instrumenting through the direct lateral or soft spot portal.[7]

Specific Steps

Specific steps of this procedure are outlined in Box 44-1.

Arthroscopic debridement of an osteoarthritic elbow begins in the posterior aspect of the joint when the

---

BOX 44-1 Surgical Steps

1. Mark all portal sites and surface anatomy.
2. Perform elbow distention.
3. Establish portals.
4. Begin work in posterior compartment.
5. Perform capsular release (posterior capsule first if patient lacks flexion).
6. Remove osteophytes along olecranon and olecranon fossa.
7. Move to anterior compartment.
8. Remove all obvious loose bodies; remove radial and coronoid osteophytes.
9. Perform anterior capsulectomy off humerus (lateral viewing portal).
10. Viewing from the medial portal, perform capsulectomy from radial head and capitellum.

---

patient predominantly lacks flexion and in the anterior aspect of the joint when the patient predominantly lacks extension (see Box 44-1). For greater flexion to be achieved at surgery, the posterior aspect of the capsule needs to be released. This is easiest to perform early in the procedure, before any swelling or fluid extravasation has occurred. In particular, release of the postero-medial aspect of the capsule requires identification of the ulnar nerve so that the nerve will not be injured (Fig. 44-5). If the greatest limitation of motion is in extension, the procedure should begin in the anterior compartment.

The posterior compartment is visualized well from the posterolateral portal, and the directly posterior portal can be used as a working portal. Osteophytes develop both on the tip of the olecranon and along the medial and lateral sides of the ulna. It is important to check for osteophytes on the sides of the olecranon; often they are overlooked and only the one on the tip of the olecranon is addressed. In addition, the olecranon fossa should be checked for osteophytes along the rim on the posterior aspect of the humerus. These osteophytes often match arthritic osseous formation on the olecranon, and both sites of bone formation need to be excised for normal joint motion to be restored.

After initial joint inspection from an anterior portal and removal of obvious loose bodies, all work on bone is performed (Fig. 44-6). A shaver or bur can be used to remove osteophytes from the radial and coronoid fossae of the humerus. Often, these osteophytes are neglected, and only the tip of the coronoid is excised (Fig. 44-7). The medial aspect of the coronoid should

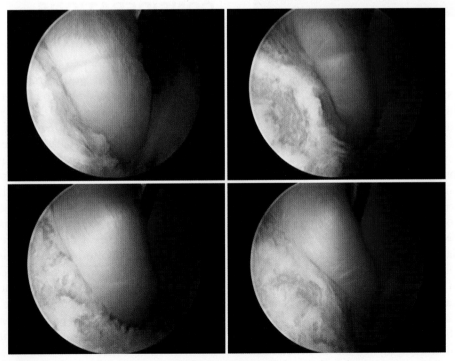

Figure 44-5. Arthroscopic views of the ulnar nerve after posteromedial capsular release.

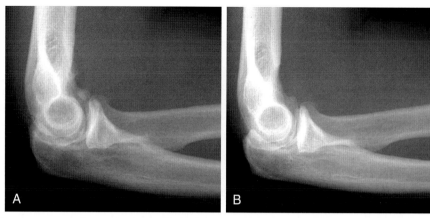

Figure 44-6. A, Preoperative radiograph demonstrating anterior and posterior osteophytes. **B,** Postoperative radiograph demonstrating osteophyte excision around the elbow joint.

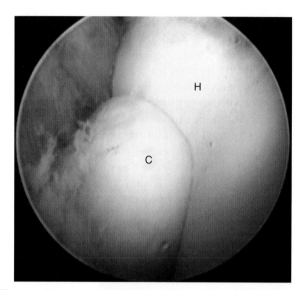

Figure 44-7. Arthroscopic view of the tip of the coronoid *(C)* and distal humerus *(H).*

also be examined for osteophytes, which may be missed if they are not specifically sought. Use of motorized instruments without a suction device attached allows adequate tissue removal and reduces the risk of inadvertent neurovascular injury.

Once all osteophytes have been excised, the anterior aspect of the capsule can be removed. It helps initially to take the capsule off the humerus. This tends also to increase the working space in the anterior compartment. While viewing from the lateral side, the surgeon excises the anterior aspect of the capsule with a shaver or punch. The median nerve is the closest important structure, but it is behind the brachialis muscle. After the capsule has been excised to the midline of the joint, the viewing portal is changed to the medial side, and the shaver is placed through the lateral portal. Care must be taken when the capsule is excised just anterior to the radial head and the capitellum. The radial nerve is at great risk for injury at this location. Often a small

fat pad can be visualized in this area. The radial nerve lies just anterior to this fat pad.

At the end of the procedure, the maximum range of motion of the elbow is evaluated and documented (Fig. 44-8). The elbow should then be placed in an extended position with a compressive dressing. The extended position limits the amount of swelling and accumulation of intra-articular fluid, in contrast to a flexed posture as flexion allows a maximal amount of fluid to collect in the elbow joint. Patients are examined immediately after the surgical procedure, when they are awake in the recovery room, to confirm that the neurovascular status is intact postoperatively.

POSTOPERATIVE CONSIDERATIONS

Rehabilitation

Elevation of the arm into a "Statue of Liberty" position overnight helps limit postoperative swelling. Motion can be delayed for 24 hours to allow edema to resolve. Continuous passive motion (CPM) or splinting can then be started to help maintain the arc of motion achieved in the operating room. CPM is often prescribed for patients who have severely restricted motion preoperatively, and may not be needed for those with a minimal loss of motion. However, there is little evidence to confirm that CPM restores motion better than splints alone or physical therapy. If CPM is used, it is typically applied for 23 hours a day, with breaks for cleaning and eating. The motion setting is started at the same maximum motion achieved in the operating room. We do not start with a gentle range of motion and work up to the range of motion restored in the operating room. CPM can be used with an indwelling axillary block for paralysis and pain control for the first 24 hours, or intravenous narcotics can be used for pain control. One concern over use of CPM under the setting of a regional

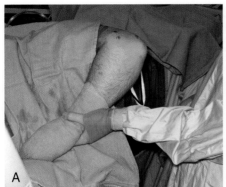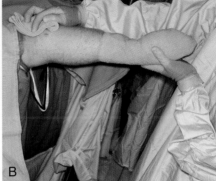

Figure 44-8. A, Intraoperative view demonstrating full flexion after arthroscopic release. **B,** Intraoperative view demonstrating full extension after arthroscopic debridement and release.

TABLE 44-1. Results of Arthroscopic Debridement of the Osteoarthritic Elbow

Study	Population	Results
Cohen et al[15] (2000)	26 Patients	Excellent pain relief, no major complications
Savoie et al[1] (1999)	24 Patients	All had decrease in pain, 81-degree increase in arc of motion
Phillips and Strasburger[16] (1998)	25 Patients	Satisfactory results, increase of 41 degrees in total arc of motion
Kim and Shin[17] (2000)	30 Patients	92% improvement in the range of motion, from a mean of 81 degrees preoperatively to a mean of 121 degrees postoperatively
Adams et al[18] (2007)	41 Patients	81% good to excellent results Postoperative range of motion 8.4 to 131.6 degrees
DeGreef et al[19] (2010)	20 Elbows	Arc of motion improved from 94 to 123 degrees 85% of patients had improvement in symptoms Pain relief was better in mild to moderate arthritis than in severe arthritis

block is potential for nerve injury, particularly referable to the ulnar nerve. We are not aware of any reports on the use of intra-articular catheters to deliver lidocaine or narcotics. CPM, when used, is typically continued for the first 3 or 4 weeks after surgery.

Splinting is also an effective option, and it typically involves alternating periods of extension and flexion. In our practice, static splints are preferred. The patient is taught to alternate periods of flexion and extension, typically for an hour at each end of the range of motion achieved at surgery. The neurovascular status—in particular, the ulnar nerve—should be evaluated at regular intervals during postoperative rehabilitation, especially in patients in whom a significant amount of motion has been restored. Ulnar neuropathy has been noted after arthroscopic or open release in some patients who had 90 degrees or less of flexion preoperatively and in whom surgery restored substantially greater flexion.[8-10]

Complications

Complications of elbow arthroscopy include compartment syndrome, septic arthritis, and nerve injury. In a report of 473 elbow arthroscopies performed by experienced elbow arthroscopists, four types of minor complications, including infection, nerve injury, prolonged drainage, and contracture, were identified in 50 cases.[9] The most common complication was persistent portal drainage, and the most serious was deep infection. Neurologic complications were limited to transient nerve palsies; there were no permanent nerve injuries. Savoie and Field[11] reported a 3% prevalence of neurologic complications in a review of the results of 465 arthroscopy procedures presented in the literature. The rate of permanent neurologic injury appears to be higher in the elbow than in the knee or shoulder, and the risk of nerve injury at the elbow is higher in patients with rheumatoid arthritis or in those undergoing a capsular release.[9] Substantial injury involving the radial, median, and ulnar nerves has been reported during elbow arthroscopy.[12-14] In some cases, arthroscopic identification of nerves allows safe capsulectomy. This is particularly true with regard to the ulnar nerve.

Results

Few reports of arthroscopic debridement for treatment of osteoarthritis or rheumatoid arthritis of the elbow

TABLE 44-2. Results of Arthroscopic Debridement of the Rheumatoid Elbow

Study	Population	Results
Lee and Morrey[20] (1997)	14 Patients	93% good to excellent MEP scores At longer follow-up (average, 42 months) results deteriorated, with only 57% good to excellent
Horiuchi et al[21] (2002)	21 Elbows followed for >42 months	Most favorable results seen in Larsen grades 1 and 2 elbows
Nemoto et al[22] (2004)	11 Patients followed after arthroscopic synovectomy (mean 37 months)	Pain relief and satisfactory functional results noted in all Larsen grades
Kang et al[23] (2010)	26 Elbows with Larsen grade ≤3 changes underwent arthroscopic synovectomy, followed for 34 months	Improvements in pain, MEP scores, and motion noted Some patients experienced recurrence of synovitis
Chalmers et al[4] (2011)	Comparison of arthroscopic and open synovectomy in the setting of rheumatoid arthritis	Similar improvements postoperatively in pain between the two groups, but recurrent synovitis and progression of radiographic findings occurred more often in the arthroscopic cohort

MEP, Mayo Elbow Performance.

are available (Tables 44-1 and 44-2). The current literature has shown satisfactory results with increases in range of motion and improvement of pain. With rheumatoid arthritis, recurrent synovitis and radiographic progression may occur, and results may be poorer with more advanced Larsen grades. Nevertheless, these studies suggest that arthroscopic debridement of the arthritic elbow is a reasonable option.[4,5,7,19-24]

REFERENCES

1. Savoie F, Nunley PD, Field LD. Arthroscopic management of the arthritic elbow: indications, technique, and results. *J Shoulder Elbow Surg.* 1999;8:214-219.
2. Steinmann SP. Elbow arthroscopy. *J Am Soc Surg Hand.* 2003;3:199-207.
3. O'Driscoll SW. Elbow arthritis. *J Am Acad Orthop Surg.* 1993;1:106-116.
4. Chalmers PN, Sherman SL, Raphael BS, et al. Rheumatoid synovectomy: does the surgical approach matter? *Clin Orthop Relat Res.* 2011;469(7):2062-2071.
5. Yeoh KM, King GJ, Faber KJ, et al. Evidence-based indications for elbow arthroscopy. *Arthroscopy.* 2012;28(2):272-282.
6. Adams JE, Reding MT. Hemophilic arthropathy of the elbow. *Hand Clin.* 2011;27(2):151-163.
7. van den Ende KI, McIntosh AL, Adams JE, et al. Osteochondritis dissecans of the capitellum: a review of the literature and a distal ulnar portal. *Arthroscopy.* 2011;27(1):122-128.
8. Aldridge JM 3rd, Atkins TA, Gunneson EE, et al. Anterior release of the elbow for extension loss. *J Bone Joint Surg Am.* 2004;86:1955-1960.
9. Kelly EW, Morrey BF, O'Driscoll SW. Complications of elbow arthroscopy. *J Bone Joint Surg Am.* 2001;83:25-34.
10. Wright TW, Glowczewskie F Jr, Cowin D, et al. Ulnar nerve excursion and strain at the elbow and wrist associated with upper extremity motion. *J Hand Surg Am.* 2001;26:655-662.
11. Savoie F, Field LD. Complications of elbow arthroscopy. In: Savoie F, Field LD, eds. *Arthroscopy of the Elbow.* New York: Churchill Livingstone; 1996:151-156.
12. Hahn M, Grossman JA. Ulnar nerve laceration as a result of elbow arthroscopy. *J Hand Surg Br.* 1998;23:109.
13. Papilion JD, Neff RS, Shall LM. Compression neuropathy of the radial nerve as a complication of elbow arthroscopy: a case report and review of the literature. *Arthroscopy.* 1998;4:284-286.
14. Thomas MA, Fast A, Shapiro D. Radial nerve damage as a complication of elbow arthroscopy. *Clin Orthop Relat Res.* 1987;215:130-131.
15. Cohen AP, Redden JF, Stanley D. Treatment of osteoarthritis of the elbow: a comparison of open and arthroscopic debridement. *Arthroscopy.* 2000;16:701-706.
16. Phillips BB, Strasburger S. Arthroscopic treatment of arthrofibrosis of the elbow joint. *Arthroscopy.* 1998;14:38-44.
17. Kim SJ, Shin SJ. Arthroscopic treatment for limitation of motion of the elbow. *Clin Orthop Relat Res.* 2000;375:140-148.
18. Adams JE, Wolff LH III, Merten SM, et al. *Osteoarthritis of the elbow: results of arthroscopic osteophyte resection and capsulectomy.* Podium Presentation, Twenty-Third Annual Open Meeting of the American Shoulder and Elbow Surgeons, February 17, 2007, San Diego, California.
19. DeGreef I, Samorjai N, De Smet L. The Outerbridge-Kashiwaghi procedure in elbow arthroscopy. *Acta Orthop Belg.* 2010;76(4):468-471.
20. Lee BP, Morrey BF. Arthroscopic synovectomy of the elbow for rheumatoid arthritis. A prospective study. *J Bone Joint Surg Br.* 1997;79(5):770-772.

21. Horiuchi K, Momohara S, Tomatsu T, et al. Arthoscopic synovectomy of the elbow in rheumatoid arthritis. *J Bone Surg Am.* 2002;84(3):342-347.

22. Nemoto K, Arino H, Yoshihara Y, et al. Arthroscopic synovectomy for the rheumatoid elbow: a short-term outcome. *J Shoulder Elbow Surg.* 2004;13(6):652-655.

23. Kang HJ, Park MJ, Ahn JH, et al. Arthroscopic synovectomy for the rheumatoid elbow. *Arthroscopy.* 2010;26(9):1195-1202.

24. Savoie FH 3rd, O'Brien MJ, Field LD. Arthroscopy for arthritis of the elbow. *Hand Clin.* 2011;27(2):171-178.

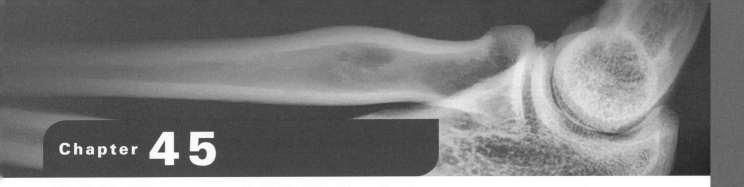

Arthroscopic Treatment of Lateral Epicondylitis

Christian Lattermann, Anthony A. Romeo, Brian J. Cole, and D. Jeff Covell

Chapter Synopsis

- Lateral epicondylitis refractory to conservative management may benefit from arthroscopic release of the extensor carpi radialis brevis (ECRB) origin. This more recently described technique offers the benefit of direct visualization of the pathologic process, addresses concomitant intra-articular disease, is minimally invasive, and is well tolerated by patients. This chapter discusses the approach, relevant anatomy, and technique for arthroscopic release of the ECRB tendon, as well as postoperative management and outcomes.

Important Points

- Debridement is indicated for patients refractory to conservative therapy who have no contraindications to elbow arthroscopy.
- The ECRB tendon inserts on the superior aspect of the capitellum and extends distally to the midline of the radiocapitellar joint.
- Care must be taken during debridement to avoid accidental resection of the lateral collateral ligament and extensor digitorum communis.

Clinical and Surgical Pearls

Visualization

- In case of a capacious anterior capsule that tends to obstruct viewing from the medial portal, a small key elevator can be inserted through a high anterolateral accessory portal to elevate the anterolateral capsule, greatly enhancing visualization from the medial portal.

Clinical and Surgical Pitfalls

Debridement

- The resection of the capsule and the ECRB should not extend farther distally than the midline of the radiocapitellar joint. Resection past this landmark puts the lateral collateral ligament at risk.
- Once the debridement of the ECRB has been performed, do not debride the extensor digitorum communis. Debridement of the extensor digitorum communis and extensor aponeurosis can result in synovial fistula.

Lateral epicondylitis is a well-known musculoskeletal phenomenon that can occur after minor trauma or chronic overuse. In general, lateral epicondylitis responds well to nonoperative management, including activity modification, counterforce bracing, physical therapy, and corticosteroid injections. A relatively small number of patients, however, have refractory symptoms. In such situations an operative procedure may be warranted. Many different operative techniques have been developed for the treatment of lateral epicondylitis. The goal of this chapter is to describe a more recent technique—arthroscopic extensor carpi radialis brevis (ECRB) release. We believe that this technique is advantageous because it offers direct visualization of the pathologic process, enables the surgeon to concomitantly address intra-articular disease, and is minimally invasive in nature and thus well tolerated by the patient.

PREOPERATIVE CONSIDERATIONS

History

Typical History

- Traumatic onset (usually minor trauma) aggravated by repetitive motion.
- Insidious onset—chronic repetitive wrist and elbow motion at work or recreationally.
- Tenderness directly over the origin of the ECRB on the lateral epicondyle.
- Aggravation of symptoms with active resisted wrist extension and passive wrist flexion.
- Often previously treated with nonoperative measures.
- Pain with range of motion of the elbow and clicking may point to associated joint disease.

Physical Examination

Factors Affecting Surgical Indication

- Range of motion—should be normal
- Clicking with range of motion (synovial plica)
- Effusion (intra-articular disease)

Factors Affecting Surgical Planning

- Previous ulnar nerve transposition
- Ulnohumeral or radiocapitellar arthritis
- Previous distal humerus or olecranon fracture

It is important to perform a thorough neurovascular examination to rule out entrapment of the posterior interosseous nerve, subluxation of the ulnar nerve, or degenerative changes in the radiocapitellar joint.

Imaging

Radiography

- Anteroposterior view of the elbow in full extension
- Lateral view of the elbow in 90 degrees of flexion

Optional Views

- Axial view to outline the olecranon and its articulations
- Radial head view

Other Modalities

- Magnetic resonance imaging with or without the administration of gadolinium

Magnetic resonance imaging will demonstrate degenerative changes in the origin of the ECRB; it may show a synovial plica in the radiocapitellar joint when it is performed with the administration of contrast material. Visualization of loose bodies is generally better with magnetic resonance images than with plain radiographs, which will display loose bodies in only 25% of patients.

Indications and Contraindications

The ideal patient has localized symptoms directly anterior and inferior to the lateral epicondyle at the origin of the ECRB and has full range of motion. Conservative treatment options have failed.

Contraindications are those generally associated with elbow arthroscopy. These include significant alterations of the normal bone anatomy, previous placement of hardware, ankylosis of the elbow joint, acute or chronic soft tissue infections, and osteomyelitis of the elbow.

SURGICAL TECHNIQUE

Anesthesia and Positioning

The patient is placed in the supine, prone, or lateral decubitus position, according to the surgeon's preference for elbow arthroscopy. The procedure can be performed with the patient under general anesthesia or with regional block with simple sedation. However, some patients may not tolerate the prone position under sedation alone because of unrelated issues, such as shoulder pain in the ipsilateral or contralateral shoulder.

The patient is positioned prone with the arm hanging over the side in 90 degrees of abduction and neutral rotation (Fig. 45-1). Care needs to be taken that the arm is not abducted more than 90 degrees and that the shoulder is not hyperextended, to minimize the risk of neurovascular complications. A nonsterile tourniquet is used with inflation pressures of 200 to 250 mm Hg

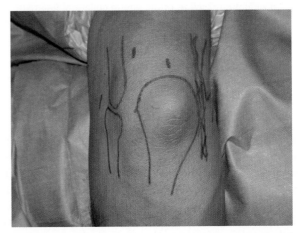

Figure 45-1. Patient in the prone position. Note that the arm is hanging down, thus avoiding hyperextension of the shoulder.

according to the size of the arm and systolic blood pressure. The procedure can be performed with the surgeon either standing or seated, and the operating table is adjusted accordingly.

Surgical Landmarks, Incisions, and Portals

Landmarks

- Tip of olecranon process
- Lateral epicondyle
- Medial epicondyle
- Ulnar nerve (test for subluxation)
- Radial head and radiocapitellar joint

Portals and Approaches

- Insufflation of joint with 30 mL of saline by use of a spinal needle
- Proximal medial viewing portal
- Proximal lateral portal
- Posterior superior portal (optional if there is posterior synovitis)
- Direct lateral (soft-spot) portal (optional if there is radial head or capitellar disease)

Structures at Risk

- Proximal medial portal: ulnar nerve
- Proximal lateral portal: lateral antebrachial cutaneous nerve
- Excessive release: lateral ulnar collateral ligament, posterior interosseous nerve

Examination Under Anesthesia and Diagnostic Arthroscopy

Examination under anesthesia should evaluate range of motion and ligamentous stability. Diagnostic arthroscopy is useful to evaluate other intra-articular disease, such as loose bodies, ligamentous deficiency, or chondral defects.

Specific Steps

Specific steps of this procedure are outlined in Box 45-1.

BOX 45-1 Surgical Steps

1. Portal placement
2. Diagnostic arthroscopy
3. Debridement of (ECRB) origin and release of ECRB
4. Closure

ECRB, Extensor carpi radialis brevis.

---

1. Portal Placement

Before any portals are placed, a thorough manual palpation of the olecranon tip, the radiocapitellar joint, the lateral medial epicondyle, and the ulnar nerve is performed. Particular attention is needed to determine whether the patient has ulnar nerve subluxation. The landmarks are marked clearly (Fig. 45-2). A sterile or nonsterile tourniquet is necessary and should be inflated before any portals are placed.

Then saline solution, 30 mL, is instilled into the soft spot of the triangle formed among the tip of the olecranon, the lateral epicondyle, and the radial head. Visible distention of the joint and backflow through the injection needle (18 gauge) confirm intra-articular instillation.

For the proximal medial viewing portal, the medial epicondyle and the medial intermuscular septum are directly palpated. At approximately 2 cm proximal to the medial epicondyle and 1 cm anterior to the medial intermuscular septum, a small skin incision is made with a No. 15 blade. A small hemostat is used to spread carefully down to the capsule, thus avoiding injury to the cutaneous sensory nerves. With the elbow maintained in 90 degrees of flexion and neutral rotation, the cannula with a blunt trocar is then introduced by sliding along the anterior surface of the distal humerus, aiming toward the radiocapitellar joint. Subsequently the proximal lateral portal is established approximately 2 cm proximal and 2 cm anterior to the lateral epicondyle. The correct position of the portal is verified under direct vision by use of a spinal needle. Once the position has been verified, the "nick and spread" technique is again used, and a blunt Wissinger rod is positioned to serve as a guide for a small 5-mm threaded arthroscopic cannula. An additional superior lateral portal can be helpful if the anterior capsule is capacious. A small key elevator can be inserted through this accessory portal

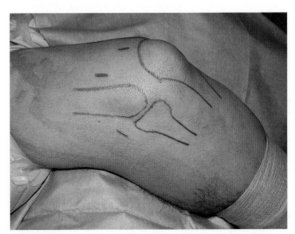

Figure 45-2. The portals and landmarks are clearly marked. The elbow can be accessed freely from the medial, lateral, and posterior directions.

and used to elevate the anterolateral capsule, greatly enhancing visualization from the medial portal.

2. Diagnostic Arthroscopy

Routine diagnostic arthroscopy is performed. If any pathologic process is suspected in the ulnohumeral joint, a posterior portal is established to evaluate the ulnar and radial recesses. The radiocapitellar joint is evaluated for, among other entities, a soft tissue band or plica overriding the radius with pronation and supination, because this can be a cause of impingement. The lateral joint capsule and the insertion of the ECRB are assessed under direct vision. We prefer to grade ECRB involvement according to the grading suggested by Baker and colleagues.[1]

3. Debridement of ECRB Origin and Release of ECRB

A thorough appreciation of the anatomy of the elbow, and of the ECRB in particular, is paramount to mastering this arthroscopic technique. The ECRB origin is extra-articular, thus necessitating the resection of the capsule adjacent to the capitellum for visualization of the ECRB origin. We prefer to perform the resection sequentially in four steps, resulting in a diamond-shaped resection zone (Fig. 45-3).[2,3]

Step 1

For visualization of the ECRB, the overlying anterolateral capsule must be removed, although in some patients the capsule will already be torn, revealing the origin. The margins of the resection extend superiorly from the top of the capitellum to distally at the level of the

midline of the radiocapitellar joint. If the resection extends farther distal than the midline of the radiocapitellar joint, the lateral collateral ligament is at risk.

Step 2

After adequate exposure has been obtained, we turn our attention to resection of the ECRB origin. We start at the superior aspect of the capitellum, which represents the proximal and anterior margin of the resection. In a probing motion with a monopolar or bipolar radiofrequency probe, we resect the tendinous bands that represent the ECRB origin until we expose the red muscle fibers of the extensor carpi radialis longus.

Step 3

We then continue the resection anteroinferiorly. The posteroinferior border of the resection is marked by the lateral collateral ligament. One has to be careful to visualize the lateral collateral ligament. This is often easier once the semicircular fibers that cross from the lateral collateral to the annular radial ligament are visualized. Gravity inflow or the pump pressure can help with joint distention that separates the tendon from the lateral collateral ligament. The resection is performed under direct vision with the scope in the anteromedial portal (Fig. 45-4).

Step 4

The posterior aspect of the diamond-shaped resection zone is formed by the tendon of the extensor digitorum communis. The resection is carried up to the extensor digitorum communis tendon but not past it. There is a distinct fibrous band curving over top of the ECRB that constitutes the extensor aponeurosis. This band must

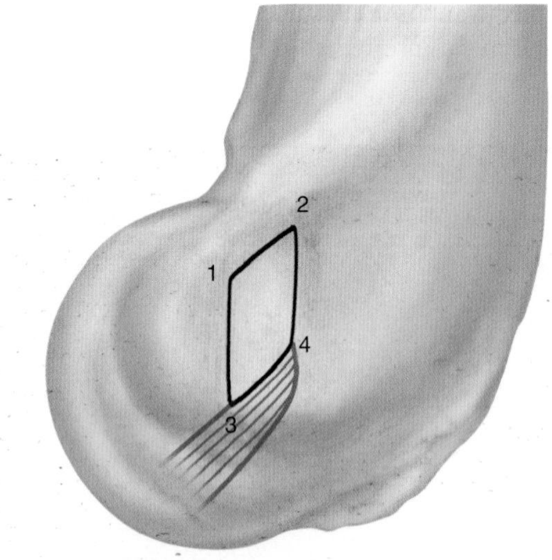

Figure 45-3. A diamond-shaped resection zone on the lateral epicondyle is debrided to perform a full resection of the extensor carpi radialis brevis origin. The lateral border is taken down to but not into the lateral collateral ligament. Steps 1 to 4 mark the sequence of the debridement zone.

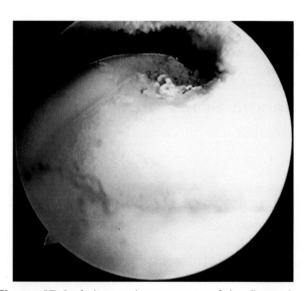

Figure 45-4. Arthroscopic appearance of the diamond-shaped resection zone after debridement.

not be cut because this could result in a subcutaneous fistula. The total area of debridement is approximately 13 × 7 mm.[4] The capsule is not repaired.

4. Closure

Standard closure of the portals is performed.

POSTOPERATIVE CONSIDERATIONS

Rehabilitation

- Sling for comfort
- Finger, wrist, and elbow motion as tolerated

- No lifting or gripping activities until follow-up (7 to 10 days)
- Continued range-of-motion and very light gripping exercises at 10 days
- No resistive exercises until after 3 or 4 weeks, if pain free
- Full use of the arm without restrictions at 6 to 12 weeks

Complications

Complications are those of elbow arthroscopy:

- Ulnar or lateral antebrachial cutaneous nerve damage caused by portal placement

TABLE 45-1. Clinical Results of Arthroscopic Treatment of Lateral Epicondylitis

Study	Follow-up	Population	Outcome
Baker et al[1] (2000)	2.8 years	42 patients	VAS pain: 0.9/10 Grip strength: 96% Return to work at 2.2 weeks
Baker and Baker[5] (2008)	10.8 years	30 patients	63% intra-articular pathology Nirschl pain phase scale: 0 (rest) Mayo score: 11.7/12 87% satisfied with results at long-term follow-up
Cummins[9] (2006)	1.8 years	18 patients	VAS pain: 1.6/10 (rest) Completeness of arthroscopic ECRB debridement comparable to that of open procedure
Grewal et al[10] (2009)	3.5 years	36 patients	VAS satisfaction: 8/10 Average total PRTEE score: 26.2/100 ASES-e score: 16.1/50 (pain), 27.9/50 (function) Grip strength improvement of 27.3%
Jerosch and Schunck[2] (2006)	1.8 years	20 patients	VAS pain: 0.5 (rest) Mayo score: 10.9/12 Average return to work after 3.2 weeks
Lattermann et al[11] (2010)	3.5 years	36 patients	VAS pain: 1.9/10 Mayo score: 11.1 Grip strength: 91% 88% reported satisfactory outcome Average return to work: 3.8 weeks
Orthman et al[12] (2011)	1 year	14 patients treated by arthroscopy	VAS pain: 2/10 DASH Outcome Measure score: 48/100 92.85% pleased or satisfied
Owens et al[13] (2001)	2 years	16 patients	VAS pain: 0.59/10 Average return to work at 6 days
Peart et al[14] (2004)	2 years	33 patients treated arthroscopically	72% good and excellent results compared with 69% by open treatment Earlier return to work for arthroscopically treated patients
Szabo et al[8] (2006)	4 years	41 patients	44% of arthroscopically treated patients had intra-articular pathology Andrews-Carson elbow score: 195.4
Wada et al[15] (2009)	2.3 years	18 patients, 20 elbows	VAS pain: 0.3/10 (rest) DASH Outcome Measure score: 10.6/100 JOA score: 90/100 Average return to work: 3.4 weeks

ASES-e, American Shoulder and Elbow Surgeons Elbow form; *DASH,* Disabilities of the Arm, Shoulder and Hand; *ECRB,* extensor carpi radialis brevis; *JOA,* Japanese Orthopedic Association; *Mayo score,* Mayo Clinic Elbow Performance Index; *PRTEE,* Patient-Rated Tennis Elbow Evaluation; *VAS,* visual analogue scale.

- Posterior interosseous nerve or collateral ligament damage caused by excessive release
- Infection
- Synovial fistula

RESULTS

After debridement for lateral epicondylitis, good to excellent results are achieved in 85% to 90% of patients. The results of arthroscopic debridement are certainly comparable, and the arthroscopic approach has the additional benefit of being able to address concomitant disease that does exist in approximately 30% of patients, with higher incidence reported in some studies.[1,5-8] Patients often are immediately pain free and can return to work in 1 to 3 weeks, depending on their physical category of work (Table 45-1).

REFERENCES

1. Baker CL Jr, Murphy KP, Gottlob CA, et al. Arthroscopic classification and treatment of lateral epicondylitis: two-year clinical results. *J Shoulder Elbow Surg.* 2000;9: 475-482.
2. Jerosch J, Schunck J. Arthroscopic treatment of lateral epicondylitis: Indication, technique and early results. *Knee Surg Sports Traumatol Arthrosc.* 2006;14:379-382.
3. Cohen M, Romeo AA. Lateral epicondylitis: open and arthroscopic treatment. *J Am Soc Surg Hand.* 2001;3: 172-176.
4. Cohen MS, Romeo AA, Hennigan SP, et al. Lateral epicondylitis: Anatomic relationships of the extensor origins and implications for arthroscopic treatment. *J Shoulder Elbow Surg.* 2008;17:954-960.
5. Baker CL Jr, Baker CL 3rd. Long-term follow-up of arthroscopic treatment of lateral epicondylitis. *Am J Sports Med.* 2008;36:254-260.
6. Kuklo TR, Taylor KF, Murphy KP, et al. Arthroscopic release for lateral epicondylitis: a cadaveric model. *Arthroscopy.* 1999;15:259-264.
7. Mullett H, Sprague M, Brown G, et al. Arthroscopic treatment of lateral epicondylitis: clinical and cadaveric studies. *Clin Orthop Relat Res.* 2005;439:123-128.
8. Szabo SJ, Savoie FH 3rd, Field LD, et al. Tendinosis of the extensor carpi radialis brevis: an evaluation of three methods of operative treatment. *J Shoulder Elbow Surg.* 2006;15:721-727.
9. Cummins CA. Lateral epicondylitis: in vivo assessment of arthroscopic debridement and correlation with patient outcomes. *Am J Sports Med.* 2006;34:1486-1491.
10. Grewal R, MacDermid JC, Shah P, et al. Functional outcome of arthroscopic extensor carpi radialis brevis tendon release in chronic lateral epicondylitis. *J Hand Surg Am.* 2009;34:849-857.
11. Lattermann C, Romeo AA, Anbari A, et al. Arthroscopic debridement of the extensor carpi radialis brevis for recalcitrant lateral epicondylitis. *J Shoulder Elbow Surg.* 2010;19:651-656.
12. Othman AM. Arthroscopic versus percutaneous release of common extensor origin for treatment of chronic tennis elbow. *Arch Orthop Trauma Surg.* 2011;131: 383-388.
13. Owens BD, Murphy KP, Kuklo TR. Arthroscopic release for lateral epicondylitis. *Arthroscopy.* 2001;17:582-587.
14. Peart RE, Strickler SS, Schweitzer KM Jr. Lateral epicondylitis: a comparative study of open and arthroscopic lateral release. *Am J Orthop.* 2004;33:565-567.
15. Wada T, Moriya T, Iba K, et al. Functional outcomes after arthroscopic treatment of lateral epicondylitis. *J Orthop Sci.* 2009;14:167-174.

Chapter 46

Ulnar Collateral Ligament Repair and Reconstruction

| Part **1** | **Ulnar Collateral Ligament Repair** |

Champ L. Baker Jr and Champ L. Baker III

Chapter Synopsis

- Traditional operative treatment of ulnar collateral ligament (UCL) injury in the throwing athlete consists of reconstruction with autogenous graft. However, some athletes can have UCL injury isolated to either the humeral or ulnar insertion without significant attritional, degenerative changes. Such patients may be candidates for a direct, primary ligament repair, which could allow earlier return to competition than a reconstruction with similar high rates of success.

Important Points

- For repair, patients must have injury isolated to either the humeral or the ulnar insertion or both, with no significant ligament damage.

- The surgeon and patient should both be alert to the possibility of a reconstruction based on intraoperative findings.

- The surgeon should assess the patient for concurrent pathology, such as ulnar nerve irritation and posteromedial impingement.

Clinical and Surgical Pitfalls

- To avoid compression of the ulnar nerve when the flexor muscle tendon split is performed, do not use a retractor against the bone inferiorly.

- When sutures are passed through the ligament proper posteriorly, care should be taken to avoid the ulnar nerve.

- The ligament may also be repaired back to the humeral insertion through drill holes. An adequate bone bridge should be maintained to avoid fracture and inadequate fixation.

Injury to the medial side of the elbow is common in overhead athletes, such as baseball pitchers, tennis players, and javelin throwers. The overhead throwing motion places tremendous valgus stress on the elbow that is resisted by the medial structures. The anterior bundle of the ulnar collateral ligament (UCL) has been shown to be the primary restraint to valgus stress about the elbow.[1] Repeated high valgus stresses imparted from the repetitive act of throwing can result in chronic attenuation or acute rupture of the UCL. In the throwing athlete, UCL insufficiency can manifest as disabling elbow pain with the inability to compete effectively. Various techniques of UCL reconstruction have been reported with high rates of success in returning the athlete to competition; however, an increased incidence of UCL injuries in younger patients has led to consideration of primary repair as a surgical option. Many young athletes may have injury that is isolated to either the humeral or the ulnar insertion and thus is amenable to direct repair, perhaps allowing earlier return to sport. Recent reports have detailed high rates of success in early follow-up.[2,3] Constants in operative management include an accurate diagnosis, careful patient selection, anatomic repair of the UCL insertion, and maintenance of a specific rehabilitation program to allow the athlete to return successfully to sport.

PREOPERATIVE CONSIDERATIONS

History

The typical history in a throwing athlete with UCL injury is episodic medial elbow pain that prevents him or her from competing effectively. Pain is usually elicited in the early acceleration phase of throwing. Affected pitchers complain of loss of velocity or accuracy. On occasion the athlete will sustain an acute injury with sudden onset of medial pain accompanied by a "pop" followed by an inability to continue throwing. Less commonly, patients report a history of a fall on an outstretched hand or direct trauma to the elbow followed by medial elbow pain and swelling.[2] Symptoms of ulnar nerve irritability, such as paresthesias, in the little and ring fingers can also be present.

Physical Examination

A thorough physical examination of the throwing athlete includes the following:

- Evaluation of the neck and entire upper extremity
- Direct assessment of the ulnar nerve for subluxation, irritability (presence of Tinel sign), and integrity of distal motor and sensory function in the hand

Tenderness may be present and elicited over the UCL ligament slightly distal and posterior to the flexor-pronator muscle origin.

Several tests have been described to evaluate the integrity of the UCL:

- Manual valgus stress test performed at 30 degrees of elbow flexion
- "Milking maneuver"[4]
- Moving valgus stress test[5]

These tests may elicit medial elbow pain with valgus stress, or the examiner may appreciate medial joint line opening with stress especially in comparison with the contralateral elbow. The possible presence of concurrent posteromedial impingement in the thrower's elbow can be evaluated with the valgus extension overload test.[6]

Imaging

Radiography

- Anteroposterior, lateral, and axial views of the elbow

Plain radiographs are inspected for loose bodies; evidence of degenerative changes, such as posteromedial osteophytes of the olecranon; medial joint line spurring; and possible calcifications in the UCL that are indicative of a chronic injury.

Other Modalities

- Computed tomographic arthrography
- Magnetic resonance imaging

We prefer magnetic resonance imaging for detailed characterization of the integrity of the UCL and evaluation of other soft tissue structures.

Indications and Contraindications

The indication for UCL repair in a throwing athlete is medial elbow pain associated with UCL insufficiency that prevents the athlete from competing effectively. Injury isolated to either the UCL humeral or ulnar insertion without other ligament damage on inspection may be effectively treated with repair. If at the time of surgery the ligament is found to have chronic attenuation or damage, then a reconstruction rather than repair should be performed. Athletes who do not plan on returning to sport and those who are able to return to sport after rehabilitation and do not subject their elbows to repeated valgus stress are not generally considered candidates for operative intervention.

SURGICAL TECHNIQUE
Anesthesia and Positioning

We prefer to perform the procedure with the patient under general anesthesia, although, based on the preferences of the surgeon, patient, and anesthesiologist, regional anesthesia or a combination of general and regional anesthesia can be used. The patient is placed supine on the operating table with the affected extremity abducted and placed on an attached hand table. A sterile or nonsterile pneumatic tourniquet is placed about the arm as proximal as possible for exposure. The arm is then prepared and draped in the usual sterile fashion.

If an arthroscopic procedure is required for concurrent posterior impingement or posteromedial ulnar osteophyte excision, we perform arthroscopy first with the patient in the supine position with the arm suspended by a commercially available arm holder.

Surgical Landmarks and Incision

The palpable medial epicondyle is identified, and an approximately 8- to 10-cm curvilinear incision is centered over the medial epicondyle. During the exposure, care is taken to identify and to protect the branches of the medial antebrachial cutaneous nerve that cross the operative field. Injury to these nerves can result in either sensory loss along the medial aspect of the forearm or a painful neuroma.

Specific Steps

See Box 46-1.

1. Exposure

Dissection is carried down to the level of the forearm fascia and the flexor-pronator aponeurosis (Fig. 46-1). We prefer the muscle-splitting approach[7] for exposure of the UCL. A fascial raphe can usually be identified in the flexor-pronator mass at the junction of the anterior two thirds and posterior third of the muscle group. This raphe represents an internervous plane between the median nerve–innervated palmaris longus and deeper flexor digitorum superficialis and the ulnar nerve–innervated flexor carpi ulnaris. The fascia is split through the raphe from the medial epicondyle to a point

approximately 1 cm distal to the sublime tubercle. The sublime tubercle can be palpated deep under the flexor mass. More distal dissection risks denervation of the surrounding musculature from crossing nerve branches. The muscle is then bluntly divided down to the level of the underlying UCL (Fig. 46-2). Care is taken during the split and division of the muscle because the ulnar nerve lies just posterior to the approach. A blunt self-retainer is used to retract the musculature, and a small periosteal elevator can be used to clean any remaining muscle fibers from the UCL.

2. Ligament Assessment

The UCL is thoroughly inspected for tearing and overall tissue quality. The humeral and ulnar insertions are carefully evaluated based on preoperative imaging (Fig. 46-3). After external inspection of the ligament, a longitudinal incision is made in the direction of its fibers to assess undersurface tears and degeneration. If the ligament is found to have midsubstance tearing, significant degeneration, or poor tissue quality, a reconstruction should be performed instead of repair.

BOX 46-1 Surgical Steps

- Exposure
- Ligament assessment
- Ligament repair
- Closure

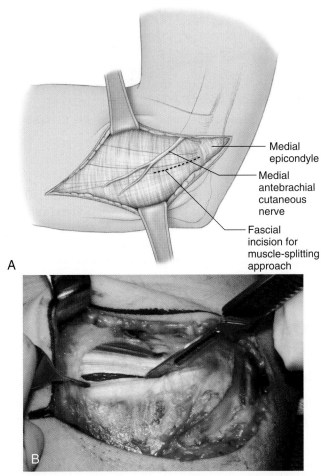

Figure 46-1. Muscle-splitting incision through fascia to expose the ulnar collateral ligament.

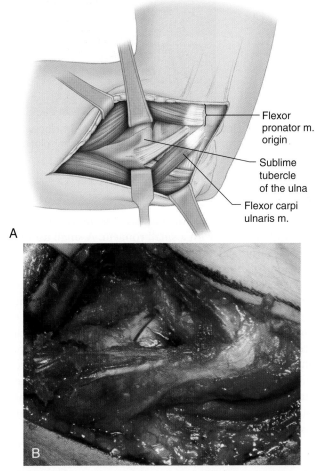

Figure 46-2. Approach to the ulnar collateral ligament. Application of valgus stress demonstrates medial joint line opening.

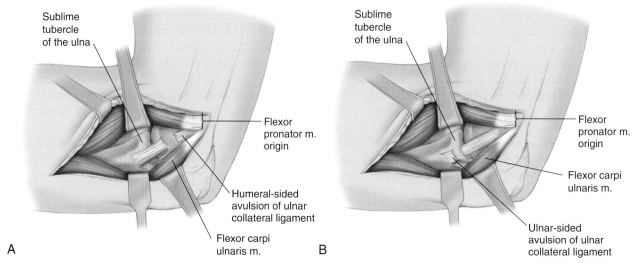

Figure 46-3. Humeral disruption **(A)** and ulnar disruption **(B)** of the ulnar collateral ligament. Medial aspect of the joint is exposed.

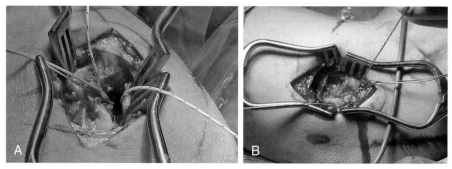

Figure 46-4. Intraoperative images **(A)** of right elbow with suture anchor placed in the humeral insertion site to repair humeral-sided avulsion and **(B)** after suture anchor placement of humeral avulsion is complete.

3. Ligament Repair

For humeral avulsions, the native ligament insertion site is gently prepared with a small rongeur. A small double-loaded suture anchor is placed at the apex of the V junction of the trochlea and medial epicondyle as described by Savoie and colleagues[3] (Fig. 46-4A). Currently we use 2.9-mm Bioraptor suture anchors (Smith & Nephew Endoscopy, Andover, MA). Both sets of sutures are placed in horizontal mattress fashion in the proximal ligament and tied (Fig. 46-4B). Similarly, for ulnar avulsions the sublime tubercle is gently prepared with a small rongeur. A double-loaded anchor is placed into the sublime tubercle, and both sets of sutures are passed in mattress fashion in the most distal aspect of healthy ligament and tied.

4. Closure

The tourniquet is deflated, and meticulous hemostasis is obtained to prevent a postoperative hematoma. The wound is thoroughly irrigated before closure. The flexor-pronator mass is closed with No. 0 Vicryl suture, followed by routine skin closure. A sterile dressing is applied, and the arm is splinted in approximately 90 degrees of flexion with the forearm in neutral rotation.

POSTOPERATIVE CONSIDERATIONS

Rehabilitation

The splint is removed after 1 week, and the elbow is placed in a hinged brace to initially allow 30 degrees of extension. Range of motion is progressed to full motion over the next month. Light resistance exercises are instituted for the wrist and forearm, along with initiation of core strengthening, scapular stabilization,

TABLE 46-1. Results of Ulnar Collateral Ligament (UCL) Repair

Author	Follow-Up	Results	Comments
Azar et al[8] (2000)	Average 35 months	5/8 (63%) patients returned to same or higher level of competition	Authors do not recommend isolated UCL repair.
Conway et al[9] (1992)	Average 6.3 years	7/14 (50%) patients returned to same or higher level of competition	Authors more confident of a satisfactory result after reconstruction than after repair.
Richard et al[2] (2008)	Minimum 16 months	9/11 (82%) athletes with acute traumatic valgus instability treated with direct UCL and flexor pronator repair returned to athletics	All patients had humeral-side avulsion of UCL and flexor-pronator disruption.
Norwood et al[10] (1981)	20-26 months	4 patients with acute valgus traumatic instability treated with direct UCL and flexor pronator repair	All patients returned to full activities with normal motion and no symptoms of residual instability.

and rotator cuff strengthening exercises. Internal rotation strengthening is avoided until approximately 10 weeks. Patients begin sport-specific rehabilitation and light plyometrics at this time. Patients are allowed to throw beginning at 12 weeks. Throwing is advanced, with return to sport typically at 6 months after surgery.

Complications

- Ulnar nerve irritation
- Hematoma
- Superficial or deep infection
- Loss of motion

RESULTS

There are limited reports in the literature regarding outcomes after UCL repair (Table 46-1), especially in comparison to results after UCL reconstruction. Several reports detailing results after UCL reconstruction have included small numbers of patients treated with repair.[8,9] In the largest series to date, Savoie and colleagues[3] reported on 60 patients with a mean age of 17.2 years who underwent repair of the UCL and were followed for an average of 59 months after surgery. Based on the Andrews-Carson rating, good to excellent results were found in 93% of patients, and 58 patients were able to return to the same or a higher level of sport. The results of UCL repair are best measured by the athlete's return to sport.

REFERENCES

1. Callaway GH, Field LD, Deng XH, et al. Biomechanical evaluation of the medial collateral ligament of the elbow. *J Bone Joint Surg Am*. 1997;79:1223-1231.
2. Richard MJ, Aldridge 3rd JM, Wiesler ER, et al. Traumatic valgus instability of the elbow: pathoanatomy and results of direct repair. *J Bone Joint Surg Am*. 2008;90:2416-2422.
3. Savoie 3rd FH, Trenhaile SW, Roberts J, et al. Primary repair of ulnar collateral ligament injuries of the elbow in young athletes: a case series of injuries to the proximal and distal ends of the ligament. *Am J Sports Med*. 2008;36:1066-1072.
4. Veltri DM, O'Brien SJ, Field LD, et al. The milking maneuver: a new test to evaluate the MCL of the elbow in the throwing athlete [abstract]. *J Shoulder Elbow Surg*. 1995;4:S10.
5. O'Driscoll SW, Lawton RL, Smith AM. The "moving valgus stress test" for medial collateral ligament tears of the elbow. *Am J Sports Med*. 2005;33:231-239.
6. Andrews JR, Whiteside JA, Buettner CM. Clinical evaluation of the elbow in throwers. *Oper Tech Sports Med*. 1996;4:77-83.
7. Smith GR, Altchek DW, Pagnani MJ, et al. A muscle splitting approach to the ulnar collateral ligament of the elbow: neuroanatomy and operative technique. *Am J Sports Med*. 1996;24:575-580.
8. Azar FM, Andrews JR, Wilk KE, et al. Operative treatment of ulnar collateral ligament injuries of the elbow in athletes. *Am J Sports Med*. 2000;28:16-23.
9. Conway JE, Jobe FW, Glousman RE, et al. Medial instability of the elbow in throwing athletes: treatment by repair or reconstruction of the ulnar collateral ligament. *J Bone Joint Surg Am*. 1992;74:67-83.
10. Norwood LA, Shook JA, Andrews JR. Acute medial elbow ruptures. *Am J Sports Med*. 1981;9:16-19.

Part 2 Docking Technique

Christopher C. Dodson, Joshua S. Dines, and David W. Altchek

Chapter Synopsis
- The docking technique has resulted in excellent outcomes for athletes at all levels of play and has proven to be a minimally invasive and reliable method of reconstruction of the ulnar collateral ligament (UCL).

Important Points
- The palmaris longus and gracilis tendons are ideal grafts for UCL reconstruction.
- Perform arthroscopy before UCL reconstruction to address common pathologies seen in the throwing athlete.

Clinical and Surgical Pearls
- Use a muscle splitting approach to the UCL
- The optimal length of the graft is determined by placing the second limb of the graft adjacent to the humeral tunnel, avoid undertensioning.

Clinical and Surgical Pitfalls
- Aggressive retraction of the medial antebrachial cutaneous nerve and the ulnar nerve can lead to postoperative neuropathies.
- A bone bridge of less than 2 cm can lead to fracture of graft tunnels.

The anterior bundle of the ulnar collateral ligament (UCL) of the elbow is the primary restraint to valgus load. It has been well documented that throwing athletes are prone to injury of this structure secondary to the repetitive valgus loads to which the elbow is subjected with overhead pitching.[1-6] Originally described in javelin throwers, this injury is almost exclusively seen in overhead throwing athletes, with baseball pitchers being the most prevalent group of patients. Injury to the UCL has also been shown in wrestlers, tennis players, professional football players, and arm wrestlers. Symptomatic valgus instability can arise in these athletes after a UCL injury, necessitating operative intervention.[1-6] Although injury to the UCL in the nonthrowing athlete can have excellent results with nonoperative intervention, the overhead throwing athlete may find an injury to the UCL of the elbow to be a career-ending event if surgical intervention is not employed.

BIOMECHANICS AND ANATOMY

The UCL complex is composed of an anterior bundle, a posterior bundle, and a transverse bundle[7,8] (Fig. 46-5). The anterior bundle has been shown to be the primary restraint to valgus stress at the elbow. Injury to the anterior bundle can cause instability of the elbow with subsequent disabling pain in overhead throwing athletes. The humeral origin of both the anterior and the posterior bundles is the medial epicondyle. The anterior bundle originates from the anteroinferior aspect of the medial epicondyle and inserts at the sublime tubercle of the ulna. The posterior bundle is triangular, smaller, and fanlike in nature; it originates from the posteroinferior aspect of the medial epicondyle and attaches to the medial olecranon margin.[7,8]

The anterior bundle has separate bands that function as a cam, tightening in a reciprocal fashion as the elbow is flexed and extended. In a cadaveric study, Callaway and colleagues[7] performed sequential cutting of the medial collateral ligament (MCL) while a valgus torque was applied. The anterior band of the anterior bundle

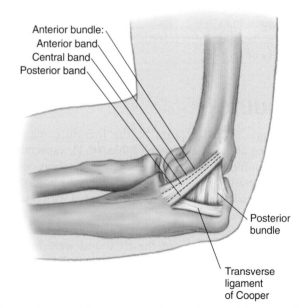

Figure 46-5. Schematic drawing of the medial collateral ligament (MCL) complex. Note that the anterior bundle is composed of three bands. The anterior band of the anterior bundle is the primary restraint to valgus stress.

was the primary restraint to valgus rotation at 30, 60, and 90 degrees of flexion. The posterior band of the anterior bundle was a co-primary restraint with the anterior band at 120 degrees.[7] In a separate study, Field and colleagues[9] evaluated the laxity seen with UCL injury when viewed through the arthroscope. They found that ulnohumeral joint opening was not visualized in any specimen until complete sectioning of the anterior bundle had been performed. However, only 1 to 2 mm of joint opening was present with complete transaction of the anterior bundle, emphasizing the subtle examination findings in these athletes. It was shown that the maximum amount of valgus laxity was seen best at 60 to 75 degrees of flexion.

The flexor carpi ulnaris (FCU) is the predominant muscle overlying the UCL. It is the most posterior structure of the flexor-pronator mass, which places it directly overlying the anterior bundle of the UCL.[8] Thus the FCU is optimally positioned to provide direct support to the UCL with regard to valgus stability. Preservation of the FCU is important during reconstruction of the UCL, to maintain one of the secondary restraints to valgus stress. This is further discussed later, when the surgical technique we currently use is described.

The ulnar nerve lies in close proximity to the UCL. It courses from a point posterior to the medial intermuscular septum above the medial epicondyle toward the anterior aspect of the medial elbow. Once it passes anterior to the intermuscular septum, the ulnar nerve then courses posterior to the medial epicondyle within the cubital tunnel. It then progresses distally to a point just posterior to the sublime tubercle. At this point the ulnar nerve dives into the FCU, which it innervates. It is important to be familiar with the anatomy of this vulnerable structure during UCL reconstruction, to avoid an iatrogenic injury.

PREOPERATIVE CONSIDERATIONS

History and Physical Examination

In the evaluation of overhead athletes with medial-sided elbow complaints, it is important to first obtain a detailed history. Questions should be posed regarding the chronicity of the symptoms as well as their effect on overhead activity. Issues regarding velocity, accuracy, and stamina are important to the throwing athlete and should therefore be addressed. It is important to note that many of these athletes will modify their pitching techniques to compensate for the pain; however, these athletes will not be able to reach their maximal throwing velocity secondary to the altered mechanics being implemented. The phase of throwing in which the pain

occurs is another important aspect. Conway and colleagues[2] have shown that nearly 85% of athletes with medial elbow instability report discomfort during the acceleration phase of throwing, in contrast to less than 25% of athletes who will experience pain during the deceleration phase. This same study also showed that up to 40% of patients with MCL injuries may also have ulnar neuritis; therefore a history of ulnar nerve symptoms should be ascertained as well as information pertaining to the position in which these symptoms are most prevalent.[2]

Presentation will be with either an acute event or an acute-on-chronic episode. In an acute event the patient reports having heard a "pop" and subsequently experiencing acute medial pain with the inability to continue pitching. In an acute-on-chronic event the patient will have experienced an innocuous onset of medial-sided elbow pain over an extended period of time with overhead throwing. This would preclude the acute event as described previously with an inability to continue with full-velocity pitching.

Both passive and active range of motion of the elbow should be documented. During the range-of-motion testing, attention should be turned to the detection of any crepitus, pain, or mechanical blocks. Patients with valgus overload frequently develop posteromedial osteophytes that manifest as a bony block to full extension. A loose body may also cause similar examination findings.

Direct palpation of the origin of the UCL is unreliable secondary to the overlying flexor-pronator mass. However, an attempt should be made to elicit discomfort in this region with palpation. The ulnar nerve should be palpated (e.g., Tinel sign) to assess for ulnar neuritis or subluxation of the nerve resulting in paresthesias. The medial epicondylar insertion of the flexor pronator mass should also be palpated for tenderness. If the flexor pronator tendon is involved, pain will be reproduced with resisted forearm pronation. This resisted maneuver can help distinguish a UCL injury from flexor pronator tendonitis.

Several tests for the UCL have been described. In general, we typically find the valgus stress test and the moving valgus stress test to be the most specific. To perform the valgus stress test, the examiner places the patient's distal forearm under the axilla and applies a valgus load to the elbow in 30 degrees of flexion while palpating the MCL (Fig. 46-6). If the patient reports increased medial-sided elbow pain or if valgus instability is present, then the test result is considered positive. However, it must be noted that the amount of instability present in these patients is sometimes too small to be picked up by this maneuver. Therefore pain may be the only indication of a UCL injury with this test. The moving valgus stress test was originally described by O'Driscoll.[10] This test is performed by applying a valgus

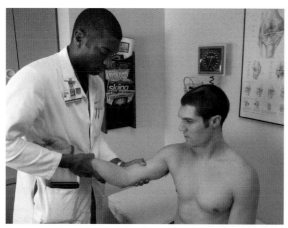

Figure 46-6. Valgus stress test. While one hand of the examiner supports the elbow, valgus stress is applied with the elbow in approximately 30 degrees of flexion. Tenderness to palpation over the medial collateral ligament and valgus laxity are assessed.

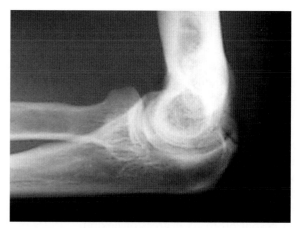

Figure 46-8. Lateral radiograph of the elbow showing a prominent osteophyte at the tip of the olecranon. Patients who have x-ray films consistent with valgus extension overload need to undergo magnetic resonance imaging for assessment of the medial collateral ligament.

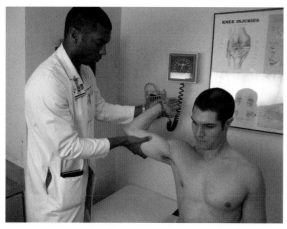

Figure 46-7. The moving valgus stress test is performed by applying a valgus stress to the maximally flexed elbow and then quickly extending the elbow. A positive test result is usually pain produced between 120 and 70 degrees of flexion.

stress to the elbow in the flexed position and then quickly extending the elbow (Fig. 46-7). A positive test result occurs when medial pain is produced, typically between 120 and 70 degrees of flexion, as a result of shear stress on the UCL. Finally, we also sometimes use the "milking maneuver," which is performed by pulling on the patient's thumb with the forearm supinated, the shoulder extended, and the elbow flexed to 90 degrees. A feeling of instability and apprehension along with pain is a positive finding and indicates insufficiency of the posterior band of the anterior bundle.

Posterior impingement secondary to posteromedial olecranon osteophytes should also be assessed. This is accomplished through the valgus extension overload test. The examiner uses one hand to apply a valgus force across the elbow while stabilizing the elbow joint with

the opposite hand. The forearm is placed in a pronated position and the elbow is then quickly brought to full extension while the valgus load is applied. A positive test result is indicated by pain in the posteromedial aspect of the elbow.

Imaging

Plain radiographs remain the gold standard for initial evaluation of the elbow. Routine anteroposterior (AP), lateral, and oblique views should be obtained. These standard radiographic views may reveal calcifications in the UCL, medial spurs on the humerus and ulna at the joint line, spurs on the posterior olecranon tip, or loose bodies in the olecranon fossa (Fig. 46-8). Stress radiographs have been advocated to aid in the diagnosis of UCL tears, but we do not routinely use them.

We recommend magnetic resonance imaging (MRI) for every patient with a suspected UCL tear. Both contrast and noncontrast MRI sequences can be used with success. When available, we use three-dimensional volumetric gradient echo and fast spin echo techniques, which enable thin-section (<3 mm) imaging of the elbow, thus improving visualization of partial tears of the UCL and obviating the need for contrast injection.[11] Partial tears can be seen on MRI as areas of focal interruption that do not extend through the full thickness of the ligament. Complete tears can be seen on coronal MRI scans as increased signal intensity and focal disruption of the normally hypointense, vertically oriented ligament (Fig. 46-9). In chronic ligament injuries without tears, the UCL will appear thickened without focal discontinuity, but with global increased signal intensity. Because arthroscopic evaluation of the UCL is limited in its ability to visualize the anterior bundle and humeral or ulnar insertions, MRI is an effective technique for

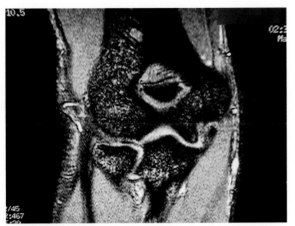

Figure 46-9. Coronal magnetic resonance image shows abnormal signal intensity and structure of the humeral insertion of the medial collateral ligament, indicating a complete tear.

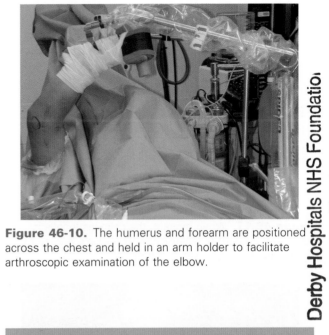

Figure 46-10. The humerus and forearm are positioned across the chest and held in an arm holder to facilitate arthroscopic examination of the elbow.

distinguishing ligament tears from flexor or pronator tendinopathy. Osteochondral impaction injuries to the radiocapitellar joint may also be seen, which emphasizes the importance of obtaining appropriate cartilage pulse sequencing.

Development of the Docking Procedure

Early experience with MCL reconstruction at the Hospital for Special Surgery (HSS) led to some concerns about the original procedure as described by Jobe.[2] These concerns included the ability to adequately tension the graft at the time of final fixation; potential complications from detachment of the flexor origin; potential complications from the placement of three large drill holes in a limited area on the epicondyle; complications from routine ulnar nerve transposition; and the strength of suture fixation of the free tendon graft. Therefore in 1996 the senior author (D.W.A.) began to look for alternative methods to reconstruct the UCL to address these concerns. The resulting procedure is referred to as the *docking technique* and highlights the following: use of a muscle splitting safe zone approach; avoidance of routine transposition of the ulnar nerve; reduction in the number of large drill holes from three to one in the medial epicondyle; and addressing of tendon length to ensure proper tensioning and fixation in bony tunnels.

SURGICAL TECHNIQUE
Anesthesia and Positioning

At our institutions the procedure is generally performed with use of regional anesthesia. After the block has been administered the patient remains in the supine position,

---

BOX 46-2 Surgical Steps

- Arthroscopic examination
- Harvesting of the palmaris longus for graft reconstruction
- Exposure of the sublime tubercle subperiosteally in preparation for drilling ulnar tunnels
- Passage of the graft through the ulnar tunnel from anterior to posterior and docking of the limb with sutures into the humerus
- Tie-down of the graft sutures

---

a tourniquet is placed, and the involved upper extremity is prepared and draped in the usual sterile fashion. Some situations require arthroscopic evaluation and treatment of certain intra-articular pathologies (loose bodies, posterior medial impingement). Such procedures are performed before the UCL reconstruction. With use of an arm holder (Spider, Tenet Medical Engineering, Calgary, Alberta, Canada), the humerus and forearm are positioned across the patient's chest for the arthroscopic evaluation of the elbow (Fig. 46-10). The supine position allows for easy conversion to the open UCL procedure once arthroscopy has been completed.

Surgical Steps

See Box 46-2.

Once the arthroscopy has been completed, the arm is released from the arm holder and placed on the hand table. When the palmaris longus tendon is absent, the gracilis tendon is harvested at this time. Otherwise, the ipsilateral palmaris longus tendon is harvested through a 1-cm incision in the volar wrist flexion crease over the

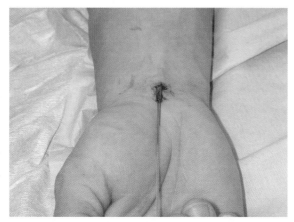

Figure 46-11. When present, the palmaris longus is harvested for graft reconstruction. The visible portion of the tendon is tagged with a suture.

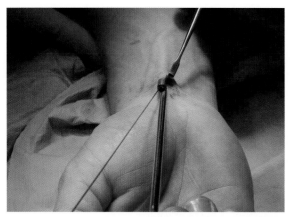

Figure 46-12. A tendon stripper is used to harvest the remaining tendon once it has been identified and tagged.

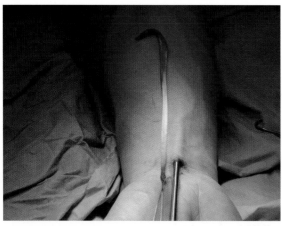

Figure 46-13. Final picture demonstrating complete harvest of the palmaris tendon.

tendon. At the time of harvest, the visible portion of the tendon is tagged with a No. 1 Ethibond suture (Ethicon, Johnson & Johnson) in a Krackow fashion, and the remaining tendon is then harvested with a tendon stripper (Figs. 46-11 to 46-13). The incision is then closed

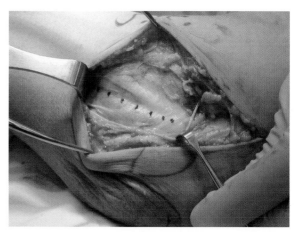

Figure 46-14. A muscle splitting approach is used through the posterior one third of the common flexor pronator mass within the most anterior fibers of the flexor carpi ulnaris muscle *(dotted line).*

with interrupted nylon sutures, and the tendon is placed in a moist sponge on the back table.

After the arm has been exsanguinated to the level of the tourniquet, an 8- to 10-cm incision is created from the distal third of the intermuscular septum across the medial epicondyle to a point 2 cm beyond the sublime tubercle of the ulna. In exposing the fascia of the flexor-pronator mass, care is taken to identify and preserve the antebrachial cutaneous branch of the medial nerve, which frequently crosses the operative field. A muscle splitting approach is then used through the posterior one third of the common flexor pronator mass within the most anterior fibers of the FCU muscle (Fig. 46-14). This approach is beneficial because it uses a true inter-nervous plane, allows for adequate exposure of the native UCL, and is less traumatic than detachment of the entire flexor-pronator mass from its origin. The anterior bundle of the UCL is then incised longitudinally to expose the joint.

The tunnel positions for the ulna are exposed first. The posterior tunnel requires that the surgeon subperi-osteally expose the ulna 4 to 5 mm posterior to the sublime tubercle while meticulously protecting the ulnar nerve (Fig. 46-15). With use of a 3-mm bur, tunnels are made anterior and posterior to the sublime tubercle such that a 2-cm bridge exists between them. The tunnels are connected with use of a small, curved curette, with care taken not to violate the bony bridge. A suture passer is used to pass a looped suture through the tunnel. For the humeral tunnel position to be exposed, the incision within the native UCL is extended proximally to the level of the epicondyle. A longitudinal tunnel is then created along the axis of the medial epicondyle with a 4-mm bur; care is taken not to violate the posterior cortex of the proximal epicondyle. The upper border of the epicondyle, just anterior to the

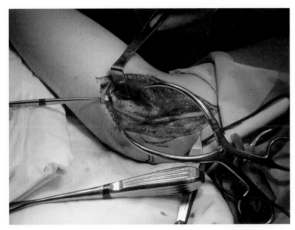

Figure 46-15. The sublime tubercle is exposed subperiosteally in preparation for drilling ulnar tunnels.

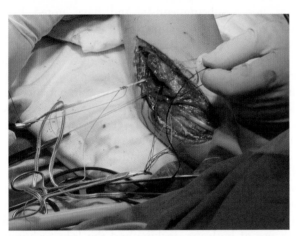

Figure 46-16. The graft is passed through the ulnar tunnel from anterior to posterior; the limb with sutures is ultimately docked into the humerus.

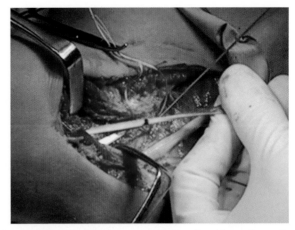

Figure 46-17. Final length is determined by referencing the graft to the exit hole in the humeral tunnel. This point is marked on the graft, and a No. 1 Ethibond suture is placed in a Krackow fashion.

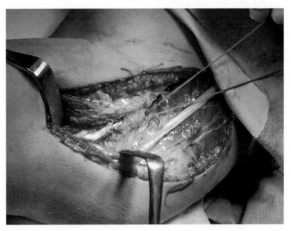

Figure 46-18. Once both limbs of the graft have been successfully docked into the humeral tunnel, the graft sutures are tied down.

intramuscular septum, is then exposed, and two small anterior exit punctures are made with a 1.5-mm bur. They should be approximately 5 mm to 1 cm apart from each other. Again, a suture passer is used from each of the two exit punctures to pass a looped suture, which will be used later for graft passage. With the elbow reduced, the incision in the native UCL is repaired with a 2-0 absorbable suture.

With the forearm supinated and a mild varus stress applied to the elbow, the graft is then passed through the ulnar tunnel from anterior to posterior (Fig. 46-16). The limb of the graft on which sutures have already been placed is passed into the humeral tunnel with the sutures exiting one of the small humeral exit punctures. This first limb of the graft is now securely docked in the humerus. With the elbow reduced, the graft is tensioned in flexion and extension to determine what length would be optimal by placement of the second limb of the graft adjacent to the humeral tunnel. Final length is determined by referencing the graft to the exit

hole in the humeral tunnel. This point is marked on the graft, and a No. 1 Ethibond suture is placed in a Krackow fashion (Fig. 46-17). The excess graft is then excised immediately above the Krackow stitch; this end of the graft is then docked securely in the humeral tunnel, with the sutures exiting the free exit puncture.

Final graft tensioning is performed by taking the elbow through a full range of motion. Once the surgeon is satisfied, the two sets of graft sutures are tied over the bony bridge on the humeral epicondyle (Figs. 46-18 and 46-19). After the tourniquet has been deflated and hemostasis achieved, an ulnar nerve transposition is performed if indicated. We do this only when the preoperative examination findings are consistent with ulnar neuritis. Otherwise, the fascia over the flexor pronator mass is reapproximated, and the remaining wound is closed in layers. The elbow is then placed in a plaster splint at 45 degrees of flexion and neutral rotation with the hand land wrist free.

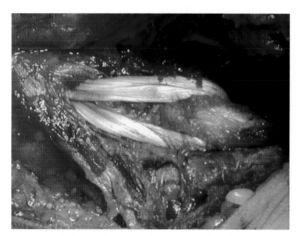

Figure 46-19. Final image demonstrating the completed ulnar collateral ligament reconstruction.

POSTOPERATIVE MANAGEMENT

Immediately after surgery, the patient's arm is placed in a plaster splint for approximately 1 week. At the first postoperative visit, the sutures are removed and the elbow is placed in a hinged brace. Initially, motion is allowed only from 30 degrees of extension to 90 degrees of flexion. In the third to fifth week, motion is advanced to 15 degrees of extension and 105 degrees of flexion. Wrist flexion of the contralateral limb is also encouraged if the palmaris longus was harvested from that forearm. At 6 weeks, the brace is discontinued and formal physical therapy is begun, focusing on shoulder and forearm strengthening as well as elbow range of motion. By 12 weeks the patient is advanced to an aggressive physical therapy program that includes trunk strengthening as well as shoulder and scapula strengthening. A formal tossing program is begun at 16 weeks. Initially, throwing starts at a distance of 45 feet and is advanced at regular stages. If pain occurs during any stage, the patient is instructed to back up to the previous stage of therapy. If at 9 months the patient can throw pain free from 180 feet, he or she is allowed to begin pitching from a mound. We generally discourage competitive pitching until 1 year postoperatively.

The most common postoperative complications are medial forearm numbness secondary to injury to the medial antebrachial cutaneous nerve and ulnar neuropathy. Fortunately, both issues are typically traction injuries related to retractor placement and usually resolve on their own. Much less common is fracture at the sublime tubercle or medial epicondyle secondary to inadequate spacing of tunnel placement.

RESULTS

Conway and colleagues[2] conducted the first outcome study on the original procedure, as described by Jobe, which included detachment of the flexor-pronator mass and routine transposition of the ulnar nerve. Only 68% of the athletes in that series were able to return to either their previous or a higher level of competition. In addition, 21% of the patients were observed to develop postoperative ulnar nerve neuropathies.

Thompson and colleagues[5] were the first to report on 83 athletes who underwent UCL reconstruction with use of a muscle splitting approach without transposition of the ulnar nerve. Of these 83 patients, 33 were followed for at least 2 years. The surgical result was excellent in 27 of 33 patients (82%), good in four (12%), and fair in two (6%). These results improved to 93% excellent when those patients who had had a prior procedure were excluded. Several authors have since reported on UCL reconstruction with use of a muscle splitting approach or transposition of the ulnar nerve subcutaneously and have noted lower ulnar nerve–related complication rates ranging from 8% to 9%.

We have reported on 100 consecutive UCL reconstructions in which the docking technique was used, with an average follow-up of 3 years.[3] No patients were lost to follow-up. Ninety of 100 patients (90%) returned to or exceeded their previous level of competition for at least 1 year, meeting the Conway-Jobe classification of excellent. In addition, seven patients had a good result, which means that they were able to compete at a lower level for at least 12 months. Two patients (2%) had poor results and were not able to return to throwing. Other authors have also reported excellent results with use of both the docking and the Jobe techniques (Table 46-2).[1,12]

In our series, 22% of patients underwent a subcutaneous transposition with fascial sling at the time of surgery. None of these patients developed postoperative complications. Two athletes (2%) required transposition postoperatively after they had returned to throwing for at least 1 year. Neither patient had preoperative symptoms, and both had excellent results at the time of follow-up.

As previously stated, we sometimes find it necessary to perform arthroscopic evaluation both anteriorly and posteriorly of all patients before reconstruction. It is not unusual for this patient group to develop intra-articular pathology secondary to the mechanic of valgus extension overload. In our series, 45 of 100 patients (45%) had associated intra-articular pathology; all were managed arthroscopically just before reconstruction.[3] Detection of the lesions on preoperative imaging studies occurred in only 25 of the 45 patients. Without arthroscopy, a posterior arthrotomy is necessary to treat such pathology and necessitates transposition of the ulnar nerve. Arthroscopy is a more minimally invasive approach and has the added benefit of avoiding obligatory transposition of the nerve.

TABLE 46-2. Results of Studies of the Docking Technique

Authors	No. of Patients	FPM Approach	Fixation	Obligatory UNT	UNT Tech	Excellent Results	Complications
Conway et al[3] (1992)	71	Detach	Figure-of-eight	Yes	SM	68%	21% UN 27% total
Cain[1] (2010)	72	Detach	Figure-of-eight	Yes	SC	78%	11% UN
Azar[12] (2000)	91	Retract	Figure-of-eight	Yes	SC	81%	1% UN 9% total
Thompson et al[12] (2001)	83	Split	Figure-of-eight	No	None	82%	5% UN 10% total
Petty[13] (2004)	31	Split	Figure-of-eight	Yes	SC	74%	7% UN 11% total
Paletta[14] (2006)	25	Split	Docking	No	SC	92%	4% UN 8% total
Dodson[6] (2006)	100	Split	Docking	No	SC	90%	2% UN 3% total
Koh[15] (2006)	20	Split	Docking	No	SC	95%	5% UN
Cain[1] (2010)	743	Retract	Figure-of-eight	Yes	SC	83%	20%

FPM, Flexor pronator mass; *SM,* submuscular transposition; *SC,* subcutaneous; *UN,* ulnar nerve; *UNT,* ulnar nerve transposition.

SUMMARY

We believe that the modifications described in the docking technique have resulted in excellent outcomes for athletes at all levels of play and that the technique has proven to be a minimally invasive and reliable method of reconstruction of the UCL.

REFERENCES

1. Cain Jr EL, Andrews JR, Dugas JR, et al. Outcome of ulnar collateral ligament reconstruction of the elbow in 1281 athletes: Results in 743 athletes with minimum 2 year follow-up. *Am J Sports Med.* 2010;38(12):2426-2434.
2. Conway JE, Jobe FW, Glousman RE, et al. Medial instability of the elbow in throwing athletes. Treatment by repair or reconstruction of the ulnar collateral ligament. *J Bone Joint Surg Am.* 1992;74(1):67-83.
3. Dodson CC, Thomas A, Dines JS, et al. Medial collateral ligament reconstruction of the elbow in throwing athletes. *Am J Sports Med.* 2006;34(12):1926-1932.
4. Jobe FW, Stark H, Lombardo SJ. Reconstruction of the ulnar collateral ligament in athletes. *J Bone Joint Surg Am.* 1986;68(8):1158-1163.
5. Thompson WH, Jobe FW, Yocum LA, et al. Ulnar collateral ligament reconstruction in athletes: muscle-splitting approach without transposition of the ulnar nerve. *J Shoulder Elbow Surg.* 2001;10(2):152-157.
6. Dodson CC, Thomas A, Dines JS, et al. Medial collateral ligament reconstruction of the elbow in throwing athletes. *Am J Sports Med.* 2006;34(12):1926-1932.
7. Callaway GH, Field LD, Deng XH, et al. Biomechanical evaluation of the medial collateral ligament of the elbow. *J Bone Joint Surg Am.* 1997;79(8):1223-1231.
8. Davidson PA, Pink M, Perry J, et al. Functional anatomy of the flexor pronator muscle group in relation to the medial collateral ligament of the elbow. *Am J Sports Med.* 1995;23(2):245-250.
9. Field LD, Callaway GH, O'Brien SJ, et al. Arthroscopic assessment of the medial collateral ligament complex of the elbow. *Am J Sports Med.* 1995;23(4):396-400.
10. O'Driscoll SW, Lawton RL, Smith AM. The "Moving Valgus Stress Test" for Medial Collateral Ligament Tears of the Elbow. *Am J Sports Med.* 2005;33(2):231-239.
11. Gaary EA, Potter HG, Altchek DW. Medial elbow pain in the throwing athlete: MR imaging evaluation. *AJR Am J Roentgenol.* 1997;168(3):795-800.
12. Azar FM, Andrews JR, Wilk KE, et al. Operative treatment of ulnar collateral ligament injuries of the elbow in athletes. *Am J Sports Med.* 2000;28:16-23.
13. Petty DH, Andrews JR, Fleisig GS, et al. Ulnar collateral ligament reconstruction in high school baseball players: clinical results and injury risk factors. *Am J Sports Med.* 2004;32:1158-1164.
14. Paletta GA Jr, Wright RW. The modified docking procedures for elbow ulnar collateral ligament reconstruction: 2-year follow-up in elite throwers. *Am J Sports Med.* 2006;34:1594-1598.
15. Koh JL, Schaefer MF, Keuter G, et al. Ulnar collateral ligament reconstruction in elite throwing athletes. *Arthroscopy.* 2006;22:1187-1191.

Part 3   Modified Jobe Technique

Andrew J. Blackman and Matthew V. Smith

Chapter Synopsis
- The Jobe technique was the first technique reported for ulnar collateral ligament (UCL) reconstruction, and several subsequent modifications have been described. The procedure involves passage of a graft, most commonly the palmaris longus tendon, through the ulnar and humeral tunnels in a figure-of-eight fashion. More than 80% of athletes return to their previous level of sport.

Important Points
- Accurate diagnosis is paramount.
- Medial elbow pain during late cocking or early acceleration phase of throwing is hallmark of UCL insufficiency.
- Surgery indicated after failure of nonoperative treatment.
- Prolonged rehabilitation period must be discussed with patient.

Clinical and Surgical Pearls
- A muscle splitting approach or elevation of the flexor-pronator mass without detachment from the medial epicondyle can be used to expose the UCL.
- Identify and protect the ulnar nerve while drilling the tunnels.
- Tension graft with elbow flexed to 30 degrees, forearm supinated, and varus stress applied to elbow.
- Identify valgus extension overload with olecranon osteophytes preoperatively because recognition and treatment can prevent persistent pain postoperatively.

Clinical and Surgical Pitfalls
- Ulnar or medial antebrachial cutaneous nerve neurapraxia is the most common complication. Identify and protect these nerves during surgery.
- Fractures through bone tunnels can occur. Place tunnels 10 mm apart to minimize risk.

The anterior bundle of the ulnar collateral ligament (UCL) is the primary restraint to valgus forces at the elbow.[1] Injury to this structure can occur in individuals whose elbows are subjected to large valgus loads, as in throwing or as a result of elbow dislocation. Injury to the UCL is most commonly seen in overhead or throwing athletes whose elbows are subjected to repetitive valgus loads during the late cocking and early acceleration phases of throwing. Once injured, throwing athletes with UCL insufficiency often experience disabling elbow pain and are unable to compete at a high level. Jobe and colleagues provided the first description of surgical reconstruction of the UCL in 1986.[2] Since that time, this procedure has become the gold standard for surgical treatment of UCL deficiency. Several modifications have been made to the original technique to decrease the amount of soft tissue dissection required and lessen the technical demands of the operation. Reports have shown patients who have undergone this operation to return to their previous level of competition or a higher level more than 80% of the time.[3-5] This chapter describes the modified Jobe technique for UCL reconstruction, as well as discussing preoperative considerations and offering a brief review of reported results.

PREOPERATIVE CONSIDERATIONS

History

UCL insufficiency can manifest as either an acute or a chronic injury. The hallmark symptom is medial elbow pain during the late cocking and early acceleration phases of the throwing motion, which is present in 85% of patients.[6] Acute injuries can be accompanied by a "pop," acute pain, and inability to continue throwing. Chronic injuries typically involve an insidious onset of medial elbow pain associated with loss of velocity or accuracy. It is important to solicit a history of pain or paresthesias in the ulnar two digits that may indicate associated ulnar neuritis. Valgus extension overload (VEO), a clinical entity often related to UCL insufficiency, can cause posteromedial elbow pain in the deceleration phase (or follow-through phase) of the throwing motion, limited extension, and mechanical symptoms. Occasionally, symptoms of VEO may overshadow those of UCL insufficiency at initial presentation.

Signs and Symptoms

- Medial elbow pain during late cocking and/or early acceleration

- Loss of accuracy or velocity of throws
- Feeling of a "pop" in acute injuries
- Ulnar nerve symptoms—paresthesias, radiating pain, weakness
- VEO symptoms—posteromedial pain, loss of extension, mechanical symptoms

Physical Examination

Tenderness over the UCL or its insertions at the base of the medial humeral epicondyle and the sublime tubercle of the proximal medial ulna may be present, especially if the ligament is acutely injured. Several special tests for UCL injury have been described. Applying a valgus stress with the elbow flexed to 25 degrees may elicit medial pain or excessive gapping.[7] The moving valgus stress test begins with the application of a valgus force to the maximally flexed elbow. While the valgus torque is maintained, the elbow is rapidly extended to 30 degrees. Reproduction of the patient's medial elbow pain is a positive test result.[8] With the milking maneuver, the examiner places valgus stress on the flexed elbow by grasping and pulling on the thumb of the affected hand.[9] Reproduction of the patient's medial elbow pain is a positive test result, as with the moving valgus stress test. A positive Tinel sign at the cubital tunnel may be present in patients with associated ulnar neuritis. A thorough neurovascular examination, with special focus on the sensorimotor function of the ulnar nerve, should be completed. Palpation of the ulnar nerve at the cubital tunnel through the elbow's full range of motion should be performed to identify concomitant ulnar nerve subluxation. Patients with associated VEO will have pain and tenderness over the posteromedial olecranon tip. They also may have pain with valgus stress and rapid hyperextension simulating the follow-through phase of the throwing motion.

Imaging

Evaluation begins with anteroposterior, lateral, and oblique plain radiographs, which are often unremarkable. Valgus stress radiographs with the elbow in 30 degrees of flexion may demonstrate ulnohumeral joint widening medially. Comparison stress views of the uninjured side may be helpful in some patients. An oblique axial radiograph with the elbow flexed to 120 degrees helps to visualize posteromedial olecranon osteophytes, which are often seen in VEO and may require excision at the time of surgery. The advanced imaging modality of choice at our institution is magnetic resonance arthrography (MRA), which improves diagnostic accuracy compared with noncontrast magnetic resonance imaging (MRI).[10] MRA findings can include thickening of the UCL, partial-thickness articular-sided tears, and full-thickness ligament tears (Fig. 46-20).

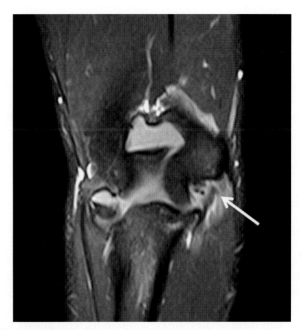

Figure 46-20. Magnetic resonance arthrogram demonstrating a tear of the ulnar collateral ligament *(arrow)*.

Indications and Contraindications

Initial treatment often begins with a 2- to 3-month period of active rest. During this period, icing and anti-inflammatory medications are used, as well as physical therapy for flexor-pronator strengthening, range of motion, and scapular stabilization. Once the patient is asymptomatic and the physical examination findings are normal, an interval throwing program is begun. Forty-two percent of patients have been reported to return to their previous level of sports participation after nonoperative treatment.[11] A relative indication to acutely reconstruct the UCL is a UCL tear that occurs in a pitcher at the beginning of a baseball season. Rehabilitation for 2 to 3 months may jeopardize return for the following season because the average time it takes to return to pitching is approximately 11 months. Otherwise, failure of nonoperative management, ability to participate in the long rehabilitation, and desire to continue overhead sports are indications for UCL reconstruction. Relative contraindications include patients with little valgus demand on the elbow and those not intending to return to throwing.

SURGICAL TECHNIQUE

Anesthesia and Positioning

The procedure is performed typically with the patient under general anesthesia without regional block so a reliable postoperative examination of ulnar nerve function can be performed. The patient is positioned supine on the operating table with the operative extremity placed on a radiolucent hand table or arm board. A nonsterile pneumatic tourniquet is placed on the brachium. The palmaris longus tendon is our first choice for the graft. If the palmaris tendon is not available, a pneumatic tourniquet is also placed on a lower extremity for gracilis or plantaris tendon harvest. The operative limb or limbs are then prepared and draped in the usual sterile fashion.

Specific Steps

Box 46-3 outlines the specific steps of this procedure.

1. Graft Harvest

Graft choices include the ipsilateral palmaris longus, plantaris, and gracilis. Our graft of choice is the ipsilateral palmaris longus tendon. This tendon is harvested through three small transverse incisions. This allows for clear identification of the palmaris tendon and minimizes the risk of erroneously harvesting the median nerve. The most distal incision is made at the proximal wrist flexor crease. The second incision is made 7.5 cm proximal to the first. The most proximal incision is 15 cm proximal to the distal incision. Identify the palmaris longus tendon just beneath the skin distally. Pulling tension on the palmaris longus tendon, identify the tendon in the middle incision and again in the proximal incision. Once it is clearly identified, the tendon is sharply released distally and is pulled out through the proximal wound. It may be necessary to bluntly release adjacent soft tissue. Alternatively, a tendon stripper can be used. A graft length of approximately 15 cm is preferred. Prepare the graft by whipstitching a No. 2 nonabsorbable braided suture into both ends of the graft.

BOX 46-3 Surgical Steps

Exposure: Center 10-cm incision over medial epicondyle; muscle splitting approach or retraction of flexor-pronator mass anteriorly.

Graft harvest: Palmaris longus tendon preferred; plantaris, gracilis also described.

Ulnar tunnels: Anterior and posterior to sublime tubercle; 10-mm bone bridge.

Humeral tunnels:
1. Isometric point on anteroinferior medial epicondyle.
2. Just anterior to attachment of intermuscular septum on medial epicondyle.
3. 10 mm inferior to second tunnel, on medial epicondyle.

Graft passage: Figure-of-eight configuration through ulnar and humeral tunnels.

Graft tensioning: Apply 30 degrees of elbow flexion, full forearm supination, varus force to elbow.

---

2. Incision and Exposure

Surgical Landmarks and Incisions

After exsanguination of the limb and elevation of the tourniquet, make a curvilinear incision centered over the medial epicondyle and extending proximally and distally (Fig. 46-21). Make a 10-cm incision centered over the medial epicondyle. Bluntly dissect through the subcutaneous tissues with Metzenbaum scissors to identify and protect branches of the medial antebrachial cutaneous nerve. Then identify and protect the ulnar nerve as it courses posterior to the medial epicondyle. Of note, the senior author (M.V.S.) does not routinely perform ulnar nerve transposition in conjunction with a UCL reconstruction unless the patient demonstrates preoperative sensory ulnar neuritis at rest, symptomatic ulnar nerve subluxation, or ulnar nerve motor dysfunction. Identify the fascia overlying the flexor-pronator mass (Fig. 46-22). The flexor-pronator mass can be managed either with a muscle splitting approach[6] or by retracting the entire flexor-pronator mass anteriorly[3] while leaving the flexor-pronator mass attached to the medial epicondyle. If the flexor-pronator mass is elevated anteriorly, a small wide Hohmann retractor can be placed around the anterior proximal ulna to improve retraction. To use the muscle splitting approach, incise the flexor-pronator fascia longitudinally at the junction of its anterior two thirds and posterior one third. A fascial raphe is typically present at this level, which can be bluntly dissected down to the level of the UCL. In either approach, a periosteal elevator is used to reflect the deep muscle off of the UCL, exposing the ligament in its entirety, as well as the sublime tubercle and the medial epicondyle (Fig. 46-23). Most commonly, a

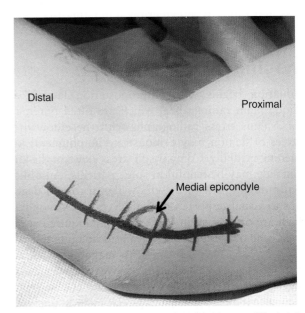

Distal

Proximal

Medial epicondyle

Figure 46-21. Recommended incision for modified Jobe ulnar collateral ligament reconstruction.

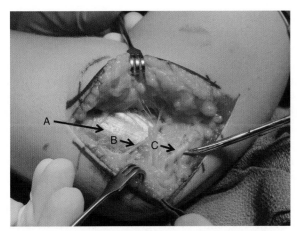

Figure 46-22. Exposure for ulnar collateral ligament reconstruction. **A,** Flexor-pronator fascia; **B,** branch of medial antebrachial cutaneous nerve; and **C,** ulnar nerve.

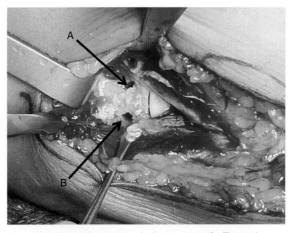

Figure 46-24. Ulnar tunnel placement. **A,** Tunnel on anterior aspect of sublime tubercle; **B,** tunnel on posterior aspect of sublime tubercle.

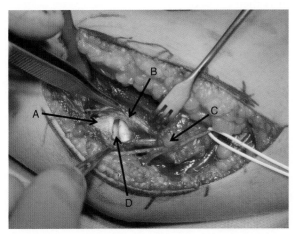

Figure 46-23. Deep exposure for ulnar collateral ligament (UCL) reconstruction with flexor-pronator mass retracted anteriorly. **A,** Sublime tubercle; **B,** anterior half of native UCL retracted anteriorly; **C,** medial epicondyle; and **D,** ulnohumeral joint space.

thickened, scarred, and attenuated UCL is encountered, but full-thickness tears may also be found. Make a longitudinal incision through the UCL, revealing the ulnohumeral joint. Application of valgus stress with the elbow flexed to 30 degrees should reveal widening of the joint in patients with UCL insufficiency.

3. Ulnar Tunnels

Use a 3.5-mm (or 4-mm for gracilis) drill bit to create converging tunnels just posterior and anterior to the sublime tubercle, leaving a 10-mm bone bridge between the tunnels (Fig. 46-24). After the first tunnel has been drilled, place a small straight curette into the tunnel to give a reference angle for drilling the second tunnel. Use a small curved curette to remove bony debris from the tunnels and to confirm that the tunnels connect. Thread a passing suture through the ulnar tunnels.

4. Humeral Tunnels

Place the two limbs of the suture that was passed through the ulnar tunnels on the anteroinferior surface of the medial epicondyle at the anatomic humeral insertion of the UCL, and take the elbow through a range of motion to verify the isometric point. Use a 4-mm (4.5-mm for gracilis) drill bit to create a tunnel beginning at the isometric point, directed posteriorly toward the back of the epicondyle. Do not penetrate the posterior cortex. Place a straight curette in the tunnel as a marker. Drill a 3.5-mm tunnel in the medial epicondyle beginning just anterior to the attachment of the intermuscular septum, directed distally toward the midportion of the first tunnel, which has been marked with the straight curette. Drill another 3.5-mm tunnel in the medial epicondyle beginning 10 mm inferior to the second tunnel, directed distally again toward the midportion of the first tunnel (Fig. 46-25). The three humeral tunnel entry points should be positioned at least 10 mm from each other to avoid fracture of the bone bridges. Use a small curette to remove bony debris from the tunnels and confirm that they connect.

5. Graft Passage

Use the previously placed passing suture to pass the graft from anterior to posterior through the ulnar tunnel. Then pass the graft through the humeral tunnels in a figure-of-eight configuration. Use a Hewson suture passer to pass the anterior end of the graft from distal to proximal through the more inferior humeral tunnel. Reverse the suture passer and pass the same end of the graft from proximal to distal through the other tunnel (Fig. 46-26A).

6. Graft Tensioning

Before tensioning the graft, close the arthrotomy with No. 0 Vicryl. This may be done before graft passage for

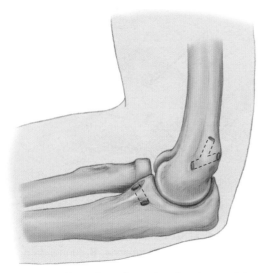

Figure 46-25. Tunnel configuration for ulnar collateral ligament reconstruction.

better visualization. Place the elbow in 30 degrees of flexion, fully supinate the forearm, and apply a varus stress to the elbow. Apply tension to both ends of the graft while maintaining the position of the arm, and suture the graft to itself—side to side, proximally, and distally—with No. 2 FiberWire (Fig. 46-26B). We typically suture the two limbs of the graft together, side to side, along their entire length to make a single-limbed graft. Take the elbow through a full range of motion to verify isometry and ensure that no undue tension is placed on the reconstruction.

Alternatively, the graft can be passed so that each end exits one of the humeral tunnels posteriorly (Fig. 46-27A). The ends of the graft are crossed over each other while the graft is tensioned and the elbow is positioned as noted previously. The two ends of the graft are then sutured together, side to side, over the posterior aspect of the medial epicondyle (Fig. 46-27B). Excess graft is then excised.

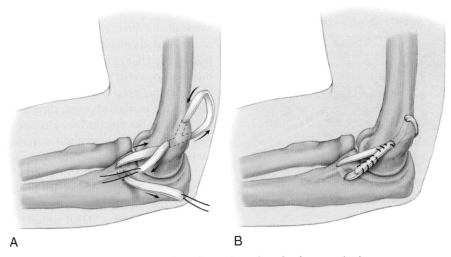

A   B

Figure 46-26. Figure-of-eight graft placement and configuration of graft after tensioning.

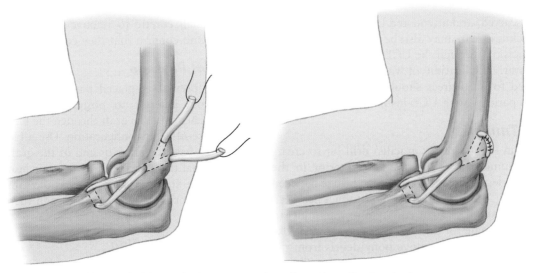

Figure 46-27. Alternative figure-of-eight graft placement and configuration after tensioning.

7. Closure

After thorough irrigation of the wound, close the flexor-pronator fascia with No. 0 Vicryl, the subcutaneous tissues with inverted 3-0 Monocryl simple stitches, and the skin with a running 4-0 Monocryl subcuticular closure. Graft harvest wounds are closed either with 4-0 subcuticular Monocryl or with 4-0 nylon. Sterile dressings are applied. The patient is placed into a long-arm posterior splint for 10 to 14 days after surgery.

POSTOPERATIVE CONSIDERATIONS

Rehabilitation

The procedure is typically performed in an outpatient setting. The patient is then seen 10 to 14 days postoperatively for splint removal and wound check. He or she is placed in a hinged elbow brace to protect against valgus stress. Physical therapy commences at that point, with range of motion limited initially to 25 to 110 degrees. Five degrees of extension and 10 degrees of flexion are added per week so that full motion is achieved at 6 weeks. Light resistance exercises are introduced at 4 weeks. Resisted shoulder internal rotation is avoided until week 6. The brace is discontinued at 5 weeks. The Thrower's Ten Program is initiated during week 6. At 8 weeks, plyometric exercises are initiated including chest pass and side throw. Week 14 marks the beginning of sport-specific rehabilitation with one-hand plyometric exercises, followed by initiation of a two-phase interval throwing program at week 16. Phase I involves long tossing with throwing every other day and progression to the next stage only if the athlete is pain free. Phase II is typically reached at 22 to 24 weeks and involves throwing from the mound with a gradual progression to competitive throwing and sports, which is allowed at week 32 at the earliest. Scapular stabilization and rotator cuff strengthening are emphasized throughout the rehabilitation program and should be continued after the athlete has returned to competitive sports.

Complications

Postoperative complications occur in 20% of patients.[4] The most common complication is minor postoperative ulnar nerve neurapraxia (16% of patients), which typically resolves within 6 weeks. Ulnar nerve palsy requiring surgical intervention has been reported.[2,4,6] Neurapraxia of the medial antebrachial cutaneous nerve can occur as well. Superficial or deep infections requiring treatment ranging from oral antibiotics to operative debridement are possible. Loss of terminal extension is expected, with reported deficits ranging from 3 to 17 degrees.[12] The need for additional elbow surgery is relatively uncommon, but arthroscopic debridement of an olecranon osteophyte (7%) and revision UCL reconstruction (1%)[4] can occur. Fracture of the medial epicondyle at a tunnel site is rare but can require open reduction and internal fixation if it happens.

RESULTS

Results after the modified Jobe technique for UCL reconstruction are generally favorable and are usually measured by ability to return to sporting activities (Table 46-3). With larger series, it has been reported that more than 80% of athletes are able to return to their previous level of competition or higher, although their rehabilitation commonly takes a year or more. Variables such as graft choice, concomitant olecranon osteophyte debridement, and presence of postoperative

TABLE 46-3. Results of Jobe and Modified Jobe Techniques for Ulnar Collateral Ligament Reconstruction

Author	No. of Patients	Average Follow-Up	Surgical Technique	Results
Azar et al[3] (2000)	59	35.4 months	Modified Jobe technique: Muscle splitting approach Subcutaneous ulnar nerve transposition (UNT) in all patients	81% return to previous level of competition 8.8% complications
Cain et al[4] (2010)	743	37 months	Modified Jobe technique as in Azar (2000)	83% return to previous level of competition 20% complications
Conway et al[6] (1992)	68	6.3 years	Original Jobe technique Detachment of flexor-pronator origin Submuscular UNT in all patients	68% return to previous level of competition Average 3-mm widening on valgus-stress radiograph 21% complications
Jobe et al[2] (1986)	16	47 months	Original Jobe technique	63% return to previous level of competition 37% complications
Thompson et al[5] (2001)	33	3.1 years	Modified Jobe technique: Muscle splitting approach No UNT	82% return to previous level of competition 12% complications

ulnar nerve symptoms have not been shown to affect ability to return to sports.[4] The modified Jobe technique is still the gold standard to which other UCL reconstruction techniques are held.

REFERENCES

1. Callaway GH, Field LD, Deng XH, et al. Biomechanical evaluation of the medial collateral ligament of the elbow. *J Bone Joint Surg Am.* 1997;79:1223-1231.
2. Jobe FW, Stark H, Lombardo SJ. Reconstruction of the ulnar collateral ligament in athletes. *J Bone Joint Surg Am.* 1986;68:1158-1163.
3. Azar FM, Andrews JR, Wilk KE, et al. Operative treatment of ulnar collateral ligament injuries of the elbow in athletes. *Am J Sports Med.* 2000;28:16-23.
4. Cain EL, Andrews JR, Dugas JR, et al. Outcome of ulnar collateral ligament reconstruction of the elbow in 1281 athletes: results in 743 athletes with minimum 2-year follow-up. *Am J Sports Med.* 2010;38:2426-2434.
5. Thompson WH, Jobe FW, Yocum LA, et al. Ulnar collateral ligament reconstruction in athletes: muscle-splitting approach without transposition of the ulnar nerve. *J Shoulder Elbow Surg.* 2001;10:152-157.
6. Conway JE, Jobe FW, Glousman RE, et al. Medial instability of the elbow in throwing athletes: treatment by repair or reconstruction of the ulnar collateral ligament. *J Bone Joint Surg Am.* 1992;74:67-83.
7. Andrews JR, Wilk KE, Satterwhite YE, et al. Physical examination of the thrower's elbow. *J Orthop Sports Phys Ther.* 1993;17:296-304.
8. O'Driscoll SW, Lawton RL, Smith AM. The "moving valgus stress test" for medial collateral ligament tears of the elbow. *Am J Sports Med.* 2005;33:231-239.
9. Veltri DM, O'Brien SJ, Field LD, et al. The milking maneuver: a new test to evaluate the MCL of the elbow in the throwing athlete. *J Shoulder Elbow Surg.* 1995;4:S10.
10. Carrino JA, Morrison WB, Zou KH, et al. Noncontrast MR imaging and MR arthrography of the ulnar collateral ligament of the elbow: prospective evaluation of two-dimensional pulse sequences for detection of complete tears. *Skeletal Radiol.* 2001;30:625-632.
11. Rettig AC, Sherrill C, Snead DS, et al. Nonoperative treatment of ulnar collateral ligament injuries in throwing athletes. *Am J Sports Med.* 2001;29:15-17.
12. Vitale MA, Ahmad CS. The outcome of elbow ulnar collateral ligament reconstruction in overhead athletes: a systematic review. *Am J Sports Med.* 2008;36:1193-1205.

Part 4 DANE Technique

Joshua S. Dines and Neal S. ElAttrache

Chapter Synopsis
- Elbow ulnar collateral ligament (UCL) injuries are potentially career ending. The DANE technique is an effective way to reconstruct the ligament. It is performed through a muscle splitting approach and employs a combination of interference screw fixation on the ulna and the docking technique on the humerus. Clinical outcomes are excellent in about 90% of patients.

Important Points
- Ligament reconstruction can be considered in patients with medial-sided elbow pain who have examination findings and imaging studies consistent with UCL tear and in whom conservative management has failed.
- It is important to identify associated pathology, such as ulnar nerve injuries and/or symptoms consistent with valgus extension overload.
- Postoperatively, patients should not start a throwing program until the 4-month mark, and return to competition should not occur before 9 to 12 months after surgery.

Clinical and Surgical Pearls
- To reconstruct the ligament, a muscle splitting approach should be used.

- With use of an interference screw for fixation on the ulna, only one socket is needed distally, potentially decreasing risk to the ulnar nerve.
- The native ligament should be repaired after the graft is secured in the ulnar socket, before docking of the graft into the humerus.
- The graft should be tensioned with the elbow flexed 30 degrees, the forearm supinated, and a varus stress applied.

Clinical and Surgical Pitfalls
- Protect the graft when inserting the interference screw.
- Make sure the ulnar socket is distal enough to avoid penetration into the joint.
- Cycle the graft before determining the appropriate amount to dock into the humeral socket.

Video
- Video 46-1: Elbow ulnar collateral ligament reconstruction by the DANE technique

Elbow medial ulnar collateral ligament (UCL) reconstruction is the treatment of choice for overhand athletes with symptomatic ligament insufficiency who want to return to their previous level of sport. UCL injuries are the result of the extreme valgus forces generated during the late cocking and early acceleration phases of throwing. The primary restraint to these forces is the anterior bundle of the UCL; however, each throw approaches the ultimate tensile strength of the ligament. Shoulder internal rotation and the forearm flexors help stabilize the elbow, but repeated throwing can lead to microtrauma and eventual ligament failure.

Before Jobe's description of a reconstruction technique for UCL insufficiency, the injury was career ending.[1] Despite successful results in about 70% of patients, concerns with elevation of the flexor-pronator mass, ulnar nerve complications, and relatively large bone tunnels in the medial epicondyle of the humerus led to modifications to Jobe's technique. A novel modification was the docking technique, which relied on smaller holes in the relatively small medial epicondyle and simplified graft tensioning.[2] Based on the clinical success of the docking technique[2-4] combined with biomechanical studies that showed improved construct strength with interference screws, the DANE technique was developed (Table 46-4).[5,6] It relies on proximal docking of the graft, as described by David Altchek (DA) and distal interference screw fixation on the ulna based on work by Neal ElAttrache (NE).

Additional benefits of the DANE technique include better restoration of native ligament anatomy (based on cadaver studies showing that the UCL tapers to a narrower insertion on the ulna)[7]; decreased risk of ulnar nerve injury by obviating the need for a posterior ulnar tunnel; decreased risk of ulnar bone bridge fracture; and improved tendon-to-bone healing in the ulnar socket because of compression with the interference screw and aperture fixation. The technique is particularly useful with sublime tubercle insufficiency and for certain revision UCL procedures. The DANE technique is described in the following sections.

PREOPERATIVE CONSIDERATIONS

History

Athletes with injury to the UCL will report medial-sided elbow pain. With regard to baseball players, the pain typically occurs during the late cocking and early acceleration phases of throwing. Occasionally the injury will be acute, as evidenced by a "pop" during throwing, but more commonly it is a chronic or acute-on-chronic scenario. In these situations the athletes may report decreased pitch velocity or control and they may find it difficult to warm up. It is important to ask about ulnar nerve symptoms, because these are commonly associated with UCL tears. Transient ulnar paresthesias that occur during throwing are likely a result of the valgus instability. These typically resolve after reconstruction of the ligament. More persistent sensory symptoms, or motor symptoms, indicate intrinsic pathology to the nerve. These patients require transposition at the time of UCL reconstruction. Mechanical symptoms such as catching or locking may be a result of posteromedial olecranon osteophytes and/or loose bodies. It is important to realize that not all medial-sided elbow pain is caused by UCL insufficiency. A thorough differential diagnosis includes flexor-pronator tendinosis, ulnar neuritis, stress fractures of the olecranon or ulna, and posteromedial osteophytes.

Physical Examination

A thorough physical examination of an athlete with elbow pain begins with an assessment of the proximal components of the kinetic chain, including the shoulder, scapula, core, and lower extremities, because injuries to these areas can lead to changes in throwing biomechanics and subsequent elbow injury. The medial and lateral recesses should be performed to detect the presence of an effusion. Patients often have tenderness along the course of the ligament. Focal tenderness in the area of the flexor-pronator mass or various bony landmarks, including the posterior olecranon or radial head, may signify associated pathology. A positive compression test result or positive Tinel sign at the cubital tunnel may suggest the presence of ulnar neuropathy.

UCL competency is assessed with several specific physical examination maneuvers. The valgus stress test is performed with the elbow flexed 30 degrees and the forearm pronated. A valgus stress is applied to detect any widening at the ulnohumeral joint. Even in the absence of frank instability, some patients report pain with this maneuver. The moving valgus stress test, as described by O'Driscoll, is extremely sensitive for UCL tears.[7] The patient is seated upright with the arm placed in the abducted and externally rotated position to

TABLE 46-4. Results of Studies of the DANE Technique		
Author	No. of Patients	Outcome
Conway[5] (2006)	7	Excellent outcome in 6 of 7 (85%)
Dines et al[6] (2007)	22	Excellent results in 19 of 22 (86%); fair result in 2; poor result in 1

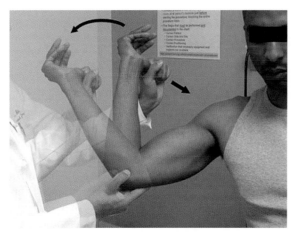

Figure 46-28. Moving valgus stress test as described by O'Driscoll.[2]

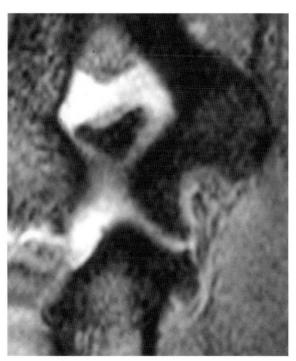

Figure 46-29. Coronal magnetic resonance imaging scan showing complete tear of ulnar collateral ligament.

simulate the throwing position. A valgus stress is applied to the elbow, which is ranged quickly from full flexion to extension. The maneuver is designed to simulate the valgus forces experienced during the overhead throw. For a positive test result, a patient reports pain at 70 to 120 degrees of the flexion arc (Fig. 46-28). Despite O'Driscoll's report of 100% sensitivity, in our experience, even in patients with UCL tears, the result of this test is often dependent on when the player last threw. Occasionally, players with UCL insufficiency who have been resting for weeks can have a negative moving valgus stress test result, whereas those with tears who have thrown within a few days before being examined almost always have a positive test result.

Imaging

Imaging evaluation includes standard anteroposterior (AP) and lateral radiographs of the elbow. With chronic valgus loading of the UCL, varying degrees of ligamentous ossification may be observed. At our institution we routinely use noncontrast magnetic resonance imaging (MRI) to diagnose UCL pathology (Fig. 46-29). It can also help identify other signs of valgus extension overload. Reported sensitivity for noncontrast MRI approaches 75%, and specificity has been reported to be 100% for UCL tears.

Indications and Contraindications

We reserve ligament reconstruction for athletes with medial-sided elbow pain consistent with UCL insufficiency who have failed conservative treatment. In addition, they must be willing to be compliant with the year-long rehabilitation process typically required after reconstruction.

The DANE technique may have particular utility with sublime tubercle insufficiency and/or revision UCL reconstructions.

Ulnar nerve transposition is indicated for athletes with motor changes resulting from ulnar nerve pathology or persistent sensory deficits. We prefer to use an anterior subcutaneous ulnar nerve transposition technique.

Preoperatively, we identify the source of our graft for ligament reconstruction. Gracilis or palmaris grafts are our preferred choices.

UCL reconstruction is contraindicated in patients unwilling to go through the prolonged postoperative rehabilitation course. In addition, if the athlete will not have the opportunity to play baseball again, the surgery is likely unnecessary. An example of this would be the high school athlete who is not talented enough to play in college. Clearly, active infection is a contraindication.

SURGICAL TECHNIQUE
Anesthesia and Positioning

The procedure is performed with the patient under regional anesthesia and supine and the injured arm on an arm board. We apply a nonsterile tourniquet to the upper arm, and the arm is prepared and draped in a sterile fashion.

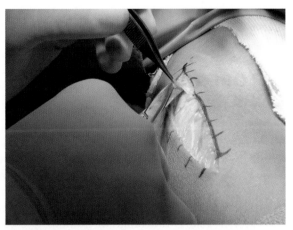

Figure 46-30. Medially based incision beginning just proximal to the medial epicondyle and extending distally past the sublime tubercle.

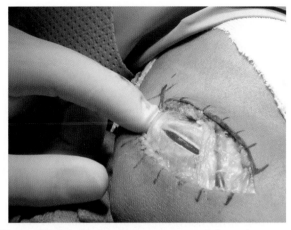

Figure 46-31. Native ligament exposed through a muscle splitting approach, then incised in line with its fibers.

BOX 46-4 Surgical Steps

- Incision
- Exposure and harvest of native ligament
- Creation of ulnar socket
- Creation of humeral socket
- Fixation of graft into the ulnar socket

Surgical Landmarks and Incisions

See Box 46-4.

At this point, the previously determined graft is harvested. If the Palmaris longus tendon is to be used, we make a small transverse incision just proximal to the wrist flexor crease. A No. 1 braided, nonabsorbable suture is placed in a Krackow fashion in the tendon before a tendon stripper is used to harvest the graft. The graft is then folded onto itself, and No. 2 nonabsorbable suture is used to run a locking Krackow stitch in the folded 25 mm of the graft. We then exsanguinate the arm and inflate the tourniquet. A medial incision is made starting 1 cm proximal to the medial epicondyle and extending distally over the UCL to a point about 2 cm past the sublime tubercle (Fig. 46-30).

A muscle splitting approach through the posterior third of the common flexor mass within the anterior fibers of the flexor carpi ulnaris is used. A submuscular dissection is used to expose the anterior bundle of the ligament. The joint is exposed by incision of the native ligament in line with its fibers (Fig. 46-31). UCL laxity can be confirmed by joint surface separation of 3 mm or more with the application of a valgus stress. We place a 2-0 Vicryl suture on each side of the ligament to be used for repair later in the procedure.

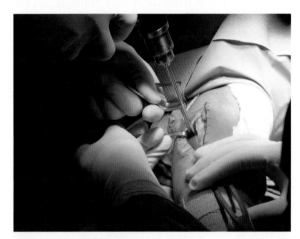

Figure 46-32. Ulnar socket created in the sublime tubercle.

The ulnar socket is centered on the sublime tubercle and angled just distally toward the supinator crest on the lateral aspect of the ulna. It is drilled to a depth of 15 mm (Fig. 46-32). The diameter is based on the size of the folded end of the graft.

On the humeral side, a 4.5-mm bur is used to create the humeral tunnel in the origin of the UCL on the anterior-distal aspect of the medial epicondyle (Fig. 46-33). Care should be taken to avoid a position that is too shallow in the epicondyle, leaving only a thin roof of bone over the graft. The tunnel is drilled longitudinally along the axis of the medial epicondyle to a depth of 15 mm. Two connecting puncture holes are made with a dental bur. These exit punctures should be located about 10 mm apart on the anterior surface of the epicondyle. Shuttling sutures are then brought through the humeral tunnel out each exit puncture and clamped for later use.

At this point, an appropriately sized Bio-Tenodesis Screw (Arthrex, Naples, FL) is used to secure the folded end of the graft in the ulnar socket (Fig. 46-34). We prefer to use a screw diameter that is the same size or slightly smaller than the tunnel. The native ligament is repaired with use of the previously placed sutures while the elbow is flexed 30 degrees, the forearm is supinated, and a varus stress is applied. The two limbs of the graft are measured for the appropriate length, and locking Krackow stitches are placed at each end. The anterior and posterior limbs are shuttled into the medial epicondylar tunnel. Application of tension through the grasping suture keeps the limbs of graft docked in the humeral tunnel. The elbow is again reduced with a varus force, and the forearm is supinated for cycling and tensioning of the graft. Final graft tensioning is verified, and the grasping sutures are tied over a bone bridge (Fig. 46-35).

The tourniquet is deflated, and hemostasis is achieved. The fascia from the muscle splitting approach is reapproximated. The wound is closed in layers; the patient is placed in a posterior splint with the elbow flexed about 50 degrees and the forearm is supinated to reduce the joint.

POSTOPERATIVE CONSIDERATIONS

Patients are switched to a hinged elbow brace at 1 week postoperatively. Because the anterior and posterior bands of the reconstructed ligament are not isometric, bracing is used to prevent excessive strain on the graft at extremes of range of motion. Motion is allowed from 60 to 100 degrees and advanced by about 15 degrees per week. The goal is full range of motion by 6 to 8 weeks after surgery, at which point the use of the brace is discontinued. Physical therapy is instituted to work on rotator cuff, forearm, core, and lower extremity strengthening. Any residual loss of elbow motion is addressed. Most baseball players start an interval throwing program at about 4 months after surgery and progress to throwing off a mound at about 8 months. Return to competitive pitching is allowed 9 to 12 months after surgery.

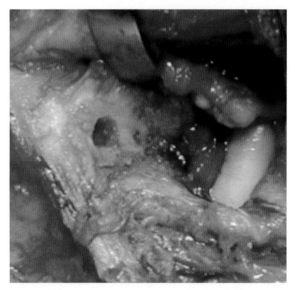

Figure 46-33. Humeral socket drilled to a depth of about 15 mm in the medial epicondyle.

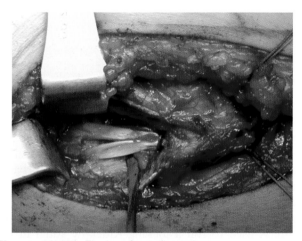

Figure 46-35. Final graft configuration.

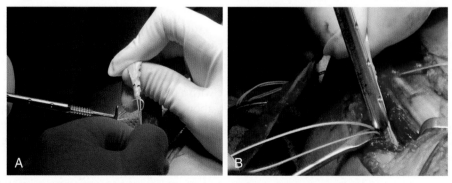

Figure 46-34. Graft fixed into ulnar socket with Bio-Tenodesis Screw *(Arthrex, Naples, FL)*.

RESULTS

The reported results of the DANE technique compare favorably with other reported outcomes of UCL reconstruction.[1-4,8] Conway initially described the DANE technique and reported his preliminary results.[5] He followed seven pitchers for more than 2 years after UCL reconstruction with the DANE technique; six of the seven had an excellent outcome (85%).

In a larger series, we reported on the outcomes of our first 22 athletes treated with the DANE technique.[6] Nineteen of 22 had excellent results (86%). There were two fair results and one poor outcome. The poor result was in a revision procedure. Impressively, in two other revision procedures, the players returned to their previous level of play, consistent with excellent outcomes.

SUMMARY

In conclusion, the DANE technique is the novel modification of the docking technique for UCL reconstruction. It incorporates the benefits of the docking technique, including smaller drill holes on the humerus and simplified tensioning, while adding the benefits of improved tendon-to-bone healing, better re-creation of the normal anatomy, and decreased risk of ulnar bone bridge fracture. In addition, it offers particular utility in revision UCL surgeries and in patients with sublime tubercle fracture or insufficiency.

REFERENCES

1. Jobe FW, Stark H, Lombardo SJ. Reconstruction of the ulnar collateral ligament in athletes. *J Bone Joint Surg Am*. 1986;68:1158-1163.
2. Rohrbough JT, Altchek DW, Hyman J, et al. Medial collateral ligament reconstruction of the elbow using the docking technique. *Am J Sports Med*. 2002;30:541.
3. Bowers A, Dines J, Dines D, et al. Elbow medial ulnar collateral ligament reconstruction: clinical relevance and the docking technique. *J Shoulder Elbow Surg*. 2010; 19(2S):110-117.
4. Dodson CC, Thomas A, Dines JS, et al. Medial ulnar collateral ligament reconstruction of the elbow in throwing athletes. *Am J Sports Med*. 2006;34(12):1926-1932.
5. Conway J. The DANE TJ. Procedure for Elbow Medial Ulnar Collateral Ligament Insufficiency. *Tech Shoulder Elbow Surg*. 2006;7(1):36-43.
6. Dines JS, ElAttrache NS, Conway J, et al. Clinical outcomes of the DANE TJ technique to treat medial ulnar collateral ligament insufficiency of the elbow. *Am J Sports Med*. 2007;35(12):2039-2044.
7. O'Driscoll S, Lawton R, Smith A. The moving valgus stress test for medial collateral ligament tears of the elbow. *Am J Sports Med*. 2005;33(2):231-239.
8. Vitale MA, Ahmad CS. The outcome of elbow ulnar collateral ligament reconstruction in overhead athletes: a systematic review. *Am J Sports Med*. 2008;36(6): 1193-2005.
9. Ochi N, Ogura T, Hashizume H, et al. Anatomic relation between the medial collateral ligament of the elbow and the humero-ulnar joint axis. *J Shoulder Elbow Surg*. 1999; 8:6-10.

Chapter 47

Surgical Treatment of Posterolateral Instability of the Elbow

Emilie Cheung, Eric Rightmire, and Marc R. Safran

Chapter Synopsis

- The pathoanatomy leading to chronic posterolateral rotatory instability of the elbow has become better understood in the last two decades owing to biomechanical and clinical studies. The results of surgical techniques to reconstruct or repair the lateral collateral ligament (LCL) complex have been favorable. Concomitant complex elbow trauma (fractures of the coronoid and radial head) is associated with more unpredictable results than isolated ligamentous injury. Recent advances in arthroscopic repair with promising outcomes have been described.

Important Points

- Posterolateral rotator instability is clinically evident when the elbow is loaded in the terminally extended and supinated position.
- Useful clinical tests are the posterolateral pivot test, posterolateral drawer test, prone pushup test, and armchair pushup test.

Clinical and Surgical Pearls

- Primary repair is preferable in acute situations when patients demonstrate recurrent instability refractory to an initial period of conservative treatment. This is performed by reattachment of the ligament to the anterior-inferior portion of the lateral epicondyle with suture anchor or transosseous fixation.
- In the setting of chronic ligamentous insufficiency for longer than 6 months, reconstruction of the deficient LCL complex with a free tendinous autograft or allograft is recommended.

Clinical and Surgical Pitfalls

- During surgical reconstruction of the LCL complex, the forearm should be pronated and flexed to approximately 60 degrees before final tying of the suture to secure the tendon graft.
- The humeral fixation point for the graft is usually more anterior than one would anticipate.
- Because instability occurs with the elbow in extension, it is important to ensure that the graft is placed taut enough in extension.

The term *posterolateral rotatory instability* (PLRI) was coined by O'Driscoll and colleagues[1] in 1991, though it was probably first recognized in 1966 (Osbourne-Cotterill). PLRI is now considered to be the most common pattern of recurrent elbow instability. Furthermore, it is currently accepted that chronic lateral collateral ligament (LCL) injury or laxity is the primary pathologic finding in the development of the unstable elbow in the absence of fracture, and it is this injury that is clinically found in PLRI.

The elbow is considered to be one of the most inherently stable, constrained joints in the body. Elbow stability is maintained by bony anatomy as well as by the medial and lateral ligamentous complexes and balanced muscle forces. The ulnohumeral, radiohumeral, and radioulnar joints are the three articulations that compose the bony anatomy of the elbow joint.

The lateral and medial sides of the elbow have distinct ligamentous complexes. The medial, or ulnar, collateral ligament complex has three components: the anterior oblique ligament, also known as the *anterior bundle;* the posterior oblique ligament, also known as the *posterior bundle;* and the transverse ligament, also known as the *Cooper ligament.* The anterior oblique ligament is functionally subdivided into anterior and posterior bands; it is widely considered to be the primary restraint to valgus stress.

The lateral or radial side, known as the *lateral collateral ligament complex,* has four components: the lateral (or radial) ulnar collateral ligament, the radial collateral ligament (RCL), the annular ligament, and the accessory LCL. Deficiency of the lateral ulnar collateral ligament (LUCL) is widely believed to be the primary component in PLRI, as demonstrated by O'Driscoll and colleagues.[1,2] Studies have shown that LUCL is the essential lesion in PLRI, but clinically the RCL and lateral capsule are also important stabilizing structures.[3-5] Cadaveric studies have demonstrated that PLRI is evident only when both the LUCL and RCL are injured, but not when they are cut in isolation.[6,7]

The LUCL originates proximally on the lateral epicondyle of the humerus and attaches distally to the tubercle of the supinator crest of the ulna. The humeral attachment is historically considered to be the isometric point on the lateral side of the elbow. However, recently it has been elucidated that there is no "true" isometric point because the ligament length changes with flexion and extension.[8] The distal attachment is a broad fan-shaped thickening of the capsule that blends with and arches superficial and distal to the annular ligament to insert onto the ulna.[3,4] The LCL complex also serves as a posterior sling to prevent posterior subluxation of the radial head.

PLRI can be considered a spectrum of instability, consisting of three stages ranging from instability to frank dislocation, according to the degree of soft tissue disruption.[1,2] In PLRI the proximal radioulnar joint relationship is maintained, and both the ulna and radius move together as one unit relative to the humerus. This begins with injury to the LCL complex. First, there is subluxation of the elbow in a posterolateral direction such that there is posterior radial head subluxation underneath the humerus. Second, as soft tissue disruption continues to involve the anterior and posterior capsule, there is incomplete dislocation with the coronoid perched underneath the trochlea. Third, there is complete dislocation of the elbow with the coronoid resting behind the humerus. Again, in this spectrum of instability the radioulnar relationship is maintained.

In the setting of trauma, the lateral ligamentous injury that results in PLRI usually occurs proximally, at the lateral epicondyle. After an elbow dislocation there is usually a "bare area" visible at the lateral epicondyle where the LCL complex has become avulsed with associated involvement of the RCL and the common extensor tendon origin (Fig. 47-1).

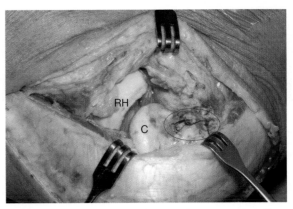

Figure 47-1. Intraoperative image demonstrating "bare area" (within the black circle) at the region of the lateral epicondyle on the left elbow. This patient had a history of recurrent posterolateral rotatory instability after traumatic dislocation of the elbow.

PREOPERATIVE CONSIDERATIONS

History

Patients have symptoms of pain, locking, snapping, clicking, or recurrent instability, usually preceded by trauma to the elbow or a fall on an outstretched hand (50% to 75%) or, less commonly, a history of previous elbow surgery.[5] A history of elbow dislocation is common, although some patients may report recurrent elbow sprains.[9] Ligamentous laxity and childhood elbow fracture with a resultant cubitus varus deformity have also been reported to be predisposing factors.[10] PLRI can also occur iatrogenically through lateral elbow surgical approaches that disrupt the ligament, arthroscopic elbow procedures, or multiple steroid injections into the region.[5,11]

In the case of traumatic injury, the mechanism usually involves axial compression, hyperextension, and external rotation (supination) of the elbow (Fig. 47-2). Direct varus stress injuries are a less common cause. These usually occur with a fall onto an outstretched hand. In general, injury to the lateral ligamentous structures is considered the initial stage in a continuum of instability[1] (Fig. 47-3). This begins with injury to the LUCL, followed by injury to the entire LCL complex, to the anterior and posterior capsule, and finally to the posterior and anterior bands of the ulnar collateral ligament complex, leading to frank dislocation.

Physical Examination

In cases of chronic LUCL insufficiency, physical examination will elicit symptoms of apprehension when the elbow is loaded in the terminally extended and supinated position. The PLRI test (lateral pivot shift test)

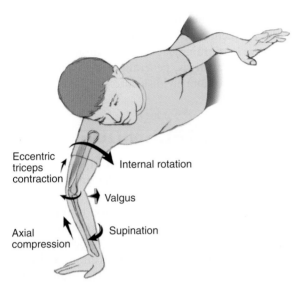

Figure 47-2. Axial compression, hyperextension, and external rotation (supination) mechanism of injury.

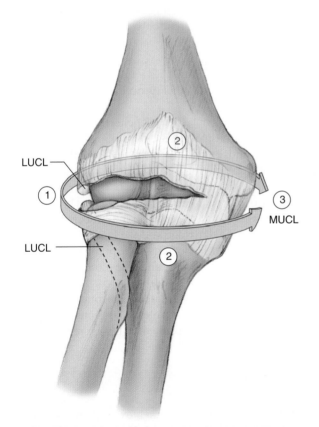

Figure 47-3. Continuum of instability. *LUCL,* Lateral ulnar collateral ligament; *MUCL,* medial ulnar collateral ligament.

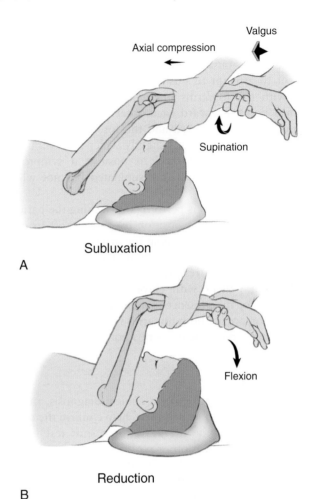

Figure 47-4. Posterolateral rotatory instability test.

has been described for the diagnosis of PLRI.[1,2] The test is easiest to perform with the patient in a supine position (Fig. 47-4). With the shoulder forward flexed, the forearm is placed in full supination and extension. The elbow is then gently flexed while the examiner applies a slight valgus force and axial load. The radial head is subluxed in the starting (extended) position. Posterior subluxation of the radial head can be palpated as a posterior prominence and dimple in the skin. With further flexion beyond 40 degrees, the radial head spontaneously reduces with a "clunk," reproducing the patient's symptoms. With more significant injury and laxity, the clunk of reduction occurs in greater degrees of elbow flexion. This maneuver may be difficult to perform in an awake patient, and thus guarding and apprehension alone are suggestive of a positive test result. Because of guarding, demonstration of the pivot shift may require local (intra-articular) anesthetic or general anesthesia. The test may also be done under live fluoroscopic visualization.

Other tests are the posterolateral drawer test, the prone pushup test, and the chair pushup test.[12] The posterolateral drawer test is analogous to the drawer or Lachman test of the knee. The patient is placed supine with the arm in the overhead position, such that it represents a leg, and the elbow resembles a knee. The elbow is flexed 90 degrees and supinated. With terminal supination the lateral side of the forearm is rotated away from the humerus, so that the radius and ulna subluxate away from the humerus, leaving a dimple in the skin behind the radial head.

The prone pushup test is performed by asking the patient to attempt to push up from a prone position, first with the forearms maximally pronated and the thumbs pointed toward each other and then with the thumbs pointed outward and the forearms maximally supinated, with the hands slightly wider than shoulder width apart. The test result is positive if symptoms occur when the forearms are supinated but not when they are pronated.

The chair pushup is performed by asking the patient to stand from a sitting position by pushing off from a chair with the hands grasping the armrests with palms facing inward (forearm supination). Pain on this maneuver is a positive test result.

When a patient with chronic PLRI is examined, evaluation for the presence of a palmaris longus tendon in either forearm or both forearms is important to determine whether the patient has this potential graft source.

Imaging

Although PLRI is primarily a clinical diagnosis, radiologic evaluation can be helpful to help confirm the diagnosis. Studies include the PLRI pivot shift test under fluoroscopic visualization or with stress radiographs to demonstrate radial head subluxation and ulnohumeral joint widening. Plain films can show bony avulsions or subtle signs of subluxation. Magnetic resonance imaging has been shown to be useful in identifying components of the lateral collateral complex with the appropriate thin-cut pulse sequences and an experienced radiology staff.[13] Arthroscopy is a useful adjunct to help identify radial head subluxation or lateral joint widening with stress testing and to assess any intra-articular disease.[14,15]

Indications and Contraindications

Acute, simple elbow dislocations are best treated non-surgically with a splint for approximately 1 to 2 weeks. The forearm should be kept in pronation. However, if there is a bony avulsion, primary surgical repair may provide reliably consistent good results and prevent chronic instability. Surgery is indicated for patients who have recurrent instability of the elbow after the initial 2-week period of conservative treatment. For example, if a patient experiences recurrent instability after the splint has been removed, then he or she would be a candidate for repair of the LCL complex back to the lateral epicondyle. Patients with associated fractures of the radial head and coronoid should also be treated with fracture fixation if the respective fractures are displaced. If the injury is over 6 months old, then such a patient would possibly be a candidate for ligamentous

reconstruction rather than repair because it is thought that the ligament tends to attenuate with time.

Relative contraindications to surgery are open physes, elbow arthritis, generalized ligamentous laxity, and ability to voluntarily dislocate. No absolute contraindications exist.

SURGICAL TECHNIQUE

General anesthesia with the patient in the supine position is preferred. Examination under anesthesia is performed to include medial and lateral stability testing and posterolateral rotatory stability testing. Fluoroscopic visualization is performed during stability testing if the diagnosis is in question. The upper extremity is prepared and draped in the usual fashion, and a tourniquet is applied to the upper arm. The graft of choice is an autogenous palmaris longus, with ipsilateral being the first choice and contralateral the second. If no palmaris longus is present, a lower extremity is prepared and draped for semitendinosus or gracilis harvesting. Alternatively, allograft tendon can be used.

Specific Steps

The specific steps of this procedure are outlined in Box 47-1.

An 8- to 10-cm lateral (Kocher) incision is made beginning approximately 3 cm proximal to the lateral epicondyle and extending over the lateral epicondyle and along the anterior border of the anconeus distally (Fig. 47-5). The interval between the anconeus and the extensor carpi ulnaris is developed. The proximal anconeus and distal triceps can be reflected from the lateral supracondylar ridge and the lateral epicondyle to improve exposure. The extensor carpi ulnaris is elevated off the annular ligament and the common extensor tendon–extensor carpi radialis brevis is elevated off the anterior aspect of the lateral epicondyle to expose the lateral ligamentous complex. Care must be taken to preserve the anterior capsule and LUCL remnant. This

---

BOX 47-1 Surgical Steps

1. Lateral (Kocher) incision 3 cm proximal to the lateral epicondyle and extending over the lateral epicondyle and along the anterior border of the anconeus distally
2. Primary repair: reattachment of the intact ligament to the anterior-inferior portion of the lateral epicondyle
3. Reconstruction of the deficient lateral ulnar collateral ligament with a free ligamentous autograft
4. Tensioning and suturing of the graft
5. Plication of the capsule over the graft
6. Final tensioning of the graft

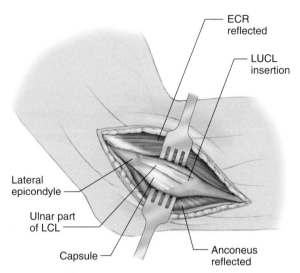

Figure 47-5. Surgical approach (Kocher). *ECR,* extensor carpi radialis; *LCL,* lateral collateral ligament; *LUCL,* lateral ulnar collateral ligament.

is most easily accomplished by beginning the dissection distally in the interval. Use of a periosteal or Freer elevator rather than a knife may facilitate dissection while reducing the risk of further injury to the underlying LCL complex.

A modified PLRI pivot test can be performed again at this time to identify ligament and capsular deficiencies. This may be performed by placing the elbow in terminal extension and supination. The position of the radial head in relation to the capitellum can be visualized. The radial head is usually noted to rotate posterolaterally away from the capitellum as the elbow is placed in this position of terminal extension and supination. The LUCL is examined and assessed for primary repair. If adequate tissue is not available, a ligamentous graft reconstruction is indicated.

Primary repair is performed by reattachment of the intact ligament to the anterior-inferior portion of the lateral epicondyle with suture anchors or transosseous sutures. This is usually performed with capsular plication. Two drill holes are placed in the midportion of the lateral epicondyle at the anatomic origin of the LUCL. A nonabsorbable suture is placed through a drill hole, and a running locked stitch is placed along the path of the ligament. The suture is then tied over the bone bridge. Alternatively, a suture anchor is placed at the origin of the LUCL, and a locked running suture is placed in the LUCL remnant for the primary repair. The humeral fixation point for the graft is usually more anterior than one would anticipate. Because instability occurs with the elbow in extension, it is important to ensure that the graft is placed taut enough in extension. The forearm is pronated and flexed to approximately 60 to 70 degrees before final tying of the suture. The elbow is then splinted at 90 degrees of flexion and pronation.

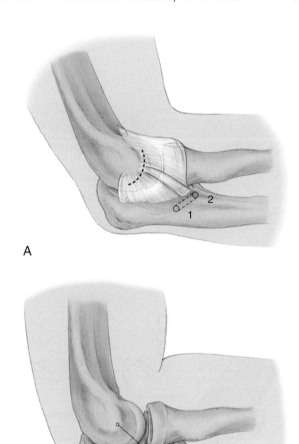

Figure 47-6. Two drill holes in the ulna in the supinator tubercle and 1 to 1.5 cm posterior and perpendicular to the axis of the lateral ulnar collateral ligament.

Reconstruction of the deficient LUCL is performed with a free ligamentous graft, such as the palmaris longus tendon, semitendinosus, or gracilis. Required graft length is approximately 20 cm. The palmaris longus can be harvested through a 1-cm incision at the distal volar wrist crease with a standard tendon stripper. A capsular incision of the lateral elbow is made anterior to the lateral ligamentous complex for joint inspection and later imbrication. The graft should be reconstructed superficial to the deep capsular layer to avoid any potential abrasion of the cartilage by the sutures within the graft. Two 3.5-mm drill holes are placed in the ulna, one into the supinator tubercle just distal to the lateral attachment of the capsule and the other approximately 1 to 1.5 cm posterior in a perpendicular line to the axis of the LUCL. The underlying bone is channeled with a curved awl connecting the two holes (Fig. 47-6).

A suture is passed through the drill holes, and a hemostat is attached to help identify the isometric attachment of the LCL complex on the lateral epicondyle.

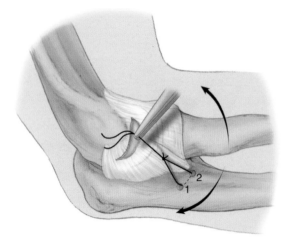

Figure 47-7. Determination of the isometric point.

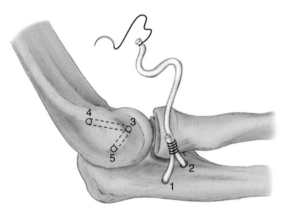

Figure 47-8. Drilling of the humeral tunnels.

The hemostat is placed on the lateral epicondyle, and the elbow is flexed and extended to identify the ideal isometric point at which both limbs of the suture remain taut (Fig. 47-7). This point should correspond to the middle of the capitellum on a lateral radiograph.

A 4.5-mm drill hole is placed at the isometric point angled medially and proximally toward the supracondylar ridge and burred to a size of 5 or 6 mm. This hole should tend anterior and proximal to the established isometric point, especially during enlargement, to ensure that the graft is tight in extension. A second hole is made just posterior to the supracondylar ridge, about 1.5 cm proximally, and a tunnel is developed between the two. A second tunnel is made from the same isometric entry point by drilling a third hole 1 to 1.5 cm distal to the second hole so that a bridge of bone remains between it and the first tunnel (Fig. 47-8).

The graft is passed through the ulnar tunnel from anterior to posterior. One end of the graft is passed into the isometric hole in the humerus, out the proximal tunnel, along the posterior humeral cortex, and back in the distal tunnel, emerging through the isometric hole (Fig. 47-9).

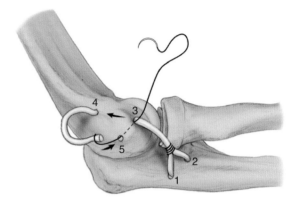

Figure 47-9. Passing of the graft.

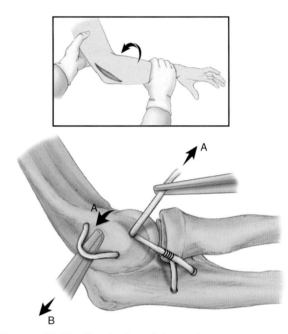

Figure 47-10. Tensioning of the graft.

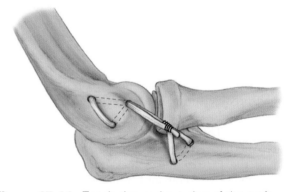

Figure 47-11. Tensioning and suturing of the graft.

The graft is tensioned with the arm maximally pronated in about 60 to 70 degrees of flexion and sutured to itself in a figure-of-eight configuration (Figs. 47-10 and 47-11).

Alternatively, interference screw fixation with screw-in suture anchors may be used instead of the

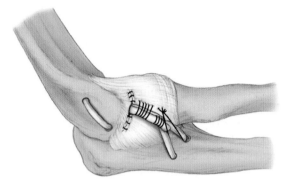

Figure 47-12. Plication of the capsule over the graft.

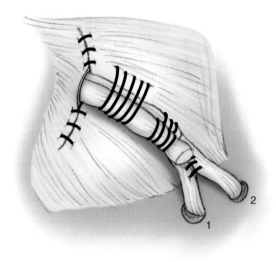

Figure 47-13. Final tensioning of the graft.

transosseous tunnel technique. The appropriate length required for the graft is measured, taking into account the desired graft length that will be needed to occupy the length of each of the bone tunnels. A blind-ended tunnel in the lateral epicondyle is created at the isometric point, and the graft is secured with an interference screw. This eliminates the need for three holes and two tunnels in the lateral epicondyle. The resultant graft may be double-stranded instead of a three-ply reconstruction with the figure-of-eight graft originally described. If a semitendinosus or gracilis graft is used, the thickness of a single-ply graft may be sufficient. Another blind-ended tunnel is then created at the supinator crest, and the graft is secured with an interference screw. The interference screw technique can be used on either end or on both ends (humeral and ulnar) for fixation. The capsule is plicated as necessary beneath the graft and sutured to the graft for augmentation (Fig. 47-12). One disadvantage of the interference screw technique is that there is limited ability to fine-tune the tensioning of the graft with the placement of the screws.

The graft is tensioned further by pulling it anteriorly and suturing it to the capsule and by closing the distal loop of the figure-of-eight construct (Fig. 47-13). The overlying soft tissues are closed in layers.

POSTOPERATIVE CONSIDERATIONS

Rehabilitation

An above-elbow splint is placed postoperatively with the forearm in pronation and the elbow at 90 degrees of flexion. It is removed at 1 week, and a 30-degree extension block splint or hinged brace is applied for 6 weeks. Full range of motion in a hinged elbow brace is initiated at 6 weeks. Bracing is usually discontinued after 2 to 3 months, at which point the patient begins a strengthening program within pain-free limits. This can be variable on the basis of the patient's compliance and the strength of the repair. Full recovery is expected after 6 to 9 months.

Complications

Potential complications include cutaneous nerve damage (from incision or tendon harvesting), persistent flexion contracture, and persistent instability. Care is required to prevent fracturing through bone bridges. Persistent instability can often be attributed to a posteriorly placed tunnel on the humerus that leaves the graft lax in extension, the position in which PLRI occurs. Persistent flexion contracture of about 10 degrees has often been reported after surgical reconstruction, but this can be protective against recurrent instability because PLRI occurs in terminal extension.

RESULTS

Primary repair of the LUCL in the acute setting, when possible, has excellent results. Osborne and Cotterill[16] reported excellent results in eight patients with transosseous repair, and Nestor and colleagues[17] reported excellent results in three patients. Ligamentous reconstruction results have been mixed (Table 47-1). Sanchez-Sotelo and colleagues[18] reported that 86% of 44 of patients had a satisfactory outcome after reconstruction or repair of the LUCL, and the mean Mayo Clinic Elbow Performance Index score was 85 at a mean of 6 years. Five of the 44 patients had recurrence of instability after the index surgery. Significantly better results were reported in patients with a posttraumatic cause, in those with subjective symptoms of instability, and in those who had an augmented reconstruction with use of a tendon graft.

Rhyou and Park[21] reported on preliminarily favorable results in a small case series of three patients who had a novel technique of dual reconstruction of both the RCL and LUCL with use of the palmaris or a half-slip of the flexor carpi radialis tendon. The authors

TABLE 47-1. Results after Reconstruction of the Lateral Ulnar Collateral Ligament

Study	Mean Follow-up	Outcome
Sanchez-Sotelo et al[18] (2005)	6 years	40 (89%) of 45 stable 38 (84%) of 45 satisfied
Olsen and Søjbjerg[19] (2003)	44 months	14 (78%) of 18 stable 17 (94%) of 18 satisfied
Nestor et al[17] (1992)*	42 months	10 (91%) of 11 stable 7 (64%) of 11 excellent
Lee and Teo[20] (2003)*	24 months	10 (100%) of 10 stable 10 (100%) of 10 satisfied

*Study group included direct repair and ligament reconstruction.

modified the original technique by placing the graft insertion site through the annular ligament instead of through the supinator crest of the ulna with the intention of producing a more flexible isometric point setting. The graft was passed outward to inward through two slits in the annular ligament: one just distal to the insertion site of the annular ligament near the proximal ulna, and the other just distal to the equator of the annular ligament. The two limbs of the graft were tightened and secured to the isometric point on the lateral epicondyle. They attempted to reconstruct both the RCL and the LUCL simultaneously and to incorporate them into the annular ligament to simulate the normal LCL complex. The authors reported that the patients had complete resolution of PLRI after this procedure but acknowledged that the report was very limited in the level of clinical follow-up, and the actual length of follow-up was not reported.

Arthroscopy

Arthroscopic techniques for diagnosis of PLRI have been described.[14,15] While the surgeon views from an anteromedial portal, a pivot-shift maneuver is performed, and the radial head may be seen rotating and translating posteriorly if PLRI is present. While the surgeon views from a posterolateral portal, the arthroscope can be easily driven through the lateral gutter and into the lateral aspect of the ulnohumeral joint. This has been called the *elbow drive-through sign*, analogous to the drive-through sign in shoulder instability. In addition, in viewing from the posterolateral portal or the direct lateral portal, the radial head can be seen subluxating posteriorly with supination with the elbow near extension, and occasionally in flexion.

Arthroscopic techniques for plication of the LCL complex have been described by Smith and colleagues.[14,15] Sutures are placed arthroscopically into the lateral gutter, tightening the posterolateral structures. The capsular plication can be augmented by percutaneous placement of a suture anchor at the lateral epicondyle, lassoing the plication sutures arthroscopically and in effect reattaching the ligament complex to the lateral epicondyle. With this technique, Smith and colleagues[14,15] found that results were equally as effective as open techniques in improving elbow function. In addition to capsular plication, arthroscopic electrothermal shrinkage of the ligamentous structures for recurrent PLRI has also been reported by Spahn and colleagues.[22] They documented good to moderate results with this technique, with a mean improvement in MEPS score from 40 preoperatively to 77 postoperatively, at a mean of 2.5 years.

CONCLUSION

The pathoanatomy leading to chronic lateral instability of the elbow has become better understood in the last two decades owing to biomechanical and clinical studies investigating this complex injury. The results of surgical techniques that reconstruct or repair the LUCL have been favorable. Newer arthroscopic techniques to reconstruct the LCL complex have been shown to have promising outcomes.

REFERENCES

1. O'Driscoll SW, Bell DF, Morrey BF. Posterolateral rotatory instability of the elbow. *J Bone Joint Surg Am.* 1991;73:440-446.
2. O'Driscoll SW, Morrey BF, Korinek S, et al. Elbow subluxation and dislocation. A spectrum of instability. *Clin Orthop Relat Res.* 1992;280:186-197.
3. Cohen MS, Hastings II H. Rotatory instability of the elbow: the anatomy and role of the lateral elbow stabilizers. *J Bone Joint Surg Am.* 1997;79:225-233.
4. Dunning CE, Zarzour ZD, Patterson SD, et al. Ligamentous stabilizers against posterolateral rotatory instability of the elbow. *J Bone Joint Surg Am.* 2001;83:1823-1828.
5. Hall JA, McKee MD. Posterolateral rotatory instability of the elbow following radial head resection. *J Bone Joint Surg Am.* 2005;87:1571-1579.
6. McAdams TR, Masters GW, Srivastava S. The effect of arthroscopic sectioning of the lateral ligament complex of the elbow on posterolateral rotatory stability. *J Shoulder Elbow Surg.* 2005;14(3):298-301.
7. Regan WD, Korinek SL, Morrey BF, et al. Biomechanical study of ligaments around the elbow joint. *Clin Orthop Relat Res.* 1991;271:170-179.
8. Morimoto H, Murase T, Arimitsu S, et al. The in vivo isometric point of the lateral ligament of the elbow. *J Bone Joint Surg Am.* 2007;89:2011-2017
9. Ball CM, Galatz LM, Yamaguchi K. Elbow instability: treatment strategies and emerging concepts. *Instr Course Lect.* 2002;51:53-61.
10. O'Driscoll SW, Spinner RJ, McKee MD, et al. Tardy posterolateral rotatory instability of the elbow due to cubitus varus. *J Bone Joint Surg Am.* 2001;83:1358-1369.

11. Mehta JA, Bain GI. Posterolateral rotatory instability of the elbow. *J Am Acad Orthop Surg.* 2004;12:405-415.

12. Regan W. Lapner PC. Prospective evaluation of two diagnostic apprehension signs for posterolateral instability of the elbow. *J Shoulder Elbow Surg.* 2006;13:344-346.

13. Potter HG, Weiland AJ, Schatz JA, et al. Posterolateral rotatory instability of the elbow: usefulness of MR imaging in diagnosis. *Radiology.* 1997;204:185-189.

14. Smith JP 3rd, Savoie FH 3rd, Field LD. Posterolateral rotatory instability of the elbow. *Clin Sports Med.* 2001;20:47-58.

15. Yadao MA, Savoie FH 3rd, Field LD. Posterolateral rotatory instability of the elbow. *Instr Course Lect.* 2004;23:629-642.

16. Osborne G, Cotterill P. Recurrent dislocation of the elbow. *J Bone Joint Surg Br.* 1966;48:340-346.

17. Nestor BJ, O'Driscoll SW, Morrey BF. Ligamentous reconstruction for posterolateral rotatory instability of the elbow. *J Bone Joint Surg Am.* 1992;74:1235-1241.

18. Sanchez-Sotelo J, Morrey BF, O'Driscoll SW. Ligamentous repair and reconstruction for posterolateral rotatory instability of the elbow. *J Bone Joint Surg Br.* 2005;87:54-61.

19. Olsen BS, Søjbjerg JO. The treatment of recurrent posterolateral instability of the elbow. *J Bone Joint Surg Br.* 2003;85:342-346.

20. Lee BP, Teo LH. Surgical reconstruction for posterolateral instability of the elbow. *J Shoulder Elbow Surg.* 2003;12:476-479.

21. Rhyou H, Park MJ. Dual reconstruction of the radial collateral ligament and lateral ulnar collateral ligament in posterolateral rotator instability of the elbow. *Knee Surg Sports Trauma Arthrosc.* 2011;19:1009-1012.

22. Spahn G, Kirschbaum S, Klinger HM, et al. Arthroscopic electrothermal shrinkage of chronic posterolateral elbow instability: good or moderate outcome in 21 patients followed for an average of 2.5 years. *Acta Orthop.* 2006;77:285-289.

Chapter 48

Open Elbow Contracture Release

David Ring and Diego Fernandez

Chapter Synopsis

- Elbow stiffness is common after injury.
- A stiff capsule can usually be stretched with confident exercises; patience is warranted, because intentionally hurting one's elbow after injury or surgery can be counterintuitive.
- Operative treatment is necessary when heterotopic ossification, implants, malunion, nonunion, or articular damage hinders motion and when there is compression of the ulnar nerve.
- Knowledge of both the medial and the lateral approaches to elbow contracture release allows the surgeon to address all forms of posttraumatic elbow stiffness.

Important Points

- Have patience with pure capsular contracture.
- Examine closely for signs of ulnar nerve compression.
- Heterotopic ossification has a better prognosis than pure capsular contracture. It is probably best to plan surgery for 3 to 4 months after injury to allow the bone to mature and the soft tissues to become more mobile.

Clinical and Surgical Pearls

- A single posterior skin incision gives access to the entire elbow.
- Good anterior exposure is possible through either lateral or medial muscle intervals.
- The anterior interval on the lateral side is roughly between the extensor carpi radialis brevis (ECRB) and the extensor digitorum communis (EDC) (it is difficult to be precise). On the medial side the anterior interval is a 50:50 split of the flexor pronator mass anterior to the ulnar nerve.

Clinical and Surgical Pitfalls

- For release of capsular contracture, remove the implants *after* having pushed the elbow into maximum flexion and extension.
- It is better to keep the implants used to repair the fracture in place when heterotopic bone is removed. The combined removal of bone and implants creates a notable risk of fracture.
- The better one understands where the pathology is, the easier the surgery (i.e., the better the planning). Three-dimensional computed tomography should be performed to allow study of the precise location of the heterotopic bone that is blocking motion.

Elbow motion can be restricted by contracture of the skin, capsule, and muscles; heterotopic ossification, osteophytes, or implants; articular incongruity or damage; and malunion or nonunion.[1] Ulnar neuropathy is commonly associated with elbow contracture and can be precipitated or exacerbated by surgeries that increase mobility.[2] The best candidate for an arthroscopic elbow contracture release is a patient with capsular contracture with or without osteophytes. Most patients with pure capsular contractures after trauma can achieve functional motion with time and exercises (including static progressive or dynamic elbow splinting).[3,4] Primary elbow arthritis is uncommon. Ulnar nerve decompression is worth considering in patients with less than 100 degrees of flexion even when there are no signs or symptoms of ulnar neuropathy.[2] Once the ulnar nerve has been released, performance of a capsular excision from the medial side is straightforward.[5] Arthroscopic elbow contracture release is more difficult and more dangerous than open contracture release, particularly because elbow arthroscopy is an uncommon procedure at which most of us are not well practiced.[6-10] For all of these reasons, operative treatment of elbow stiffness is best reserved for patients with heterotopic bone, errant implants, or ulnar neuropathy—situations in which an open procedure is preferable.

PREOPERATIVE CONSIDERATIONS

History

It is helpful to be aware of the details of prior trauma, burn, or central nervous system injury, prior surgeries in particular. In patients with prior central nervous system injury, one must determine the ability of the patient to participate in a postoperative rehabilitation protocol.[11] A painful contracture suggests arthritis or ulnar neuropathy. Numbness and dexterity problems suggest ulnar neuropathy.

Physical Examination

The quality of the skin is important, particularly in postburn contractures.[12] The status of the skin with respect to prior injury and operative treatment will influence the operative tactics. When planning operative treatment of a posttraumatic contracture, we prefer to wait until the skin and scar are mobile and soft and no longer edematous or adherent. A complete motor and sensory examination of the ulnar nerve is performed, along with evaluation for a Tinel sign and an elbow flexion test.

Imaging

Standard anteroposterior and lateral radiographs of the elbow are usually sufficient to identify and to characterize arthritis, heterotopic ossification, and nonunions, but computed tomography is occasionally of use. In more complex cases the computed tomographic scan can help with preoperative planning.[11] Three-dimensional reconstructions are particularly easy to interpret. Computed tomographic scans may be particularly useful for characterizing malunion of the articular surface of the distal humerus.[13]

Neurophysiologic testing should be considered when there is any possibility of preoperative ulnar neuropathy.

Indications and Contraindications

Morrey and colleagues[14] found that 15 daily activities could be accomplished with an arc of ulnohumeral motion of 30 to 130 degrees of flexion and an arc of forearm rotation of 50 degrees of pronation to 50 degrees of supination. However, these numbers should not be used to decide when to operate for elbow stiffness. Patients can adapt to and function well with much less motion,[15] perhaps more so when the stiffness is in the nondominant elbow. Therefore the indication for operative contracture release is a combination of diminished elbow motion and disability directly related to stiffness.

Simple capsular contracture (no heterotopic bone, no malunion or nonunion, no implants blocking motion, no ulnar neuropathy) usually responds to reassurance and encouragement of exercises, time, and static progressive or dynamic elbow splinting.[3] Therefore one should never rush into operative treatment of capsular contracture; patience and frequent visits for reassurance and encouragement are worthwhile.

Obvious hindrances to motion, including heterotopic bone, malunion, nonunion, prominent implants, and ulnar neuropathy, merit operative treatment. Heterotopic ossification can be resected within 3 or 4 months of injury (when it is radiographically mature and the skin is mobile with little or no edema) regardless of activity on bone scans.[11,12,16,17] Stiffness associated with advanced arthrosis or unsalvageable nonunion or malunion should be treated by interpositional or prosthetic elbow arthroplasty.[18,19]

Surgical Planning

Elbow capsulectomy can be performed simultaneously with debridement of a deep infection. It also forms an integral part of the treatment of malunion,[13] nonunion,[19] and instability.[20] Unstable skin can be treated with either prior or concomitant procedures to improve soft tissue coverage.[12]

Patients with capsular contracture who desire extension can be treated with lateral capsulectomy (Fig. 48-1).[21,22] Patients with concomitant ulnar neuropathy or limitation of elbow flexion are best treated with medial capsulectomy (Fig. 48-2).[5,23] Patients with heterotopic bone, prominent implants, or complex contracture that cannot be adequately released from medial or lateral alone may benefit from a combined release.[5,12] Preoperative (within 24 hours) radiation therapy (a single 7-Gy dose) is administered to patients with heterotopic bone to be excised.

Direct anterior release[24] is rarely necessary because the anterior capsule can be more safely excised from medial or lateral. A posterior release with splitting of the triceps and fenestration of the olecranon fossa for access to the anterior elbow is used primarily for debridement of primary elbow arthrosis.[2]

This chapter describes elbow capsulectomy through lateral (see Fig. 48-1) and medial (see Fig. 48-2) intervals.

Text continued on p. 515

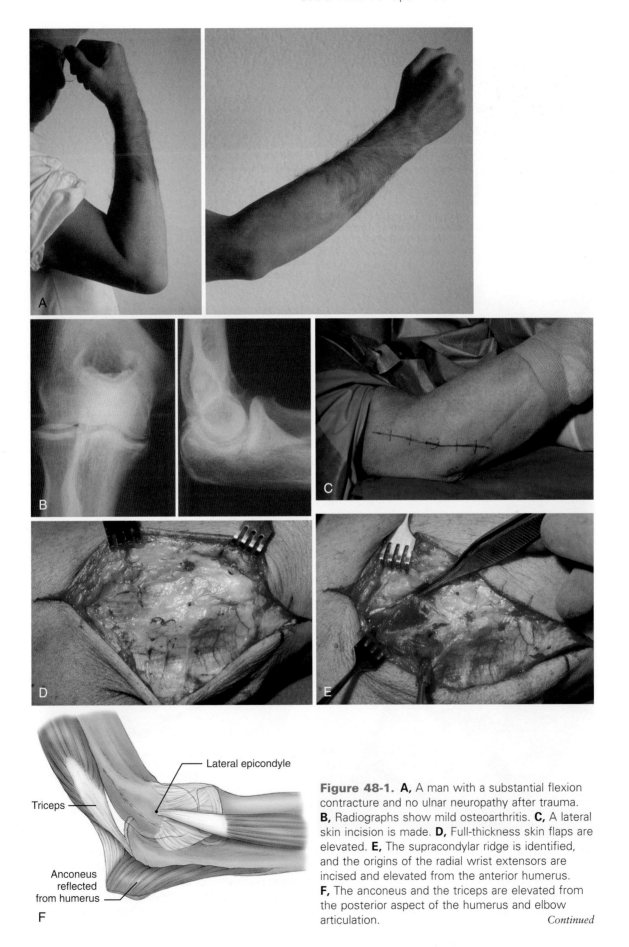

Figure 48-1. A, A man with a substantial flexion contracture and no ulnar neuropathy after trauma. **B,** Radiographs show mild osteoarthritis. **C,** A lateral skin incision is made. **D,** Full-thickness skin flaps are elevated. **E,** The supracondylar ridge is identified, and the origins of the radial wrist extensors are incised and elevated from the anterior humerus. **F,** The anconeus and the triceps are elevated from the posterior aspect of the humerus and elbow articulation. *Continued*

Lateral epicondyle

Triceps

Anconeus reflected from humerus

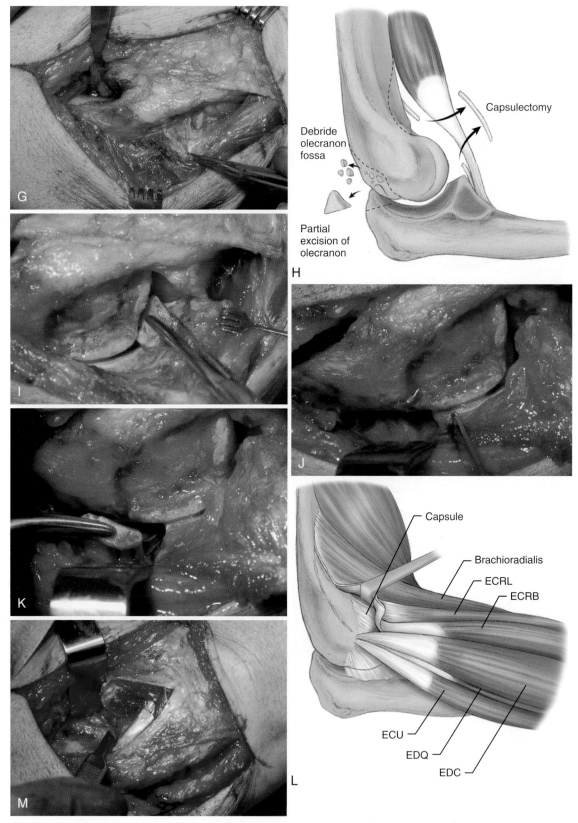

Figure 48-1. cont'd. G, The posterolateral capsule *(forceps)* is excised. **H,** Osteophytes are removed from the tip of the olecranon, and the olecranon fossa is cleared. **I,** Loose bodies *(forceps)* are often found in the posterolateral gutter. **J,** An osteotome is poised to cut the olecranon tip. **K,** Removal of the olecranon tip. **L,** Anteriorly, the interval between the extensor carpi radialis brevis *(ECRB)* and the extensor digitorum communis *(EDC)* is developed to better expose the anterior elbow capsule. **M,** The anterior elbow capsule is excised. *ECRL,* Extensor carpi radialis longus; *ECU,* extensor carpi ulnaris; *EDQ,* extensor digiti quinti.

Continued

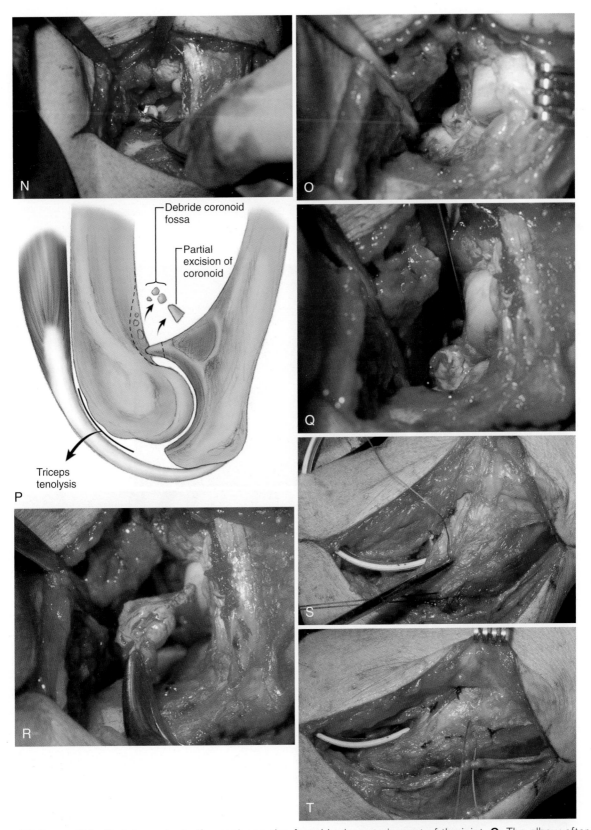

Figure 48-1. cont'd. **N,** A loose body *(forceps)* was also found in the anterior part of the joint. **O,** The elbow after excision of the anterior capsule. **P,** At this point, the coronoid tip is excised and the coronoid fossa is cleared out. **Q,** An osteotome is poised to cut the coronoid tip. **R,** Removal of the olecranon tip *(forceps)*. **S,** The anterior interval is closed, in this case over a suction drain. **T,** Closure of the posterior interval.

Continued

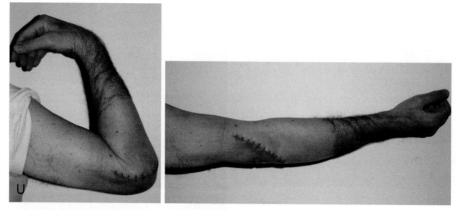

Figure 48-1. cont'd. U, Final motion was excellent.

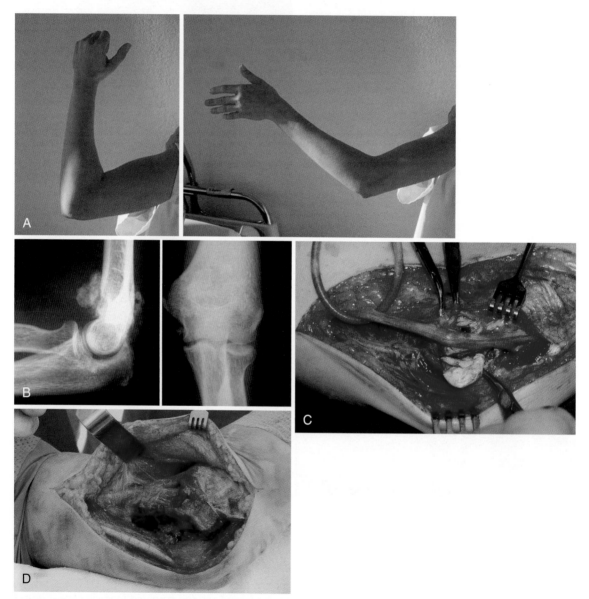

Figure 48-2. A, A patient with severe elbow contracture and ulnar nerve dysfunction. **B,** Lateral and anteroposterior radiographs demonstrate synovial chondromatosis. **C,** A complete release of the ulnar nerve is performed. The nerve is transposed anteriorly in the subcutaneous tissues at the end of the surgery. **D,** The flexor-pronator mass is split, and the anterior half is elevated off elbe anterior humerus and capsule along with the brachialis.

Continued

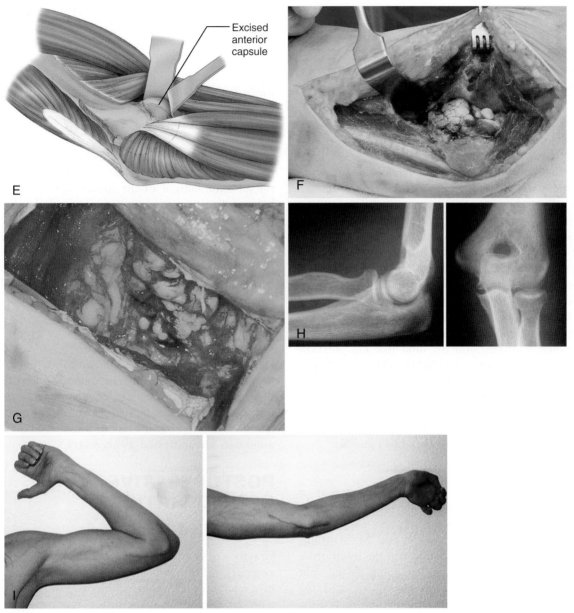

Figure 48-2. cont'd. E, A schematic drawing of the muscle interval and exposure of the anterior capsule. **F,** After capsular excision, the synovial chondromatosis is apparent. **G,** More synovial chondromatosis is seen after elevation of the triceps off the distal humerus and posterior capsule and excision of the posterior capsule. **H,** Final lateral and anteroposterior radiographs demonstrate resection of the synovial chondromatosis. **I,** Flexion and extension were improved.

SURGICAL TECHNIQUE

Open elbow contracture release can be performed with the patient under general anesthesia or with use of a brachial plexus block. The patient is supine, and the arm is supported on a hand table. A sterile tourniquet is applied to the upper arm.

The skin incision can be straight and directly over the muscle interval to be used or posterior with a skin flap elevated to expose the muscle interval (see Fig. 48-1C). If both medial and lateral intervals are to be used, a single posterior incision or both medial and lateral incisions can be made. In the unusual case of a direct anterior release, a direct anterior skin incision that crosses the flexion creases obliquely is made.

Specific Steps

Lateral Elbow Capsulectomy

The specific steps of this procedure are outlined in Box 48-1.

BOX 48-1 Surgical Steps for Lateral Capsulectomy

1. Lateral approach and posterior dissection
2. Anterior dissection
3. Medial dissection

1. Lateral Approach and Posterior Dissection

Release of elbow stiffness from the lateral side preserves the common wrist and digit extensors overlying the lateral collateral ligament. The skin is mobilized off the fascia to help identify the appropriate deep muscle interval (see Fig. 48-1D). Deep dissection is begun by identifying the supracondylar ridge, dividing the overlying fascia, and exposing the ridge (see Fig. 48-1E). The triceps is elevated off the posterior humerus and elbow capsule (see Fig. 48-1F). The posterior dissection continues distally in the interval between the anconeus and extensor carpi ulnaris. The anconeus is elevated off the capsule, the humerus, and the ulna (see Fig. 48-1G). Care is taken to preserve the lateral collateral ligament complex while the posterior elbow capsule is excised. The olecranon fossa is cleared out and even burred to deepen it if necessary (see Fig. 48-1H). Loose bodies are identified and removed (Fig. 48-1I). The tip of the olecranon can also be excised (see Fig. 48-1J and K).

2. Anterior Dissection

The origin of the extensor carpi radialis and part of the origin of the brachioradialis are released and elevated along with the brachialis off the anterior humerus and elbow capsule (see Fig. 48-1L and M). Distally, an interval is developed just anterior to the midportion of the capitellum, roughly corresponding to the split between the extensor carpi radialis brevis and the extensor digitorum communis, although in practice the interval is not precise (see Fig. 48-1L, N, and O). Keeping the dissection over the anterior half of the radiocapitellar joint will protect the lateral collateral ligament complex. The anterior elbow capsule is excised (see Fig. 48-1N).

3. Medial Dissection

At the medial side of the elbow, the capsulectomy may transition to a capsulotomy for safety, depending on visualization (see Fig. 48-1O). The radial and coronoid fossae can be cleared out and deepened as needed (see Fig. 48-1P). The tip of the coronoid can be excised (see Fig. 48-1Q and R). Resection of a deformed radial head may also be helpful in some patients.

Both the anterior and the posterior muscle intervals are sutured (see Fig. 48-1S and T). Drains are used at the discretion of the surgeon. The skin is closed according to the surgeon's preference.

Medial Elbow Capsulectomy

After skin incision, the ulnar nerve is identified on the medial border of the triceps. A complete release of the nerve through the arcade of Struthers, Osborne ligament, and flexor-pronator aponeurosis is then performed, along with neurolysis of the ulnar nerve if there is extensive scarring (see Fig. 48-2C). Skin flaps can be safely elevated once the ulnar nerve is identified and protected.

The flexor-pronator mass is identified and split in half between the interval where the ulnar nerve runs and the anterior margin of the muscle mass. The anterior half of the flexor-pronator mass and the brachialis muscle are elevated off the anterior humerus and elbow capsule (see Fig. 48-2D to F). The triceps is elevated off the distal humerus and the posterior elbow capsule (see Fig. 48-2G). Capsular excision, fossae deepening, and coronoid and olecranon tip excision are as described for lateral capsulectomy.

Heterotopic Bone Excision and Other Factors

Heterotopic bone is excised piecemeal, with care taken to identify and to protect native bone and articulation. Bleeding bone surfaces are covered with bone wax. Implants are removed after capsulectomy and elbow manipulation to limit the risk of fracture. Malunion and nonunion are addressed as necessary.

POSTOPERATIVE CONSIDERATIONS

Rehabilitation

Gravity-assisted and active-assisted range of motion exercises are initiated the morning after surgery. Static progressive or dynamic splints are used in patients who have trouble maintaining motion obtained in surgery. These splints are initiated as soon as the wound is stable.

Complications

Complications include recurrent stiffness and ulnar neuropathy (caused by restoration of flexion or by handling of the nerve).

RESULTS

The majority of published case series reporting the results of open elbow contracture release describe a single technique used to treat patients with a variety of diagnoses (Table 48-1). The results of various techniques seem comparable, although few data are available about the use of a medial exposure for posttraumatic contractures.[23,26] In general, about 75% of patients

TABLE 48-1. Published Case Series Reporting the Results of Open Elbow Contracture Release

Study	No. of Patients	Diagnosis	Operative Technique	Preoperative Arc (Degrees)	Postoperative Arc (Degrees)
Tosun et al[25] (2007)	22	Posttraumatic	Combined lateral and medial	35	86
Ring et al[26] (2006)	46	Posttraumatic	Patient-specific, variable	45	103
Tan et al[27] (2006)	52	Posttraumatic	Patient-specific, variable	57	116
Ring et al[28] (2005)	42	Posttraumatic	Patient-specific, variable; 23 had hinged external fixation	21	105
Aldridge et al[29] (2004)	77	Posttraumatic	Anterior; most with continuous passive motion postoperatively	59	97
Gosling et al[30] (2004)	59	Posttraumatic	Patient-specific, variable	68	101
Wu[31] (2003)	20	Posttraumatic	Patient-specific, variable	47	118
Heirweg and De Smet[32] (2003)	16	Posttraumatic	Patient-specific, variable	47	87
Stans et al[33] (2002)	37	Mixed; age younger than 21 years	Patient-specific, variable	66	94
Wada et al[34] (2000)	13	Posttraumatic	Medial	46	110
Kraushaar et al[35] (1999)	12	Posttraumatic	Lateral	70	117
Mansat and Morrey[22] (1998)	37	Mixed	Lateral	49	94
Cohen and Hastings[21] (1998)	22	Posttraumatic	Lateral	74	129
Hertel et al[36] (1997)	26	Mixed	Patient-specific, variable	66	100

regain at least an 80-degree arc of flexion.[26] Patients with limited flexion—particularly because of primary osteoarthritis—may be susceptible to ulnar neuropathy after release.[2] The results of excision of subtotal heterotopic ossification may be superior to the results of capsular contracture release alone,[37] but the results of excision of complete bone ankylosis, although generally rewarding, are less predictable.[12]

REFERENCES

1. Morrey BF. Post-traumatic contracture of the elbow. Operative treatment, including distraction arthroplasty. *J Bone Joint Surg Am.* 1990;72:601-618.
2. Antuna SA, Morrey BF, Adams RA, et al. Ulnohumeral arthroplasty for primary degenerative arthritis of the elbow: long-term outcome and complications. *J Bone Joint Surg Am.* 2002;84:2168-2173.
3. Doornberg JN, Ring D, Jupiter JB. Static progressive splinting for posttraumatic elbow stiffness. *J Orthop Trauma.* 2006;20:400-404.
4. Green DP, McCoy H. Turnbuckle orthotic correction of elbow-flexion contractures after acute injuries. *J Bone Joint Surg Am.* 1979;61:1092-1095.
5. Hotchkiss RN. Elbow contracture. In: Green DP, Hotchkiss RN, Pederson WC, eds. *Green's Operative Hand Surgery.* Philadelphia: Churchill Livingstone; 1999:667-682.
6. Ball CM, Meunier M, Galatz LM, et al. Arthroscopic treatment of post-traumatic elbow contracture. *J Shoulder Elbow Surg.* 2002;11:624-629.
7. Haapaniemi T, Berggren M, Adolfsson L. Complete transection of the median and radial nerves during arthroscopic release of posttraumatic elbow contracture. *Arthroscopy.* 1999;15:784-787.
8. Jones GS, Savoie 3rd FH. Arthroscopic capsular release of flexion contractures (arthrofibrosis) of the elbow. *Arthroscopy.* 1993;9:277-283.
9. Kim SJ, Kim HK, Lee JW. Arthroscopy for limitation of motion of the elbow. *Arthroscopy.* 1995;11:680-683.
10. Phillips BB, Strasburger S. Arthroscopic treatment of arthrofibrosis of the elbow joint. *Arthroscopy.* 1998;14:38-44.
11. Viola RW, Hastings H. Treatment of ectopic ossification about the elbow. *Clin Orthop Relat Res.* 2000;370:65-86.
12. Ring D, Jupiter J. The operative release of complete ankylosis of the elbow due to heterotopic bone in patients without severe injury of the central nervous system. *J Bone Joint Surg Am.* 2003;85:849-857.
13. McKee M, Jupiter J, Toh CL, et al. Reconstruction after malunion and nonunion of intra-articular fractures of the distal humerus. *J Bone Joint Surg Br.* 1994;76:614-621.
14. Morrey BF, Askew LJ, Chao EY. A biomechanical study of normal functional elbow motion. *J Bone Joint Surg Am.* 1981;63:872-880.

15. Doornberg JN, Ring D, Fabian LM, et al. Pain dominates measurements of elbow function and health status. *J Bone Joint Surg Am.* 2005;87:1725-1731.

16. Jupiter JB, Ring D. Operative treatment of post-traumatic proximal radioulnar synostosis. *J Bone Joint Surg Am.* 1998;80:248-257.

17. Viola RW, Hanel DP. Early "simple" release of posttraumatic elbow contracture associated with heterotopic ossification. *J Hand Surg Am.* 1999;24:370-380.

18. Morrey BF, Adams RA, Bryan RS. Total elbow replacement for post-traumatic arthritis of the elbow. *J Bone Joint Surg Br.* 1991;73:607-612.

19. Helfet DL, Kloen P, Anand N, et al. Open reduction and internal fixation of delayed unions and nonunions of fractures of the distal part of the humerus. *J Bone Joint Surg Am.* 2003;85:33-40.

20. Ring D, Hannouche D, Jupiter JB. Surgical treatment of persistent dislocation or subluxation of the ulnohumeral joint after fracture-dislocation of the elbow. *J Hand Surg Am.* 2004;29:470-480.

21. Cohen MS, Hastings H. Post-traumatic contracture of the elbow: operative release using a lateral collateral ligament sparing approach. *J Bone Joint Surg Br.* 1998;80:805-812.

22. Mansat P, Morrey BF. The column procedure: a limited lateral approach for extrinsic contracture of the elbow. *J Bone Joint Surg Am.* 1998;80:1603-1615.

23. Wada T, Isogai S, Ishii S, et al. Debridement arthroplasty for primary osteoarthritis of the elbow. Surgical technique. *J Bone Joint Surg Am.* 2005;87(suppl 1, pt 1):95-105.

24. Urbaniak JR, Hansen PE, Beissinger SF, et al. Correction of post-traumatic flexion contracture of the elbow by anterior capsulotomy. *J Bone Joint Surg Am.* 1985;67:1160-1164.

25. Tosun B, Gundes H, Buluc L, et al. The use of combined lateral and medial releases in the treatment of post-traumatic contracture of the elbow. *Int Orthop.* 2007;31(5):635-638.

26. Ring D, Adey L, Zurakowski D, et al. Elbow capsulectomy for posttraumatic elbow stiffness. *J Hand Surg Am.* 2006;31:1264-1271.

27. Tan V, Daluiski A, Simic P, et al. Outcome of open release for post-traumatic elbow stiffness. *J Trauma.* 2006;61:673-678.

28. Ring D, Hotchkiss RN, Guss D, et al. Hinged elbow external fixation for severe elbow contracture. *J Bone Joint Surg Am.* 2005;87:1293-1296.

29. Aldridge 3rd JM, Atkins TA, Gunneson EE, et al. Anterior release of the elbow for extension loss. *J Bone Joint Surg Am.* 2004;86:1955-1960.

30. Gosling T, Blauth M, Lange T, et al. Outcome assessment after arthrolysis of the elbow. *Arch Orthop Trauma Surg.* 2004;124:232-236.

31. Wu CC. Posttraumatic contracture of elbow treated with intraarticular technique. *Arch Orthop Trauma Surg.* 2003;123:494-500.

32. Heirweg S, De Smet L. Operative treatment of elbow stiffness: evaluation and outcome. *Acta Orthop Belg.* 2003;69:18-22.

33. Stans AA, Maritz NG, O'Driscoll SW, et al. Operative treatment of elbow contracture in patients twenty-one years of age or younger. *J Bone Joint Surg Am.* 2002;84:382-387.

34. Wada T, Ishii S, Usui M, et al. The medial approach for operative release of post-traumatic contracture of the elbow. *J Bone Joint Surg Br.* 2000;82:68-73.

35. Kraushaar BS, Nirschl RP, Cox W. A modified lateral approach for release of posttraumatic elbow flexion contracture. *J Shoulder Elbow Surg.* 1999;8:476-480.

36. Hertel R, Pisan M, Lambert S, et al. Operative management of the stiff elbow: sequential arthrolysis based on a transhumeral approach. *J Shoulder Elbow Surg.* 1997;6:82-88.

37. Lindenhovius AL, Linzel DS, Doornberg JN, et al. Comparison of elbow contracture release in elbows with and without heterotopic ossification restricting motion. *J Shoulder Elbow Surg.* 2007;16:621-625.

Chapter 49

Open Treatment of Lateral and Medial Epicondylitis

Michael W. Kessler and Neal C. Chen

Chapter Synopsis

- Surgical intervention for medial and lateral epicondylitis should be performed only after a year of conservative, nonoperative management has failed. Methods consist of anti-inflammatories, bracing, injections, and physical therapy. If a patient continues to have pain and loss of function after failing conservative management, open treatment of medial and lateral epicondylitis is appropriate. Debridement of the devitalized tendon to its bony insertion and creation of a bleeding vascular bed are imperative to successful outcomes.

Important Points

Lateral Epicondylitis

- Identify the exact area of pathologic change by palpation preoperatively.

Medial Epicondylitis

- Differentiate cubital tunnel syndrome from medial epicondylitis.
- If a patient has signs and symptoms of cubital tunnel syndrome, the ulnar nerve should be addressed, as well as the medial epicondylitis.

Clinical and Surgical Pearls

Lateral Epicondylitis

- Completely release or excise diseased tissue.
- Decorticate the lateral epicondyle.
- If the joint is exposed, repair the capsule to prevent fistula formation.

Medial Epicondylitis

- Protect the fibers of the medial collateral ligament during debridement.
- Identify and protect the ulnar nerve.
- Debride the degenerative tissue on the undersurface of the flexor-pronator mass.

Clinical and Surgical Pitfalls

Lateral Epicondylitis

- Avoid excessive resection to minimize injury to the lateral collateral ligament.

Medial Epicondylitis

- Avoid excessive resection to minimize injury to the medial collateral ligament.

LATERAL EPICONDYLITIS

Elbow pain is an extremely common problem in the general population, with lateral epicondylitis occurring in up to 4% of the general population. This condition can be exacerbated by athletic endeavors or activities involving heavy labor. Forceful activities and those with high forces combined with high repetition or awkward posture have been shown to increase the likelihood of development of lateral epicondylitis.[1] Both in vivo and in vitro studies histologically illustrate an ongoing degenerative process followed by a reparative cycle.[2] It is infrequent that a singular incident initiates a visit to the physician; rather, patients experience a chronic sequence of injury, pain, healing and resolution, followed by another inciting event. Prior investigations found that up to 26% of patients with this diagnosis have chronic symptoms and up to 40% have prolonged minor discomfort.[3] In a review, Faro and Wolf found that "the vast majority of cases respond to conservative therapy...although it may take up to 18 months to attain full recovery."[4]

Numerous studies have reported 75% to 90% cure rates with a sufficient trial of nonoperative therapy. Initial treatment of lateral epicondylitis begins with activity modification. Patients are instructed to avoid lifting with the wrist extended and to lift objects with the elbow in flexion as close to the body as possible with the hand in supination or neutral position to avoid applying stresses to the wrist extensor muscles. Patients who actively participate in racket sports should consider rackets with better shock absorption and consult with their instructor on optimal mechanics to minimize persistent problems. Conservative treatment also includes physical therapy focusing initially on stretching and progressive light eccentric strengthening of the forearm wrist extensors. Use of orthotics, such as nighttime wrist extension splinting, may be helpful for controlling pain.[5] However, if nonoperative treatment for a period of 12 to 18 months fails, operative treatment is indicated for persistent pain and disability.

Many techniques have been described for release of the extensor carpi radialis brevis (ECRB) that use open, percutaneous, and arthroscopic approaches. Recent research has shown no significant difference in outcomes between open and arthroscopic release.[6] We prefer open excision of the pathologic portion of the ECRB tendon with subsequent stimulation of bleeding bone and repair of the defect, given the reproducibility of the postoperative results and relative straightforwardness of the procedure.

PREOPERATIVE CONSIDERATIONS

History and Physical Examination

Evaluation of the athlete with lateral elbow pain begins with a thorough history. The history focuses on types of racket sports as well as any recent changes in equipment. A history of repetitive activity or overuse can often be elicited.

Athletes typically have lateral elbow pain, frequently extending into the dorsal forearm, and decreased grip strength. Symptoms are exacerbated by activities involving wrist extension against gravity. The key finding during physical examination is localized tenderness at the origin of the ECRB. In addition, there is pain with wrist extension and long finger extension when the elbow is maintained in an extended position owing to the fact that the ECRB origin is at the base of the long finger metacarpal.[7]

Key Physical Findings

- Pain at the lateral elbow
- Exacerbation of pain with resisted wrist extension
- Pain localized to the anterior portion of the lateral epicondyle, which is the ECRB origin
- Decreased grip strength with the elbow fully extended compared with the elbow flexed
- Pain that occasionally radiates along the dorsum of the forearm

Radiography

- Standard radiographs of elbow (anteroposterior, lateral, oblique views)
  - Evaluate for calcifications, osteochondral defect, exostosis, and degenerative changes of the radiocapitellar joint

Indications

The best candidate for operative intervention has had approximately 12 months of conservative treatment. This includes rest, nonsteroidal anti-inflammatory medication, bracing, and therapy.[8] Other modalities such as extracorporeal shock wave therapy, botulinum toxin injection, corticosteroid injection, and platelet-rich plasma injection have been reported, but the evidence that these interventions are successful is limited. Other causes of lateral elbow pain such as radiocapitellar arthritis should be considered. Results after surgical intervention reveal that 40% to 97% of patients who undergo open ECRB release or debridement have decreased pain and improved function.[4]

Key Indications

- Failure of conservative treatment for 12 months
- Highly competitive athletes
- Multiple cortisone injections (more than two)
- Lateral epicondyle bone exostosis or calcification of the common extensor tendon

SURGICAL TECHNIQUE

Several surgical techniques have been described for the treatment of lateral epicondylitis. Surgical treatment ranges from resection of the epicondyle to percutaneous or open division of the common extensor origin to tendon-lengthening techniques. The most common technique involves identification and excision of the abnormal ECRB origin with creation of a vascular bone bed to promote healing.[9]

The authors prefer open excision of the pathologic portion of the ECRB tendon with stimulation of bleeding bone and repair of the defect for initial surgical management. Retrospective results have revealed high success rates, with 83% to 94% of patients experiencing pain relief.[4]

Anesthesia and Positioning

On the basis of the preferences of the surgeon and anesthesiologist, the procedure can be performed with use of regional axillary block, Bier block, or local anesthetic with sedation. However, tourniquet pain may become difficult for the patient to tolerate if the procedure takes more than 10 to 15 minutes. The patient is positioned supine on the operating room table with the arm on a standard hand table. A nonsterile tourniquet is placed around the upper arm.

Surgical Landmarks and Incisions

Landmarks

- Lateral epicondyle
- Radial head
- Olecranon

Skin Incision

- Centered slightly anterior to the lateral epicondyle
- Extend 1 cm proximal to the lateral epicondyle to 2 to 3 cm distally toward the radial head

Specific Steps

The specific steps of this procedure are outlined in Box 49-1.

The skin incision is marked slightly anterior to the lateral epicondyle (Fig. 49-1) in a curvilinear pattern. Important landmarks to be outlined are the lateral epicondyle, radial head, and olecranon. Thick skin flaps are developed sharply down to the fascial layer. Typically, no significant cutaneous nerves are present in this area because it is a watershed region between the posterior antebrachial cutaneous nerve and the lateral antebrachial cutaneous nerve (Fig. 49-2).

The ECRB is identified by locating the interval between the muscle and tendon at the lateral epicondyle. The tendinous edge marks the overlapping extensor

digitorum communis and underlying ECRB (Fig. 49-3). Sharply incise the fascia between the extensor carpi radialis longus and extensor digitorum communis aponeurosis. Expose the ECRB origin, deep to the extensor digitorum communis. The ECRB is often friable and amorphic, lacking the longitudinal fibers of the normal adjacent tendon.

The degenerated tendon is identified and then sharply divided (Figs. 49-4 to 49-6). To avoid injury to the lateral collateral ligament, stay anterior to the epicondyle. The lateral collateral ligament originates on the distal portion of the epicondyle. Once the tendon has been adequately debrided, a rongeur or curette is used to decorticate the lateral epicondyle and enhance the blood supply to the tendon (Fig. 49-7).

After adequate debridement, the capitellum may be partially visible (Fig. 49-8). Close the capsule to prevent fistula formation. A side-to-side repair of the extensor mechanism is achieved with interrupted 2-0 absorbable sutures.

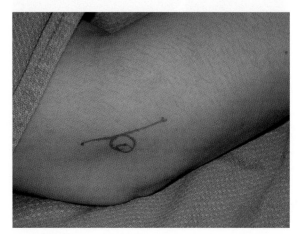

Figure 49-1. Curvilinear skin incision slightly anterior to the lateral epicondyle.

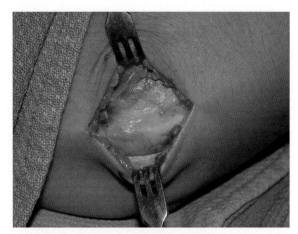

Figure 49-2. Thick skin flaps are developed down to the layer of the extensor carpi radialis longus and extensor digitorum communis aponeurosis.

BOX 49-1 Surgical Steps: Lateral Epicondylitis

1. Exposure
2. Identification of ECRB
3. Debridement of ECRB
4. Decortication of lateral epicondyle
5. Capsular and fascial closure
6. Skin closure

ECRB, Extensor carpi radialis brevis.

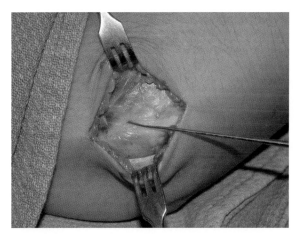

Figure 49-3. Fascial interval between the extensor carpi radialis longus and extensor digitorum communis aponeurosis.

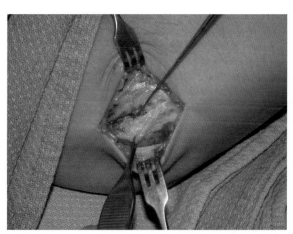

Figure 49-4. Forceps retracting extensor digitorum communis to reveal degenerated extensor carpi radialis brevis tendon.

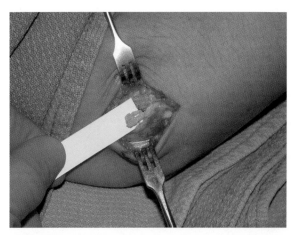

Figure 49-5. The friable and amorphic extensor carpi radialis brevis tendon is identified.

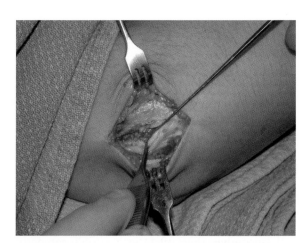

Figure 49-6. After debridement of the extensor carpi radialis brevis, forceps grasping more normal tendon striations of extensor origin.

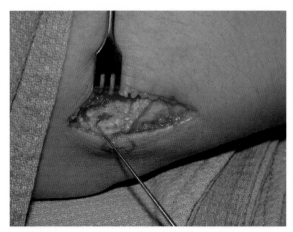

Figure 49-7. Lateral epicondyle decorticated.

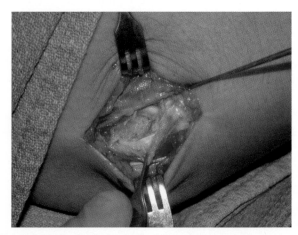

Figure 49-8. Radiocapitellar joint after adequate debridement of the extensor carpi radialis brevis.

The wound is copiously irrigated with antibiotic solution. The tourniquet is released, and adequate hemostasis is achieved. The subcutaneous tissues are closed with an absorbable suture, and the skin is closed with a 4-0 subcuticular stitch. The patient's elbow is then placed into a soft dressing.

POSTOPERATIVE CONSIDERATIONS

Follow-up

At 10 to 14 days postoperatively, the soft dressing is taken down and the wound is checked.

Rehabilitation

- 2 weeks: Active range of motion exercises are begun for the elbow, wrist, and forearm; progressive passive range of motion is instituted as necessary.
- 6 weeks: Gentle strengthening begins with light repetition.
- 3 months: Increased strengthening exercises are initiated. Return to competitive sports is permitted once strength has returned to 85% of the contralateral arm.

Complications

- Elbow instability secondary to excessive resection of lateral collateral ligament
- Joint fistula formation

RESULTS

Results of this procedure are summarized in Table 49-1.

ECRB release and lateral epicondyle drilling were shown by Das and Maffulli to have good or excellent results in 75% of patients studied.[13] Nirschl's original work revealed 97.7% improvement and 85.2% return to work rates compared with preoperative status,[10] and follow-up studies showed 83% to 94% pain relief.[11,12] Coleman and Matheson found 95% good to excellent results with average follow-up of 9.8 years after open treatment for lateral epicondylitis.[14]

Although these results are encouraging, they should be approached with some caution. Patients who undergo surgical intervention with a brief period of nonoperative treatment are likely to improve regardless, which presents some degree of selection bias if the surgical indications are particularly aggressive. In addition, these reports are uncontrolled retrospective series without validated outcomes, which presents inherent limitations for interpreting the results.

MEDIAL EPICONDYLITIS

Medial epicondylitis occurs at least five times less frequently than lateral epicondylitis; however, it is also associated with sports overuse activities.[9] This disorder is an injury that affects many athletes at all levels, especially throwing athletes, and is also known as *golfer's elbow* and *pitcher's elbow*. The primary cause is an overuse syndrome of the flexor-pronator mass, or conjoined tendon of the pronator teres, flexor carpi radialis, palmaris longus, and flexor carpi ulnaris tendons.[15] The most commonly affected tendon is the flexor carpi radialis, followed by the pronator teres, primarily owing to their anterior attachment on the medial epicondyle.[16] The pathophysiologic process of medial epicondylitis represents a microtearing of the medial tendon and ligaments. Pain is the main presenting symptom; however, the athlete may also have ulnar nerve symptoms of numbness and tingling in the small and ring fingers. The pain is localized to the medial aspect of the elbow. On occasion, pain may be distal to the medial epicondyle and radiate into the flexor-pronator mass. Activities that require pronation and flexion of the elbow and wrist exacerbate symptoms.

Nonoperative treatment begins with activity modification, including changing racket grip size for athletes playing racket sports. Athletes are encouraged to avoid constant activities that require pushing the hand with the forearm in pronation. Athletes are also educated in proper warm-up technique and conditioning. Anti-inflammatory medications, stretching, and counterforce bracing may also be helpful. Anti-inflammatory medication is administered for a period of 10 to 14 days. When the athlete does not respond to conservative treatment for a period of 12 months, operative intervention is discussed. Open surgical release of the flexor-pronator origin remains the mainstay of operative treatment.

TABLE 49-1. Results of Surgical Treatment of Lateral Epicondylitis

Study	Follow-up	Outcome
Nirschl and Pettrone[10] (1979)	6 years	85% complete relief of symptoms and no activity restrictions
Organ et al[11] (1997)	64 months	83% good to excellent results
Rosenberg and Henderson[12] (2002)	2 years	95% satisfactory results
Das and Maffulli[13] (2002)	4 years	75% excellent or good
Coleman et al[14] (2010)	9.8 years	97% good to excellent results

PREOPERATIVE CONSIDERATIONS

History and Physical Examination

The diagnosis of medial epicondylitis requires a thorough history and physical examination. Athletes have tenderness over the medial epicondyle and pain with resisted pronation or wrist flexion. On occasion the pain may radiate into the forearm. Athletes usually have a full range of motion at the elbow; however, they should be monitored for development of a flexion contracture. The findings on neurovascular examination are usually normal.

It is important to differentiate between ulnar neuropathy (cubital tunnel syndrome) and medial epicondylitis. Ulnar neuropathy usually manifests on physical examination with a positive Tinel sign or a positive elbow flexion test result—numbness and tingling in the ring and small fingers.

Radiographs are usually normal but should be obtained to check for calcification of the flexor-pronator mass or evidence of previous injury to the medial epicondyle, such as an avulsion. Calcification may suggest a previous injury to the ulnar collateral ligament.

Key Physical Findings

- Point tenderness at the medial epicondyle
- Pain exacerbated with resisted wrist flexion and pronation
- Tinel sign and positive compression test result at elbow

Evaluate for ulnar nerve subluxation.

Radiography

- Standard radiographs of elbow (anteroposterior, lateral, oblique views)

Evaluate for medial ulnohumeral osteophytes, medial collateral ligament calcification, and evidence of previous injury to the medial epicondyle, such as a malunited avulsion fracture.

Indications

- Failure of nonoperative treatment for approximately 12 months
- Exclusion of other pathologic causes of medial-sided elbow pain

SURGICAL TECHNIQUE

Surgical treatment of medial epicondylitis is not as well understood as that of lateral epicondylitis. Procedures for medial epicondylitis range from percutaneous epicondylar release to epicondylectomy. Most have agreed that standard surgical treatment of medial epicondylitis involves excision of the pathologic portion of the tendon and repair of the defect, similar to treatment of lateral epicondylitis.

Anesthesia and Positioning

- Regional axillary or Bier block anesthesia
- Patient supine on operating room table with upper arm on a hand table
- Nonsterile upper arm tourniquet

Surgical Landmarks and Incisions

Landmarks

- Medial epicondyle
- Flexor-pronator mass
- Ulnar nerve

Skin Incision

- Gently curved 3- to 4-cm incision along the medial epicondyle

Specific Steps

Specific steps of this procedure are outlined in Box 49-2.

The patient is placed supine on a standard operating room table with the arm on an arm board. A nonsterile tourniquet is placed on the upper arm. The arm is exsanguinated with an Esmarch band, and the tourniquet is inflated. A 3- to 4-cm oblique skin incision is made just anterior to the medial epicondyle, and the dissection is carried down through the subcutaneous tissue (Fig. 49-9).

Thick skin flaps are developed down to the flexor-pronator origin. Branches of the medial antebrachial cutaneous nerve, which are typically 1 inch distal to the medial epicondyle, should be identified and protected during this part of the surgical exposure (Fig. 49-10).

BOX 49-2 Surgical Steps: Medial Epicondylitis

1. Exposure
2. Identification of flexor-pronator mass
3. Identification and protection of ulnar nerve
4. Incision of common flexor origin fascial interval
5. Debridement of degenerative tissue on undersurface of flexor-pronator mass
6. Decortication of medial epicondyle
7. Repair of flexor-pronator mass
8. Skin closure

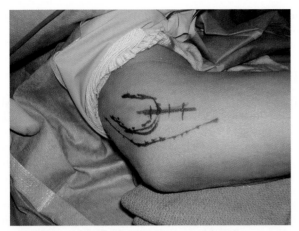

Figure 49-9. Medial epicondyle skin incision.

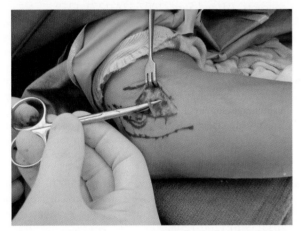

Figure 49-10. Skin incision and branch of the medial antebrachial cutaneous nerve.

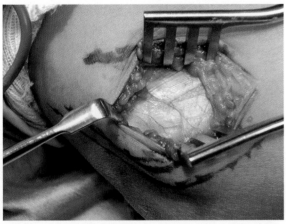

Figure 49-11. Fascial interval between the flexor carpi radialis and pronator teres.

The anterior skin flap is mobilized, and the flexor-pronator mass is identified. The ulnar nerve is identified and protected throughout the procedure. Once the common flexor origin has been identified, the fascial interval between the flexor carpi radialis and pronator teres is sharply incised (Fig. 49-11).

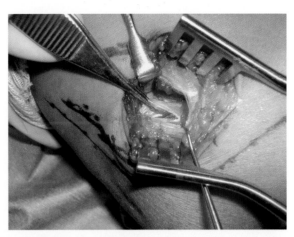

Figure 49-12. Degenerative tissue on the undersurface of the flexor-pronator mass debrided.

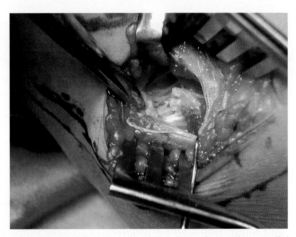

Figure 49-13. Rongeur used to decorticate the medial epicondyle.

The degenerative tissue on the undersurface of the flexor-pronator mass is identified and debrided (Fig. 49-12). Deep to the flexor-pronator mass lies the ulnar collateral ligament. Special attention should be paid to protection of the medial collateral ligament during debridement. A rongeur or rasp is used to decorticate the medial epicondyle and create a vascular bed (Fig. 49-13).

The common flexor-pronator mass is repaired with an absorbable 2-0 suture (Fig. 49-14). The subcutaneous tissues are closed with 4-0 absorbable suture, and skin is closed with 4-0 subcuticular suture. The arm is placed into a well-padded sterile dressing. A posterior splint may be used if the patient was particularly uncomfortable preoperatively.

POSTOPERATIVE CONSIDERATIONS

Follow-up

The dressings are removed 10 to 14 days postoperatively.

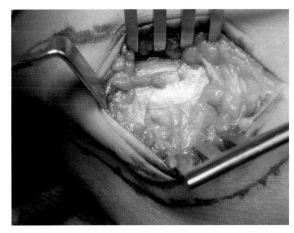

Figure 49-14. Common flexor-pronator mass repaired.

TABLE 49-2. Results of Operative Treatment of Medial Epicondylitis

Study	Follow-up	Results
Vangsness and Jobe[17] (1991)	6 years	97% good to excellent results

Rehabilitation

- Days 10-14: Gentle active range-of-motion exercises are begun for the elbow as well as for the wrist and hand, followed by progressive passive range of motion. A stretching program is resumed.
- 4-6 weeks: Strengthening program starts.
- 12 weeks: Return to play is permitted once strength is 85% that of the contralateral extremity.

Complications

- Residual pain
- Valgus instability
- Unaddressed cubital tunnel syndrome
- Hypoesthesia along proximal forearm
- Medial antebrachial cutaneous neuroma

RESULTS

Results of this procedure are summarized in Table 49-2.

In a review of 35 patients with recalcitrant medial epicondylitis treated surgically, Vangsness and Jobe noted an improvement in subjective elbow function from 38% to 98% of normal.[17] Of these patients, 97% exhibited excellent results and 86% were able to use the elbow without physical limitations. Again, the same caveats for the results of lateral epicondylitis

are present for the results of debridement of medial epicondylitis.

REFERENCES

1. Shiri R, Viikari-Juntura E. Lateral and medial epicondylitis: Role of occupational factors. *Best Pract Res Clin Rheumatol.* 2011;25:43-57.
2. Kim JW, Chun CH, Shim DM, et al. Arthroscopic treatment of lateral epicondylitis: comparison of the outcome of ECRB release with and without decortications. *Knee Surg Sports Traumatol Arthrosc.* 2011;19:1178-1183.
3. Binder AI, Hazelman BL. Lateral humeral epicondylitis: a study of natural history and the effect of conservative therapy. *Br J Rheumatol.* 1983;22:73-76.
4. Faro F, Wolf JM. Lateral epicondylitis: review and current concepts. *J Hand Surg.* 2007;32A:1271-1279.
5. Struijs PA, Kerkhoffs GM, Assendelft WJ, et al. Conservative treatment of lateral epicondylitis: brace versus physical therapy or a combination of both—a randomized clinical trial. *Am J Sports Med.* 2004;32:462-469.
6. Peart RE, Strickler SS, Schweitzer Jr KM. Lateral epicondylitis: a comparative study of open and arthroscopic lateral release. *Am J Orthop.* 2004;33:565-567.
7. Walton MJ, Mackie K, Fallon M, et al. The reliability and validity of magnetic resonance imaging in the assessment of chronic lateral epicondylitis. *J Hand Surg.* 2011;36A:475-479.
8. Gosens T, Peerbooms JC, van Laar W, et al. Ongoing positive effect of platelet-rich plasma versus corticosteroid injection in lateral epicondylitis. *Am J Sports Med.* 2011;39(6):1200-1208.
9. Schipper ON, Dunn JH, Ochiai DH, et al. Nirschl surgical technique for concomitant lateral and medial elbow tendinosis. *Am J Sports Med.* 2011;39(5):972-976.
10. Nirschl RP, Pettrone FA. Tennis elbow. The surgical treatment of lateral epicondylitis. *J Bone Joint Surg Am.* 1979;61:832-839.
11. Organ SW, Nirschl RP, Kraushaar BS, et al. Salvage surgery for lateral tennis elbow. *Am J Sports Med.* 1997;25:746-750.
12. Rosenberg N, Henderson I. Surgical treatment of resistant lateral epicondylitis. Follow-up study of 19 patients after excision, release and repair of proximal common extensor tendon origin. *Arch Orthop Trauma Surg.* 2002;122:514-517.
13. Das D, Maffulli N. Surgical management of tennis elbow. *J Sports Med Phys Fitness.* 2002;42:190-197.
14. Coleman B, Quinlan JF, Matheson JA. Surgical treatment for lateral epicondylitis: a long-term follow-up of results. *J Shoulder Elbow Surg.* 2010;19(3):363-367.
15. Ciccotti MC, Schwartz MA, Ciccotti MG. Diagnosis and treatment of medial epicondylitis of the elbow. *Clin Sports Med.* 2004;23:693-705.
16. Leach RE, Miller JK. Lateral and medial epicondylitis of the elbow. *Clin Sports Med.* 1987;6:259-272.
17. Vangsness C, Jobe FW. Surgical treatment of medial epicondylitis: results in 35 elbows. *J Bone Joint Surg Br.* 1991;73:409-411.

Chapter 50

Distal Biceps Repair

Peter N. Chalmers, Geoffrey S. Van Thiel, John J. Fernandez, and Nikhil N. Verma

Chapter Synopsis
- This chapter describes the technique for completing a distal biceps tendon repair and provides an overview of the contemporary results.

Important Points
- There are two predominant techniques—the one-incision and the two-incision approaches—to repair of the distal biceps.
- The one-incision technique is described in detail in this chapter. The theoretical benefit is a less-invasive approach with the added risk of dissection in the anterior elbow.
- The two-incision approach has traditionally been described as carrying a higher risk of heterotopic ossification and being a larger approach; however, recent research has shown low rates of ossification with newer techniques.
- It is essential to identify and protect the lateral antebrachial cutaneous nerve.
- The biceps tendon should be placed on the ulnar side of the radial tuberosity.

Clinical and Surgical Pearls
- The supine position with a radiolucent hand table is used.

- A transverse incision is made at the distal aspect of the flexion crease in the elbow with an L component that overlies the brachioradialis; this can also be extended proximally if needed with a vertical component on the medial aspect of the arm.
- After incision, identify the lateral antebrachial cutaneous nerve. Injury to the nerve can cause paresthesias in the forearm.
- The biceps tendon may be retracted proximally.
- During exposure of the radial tuberosity, the arm should be in supination to protect the posterior interosseus nerve.

Clinical and Surgical Pitfalls
- Injury to the lateral antebrachial cutaneous nerve can result in paresthesias in the forearm.
- Injury to the posterior interosseus nerve can cause significant functional complications.
- There can be many recurrent vessels from the radial artery in the field of exposure. These should be meticulously coagulated to prevent postoperative bleeding.

The distal, insertion, bicipital tendon ruptures relatively infrequently, with an incidence of 1.2 ruptures per 100,000 person-years.[1] Proximal tendon ruptures are far more common, accounting for 97% of all biceps tendon ruptures.[1] However, when distal ruptures do occur, they affect the dominant arms of highly functioning men aged 40 to 60 and can be associated with substantial functional and financial disability owing to

chronic pain and weakness in forearm supination and elbow flexion.[2,3]

Although nonoperative treatment[2,3] and tenodesis to the brachialis originally were suggested as treatment options for distal biceps ruptures,[4] anatomic reconstruction with repair of the biceps to the bicipital tuberosity on the proximal radius has led to excellent functional outcomes, high patient satisfaction, and restoration of strength and endurance in forearm supination and elbow flexion in numerous clinical series.[1-14] Boyd and Anderson's original description of such a repair involved two incisions and fixation via an osseous bridge.[15] However, whereas injury to the posterior interosseous nerve (PIN) may have been lessened with this technique, this method led to an unacceptably high incidence of heterotopic ossification and synostosis of the radius and ulna.[3,4,13,16] Thus the anterior, single-incision procedure has risen in popularity.[7,10,11,14] Fixation methods have also evolved, first with the use of suture anchors[11,14] and more recently with the EndoButton (Acufex, Smith & Nephew, Andover, MA).[6,12,17,18] The EndoButton has been demonstrated to be biomechanically superior to suture anchors by a factor of two and to an osseous bridge by a factor of three, and allows construct "prefabrication" outside of the wound.[11] In addition to success with repair of acute lesions, recently good outcomes have been demonstrated in the repair of chronic ruptures with grafting for the gap between the shortened tendon and the anatomic insertion.[8,10,12]

PREOPERATIVE CONSIDERATIONS

History

Distal biceps tendon rupture most frequently occurs in the dominant extremity in men aged 40 to 60 after a sudden eccentric extension load on an unsuspecting flexed elbow. At the time of injury patients commonly report a ripping sensation or a sudden "snap" in the anterior elbow with associated progressively worsening anterior elbow pain the day of the injury. Over the course of days to hours, edema and red-purple skin discoloration caused by subcutaneous hemorrhage develop. The presence of ecchymoses implies concomitant rupture of the lacertus fibrosus, allowing extravasation of blood from the rupture site into the subcutaneous tissues. Untreated, the patient may then develop pain in the anterior elbow with activities associated with repetitive or forceful elbow flexion or forearm supination with associated weakness in these movements. However, patient presentation is variable, and this complete constellation of findings is present only in a minority of patients.

Whereas complete ruptures are more common, not all injuries to the distal tendon involve a complete discontinuity, and some injuries may involve partial residual continuity of the tendon.[17] Although similar in symptomatology, these "partial" injuries are considerably more difficult to diagnose. Diagnosis relies on advanced imaging modalities such as magnetic resonance imaging (MRI).[17] Partial rupture exists on a spectrum with several poorly understood diagnoses including cubital bursitis, bicipital tendinosis, and biceps

paratendinitis, each of which can exist in isolation or can coexist with a distal biceps tendon rupture.[17]

Physical Examination

In the acutely ruptured distal biceps tendon, the examiner may observe diffuse swelling and ecchymoses radiating from the antecubital fossa. Acutely, guarding caused by pain may make provocative testing difficult. Once the acute inflammation has resolved, the patient may notice a change in the contour of the arm (Fig. 50-1) resulting from proximal retraction of the biceps.[1]

Several physical examination maneuvers rely on palpation of the distal biceps tendon. The examiner may be able to palpate a defect within the tendon by attempting to "hook" an index finger around the distal biceps tendon in the flexed and supinated arm. This "hook" sign can be more difficult to elicit if the lacertus fibrosus remains intact. While palpating, the examiner can then supinate and pronate the patient's arm with the other hand, which should cause proximal and distal movement, respectively, of the junction of the distal biceps tendon and the biceps muscle belly. If no motion of this junction can be appreciated with forearm rotation, the examiner should consider a distal biceps rupture. In a similar test of the "tenodesis effect" of the tendon distally and the muscle belly proximally, the examiner may manually compress the biceps muscle with the arm relaxed in 90 degrees of elbow flexion and neutral forearm rotation to slight pronation to place the biceps muscle under tension. This "squeeze" should cause an obligate supination of the forearm, analogous to the Thompson test in the calf for Achilles tendon rupture. This test has been shown to have a high sensitivity and a low false-positive rate, although its specificity is as yet undetermined.[19]

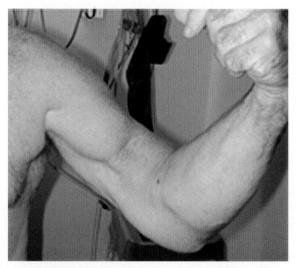

Figure 50-1. Left upper extremity in a patient with chronic distal biceps rupture demonstrating proximal retraction of the muscle belly and resultant "Popeye" sign.

Whereas active, resisted forearm supination and elbow flexion will often be objectively weak compared with the contralateral uninjured side, a lack of weakness does not exclude tendon rupture, because other muscles such as the supinator and brachialis can also account for these motions.[1]

Imaging

Radiographic imaging infrequently contributes to the diagnosis, although obtaining anteroposterior, lateral, and oblique views is crucial for exclusion of other osseous pathology. In addition, radial tuberosity avulsion fracture can have a similar presentation, and therefore the examiner must scrutinize the images closely for this easily missed diagnosis. With chronic distal biceps tendon ruptures, the radial tuberosity may undergo hypertrophic changes.[1]

In patients in whom the history and physical examination findings convincingly yield a diagnosis of distal biceps tendon rupture, no further imaging need be obtained. However, MRI can be helpful when the diagnosis is unclear or when a partial rupture is suspected.[17,20] These images can also aid surgical planning, because a proximal rupture may indicate a more proximal approach. Common MRI findings include discontinuity of the tendon with distal absence, increased T2 signal in the sheath indicating inflammatory fluid, increased T2 signal within the muscle, and a mass within the antecubital fossa resulting from the retracted proximal tendon end (Fig. 50-2). In more chronic setting, atrophy of the biceps muscle may be seen, as well as thinning or thickening of the remainder of the tendon.[17,20] Because this tendon does not travel in the traditionally defined anatomic axes, MRI in the flexed, abducted, and supinated position can be a useful adjunct.[17] In the setting of a partial tear, MRI can be used to determine the extent of the tear. MRI may lack sensitivity and not correlate with intraoperative findings. In persistently symptomatic patients with strong clinical findings, MRI should be used as an adjunct to decide the course of treatment. Anecdotally, intraoperative findings have revealed larger tears than otherwise appreciated on MRI. MRI can also be useful to assess for associated pathology such as bicipital tendinosis, bursitis, paratendinitis, hematoma, or contusion. Ultrasound may play a role in diagnosis owing to its cost-effectiveness and reliability. However, this technique is operator dependent and thus continues to be institution specific.

Indications and Contraindications

Nonoperative treatment consistently leads to persistent functional deficit and anterior elbow pain.[2,3] Such deficits may be well tolerated in low-demand individuals

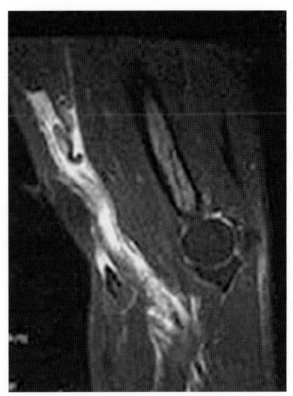

Figure 50-2. Sagittal T2-weighted magnetic resonance image demonstrating complete rupture of the distal biceps tendon with proximal retraction and significant fluid within the biceps sheath.

such as the elderly and the sedentary, particularly in the nondominant extremity. In some individuals with extensive medical comorbidities, the risk of operative intervention may outweigh these known functional deficits. However, in the majority of young, healthy, active individuals who sustain distal biceps ruptures, surgical repair should be strongly considered.[1-14]

Preoperatively, the surgeon must identify (1) whether the injury is acute or chronic, (2) whether the lacertus fibrosus is intact, (3) whether the tear is complete or partial, and (4) whether the discontinuity is at the myotendinous junction, tendon midsubstance, or bicipital tuberosity. Chronic tears not infrequently present a surgical challenge owing to retraction of the tendon and scarring of the peritendinous tissues (which may include the lateral antebrachial cutaneous nerve), alteration of the anatomy, and decreased tensile properties of the tissue after extended lack of use. In this setting the surgeon must either have a plan for the harvest of autograft tendon tissue or have allograft tissue available for reconstruction.[8,10,12]

Partial tears warrant a trial of conservative therapy with nonsteroidal anti-inflammatory medication, immobilization, and rehabilitation. However, the surgeon may wish to determine the extent of the tear with MRI, ultrasound, or, as has been reported, bursoscopy.[17]

Distal biceps tendon tears that involve more than 50% of the tendon may be indicated for completion of the tear and anatomic repair to the bicipital tuberosity, whereas tears with more than 50% of the tendon in continuity can be considered for debridement.[17] The most accurate method to determine the extent of the repair remains a subject of debate.[17]

SURGICAL TECHNIQUE

Anesthesia and Positioning

Regional anesthesia with either an axillary or a supraclavicular block minimizes anesthetic morbidity and improves immediate postoperative patient comfort and is therefore preferred. We prefer supine positioning with the arm abducted and extended onto a hand table.

Surgical Landmarks, Incisions, and Portals

Although transverse and longitudinal incisions can be used to approach the distal biceps tendon,[10] we find an L incision provides the best aspects of both (Fig. 50-3). The longitudinal aspect of the incision extends along the medial border of the brachioradialis, and the transverse aspect extends medially at the elbow crease.

Single-Incision Technique with EndoButton Fixation

The technique for this procedure is outlined in Box 50-1.

1. Approach

After incision, the surgeon must carefully dissect in the layer immediately deep to the subcutaneous veins for the lateral antebrachial cutaneous nerve, which must be protected to prevent lateral forearm paresthesias. Once this structure has been identified and protected, dissection should proceed bluntly toward the radial tuberosity (Fig. 50-4). The proximal aspect of the supinator may

cover a portion of the tuberosity and should be elevated with blunt dissection. If fibrous tissue covers the tuberosity, a Cobb elevator may assist in cleaning the cortex.

Once the tuberosity has been identified (Fig. 50-5), the brachioradialis and the lateral antebrachial cutaneous nerve are gently retracted laterally. Although visualization can be difficult, excessive retraction on the

BOX 50-1 Surgical Steps: Distal Biceps Repair

1. Approach
2. Tuberosity preparation
3. Tendon preparation
4. Fixation
5. Closure

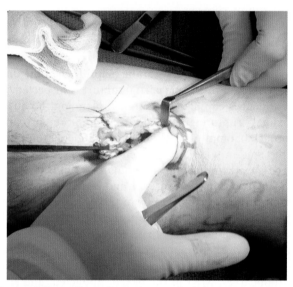

Figure 50-4. Blunt dissection carried down to expose the radial tuberosity.

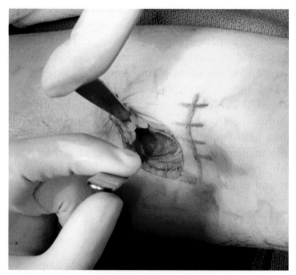

Figure 50-5. Radial tuberosity exposed at the distal aspect of the incision.

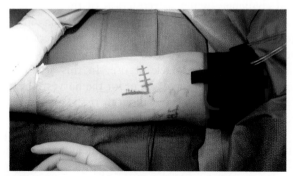

Figure 50-3. Typical anterior incision for the single-incision approach to acute biceps tendon rupture.

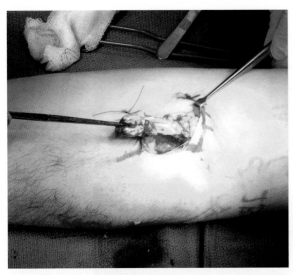

Figure 50-6. Retrieved proximal tendon stump.

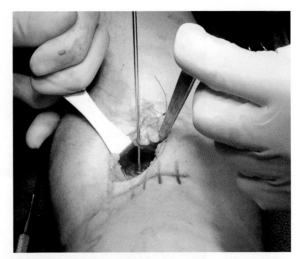

Figure 50-7. Guidewire drilled into the radial tuberosity with the arm in supination. This guidewire will then be used for preparation of the EndoButton tunnel (Acufex, Smith & Nephew, Andover, MA).

lateral structures must be avoided to prevent injury to the PIN. Supination can aid in visualization and serves to move the PIN farther laterally. The PIN is only 9 to 14 mm from the bicipital tuberosity and is thus at risk.[6,11,18] Neurapraxia has been reported in up to 10% of patients.[9,10]

The surgeon must then identify the biceps tendon sheath (Fig. 50-6). Significant inflammation may be encountered in the acute phase, as well as a reactive fluid-filled bursal sac at the radial tuberosity. Numerous veins and recurrent branches of the radial artery can be encountered with dissection in the antecubital fossa, and the surgeon must maintain meticulous hemostasis. Division of the lacertus fibrosus may be necessary for full access to the retracted biceps tendon.

2. Tuberosity Preparation

Once the exposure is complete, the tuberosity tunnel must be created. The tunnel should be located as ulnarly in the radial tuberosity as possible with the forearm supinated to re-create the most anatomic location for the tendon. The footprint of the biceps tendon on the bicipital tuberosity is in a ribbon at the ulnar side of the tuberosity encompassing 63% of the length and 13% of the width of the tuberosity.[21,22] All attempts should be made to re-create the anatomy. Initially, a guide pin is placed through the radial tuberosity at the center of the footprint were the tendon will be reattached. A 6- or 7-mm cannulated acorn reamer is then used to create a unicortical docking tunnel for the biceps tendon. The posterior (second) cortex is then overdrilled with an EndoButton drill (Fig. 50-7).[16] Attention is then turned toward preparation of the tendon.

3. Tendon Preparation

Next, the tendon stump is prepared. After the distal end of the biceps tendon has been completely freed and the

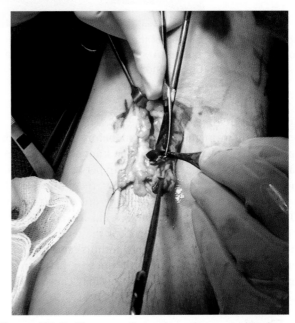

Figure 50-8. The necrotic tendon edges are sharply debrided back to healthy-appearing tissue.

degenerated or necrotic portion has been resected (Fig. 50-8), a running locking type of suture is placed with a strong, braided No. 2 or No. 5 equivalent nonabsorbable suture. Although either Krackow- or Bunnell-type stitches are acceptable, some authors prefer to combine the former proximally with the latter distally to allow excellent bite and some pliability of the distal tendon.[10] The starting point, and thus the location of the knot, should be about 2 to 3 cm proximal to the distal end of the tendon, allowing for adjustment of the knot later if needed. Each suture passage must be tensioned in the tendon to prevent later elongation. The suture is advanced proximally on the tendon for about 2 cm and

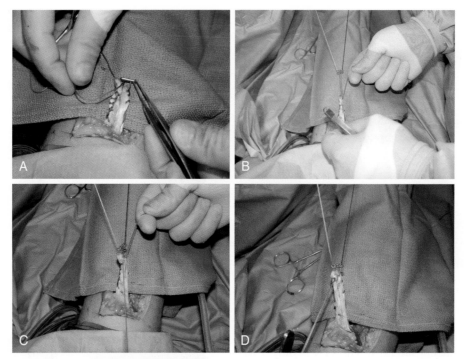

Figure 50-9. Preparation of the tendon. After the running suture finishes 2 to 3 cm proximal to the distal edge and is looped through the button (**A**), the two ends are held and tensioned (**B**) so that the button is brought to within 2 to 3 mm of the tendon end (**C**), and the knot is tied (**D**).

then distally exits the tendon end. The suture limb is then passed through the button before reentering the tendon to complete the loop. The knot should be tied, leaving a maximum 2- to 3-mm gap between the button and the free tendon end to allow the button to be manipulated and "flipped" over the dorsal cortex (Fig. 50-9). In general, the surgeon should leave as small a gap as possible between the end of the tendon and the button to prevent gapping; some authors have described performing this technique with no gap between the tendon and the button, although this may cause difficulties in "flipping" the button.[18,23]

4. Fixation

The two outer holes of the EndoButton are threaded with a different-colored sutures (Fig. 50-10), commonly referred to as the "kite strings," to identify the sutures as they draw the EndoButton into the socket and onto the posterior cortex. A Beath pin is advanced through the hole at the base of the tuberosity socket from anterior to posterior; the four suture ends (two ends of two sutures of different colors) are threaded through the eyelet, and the pin is withdrawn out the skin of the posterior forearm with the elbow in 90 degrees of flexion (Fig. 50-11). The two sutures are separated (with two strands each). One suture can be used to draw the button through the posterior cortex, and once the button is clear of the posterior cortex the other suture can be tensioned to cause the button to rotate 90 degrees

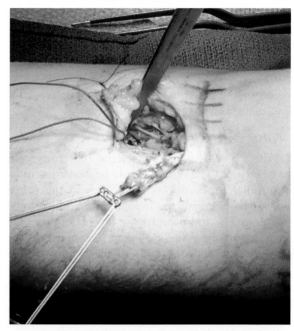

Figure 50-10. The EndoButton (Acufex, Smith & Nephew, Andover, MA) should be loaded with a suture on each end of different colors, like "kite strings," such that one can be tensioned to pass the button out of the posterior cortex and the other can be used to "flip" the button once it has cleared the posterior cortex.

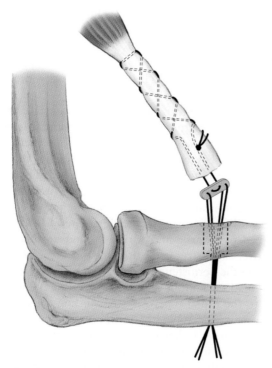

Figure 50-11. Diagram depicting single-incision EndoButton technique (Acufex, Smith & Nephew, Andover, MA). The EndoButton is secured to the tendon, and passing sutures are placed through the posterior cortical tunnel ready for tendon passage. *(Modified from Greenberg JA, Fernandez JJ, Wang T, et al. EndoButton-assisted repair of distal biceps tendon ruptures. J Shoulder Elbow Surg. 2003;12:484-490.)*

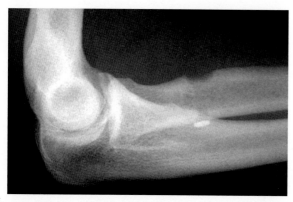

Figure 50-12. Lateral postoperative radiograph. Note the anterior cortical tunnel and the EndoButton (Acufex, Smith & Nephew, Andover, MA) securely seated in a horizontal fashion directly against the posterior cortex. *(Modified from Greenberg JA, Fernandez JJ, Wang T, et al. EndoButton-assisted repair of distal biceps tendon ruptures. J Shoulder Elbow Surg. 2003;12:484-490.)*

such that it cannot pass back through the hole in the posterior cortex, "flipping" the button. This process of button passage can be facilitated with fluoroscopic guidance (Fig. 50-12). The sutures are carefully removed by pulling them out through the posterior stab wound.

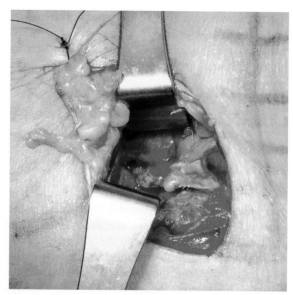

Figure 50-13. The final EndoButton (Acufex, Smith & Nephew, Andover, MA) construct, with the tendon passing through the anterior cortex, allowing direct tendon-to-bone healing.

Inspection of the tuberosity should now reveal the tendon diving into the anterior cortex (Fig. 50-13). This technique allows healing between the anterior cortex and the more proximal portion tendon tissue, which is farther from the rupture and therefore may be less likely to have intrinsic tendinosis predisposing to rerupture.

5. Closure

After thorough irrigation, the skin is closed with interrupted 2-0 absorbable subcutaneous sutures and a running 3-0 absorbable subcuticular stitch. The arm is placed in a posterior splint with the elbow in 90 degrees of flexion and neutral rotation. We generally perform these procedures on an outpatient basis.

POSTOPERATIVE CONSIDERATIONS

Follow-up

Patients are seen in the office 7 to 10 days postoperatively for suture removal and wound evaluation.

Rehabilitation

In general, we maintain the arm immobilized at 90 degrees of elbow flexion and neutral forearm rotation until the first postoperative evaluation at 7 to 10 days. At that point, assuming the wound appears to be healing well, the arm is placed in either a hinged elbow brace or a removable posterior mold at 90 degrees of flexion, to initiate passive and active-assisted range of motion from 30 degrees of flexion to maximal flexion, increasing slowly to a goal of full extension by 6 weeks postoperatively. At that point, patients are allowed unrestricted motion and strengthening. Full activities, including lifting, are allowed at 4 to 5 months postoperatively.

ALTERNATIVE TECHNIQUES

Modified Two-Incision Technique

The original Boyd-Anderson technique describes a primary incision in the antecubital fossa and a secondary incision in the posterolateral forearm.[15] This technique, although effective, was found to be complicated by radioulnar synostosis attributed to aggressive elevation of the anconeus off the proximal ulna, with damage to the proximal interosseous membrane.[3,4,13,16] Agins and colleagues[5] modified the original procedure first by a smaller anterior transverse incision and use of a small osteotome through a small posterior incision rather than a bur to form a trough for reattachment of the biceps tendon.

Bourne and Morrey[24] suggested passing a blunt hemostat through the usual path of the biceps tendon until it is palpable on the posterior skin, then making the posterior incision over the instrument's tip (Fig. 50-14). Rather than taking the supinator off the ulna, this technique allows the radial tuberosity to be exposed

from the posterior incision by splitting the supinator and common extensor, requiring no muscle to be taken off the ulna and theoretically decreasing the risk of radioulnar synostosis. During this posterior approach, the forearm is pronated to bring the tuberosity into view and to protect the PIN.

Currently the most common technique is either a transverse or longitudinal (Henry) 3- to 5-cm incision anteriorly over the antecubital fossa to retrieve and debride the biceps tendon. As mentioned earlier, Bunnell-type or other running grasping sutures are used to secure the distal end of the tendon. With the forearm supinated, a hemostat is advanced along the medial border of the radial tuberosity to the dorsolateral forearm as described by Bourne and Morrey,[24] and an incision is made over the instrument's tip. One must be careful not to violate the periosteum of the ulna. With the forearm in maximal pronation, this posterior incision is carried down to the radial tuberosity by splitting the extensor muscle mass and supinator in line with their fibers. A bur or osteotome is then used to make a cavitary opening in the tuberosity large enough to pass the tendon through. Small drill holes are then made along the margin of the cavitary opening unicortically, one for each Bunnell strand. Once the biceps tendon has been passed into the tunnel, the suture ends are passed back up through the drill holes and tied over a bone bridge. Rehabilitation is similar to that for the single-incision technique.

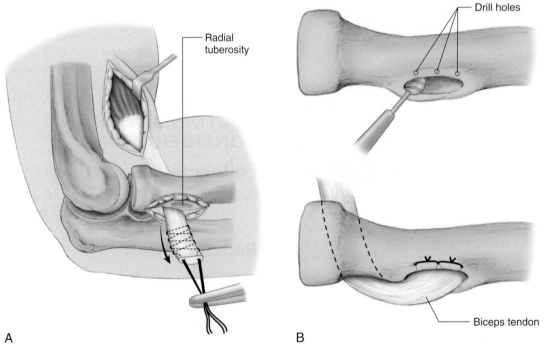

Figure 50-14. Modified technique for two-incision repair with a bone tunnel. *(Modified from Morrey BF, Askew LJ, An KN, et al. Rupture of the distal tendon of the biceps brachii. A biomechanical study. J Bone Joint Surg Am. 1985;67:418-421.)*

Delayed Treatment with Hamstring Allograft

Delayed treatment of distal biceps rupture is not uncommon and is complicated by tendon retraction, scarring to the brachialis, distorted anatomy, and poor-quality tissue. Especially when the bicipital aponeurosis is torn, the tendon may be retracted to the degree that a primary repair to the radial tuberosity either is impossible or would leave the patient with an unacceptable flexion contracture. In such cases supplementary grafts are often needed, and grafting with fascia lata, palmaris longus, Achilles tendon, and flexor carpi radialis has been described.[8,10,12]

Our preferred grafting technique uses either allograft or autologous semitendinosus tendon for reconstruction. This technique combines the EndoButton principle with hamstring allograft for late reconstruction.[8,10,12] The initial stages are as described earlier for the Endo-Button technique to prepare the tuberosity. The autograft tendon is then weaved through the distal biceps tendon with the free ends proximal so that they can be tensioned and shortened for appropriate graft length (Fig. 50-15).[12] Once the appropriate length has been confirmed, the free ends are sutured together with nonabsorbable braided suture. Similar suture is passed through the two center holes of the EndoButton and sutured in a running fashion to the medial and lateral arms of the graft to provide fixation of the biceps-graft complex to the button. As previously described for acute rupture, the graft complex with the EndoButton is then passed through the radial tuberosity and flipped over the posterior cortex.

RESULTS

Good to excellent results with regard to both elimination of pain and recovery of strength and function have been reported after single-incision and two-incision techniques for distal biceps tendon repair.[1-14] Although randomized comparative trials are lacking, a comparison of one- and two-incision repairs found that single-incision repairs resulted in better elbow flexion at final follow-up but a higher rate of transient paresthesias, although the techniques were overall very similar in their results.[9] In the largest single-surgeon series, McKee and colleagues (2005) reported their outcomes in 53 patients with a mean follow-up of 29 months. No patient developed a loss of range of motion of greater than 5 degrees, and the mean Disability of the Arm, Shoulder, and Hand score was 8.2 out of 10, with high patient satisfaction scores.[14] Other authors have replicated these findings with similar techniques.[6,10] Potential complications include radioulnar synostosis with the two-incision technique and injury to the lateral antebrachial cutaneous nerve or PIN with the single-incision techniques.[16] With either type of technique, recurrent rupture is a rare but possible occurrence.[16]

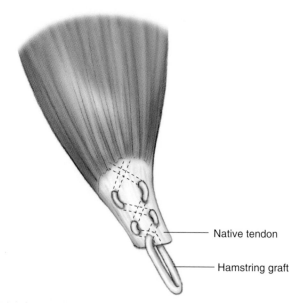

Figure 50-15. Diagram depicting technique for weaving allograft tendon through the native biceps muscle in cases of delayed reconstruction. *(Modified from Hallam P, Bain GI. Repair of chronic distal biceps tendon ruptures using autologous hamstring graft and the EndoButton. J Shoulder Elbow Surg. 2004;13:648-651.)*

— Native tendon

— Hamstring graft

REFERENCES

1. Ramsey ML. Distal biceps tendon injuries: diagnosis and management. *J Am Acad Orthop Surg.* 1999;7(3): 199-207.
2. Baker BE, Bierwagen D. Rupture of the distal tendon of the biceps brachii. Operative versus non-operative treatment. *J Bone Joint Surg Am.* 1985;67(3):414-417.
3. Chillemi C, Marinelli M, De Cupis V. Rupture of the distal biceps brachii tendon: conservative treatment versus anatomic reinsertion—clinical and radiological evaluation after 2 years. *Arch Orthop Trauma Surg.* 2007;127(8): 705-708.
4. Morrey BF, Askew LJ, An KN, et al. Rupture of the distal tendon of the biceps brachii. A biomechanical study. *J Bone Joint Surg Am.* 1985;67(3):418-421.
5. Agins HJ, Chess JL, Hoekstra DV, et al. Rupture of the distal insertion of the biceps brachii tendon. *Clin Orthop Relat Res.* 1988;234:34-38.
6. Bain GI, Prem H, Heptinstall RJ, et al. Repair of distal biceps tendon rupture: a new technique using the Endo-button. *J Shoulder Elbow Surg.* 2000;9(2):120-126.
7. Barnes SJ, Coleman SG, Gilpin D. Repair of avulsed insertion of biceps. A new technique in four cases. *J Bone Joint Surg Br.* 1993;75(6):938-939.

8. Bosman HA, Fincher M, Saw N. Anatomic direct repair of chronic distal biceps brachii tendon rupture without interposition graft. *J Shoulder Elbow Surg.* 2012;21:1342-1347.

9. El-Hawary R, Macdermid JC, Faber KJ, et al. Distal biceps tendon repair: comparison of surgical techniques. *J Hand Surg.* 2003;28(3):496-502.

10. Greenberg JA. Endobutton repair of distal biceps tendon ruptures. *J Hand Surg.* 2009;34(8):1541-1548.

11. Greenberg JA, Fernandez JJ, Wang T, et al. EndoButton-assisted repair of distal biceps tendon ruptures. *J Shoulder Elbow Surg.* 2003;12(5):484-490.

12. Hallam P, Bain GI. Repair of chronic distal biceps tendon ruptures using autologous hamstring graft and the EndoButton. *J Shoulder Elbow Surg.* 2004;13(6):648-651.

13. Karunakar MA, CHA P, Stern PJ. Distal biceps ruptures. A followup of Boyd and Anderson repair. *Clin Orthop Relat Res.* 1999;363:100-107.

14. McKee MD, Hirji R, Schemitsch EH, et al. Patient-oriented functional outcome after repair of distal biceps tendon ruptures using a single-incision technique. *J Shoulder Elbow Surg.* 2005;14(3):302-306.

15. Boyd HB, Anderson LD. A method for reinsertion of the distal biceps brachii. *J Bone Joint Surg Am.* 1961;43(7):1041-1043.

16. Cohen MS. Complications of distal biceps tendon repairs. *Sports Med Arthrosc Rev.* 2008;16(3):148-153.

17. Bain GI, Johnson LJ, Turner PC. Treatment of partial distal biceps tendon tears. *Sports Med Arthrosc Rev.* 2008;16(3):154-161.

18. Patterson RW, Sharma J, Lawton JN, et al. Distal biceps tendon reconstruction with tendoachilles allograft: a modification of the EndoButton technique utilizing an ACL reconstruction system. *J Hand Surg.* 2009;34(3):545-552.

19. Ruland RT, Dunbar RP, Bowen JD. The biceps squeeze test for diagnosis of distal biceps tendon ruptures. *Clin Orthop Relat Res.* 2005;437:128-131.

20. Falchook FS, Zlatkin MB, Erbacher GE, et al. Rupture of the distal biceps tendon: evaluation with MR imaging. *Radiology.* 1994;190(3):659-663.

21. Mazzocca AD, Cohen M, Berkson E, et al. The anatomy of the bicipital tuberosity and distal biceps tendon. *J Shoulder Elbow Surg.* 2007;16(1):122-127.

22. Hutchinson HL, Gloystein D, Gillespie M. Distal biceps tendon insertion: an anatomic study. *J Shoulder Elbow Surg.* 2008;17(2):342-346.

23. Sethi P, Obopilwe E, Rincon L, et al. Biomechanical evaluation of distal biceps reconstruction with cortical button and interference screw fixation. *J Shoulder Elbow Surg.* 2010;19(1):53-57.

24. Bourne MH, Morrey BF. Partial rupture of the distal biceps tendon. *Clin Orthop Relat Res.* 1991;271:143-148.

The Knee

Chapter 51

Patient Positioning, Portal Placement, and Normal Arthroscopic Anatomy

Robin V. West and Keerat Singh

Chapter Synopsis
- Before arthroscopic knee surgery, correct identification of the surgical site is imperative. The type of anesthesia administered and the surgical positioning of the patient vary according to patient tolerance, specific surgery, and physician preference. A variety of portals exist, with the inferolateral portal often used as a viewing portal and the inferomedial portal as a working portal. The description and usefulness of additional portals is presented. A systematic and comprehensive examination of the knee intra-articular structures is described, followed by a discussion of postoperative course.

Important Points
- Correct identification of the surgical site is imperative.
- The surgeon should be familiar with various arthroscopes and associated instruments.
- Portals should be created with proper identification of anatomic landmarks to avoid injury and complications.

- A systematic, reproducible method of examination should be developed.

Clinical and Surgical Pearls
- Establish a standard surgical technique for portal placement and a systematic diagnostic examination so that pathology is not missed.
- Create additional portals as needed to make the procedure technically less demanding and to avoid articular cartilage injury.

Clinical and Surgical Pitfalls
- Avoid an extensive fat pad debridement, which can lead to postoperative hemarthrosis and fibrosis.
- Deep vein thrombosis (DVT) is not uncommon after simple arthroscopy. Consider postoperative anticoagulation or preoperative and postoperative Doppler in sedentary patients, those with a complex knee injury, and individuals with a genetic predisposition for DVT.

IDENTIFICATION

Proper identification of the patient and surgical site should be established before any operation. To prevent wrong-site surgery—an issue on which the American Academy of Orthopaedic Surgeons has been working since 1997—the Joint Commission on Accreditation of Healthcare Organization (JCAHO) adopted a protocol in 2004. Implementation varies from hospital to hospital, but in general, the surgeon or a "credentialed provider" on the surgical team places his or her initials on the operative site in indelible ink before administration

of anesthesia. No other marking, such as an X, is recommended because it may be misinterpreted. The initials should be located in a region that remains visible after preparation and draping. Finally, during a "time-out" with the surgical team and operating room nurse, the site is confirmed again with the surgeon and the consent before an incision in made.

ANESTHESIA

Several factors contribute to the decision of which type of anesthesia is most appropriate for a given patient.

The decision to use local, regional, or general anesthesia depends on the planned procedure, the general health of the patient, and the preference of the patient, anesthesiologist, and surgeon.

Local Anesthesia

Before knee arthroscopy is performed with use of local anesthetic with or without intravenous sedation, several factors are considered. The anesthesia team may need to convert to an alternative form of anesthesia if airway management becomes difficult. With this technique, patients generally do not tolerate use of a tourniquet. Some patients may experience discomfort during manipulation of the leg and introduction of instruments into the knee. For these reasons, short procedures that do not require excessive manipulation or bone work are most suitable for local anesthesia. Suitable procedures include diagnostic arthroscopy, synovial biopsy, removal of loose bodies, and partial meniscectomy. Advantages of this technique are low morbidity, low cost, and ease of recovery. A combination of lidocaine and bupivacaine is typically used to provide short-term and long-term pain relief. Epinephrine can be used in combination with the anesthetic to aid in hemostasis.

Regional Anesthesia

Regional anesthetic options include spinal, epidural, and peripheral nerve (femoral and sciatic) anesthesia. For patients whose medical issues put them at increased risk with general anesthesia, regional anesthesia provides satisfactory anesthesia for most arthroscopic knee procedures. Tourniquet use is generally well tolerated with these techniques. Possible complications are femoral or sciatic nerve palsy, delayed onset of motor function, spinal puncture, and spinal headache.

General Anesthesia

Newer anesthetic agents continue to make general anesthesia safer with easier recovery. Complete muscle relaxation with general anesthesia allows better visualization of the joint, and the tourniquet as well as bone work are better tolerated by the patient. A consequence of endotracheal tube use is throat irritation.

PATIENT POSITIONING

The patient is positioned supine on a standard operating table. If a tourniquet is used, a layer of padding is placed on the thigh before its application. The decision to use a tourniquet should be based on surgeon preference. In our institution we rarely use a tourniquet, relying instead on the pump pressure to ensure adequate visualization during the procedure.

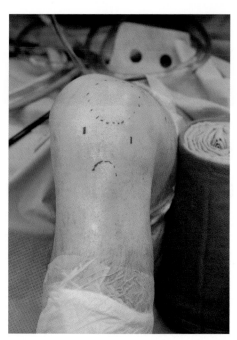

Figure 51-1. Anterior portals.

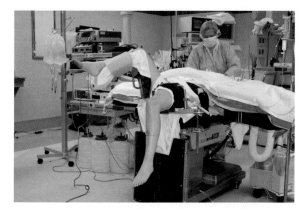

Figure 51-2. Placement of the thigh in a leg holder and flexion of the foot of the table.

On the basis of the surgeon's preference, one of two setups is used at our hospital. In the first, the patient lies supine on the table with the feet just short of the end of the table. The nonoperative leg is protected with foam padding. The operative leg is flexed to 90 degrees. A sandbag is taped to the table for the foot to rest on when the knee is flexed. A lateral post is attached the table at the level of the midthigh. The post helps stabilize the leg when a valgus force is applied to visualize the medial compartment. This method allows easy access to all aspects of the knee. However, an assistant may be required to manipulate the leg during the procedure (Fig. 51-1).

The other option entails placement of the thigh in a leg holder and flexion of the foot of the table (Fig. 51-2). On the table, the patient's operative knee must be just distal to the level of the break in the bed. The operative leg is placed into a leg holder that encompasses the proximal thigh. The opposite leg is placed into a well-leg holder and protected with foam under the knee. The operative leg is manipulated by placing it on the surgeon's pelvis or thigh and applying a varus or valgus stress at the knee. If the leg holder is too tight, it can act as a venous tourniquet and cause bleeding during surgery. Whereas this method eliminates the need for an assistant, there is no support for the leg when it is in extension. Also, larger thighs may not fit well in the leg holder.

EXAMINATION UNDER ANESTHESIA

After the administration of anesthesia, a thorough examination is performed, including range of motion, a complete patellar assessment, instability tests, and documentation of an effusion. The contralateral knee is used for comparison. Certain tests, such as a pivot shift, are better tolerated when the patient is completely relaxed. The findings of the examination are documented in the operative report. The surgeon also correlates the examination with the arthroscopic findings.

ARTHROSCOPIC EQUIPMENT

Arthroscopic equipment has continually improved in the years since its introduction. Better optical systems and the introduction of new instruments have broadened the number of ailments that can be treated arthroscopically. The scope of this chapter does not allow a comprehensive overview of all possible equipment.

Arthroscopes are described by their angle of inclination. A 0-degree scope looks straight ahead; a 30-degree scope views at a 30-degree angle from the axis of the arthroscope. Rotation of the arthroscope increases the field of view compared with the straight-ahead view from a 0-degree scope. The 30-degree scope is used most commonly; a 70-degree scope is used for added visualization in tight spaces.

A surgeon uses the arthroscopic probe as an extension of his or her finger. The probe palpates various structures and provides tactile assessment of their condition. The probe can also be used as a measuring device for lesions in the joint. Most probe tips are calibrated to a known length, typically 3 mm. Besides allowing assessment of the menisci, articular cartilage, and ligaments, a probe can maneuver loose bodies into positions that facilitate their retrieval.

Arthroscopic biters are used to remove soft tissues, such as a torn meniscus or an anterior cruciate stump. These instruments come in a variety of shapes and sizes. The heads are angled in different directions to facilitate

removal from areas that are difficult to reach. Use of an angled up-biter in the medial compartment helps the surgeon to reach the posterior meniscus by taking advantage of the convex nature of the medial tibial plateau and the concave shape of the medial femoral condyle.

Other instruments include graspers, scissors, motorized shavers and burs, and electrocautery devices. Various procedure-specific guides have been developed to assist in surgeries such as ligament reconstruction. The surgeon should take some time to become familiar with the instruments available from the hospital and various companies.

ARTHROSCOPY PORTALS

Inferolateral Portal

The inferolateral portal, or anterolateral portal, is traditionally used as the viewing portal through which the camera is inserted. The portal is made in the palpable soft spot just off the lateral border of the patellar tendon at the level of the inferior border of the patella. Especially during anterior cruciate ligament (ACL) reconstruction, we prefer to keep this portal "high and tight" to aid in visualization of the ACL tibial and femoral footprints. The anterior portion of the lateral meniscus is also at risk with inferior placement of this portal. Excessive medial placement of the portal risks injury to the patellar tendon.

Inferomedial Portal

The inferomedial (or anteromedial) portal is used primarily as a working portal. The incision is made in the medial soft spot, just medial to the patellar tendon approximately 1 cm below the inferior border of the patella. To prevent injury to the medial meniscus when the portal is established, the incision can be made under direct visualization after localization with a spinal needle.

Superomedial Portal

Historically, the superomedial portal was used for inflow or outflow of arthroscopy fluid. The portal is made 2 cm proximal to the superomedial border of the patella. The incision should be next to but not through the quadriceps tendon. During insertion, the trocar is angled into the suprapatellar pouch to avoid damage to the articular cartilage of the patella. If multiple passes are made through the soft tissues during insertion, fluid leak may occur and prevent adequate joint distention. To avoid trauma to the vastus medialis obliquus muscle, we do not routinely use this portal. Instead, we prefer to use a double-port cannula that allows controlled inflow and outflow. Studies have shown that use of the superomedial portal results in longer return of quadriceps strength and less total strength than does the standard two-portal technique.

Superolateral Portal

The superolateral portal (Fig. 51-3) allows visualization of the patellofemoral articulation, use for inflow or outflow, and removal of loose bodies from the suprapatellar pouch. This portal is made 2 cm proximal to the superolateral border of the patella. Entry through the interval between the vastus lateralis and the iliotibial band avoids injury to these structures. Use of the

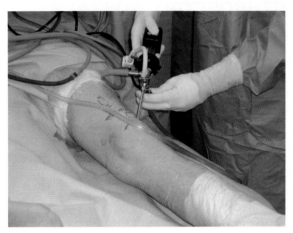

Figure 51-3. Arthroscope in the superolateral portal. View of the patellofemoral articulation.

70-degree arthroscope through the superolateral portal gives an excellent view of the patellofemoral articulation (Fig. 51-4).

Posterolateral Portal

Although the posterolateral portal is rarely used, knowledge of this portal can facilitate repair of the posterior horn of the lateral meniscus, removal of loose bodies, and synovectomy. The portal is made posterior to the lateral collateral ligament and anterior to the biceps tendon and common peroneal nerve.

Posteromedial Portal

The posteromedial portal is established to view and to access the posterior portion of the medial compartment. This portal provides access to the tibial insertion of the posterior cruciate ligament and the posterior horn of the medial meniscus. The portal is marked preoperatively before the joint distends. The portal lies 2 cm above the joint line and 1 to 2 cm posterior to the medial femoral epicondyle. Because establishment of this portal carries a high risk of chondral or meniscal damage, we recommend use of a spinal needle under direct visualization to ensure accurate placement.

Transpatellar Tendon Portal

To establish the transpatellar tendon portal, a vertical slit is made in the central portion of the patellar tendon.

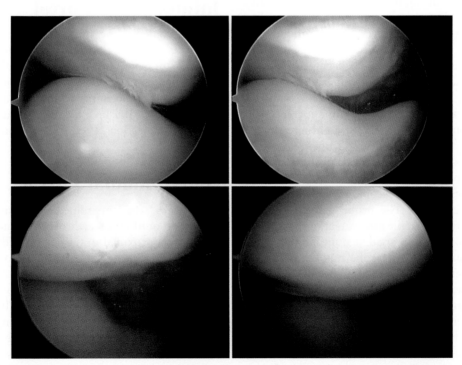

Figure 51-4. Use of the 70-degree arthroscope through the superolateral portal gives an excellent view of the patellofemoral articulation.

This portal provides access to the intracondylar notch for visualization, or it can be used as a working portal during ACL reconstruction.

ARTHROSCOPIC EVALUATION

Each surgeon needs to develop a systematic, reproducible method of examining the intra-articular structures of the knee. Multiple pictures are taken throughout the examination to document the findings of the procedure. Our systematic approach is described.

As the knee is extended, the blunt trocar is introduced into the suprapatellar pouch through the inferolateral portal. The pouch is inspected for loose bodies and adhesions from previous surgery. The camera is slowly pulled back until the undersurface of the patella comes into view. The degree of chondrosis is assessed. The camera is rotated so the trochlea can be viewed. Chondrosis is noted, and patellar tracking in the trochlear groove is assessed. However, the superolateral portal with a 70-degree arthroscope provides the best view of the patellofemoral joint.

The lateral and medial gutters are visualized by passing the arthroscope across each condyle. The gutters are visualized all the way down to the joint line. On the lateral side, loose bodies may settle in the popliteal hiatus, so this area must be inspected.

The medial compartment is entered by following the trochlea down into the intercondylar notch. A veil of tissue, the ligamentum mucosum, often covers the cruciate ligaments (Fig. 51-5). This tissue is either pulled aside with a probe or removed with a motorized shaver. The substance of the cruciates and their visible insertions are carefully inspected. Again, a probe is valuable in assessing the tension of the ligaments.

For entrance into the lateral compartment, a triangular space formed by the lateral border of the ACL, the anterior horn of the lateral meniscus, and the lateral femoral condyle is identified. The arthroscope is directed into this space while the leg is placed into a figure-of-four position. An assistant can apply a varus stress by placing pressure on the medial aspect of the knee to open the joint further. The lateral meniscus is inspected and probed (Fig. 51-6). The popliteal tendon is visible passing through the popliteal hiatus and can be traced all the way up to its femoral insertion. The leg is fully extended and flexed for assessment of the articular cartilage of the lateral compartment. If the scope is backed into the intercondylar notch with the knee in the figure-of-four position, the posterolateral bundle of the ACL can be well visualized (Fig. 51-7).

The medial compartment is then entered. With varying degrees of flexion and valgus stress, the majority of the medial meniscus is clearly visualized. The camera is rotated so the posterior horn can be seen more clearly. A probe is used to further assess the stability of the meniscus (Fig. 51-8). The cartilage of the medial femoral condyle and the medial tibial plateau is examined for degeneration. The knee is flexed and extended for full visualization of the entire condyle.

In certain procedures, the posteromedial compartment needs to be assessed. Either the posteromedial portal or the Gilchrist view can be used to assess the posterior compartment. With the Gilchrist view the posterior compartment can be viewed with the arthroscope in the anterolateral portal. The knee is flexed to 90 degrees, and a 30-degree or 70-degree arthroscope is carefully advanced between the medical femoral

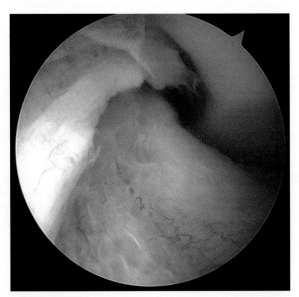

Figure 51-5. The ligamentum mucosum covering the cruciate ligaments.

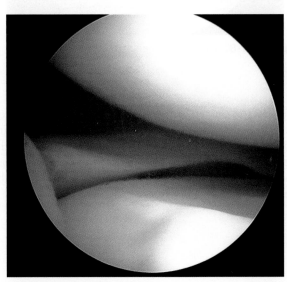

Figure 51-6. The lateral compartment.

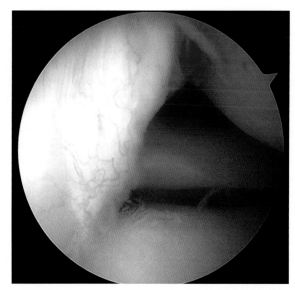

Figure 51-7. The anterior cruciate ligament visualized with the knee in the figure-of-four position.

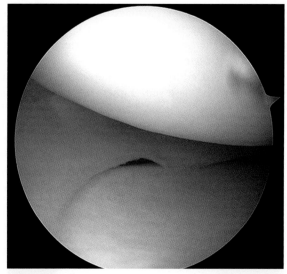

Figure 51-8. The medial meniscus.

condyle and the femoral insertion of the posterior cruciate ligament. Rotation of the arthroscope downward brings the posterior horn and root insertion of the medial meniscus into view. This view also locates loose bodies in the posterior compartment and shows the tibial insertion of the posterior cruciate ligament.

POSTOPERATIVE COURSE

The portals can be closed with either a nonabsorbable or an absorbable monofilament suture. An ice machine is used to help provide postoperative hemostasis and to decrease inflammation. Exercises, including quadriceps sets, straight-leg raises, heel slides, and calf pumps are started immediately after surgery. Crutches are used initially until the quadriceps function returns (typically a few days). Physical therapy is generally started a week after surgery. Narcotic pain medication is prescribed and selected on the basis of the procedure, the patient's allergies, and the surgeon's preference. An anti-inflammatory agent can be used to potentiate the narcotic medication. Preoperative intravenous antibiotics are routinely administered at our institution, and postoperative oral antibiotics are rarely prescribed.

SUGGESTED READINGS

Brophy RH, Dunn WR, Wickiewicz TL. Arthroscopic portal placement. *Tech Knee Surg.* 2004;3:2-7.

Chu CR, Izzo NJ, Papas NE, et al. In vitro exposure to 0.5% bupivacaine is cytotoxic to bovine articular chondrocytes. *Arthroscopy.* 2006;7:693-699.

Iossifinidis A. Knee arthroscopy under local anesthesia: results and evaluation of patients' satisfaction. *Injury.* 1996;27: 43-44.

Joint Commission on Accreditation of Healthcare Organizations (JCAHO). *Universal Protocol for Preventing Wrong Site, Wrong Procedure, Wrong Person Surgery,* JCAHO; 2003.

Kim SJ, Kim HJ. High portal: practical philosophy for positioning portals in knee arthroscopy. *Arthroscopy.* 2001; 17:333-337.

Ochi M, Adachi N, Sumen Y, et al. A new guide system for posteromedial portal in arthroscopic knee surgery. *Arch Orthop Trauma Surg.* 1998;118:25-28.

Ogilvie-Harris DJ, Biggs DJ, Mackay M, Weisleder L. Posterior portal for arthroscopic surgery of the knee. *Arthroscopy.* 1994;10:608-613.

Ong BC, Shen FH, Musahl V, et al. Knee: patient positioning, portal placement, and normal arthroscopic Anatomy. In: Miller MD, Cole BJ, eds. *Textbook of Arthroscopy.* Philadelphia: Elsevier; 2004:463-469.

Stetson WB, Templin K. Two-versus three-portal technique for routine knee arthroscopy. *Am J Sports Med.* 2002;30: 108-111.

Wu WH, Richmond JC. Arthroscopy of the knee: basic setup and technique. In: McGinty JB, Burkhart SS, Jackson RW, et al, eds. *Operative Arthroscopy.* Philadelphia: Lippincott Williams & Wilkins; 2003:211-217.

Chapter 52

Arthroscopic Meniscectomy

David C. Flanigan and Christopher C. Kaeding

Chapter Synopsis
- Meniscal tears are common. Partial meniscectomy is indicated when patients have persistent mechanical symptoms. Proper use of arthroscopic tools and portals allows for successful meniscectomy. Good to excellent results can be achieved in the appropriately indicated patient.

Important Points
- Repair the meniscus if possible

Indications
- Symptomatic meniscal tears that have failed conservative measures

Contraindications
- Septic knee
- Significant medical comorbidities

Classification
- Description of meniscus tear by tear location and tear pattern

Surgical Technique
- Proper arthroscopic setup
- Be comfortable with a variety of portals or viewing angles

- Have a complete set of meniscal biters
- Variety of shavers

Clinical and Surgical Pearls
Viewing of Meniscus
- May need to view from various portals or through the notch for complete resection

Use of Instruments
- Keep meniscal baskets in contact with meniscus at all times for consistent resection
- Appropriate resection may require use of other portals or 90-degree side-biters or back-biters

Resection of Meniscus
- Preserve the meniscocapsular junction
- Smooth edges
- Conservative resection

Clinical and Surgical Pitfalls
- Prevent iatrogenic cartilage injury
  - Make sure you have adequate visualization
  - Ensure controlled entry and removal of instruments

Tears of the meniscus have been known to cause pain and mechanical symptoms of the knee. Historically, open meniscectomy has been shown to lead to the development of progressive radiographic signs (Fairbank changes) of osteoarthritis in the meniscus-deficient compartment. With the advent of arthroscopy, partial, subtotal, or total meniscectomy can be performed with minimal incisions and on an outpatient basis. In fact, arthroscopic meniscectomy is the most commonly performed orthopedic procedure in the United States. Despite the minimally invasive nature of arthroscopy and the faster recovery afterward, radiographic changes can still be seen with partial meniscectomies because of the increased articular contact pressures. The goal of arthroscopic meniscectomy today is to remove as little meniscal tissue as possible to achieve a pain-free, stable meniscus.

PREOPERATIVE CONSIDERATIONS

History

Patients typically recall an acute sudden twisting mechanism that caused the onset of pain. Degenerative tears may be more subacute in nature and subtle in onset with underlying arthritic or baseline pain that has now become localized and sharp. A detailed history of previous knee pain, previous surgeries in the knee, and other injuries (ligament injury, fracture) should be elicited.

Symptoms

- Medial or lateral compartment pain, often posteriorly
- Pain with deep knee bending, walking, twisting mechanisms, activity
- Sensation of "giving way"
- Mechanical symptoms: catching, locking, clicking
- Continuous or recurrent effusions

Physical Examination

A thorough knee examination is crucial because meniscal tears are commonly associated with other injuries, such as anterior cruciate ligament injuries and tibial plateau fractures. A detailed knee examination has been consistently shown to be reliable in diagnosis of a meniscal tear.

Specific findings for meniscal tears may include the following:

- Antalgic gait
- Pain with squatting
- Loss of motion
- Locked knee
- Effusion
- Joint line tenderness
- Pain with hyperflexion or hyperextension
- Positive result of McMurray test
- Perimeniscal cysts or Baker cyst

Imaging

Baseline plain radiography is of limited importance for diagnosis of meniscal disorders but is necessary to rule out other pathologic processes such as stress fracture, avascular necrosis, tumor, and arthritis that may mimic meniscal signs and symptoms. Standard radiographs include a 45-degree flexed posteroanterior view, weight-bearing anteroposterior view, lateral view, and Merchant view.

Magnetic resonance imaging is not a substitute for a good examination, but it can be a useful tool to confirm the diagnosis or to differentiate pathologic changes in difficult cases. Meniscal tears on magnetic resonance imaging are described as abnormal meniscal signal that extends to the articular surface of the meniscus (grade 3 meniscal signal). Numerous studies have shown that the accuracy of magnetic resonance imaging is 95% or greater for meniscal tears.

Classification

Arthroscopic evaluation has aided in the classification of meniscal tears. Meniscal tears can be classified by vascular zone or tear patterns. Both classification systems are often used in determining whether a tear is favorable for repair.

Arnoczky and Warren[1] reported on the vascularity of the meniscus, which is divided into three zones: red-red (peripheral 25% to 33%), red-white, and white-white (central 33%). Healing has been found to be more favorable in the vascular zones (i.e., red-red and red-white).

Meniscal tears are commonly described by tear pattern. Examples of common tear patterns are illustrated in Figure 52-1.

Indications and Contraindications

Meniscectomy is indicated for any symptomatic meniscal tear that is abnormally mobile or not conducive to repair and in which conservative measures have failed.

Contraindications are active septic arthritis and significant medical comorbidities.

Instruments

Multiple manufacturers have produced meniscal baskets, biters, graspers, scissors, and arthroscopic shavers. Common instruments needed for arthroscopic meniscectomy are illustrated in Figure 52-2. These include the following:

- Meniscal biters or baskets: straight, up-going, 90-degree right and left, back-biting
- Meniscal scissors
- Meniscal grasper
- Arthroscopic shaver: 3.5- to 4.5-mm full radius

SURGICAL TECHNIQUE
Anesthesia and Positioning

The operative leg is marked in the holding area, and preoperative antibiotics are administered 30 minutes before the procedure is begun. The procedure can be performed with the patient under general, regional, spinal, or, in some cases, local anesthesia. The patient is positioned supine with all bone prominences well padded. A tourniquet is placed high on the operative thigh, and the leg is positioned in a standard leg holder. The nonoperative leg is placed in the lithotomy position, well padded. The foot of the table is then flexed down, allowing full flexion of the operative leg. The leg is prepared and draped in a standard fashion (Fig. 52-3).

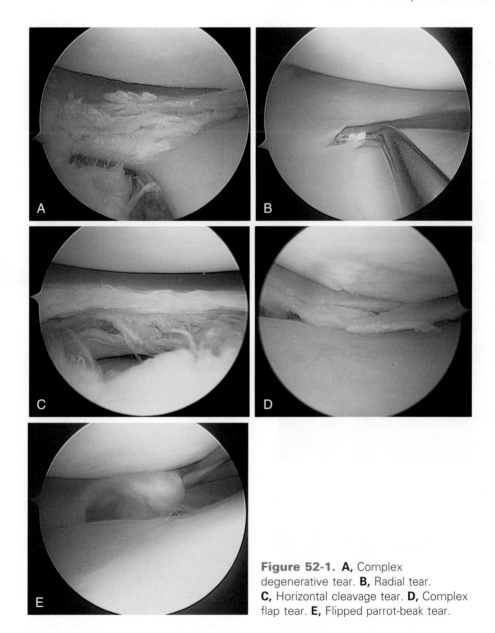

Figure 52-1. **A,** Complex degenerative tear. **B,** Radial tear. **C,** Horizontal cleavage tear. **D,** Complex flap tear. **E,** Flipped parrot-beak tear.

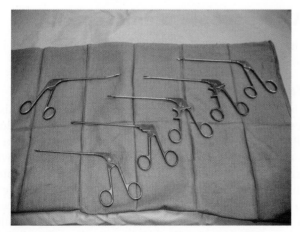

Figure 52-2. Standard arthroscopic meniscectomy instruments.

The tourniquet can be inflated per the surgeon's preference. A surgical time-out should be performed per hospital and American Academy of Orthopaedic Surgeons (AAOS) guidelines.

Portals

Portals include the following (Fig. 52-4):

- Inferomedial portal: just medial to the patellar tendon at the joint line
- Inferolateral portal: just lateral to the patellar tendon at the joint line
- Superomedial or superolateral portal: for inflow or outflow as needed, placed approximately 1 cm proximal to the superior pole of the patella, entering just posterior to the quadriceps tendon

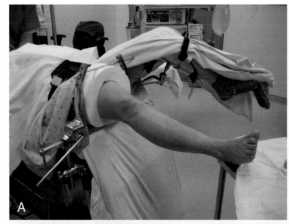

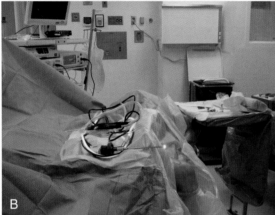

Figure 52-3. A, Patient positioning with a leg holder. **B,** Knee arthroscopy setup after sterile preparation and draping.

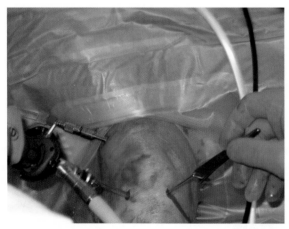

Figure 52-4. Standard arthroscopic portals. For this procedure a superolateral portal was used for inflow, the inferolateral portal for the arthroscope, and the inferomedial portal for instrumentation.

Arthroscopic Evaluation

A thorough arthroscopic evaluation of the knee is performed. The meniscus should be visually inspected and probed to determine the zone, pattern, and length of the tear and whether it is stable or unstable. Flipped

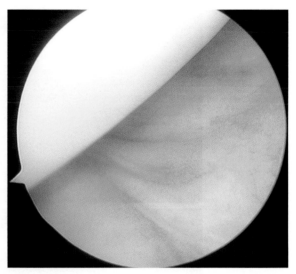

Figure 52-5. View of the posteromedial compartment by placement of the arthroscope through the notch just medial to the posterior cruciate ligament.

BOX 52-1 Key Principles of Arthroscopic Meniscectomy

- Repair of meniscus, if possible
- Resection of any abnormal mobile meniscal fragments
- Smooth transition without abrupt edges
- Preservation of the meniscocapsular junction
- Conservative resection of meniscal tissue
- Minimization of trauma to chondral surfaces

---

meniscal segments or bucket-handle tears should be reduced for meniscal evaluation.

At times, placement of the scope through the notch is necessary to determine the extent of the tear at its posterior horn or to visualize any flipped segment or loose piece posteriorly (Fig. 52-5).

Arthroscopic Meniscectomy

The key principles of this procedure are listed in Box 52-1.

Radial Tears

The goal is to saucerize the tear from the native meniscus. With use of the meniscal scissors or basket, gradually start to remove normal meniscal tissue and taper it toward the apex of the tear. It is important to move arthroscopic instruments in a controlled fashion to minimize iatrogenic cartilage damage. Care should be taken to keep the meniscal basket in contact with the meniscus at all times to allow consistency of meniscal tissue removal. For a smooth transition to be ensured, the anterior aspect of the tear may require resection with a 90-degree basket if the ipsilateral portal is used or a straight basket if the contralateral portal is used. An arthroscopic shaver can smooth any edges.

Bucket-Handle Tears

Bucket-handle tears that are irreparable because of tissue quality, deformation, or zone of injury should first be reduced to assess the length of the tear. Visualization of the extent of the posterior aspect of the tear may be improved by assessment of the meniscus through the notch. Appropriate planning to truncate the posterior attachment without leaving an abrupt edge is needed. This may require rotation of the meniscal basket or scissors more centrally and posteriorly to make a proper transition to the tear. It is typically easier to remove most of the posterior attachment first, leaving just a few strands of tissue that can easily be torn by rotating the meniscus for removal. This will prevent the meniscus from becoming a loose body when the anterior aspect is removed. The anterior aspect of the tear can then be addressed through the ipsilateral or contralateral portal as discussed earlier. After the ipsilateral portal has been enlarged with a hemostat, a grasper can be used to firmly grab the meniscus. Enlargement of the portal by several millimeters is often needed to ensure that the resected fragment is not dislodged from the grasper during extraction. Rotation of the meniscus should avulse the remaining strands of the posterior meniscus, and the meniscus can be removed en bloc through the portal. Care must be taken not to allow the resected fragment to become a loose body. A meniscal shaver can smooth any edges as necessary. Alternatively, for small bucket-handle tears, the anterior edge can be removed as detailed earlier, and the meniscal shaver can be used to debride the meniscus to its posterior base.

Horizontal Cleavage Tears

Controversy still exists about how to properly approach a horizontal cleavage tear. Options include removal of the most unstable leaf (superior or inferior) and removal of both leaves of the tear. Cleavage tears often make a flap on one of the leaflets that causes pain and mechanical symptoms. Although horizontal cleavage tears typically extend to the peripheral margin, it is not necessary to remove all of the meniscal tissue to make a stable tear and smooth transition.

Our bias is to remove the most unstable leaf, retaining part of the meniscus for function. The approach is similar to removal of a bucket-handle tear. The majority of the posterior attachment is removed through the ipsilateral portal, then the anterior attachment is removed through the contralateral portal. Finally, with use of a basket or meniscal scissors, the peripheral attachment is resected, leaving some pericapsular meniscal tissue. The leaf is removed either en bloc with the grasper or piecemeal with a shaver. The arthroscopic shaver is used to smooth any edges, but care must be taken with the thinned meniscus because the shaver may aggressively remove the tissue that is to be preserved. The stable leaf should then be assessed for the integrity of the meniscal tissue, because often some of the meniscal tissue in the white-white zone will need to be excised for a stable rim.

Meniscal Cysts

Meniscal cysts are common findings that typically indicate intra-articular disease. Meniscal tears commonly make a rent in the capsular tissue and a one-way valve occurs, allowing synovial fluid to collect extra-articularly. Lateral meniscal cysts are located off the lateral joint line associated with a midportion lateral meniscus tear. Posterior medial cysts (Baker cyst) commonly associated with a posterior medial meniscus tear dissect between the medial head of the gastrocnemius and the semimembranosus. The meniscal cyst is often decompressed with treatment of the intra-articular meniscal tear. Commonly with a lateral meniscal cyst a spinal needle can be inserted percutaneously at the lateral joint line level through the meniscal tear to aid in decompression of the cyst.

Discoid Meniscus Tears

Discoid meniscus tears commonly occur during the second to fifth decades of life. Tears often become degenerative in nature, causing both horizontal cleavage and radial components. The goal is to saucerize the meniscus to form a normal C-shaped meniscus. With a meniscus biter from the contralateral portal, start the resection anteriorly and work posteriorly; often the posterior aspect is finished from the ipsilateral portal. Careful examination and probing of the meniscus after saucerization are required, because some variants of discoid meniscus tears may require repair of the periphery as well.

POSTOPERATIVE CONSIDERATIONS

Follow-up

Patients are seen 1 week postoperatively for a wound check and suture removal. Subsequent follow-up is scheduled for 1 month postoperatively for evaluation of knee symptoms, range of motion, and strength.

Rehabilitation

Goals are to reduce pain, inflammation, and swelling and to restore motion and strength. These goals can typically be accomplished with a home exercise program. Formal physical therapy can assist older patients. A standard protocol consists of the following:

TABLE 52-1. Results of Studies of Arthroscopic Meniscectomy

Study	Medial or Lateral	Type of Tear	Follow-up	Results	Symptoms	Radiographic Changes	Notes
Bin et al[2] (2008)	Medial	Degenerative	4 years	82% had reduced pain		Preexisting grade IV OA	
Kuraishi et al[3] (2006)	Lateral	Mixed	5 years	92% had improved function		Preexisting OA OA progressed in 52%	More valgus alignment associated with poorer results
Fabricant et al[4] (2008)	Both	Mixed	1 year				Female gender and worse osteoarthritis associated with worse short-term outcomes
Chatain et al[5] (2003)	Both	Mixed	10 years	95% satisfied	14% medial; 20% lateral	22% medial; 38% lateral	Better prognosis with medial tears, age younger than 35 years, vertical tear, no cartilage damage, intact peripheral rim
Hulet et al[6] (2004)	Lateral with cyst	Mixed (57% horizontal cleavage)	5 years	87% good to excellent			
Pearse and Craig[7] (2003)	Both	Mixed (degenerative)	1 year	65% improvement			At 4 years, 32% with further surgery
Bonneux and Vandekerckhove[8] (2002)	Lateral	Mixed	8 years	64.5% good to excellent			Amount of resection correlates with results
Menetrey et al[9] (2002)	Medial	Mixed	3-7 years	90% NDM 20% DM			
Andersson-Molina et al[10] (2002)	Both	Mixed	14 years	70%			
Scheller et al[11] (2001)	Lateral	Mixed	10 years	77%			Results decrease over time
Crevoisier et al[12] (2001)	Both	Degenerative, mixed	4 years	80% satisfied 55% satisfied			Age older than 70 years
Hoser et al[13] (2001)	Lateral	Mixed	10 years	58% good to excellent			
Hulet et al[14] (2001)	Medial	95% vertical; 5% complex	12 years	95% very satisfied or satisfied			29% reoperation

Study	Side	Type	Follow-up	Results			Conclusion
Krüger-Franke et al[15] (1999)	Medial	Mixed	7 years	96%			Women at greater risk of degenerative changes
Barrett et al[16] (1998)	Lateral	Mixed	3 years	94% (grade 0-2 arthritis) and 80% (grade 3-4 arthritis) improvement	Grade 0-II Grade III or IV 14% failure		
Schimmer et al[17] (1998)	Both	Mixed	4 and 12 years	92% at 4 years, 78% at 12 years good to excellent			Underlying cartilage damage faired worse
Burks et al[18] (1997)	78% medial; 19% lateral	Mixed	14 years	88% good to excellent			No difference medial vs. lateral; ACL-deficient and female patients had worse outcomes
Matsusue and Thomson[19] (1996)	Medial	Mixed	7.8 years	83% good to excellent	Worse at 5 years if cartilage damage		Worse outcomes with grade III or IV OA
Bonamo et al[20] (1992)	Both	Mixed	3 years	83% satisfied	Preexisting grade III or IV		Worse outcomes with women, age above 60 years, grade IV changes
Lee et al[21] (2009)	Lateral	Discoid	4 years	83.7% good to excellent results		More severe osteoarthritic changes in subtotal meniscectomy vs. partial meniscectomy groups	Evidence of chondromalacia on tibial plateau at index procedure associated with more symptoms
Stilli et al[22] (2011)	Lateral	Discoid	8 years	95% good to excellent results	Pediatric patients		Preserve meniscal tissue in older patients; Younger patients may have stress adaptation
Wasser et al[23] (2011)	Lateral	Discoid	3 years	65% good to excellent results	Pediatric patients	No signs of arthritis	Saucerization with repair resulted in best results
Kim[24] (2007)	Lateral	Discoid	4 years 8 years	69.5% good to excellent results 24% good results		Worsening arthritic changes over time in subtotal meniscectomy	Long-term prognosis related to amount of resection
Okazaki et al[25] (2006)	Lateral	Discoid	10 years			Progressive changes in older patients at time of surgery	More successful for patients under the age of 25

ACL, Anterior cruciate ligament; DM, degenerative meniscus; NDM, nondegenerative meniscus; OA, osteoarthritis.

- Crutches as needed for 24 to 72 hours
- Ice for 20 minutes three to six times a day
- Immediate progression of unrestricted range-of-motion exercises (passive, active-assisted, and active), quadriceps exercises, and straight-leg raises
- No impact activities for 4 weeks
- Return to play with no inflammation, full motion, and 80% of strength of contralateral extremity

Complications

- Infection
- Deep venous thrombosis
- Arthrofibrosis
- Portal herniation or fistula
- Neuroma at portal site
- Retained meniscal fragment (loose body)
- Repeated tear of meniscus
- Continued pain in the compartment (chondral erosions)

RESULTS

Results of studies of arthroscopic meniscectomy are shown in Table 52-1.

REFERENCES

1. Arnoczky SP, Warren RF. Microvasculature of the human meniscus. *Am J Sports Med.* 1982;10:90-95.
2. Bin SI, Lee SH, Kim CW, et al. Results of arthroscopic medial meniscectomy in patients with grade IV osteoarthritis of the medial compartment. *Arthroscopy.* 2008; 24(3):264-268.
3. Kuraishi J, Akizuki S, Takizawa T, et al. Arthroscopic lateral meniscectomy in knees with lateral compartment osteoarthritis: a case series study. *Arthroscopy.* 2006; 22(8):878-883.
4. Fabricant PD, Rosenberger PH, Jokl P, et al. Predictors of short-term recovery differ from those of long-term outcome after arthroscopic partial meniscectomy. *Arthroscopy.* 2008;24(7):769-778.
5. Chatain F, Adeleine P, Chambat P, et al. A comparative study of medial versus lateral arthroscopic partial meniscectomy on stable knees: 10-year minimum follow-up. *Arthroscopy.* 2003;19:842-849.
6. Hulet C, Souquet D, Alexandre P, et al. Arthroscopic treatment of 105 lateral meniscal cysts with 5-year average follow-up. *Arthroscopy.* 2004;20:831-836.
7. Pearse EO, Craig DM. Partial meniscectomy in the presence of severe osteoarthritis does not hasten the symptomatic progression of osteoarthritis. *Arthroscopy.* 2003;19: 963-968.
8. Bonneux I, Vandekerckhove B. Arthroscopic partial lateral meniscectomy long-term results in athletes. *Acta Orthop Belg.* 2002;68:356-361.
9. Menetrey J, Siegrist O, Fritschy D. Medial meniscectomy in patients over the age of fifty: a six year follow-up study. *Swiss Surg.* 2002;8:113-119.
10. Andersson-Molina H, Karlsson H, Rockborn P. Arthroscopic partial and total meniscectomy: a long-term follow-up study with matched controls. *Arthroscopy.* 2002;18:183-189.
11. Scheller G, Sobau C, Bulow JU. Arthroscopic partial lateral meniscectomy in an otherwise normal knee: clinical, functional, and radiographic results of a long-term follow-up study. *Arthroscopy.* 2001;17:946-952.
12. Crevoisier X, Munzinger U, Drobny T. Arthroscopic partial meniscectomy in patients over 70 years of age. *Arthroscopy.* 2001;17:732-736.
13. Hoser C, Fink C, Brown C, et al. Long-term results of arthroscopic partial lateral meniscectomy in knees without associated damage. *J Bone Joint Surg Br.* 2001;83: 513-516.
14. Hulet CH, Locker BG, Schiltz D, et al. Arthroscopic medial meniscectomy on stable knees. *J Bone Joint Surg Br.* 2001;83:29-32.
15. Krüger-Franke M, Siebert CH, Kugler A, et al. Late results after arthroscopic partial medial meniscectomy. *Knee Surg Sports Traumatol Arthrosc.* 1999;7:81-84.
16. Barrett GR, Treacy SH, Ruff CG. The effect of partial lateral meniscectomy in patients ≥60 years. *Orthopedics.* 1998;21:251-257.
17. Schimmer RC, Brulhart KB, Duff C, et al. Arthroscopic partial meniscectomy: a 12-year follow-up and two-step evaluation of the long-term course. *Arthroscopy.* 1998; 14:136-142.
18. Burks RT, Metcalf MH, Metcalf RW. Fifteen-year follow-up of arthroscopic partial meniscectomy. *Arthroscopy.* 1997;13:673-679.
19. Matsusue Y, Thomson NL. Arthroscopic partial medial meniscectomy in patients over 40 years old: a 5- to 11-year follow-up study. *Arthroscopy.* 1996;12:39-44.
20. Bonamo JJ, Kessler KJ, Noah J. Arthroscopic meniscectomy in patients over the age of 40. *Am J Sports Med.* 1992;20:422-428; discussion 428-429.
21. Lee DH, Kim TH, Kim JM, et al. Results of subtotal/total or partial meniscectomy for discoid lateral meniscus in children. *Arthroscopy.* 2009;25(5):496-503.
22. Stilli S, Marchesini Reggiani L, Marcheggiani Muccioli GM, et al. Arthroscopic treatment for symptomatic discoid lateral meniscus during childhood. *Knee Surg Sports Traumatol Arthrosc.* 2011;19(8):1337-1342.
23. Wasser L, Knörr J, Accadbled F, et al. Arthroscopic treatment of discoid meniscus in children: clinical and MRI results. *Orthop Traumatol Surg Res.* 2011;97(3): 297-303.
24. Kim SJ, Chun YM, Jeong JH, et al. Effects of arthroscopic meniscectomy on the long-term prognosis for the discoid lateral meniscus. *Knee Surg Sports Traumatol Arthrosc.* 2007;15(11):1315-1320.
25. Okazaki K, Miura H, Matsuda S, et al. Arthroscopic resection of the discoid lateral meniscus: long-term follow-up for 16 years. *Arthroscopy.* 2006;22(9): 967-971.

Chapter 53

Arthroscopic Meniscus Repair: Inside-Out Technique

Jeffrey M. Tuman and Mark D. Miller

Chapter Synopsis
- The inside-out meniscus repair technique remains the gold standard against which other repair modalities are compared. This is ideal for posterior meniscus tears, allowing for capture of multiple, longitudinally oriented collagen cables when a vertical suture technique is used. Patient selection remains critical to acceptable outcomes.

Important Points
- Tear location and knee ligamentous stability are the most important factors that determine successful meniscus repair outcome.
- The anteromedial working portal should be made based on meniscus repair location.

Clinical and Surgical Pearls
- The use of double-loaded 2-0 or 0 nonabsorbable sutures with long flexible needles is recommended.
- The posterior capsular incision should be made such that the length of the incision starts at the level of the joint line. Placement of the incision here facilitates capture of the flexible needles during suture passage.

Clinical and Surgical Pitfalls
- Beware of the infrapatellar branch of the saphenous nerve during medial meniscal repairs. Entrapment of this nerve is possible during tying of the passed sutures. Such nerve entrapment is a possible cause of acute postoperative pain and formation of a neuroma.
- Beware of the peroneal nerve during lateral repairs. This nerve can be entrapped by meniscal sutures if the deep retractor is not placed deep to the gastrocnemius. Confirm that the retractor sits directly behind the capsule before suture passage. The posterior capsule should be directly visualized before sutures are tied laterally.
- Once the sutures have been passed, each suture should be sequentially tied (central to peripheral) with the leg in extension. This prevents tethering of the posterior capsule by the meniscal sutures and decreases the likelihood of a postoperative flexion contracture.

Numerous studies have confirmed the biomechanical importance of the meniscus and its relation to the development of early degenerative changes in the knee with its incompetency.[1-5] Thus meniscal repair is preferable to meniscectomy whenever feasible. Since the introduction of meniscus repair in 1885 by Annandale,[6] multiple repair techniques have been developed, both open and arthroscopic. The development of inside-out repair techniques and devices revolutionized the management of repairable meniscus tears, and use of such techniques and devices is currently the gold standard for meniscus repair. Such repair techniques are ideal for posterior meniscus tears and allow for the capture of multiple, longitudinally oriented collagen cables when a vertical suture technique is used. This chapter discusses the inside-out meniscus repair technique in detail.

PREOPERATIVE CONSIDERATIONS

History

A detailed history remains critical to the accurate diagnosis of a meniscus tear. The timing of injury and the exact mechanism, associated injuries, duration of symptoms, previous treatments, and exacerbating and alleviating factors are important points of discussion at the time of the initial visit.

Signs and Symptoms

The typical presentation of meniscal pathology includes the following:

- Acute noncontact twisting injury to the knee.
- Effusion that develops immediately after injury, as well as subsequent activity-related swelling.
- Mechanical symptoms, such as locking, catching, or clicking, may be present.
- Occasional episodes of giving way are often reported. Symptoms of instability are important to consider, especially when concomitant ligamentous injury is a concern.

Physical Examination

Typical physical examination findings of a meniscus tear include the following:

- Gait is usually normal, although there may be an antalgic gait if the presentation is acute or if a displaced or bucket-handle tear is present.
- Effusion is frequently present.
- Range of motion is usually limited if the patient is seen early with an effusion or with a displaced or bucket-handle tear. Often this will manifest as a loss of extension or a flexion contracture if chronic in nature. Range of motion may be normal if the patient is seen late or after an initial course of physical therapy.
- A positive "bounce home" test result (inability to tolerate full extension passively "bounced" from a flexed position) is present.
- Joint line tenderness is often noted.
- A positive McMurray test result may be present.
- Ligamentous stability is tested to assess for concomitant injury (e.g., Lachman, posterior drawer, and pivot-shift tests).
- Mild quadriceps atrophy may be present.

Imaging

Four plain radiographic views of the knee are typically obtained, including the following:

- Weight-bearing anteroposterior radiograph in full extension
- Weight-bearing posteroanterior 45-degree flexion radiograph (i.e., notch view)
- Non–weight-bearing 45-degree flexion lateral radiograph
- Patella sunrise radiograph

Magnetic resonance imaging (MRI) is often used in conjunction with plain radiographs to aid in the clinical diagnosis of meniscal pathology and to assess for other, associated injuries including anterior cruciate ligament (ACL) and posterior cruciate ligament (PCL) tears. The sensitivity of MRI for the detection of meniscus tears is reported to be as high as 96%, with a specificity of 97%.[7] MRI is helpful in depicting the following:

- Tear pattern, including a bucket-handle tear seen as a "double-PCL sign"
- Discoid meniscus
- Tear location
- Associated chondral injury

Indications and Contraindications

Indications for meniscus repair have remained constant throughout the evolution of repair techniques. The vascularity of the meniscus has been well described and remains critical to the treatment algorithm. Only the peripheral 10% to 30% of the meniscus is vascularized, supplied by the medial and lateral genicular arteries.[8] DeHaven classified tears in the peripheral 3 mm as vascular (referred to as the *red-red zone*), those more than 5 mm from the meniscocapsular junction as avascular *(white-white zone)*, and those in between as variable *(red-white zone)*.[9] Meniscus tears in the red-red zone have the best ability to heal because of the vascularity of the meniscus and thus are often repairable. However, reports have documented successful repair of tears in the avascular zone in young patients.[10,11] In addition, orientation of the tear must be considered. Typically, longitudinal vertical tears and bucket-handle tears are most amenable to repair. Degenerative tears or those with multiple horizontal cleavage planes are indications for partial meniscectomy.[12] Often, undersurface tears that are oblique in orientation extend from a vascular to an avascular zone and are problematic with regard to complete healing after repair. Patient compliance with the required rehabilitation course and initial limited weight-bearing status remain important for a successful outcome after meniscus repair. Finally, an intact ACL, whether reconstructed or native, has been shown to be critical to the success of the meniscus repair.[13]

SURGICAL TECHNIQUE

Anesthesia and Positioning

General, regional, or spinal anesthesia on the basis of the patient's, anesthesiologist's and surgeon's preferences is discussed preoperatively. The patient is placed supine on a standard operating room table, and a thigh tourniquet is applied. A leg holder or lateral post is applied depending on surgeon preference. If a leg holder is selected, the patient should be positioned with the knee distal to the break in the bed to allow full flexion of the knee when the table is dropped below 90 degrees from horizontal. This will also ensure circumferential access for the posterolateral or posteromedial approaches required for meniscal suturing. If a lateral post is selected, it should be placed at the level of the tourniquet and angled outwardly to allow for valgus force.

Surgical Landmarks, Incisions, and Portals

Important surgical landmarks include the following:

- Superior and inferior poles of the patella
- Medial and lateral edges of the patella tendon
- Tibial plateau
- Fibular head
- Medial and lateral joint line

Incisions and approaches include the following:

- Posterolateral approach
- Posteromedial approach

Typical portals used include the following:

- Anteromedial—the working portal for insertion of instruments; correct placement often varies depending on repair location
- Anterolateral—the viewing portal for insertion of the arthroscope, typically 1 cm lateral to the patella tendon and 1 cm proximal to the lateral joint line
- Outflow portal as needed (superolateral or superomedial)

Examination Under Anesthesia and Arthroscopic Examination

Examination under anesthesia before the start of the procedure is performed to evaluate range of motion and assess for ligamentous instability that may not be appreciated during an examination on an awake patient. A standard complete diagnostic arthroscopy is always performed before any meniscal pathologic process is addressed. Injuries to the chondral surfaces or intraarticular ligaments may need to be addressed in conjunction with the meniscal repair.

Specific Steps

The specific steps of this procedure are outlined in Box 53-1.

1. Diagnostic Arthroscopy

The patient is placed supine on the operating table, and a tourniquet is applied to the upper thigh. Arthroscopy

---

> **BOX 53-1** Specific Steps to Inside-Out Meniscus Repair
>
> 1. Diagnostic arthroscopy
> 2. Meniscal preparation
> 3. Planning of the incision
> 4. Exposure
> 5. Suture placement
> 6. Suture tying
> 7. Closure

is performed with a lateral post or a leg holder on the basis of the surgeon's preference. An initial inferolateral portal is made adjacent to the patellar tendon, and the arthroscope is inserted. Complete arthroscopy is performed to visualize the knee and to identify any associated concomitant pathology. Correct placement of the inferomedial portal is critical in addressing a meniscal tear. The location of the portal can be visualized directly by insertion of a spinal needle medial to the patellar tendon. The spinal needle should enter the medial compartment superior to the medial meniscus and parallel to the tibial plateau. The location of the portal needs to be tailored to the location of the tear. To have access to the posterior horn of the lateral meniscus, for example, the portal may need to be placed slightly more proximal and immediately adjacent to the patellar tendon for access to be gained above the tibial spine. An arthroscopic probe is then placed within the working portal, and the reparability of the meniscus tear is assessed.

2. Meniscal Preparation

The torn meniscus amenable to repair is prepared with a hand-held rasp or mechanical shaver to stimulate vascularity within the tear (Fig. 53-1). Trephination of the meniscus tear can also be completed, thought to create vascular channel formation. This is typically accomplished with a long 18-gauge needle, with care taken not to perforate the meniscal surface to avoid further injury.

3. Planning of the Incision

An arthroscopic probe may be pressed against the capsule at the junction of the middle and posterior portions of the meniscus to facilitate accurate placement of the posteromedial or posterolateral incision. The tip of the probe can usually be palpated at the posterior aspect of the joint line before an incision is made.

4. Exposure

Posteromedial

A vertical 3- to 4-cm incision is made posterior to the medial collateral ligament, extending one third above

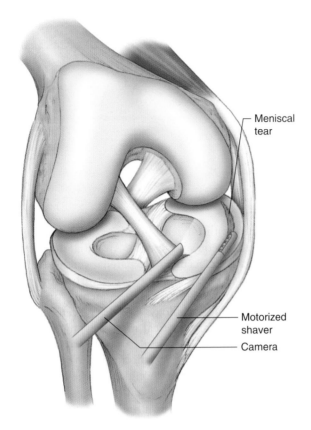

Figure 53-1. The meniscal tear is prepared with a motorized shaver to stimulate bleeding within the tear.

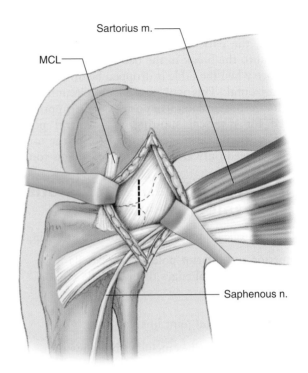

Figure 53-2. Posteromedial exposure. *m*, Muscle; *MCL*, medial collateral ligament; *n*, nerve.

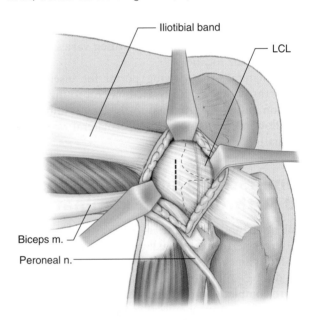

Figure 53-3. Posterolateral exposure. *m*, Muscle; *LCL*, lateral collateral ligament; *n*, nerve.

and two thirds below the joint line, with the knee flexed 60 to 90 degrees (Fig. 53-2). The incision is carried through the skin, and Metzenbaum scissors are used for subcutaneous dissection. The greater saphenous nerve lies posterior to the skin incision; thus a more posterior incision should be avoided. Dissection continues to the level of the sartorial fascia. The fascia is incised sharply with a scalpel at the superior and anterior margin of the sartorius, and the pes tendons are identified and retracted posteriorly. Blunt dissection is used to develop an interval created by the posteromedial capsule anteriorly, the semimembranosus inferiorly, and the medial head of the gastrocnemius posteriorly. A popliteal retractor is then placed within the interval for protection of the popliteal neurovascular structures.

Posterolateral

With the knee flexed 90 degrees, a vertical 3- to 4-cm incision is made over the posterolateral joint line, just posterior to the lateral collateral ligament (LCL), with one third of the incision above and two thirds below the joint line (Fig. 53-3). Flexion of the knee to 90 degrees allows the peroneal nerve, popliteus artery and inferior lateral geniculate artery to fall posteriorly. Dissection is carried through the skin, and Metzenbaum scissors are used to dissect the subcutaneous tissues. The interval between the iliotibial band and the biceps

femoris tendon is identified and sharply incised with a scalpel. Care must be taken to avoid injury to the inferior lateral genicular artery, which runs in this area. The biceps tendon is retracted posteriorly and serves to protect the peroneal nerve. Blunt dissection with the surgeon's finger allows direct palpation of the posterolateral capsule and the lateral head of the gastrocnemius. The lateral gastrocnemius is often more adherent to the posterolateral joint capsule than on the medial

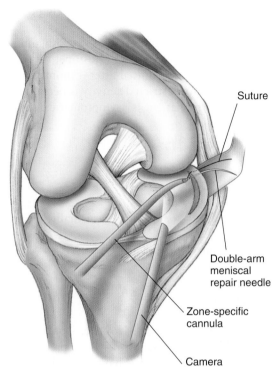

Figure 53-4. The remaining limb of the double-arm meniscal repair suture is passed to form a vertical mattress stitch.

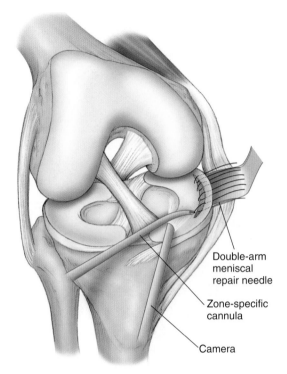

Figure 53-5. Sutures are placed from posterior to anterior at 3- to 5-mm intervals until the full extent of the tear has been addressed.

side. A popliteal retractor is placed at the posterior margin of the capsule and separates the posterolateral capsule medially from the lateral head of the gastrocnemius laterally. The remainder of the lateral meniscal repair is usually performed in the figure-of-four position.

5. Suture Placement

The meniscal body fragment is reduced with a probe in preparation for suture repair. Curved, zone-specific cannula systems are available, along with many other varieties of suture repair systems. The arthroscope remains in the ipsilateral portal for viewing; the contralateral portal is used for suture placement in the anterior and central horns of the meniscus during repair. Viewing and working portals may need to be switched for placement of posterior horn sutures. Suture placement begins at the posterior extent of the identified tear and gradually extends to the anterior margin. Double-arm meniscal repair needles are delivered into the joint and guided into position with the zone-specific cannula system. The curve of the cannula should be directed medially for a medial meniscus tear and laterally for a lateral meniscus tear to facilitate exit into the popliteal retractor. A single limb of the suture is initially passed through the meniscus above the tear and retrieved as it exits within the popliteal retractor. The remaining limb of the suture is placed in a similar manner, below the tear, to form a vertical mattress stitch (Fig. 53-4). The suture pair is

held with a clamp to facilitate suture management. Sutures are placed sequentially from posterior to anterior until the full extent of the tear has been addressed. Sutures are placed at 3- to 5-mm intervals (Fig. 53-5).

6. Suture Tying

The sutures are serially tied from posterior to anterior against the capsule, with care taken not to overtighten or to deform the meniscal body (Fig. 53-6). A fibrin clot may be placed within the meniscal tear, particularly for tears that extend to the avascular zone (e.g., complete radial tear in a young patient), before the sutures are tied. The knee is taken through a full range of motion and visualized for gap formation or suture breakage.

7. Closure

The arthroscopic portals are closed in the standard fashion, and the accessory wound is closed in layers with suture material according to surgeon preference.

POSTOPERATIVE CONSIDERATIONS

Rehabilitation

- Immediate toe-touch weight bearing is allowed in a hinged knee brace with range of motion limited to 0 to 90 degrees of flexion.

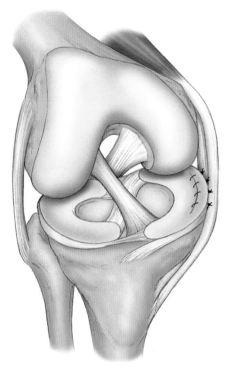

Figure 53-6. Sutures are tied from posterior to anterior over the joint capsule to complete the repair.

- Straight-leg raises are begun immediately postoperatively.
- Full weight bearing and gradual strengthening exercises are instituted at 6 weeks postoperatively.
- In-line running is permitted after 4 months.
- Return to full, unrestricted activity is permitted after 6 months if the patient is asymptomatic.

Complications

- Infection
- Arthrofibrosis
- Failure of meniscus to heal
- Nerve injury (saphenous medially, peroneal laterally)
- Vascular injury (popliteal fossa)
- Chondral injury

RESULTS

After meniscal repair, good to excellent results can be expected in approximately 85% of patients (Table 53-1). Inside-out techniques have also demonstrated good results on second-look arthroscopy.[15,17] A recent systematic review comparing inside-out and all-inside

TABLE 53-1. Results of Inside-out Meniscal Repair

Study	No. of Repairs	Criteria	Follow-up	Concomitant ACL Tear	Results
Johnson et al[14] (1999)	38	Clinical	10 years, 9 months (average)	None	76% successful
Cannon and Vittori[15] (1992)	90	Arthroscopy or arthrography	7 months (mean): isolated repairs 10 months (mean): concurrent ACL reconstructions	68 ACL tears (76%) All reconstructed	93% success with ACL reconstruction 50% success of isolated repair
Miller[16] (1988)	79	Arthroscopy or arthrography	3.25 years (mean)	68 reconstructions 22 stable ACLs	93% healed with ACL reconstruction 84% healed with isolated meniscal repair
Tenuta and Arciero[17] (1994)	54	Clinical and arthroscopy	11 months (mean)	40 reconstructions 14 stable ACLs	Arthroscopy: 90% healed with ACL reconstruction 57% healed with isolated meniscal repair Better with rim width <4 mm, age below 30 years
Rubman et al[18] (1998)	198	Clinical with or without arthroscopy	Clinical examination: 42 months (23-116) 180 meniscal repairs (91%) in 160 patients Arthroscopy: 18 months (2-81) 91 meniscal repairs (46%) in 79 patients	128 ACL tears (72%) 126 reconstructed 96 concurrent 30 delayed	80% asymptomatic (clinically) 20% (39) repeated arthroscopy for symptoms 2 (5%) healed 13 (33%) partially healed 24 (62%) failed Arthroscopy (91 repairs) 23 (25%) completely healed 35 (38%) partially healed 33 (36%) failed

Continued

TABLE 53-1 Results of Inside-out Meniscal Repair—cont'd

Study	No. of Repairs	Criteria	Follow-up	Concomitant ACL Tear	Results
Eggli et al[19] (1995)	54	Clinical with or without magnetic resonance imaging	7.5 years (average)	None	73% success 64% of failures in first 6 months Better with acute injury (<8 weeks), age younger than 30 years, tear length <2.5 cm Worse with rim width >3 mm, absorbable sutures
Albrecht-Olsen and Bak[20] (1993)	27	3 clinical	3 years (median)	None	63% success

ACL, Anterior cruciate ligament.

repair techniques demonstrated a clinical failure rate of 17% for inside-out techniques.[19] Results are best for traumatic vertical tears in young patients who undergo concomitant ACL reconstruction. However, excellent results have also been reported for isolated meniscal repairs, as well as for complex tears extending to the avascular portion of the meniscus.

REFERENCES

1. Alford JW, Lewis P, Kang RW, et al. Rapid progression of chondral disease in the lateral compartment of the knee following meniscectomy. *Arthroscopy.* 2005;21:1505-1509.
2. Allen PR, Denham RA, Swan AV. Late degenerative changes after meniscectomy: Factors affecting the knee after operation. *J Bone Joint Surg.* 1984;66:666-671.
3. Fairbank TJ. Knee joint changes after meniscectomy. *J Bone Joint Surg Br.* 1948;30:664-670.
4. Fithian DC, Kelly MA, Mow VC. Material properties and structure-function relationship in the menisci. *Clin Orthop Relat Res.* 1990;252:19-31.
5. Levy IM, Torzilli PA, Warren RF. The effect of medial meniscectomy on anterior-posterior motion of the knee. *J Bone Joint Surg Am.* 1982;64:883-888.
6. Annandale T. An operation for displaced semilunar cartilage. *Br Med J.* 1885;1:779.
7. Magee T, Williams W. 3.0-T MRI of meniscal tears. *Am J Radiol.* 2006;187:371-375.
8. Arnoczky SP, Warren RF. The microvasculature of the human meniscus. *Am J Sports Med.* 1982;10:90-95.
9. DeHaven KE. Decision-making features in the treatment of meniscal lesions. *Clin Orthop Relat Res.* 1990;252:49-54.
10. Noyes FR, Barber-Westin SD. Arthroscopic repair of meniscal tears extending into the avascular zone in patients younger than twenty years of age. *Am J Sports Med.* 2002;30:589-600.
11. Rubman MH, Noyes FR, Barber-Westin SD. Arthroscopic repair of meniscal tears that extend into the avascular zone: a review of 198 single and complex tears. *Am J Sports Med.* 1998;26:87-95.
12. Schmitz MA, Rouse Jr LM, DeHaven KE. The management of meniscal tears in the ACL-deficient knee. *Clin Sports Med.* 1996;15:573-593.
13. Hanks GA, Gause TM, Handal JA, et al. Meniscus repair in the anterior cruciate deficient knee. *Am J Sports Med.* 1990;18:606-611.
14. Grant JA, Wilde J, Miller BS, et al. Comparison of inside-out and all-inside techniques for the repair of isolated meniscal tears: A systemic review. *Am J Sports Med.* 2011.
15. Cannon WD, Vittori, JM. The incidence of healing in arthroscopic meniscal repairs in anterior cruciate ligament-reconstructed knees versus stable knees. *Am J Sports Med.* 1992;20:176-181.
16. Tenuta JJ, Arciero RA. Arthroscopic evaluation of meniscal repairs. Factors that affect healing. *Am J Sports Med.* 1994;22:797-802.
17. Tenuta JJ, Arciero RA. Arthroscopic evaluation of meniscal repairs. Factors that affect healing. *Am J Sports Med.* 1994;22:797-802.
18. Rubman MH, Noyes FR, Barber-Westin SD. Arthroscopic repair of meniscal tears that extend into the avascular zone: a review of 198 single and complex tears. *Am J Sports Med.* 1998;26:87-95.
19. Eggli S, Wegmuller H, Kosina J, et al. Long-term results of arthroscopic meniscal repair: an analysis of isolated tears. *Am J Sports Med.* 1995;23:715-720.
20. Albrecht-Olsen PM, Bak K. Arthroscopic repair of the bucket-handle meniscus: 10 failures in 27 stable knees followed for 3 years. *Acta Orthop Scand.* 1993;64:446-448.

Chapter 54

Arthroscopic Meniscus Repair: Outside-in Technique

Marc Korn, Asheesh Bedi, and Answorth A. Allen

Chapter Synopsis
- In attempting meniscal repair, the outside-in technique is a successful arthroscopic approach that has gained popularity for reparable lesions of the anterior horn and body. Owing to the importance of the meniscus in proper function of the knee, a detailed understanding of this surgical option is essential. This chapter provides important clinical and surgical details that should be considered in addressing a meniscal tear with the outside-in technique.

Important Points
- Ideal candidate—Young, compliant patient with short history of pain.
- Ideal tear—Vertical, longitudinal tear in red-red zone of the anterior horn or body of the meniscus
- Contraindications—Older patients with unstable or anterior cruciate ligament (ACL)–deficient knee, horizontal cleavage tears, partial-thickness tears, stable tears, white-white zone tears, osteoarthritic changes, posterior horn and root injury.
- Classification—Arthroscopic surgical technique for addressing meniscal tears.
- Symptoms—Often occur after a traumatic event of the knee; include locking or catching of the knee, effusion, focal tenderness, pain during deep flexion and meniscal compression.
- Surgical technique—Anesthesia determined by patient and anesthesiologist. Leg position should allow for access to posteromedial and posterolateral corners of

knee, and position will be modified depending on target region of meniscus.

Clinical and Surgical Pearls
- Proper counseling is essential to ensure compliance and proper rehabilitation.
- Abrasion of the meniscal surface and adjacent synovium is recommended.
- Abrasion notchplasty and microfractures in the notch can provide access to marrow-derived mesenchymal cells to augment healing of isolated meniscal repairs.
- Vertically oriented sutures allow for improved biomechanical strength of the repair construct.
- Fibrin clots can function as scaffold and also serve as a source of chemotactic and mitogenic stimuli.

Clinical and Surgical Pitfalls
- Tears in the posterior horn of the medial meniscus are difficult to repair with the outside-in technique without considerable risk of neurovascular injury.
- The peroneal nerve is at risk with lateral meniscus repair; stay anterior to the biceps tendon to avoid damage.
- The saphenous nerve is at risk with medial meniscus repair; stay anterior to the sartorius fascia.
- Compliance with a protected rehabilitation program and restriction of terminal flexion in the early postoperative period may be critical to favorably influence healing after surgical repair.

The menisci are of paramount importance to knee function and play critical roles in load transmission, shock absorption, secondary knee stabilization, and joint lubrication. Numerous studies have established the unfavorable natural history and progression to osteoarthritis associated with removal of meniscal tissue, resulting in decreased femoral contact area and significant increases in contact stresses and chondral overload.[1,2] Therefore meniscus preservation in the young, prearthritic knee should be prioritized for all tears with patterns, tissue quality, and vascularity that are amenable to repair.

The evolution and advancement of arthroscopic surgical techniques have improved the ability to access and repair meniscal lesions. The outside-in technique was first described by Warren as an alternative method to decrease the risk of neurovascular injury with repair.[3] Whereas inside-out and all-inside techniques have evolved for meniscal repair and are particularly useful to address posterior horn lesions, the outside-in technique is a powerful and invaluable approach for repairable tears of the body and anterior horn. It is also useful to repair the anterior extension of bucket-handle tears or meniscus transplants.

PREOPERATIVE CONSIDERATIONS

A meniscal tear is one of the most common orthopedic injuries, often resulting from a traumatic event such as forceful twisting or pivoting (resulting in a "popping sensation"). Patients often report swelling and localized pain in the knee on the side of the tear. Depending on the size of the tear, patients will have varying ability to bear weight on the affected side. Patients may also report locking or catching of the knee, which is most likely caused by entrapment of the meniscus in the notch or between articular surfaces.[4]

Typical examination findings of a meniscus tear include the following:

- Effusion
- Quadriceps weakness and atrophy
- Focal joint-line tenderness
- Pain with terminal flexion (posterior horn) and/or extension (anterior horn)
- Locked knee (bucket-handle tears)
- Pain with provocative maneuvers such as the Apley grind or McMurray test, in which an axial load and twisting moment are applied to the knee to precipitate symptoms from a meniscal lesion

These physical examination findings are sensitive but not specific for meniscal pathology. Chondral injury, subchondral fractures, bone contusions, collateral ligament injury, or symptomatic plicas of the knee may cause an overlapping constellation of examination findings. It is also critical to assess the knee for stability of the cruciate ligaments, collateral ligaments, and posterolateral complex. Although meniscal injuries can occur in isolation, they are frequently accompanied by ligamentous injury. Concomitant anterior cruciate ligament (ACL) reconstruction is favorable in the setting of combined ACL and meniscal injury and has been shown to improve the rates of successful healing after meniscal repair.[5]

The diagnosis of a meniscus tear based on history and physical examination is often confirmed with imaging modalities. Plain radiographs, including anteroposterior (AP), posteroanterior flexion weight-bearing, and lateral radiographs are obtained to assess for occult fractures and osteoarthritic changes. Hip-to-ankle, standing long-leg radiographs may be critical to evaluate meniscus tears in the setting of malalignment. In these situations, restoration of normal alignment is of tantamount importance to treatment of the meniscus tear for favorable long-term outcomes and healing. Magnetic resonance imaging, with meniscus-specific sequences, can be confirmatory of the diagnosis. Important findings may include the following:

- Recognition of the meniscus tear, location, and pattern. The peripheral third of the meniscus ("red-red") zone offers the greatest vascularity and the most favorable prognosis for healing after a repair. Recognition of pattern is also critical, because vertical, longitudinal tears may be more amenable to repair, whereas radial, complex, and horizontal cleavage tears are often treated more effectively with partial meniscectomy. This preoperative information allows for more effective counseling with the patient regarding intraoperative expectations, postoperative rehabilitation, and the natural history of the injury.
- Associated chondral injury or bone contusion. Focal chondral defects may mimic meniscal pathology or be present in combination with a meniscus tear and may be treated simultaneously with a marrow stimulation (microfracture) or whole-tissue transplantation procedure. In contrast, diffuse chondral degeneration may be a relative contraindication to surgical intervention and may compromise the outcomes of surgical treatment of meniscal injury.
- Integrity of the cruciate, collateral, posterolateral corner ligament complexes.

The outside-in repair is an ideal choice for a young, compliant patient with a meniscal injury in the absence of significant chondral degeneration. Favorable prognostic factors and indications for an outside-in repair include the following:

- Peripheral "red-red" or "red-white" zone tears
- Longitudinal ("vertical") tear pattern
- Tears of the body or anterior horn that are accessible via an outside-in trajectory without significant risk of neurovascular injury
- Bucket-handle meniscus tears with anterior horn extension
- Acute injury with reducible tear pattern
- Associated ACL reconstruction

Relative contraindications to meniscal repair with an outside-in technique include the following:

- Diffuse chondral degeneration or injury
- Irreparable, complex tear patterns
- Chronic tears with compromised tissue quality for suture fixation
- Posterior horn or root injuries with significant risk for neurovascular injury with an outside-in approach
- Tears in the central "red-white" or "white-white" zones
- An unstable knee with cruciate, collateral, or posterolateral corner insufficiency

SURGICAL TECHNIQUE

Patient Education

Patient education and counseling are essential before surgical treatment of any meniscal tear. The appropriate treatment must be individualized and is a function of tear pattern, chronicity, associated knee injuries, and patient goals and expectations. Full understanding of and compliance with the protected rehabilitation after meniscal repair are also necessary for a favorable outcome to be achieved, even in the setting of a robust repair construct. The natural history of a failed meniscus repair or meniscectomy should also be reviewed.

Anesthesia

The choice of anesthesia is typically made based on discussion between the anesthesiologist and the patient. Spinal anesthesia is very effective for arthroscopy and meniscal repair in the outpatient surgical setting. Although femoral nerve blocks can be used, they can delay rehabilitation and a complete return of quadriceps function.

Surgical Steps

The surgical steps for this procedure are outlined in Box 54-1.

An examination under anesthesia of the involved and contralateral knee is performed to assess for

---

BOX 54-1 Surgical Steps: Arthroscopic Meniscus Tear

1. Perform examination under anesthesia.
2. Determine pattern and extent of meniscal tear.
3. Rasp and debride edges and synovium.
4. Introduce spinal needle into joint.
5. Incise around the needle.
6. Introduce second needle through same incision.
7. Place sutures, alternating between tibial and femoral surfaces of meniscus.

---

effusion, range of motion, and ligamentous stability. The patient's leg should be positioned with the distal thigh extended over the break in the table, and the leg holder should be positioned proximally to allow access to the posterior knee. An unsterile tourniquet is often applied but may be variably inflated during the surgical procedure to control bleeding. An arthroscope is then inserted into the knee through an anterolateral portal for performance of a complete diagnostic examination of the knee, including an assessment of chondral and meniscal status in both compartments. The medial and lateral meniscus should be carefully inspected and probed throughout the superior and inferior surfaces to assess for unstable partial-thickness or full-thickness injury. In varus knees with difficult access or visualization, the deep MCL may be carefully released or fenestrated to improve the inspection. The meniscal roots should also be directly visualized in the posteromedial and posterolateral recesses to assess for occult injury or insufficiency warranting repair.

If a meniscus tear is identified, the pattern and extent of the lesion are defined. Outside-in repairs may be most useful in the management of anterior body and anterior horn tears that cannot be safely accessed with the trajectory of an inside-out cannula or all-inside device. Reparable lesions that are unstable or evertable in these locations and in the red-white zone or red-red zone should be repaired. Care must be taken to protect the saphenous nerve and its associated branches with spinal needle passage and skin incisions along the medial joint line. Correspondingly, needle passage and dissection must be avoided posterior to the biceps tendon laterally to minimize risk to the peroneal nerve. The tear edges are debrided and rasped, as is the adjacent synovium at the meniscocapsular junction. Under direct arthroscopic visualization, a spinal needle (18 gauge) is placed into the joint and penetrates the inner portion of the superior or inferior meniscal surface (Fig. 54-1). The needle should avoid the inner rim, because this thin region is avascular and likely to tear under tension. After the needle has penetrated the meniscus, a superficial incision is made around the needle and subcutaneous tissue is spread down to the capsule with a hemostat (Fig. 54-2). Nerves, veins, and tendons should also be cleared. A second needle is inserted through the same incision, into an adjacent part of the meniscus (Fig. 54-3). Ideally, the position of the second needle should allow for the vertical mattress configuration of the suture. Though other suture orientations have been used successfully, studies have demonstrated that vertical mattress sutures allow the least residual displacement and the highest strength by wrapping perpendicular to circumferential collagen bundles.[6] Suture placement should alternate between tibial and femoral surfaces of the meniscus to ensure approximation in the capsule.

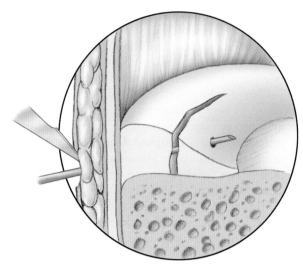

Figure 54-1. Once you are satisfied with needle position, make a small skin incision.

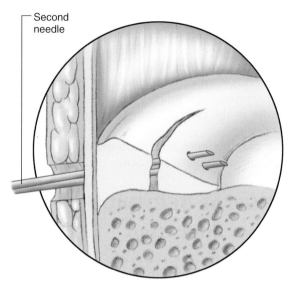

Figure 54-3. A second needle is introduced through the skin incision and across the tear.

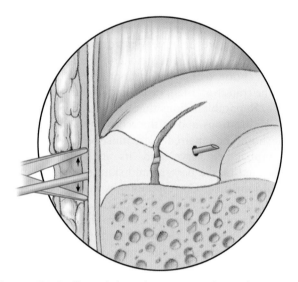

Figure 54-2. Spread the subcutaneous tissue down to the capsule by use of a hemostat.

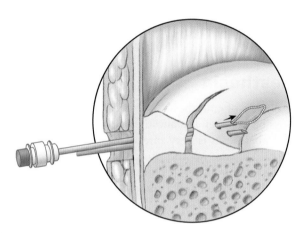

Figure 54-4. Pass the cable loop through one needle.

Suturing Options

Sutures are secured with a variety of possible techniques. The cable loop pull-through technique requires passage of a cable loop through the spinal needles.[7] The absorbable suture is pushed through the anterior portal and threaded through the cable loop. The loop is then withdrawn and the suture is pulled through the meniscus. It is important to pull the needle and cable loop together to avoid suture entrapment and breakage in the spinal needle. The other end of the suture is then threaded through a cable loop in the other needle. The cable loop and the needle are withdrawn from the meniscus together (Figs. 54-4 to 54-8). After both ends of the suture have been threaded through the meniscus, the needles are withdrawn and the suture ends are tied together over the capsule.

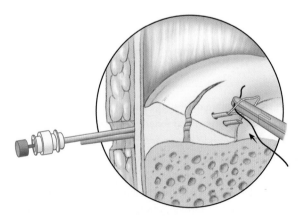

Figure 54-5. Place an absorbable suture with the grasper through the anterior portal into the wire loop.

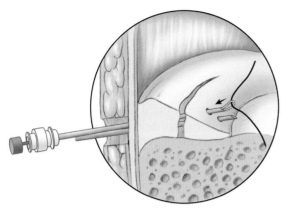

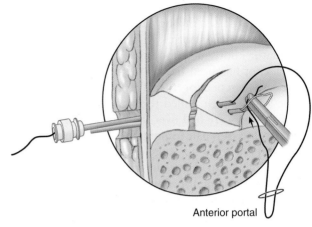

Figure 54-6. The cable loop is withdrawn out the needle with the suture.

Anterior portal

Figure 54-7. The procedure is repeated for the second needle, feeding the other end of the suture through the cable loop.

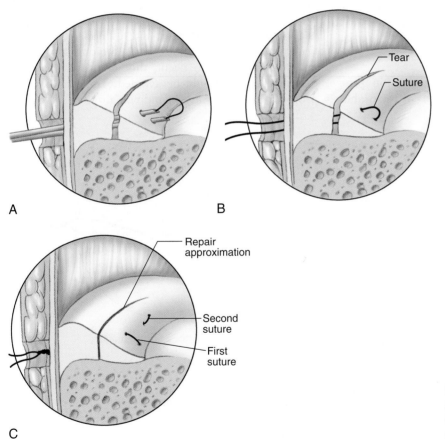

A

B

Tear
Suture

Repair approximation

Second suture

First suture

C

Figure 54-8. A and **B,** Both needles are withdrawn from the incision. **C,** The single suture is tied down subcutaneously over the capsule.

In the cable loop capture technique, a suture is placed through one of the needles. The cable loop is then used in the other needle to pull the free end of the suture back through. It may sometimes be necessary to assist guidance of the free end of the suture into the cable loop with a probe or grasper in the medial or lateral portals. Once again, the needles are withdrawn and the ends are secured over the capsule (Fig. 54-9).[8]

In the Mulberry knot technique, two sutures are used (one for each needle) and then fastened together. The first suture is passed through the spinal needle and pulled through the anterior portal. The process is repeated for the second suture. A knot (three or four throws) is then tied at the end of each suture. Once the two knots are in place internally, the two sutures are tied together over the capsule (Fig. 54-10).[9]

The dilator knot technique also requires two sutures. Each suture is passed through a spinal needle and pulled through the anterior portal. At this point a small knot, the "dilator knot," is tied on one suture (two throws). After a knot has been tied in the first suture, the two sutures are then tied together. The suture containing the dilator knot is then pulled through the meniscus, and the two sutures are tied over the capsule (Fig. 54-11).[8]

Regardless of repair technique, it has been the senior authors' preference to augment healing of isolated outside-in meniscal repairs in the red-red or red-white zones. This is accomplished with fibrin clot and/or abrasion notchplasty or microfracture of the notch. We also commonly replace the monofilament suture by shuttling in exchange for a nonabsorbable suture, which may offer greater biomechanical strength and tensioning during knot fixation.

POSTOPERATIVE CONSIDERATIONS

Rehabilitation

Compliance with a postoperative rehabilitation protocol is critical to maximize chances of favorable healing after outside-in meniscal repair. Studies have demonstrated that prolonged immobilization can lead to decreased collagen content in the recovering meniscus.[10] As a result, compliance with a methodic and incremental regimen is important for patients. Immediately after the procedure, weight bearing should be limited and the patient fitted for a double upright hinge brace. During the first few postoperative days, the patient should focus on effusion control, quadriceps strengthening, and ankle pump exercises. With improving quadriceps strength and control, progressive weight bearing is permitted. For the first 3 to 4 weeks, full weight bearing is allowed with the brace locked in full extension. If the patient is recovering from a radial or complex horizontal tear pattern, only toe-touch weight bearing is recommended during the first 3 weeks. During the first 4 weeks, flexion is limited to 90 degrees to minimize shear forces and displacement with terminal flexion. Full motion and weight bearing without the brace are typically permissible at 4 to 6 weeks. Running is allowed at 3 to 4 months, and full athletic participation can begin at 5 to 6 months. At 6 months, squatting and hyperflexion can occur, though up to this point extreme flexion should be avoided. The rehabilitation protocol, however, must be individualized based on tear

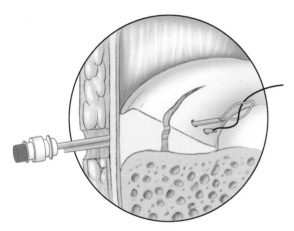

Figure 54-9. The cable loop capture technique.

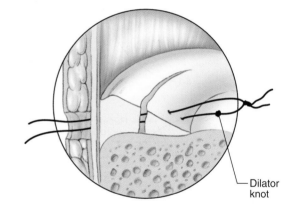

Dilator knot

Figure 54-11. The dilator knot technique.

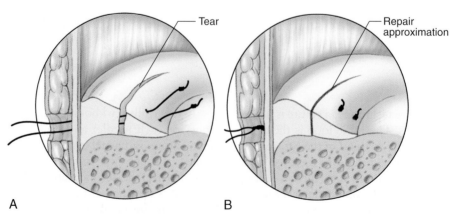

Tear

Repair approximation

A   B

Figure 54-10. The Mulberry knot technique.

pattern, severity, repair quality, and functional demands of the patient.

Complications

Patients should be informed of the potential for neurovascular injury and loss of motion as a result of outside-in meniscal repair. The peroneal nerve is at risk during repairs of the lateral meniscus, and the saphenous nerve is at risk during medial repairs. However, transillumination, proper orientation of the knee, attentive needle placement, and careful blunt dissection down to the capsule before sutures are tied can minimize the risk of these injuries. Vascular injury is more likely in tears of the far posterior horn of the meniscus and is a relative contraindication to the outside-in technique.[11] These posterior lesions are better approached with an inside-out repair with posteromedial or posterolateral safety incisions. The meniscal repair may fail owing to reinjury, inadequate protection of the repair, poor indication, occult instability of the knee, or poor surgical technique.[12] Competitive athletes in unique sports such as wrestling, with high demands of deep flexion and twisting, may also have retears with return to high-level sports, despite a favorable repair construct and tear pattern.[13] Patients with locked bucket-handle repairs and concurrent ACL reconstructions have been found to be at higher risk for loss of motion postoperatively.[14]

RESULTS

Hantes and associates[15] compared outside-in, inside-out, and all-inside techniques with clinical evaluations in a recent study. In randomly determined meniscal repairs of 57 patients, 17 were performed with the outside-in technique (group A), 20 with the inside-out technique (group B), and 20 with all-inside procedures (group C). Researchers followed up with the patients and evaluated their condition based on several clinical criteria (joint-line tenderness, locking, swelling, and McMurray test result). According to these examinations, 100% of group A repairs were considered healed, 95% of group B repairs were considered healed, and 65% of group C repairs were considered healed. For groups A, B, and C, the average follow-up times were 23 months, 22 months, and 22 months, respectively. Hantes and colleagues also evaluated the time required for meniscal repair with each of the three techniques. The outside-in technique averaged 38.5 minutes, the inside-out technique averaged 18.1 minutes, and the all-inside technique averaged 13.6 minutes.[15]

Though many studies look at clinical symptoms to classify healing, other studies have implemented second-look arthroscopy to verify that complete healing has occurred. In many cases a patient can be asymptomatic

TABLE 54-1. Outside-in Meniscus Repair Results

Study	No. of Patients	Follow-up	Outcome
Morgan et al[17] (1991)	74	2 months to 4 years	84% asymptomatic (62/74) 65% complete healing (48/74) 19% complete healing (14/74) 16% failed (12/74)
van Trommel et al[16] (1998)	51	3-80 months	45% complete healing (23/51) 31% partial healing (16/51) 24% no healing (12/51)
Hantes et al[15] (2006)	20	Mean, 23 months	100% healed (20/20)

despite the fact that the meniscus is incompletely healed.[16] A study by Morgan and colleagues[17] followed up on 74 patients of an earlier study with second-look arthroscopy to visualize meniscal healing. The time between repair and second look ranged from 2 months to 4 years, with an average of 8.5 months. Eighty-four percent of patients were asymptomatic at their follow-up evaluation (65% completely healed, 19% incompletely healed). Sixteen percent of the patients (12) had failed surgeries. Eleven of the 12 failures occurred after repair of the posterior horn of the medial meniscus, and all 12 failures occurred in patients with concurrent ACL injury. The study also revealed that 3 to 4 months were required for complete fibroblastic repair and disappearance of the absorbable sutures.[17] The more recent findings of van Trommel and co-workers[16] evaluated the outside-in technique in meniscal repairs in different regions of the medial and lateral meniscus, with follow-up ranging from 3 to 80 months. In all 15 partially healed patients with tears extending from the posterior to the middle third of the meniscus, the posterior third was always the unhealed portion.[16] The findings reinforced the belief that the outside-in technique is an effective treatment for lateral meniscus tears as well as anterior and middle tears of the medial meniscus. The aforementioned techniques (inside-out, all-inside) are preferred for posterior tears of the medial meniscus. These three studies are summarized in Table 54-1.

REFERENCES

1. Fukubayashi T, Kurosawa H. The contact area and pressure distribution pattern of the knee. A study of normal and osteoarthrotic knee joints. *Acta Orthop Scand.* 1980; 51(6):871-879.

2. Kettelkamp DB, Jacobs AW. Tibiofemoral contact area—determination and implications. *J Bone Joint Surg Am.* 1972;54(2):349-356.

3. Warren RF. Arthroscopic meniscus repair. *Arthroscopy.* 1985;1:170-172.

4. Bedi A, Feeley BT, Williams RJ 3rd. Management of articular cartilage defects of the knee. *J Bone Joint Surg Am.* 2010;92:994-1009.

5. Melton JT, Murray JR, Karim A, et al. Meniscal repair in anterior cruciate ligament reconstruction: a long-term outcome study. *Knee Surg Sports Traumatol Arthrosc.* 2011;19(10):1729-1734.

6. Rankin CC, Lintner DM, Noble PC, et al. A biomechanical analysis of meniscal repair techniques. *Am J Sports Med.* 2002;30:492-497.

7. Johnson LL. Meniscus repair: the outside-in technique. In: Jackson DW, ed. *Reconstructive Knee Surgery. Master Techniques in Orthopaedic Surgery.* Philadelphia: Lippincott Williams & Wilkins; 2003:39.

8. Cooper DE. Arthroscopic meniscus repair: outside-in technique. *Oper Tech Sports Med.* 1994;2(3):190-200.

9. Warren RF. Chronic anterior cruciate ligament injury. In: Parisien JS, ed. *Arthroscopic Surgery.* New York: McGraw-Hill; 1988:130.

10. Dowdy PA, Miniaci A, Arnoczky SP, et al. The effect of cast immobilization on meniscal healing. An experimental study in the dog. *Am J Sports Med.* 1995;23:721-728.

11. Bernard M, Grothues-Spork M, Georgoulis A, et al. Neural and vascular complications of arthroscopic meniscal surgery. *Knee Surg Sports Traumatol Arthrosc.* 1994;2(1):14-18.

12. Cohen SB, Anderson MW, Miller MD. Chondral injury after arthroscopic meniscal repair using bioabsorbable Mitek Rapidloc meniscal fixation. *Arthroscopy.* 2003;19:E24-E26.

13. Logan M, Watts M, Owen J, et al. Meniscal repair in the elite athlete: results of 45 repairs with a minimum 5-year follow-up. *Am J Sports Med.* 2009;37:1131-1134.

14. Shelbourne KD, Johnson GE. Locked bucket-handle meniscal tears in knees with chronic anterior cruciate ligament deficiency. *Am J Sports Med.* 1993;21:779-782; discussion 782.

15. Hantes ME, Zachos VC, Varitimidis SE, et al. Arthroscopic meniscal repair: a comparative study between three different surgical techniques. *Knee Surg Sports Traumatol Arthrosc.* 2006;14(12):1232-1237.

16. van Trommel MF, Simonian PT, Potter HG, et al. Different regional healing rates with the outside-in technique for meniscal repair. *Am J Sports Med.* 1998;26(3):446-452.

17. Morgan CD, Wojtys EM, Casscells CD, et al. Arthroscopic meniscal repair evaluated by second-look arthroscopy. *Am J Sports Med.* 1991;19(6):632-637; discussion 637-638.

Chapter 55

Arthroscopic Meniscus Repair: All-Inside Technique

Marc S. Haro, Jeffrey M. Tuman, and David Diduch

Chapter Synopsis

- All-inside meniscal repair offers many advantages over traditional inside-out or outside-in meniscal repairs. Benefits include decreased operative times, avoidance of the risks associated with secondary incisions, and ease of use of the implants. Implant designs have evolved since their introduction; this has allowed for safe, reliable all-inside meniscal repairs with results that compare favorably with those of more traditional open methods.

Important Points

- Need to identify meniscal tears that are amenable to repair
- Need to be familiar with the specific features of each device used for all-inside meniscal repair including possible suture configuration, deployment mechanism, tensioning method, and location of knots and backstops

Clinical and Surgical Pearls

- Use a portal that affords the most perpendicular approach to the tear.

- Change portals as necessary.
- Vertical mattress suture configurations are optimal for strength and healing.
- Leave suture attached to implants until all implants are in, to allow repeated tensioning.
- Newer, suture-based fourth-generation devices offer definite advantages over previous devices, including adjustable tension, lower profile, and lower chondral risk.

Clinical and Surgical Pitfalls

- Do not attempt all-inside repairs on tears at the meniscocapsular junction or tears that affect the anterior horn.
- Know the specifics of each device, including deployment mechanism, possible configurations of suture placement, and type and location of implants to prevent device misfire or breakage or injury to patient.

Morgan first described all-inside meniscal repair in 1991[1] when he used curved suture hooks and accessory posterior portals. Although these initial results demonstrated that all-inside meniscal repairs could be highly successful, they were technically difficult and required accessory incisions. Since this initial description, there has been a significant evolution with regard to surgical techniques and implant designs.

There are many advantages of an all-inside meniscal repair compared with the more traditional open procedures, including the avoidance of secondary incisions and their associated risks, decreased operative times, and the technical ease of insertion. However, to be considered successful, an all-inside meniscal repair must be able to restore the normal anatomy and must have outcomes that compare favorably with those of the more traditional and current gold standard inside-out meniscal repair technique.

In this chapter we briefly describe the evolution of the all-inside meniscal repair and more specifically concentrate on the surgical techniques and implants associated with the latest fourth-generation devices. We specifically describe the FasT-Fix (Smith & Nephew, Andover, MA), the RapidLoc (DePuy Mitek, Raynham, MA), the Omnispan (DePuy Mitek), and the new Sequent device (ConMed Linvatec, Largo, FL). We also briefly describe the Meniscal Cinch (Arthrex, Naples, FL), MaxFire MarXmen (Biomet, Warsaw,

IN), and CrossFix (Cayenne Medical, Scottsdale, AZ) devices.

PREOPERATIVE CONSIDERATIONS

History

Meniscal injury commonly occurs with a twisting injury to the knee and at times is seen in conjunction with a ligamentous knee injury. Frequently there are joint line tenderness and mechanical symptoms that include catching, locking, and giving way. Swelling typically occurs overnight in the acute setting and on an intermittent, activity-related basis with a chronic tear.

Physical Examination

- Perform full knee evaluation bilaterally.
- Rule out any hip, pelvic, or back disease that may be contributing to "knee" pain.
- Key examination elements for meniscal tears include:
  - Presence of an effusion
  - Extension deficit (which may indicate a locked meniscal fragment)
  - Joint line tenderness
  - Positive results of McMurray test and Apley test

Imaging

Radiography

Plain radiographs are helpful in assessing for gonarthrosis as well as limb alignment.

- Standing anteroposterior and posteroanterior flexed views
- Lateral and sunrise views

Other Imaging Modalities

Magnetic resonance imaging can be more than 96% accurate in identifying meniscal lesions and may be used to help confirm their presence.[2] However, it has not yet been shown to be helpful in predicting whether a tear is reparable.[3] The decision for repair versus partial resection usually requires arthroscopic assessment.

Indications

Many factors play a role in meniscal treatment decision making:

- Age of the patient
- Presence of meniscal degeneration, tear size, tear pattern, and vascularity
- Associated knee instability
- Chronicity of the tear
- Integrity of the meniscal body

Longitudinal, peripheral (vascular) tears in the red-red or red-white zones are the most amenable to repair. If there is ligamentous instability, it should be addressed at the time of meniscus repair, if possible, or in the near future if the procedure must be staged. As with other forms of repair, the all-inside technique yields better results with acute, traumatic tears and in those knees undergoing concomitant anterior cruciate ligament (ACL) reconstruction.[4] Tears that are stable with less than 3 mm of displacement with probing and that are less than 1 cm in length can be left in situ with predictable results.

Contraindications

Relative contraindications to an all-inside repair include the following:

- The anterior horn may not be accessible through anterior portals with any of the available all-inside devices.
- There must be a meniscal rim intact for the anchoring mechanisms of these devices to work appropriately. Hence, meniscocapsular separations are not suited for all-inside repair devices.
- Degenerative tears that have poor potential for healing may be unsuitable.

These situations may be better served with a suture technique, such as the inside-out or outside-in technique, or in the case of degenerative tears, a partial meniscectomy.

SURGICAL TECHNIQUE

Setup and Positioning

For knee arthroscopy with meniscal repair, one may use a lateral post or a leg holder. The patient is placed supine. A tourniquet of the appropriate size is placed high on the thigh according to surgeon preference. When a lateral post is to be used, the leg of the bed need not be broken, although it may improve posterior access. With a leg holder, it is important to position the patient far enough down the bed to allow adequate knee flexion for the operation.

After standard arthroscopic portals have been established, a complete diagnostic knee arthroscopy is performed. Meniscal pathology is identified, and if it is amenable to repair, the meniscus is prepared with standard techniques as appropriate, such as gentle rasping of the torn surfaces and more aggressive rasping of the adjacent synovium to stimulate proliferation. For isolated meniscal repair, one may consider biologic augmentation with a fibrin clot. Delivery of the fibrin clot to the tear can be facilitated by use of an absorbable suture. When an ACL reconstruction is performed simultaneously, fibrin clot occurs naturally.

The portal that affords the most perpendicular approach to the tear should be used to place the device. Typically, this will be the contralateral portal (i.e., introduce the device through the lateral portal for placement in the medial meniscal body). It is common to change portals for optimal access as devices are placed around the meniscal rim. If possible, leave sutures attached until all implants have been placed so that they can be retensioned if needed for optimal compression.

First-Generation Repairs

- All inside meniscal repairs were first described by Morgan in 1991.[1]
  - Curved suture hooks with accessory posterior portals were used to pass sutures across tear (Fig. 55-1).
  - Sutures were then retrieved and tied arthroscopically.
  - The procedure was very technically demanding.
  - It still placed neurovascular structures at risk.

Second-Generation Repairs

- All-inside devices were developed to be used through standard arthroscopic portals.
- T-Fix (Smith & Nephew)
  - Two sutures connected to a polyethylene bar were deployed through a needle to capture the peripheral meniscus or capsule (Fig. 55-2).
  - The procedure still required arthroscopic square knots that were pushed onto the meniscal surface

(no sliding knots), with minimal compression across the tear.
  - The surgeon was unable to tension knots after placement.

The second-generation devices had good short-term success rates of 80% to 90%[5-7] but, more important, taught surgeons it was possible to safely deliver an all-inside device through standard anterior arthroscopic portals. Unfortunately, the procedures were still somewhat challenging to perform, and the inability to adequately tension the sutures was less than ideal.

Third-Generation Repairs

- Bioabsorbable devices introduced
- Meniscal arrows, darts, staples, screws (Fig. 55-3)
  - These devices captured the torn meniscus and anchored it to the peripheral portion of the meniscus or the capsule.
  - They were mostly made of rigid poly-L-lactide-acid (PLLA).
  - Meniscal Arrow (ConMed Linvatec) most popular of the group
    - Easy to use
    - Passive deployment of implant
    - Current version of the meniscal arrow (Contour Meniscus Arrow) composed of a faster resorbing copolymer, 80L/20D, poly(L-lactide) (PLA) with a lower profile head and barbed along entire shaft to improve fixation strength
    - Good early success, short term follow-up

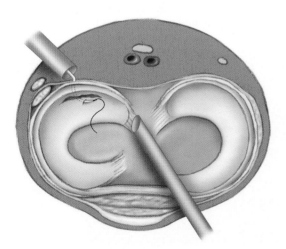

Figure 55-1. First generation all-inside meniscal repair techniques used curved suture hooks inserted through accessory posterior portals. *(Modified from Miller MD: Atlas of meniscal repair. Oper Tech Orthop. 1995;5:70-71.)*

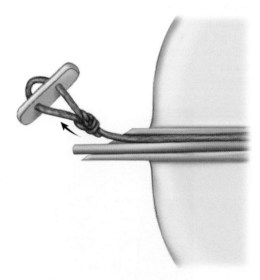

Figure 55-2. The T-Fix implant is composed of a braided suture attached to a polyethylene anchor that captures the peripheral meniscus or capsule. The anchor is deployed through a delivery needle inserted into the meniscus. This device requires arthroscopic suture tying to connect adjacent anchors securing the tear.

- Prospective randomized study demonstrated 91% healing at 2 years with ACL reconstruction[8]
  - Late failures
- Same group was evaluated at 6 years[9]
  - Success rate dropped to 71.4%.

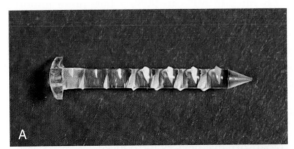
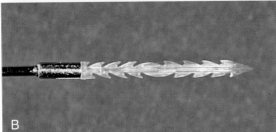
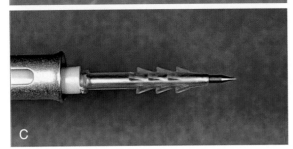

Figure 55-3. Third generation bioabsorbable all-inside meniscal repair devices. **A,** Meniscus Arrow (ConMed Linvatec, Largo, FL). **B,** Meniscal Dart (Arthrex, Naples, FL). **C,** BioStinger (ConMed Linvatec). *(From Stärke C, Kopf S, Petersen W, Becker R: Meniscal repair.* Arthroscopy. *2009;25:1033-1044.)*

- Other studies showed overall failure rate of 28% and, when an isolated meniscal repair was performed, a 42% failure rate.[10,11]
  - Many complications
    - Transient synovitis
    - Inflammatory reaction
    - Cyst formation
    - Device failure or breakage (Fig. 55-4)
    - Device migration (Fig. 55-5)
    - Chondral damage (Fig. 55-6)

Although some of the third-generation devices remain in use, most surgeons have moved away from this group owing to the high complication rate and late failures. The majority of the third-generation devices are rigid, which increases the potential for articular cartilage injury. In addition, the native meniscus moves and

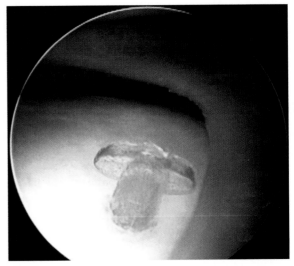

Figure 55-4. Device breakage (such as this broken arrow implant) is a potentially disastrous complication of rigid all-inside meniscal repair devices because damaging loose bodies may be trapped within the knee.

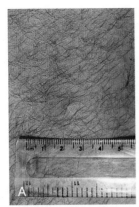
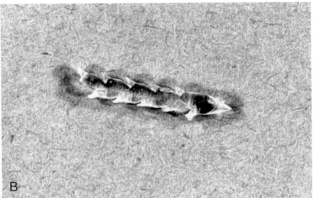

Figure 55-5. Device migration has been reported with rigid all-inside meniscal repair devices. **A,** This patient reported a painful nodule that developed at the knee joint-line after meniscal repair. **B,** Subsequent exploration of the nodule revealed a broken meniscal arrow that was excised. *(From Bonshahi AY, Hopgood P, Shepard GJ: Migration of a broken meniscal arrow: A case report and review of the literature.* Knee Surg Sports Traumatol Arthrosc. *2004;12:50-51.)*

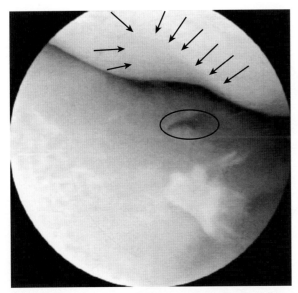

Figure 55-6. Rigid all-inside meniscal repair devices have been associated with chondral damage. Chondral grooving *(arrows)* is demonstrated during second-look arthroscopy 6 weeks after implantation of a meniscal arrow (visible within circle). *(From Ménétrey J, Seil R, Frischy D: Chondral damage after meniscal repair with the use of a bioabsorbable implant. Am J Sport Med. 2002:30;896-899.)*

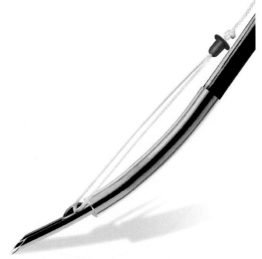

Figure 55-7. The RapidLoc (DePuy Mitek, Raynham, MA) all-inside meniscal repair device consists of a backstop anchor connected by a slipknot to an absorbable top hat, which secures the tear once tensioned. *(From Quinby JS, Golish SR, Hart JA, Diduch DR: All-inside meniscal repair using a new flexible, tensionable device. Am J Sports Med. 2006;34:1281-1286.)*

changes shape with activity. This ability may be impaired with the use of such rigid devices. Furthermore, once these devices have been placed, it is nearly impossible to modify the position if more compression is needed across the tear or if the top of the implant is proud relative to the meniscal surface. The increased risk of chondral injury and lack of adjustability led to the development of fourth-generation devices.

Fourth-Generation Repairs

The fourth-generation implants are flexible, suture-based devices and allow for variable compression and retensioning across the tear. This has made all-inside meniscal repairs a much more attractive option, and as a result, numerous new devices have been developed. In choosing a fourth-generation implant, it is important to know the specific features and characteristics of each device. Some important things to be familiar with for each device include the following:

- The various suture configurations that each device allows
  - Some devices allow a variety of suture configurations including horizontal, vertical, or oblique or a continuous running suture. Other devices allow only a specific suture configuration or only a single point of fixation.
- The location and composition of backstops, anchors, or "top hats" that the devices uses

- The type of suture material of which each device is composed
- The deployment mechanism of the device and whether this is active or passive.
  - Passively deployed devices are manually pushed into the meniscus, and the implant is left behind when the inserter is removed. Unfortunately, this can lead to implants inserted to the inappropriate depth or implants that dislodge or break during implantation. Actively deployed implants are actively inserted to a specific depth when a lever or trigger or wheel is pulled. This leads to a more consistent depth of implantation and fewer misfires.

Specific Fourth-Generation Devices

RapidLoc

- The RapidLoc is composed of a small absorbable backstop anchor made of PLA and an associated PLA or polydioxanone (PDS) top hat for meniscal compression under the pretied slipknot. A No. 2-0 absorbable Panacryl suture or a No. 2-0 Ethibond suture is used (Fig. 55-7).
- The RapidLoc is available with a 0-, 12-, or 27-degree curved inserter that is introduced into the joint through a cannula or with a malleable graft retractor and then across the meniscal tear.
- A silicone hub on the inserter limits the depth of penetration to 13 mm.

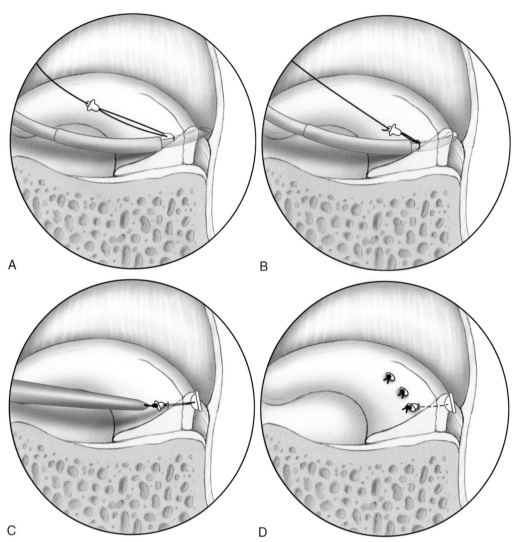

A

B

C

D

Figure 55-8. RapidLoc (DePuy Mitek, Raynham, MA) all-inside meniscus repair technique. **A,** The delivery needle is inserted into the meniscus perpendicular to the tear. A depth-limiter silicone sleeve prevents overpenetration and is typically set at 13 mm of needle penetration. **B,** The backstop anchor is deployed behind the meniscus by firing the trigger on the device handle. **C,** The knot pusher is used to advance the top hat on the slipknot, which reduces and secures the tear. **D,** Multiple devices may be inserted with this technique to secure the entirety of the meniscal tear. Once the repair is complete, the excess suture can be trimmed. *(Modified from Miller MD, Blessey PB, Chhabra A, Kline AJ, Diduch DR: Meniscal repair with the RapidLoc device: A cadaveric study. J Knee Surg. 2003;16:79-82.)*

- It is relatively easy and simple to insert.
- It cannot be applied in a variety of configurations. It applies only one point of fixation under the top hat on the single suture. Multiple implants may be used to transfix the meniscal tear in place. Second-look arthroscopy in a small group showed healing and incorporation of the top hat into the meniscal tissue and no chondral abrasion.
- The top hat is a rigid implant on the top of the meniscal surface that has the potential to cause chondral damage, although the PDS top hat is absorbable.
- Meniscal tear repair with the RapidLoc is illustrated in Figure 55-8 and summarized in Box 55-1.

FasT-Fix

- When originally introduced in 2001, the FasT-Fix was composed of two 5-mm suture bar anchors connected by a No. 0 nonabsorbable polyester suture with a pretied slipknot.
- The current version, the Ultra FasT-Fix, has 5-mm polyetheretherketone (PEEK) or bioabsorbable PLLA anchors with ultra-high-molecular-weight polyethylene (UHMWPE) high-strength sutures (Ultrabraid). This improves the device strength and ease of use (Fig. 55-10).
- Both curved and straight introducers are available.
- The FasT-Fix can be applied in a vertical, horizontal, or oblique configuration.

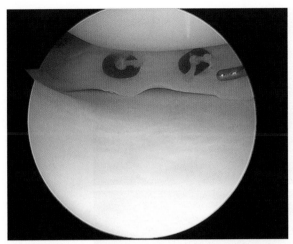

Figure 55-9. This medial meniscal tear has been repaired using two RapidLoc (DePuy Mitek, Raynham, MA) all-inside repair devices.

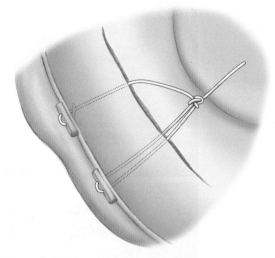

Figure 55-10. The FasT-Fix all-inside meniscal repair device (Smith & Nephew, Andover, MA) is composed of two polyetheretherketone or poly-L–lactide acid suture anchors connected by an ultra-high-molecular-weight polyethylene suture with a pretied slipknot.

BOX 55-1 Meniscal Tear Repair Using the RapidLoc*

1. The instrument is inserted into the knee through an arthroscopic portal with a graft retractor.

2. The needle should be introduced as perpendicularly as possible across the tear. Pressure is applied to reduce the tear. The needle may need to be rotated to ensure that it is perpendicular to the tear.

3. The silicone tubing provides a depth reference and limiter of 13 mm.

4. The backstop is then actively deployed when the handle on the applier is fired.

5. The applier is then removed and the pretied slipknot and backstop are advanced down to the meniscus surface with a knot pusher. This allows for variable compression across the tear

6. Multiple devices are often used to span a tear to secure it (Fig. 55-9).

*Manufactured by DePuy Mitek, Raynham, MA.

- Passive deployment of anchors is used.
- A depth-limiting sleeve on the inserter can be precut to any desired length, although 13 mm is generally recommended to protect neurovascular structures.
- No rigid structure is present on the surface of the meniscus, which minimizes the risk of chondral injury.
- Meniscal tear repair by the FasT-Fix system is illustrated in Figure 55-11 and summarized in Box 55-2.

FasT-Fix 360

- The newly released FasT-Fix 360 meniscal repair system uses an active deployment mechanism via a spring-assisted button with a 360-degree design that allows for deployment in any hand position (Fig. 55-12).
- It consists of a 2-0 Ultrabraid suture with a pretied, self-sliding knot.
- The smaller implant size reportedly allows for smaller needle insertions, thus reducing disruption to the meniscal tissue.
- It also consists of a built-in adjustable depth penetrator (from 10 to 18 mm).
- This implant offers standard straight and curved needles for insertion. In addition, it is the first to offer a reverse curve needle option (10-degree reverse curve) (Fig. 55-13) that enables the placement of undersurface sutures for alternating superior and inferior vertical mattress repairs, the strongest configuration of inside-out repairs (Fig. 55-14).

Omnispan

- The Omnispan is a newer device composed of PEEK backstops connected by No. 2-0 Orthocord (55% PDS and 45% high-molecular-weight polyethylene) high-strength suture.
- Each inserter is preloaded with two anchors that are actively deployed.
- Available in 0-, 12-, and 27-degree curved inserters.
- Both the backstops and the knot are located on the periphery of the meniscus, leaving no rigid objects or knots on the meniscal surface (Fig. 55-15).
- It can be applied in a variety of configurations including horizontal, vertical, and oblique.

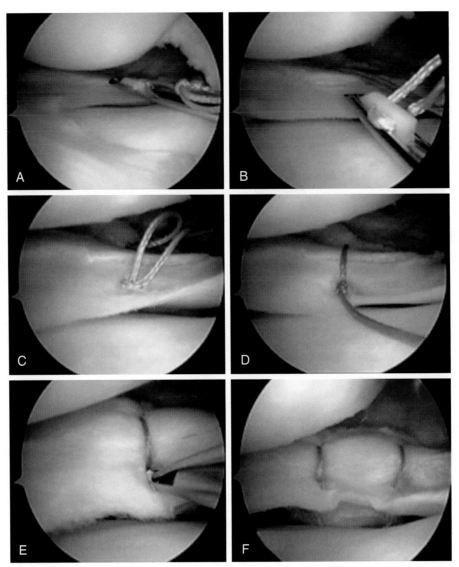

Figure 55-11. Meniscal tear repair by the FasT-Fix system (Smith & Nephew, Andover, MA). **A,** Longitudinal tear with FasT-Fix device advanced perpendicular to tear. The needle is advanced to a preset depth to safely engage the peripheral meniscal rim. The FasT-Fix needle is then pulled back while the device is left within the joint. A button on the handle adjacent to one's thumb is then advanced forward to advance the second FasT-Fix implant into place at the needle tip. **B,** The second implant may then be placed in either a horizontal or a vertical mattress configuration. Here, a vertical mattress orientation is chosen. The needle is again advanced to its preset stop. The entire device is withdrawn from the joint. **C,** The vertical mattress suture loop can be seen across the tear before tightening. **D,** The suture limb that exits the joint has a pretied slipknot that can be advanced into the joint by pulling on the free suture limb. Variable compression can be attained with the aid of a knot pusher. **E,** The excess suture is then cut. **F,** Final repair with two FasT-Fix sutures in place.

- Meniscal tear repair with the Omnispan system is illustrated in Figure 55-16 and summarized in Box 55-3.

Sequent
- The Sequent is a new fourth-generation device that allows all-inside repairs with a continuous stitching system.
- The device comes loaded with either four or seven PEEK-Optima implants connected by a No. 2-0

Hi-Fi (UHMWPE) braided suture that allows for multiple individual points of fixation and tensioning. The device does not need to be removed from the knee when multiple suture placements are made (Fig. 55-17).
- The device allows a variety of configurations of suture placement.
- Implants are located on the periphery, and the Sequent uses a knotless design.
- Implants are actively deployed.

- Meniscal tear repair with the Sequent system is illustrated in Figure 55-18 and summarized in Box 55-4.

Meniscal Cinch

- The Meniscal Cinch is composed of two PEEK implants connected by a No. 2-0 FiberWire suture with a pretied slipknot (Fig. 55-19).
- Similar to the FasT-Fix and Omnispan, it may be placed in a variety of configurations.

- There are no hard implants on the meniscal surface that might place the chondral surfaces at risk.
- Implants are actively deployed.

Maxfire MarXmen

- The Maxfire MarXmen is an all-suture-based implant with a suture coil peripheral anchor (Fig. 55-20).
- It is composed of a polyethylene suture with polypropylene (MaxBraid).

BOX 55-2 Meniscal Tear Repair with the FasT-Fix System*

- The delivery needle is inserted into the joint either through a cannula or with a graft retractor. A removable rubber sleeve provides protection of device and chondral surfaces during insertion.
- The needle is then introduced perpendicular to the meniscal tear, typically starting with the superior implant if a vertical repair is being performed (see Fig. 55-11A).
- The handle of the delivery needle is then slightly oscillated to passively deploy the first implant.
- The needle is then pulled back out of the meniscal tissue, leaving the first implant behind.
- Sliding the trigger forward advances the second anchor into the ready position. Resistance will be felt when it is fully seated into the ready position.

- The delivery needle is then inserted in the desired location of the second implant, approximately 4 to 5 mm from the first implant (see Fig. 55-11B).
- The delivery needle is then removed from the knee.
- The free suture end is then pulled to advance the pretied sliding knot onto the meniscal surface (see Fig. 55-11C).
- The knot is further tightened, then the suture is cut with the arthroscopic suture pusher/cutter (see Fig. 55-11D).
- Multiple sutures can be placed as needed to secure the tear (see Fig. 55-11E).

*Manufactured by Smith & Nephew, Andover, MA.

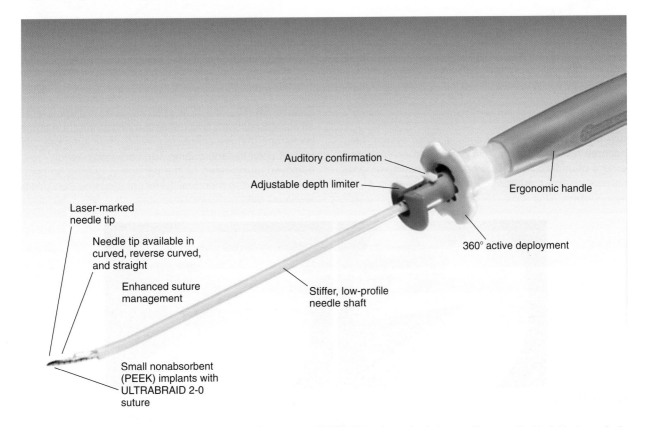

Figure 55-12. The FasT-Fix 360 meniscal repair system. *PEEK,* Polyetheretherketone. *(Courtesy Smith & Nephew, Andover, MA.)*

- It allows customized length and tension of the implant in a knotless fashion through ZipLoop Technology, a weave in which a single strand of material is woven through itself twice in opposing directions.
- It has an adjustable depth of insertion and can be placed in a variety of configurations.
- It uses active deployment of implants.

CrossFix II

- The CrossFix II is an all-suture-based device composed of 0 polyethylene suture in a double-barrel needle inserter, which is available in curved and straight forms.
- Delivery needles are placed into the meniscal tissue across the tear. The trigger is then squeezed, and a 3-mm mattress suture is deployed (Fig. 55-21).
- The inserter is then removed, and the suture end is cut off the needle tip. The surgeon then slides a pretied Westin slipknot down on the meniscal surface and tensions it by pulling on the post (white) suture. A knot pusher can be used to help tension the knot; pulling on the black suture then locks the knot. It can be further backed up with half-hitch knots if desired.

- The double-barrel needle inserter has a depth limiter but is rather bulky, which limits its ability to place sutures in a vertical position.
- Deep penetration with the needles is required to allow the suture to transfer.

POSTOPERATIVE CONSIDERATIONS
Follow-up

- 10 to 14 days for suture removal and wound check
- 6-week follow-up and progress check

Rehabilitation

Although it is unknown exactly how long it takes for the human meniscus to heal after repair, most surgeons

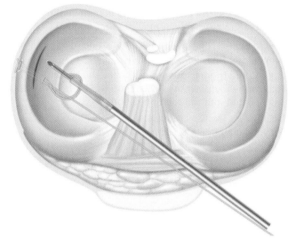

Figure 55-15. The Omnispan all-inside meniscal repair device comes with two preloaded polyetheretherketone backstops that are connected by an ultra-high-molecular-weight polyethylene suture. The backstops, when deployed, are located on the periphery, leaving no rigid materials on the meniscal surfaces. *(Courtesy DePuy Mitek, Raynham, MA.)*

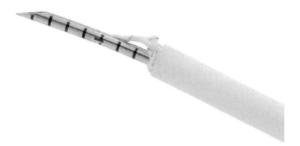

Figure 55-13. FasT-Fix 360 meniscal repair system has a 10-degree reverse-curve needle option that enables the placement of undersurface sutures for alternating superior and inferior vertical mattress repairs. *(Courtesy Smith & Nephew, Andover, MA.)*

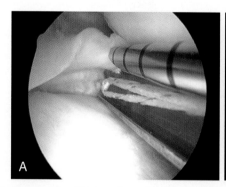
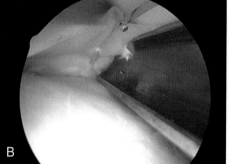

Figure 55-14. A, Repair of a tibial surface meniscus tear by placement of undersurface sutures through a slotted cannula that can be used to guide the suture and lift up the meniscus for improved visualization. **B,** Once the anchors have been deployed, the needle is removed and the knot is advanced and tensioned. *(Courtesy Smith & Nephew, Andover, MA.)*

advocate protected weight bearing and avoidance of extremes of motion for 6 weeks. Exceptions are sometimes made for weight bearing in a brace at full extension, which may apply outward compressive force to help reduce the tear. Squatting is avoided for at least 3 months, because this puts high shear forces on the posterior horn. For meniscal repair in conjunction with ACL reconstruction, the standard ACL protocol is used with the addition of the following:

- Postoperative hinged ACL brace for 6 weeks, 0 to 90 degrees of motion
- 50% weight bearing for 6 weeks

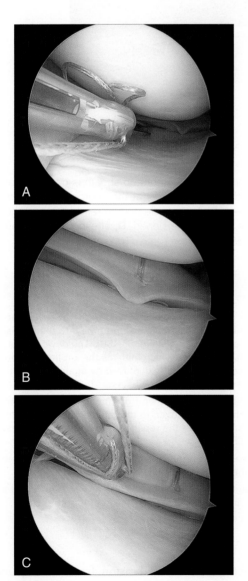

Figure 55-16. Meniscus repair using the Omnispan (DePuy Mitek, Raynham, MA). **A,** The device is inserted into the knee with a malleable graft retractor as perpendicular to the tear as possible. **B,** Final placement of initial device reapproximates the meniscal tear. **C,** Sutures can be placed in a variety of positions; often several sutures will need to be placed to reapproximate the tear.

For isolated meniscal repair without ACL reconstruction, the same weight-bearing and motion restrictions are used, with a return to sports permitted at 5 months. Compliance can be difficult because patients have minimal pain and only two small arthroscopic portals for incisions.

BOX 55-3 Meniscal Tear Repair with the Omnispan System*

- The applier is inserted into the joint with a malleable graft retractor to protect the chondral surfaces and to help prevent the devices from being caught up in soft tissues (see Fig. 55-16A).
- The needle is then advanced across the meniscal tear as perpendicularly as possible, and compression is applied to reach the desired depth, typically 13 mm, with the silicon tubing as a reference.
- Pressure is applied to prevent recoil while the large gray lever is squeezed and the first backstop is actively deployed.
- The gray lever is held down while the device is removed from the meniscal tissue, and then it is released.
- The red trigger is then compressed, which places the second backstop into the ready position.
- The meniscus is then penetrated again in the desired configuration, with 6 to 10 mm maintained between the implants, and the gray lever once again is compressed to actively deliver the second implant.
- The lever is released and the applier and needle are removed from the joint space.
- The sutures are then tensioned. Quickly pulling on the free suture limb allows both suture loops to be tensioned to stabilize the tear.
- Alternatively, if both loops do not slide when the suture is pulled, an arthroscopic probe can be placed through the first loop that tightens; then this suture loop is pulled back to tighten the other loop. Final tensioning of the free tensioning suture is then performed.
- The sutures are then cut with an arthroscopic knot pusher/cutter (see Fig. 55-16B).
- Multiple sutures can be placed in a various configurations according to the tear size and shape (see Fig. 55-16C).

*Manufactured by DePuy Mitek, Raynham, MA.

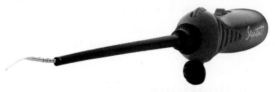

Figure 55-17. The Sequent all-inside meniscal repair device comes preloaded with four or seven polyetheretherketone Optima implants connected by an ultra-high-molecular-weight polyethylene braided suture and allows for a continuous stitch to be placed in a variety of configurations without removal of the device from the knee. *(Courtesy ConMed Linvatec, Largo, FL.)*

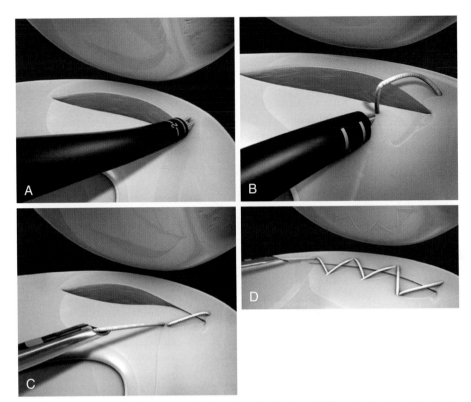

Figure 55-18. Meniscal repair using the Sequent meniscal repair device. **A,** The depth stop sheath is cut and then slid over the needle; the device is then advanced into the knee and across the meniscus tear at the appropriate location. The trigger is pulled, and the first implant is deployed across the meniscal tear. **B,** The needle is then reinserted and then the second device is actively deployed. **C,** The needle is withdrawn and the suture is tensioned. **D,** These steps are repeated an appropriate number of times to reapproximate the tear. *(Courtesy ConMed Linvatec, Largo, FL.)*

BOX 55-4 Meniscal Tear Repair with the Sequent System*

- After the approximate depth of the tear has been measured, the depth stop sheath is cut to the appropriate length. The sheath is then slid over the tip of the needle, which allows it to also serve as a protective cannula.

- The depth stop sheath is then pulled back to expose the needle once near the meniscal tissue. With the switch in the forward freewheel position, the needle is inserted into the meniscus to the appropriate depth. The trigger is pushed forward to prepare the device for deployment, then pulled back to deploy the implant (see Fig. 55-18A).

- The needle is then withdrawn from the meniscus, and the switch is placed into the ratchet position. Tension is placed up on the suture to set the implant, and the wheel is used to reel in excess suture.

- Once again the switch is moved to the freewheel position. The needle is inserted a second time into the meniscus in the new location (see Fig. 55-18B). The device is rotated two full rotations, which initiates the knotless fixation. The second implant is deployed by again pushing the trigger forward and then backward.

- The needle is withdrawn from the meniscus, and the switch is again moved to the ratchet position to allow for tensioning of the repair with the thumb wheel (see Fig. 55-18C).

- These steps are repeated to create the desired number of stitches (see Fig. 55-18D).

- Once the repair is complete, the device is removed and the suture is cut with an arthroscopic suture cutter.

*Manufactured by Linvatec ConMed, Largo, FL.

Complications

Most complications are similar to those seen in other types of meniscal repair. The complications specific to the fourth-generation devices include the following:

- Device misfire and implant breakage or migration
- Iatrogenic chondral damage
- Potential chondral abrasion from knots placed on meniscal surface[16]
- Entrapment of the popliteus, collateral ligaments, iliotibial band, and potentially neurovascular structures

Although entrapment of soft tissue structures such as the popliteus, collateral ligaments, and iliotibial band

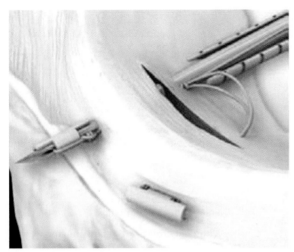

Figure 55-19. Meniscal Cinch (Arthrex, Naples, FL). *(From Barber FA, Herbert MA, Schroeder FA, Aziz-Jacobo J, Sutker MJ: Biomechanical testing of new meniscal repair techniques containing ultra-high-molecular weight polyethylene suture. Arthroscopy. 2009;25:959-967.)*

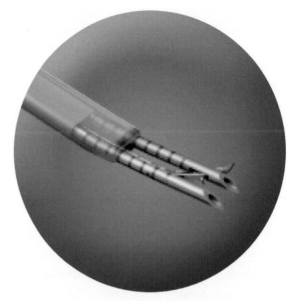

Figure 55-21. CrossFix (Cayenne Medical, Scottsdale, AZ). *(CrossFix Meniscal Repair System Surgical Technique Guide. From www.cayennemedical.com/products/crossfix.)*

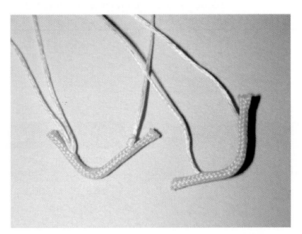

Figure 55-20. Biomet MaxFire. *(From Lawhorn K: MaxFire Meniscal Repair Device: Surgical protocol. Biomet Sports Medicine. Available at http://www.biomet.com/sportsmedicine/ productDetail.cfmcategory=28&subCategory=29&product=122.)*

can occur, it also occurs with traditional open suture meniscal repairs. It is unlikely to have any clinical significance.[13]

RESULTS

All-inside meniscal repair is an attractive option for surgeons because it is often easier and faster and can be done with fewer assistants than inside-out and outside-in techniques. Longer follow-up with third-generation rigid devices, such as the meniscal arrow, has shown decreased success rates from originally reported promising midterm results with various complications, including chondral abrasion. The fourth-generation devices are flexible and allow variable tensioning across the

repair, characteristics that are more similar to the inside-out technique. The flexibility of these devices also decreases the associated risks of the device itself on insertion. When the meniscus is repaired in isolation, success rates for inside-out meniscal repair average 60% to 80%. When the procedure is performed with a concomitant ACL reconstruction, the success rate is approximately 90%. Recent data suggest that comparable results can be achieved when all-inside techniques are used.[18] Results of all-inside techniques are listed in Table 55-1. The follow-up studies of both the FasT-Fix and RapidLoc are promising, particularly in patients with smaller tears undergoing concomitant ACL reconstruction, in whom success rates higher than 90% have been seen. Second-look arthroscopies with these implants are also promising; however, recently Tachibana and colleagues reported on a patient in whom there appeared to be chondral abrasion over the knot from a FasT-Fix device.[16] Although this is the only reported case we have seen, only further long-term studies and additional second-look arthroscopies will be able to determine if this is a more widespread problem than we currently appreciate. Inside-out meniscal repair remains the gold standard for comparison, but new all-inside repair devices, if placed correctly and vertically, appear to offer similarly excellent clinical results.

Regarding deployment mechanism, in our experience the active deployment devices are more reliable and more precise with regard to location and depth. They have less misfires compared with the passive devices, especially when tensioning of the repair is attempted. This not only increases operating room time but also cost. Active deployment devices do have a bit of

TABLE 55-1. Results of Studies of All-Inside Techniques

Author	Device	Follow-up	Success Rate	Note
Third-Generation Devices				
Gill and Diduch[8] (2002)	Arrow	2 years (average)	90.6%	With ACL reconstruction
Lee and Diduch[9] (2005)	Arrow	6.6 years (average)	71.4%	Same population with longer follow-up
Venkatachalam[12] (2001)	Suture Arrow T-Fix	21 months	78.6% 56.5% 57.1%	20/59 with concurrent ACL reconstruction Best results (71%) with concurrent ACL and medial meniscus tear
Fourth-Generation Devices				
Haas et al[4] (2005)	FasT-Fix	2 years	91% 80%	With ACL reconstruction Isolated meniscal repair
Quinby et al[13] (2005)	RapidLoc	35 months	90.7%	With concurrent ACL reconstruction
Barber[28] (2008)	FasT-Fix	30.7 month	83%	29/41 with concurrent ACL reconstruction
Barber[29] (2006)	RapidLoc	31 months	87.5%	23/32 with concurrent ACL reconstruction
Kotsovolos et al[14] (2006)	FasT-Fix	18 months	90.2%	36/58 with concurrent ACL reconstruction
Konan and Haddad[15] (2010)	Arrow, FasT-Fix	18 months	96% 86%	With ACL reconstruction In isolation Higher failure rate noted with Arrow (22.2%) than FasT-Fix (10.3%)

See text for manufacturer information.

TABLE 55-2. Biomechanics

Author	Testing Method	Vertical FasT-Fix	Horizontal FasT-Fix	Arrow	RapidLoc	Meniscal Cinch	MaxFire	Horizontal Suture	Vertical Suture
Barber et al[19] (2004)	Load to failure (N)	70.9	72.1		43.3			55.9	80.43
Fisher et al[20] (2002)	Load to failure (N)			45.89				107.65	
Durselen et al[21] (2003)	Load to failure (N) Load to failure after cyclic load (N)			52 48				103 82	
McDermott et al[22] (2003)	Load to failure (N) Gap after cycling (mm)		49.1 3.47	34.2 2.18					72.7 5.61
Dervin et al[23] (1997)	Load to failure (N)			29.6					58.3
Zantop et al[24] (2005)	Load to failure (N) Gap after cycling (mm)	94.1 5.34	80.8 6.23		30.3 6.84			50.2 6.03	71.3 5.61

TABLE 55-2. Biomechanics—cont'd

Author	Testing Method	Vertical FasT-Fix	Horizontal FasT-Fix	Arrow	RapidLoc	Meniscal Cinch	MaxFire	Horizontal Suture	Vertical Suture
Borden et al[25] (2003)	Load to failure (N) Gap after cycling (mm) Stiffness		104 5.1 7.7	49 NA 6.1					102 6 7.7
Mehta[30] (2009)	Load to failure (N) Gap after cycling (mm) 1/100/500 cycles Stiffness (N/mm)		86.1 2.46/3.59/4.74 25.2			85.3 2.12/4.07/5.94 25.5	64.5 3.65/6.70/7.19 16.3		
Aros et al[26] (2010)	Load to failure (N)	125	107		70		145 (vertical) 139 (horizontal)	183 (Fiber-Wire)	185 (Fiber-Wire)

NA, Not available. All arrows failed before completion of testing.

kickback when fired, and the user of the device must be cognizant of this before deployment to prevent inappropriate depth of placement or misfire. We have found it helpful to apply firm pressure to the device when actively deploying implants to help counteract this kickback and to allow for proper insertion of the device.

In our opinion, the ability to obtain a vertical suture configuration is ideal during concomitant ACL reconstruction and mandatory during isolated meniscal repair. The superior strength of vertical suture configuration over horizontal configuration with use of the FasT-Fix and RapidLoc constructs has previously been demonstrated.[27] Vertical mattress configuration has been shown to be the strongest construct that captures the maximum number of collagen cables. Inside-out vertical mattress sutures remain the gold standard for healing and biomechanics against which any all-inside device is compared (Table 55-2). Because some level of loosening is expected with cyclic loading of all devices, we typically recommend a slight overtightening at the time of insertion. These are important considerations for both the device engineers and clinicians to obtain maximum results with the lowest possible cost and risk to the patient.

REFERENCES

1. Morgan CD. The "all-inside" meniscal repair. *Arthroscopy.* 1991;7:120-125.
2. Magee T, Williams D. 3-0-T MRI of meniscal tears. *AJR Am J Roentgenol.* 2006;187:371-375.
3. Bernthan NM, Seeger LL, Motamedi K, et al. Can the repairability of meniscal tears be predicted with magnetic resonance imaging? *Am J Sports Med.* 2011;39:506-510.
4. Haas AL, Schepsis AA, Hornstein J, et al. Meniscal repair using the FasT-Fix all-inside meniscal repair device. *Arthroscopy.* 2005;21:167-175.
5. Asik M, Sen C, Erginsu M. Arthroscopic meniscal repair using T-fix. *Knee Surg Sports Traumatol Arthrosc.* 2002;10:284-288.
6. Escalas F, Quadras J, Caceres E, et al. T-Fix anchor sutures for arthroscopic meniscal repair. *Knee Surg Sports Traumatol Arthrosc.* 1997;5:72-76.
7. Barrett GR, Treacy SH, Ruff CG. Preliminary results of the T-fix endoscopic meniscus repair technique in an anterior cruciate ligament reconstruction population. *Arthroscopy.* 1997;13:218-223.
8. Gill SS, Diduch DR. Outcomes after meniscal repair using the meniscus arrow in knees undergoing concurrent anterior cruciate ligament reconstruction. *Arthroscopy.* 2002;18:569-577.
9. Lee GP, Diduch DR. Deteriorating outcomes after meniscal repair using the Meniscus Arrow in knees undergoing concurrent anterior cruciate ligament reconstruction: increased failure rate with long-term follow-up [see comment]. *Am J Sports Med.* 2005;33:1138-1141.
10. Gifstad T, Grontvedt T, Drogset JO. Meniscal repair with Biofix Arrows: results after 4.7 years' follow-up. *Am J Sports Med.* 2007;35(1):71-74.
11. Kurzweil PR, Tifford CD, Ignacio EM. Unsatisfactory clinical results of meniscal repair using the Meniscal Arrow. *Arthroscopy.* 2005;21(8):905.
12. Venkatachalam S, Godsiff SP, Harding ML. Review of the clinical results of arthroscopic meniscal repair. *Knee.* 2001;8:129-133.

13. Quinby J, Hart JA, Golish R, et al. *Meniscal repair using the RapidLoc in knees undergoing concurrent ACL reconstruction.* Virginia Orthopedic Society 58th annual meeting; The Homestead, Hot Springs, Va; 2005.

14. Kotsovolos ES, Hantes ME, Mastrokalos DS, et al. Results of all-inside meniscal repair with the FasT-Fix Meniscal Repair System. *Arthroscopy.* 2006;22:3-9.

15. Konan S, Haddad FS. Outcomes of meniscal preservation using all-inside meniscal repair devices. *Clin Orthop Relat Res.* 2010;468:1209-1213.

16. Tachibana Y, Sakaguchi K, Tatsuru G, et al. Repair integrity by second-look arthroscopy after arthroscopic meniscal repair with the FastT-Fix during anterior cruciate ligament reconstruction. *Am J Sports Med.* 2010:38:965-971.

17. Miller MD, Blessey PB, Chhabra A, et al. Meniscal repair with the Rapid Loc device: A cadaveric study. *J Knee Surg.* 16:79-82, 2003.

18. Choi N, Kim T, Victoroff BN. Comparison of arthroscopic medial meniscal suture repair techniques: inside-out versus all-inside repair. *Am J Sports Med.* 2009;37:2115-2150.

19. Barber FA, Herbert MA, Richards DP. Load to failure testing of new meniscal repair devices. *Arthroscopy.* 2004;20:45-50.

20. Fisher SR, Markel DC, Koman JD, et al. Pull-out and shear failure strengths of arthroscopic meniscal repair systems. *Knee Surg Sports Traumatol Arthrosc.* 2002;10:294-299.

21. Durselen L, Schneider J, Galler M, et al. Cyclic joint loading can affect the initial stability of meniscal fixation implants. *Clin Biomech.* 2003;18:44-49.

22. McDermott ID, Richards SW, Hallam P, et al. A biomechanical study of four different meniscal repair systems, comparing pull-out strengths and gapping under cyclic loading. *Knee Surg Sports Traumatol Arthrosc.* 2003;11:23-29.

23. Dervin GF, Downing KJ, Keene GC, et al. Failure strengths of suture versus biodegradable arrow for meniscal repair: an in vitro study. *Arthroscopy.* 1997;13:296-300.

24. Zantop T, Eggers AK, Musahl V, et al. Cyclic testing of flexible all-inside meniscus suture anchors: biomechanical analysis. *Am J Sports Med.* 2005;33:388-394.

25. Borden P, Nyland J, Caborn DN, et al. Biomechanical comparison of the FasT-Fix meniscal repair suture system with vertical mattress sutures and meniscus arrows. *Am J Sports Med.* 2003;31:374-378.

26. Aros BC, Pedroza A, Vasileff WK, et al. Mechanical comparison of meniscal repair devices with mattress suture devices in vitro. *Knee Surg Sports Traumatol Arthrosc.* 2010;18:1594-1598.

27. Kocabey Y, Chang HC, Brand Jr JC, et al. A biomechanical comparison of the FasT-Fix meniscal repair suture system and the RapidLoc device in cadaver meniscus. *Arthroscopy.* 2006;22:406-413.

28. Barber FA, Schroeder FA, Oro FB, et al. FasT-Fix meniscal repair: mid-term results. *Arthroscopy.* 2008;24:1342-1348.

29. Barber FA, Coons DA, Ruiz-Suarez M. Meniscal repair with RapidLoc meniscal repair device. *Arthroscopy.* 2006;22:962-966.

30. Mehta VM, Terry MA. Cyclic testing of 3 all-inside meniscal repair devices: a biomechanical analysis. *Am J Sports Med.* 2009;37:2435-2439.

Chapter 56

Allograft Meniscus Transplantation: Bridge-in-Slot Technique

Andreas A. Gomoll, Jack Farr II, and Brian J. Cole

Chapter Synopsis

- This chapter summarizes the indications for and technique and results of meniscal allograft transplantation with the bridge-in-slot technique for the treatment of symptomatic meniscal deficiency.

Important Points

- Meniscal transplants are indicated for symptomatic compartment overload caused by total or subtotal meniscectomy.
- Osteoarthritis, with the exception of very specific circumstances, is a contraindication.

Clinical and Surgical Pearls

- Ensure that the graft has been received in acceptable condition and that the size and side are correct before the patient is anesthetized.
- A transpatellar tendon approach is commonly necessary to align the slot with the anterior and posterior meniscal roots.
- Preserve a 2-mm peripheral rim of meniscal tissue if possible to facilitate the capsular repair and potentially reduce extrusion.
- Use the appropriate varus or valgus stress with hyperflexion followed by extension of the knee to reduce the transplant under the femoral condyle. Especially medially, pie-crusting of the medial collateral ligament (MCL) can occasionally become necessary if the compartment is tight.

Clinical and Surgical Pitfalls

- Make sure the graft is not undersized; this can complicate capsular repair and increases the failure rate.

It is generally believed that any significant meniscectomy alters the biomechanical and biologic environment of the normal knee, eventually resulting in pain, recurrent swelling, and effusions. Overt secondary osteoarthritis is often the endpoint.[1,2] Recognition of these consequences has led to a strong commitment within the orthopedic community to meniscus-sparing interventions. However, there are cases in which meniscal preservation is not possible. In carefully selected patients, meniscal allografts can restore nearly normal knee anatomy and biomechanics, providing excellent pain relief and improved function.[9]

Several techniques exist for allograft meniscus transplantation, including bone plugs, a keyhole technique, and a dovetail technique. We prefer the bridge-in-slot technique[4] because of its simplicity and secure bone fixation, the ability to more easily perform concomitant procedures such as osteotomy and ligament reconstruction, and the advantages of maintaining the relationship of the native anterior and posterior horns of the meniscus.

PREOPERATIVE CONSIDERATIONS

History

It is essential to elicit a thorough history, including the causative mechanism, associated injuries, and prior treatments. Operative reports are helpful to evaluate arthritic changes that could constitute a contraindication to meniscal transplantation.

Typical History

- Knee injury, often an acute traumatic event initiating meniscal treatment

- One or more meniscectomies, open or arthroscopically performed with initial improvement
- Subsequent development of ipsilateral joint line pain and activity-related swelling
- Giving way (occasionally reported)

Physical Examination

Factors Affecting Surgical Indication

- Range of motion: usually preserved
- Effusion
- Joint line or femoral condyle tenderness
- Objective evidence of joint space narrowing (magnetic resonance imaging, flexion weight-bearing radiographs); development of localized or diffuse chondral disease in the ipsilateral compartment

Factors Affecting Surgical Planning

- Preexisting incisions
- Limb malalignment (may require concomitant realignment procedure)
- Ligamentous instability (may require prior or concomitant reconstructive procedure)
- Chondral injury, typically involving the femoral condyle (may require concomitant cartilage repair procedure)

Imaging

Radiography

- Weight-bearing anteroposterior radiograph in full extension
- Weight-bearing posteroanterior 45-degree flexion radiograph
- Non–weight-bearing 45-degree flexion lateral view
- Axial view of the patellofemoral joint
- Long-cassette mechanical axis view to evaluate malalignment

Other Modalities

- Magnetic resonance imaging with or without the intra-articular administration of contrast material is performed to assess extent of meniscectomy, degree of articular cartilage damage, and presence of subchondral edema in the involved compartment.
- Technetium bone scanning may indicate stress overload in the involved compartment or overt osteoarthritis.

Indications and Contraindications

The ideal candidate has a history of prior total or subtotal meniscectomy with persistent pain localized to the involved compartment, intact articular surfaces (ideally grade I or II), normal alignment, and a stable joint.

Associated pathologic findings, such as malalignment, discrete chondral defects, and ligamentous instability, are not contraindications in an otherwise appropriate candidate because they can be addressed in either staged or concomitant procedures.

In addition to uncorrected comorbidities (malalignment, ligament deficiency, uncorrected localized chondral damage in the involved compartment), contraindications are overt arthroscopic or radiographic arthritic changes (especially associated with femoral condyle or tibial flattening), history of inflammatory arthritis, marked obesity, and previous infection.

Surgical Planning

Concomitant Procedures

Significant limb malalignment, ligamentous instability, or discrete chondral defects can be addressed either before or concomitantly with meniscus transplantation.

Allograft Sizing

Meniscal allografts are size and compartment specific. Preoperative measurements are obtained from anteroposterior and lateral radiographs with magnification markers placed on the skin at the level of the joint line. After radiographic magnification is accounted for, meniscal width is measured on the anteroposterior radiograph from the edge of the ipsilateral tibial spine to the edge of the tibial plateau. Meniscal length is calculated by multiplying the depth of the tibial plateau (as measured on lateral radiographs) by 0.8 for the medial meniscus and 0.7 for the lateral meniscus (Fig. 56-1).

Meniscal Graft Processing and Preservation

Meniscal allografts are harvested by sterile surgical technique, most commonly within 24 hours of donor asystole. Unlike with fresh osteochondral allografts, cell viability in meniscal allografts does not seem to improve the morphologic or biochemical characteristics of the grafts; thus the most commonly implanted grafts are either fresh-frozen or cryopreserved. The risk of disease transmission is minimized through rigid donor screening, graft culturing, and polymerase chain reaction testing for human immunodeficiency virus. Several tissue banks are evaluating secondary sterilization techniques to further improve the safety of meniscal allograft tissue.

SURGICAL TECHNIQUE

Anesthesia and Positioning

On the basis of the surgeon's, anesthesiologist's, and patient's preferences, the procedure can be performed with general, spinal, or regional anesthesia or a

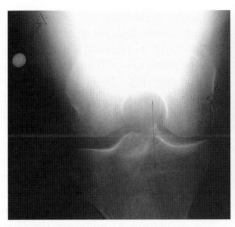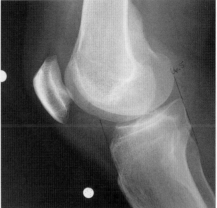

Figure 56-1. Graft sizing on anteroposterior and lateral radiographs.

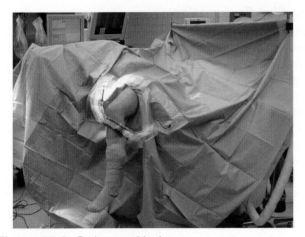

Figure 56-2. Patient positioning.

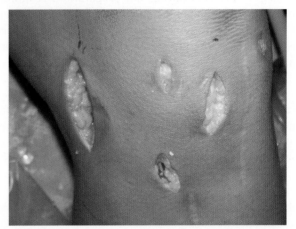

Figure 56-3. Incisions: accessory posteromedial incision *(left);* inferomedial and inferolateral arthroscopy portals, mini-arthrotomy for meniscal insertion *(between portals);* accessory incision for concomitant allograft anterior cruciate ligament reconstruction in this patient *(inferior).*

combination thereof. The patient is positioned supine on a standard operating room table, with a thigh tourniquet, and the extremity is placed in a standard leg holder allowing full knee flexion or hyperflexion (Fig. 56-2). The posteromedial or posterolateral corner must be freely accessible for inside-out meniscus suturing to be performed.

Surgical Landmarks, Incisions, and Portals

Landmarks
- Patella
- Patellar tendon
- Tibial plateau
- Fibular head

Portals and Approaches
See Fig. 56-3 for portals and approaches:

- Inferomedial portal
- Inferolateral portal
- Additional outflow portals as needed

- Posteromedial or posterolateral approach
- Mini-arthrotomy through ipsilateral side of patellar tendon

Structures at Risk
- Posterolateral approach: peroneal nerve, lateral collateral ligament, popliteus tendon
- Posteromedial approach: saphenous nerve, medial collateral ligament
- Mini-arthrotomy: patellar tendon

Examination Under Anesthesia and Diagnostic Arthroscopy

Examination under anesthesia should evaluate range of motion and ligamentous stability. Diagnostic arthroscopy is useful to evaluate for other intra-articular pathologic processes, such as loose bodies, ligamentous deficiency, and chondral defects.

Specific Steps

The specific steps of the procedure are outlined in Box 56-1.

1. Arthroscopic Preparation

The initial steps for medial and lateral meniscus transplantation are similar. The remaining meniscus is debrided to a stable, 1- to 2-mm peripheral rim until punctate bleeding occurs (Fig. 56-4). The most anterior aspect of the meniscus can be excised under direct visualization by use of a No. 11 scalpel blade placed through the ipsilateral portal followed by the use of an aggressive arthroscopic shaver. The anterior and posterior horn insertion sites should be maintained because they are helpful markers during slot preparation. A limited notchplasty along the most inferior and posterior aspect of the ipsilateral femoral condyle allows improved visualization of the posterior horn and facilitates graft passage.

2. Exposure

A mini-arthrotomy is performed in line with the anterior and posterior horn insertion sites of the involved meniscus (see Fig. 56-3). This allows correct orientation of the slot and introduction of the graft. Depending on the surgeon's preference, the arthrotomy can be performed either directly adjacent to or through the patellar tendon in line with its fibers. An ipsilateral (either posteromedial or posterolateral) approach is required for meniscal repair (see Fig. 56-3). The incision should extend approximately one third above and two thirds below the joint line and allow adequate exposure to protect the neurovascular structures during passage of the inside-out sutures. The ipsilateral gastrocnemius muscle-tendon junction is elevated off the posterior capsule, and a meniscal retractor is placed anterior to it. Elevation of either the iliotibial band–tensor fasciae latae or sartorius fascia anteriorly allows suture tying beneath these structures to minimize the chances of capturing the knee as a result of soft tissue tethering.

3. Slot Preparation

Slot orientation follows the normal anatomy of the meniscus attachment sites. By use of electrocautery, the centers of the anterior and posterior horn attachment sites are connected with a line. With this line as a guide, a 4-mm bur is used to make a reference slot in the tibial plateau. Its height and width will equal the dimensions of the bur, and its alignment in the sagittal plane should parallel the slope of the tibial plateau (Fig. 56-5). Slot dimensions should be confirmed by placement of a depth gauge in the reference slot, which also measures the anteroposterior length of the tibial plateau (Fig. 56-6). With use of a drill guide, a guide pin is placed just deep and parallel to the reference slot (Fig. 56-7) and advanced to but not through the posterior cortex. The pin is subsequently over-reamed with a 7- or 8-mm cannulated drill bit (Fig. 56-8), again with care taken to maintain the posterior cortex. A box cutter is then used to make a slot 7 to 8 mm wide by 10 mm deep (Fig. 56-9), which is smoothed and refined with a 7- to 8-mm rasp to ensure that the bone bridge will slide smoothly into the slot (Fig. 56-10).

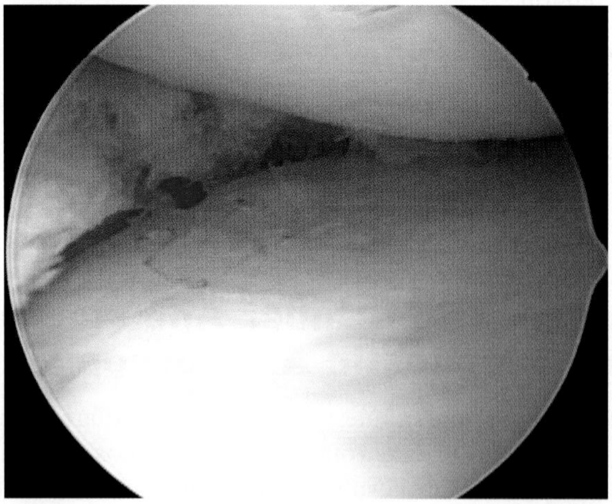

BOX 56-1 Surgical Steps

1. Arthroscopic preparation
2. Exposure
3. Slot preparation
4. Allograft preparation
5. Graft insertion and fixation
6. Closure

Figure 56-4. Meniscus debrided back to a stable and bleeding rim.

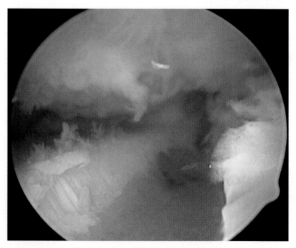

Figure 56-5. Reference slot prepared with a bur.

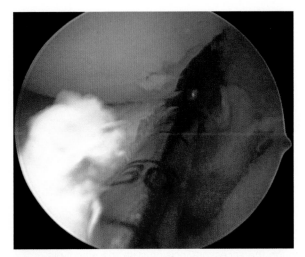

Figure 56-6. Guide probe in reference slot.

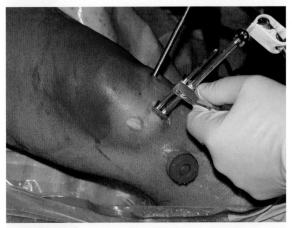

Figure 56-7. Guide pin placement.

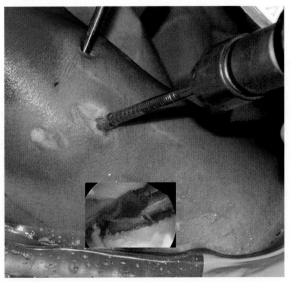

Figure 56-8. Overburring of guide pin to make the slot. *Inset:* arthroscopic view.

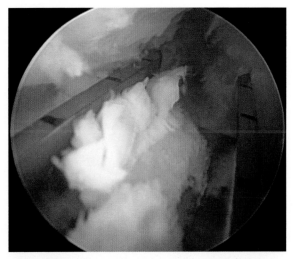

Figure 56-9. View of the box cutter connecting the superficial reference slot and deeper bur tunnel.

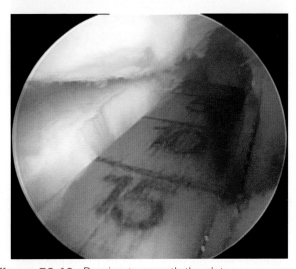

Figure 56-10. Rasping to smooth the slot.

4. Meniscal Allograft Preparation

This technique uses a bone bridge to secure the graft to the tibial plateau. The bone bridge is intentionally undersized by 1 mm to facilitate graft passage and to reduce the risk of inadvertent bridge fracture during insertion. The attachment sites of the meniscus are identified on the bone block, and the accessory attachments are debrided. Only the true attachment sites should remain, usually 5 to 6 mm wide. The bone bridge is then cut to a width of 7 mm and a height of 1 cm. Also, any bone extending beyond the posterior horn attachment site is removed; bone anterior to the attachment site of the anterior horn should be preserved to maintain graft integrity during insertion. A vertical mattress traction suture of No. 0 polydioxanone (PDS) is placed at the junction of the posterior and middle thirds of the meniscus (Fig. 56-11).

On occasion, the anterior horn attachment can be larger, up to 9 mm wide. If the anterior horn attachment

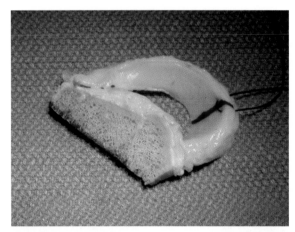

Figure 56-11. Prepared allograft with traction suture.

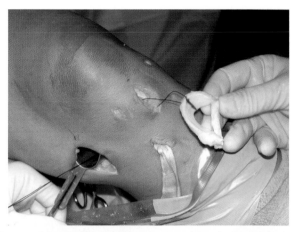

Figure 56-13. The traction sutures have been passed through the accessory incision with the nitinol pin.

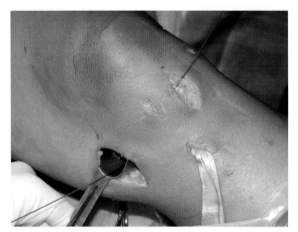

Figure 56-12. Nitinol wire in place. Also shown is an Achilles tendon allograft for anterior cruciate ligament reconstruction.

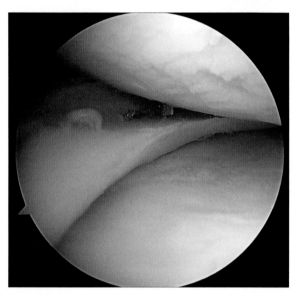

Figure 56-14. The reduced meniscus and bridge situated in the slot.

site is wider than the intended width of the bone bridge, the attachment should be left intact, and the width of the bone bridge should be increased accordingly in the area of the anterior horn insertion only; the remainder of the bone bridge should be trimmed to 7 mm as intended. To accommodate the increased width, the corresponding area of the recipient slot should be widened accordingly.

5. Meniscus Insertion and Fixation

A single-barrel, zone-specific meniscal repair cannula is placed through the contralateral portal with viewing through the ipsilateral portal. The cannula is directed toward the capsular attachment site of the junction of the posterior and middle thirds of the meniscus. A long, flexible nitinol suture-passing pin is placed through the capsule to exit the accessory posteromedial or posterolateral incision. The proximal end of the nitinol pin is then withdrawn from the anterior arthrotomy site (Fig. 56-12), the allograft traction sutures are passed through the loop of the nitinol pin, and the pin and sutures are withdrawn through the accessory incision (Fig. 56-13).

With the aid of the traction sutures, the meniscal allograft is pulled into the joint through the anterior arthrotomy while the bone bridge is advanced into the tibial slot, and the meniscus is manually reduced under the condyle with a finger placed through the arthrotomy (Fig. 56-14). Appropriate valgus or varus stress to open the ipsilateral compartment aids in graft introduction and reduction. Once the meniscus has been reduced, the knee is cycled to ensure proper placement and capturing by the tibiofemoral articulation, and the bone bridge is secured within the tibial slot with a bioabsorbable cortical interference screw.

Alternatively, the bone bridge can be secured with transosseous sutures. With this technique, two transosseous tunnels are created with an anterior cruciate ligament (ACL) tibial aimer and guide pin, starting at the anteromedial proximal tibia. One tunnel exits the floor of the tibial slot in the most posterior aspect, and the other exits anteriorly, both approximating the root

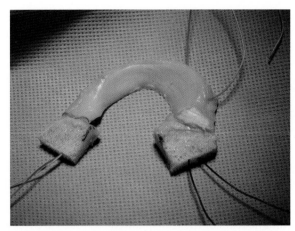

Figure 56-15. Alternate graft preparation technique for suture fixation. In this instance the central third of the bone bridge was removed to allow for concomitant revision anterior cruciate ligament reconstruction.

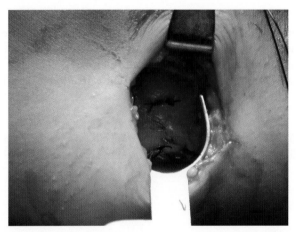

Figure 56-16. Capsular sutures for the meniscal repair as viewed through the posteromedial incision.

attachment sites. Pull sutures are placed with use of a suture passer. During preparation of the meniscal transplant, small holes are drilled through the bone bridge into the footprint of each meniscal root, with care taken not to wrap up the soft tissues with the drill bit. No. 2 nonresorbable sutures are brought through the hole, around the meniscal root, and back through the hole (Fig. 56-15). The sutures are then shuttled through the transosseous tunnels and tied over a bone bridge on the anteromedial tibia after the graft has been seated.

Finally, the graft is attached to the capsule with standard inside-out vertical mattress sutures placed equally on the dorsal and ventral meniscal surfaces (Fig. 56-16). This fixation can be supplemented with appropriate all-inside fixation devices placed most posteriorly and outside-in suture placed most anteriorly.

6. Closure

Standard closure of the arthrotomy and accessory incisions is performed.

Combined Procedures

Anterior Cruciate Ligament Reconstruction and Medial Meniscus Allograft Transplantation

- Prepare the soft tissue graft (hamstring autograft or Achilles tendon, tibialis anterior, or hamstring allograft).
- Drill the tibial tunnel for the ACL as obliquely as possible, entering the lateral aspect of the tibial footprint.
- Drill the femoral tunnel for the ACL.
- Prepare the meniscal slot as usual.
- Pass and fix the femoral side of the ACL graft.
- Pass the meniscus and reduce the soft tissue and bone components. This is facilitated by use of transosseous suture fixation with removal of the middle third of the bone bridge (see Fig. 56-15). Otherwise, the bone plug technique can be used.
- Fix the tibial side of the ACL graft.
- Place interference screw against the meniscus bridge (between the ACL and the most lateral aspect of bridge).
- Repair the meniscus.
- *Note:* Notching the bone bridge may reduce the intersection pressure of the ACL graft against the bone bridge.

Tibial Osteotomy and Medial Meniscus Allograft Transplantation

- Perform all aspects of meniscus transplantation first.
- Perform opening wedge osteotomy such that the line of the osteotomy passes at least 1.5 cm below the bottom of the tibial slot.

POSTOPERATIVE CONSIDERATIONS

Follow-up

- At 7 to 10 days for suture removal and postoperative radiographs (Fig. 56-17).

Rehabilitation

- Immediate partial weight bearing is allowed in a hinged knee brace; range of motion is limited to 0 to 90 degrees of flexion.
- Non–weight-bearing flexion beyond 90 degrees is allowed immediately.
- Full weight bearing and range of motion and gentle strengthening exercises are initiated at 4 weeks postoperatively.
- In-line running is permitted after 16 weeks.

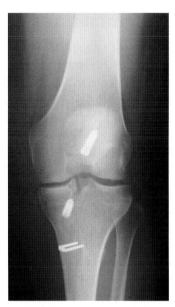

Figure 56-17. Postoperative radiograph (concomitant anterior cruciate ligament reconstruction).

- Return to full activities is permitted after 6 months, once strength has returned to more than 80% that of the contralateral leg.

Complications

Complications are those of meniscal repair:

- Incomplete healing of the meniscus repair
- Infection
- Arthrofibrosis
- Neurovascular injury (saphenous nerve medially, peroneal nerve laterally)

Traumatic tears of the transplanted meniscus are treated with standard arthroscopic meniscal repair or partial meniscectomy as indicated.

RESULTS

After meniscal allograft transplantation, good to excellent results are achieved in nearly 85% of procedures, and patients demonstrate a measurable decrease in pain and increase in activity level (Table 56-1). The risk of graft failure appears greatest with irradiated grafts,

TABLE 56-1. Clinical Results of Meniscal Allograft Transplantation		
Study	**Follow-up**	**Outcome**
Milachowski[11] (1989)	1.2 years mean	19 (86%) of 22 successful
Garrett[7] (1993)	2-7 years	35 (81%) of 43 successful
Noyes[12] (1995)	2.5 years mean	56 (58%) of 96 failed
van Arkel[16] (1995)	2-5 years	20 (87%) of 23 successful
Cameron[2] (1997)	2.5 years mean	58 (92%) of 63 successful
Goble[8] (1996)	2 years minimum	17 (94%) of 18 successful
Carter[5] (1999)	4 years mean	45 (88%) of 51 successful
Rodeo[14] (2001)	2 years minimum	22 (67%) of 33 successful 14 (88%) of 16 with bone fixation 8 (47%) of 17 without bone fixation
Rath[13] (2001)	5.4 years mean	14 (64%) of 22 successful
Verdonk[17] (2005)	7.2 years mean	10 (16%) of 61 of lateral transplants failed 11 (28%) of 39 of medial transplants failed
Cole[6] (2006)	33.5 months mean	41 (91%) of 45 successful 85% of successful transplants would have surgery again
Sekiya[15] (2006)	3.3 years mean	96% patient-reported improvement Better range of motion in patients with bony fixation
Vundelinckx[18] (2010)	8.9 years mean	45 (92%) of 49 successful Increased preoperative osteoarthritis correlated with decreased outcomes 58% of patients demonstrated no increase in osteoarthritis
LaPrade[10] (2010)	2.5 years mean	35 (88%) of 40 successful

grade III or IV osteoarthritic changes, and residual malalignment or instability.

REFERENCES

1. Alford W, Cole BJ. The indications and technique for meniscal transplant. *Orthop Clin North Am.* 2005;36: 469-484.
2. Cameron JC, Saha S. Meniscal allograft transplantation for unicompartmental arthritis of the knee. *Clin Orthop Relat Res.* 1997;337:164-171.
3. Cole BJ, Rodeo S, Carter T. Allograft meniscus transplantation: indications, techniques, results. *J Bone Joint Surg Am.* 2002;84:1236-1250.
4. Farr J, Meneghini RM, Cole BJ. Allograft interference screw fixation in meniscus transplantation. *Arthroscopy.* 2004;20:322-327.
5. Carter TR. Meniscal allograft transplantation. *Sports Med Arthrosc Rev.* 1999;7:51-62.
6. Cole BJ, Dennis MG, Lee SJ, et al. Prospective evaluation of allograft meniscus transplantation: a minimum 2-year follow-up. *Am J Sports Med.* 2006;34:919-927.
7. Garrett JC. Meniscal transplantation: a review of 43 cases with two to seven year follow-up. *Sports Med Arthrosc Rev.* 1993;1:164-167.
8. Goble EM, Kane SM, Wilcox TR, et al. Meniscal allografts. In: McGinty JB, Caspari RB, Jackson RW, Poehling GG, eds. *Operative Arthroscopy.* Philadelphia: Lippincott-Raven; 1996:317-331.
9. Graf KW, Sekiya JK, Wojtys EM. Long-term results following meniscal allograft transplantation: minimum eight and one half-year follow-up. *Arthroscopy.* 2004;20: 129-140.
10. LaPrade RF, Wills NJ, Spiridonov SI, et al. A prospective outcomes study of meniscal allograft transplantation. *Am J Sports Med.* 2010;38:1804-1812.
11. Milachowski KA, Weismeir K, Wirth CJ. Homologous meniscus transplantation: experimental and clinical results. *Int Orthop.* 1989;13:1-11.
12. Noyes FR, Barber-Westin SD. Irradiated meniscus allografts in the human knee: a two to five year follow-up. *Orthop Trans.* 1995;19:417.
13. Rath E, Richmond JC, Yassir W, et al. Meniscal allograft transplantation: two to eight year results. *Am J Sports Med.* 2001;29:410-414.
14. Rodeo SA. Current concepts: meniscus allografts-where do we stand? *Am J Sports Med.* 2001;29:246-261.
15. Sekiya JK, West RV, Groff YJ, et al. Clinical outcomes following isolated lateral meniscal allograft transplantation. *Arthroscopy.* 2006;22:771-780.
16. van Arkel ERA, de Boer HH. Human meniscal transplantation: preliminary results at 2- to 5-year follow-up. *J Bone Joint Surg Br.* 1995;77:589-595.
17. Verdonk PC, Demurie A, Almqvist KF, et al. Transplantation of viable meniscal allograft. Survivorship analysis and clinical outcome of one hundred cases. *J Bone Joint Surg Am.* 2005;87:715-724.
18. Vundelinckx B, Bellemans J, Vanlauwe J. Arthroscopically assisted meniscal allograft transplantation in the knee: a medium-term subjective, clinical, and radiographical outcome evaluation. *Am J Sports Med.* 2010;38: 2240-2247.

Chapter 57

Allograft Meniscus Transplantation: Dovetail Technique

Thomas R. Carter

Chapter Synopsis

- Meniscal allografts have been shown to provide subjective benefit in knees that have undergone meniscectomy. Various surgical techniques have been described, but basic science studies have shown that maintenance of the horn attachments with bone provides superior function. The dovetail technique is a method that provides not only a bone bridge but also a press-fit fixation.

Important Points

- Patients should be symptomatic or have radiographic evidence of stress reaction of the involved compartment.
- Rule out other possible causes of the patient's pain when considering candidates.
- Because of the higher failure rate in knees with advanced arthritis and the limited supply of grafts, meniscal allografts should not be considered a substitute for arthroplasty.
- Any additional pathology (e.g., anterior cruciate ligament [ACL] deficiency) must be corrected to improve success.
- An osteotomy should be done when the mechanical axis passes through the involved compartment, but typically only to the opposite tibial spine rather than to the extent required for an arthritic knee.

Clinical and Surgical Pearls

- Proper placement of the arthroscopic portals has a major effect on allowing complete visualization of the posterior horn, as well as ensuring that the channel is a straight line between the two meniscus attachments. The contralateral portal is made first and hugs the patellar tendon. A spinal needle is used to ensure straight alignment before the ipsilateral portal is made.

Any obliquity on the ipsilateral side can result in improper channel alignment.

- On occasion, the graft has a tendency to be pulled outward when it is sutured. Placement of the initial few sutures in horizontal fashion on the superior aspect of the meniscus can aid in maintaining proper position.
- If the meniscus excision left no meniscal rim, all-inside sutures should be used with caution. With only the capsule to secure the graft, they tend to entrap the capsule and limit full extension or result in the meniscus being pulled outward during the repair.
- It is important to have the graft-bone channel match the height of the tibial plateau. If it is too high, the bone will impinge above on the femoral condyle and make reduction into the knee difficult and also limit knee motion. If the graft-bone is recessed in the channel, it can pull the meniscus down into the channel and as a result not allow sufficient graft at the outer border to suture. In such a case the graft is removed, and slivers from the cut bone are packed at the channel base to raise the height.
- If the bone is inserted too far into the channel, a threaded K-wire can be drilled into the end to remove the graft. If the channel preparation does not result in a press-fit, a bioscrew can be used along the side of the bone to secure it.

Clinical and Surgical Pitfalls

- Although it is technically easier to implant the meniscus without bone, basic science studies show that horn attachments secured by bone better replicate the normal meniscus.
- Whereas a graft typically heals well in the host, great attention to detail for an anatomic placement of the graft is needed to provide greater function.

The meniscus performs many functions for the well-being of the knee, including load bearing, joint stability, and congruency. With so many roles in maintaining normal knee function, it is of little debate that excision results in an increased risk of arthritis. Unfortunately, the ideal replacement for the meniscus has yet to be discovered. At present, meniscal allografts have served as the most successful substitute. Whereas the durability and the ability to prevent or to delay arthritis are questioned, studies have shown that patients typically have less pain and improved function after meniscus implantation. However, the indications are narrow, and the procedure is technically challenging.

Many surgical methods have been described for meniscal allograft transplantation. They are typically classified into two broad categories on the basis of securing the meniscus at its attachment sites with bone or without bone. Although bone fixation techniques are more difficult, several basic science studies have shown that they more closely replicate normal meniscus stress force protection. Although a few clinical studies report no difference in outcome when bone fixation is not used, until comparative long-term studies have been completed, bone fixation methods are recommended.

Within the bone fixation category, several techniques are used. These include bone plugs, the keyhole method, the slot technique, and the dovetail technique. Each has its pros and cons. I prefer the dovetail technique for the lateral meniscus and bone plugs for the medial meniscus. The rationale for the medial side takes into consideration that the distance between the anterior and posterior horns is typically 2.5 to 3 cm, with a highly variable anterior attachment site. Having the horns separate (i.e., two separate bone plugs) enables placement of the bone plugs to match the native meniscus insertion sites. Because the anterior and posterior horns of the native lateral meniscus are usually only a centimeter apart, the presence of two bone tunnels in such close proximity would create a great risk that the tunnels would converge and compromise fixation. As a result, a bone bridge between the horns is recommended on the lateral side. The dovetail method enables not only preparation of the channel under direct observation but also a press-fit fixation.

PREOPERATIVE CONSIDERATIONS

History

Not all patients who have undergone meniscectomy go on to develop arthritis, and with the supply of meniscus limited to only a few thousand per year, candidates need to be selected wisely. Treatment may be considered simply as a preventative measure although the patient has no symptoms and only limited meniscectomy. At present there is general agreement that the first considerations for meniscal allograft are a history of the patient being symptomatic and confirmation that the majority of the meniscus has been excised.

Typical History

The typical history for appropriate candidates is as follows:

- Symptoms are localized to the involved compartment.
- Discomfort is commonly present with activities of daily living and enhanced activity.
- Joint effusions may occur and are commonly activity related.

Physical Examination

Possible candidates typically have minimal physical findings beyond joint line tenderness and, at most, mild joint effusions.

More often, patients have findings that may preclude surgical candidacy, such as the following:

- Evidence of diffuse arthritis: palpable osteophytes, decreased range of motion, marked crepitus
- Ligamentous instability (needs to be corrected before or at the time of implantation)
- Limb malalignment (if mechanical axis is through involved compartment, may need realignment)
- Morbid obesity
- Other limb or back abnormalities

Imaging

Radiography

Include a magnification marker for reference in graft sizing.

- Weight-bearing 45-degree posteroanterior view
- Weight-bearing anteroposterior view in full extension
- Non–weight-bearing 45-degree lateral view
- Axial view of the patellofemoral joint
- Full-length view of limb for mechanical axis evaluation

Other Modalities

Magnetic resonance imaging is performed if there is a question of degree of meniscectomy or associated pathologic change or to evaluate bone stress reaction.

Historically, bone scans can be performed if there is a question of reactive changes in the joint and if localized only to the involved knee compartment. However, magnetic resonance scans are just as useful for this purpose and have superseded the use of bone scans.

Indications and Contraindications

The ideal candidate is a patient who has had a prior meniscectomy in an otherwise normal knee and experiences pain localized to the involved compartment. The degree of articular cartilage damage is slight and is found only in the affected side. The knee is without ligament laxity, and the limb alignment is similar to that of the contralateral leg.

However such ideal patients are few. Consideration may be given to patients with grade III chondrosis but not diffuse knee involvement. Patients with grade IV chondromalacia are not candidates, unless there is a localized defect that can be corrected with joint repair or restoration-type procedures. Associated pathologic processes, such as ligament instability and limb malalignment, provided correction can be performed, do not exclude patients.

Contraindications are advanced arthrosis of the involved compartment and diffuse knee joint chondrosis. Comorbidities that are not correctable are exclusion criteria. Obesity, inflammatory arthropathy, and avascular necrosis are also contraindications. Unrealistic expectations of the patient should also be taken into consideration (the knee will not be returned to normal).

Surgical Planning

Concomitant Procedures

Ligament instability and contained chondral defects are addressed at the time of the meniscus implantation. Controversy exists as to whether limb realignment should be performed any time the mechanical axis passes through the involved compartment or only if there is a measurable difference between the two legs. I typically will perform an osteotomy when the comparative mechanical axis of the lower extremities shows more than 2 to 3 degrees toward the involved side consistent with the degeneration of the joint. Apart from this debate, limb realignment procedures are usually performed when the meniscus is implanted.

If both osteotomy and ligament reconstructions are necessary, it is common to stage the procedures because of concerns regarding tunnel or screw overlap and associated adequate fixation. My preference is to perform the osteotomy first, then after healing perform the meniscus and ligament reconstructions.

Allograft Sizing

Various methods have been used for sizing of meniscal allografts to match the host. Although magnetic resonance images and computed tomographic scans can be used, plain radiographs are the most common means. Anteroposterior and lateral views are obtained with a magnification marker placed at the level of the joint line. Any obliquity or rotation that may affect measurement of the tibial plateau is not acceptable. Regardless of the method of sizing the graft, it is prudent for the treating surgeon to verify the size match.

Meniscal Graft Processing and Preservation

Although the risk of disease transmission from meniscal allografts is minimal, it still exists. It is thus vital to ensure that the tissue bank has been certified by the American Association of Tissue Banks. To obtain the certification, the bank must follow stringent methods of procurement and processing of the allograft tissue. In addition, as with any allograft, an immune response can occur. The immune load is particularly greater with fresh tissue. Thus because of the increased risk of disease transmission and possible immune reaction, fresh meniscal allografts are not recommended.

The most commonly used grafts are cryopreserved or frozen. Whereas some degree of cell viability is able to be achieved with cryopreservation, the clinical benefit compared with frozen grafts, which are acellular, has not been determined. Lyophilization (i.e., freeze-drying) eliminates contamination, but it is not recommended because of the deleterious effect it has on the structural integrity of the meniscal allograft.

SURGICAL TECHNIQUE

Anesthesia and Positioning

The procedure is typically performed with the patient under general anesthesia. The patient's position and the setup are the same as the surgeon's preference in performing a meniscus repair.

Surgical Landmarks, Incisions, and Portals

Landmarks

- Patella
- Patellar tendon
- Tibial plateau
- Fibular head (lateral meniscus)

Portals and Approaches

- Anteromedial: border of patellar tendon
- Anterolateral: border of patellar tendon
- Outflow portal as desired
- Posteromedial or posterolateral: ipsilateral portal graft for suturing

- Mini-arthrotomy: extend ipsilateral portal for graft insertion

Structures at Risk
- Popliteal structures: nerve, artery, and vein
- Posteromedial approach: saphenous nerve
- Posterolateral approach: peroneal nerve, popliteal tendon

Examination Under Anesthesia and Diagnostic Arthroscopy

The meniscal allograft should not be opened before a complete physical examination of the knee and diagnostic arthroscopy have been performed. Their significance is to confirm that the patient is a candidate for a meniscal allograft.

Specific Steps

The specific steps of this procedure are outlined in Box 57-1.

1. Arthroscopic Host Site Preparation

The initial arthroscopic portal should be established on the side opposite the graft and immediately adjacent to the patellar tendon border. Use of this approach enables passage of the scope through the notch and visualization of the posterior horn attachment, which is vital to graft positioning. Before the involved compartment portal is made, a spinal needle is used to confirm that the portal site is directly in line with the horn attachments. Any obliquity in the skin incision to the horn attachments can cause difficulty in the proper orientation when the bone channel is prepared. Once the portals have been made, the meniscal remnant is debrided to approximately a 2-mm outer border vascular rim (Figs. 57-1 and 57-2). Rather than arthroscopically, the anterior segment can also be debrided through the arthrotomy made later to insert the graft. To ensure proper channel height and alignment, a shaver or bur is used to remove the tibial spine to a height that is equal to the level of the tibial plateau articular cartilage and straight in line with the attachment sites (Fig. 57-3). If there is still any difficulty in full visualization of the posterior horn attachment, a limited notchplasty should be performed.

BOX 57-1 Surgical Steps

1. Arthroscopic host site preparation
2. Meniscal allograft preparation
3. Arthrotomy with graft insertion
4. Securing of graft
5. Closure

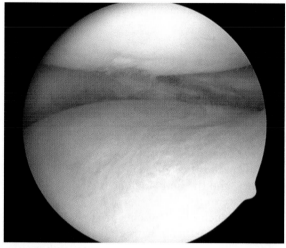

Figure 57-1. Lateral compartment showing complete meniscectomy.

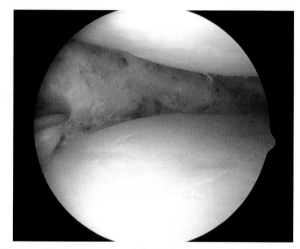

Figure 57-2. Remnant debrided to a bleeding border.

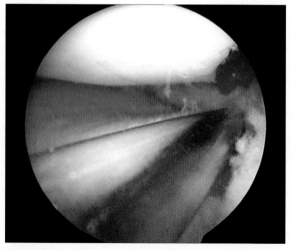

Figure 57-3. Shaver used to initial channel in-line with attachments.

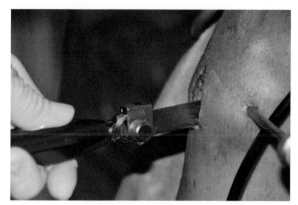

Figure 57-4. Osteotome placed into knee and used as a drill guide.

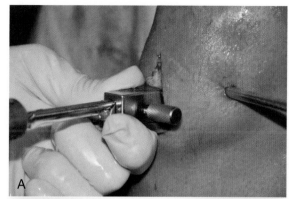

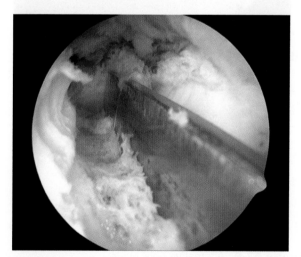

Figure 57-5. A, Drill guide attached to osteotome. **B,** View of drill following the osteotome.

Likewise, the entire anterior attachment needs to be seen to ensure that the channel is begun at the proper height. Although a tourniquet can be inflated at any time, it is typically not done so until this point. Waiting allows confirmation of a vascular rim and conserves tourniquet time. Higher pressure and inflow rates are often needed to limit bleeding during bone channel preparation, which is why the tourniquet may be required at this point in the procedure.

The ipsilateral portal is extended to approximately 3 cm in length. The osteotome is brought into the knee and used as a guide for further channel preparation (Fig. 57-4). It follows the initial trough and is placed at the most central aspect of the knee near the notch (hugging the anterior cruciate ligament [ACL] insertion) to allow room for proper drill placement. A guideline on the osteotome is followed to ensure the proper depth in the tibial plateau at all times. The osteotome should be inserted to 1 or 2 mm just short of the back of the plateau to maintain a back wall and prevent overinsertion of the graft. The initial osteotome attachment guide is placed and allows a 6-mm drill to initiate the channel under direct visualization (Figs. 57-5 and 57-6). The second osteotome attachment is used for placement of a 7-mm drill just beneath the level of the first drill. The second drill is used to deepen the channel and can also be seen at all times to ensure proper placement. A rasp and tamp dilator finish the dovetail slot by expanding the channel and compressing the cancellous bone at its borders (Figs. 57-7 and 57-8).

An alternative method for performance of the initial step for the channel preparation is to use a drill guide (Fig. 57-9). The benefits are that it is technically less challenging and less time-consuming; the downside is that the drill pins are not visualized at all times, and therefore there is an increased risk of neurovascular injury. The drill guide is placed in line with the initial burred trough and secured to the tibia, similar to a posterior cruciate ligament guide for comparison. Two drill sleeves are placed within the guide, and guidewires

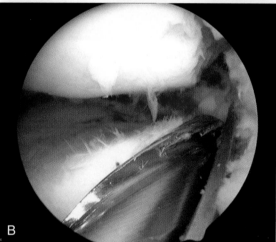

Figure 57-6. Channel after first drill.

are advanced into the sleeves, stopping just sort of the tibial cortex. Calibrations on the tibial drill guide can be used to determine the appropriate pin length. Once the guidewires have been placed, the drill sleeves are removed and the pins are drilled in a similar manner to placement of the osteotome guide.

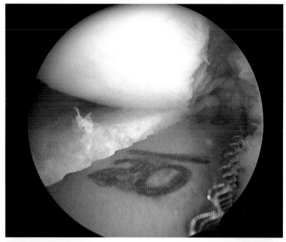

Figure 57-7. Rasp inserted to complete channel.

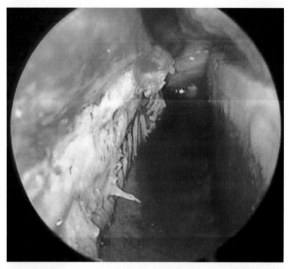

Figure 57-8. Appearance of completed dovetail slot.

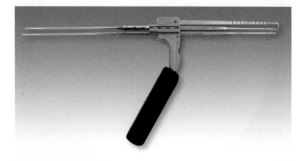

Figure 57-9. Alternative tibial guide.

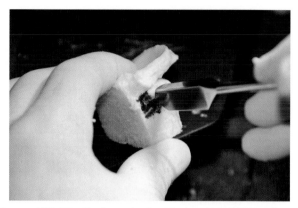

Figure 57-10. Graft marked with the dovetail template.

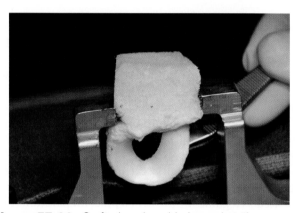

Figure 57-11. Graft placed upside in workstation.

2. Meniscal Allograft Preparation

One of the main benefits of the dovetail method is the use of cutting guides to prepare the graft, rather than preparation by a freehand technique. As a result, it not only saves time but, more important, decreases the chance of an improper match between the recipient channel and graft. The graft is initially trimmed of any bone and soft tissues so that the horn attachments are flush with the ends of the allograft bone. The trapezoidal rasp for the slot preparation is then used to mark the graft as a dovetail template (Fig. 57-10). The graft is inserted upside-down into the workstation and secured with the side attachments (Fig. 57-11). The three cutting guides are placed in sequential order, and with a sagittal saw the vertical, horizontal, and oblique cuts are made, resulting in a dovetail design (Fig. 57-12).

The dovetail graft sizer is used to confirm that the allograft will slide through the channel. The fit should be snug to allow a press fit, but not so tight that the graft does not slide through smoothly (Fig. 57-13). Any minor adjustments should be made at this time rather than attempted during insertion of the graft.

3. Arthrotomy with Graft Insertion

As with a standard meniscus repair by inside-out technique, a posteromedial or posterolateral incision is made to retrieve the meniscal sutures. A "reduction" suture is placed through the graft at the 10- or 2-o'clock position, passed into the joint, and retrieved. Proper placement of the reduction suture is important. When it is placed in the middle of the graft, there is a

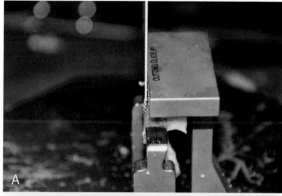

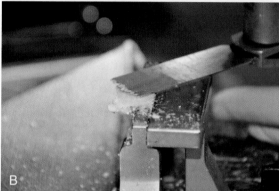

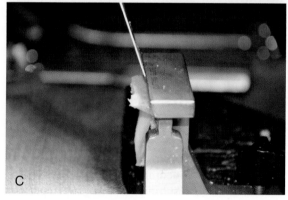

Figure 57-12. Three cutting guides complete the graft preparation.

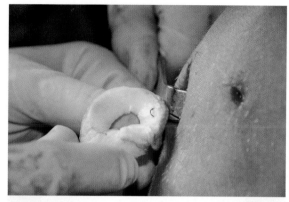

Figure 57-14. Graft brought into the knee, including the reduction suture.

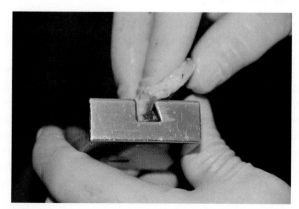

Figure 57-13. Graft sizer used to confirm size and press fit capability.

tendency for the graft to be pulled outward and not fully reduce into the knee. With the suture retrieved, the meniscus is inserted into the channel and gently pushed inward while the surgeon carefully pulls on the suture (Fig. 57-14). Extreme force should not be used because the sutures can be pulled through the graft, and the bone bridge can be either fractured or inserted too far into the channel. Provided the channel and the graft bone are of proper size, a tamp can be used to gently assist in insertion of the bone bridge. Care must be taken on insertion of the graft, because too much force may break out the posterior wall. Gentle tension on the reduction suture and application of an appropriate amount of varus or valgus stress on the knee aid in reduction of the meniscus.

Once the graft has been reduced, there is a tendency to first repair the anterior aspect of the graft under direct visualization before the arthrotomy is closed. However, to assist in anatomic placement, one or two sutures should initially be placed in the posterior then middle segments. The anterior horn, because it is more amendable to change in positioning, is secured last. If there is a graft size mismatch and the anterior horn is sutured first, the graft has a tendency to extrude when too large, and if too small to apply excessive tension on the repair sutures. Once the graft placement is complete, the arthrotomy is closed and suturing is completed.

4. Securing of Graft

Numerous methods can be used to secure the graft, but inside-out vertical mattress sutures are preferred because of greater strength.

An all-inside technique can be used, but if the remnant of the graft is small, special care must be taken to not entrap the capsule when these devices are used. Either absorbable or nonabsorbable sutures can be used; healing of the graft to the host readily occurs. Eight to 10 sutures are typically all that is needed (Fig. 57-15).

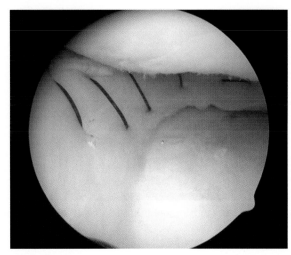

Figure 57-15. Completed meniscal allograft.

5. Closure

The wounds are closed, and a dressing is applied according to the treating surgeon's preference. A postoperative brace is applied and initially locked in full extension.

Combined Procedures

Anterior Cruciate Ligament Reconstruction and Meniscal Allograft Transplantation

- Arthroscopic preparation for both procedures is performed first, including meniscus channel and the ACL tunnels.
- The meniscus is placed and sutured.
- The ACL graft is passed and secured last.
- Proper tunnel and channel placements should not result in overlap.
- The meniscus is completed first to decrease difficulty in meniscus insertion.

Tibial Osteotomy and Meniscal Allograft Transplantation

- Meniscus implantation is completed first.
- Osteotomy is performed second for significant varus or valgus stress to open the joint, because meniscus repair can put significant stress on osteotomy.
- Perform the osteotomy line as low as possible to avoid disruption of dovetail bone.

Tibial Osteotomy, Anterior Cruciate Ligament Reconstruction, and Meniscal Allograft Transplantation

- These procedures are typically staged because of the concern for overlap of channel, tunnels, and screws resulting in poor fixation.
- Osteotomy is performed first, then ACL reconstruction and meniscus implantation after the osteotomy is healed.

POSTOPERATIVE CONSIDERATIONS

Follow-up

- The initial postoperative visit is at 7 to 10 days with anteroposterior and lateral radiographs obtained as a baseline study.
- Monthly visits are common until a stationary point has been attained.

Rehabilitation

- A brace is applied in full extension after the procedure. Range of motion is permitted once the patient is able to perform straight-leg raises.
- Partial weight bearing with the postoperative brace set at 0 to 90 degrees is permitted during the initial 4 weeks.
- Full weight bearing and unrestricted range of motion are permitted after 4 weeks.
- Progressive strengthening and functional training similar to ACL protocols are followed.
- Running is permitted at 12 weeks.
- Return to full activities is permitted at 4 months if strength is 80% or greater compared with the contralateral limb with normal functional testing. However, most patients do not achieve these goals until 5 to 6 months postoperatively.

Complications

- Infection
- Arthrofibrosis
- Neurovascular injury during implantation
- Meniscus tear or incomplete healing
- Graft extrusion resulting from improper placement or size
- Loss of bone fixation or fracture

RESULTS

The initial studies reported mixed results with meniscal allografts; however, the indications and surgical techniques were diverse.

Some series included grafts placed in severely arthritic knees; others used the inferior lyophilized grafts. As the indications and techniques have become refined, the results have improved significantly. Many long-term studies report that the majority of patients have good to excellent results, with a graft survival rate of approximately 80% at 10 years. However, the studies also show that the ability of meniscal allografts to slow the progression of arthritis is still unproven.

Although the number of short-term and midterm clinical studies are numerous, the number of long-term

TABLE 57-1. Results of Studies of Meniscal Allografts

Study	Follow-up (Mean)	Study Size	Clinical Results	Information Gained
Garrett[3] (1993)	2-7 years (unknown)	43 patients 44 grafts	35 of 43 successful 20 of 28 intact at second-look arthroscopy 8 failures related to arthrosis	Grafts can reliably heal Advanced arthrosis results in failure
Noyes and Barber-Westin[4] (1995)	22-58 months (30 months)	82 patients 96 grafts	58% of failed grafts were lyophilized Majority of patients had advanced arthrosis	Arthritic knees and lyophilized grafts have high failure rates
Carter[5] (1999)	24-73 months (35 months)	46 patients 46 grafts	45 patients had improvement in pain 38 grafts were healed at second-look arthroscopy	Successful outcome with stringent patient selection Excellent healing to host
Rodeo[6] (2001)	Range unknown (2-year minimum)	33 patients 33 grafts	22 of 33 successful: 14 of 16 with bone fixation, 8 of 17 without bone	Bone fixation results are more favorable than when horns are not secured with bone
Wirth et al[7] (2002)	12-15 years (14 years)	22 patients 23 grafts	Magnetic resonance imaging evaluation: 6 deep frozen, similar to normal meniscus; 17 lyophilized, similar to meniscectomy	Arthritis progression slowed with use of frozen grafts
Verdonk et al[8] (2005)	5-14.5 (7.2 years)	100 grafts 96 patients	Cumulative survival of 74% medial and 70% lateral at 5 years; 14 of 17 survived when osteotomy also performed	High rate of success with strict indications Need to address malalignment Results deteriorate with time
Cole et al[9] (2006)	24-57 months (33.5 months)	45 patients	41 of 45 successful	High rate of success with strict indications
Hommen et al[10] (2007)	115-167 months (141 months)	20 grafts 20 patients	18 of 20 had improvement in Lysholm and pain scores 5 complete and 2 partial meniscectomies Multiple surgical techniques Half of series had grade III or IV chondromalacia	Stringent patient selection and standardized surgical technique are important for success
van der Wal et al[11] (2009)	13.8 ± 2.8 years	57 patients 63 grafts	Cumulative survival rates of 76%, 50%, and 67% for lateral, medial, and combined, respectively 19 patients with grade IV chondromalacia and 3 with ACL deficiency had higher failure rate	Arthritic and unstable knees have decreased success Results deteriorate over time
Carter and Rabago[12] (2011)	10-year follow-up (minimum 10 years)	40 patients 41 grafts	39 of 40 improvement symptoms at 2 years 32 of 40 at 10 years 7 partial meniscectomies: IV beyond 7 years: graft survivorship (83%) at 10 years Radiographs: 14 no change, 15 mild, 5 moderate to advanced	Patient selection vital to success Grafts not able to uniformly stop progression of arthritis Ability to slow progression still unclear
Saltzman et al[13] (2012)	8.49 years (minimum 7 years)	25 patients 25 grafts	Statistically significant improvement in IKDC, Lysholm scales 3 partial meniscectomies: graft survivorship 88%	Grafts are durable Able to provide subjective improvement long term

IKDC, International Knee Documentation Committee.

studies is still small. Table 57-1 summarizes the majority of long-term studies.

REFERENCES

1. Chen MI, Branch TP, Hutton WC. Is it important to secure the horns of the lateral meniscal transplantation? A cadaveric study. *Arthroscopy*. 1996;12:174-181.

2. Pollard ME, Kang Q, Berg EE. Radiographic sizing for meniscal transplantation. *Arthroscopy*. 1995;11:684-687.

3. Garrett JC. Meniscal transplantation: a review of 43 cases with two to seven year follow-up. *Sports Med Arthrosc Rev*. 1993;2:164-167.

4. Noyes FR, Barber-Westin SD, Rankin M. Meniscal transplantation in symptomatic patients less than fifty years old. *J Bone Joint Surg Am*. 2004;86:1392-1404.

5. Carter TR. Meniscal allograft transplantation. *Sports Med Arthrosc Rev.* 1999;7:51-62.

6. Rodeo SA. Meniscal allografts: where do we stand? *Am J Sports Med.* 2001;29:246-261.

7. Wirth CJ, Peters G, Milachowski KA, et al. Long-term results of meniscal allograft transplantation. *Am J Sports Med.* 2002;30:174-181.

8. Verdonk PC, Demurie A, Almqvist KF, et al. Transplantation of viable meniscal allograft. Survivorship analysis and clinical outcome of one hundred cases. *J Bone Joint Surg Am.* 2005;87:715-724.

9. Cole BJ, Dennis MG, Lee SJ, et al. Prospective evaluation of allograft meniscus transplantation: a minimum 2-year follow-up. *Am J Sports Med.* 2006;34:919-927.

10. Hommen JP, Applegate GR, Del Pizzo W. Meniscus allograft transplantation: ten-year results of cryopreserved allografts. *Arthroscopy.* 2007;23:388-393.

11. van der Wal RJ, Thomassen BJ, van Arkel ER. Long-term clinical outcome of open meniscal allograft transplantation. *Am J Sports Med.* 2009;37:2134-2139.

12. Carter TR, Rabago M. *Meniscal allograft transplantation: ten-year follow-up.* Presented at the 78th Annual meeting of the American Academy of Orthopedic Surgeons, San Diego, CA February 2011.

13. Saltzman BM, Bajaj S, Salata M, et al. *Prospective long-term evaluation of allograft meniscus transplantation: a minimum 7-year follow-up.* Presented at the 78th Annual Meeting of the American Academy of Orthopedic Surgeons, San Diego CA, February 2011.

SUGGESTED READINGS

Cole B, Carter T, Rodeo S. Allograft meniscal transplantation: background, techniques, and results. *J Bone Joint Surg Am.* 2002;84:1236-1250.

Hergan D, Thut D, Sherman O, et al. A systemic review: meniscal allograft transplantation. *Arthroscopy.* 2011; 27:101-112.

Rijk PC. Meniscal allograft transplantation-part I: background, results, graft selection and preservation, and surgical considerations. *Arthroscopy.* 2004;20:728-743.

Chapter 58

Arthroscopic Meniscus Transplantation: Bone Plug

Alex Dukas, Michael Pensak, Zachary Stender, and Thomas DeBerardino

Chapter Synopsis

- Arthroscopic meniscal allograft transplantation (MAT) has the potential to relieve pain and increase knee function within a subset of patients with badly damaged menisci or after subtotal or total meniscectomy. The arthroscopic bone plug technique allows a surgeon to match the allograft to the patient's specific anatomy and to perform concomitant procedures while achieving the benefits of minimally invasive surgery. This chapter outlines the indications, contraindications, and surgical technique required to optimize the chances of a successful outcome.

Important Points

- Arthroscopic MAT has been shown to provide pain relief and increased function.
- Ideal candidates should be younger than 50 years.
- Articular cartilage damage must be minimal (Outerbridge grade I or II).
- Mechanical alignment and joint stability must be optimal or able to be corrected at the time of MAT.
- Bone plugs allow for allograft fixation that precisely matches the patient's own anatomy.

Clinical and Surgical Pearls

- Restore mechanical alignment and soft tissue stability to the knee.

- Use different-appearing sutures to avoid confusion.
- Mark the graft with the correct orientation to avoid any confusion should twisting or flipping occur during graft reduction.
- Mark the superior edge of the bone plug to allow for proper depth placement.
- Perform an adequate notchplasty and flattening of the tibial eminence to allow for visualization of the posterior horn socket.

Clinical and Surgical Pitfalls

- Failure to address mechanical malalignment and/or concomitant pathology will result in failure of MAT even with an anatomic reconstruction.
- Avoid meniscal extrusion by first securing the allograft to the posterior horn then to the anterior horn, followed by the body to the capsule.

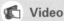 Video

- Video 58-1: Arthroscopic meniscus transplantation

The meniscus plays an important role in load transmission, shock absorption, stability, articular cartilage nutrition, and lubrication within the knee joint. Removal of this important anatomic structure results in eventual joint degeneration. Because of this, the standard of care for meniscal injuries has focused on meniscal preservation and repair techniques in an effort to safeguard joint cartilage. However, in some situations these techniques are not appropriate, and total or subtotal meniscectomy is necessary. Meniscal allograft transplantation (MAT) is a viable option in a subpopulation of these patients.

Many different techniques are used for MAT, and none has been shown to be definitively superior to the others. The senior author (T.D.) advocates an all-arthroscopic technique with use of individual bone plugs for both medial and lateral MAT for the following reasons:

1. Arthroscopic technique allows for anatomic placement of both meniscal horns, which minimizes meniscal extrusion and maximizes hoop stresses, presumably leading to enhanced knee kinematics.
2. Bone plugs can be adapted to a patient's individual anatomy.
3. Concomitant surgical procedures can be performed at the time of MAT to address ligamentous instability, mechanical malalignment, and cartilaginous defects.
4. An all-arthroscopic technique is minimally invasive and can be used in an outpatient setting.

PREOPERATIVE CONSIDERATIONS

Indications

Success of MAT hinges on proper patient selection. Prior total or subtotal meniscectomy and pain with activity localized to the meniscectomized compartment are the most common indications. Ideally patients should be younger than 50 years, have minimal Outerbridge changes to their articular cartilage (grade I or II), and possess an optimal mechanical environment from a stability and alignment perspective. Patients who do not fit all these criteria at the time of clinical presentation should not be precluded from undergoing MAT. Instead, a detailed single or staged surgical plan should be formulated to make sure that all knee abnormalities are addressed and that native knee anatomy, stability, and kinematics are restored, thereby giving the meniscal allograft the best chance of incorporation at the time of implantation.

Though beyond the scope of this chapter, concomitant procedures performed with MAT include anterior cruciate ligament (ACL) reconstruction, revision ACL reconstruction, posterolateral corner (PLC) reconstruction, osteotomies of the distal femur and proximal tibia to correct for coronal plane malalignment, and any number of procedures to address focal, cartilaginous defects (e.g., autologous chondrocyte implantation [ACI], osteochondral autograft transplantation surgery [OATS]). Patients need to be willing to comply with postoperative rehabilitation protocols and should be thoroughly counseled that the intent of the MAT is to restore knee function and decrease pain, not return patients to their peak, preinjury level of activity, especially high-performance athletes.

Contraindications

Patients should not undergo MAT if they are asymptomatic; possess overt signs of joint degeneration on plain radiographs (joint space narrowing, osteophytes, subchondral cysts, sclerosis); demonstrate diffuse, high-grade cartilage changes (Outerbridge grade III or IV) on magnetic resonance imaging (MRI); or have fixed sagittal or coronal plain deformities. In addition, muscular atrophy, history of knee sepsis, history of inflammatory arthritis, and conditions such as immune disorders, diabetes mellitus, gout, and marked obesity are relative contraindications. Last, but important, patients who are not willing to comply with the postoperative rehabilitation or who seek unrealistic outcomes are not ideal candidates for MAT.

Graft Sizing

Meniscal allografts must be appropriately sized to prevent overstuffing of the joint leading to stiffness, or conversely to prevent undersizing, which leads to poor joint surface coverage and increased forces across the graft. The senior author has consistently used one tissue bank over the course of his career and receives a size-matched meniscal allograft based on the preoperative MRI scan supplied to the tissue bank. Other surgeons use measurements made from radiographs to arrive at the appropriate graft size, but this has not been the experience of the senior author.

Imaging

A standard set of weight-bearing plain radiographs should be obtained for all patients being evaluated for MAT and should include the following views: 45-degree posteroanterior (PA), anteroposterior (AP) in full extension, 45-degree lateral, Merchant views of the patella, and full-length mechanical axis films of the lower extremity. Magnification markers placed on the skin are important for sizing of the meniscal allograft before surgery. CT scan has a limited role in preparing for MAT surgery except when a revision ACL procedure needs to be performed and there is concern for lysis around the bone tunnels. MRI is useful to assess the extent of meniscal damage and the integrity of the articular cartilage, and to identify ligamentous damage and the presence of any subchondral edema. Bone scans have been described in the literature for differentiation of compartment stress overload from overt arthritis, but they are rarely ordered in the clinical setting of patients being evaluated for MAT.

SURGICAL TECHNIQUE

Overview

Many techniques for MAT have been described in the literature. The technique the senior author has used for the past 15 years uses bone plugs to secure either the medial or the lateral meniscal allograft or both to the anatomic insertion sites of both meniscal horns. The graft is placed arthroscopically via the ipsilateral anterior portal and secured to the capsule with permanent inside-out sutures. The bone plugs roughly measure 9 mm in diameter and 7 mm in height; they are placed into 10-mm bone sockets. This particular configuration makes bone plugs a viable option for medial as well as lateral MAT despite the closer proximity of the lateral menisci's horn insertion sites. This technique has relatively low morbidity in the hands of the senior author, enabling it to be performed in the outpatient setting.

Anesthesia and Positioning

The patient is placed supine on the surgical bed with a thigh tourniquet applied, though rarely inflated. A lateral post allows for application of a valgus force to open the medial compartment. The foot of the bed is flexed maximally with enough room behind the passively flexed knee to allow a fist to be placed. Two rolled sheets placed under the pad of the bed prevent hyperextension at the hip. The contralateral lower extremity is safely cradled in a well leg holder with the hip and knee slightly flexed in an abducted position (Fig. 58-1). The graft is checked by the surgeon at least 1 day before the scheduled surgery to verify it is for the correct limb and for the correct compartment. While the patient is being brought into the room and positioned for surgery, the graft is thawed and prepared for transplantation on the back table. The graft is usually ready for implantation as the leg is being prepared and draped. Anesthesia routinely includes a regional block performed in the preoperative area once the patient's site is signed by the surgeon. A general anesthetic is used as well to help expedite the surgery.

Specific Steps

Box 58-1 outlines the specific steps of this procedure.

Graft Preparation

The size-matched meniscal allograft arrives secured to its hemiplateau. The central cut made through the tibial plateau will serve as the medial wall of the anterior and posterior bone plugs. Occasionally the entire plateau and both menisci are provided, and the central cut will have to be made. The first step in graft preparation involves freeing the body of the donor meniscus and removing any extraneous nonmeniscal tissue. With the horn insertion sites clearly identified, a microsagittal saw is used to fashion vertical box cuts around the remaining three sides of the horn insertion sites to a depth of 10 mm. A final transverse cut is made orthogonal to the vertical cuts to free the bony insertions sites from the plateau. The minimal morbidity to the donor plateau mimics the minimal morbidity to the recipient's knee (Fig. 58-2). After the plugs have been freed, a small

---

BOX 58-1 Surgical Steps

Graft Preparation
- Anchoring and vertical sutures
- Guide markings

Knee Preparation
- Removal of meniscal remnant
- Arthroscopic portals and incisions
- Posterior bone plug socket

Graft Placement
- Passage of sutures
- Reduction of graft into knee joint
- Securing of posterior third of graft
- Preparation of anterior horn socket
- Securing of anterior bone plug
- Inside-out sutures through remaining meniscal body

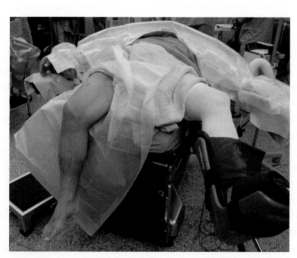

Figure 58-1. Patient positioning for meniscal allograft transplantation procedure.

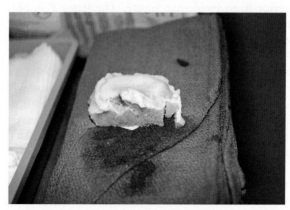

Figure 58-2. Hemiplateau appearance after removal of meniscus.

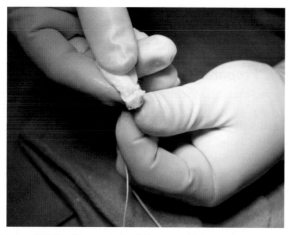

Figure 58-3. Placement of the grasping sutures.

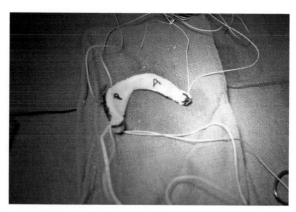

Figure 58-4. Final appearance of a prepared right lateral meniscal allograft.

rongeur is used reshape the plugs from square to cylindric. Both bone plugs are 7 mm in depth, with the anterior measuring 10 mm in diameter and the posterior 9 mm. A small central drill hole is placed through the vertical axis of each bone plug.

A permanent No. 2 suture is passed up through each bone plug from the inferior side, driven across the meniscal insertion tissue, and then passed down through the hole in the plug as illustrated in Figure 58-3. This configuration forms a solid grasping suture for anchoring into the posterior bone socket. For visual differentiation, the senior author uses a solid blue No. 2 FiberWire (Arthrex, Naples, FL) in the posterior horn and a hashmarked TigerWire (Arthrex) in the anterior horn. Two other vertical TigerWire and FiberWire sutures are placed across the full thickness of the posterior horn tissue, one approximately 1 cm from the other. The senior author routinely places a TigerWire suture in the position closest to the posterior horn. This set of sutures will be sequentially passed across the posterior capsule, and the sutures tied to each other, thus securing the posterior horn of the graft to the capsule.

A surgical marker is used to place the letter *A* (anterior) on the graft at the position of the first desired anterior horn inside-out suture. The letter *P* is placed on the superior surface of the meniscus juxtaposed to the second preplaced vertical FiberWire suture (see Fig. 58-3). The visible letters are marked on the graft to maintain visual orientation of the graft in the knee joint and outline the visible confines between which the necessary inside-out sutures will be placed for final graft fixation. An additional mark is placed along the superoposterior margin of the meniscus. These marks serve as visible cues to ensure the graft is not twisting or flipping as it is being reduced into final position across the knee joint. Finally a mark is made on the superior rim of the bone plug to visualize proper depth placement into the bone socket when seen arthroscopically (Fig. 58-4).

Knee Preparation

Any other concomitant procedures need to be planned carefully to avoid harm to the meniscal allograft transplant tissue. A high tibial osteotomy (HTO) is commonly performed in conjunction with MAT to provide for an optimal mechanical environment and to offload the medial compartment to maximize the chance of clinical success. The HTO always precedes the transplantation portion of the procedure. Initially, diagnostic arthroscopy is performed to confirm the adequacy of the lateral compartment to withstand the increased load the HTO will transfer to that compartment. If a distal femoral osteotomy (DFO) is warranted to unload the lateral compartment for a lateral meniscal transplant, the senior author usually performs the DFO as a separate procedure and allows adequate healing time before proceeding with the lateral transplantation. This is largely because of the added morbidity of the DFO as compared with an HTO. Any other planned procedures (e.g., osteochondral allografts, ACI, ACL reconstruction) are completed after the posterior horn and bone plug have been secured to their respective insertion sites. During an ACL reconstruction, the anterior horn is not secured within its anatomic bone socket until the ACL tibial tunnel is made and the ACL graft has been passed. Likewise, protecting the anterior horn in the medial gutter during osteochondral graft placement in the ipsilateral compartment keeps the meniscus out of harm's way and provides excellent exposure for cartilage lesions located on the flexion aspect of the condyle.

Standard arthroscopy portals are used for both medial and lateral MAT procedures. In addition, a posteromedial or posterolateral incision is necessary for medial and lateral MAT procedures, respectively, to allow for reception of the permanent meniscocapsular sutures via an inside-out technique. These 3-cm incisions are the same incisions used for standard arthroscopic repair of medial and lateral meniscal tears with use of inside-out sutures.

Any remnants of the old meniscus need to be carefully removed. A residual small capsular stump can serve as an excellent visible cue for securing the allograft meniscus to its proper anatomic location on the capsule. The anterior and posterior horn insertion sites are cleared of any extraneous soft tissue and residual meniscus down to bone. It is critical to place the allograft meniscus bone plugs in the exact location of the native meniscus insertions.

A 10-mm flexible silicone PassPort cannula (Arthrex) is then placed into the ipsilateral portal to maintain a clear passageway into and out of the joint. Visualization of the insertion site often requires a modest notchplasty (Fig. 58-5A). The ipsilateral tibial eminence usually requires flattening with a bur for ease of graft passage. The medial notch wall (below the posteromedial bundle of the PCL) can also be taken down with a shaver or bur to achieve better visualization of the posterior insertion site and ease of graft passage. Before the posterior horn socket is drilled and the graft is passed, a dilator can be placed along the intended course of the bone plug's passage to ensure that the graft will easily pass across the notch.

The 9-mm posterior horn socket is made with a 9-mm FlipCutter (Arthrex) to a depth of 10 mm (see Fig. 58-5). First an ACL drill guide is placed in the ipsilateral anterior portal and used to aim the FlipCutter to enter knee joint at the center of the posterior horn insertion site. The drill enters the tibia via a stab incision at an angle of approximately 50 degrees. The FlipCutter is pulled back slowly at full speed to create a 10-mm-deep socket. A passing suture is placed up the tibial socket via the drill sleeve and secured for later graft passage (Fig. 58-6).

For placement of the next passing suture, the arthroscope is positioned in the ipsilateral portal and a 90-degree SutureLasso (Arthrex) is introduced from the contralateral portal across the notch to exit the capsule just beyond the posterior horn insertion site. This exit site corresponds with the first TigerWire vertical suture placed into the posterior horn of the allograft. The lasso is then used to retrieve a looped TigerWire suture (Fig. 58-7), which is passed back across the joint to exit the contralateral portal. The arthroscope is returned to the contralateral portal. The looped portion of the Suture-Lasso is now flipped so that the looped end is left sticking out of the PassPort (Arthrex) cannula handle and the unlooped end is ready to be inserted through the posterior capsule 1 cm away from the TigerWire passing suture. The SutureLasso passing wire is left in place and

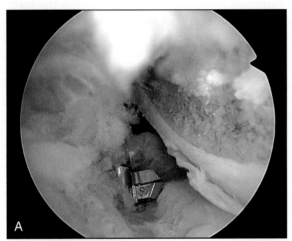

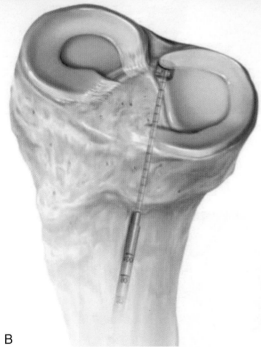

Figure 58-5. A, A 9-mm FlipCutter ready to form 10-mm deep posterior horn socket. Note the medial wall and notchplasty. **B,** FlipCutter preparing the posterior socket. *(**B,** Courtesy Arthrex, Naples, FL.)*

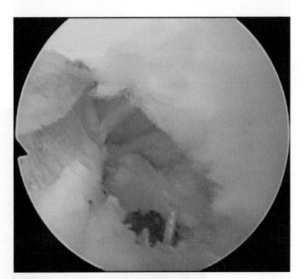

Figure 58-6. FiberStick (Arthrex, Naples, FL) placed as passing suture for posterior horn bone plug.

corresponds to the final vertical preplaced No. 2 Fiber-Wire suture juxtaposed to the letter *P* on the meniscal graft. Careful attention is needed to ensure that the three passing sutures are retrieved such that all exit the knee via the ipsilateral PassPort cannula free of any twists or crossovers (Fig. 58-8). The PassPort cannula is removed from the portal, and the knee is ready to receive the meniscus transplant. Compulsive preparation of the joint compartment takes time but will ensure safe and efficient passage of the MAT construct.

Graft Placement

The meniscal allograft is brought up to the knee and passed with use of the sutures previously placed in the posterior horn bone plug and those placed vertically in the posterior horn (Fig. 58-9).

The posterior horn bone plug is gently guided in through the portal and seated in the dilated pathway on the way to the posterior horn bone socket (Fig. 58-10). Concurrently an assistant maintains tension on the two vertical sutures and wedges the body of the meniscus into the joint space, making sure the graft does not twist. A blunt obturator can help guide the body into position from the anterior portal as well. A slight valgus force is applied to the knee to open the medial

compartment while tension is increased on the vertical sutures. This combination of maneuvers allows for efficient and gentle reduction of the body of the meniscus. The valgus force and suture tension are then relaxed and attention is focused on the final reduction of the posterior horn bone plug into the bony socket. While tension is applied to the posterior bone plug sutures, a grasping instrument may help rotate the bone plug into the correct trajectory. Once the bone plug is fully seated, final bone plug fixation is obtained by tying the sutures together at the tibial exit over a two-hole oblong metallic button (Fig. 58-11). The two vertical sutures are then tied together over the external surface of the posterior capsule. The posterior third of the meniscal graft is now secured.

Attention is then turned toward drilling the anterior horn bone socket. A trial reduction of the anterior horn bone plug into the insertion site of the resected native anterior horn is attempted. Once the appropriate location has been confirmed, a drill guide sleeve is introduced into the ipsilateral portal (contralateral portal for lateral MAT) to allow placement of the drill into the center of the desired bone plug location (Fig. 58-12). A 10-mm low-profile cannulated acorn reamer is used to drill a socket to a depth of 10 mm (Fig. 58-13). The

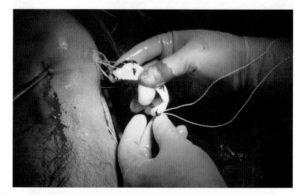

Figure 58-9. Right knee medial meniscus ready for insertion.

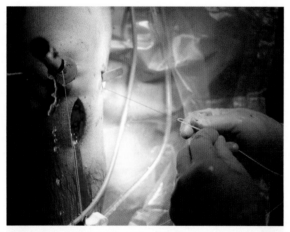

Figure 58-7. Retrieval of TigerWire (Arthrex, Naples, FL) passing suture.

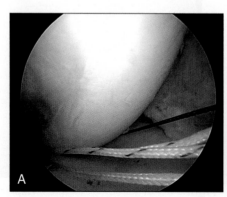
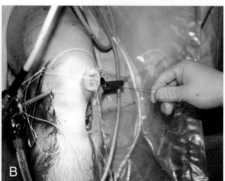

Figure 58-8. A, Passing sutures in place. **B,** Passing sutures ready for exchange of graft sutures.

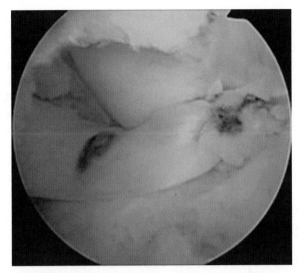

Figure 58-10. Graft ready for passage across joint.

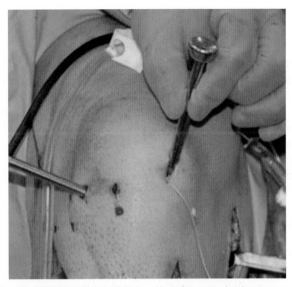

Figure 58-12. Drill guide in place for anterior horn placement.

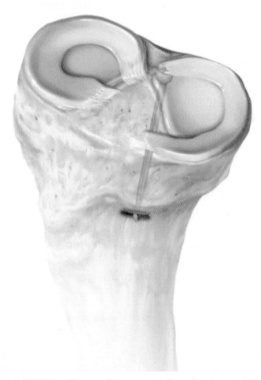

Figure 58-11. The graft is secured and sutures are tied over a button. *(Courtesy Arthrex, Naples, FL.)*

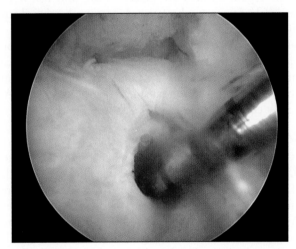

Figure 58-13. Drilling the anterior horn socket.

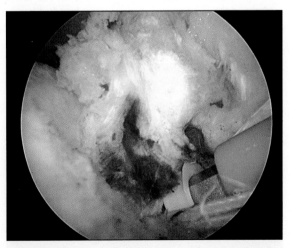

Figure 58-14. Anchoring down the anterior horn with a SwiveLock (Arthrex, Naples, FL).

anterior bone plug sutures are passed through the lead element of a SwiveLock anchor (Arthrex). The Swive-Lock anchor and the driver are introduced into the portal and positioned juxtaposed to the cancellous portion of the bone plug with the sutures under tension. The SwiveLock anchor and driver guide the bone plug into the bone socket, and the bone plug is reduced by driving the lead element of the anchor and captured sutures into the base of the bone socket (Fig. 58-14). Several taps with a mallet on the driver handle may help fully reduce the bone plug and place the trailing screw portion of the SwiveLock anchor at the opening of the bone socket. The trailing screw acts like an interference screw between the bone plug and bone socket. The driver is removed once the device is fully seated. The suture tails are cut flush with the bone. With the anterior horn and posterior third of the meniscus allograft secured, the normal hoop stresses of the meniscus are reestablished. The only remaining task is to place inside-out vertical meniscal repair sutures to secure the capsule to the periphery of the body of the meniscus. This specific order of repair helps prevent meniscal extrusion, which could happen if the meniscus were repaired to the capsule from back to front before finalization of the placement of the anterior horn bone plug.

Inside-Out Repair

Double-armed 2-0 FiberWire sutures with long meniscal repair needles are used to complete the repair of the meniscus. A SharpShooter (ConMed Linvatec, Largo, FL) needle delivery device helps speed up this portion of the repair. Sutures are placed above and below the meniscal edge from the letter *A* previously placed just off the anterior horn of the meniscus. The letter *P* denotes the posterior extent of the remaining inside-out repair and reflects the location of the second vertical suture used to pass the graft and provide initial graft fixation to the posterior capsule (Fig. 58-15). The MAT is now complete (Fig. 58-16).

Concomitant Procedures

ACL reconstruction and fresh osteochondral allograft placement may necessarily alter the final steps of the MAT technique detailed earlier. The ACL femoral and tibial sockets are routinely made with FlipCutters (Arthrex), and passing sutures are placed just after the posterior horn bone plug has been completed. The meniscus is then passed and secured posteriorly in the same fashion as described earlier. The anterior horn, however, is parked in the medial gutter until the remainder of the ACL reconstruction is completed. The anterior horn bone socket is then made in the same way as

described earlier, and the bone plug is secured with the same anchor. Inside-out sutures complete the MAT procedure. In a similar sequence of workflow, a small arthrotomy allows for medial femoral condyle exposure and osteochondral graft placement with the anterior horn temporarily parked in the medial gutter. The MAT procedure is then completed just as with an ACL reconstruction as described previously. The temporary absence of the anterior horn is especially useful when access is needed during osteochondral allograft transplantation on the high flexion aspect of the femoral condyle.

POSTOPERATIVE CONSIDERATIONS

Postoperative Rehabilitation

The rehabilitation begins on the day of surgery with ankle pumps, straight-leg raises, and thigh isometric contractions.

Bracing

Postoperatively the patient is placed in a hinged knee brace locked in full extension. Immobilization is initially important for wound healing, and the brace is adjusted only in the office or occasionally by the physical therapist. After the initial 2 to 3 days the brace is adjusted to allow motion from full extension to 60 degrees of flexion. The hinged knee brace is to be worn at all times over the first 4 postoperative weeks. At week 5 the brace may be removed while the patient is in bed or resting. Flexion is increased to 90 degrees at the eighth postoperative week, and the patient is fit for a custom knee brace to be worn for a year. Unloader braces may be worn depending on patient tolerance.

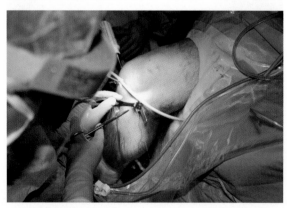

Figure 58-15. Placement of inside-out sutures.

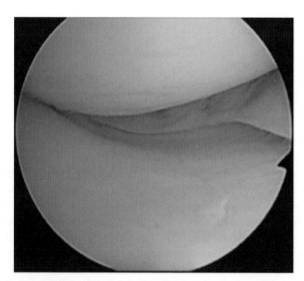

Figure 58-16. Final right medial meniscal allograft transplantation appearance.

Weight Bearing

The patient's initial weight-bearing status is foot-flat touch-down. Advancement to full weight bearing as tolerated is initiated at the first physical therapy visit, with a hinged knee brace used at all times.

Physical Therapy

Range of motion, gait, and strengthening exercises are started immediately at the first physical therapy visit.

Return to Sport

Light, sport-specific exercises are allowed at 4 months in addition to straight line running.

Concomitant Procedures

The physical therapy and rehabilitation guidelines described previously are to be limited by the restrictions of any concomitant procedure with more stringent weight-bearing, range-of-motion, or bracing limitations.

RESULTS

Assessment of the literature on MAT yields results that are not easily comparable. There have been no randomized controlled trials to date. The studies that exist on the subject often have relatively small sample numbers, consist of mostly retrospective case series, have limited follow-up, and lack universal outcome measurements. In addition, the studies vary greatly in their inclusion and exclusion criteria, concomitant procedures, methods of graft preservation, measurement, and fixation; all of these factors confound the reported outcomes even further (Table 58-1).

Many different surgical techniques have been reported. Human cadaveric studies have shown that secure anatomic fixation with bone plugs attached to the anterior and posterior horns is essential in restoring normal contact mechanics for both the medial and lateral menisci. When performed correctly in the right patient, MAT will result in pain relief and increased function. Whether these results correlate with a decreased degeneration of articular cartilage and eventual joint arthrosis has yet to be established.

TABLE 58-1. Results of Arthroscopic Meniscus Transplantation

Author	Study Size	Follow-up (Range)	Clinical Results
Cole et al[1] (2006)	36 patients 40 grafts	33.5 months (24-57 months)	77.5% of patients completely or mostly satisfied 90% of patients had normal or nearly normal IKDC examination score
Farr et al[2] (2007)	29 patients 29 grafts	4.5 years (3.2-5.8 years)	44.8% excellent or good Lysholm score
LaPrade et al[3] (2010)	40 patients 40 grafts	2.5 years (1.8-4.0 years)	72 mean IKDC score 75.3 Modified Cincinnati score 91% of patients reported improved pain and function
Zhang et al[4] (2012)	18 grafts	24.9 months (18-41 months)	67% of patients satisfied
Noyes et al[5] (2004)	38 patients 40 grafts	40 months (24-69 months)	89% pain free with ADLs 76% returned to light, low-impact sports activities
Rath et al[6] (2001)	18 patients 22 grafts	5.4 years (2-8 years)	54 mean IKDC score
Rue et al[7] (2008)	29 patients	3.1 years (1.9-5.6 years)	76% completely or mostly satisfied 90% would repeat surgery
Ryu et al[8] (2002)	25 patients 26 grafts	33 months (12-72 months)	83% patient satisfaction 68% of patients had normal IKDC score
Sekiya et al[9] (2003)	28 patients 31 grafts	2.8 years (1.8-5.6 years)	85.7% of patients had normal or near-normal IKDC score 93% of patients greatly or somewhat improved
Yoldas et al[10] (2003)	31 patients 34 grafts	2.9 years (2-5.5 years)	96.8% greatly or somewhat improved 96.8% knee function normal or nearly normal
Stollsteimer et al[11] (2000)	22 patients 23 grafts	40 months (13-49 months)	56.5% normal or near-normal IKDC score 78% of patients had pain improvement
Graf et al[12] (2004)	8 patients 8 grafts	9.7 years (8.5-10.3 years)	87.5% of patients returned to recreational sports 100% of patients satisfied 12.5% near-normal overall IKDC score; no normal scores

ADLs, activities of daily living; *IKDC,* International Knee Documentation Committee.

REFERENCES

1. Cole BJ, Dennis MG, Lee SJ, et al. Prospective evaluation of allograft meniscus transplantation: a minimum 2-year follow-up. *Am J Sports Med.* 2006;34(6):919-927.

2. Farr J, Rawal A, Marberry KM. Concomitant meniscal allograft transplantation and autologous chondrocyte implantation: minimum 2-year follow-up. *Am J Sports Med.* 2007;35(9):1459-1466.

3. LaPrade RF, Wills NJ, Spiridonov SI, et al. A prospective outcomes study of meniscal allograft transplantation. *Am J Sports Med.* 2010;38(9):1804-1812.

4. Zhang H, Liu X, Wei Y, et al. Meniscal allograft transplantation in isolated and combined surgery. *Knee Surg Sports Traumatol Arthrosc.* 2012;20(2):281-289.

5. Noyes FR, Barber-Westin SD, Rankin M. Meniscal transplantation in symptomatic patients less than fifty years old. *J Bone Joint Surg Am.* 2004;86(7):1392-1404.

6. Rath E, Richmond JC, Yassir W, et al. Meniscal allograft transplantation. Two- to eight-year results. *Am J Sports Med.* 2001;29(4):410-414.

7. Rue JP, Yanke AB, Busam ML, et al. Prospective evaluation of concurrent meniscus transplantation and articular cartilage repair: minimum 2-year follow-up. *Am J Sports Med.* 2008;36(9):1770-1778.

8. Ryu RK, Dunbar VW, Morse GG. Meniscal allograft replacement: a 1-year to 6-year experience. *Arthroscopy.* 2002;18(9):989-994.

9. Sekiya JK, Giffin JR, Irrgang JJ, et al. Clinical outcomes after combined meniscal allograft transplantation and anterior cruciate ligament reconstruction. *Am J Sports Med.* 2003;31(6):896-906.

10. Yoldas EA, Sekiya JK, Irrgang JJ, et al. Arthroscopically assisted meniscal allograft transplantation with and without combined anterior cruciate ligament reconstruction. *Knee Surg Sports Traumatol Arthrosc.* 2003;11(3): 173-182.

11. Stollsteimer GT, Shelton WR, Dukes A, et al. Meniscal allograft transplantation: a 1- to 5-year follow-up of 22 patients. *Arthroscopy.* 2000;16(4):343-347.

12. Graf Jr KW, Sekiya JK, Wojtys EM. Long-term results after combined medial meniscal allograft transplantation and anterior cruciate ligament reconstruction: minimum 8.5-year follow-up study. *Arthroscopy.* 2004;20(2): 129-140.

Chapter 59

Meniscus Substitution: The European Perspective on Scaffolds, Allografts, and Prosthetic Implants

Peter C.M. Verdonk, Aad A.M. Dhollander, Thomas Tampere, and René Verdonk

Chapter Synopsis
- In this chapter the different options for meniscus substitution are discussed and elaborated. Specific attention is paid to the important differences in indication and surgical technique. Although a number of these therapeutic options have already proven their clinical benefit in multicenter European trials, many of them have not yet been made available outside of Europe—hence the scope of this chapter.

Important Points
- Meniscus scaffolds are indicated for partial meniscus defects (ideally less than 5 cm), whereas meniscus allografts are indicated in larger defects. Prosthetic meniscus implants are a promising new tool for meniscus deficiency but are currently still under investigation (as of 2013).

Clinical and Surgical Pearls
- Meniscus substitution is a treatment option for nonarthritic, well-aligned, stable knees.

Clinical and Surgical Pitfalls
- Significant osteophytes or flattening of the femoral condyle, often observed in chronic meniscectomy, eliminates the possibility of meniscus substitution.

Treatment of meniscal lesions is the most common surgical intervention performed by orthopedic surgeons today, with more than 1 million surgical interventions involving the meniscus performed annually in the United States and approximately 400,000 in Europe. The meniscus, a semilunar, fibrocartilaginous structure, preserves a pain-free functional knee and plays an important role in the biomechanical functions of the knee, including load bearing, load and force distribution between the femoral condyles and tibial plateau, joint stabilization, lubrication, and proprioception. Over the last few decades, the understanding of meniscal functions and consequently the management of meniscal injuries has continued to evolve, with increasing commitment among physicians to preserve the meniscus whenever possible. The natural history of a meniscus-deficient knee has been shown to involve poor clinical and radiologic outcomes over time, including disruption of load-sharing and shock absorption, diminution of joint stability, and deterioration of articular cartilage with progression to arthrosis. It is now accepted that loss of all or part of the meniscus leads to long-term degenerative changes owing to higher peak stresses on the articular cartilage in the meniscectomized compartment as a result of the decreased contact area. Thus, it seems logical to regenerate or substitute lost meniscus tissue with a scaffold, allograft, or implant to restore the function of the knee joint and to possibly prevent further joint degeneration.

In this chapter, the different options for meniscus substitution are discussed and elaborated. Specific attention is paid to the important differences in indication and surgical technique. Although a number of these therapeutic options have already been proved to be of clinical benefit in multicenter European trials, many of them have not yet been made available outside of Europe—hence the scope of this chapter.

MENISCUS SCAFFOLDS FOR THE TREATMENT OF PARTIAL MENISCUS DEFECTS

Meniscal regeneration appears to require the physical presence of a scaffold to encourage successful migration and colonization with precursor cells and vessels, eventually leading to the formation of organized meniscal tissue.[1,2]

In Europe, two scaffolds for the treatment of partial meniscus defects are available. We have acquired extensive experience with a novel, biodegradable, synthetic, acellular scaffold composed of aliphatic polyurethane (Actifit, Orteq, London, United Kingdom), which was designed to fill an unmet clinical need in the treatment of patients with irreparable partial meniscal tissue lesions. The treatment objective of the scaffold is to provide pain relief and restore lost meniscus functionality.

The scaffold comes in two configurations, one for the medial indication and one for the lateral. Design criteria were biocompatibility, strength, flexibility and ease of handling (insertion and suturing with standard arthroscopic techniques), high and interconnected porosity to support tissue ingrowth, and degradation over a suitable time as new tissue forms and matures. The scaffold is highly porous, with approximately 20% of the structure being composed of biodegradable aliphatic polyurethane and the remaining 80% being the pores.

When implanted into the void created in the meniscal tissue after a standard arthroscopic partial meniscectomy and connected to the vascularized portion of the meniscus, the scaffold provides a three-dimensional matrix of interconnected pores for vascular ingrowth.

INDICATIONS

Meniscus scaffold implantation represents a novel biologic solution for the treatment of patients with symptomatic partial meniscus defects and limited signs of cartilage degeneration. Because the negative impact of meniscectomy in anterior cruciate ligament (ACL)–injured knees on long-term cartilage degeneration has recently been established, prophylactic meniscus reconstruction with use of a scaffold in the ACL-reconstructed knee with partial meniscectomy could be another indication.

The key inclusion criteria are as follows:

1. Irreparable medial or lateral meniscal tear or partial meniscus loss, with intact rim. Most important, the synthetic meniscus substitute is not intended for the treatment of total or subtotal meniscus defects. Ideally, the defect length should be limited to 5 to 6 cm.

2. Skeletally mature male or female patients.
3. Patients aged 16 to 50 years.
4. Stable knee joint or knee joint stabilization procedure within 12 weeks of index procedure.
5. International Cartilage Repair Society (ICRS) classification of 3.
6. Patient willing and able to give consent to participate in the clinical study, follow rehabilitation protocol, and attend or undergo all follow-up visits and procedures.

The key exclusion criteria are as follows:

1. Total meniscus loss or unstable segmental rim defect
2. Multiple areas of partial meniscus loss that could not be treated by a single scaffold
3. Any significant malalignment (varus or valgus)
4. ICRS classification of greater than 3
5. Body mass index of 35 or higher

SURGICAL TECHNIQUE

Anesthesia and Positioning

The Actifit meniscal scaffold is placed in the subject's knee using a standard arthroscopic surgery procedure and standard equipment. Implantation is usually performed with use of spinal or general anesthesia at the discretion of the orthopedic surgeon. The use of a tourniquet is optional. The surgeon may prefer thigh fixation to achieve appropriate valgus or varus stress positioning.

Examination

Verification of cartilage status and integrity of the meniscal rim and both the anterior and posterior horns should be performed. In the case of a tight medial compartment, distending the medial collateral ligament using the outside-in puncture method (several passes with a spinal needle from outside in) or the inside-out pie-crusting release technique described by Steadman allows the surgeon to adequately visualize both the femoral and the tibial cartilage status and to create an adequate working space for meniscus reconstructive surgery.

Portals

The implantation requires the usual small incisions for anteromedial and anterolateral portals, with an optional central transpatellar tendon portal. To allow for easy insertion of the scaffold, an enlargement of the portal used for insertion of the device may be required (the size of the little finger is typically sufficient). In addition, a posteromedial or posterolateral incision may be required if an inside-out meniscal fixation technique is used.

Additional small incisions are made around the joint line if an outside-in technique is used.

Specific Steps

The specific steps of the procedure are outlined in Box 59-1.

Preparation of the damaged meniscus includes surgical debridement and removal of all pathologic tissue and ensuring that the resulting defect site extends into the vascularized red-on-red or red-on-white zone of the damaged portion of the meniscus. Lesions situated farther away from the synovial border are known to have only very limited healing potential and therefore should be excluded from this type of meniscoplasty. For enhancement of healing, the meniscal rim may be punctured to create vascular access channels. Gentle rasping of the synovial lining may further stimulate meniscal healing (Fig. 59-1). The meniscal defect should be measured along the curvature of its inner edge using the accompanying specially designed meniscal ruler and meniscal ruler guide. Actifit is then measured and with a scalpel is cut to fit in such a place and manner as to ensure that sterility is maintained at all times. To allow

---

BOX 59-1 Steps in the Use of Two Scaffolds for the Treatment of Partial Meniscus Defects

1. Preparation of the damaged meniscus
2. Tailoring of the Actifit meniscal scaffold
3. Fixation of Actifit by suturing of the scaffold to the native meniscus tissue
4. Further trimming and fine-tuning intra-articularly with a basket punch

---

for shrinkage caused by suturing of the spongelike material and to ensure a snug optimal fit into the prepared defect, oversizing of the length by 10% is advised (3 mm for defects smaller than 3 cm and 5 mm for defects 3 cm or larger). To achieve a perfect fit of the scaffold with the native meniscus at the anterior junction, the anterior side should be cut at an oblique angle of 30 to 45 degrees (Fig. 59-2). Although the Actifit material is strong and flexible, the device should be handled with care and manipulated with a blunt-nosed grasper, such as the Acufex Grasper Tissue Tensioner (Smith & Nephew). Marking the cranial and caudal meniscal scaffold surface with a sterile marking pen avoids positioning problems. The Actifit device should be clamped at the posterior part of the scaffold and placed into the knee joint through the anteromedial or anterolateral portal. To ensure a good initial position of the meniscal scaffold and facilitate further fixation, the surgeon may place a vertical holding suture in the native meniscus tissue to bring Actifit through the eye of this holding suture.

Fixation of Actifit is achieved by suturing the scaffold to the native meniscus tissue. All standard meniscus suturing techniques may be used; the suturing technique employed depends on the location of the defect and the surgeon's experience and preference. All-inside suturing has proven effective, and this technique is commonly used for the posterior horn and posterior part of the rim. For the middle and anterior part of the rim, all-inside, inside-out, and outside-in techniques may be used. Horizontal sutures with an outside-in technique are commonly used for the anterior horn and posterior horn.

The manufacturer recommends standard commercially available size 2.0 nonresorbable sutures, such as polyester or polypropylene and braided or monofilament sutures.

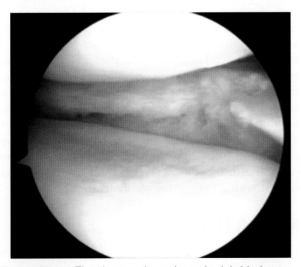

Figure 59-1. The damaged meniscus is debrided to a stable and potentially bleeding rim (tourniquet still in place at the time of this image).

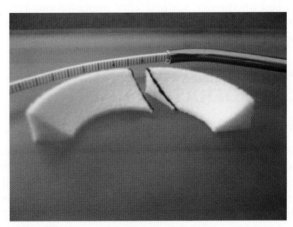

Figure 59-2. The Actifit meniscal scaffold is tailored on the surgical field with a scalpel for a perfect fit to the meniscus defect.

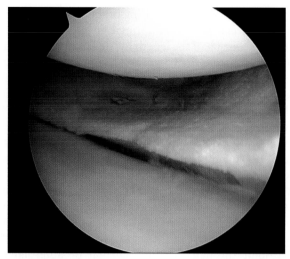

Figure 59-3. Macroscopic aspect of the scaffold 1 year after implantation showing full incorporation and integration to the rim and horns.

Fixation of the device should begin with a horizontal all-inside suture from the posterior edge of the scaffold to the native meniscus. Suturing should be secure; however, attention must be paid not to overtighten sutures, because this may alter and indent the surface of the scaffold. In line with well-known meniscal suturing techniques, the distances between the sutures should be kept to approximately 0.5 cm. Each suture should be placed at one third to one half of the scaffold's height, as determined from the lower surface of the scaffold.

After suturing, if required, the scaffold may be further trimmed and fine-tuned intra-articularly with a basket punch. Once the scaffold has been securely fixed, stability of the fixation is tested by use of the probe and movement of the knee through a range of motion (0 to 90 degrees).

To enhance the healing response, bone marrow aspiration can be performed from the notch area and directly applied on the dry scaffold after implantation. Figure 59-3 depicts a scaffold 1 year after implantation showing full peripheral integration to the meniscus rim.

POSTOPERATIVE CONSIDERATIONS
Rehabilitation Protocol

To ensure protection of the newly formed fragile tissue and to provide optimum conditions for healing, all patients are required to undergo a conservative rehabilitation program similar to that for a meniscal allograft. The rehabilitation protocol is followed for 16 to 24 weeks, with non–weight-bearing status for the first 3 weeks. Partial weight bearing is permitted from week 4 onward, with a gradual increase in loading up to 100%

load at 9 weeks postimplantation. Progressive weight bearing is initiated in stages, increasing by 10 kg per week for patients weighing 60 kg or less and by 15 kg per week for patients weighing more than 60 kg up to 90 kg. Full weight bearing with an unloader brace is allowed from week 9 onward, and without the use of the unloader brace from week 14 onward. Range-of-motion exercises are gradually initiated but limited to 90 degrees of flexion for the first 6 weeks.

Gradual resumption of sports is generally commenced at 6 months at the discretion of the responsible orthopedic surgeon; however, contact sports are recommenced only after 9 months.

RESULTS

Meniscus scaffolds are a safe and viable option for the treatment of painful partial meniscus defects. Current literature has provided short-term 2-year evidence for a continued significant improvement in pain and function.[3] In addition, a recent histologic study provides insights into the regeneration of an immature meniscus-like tissue at 1 year after implantation.[2]

MENISCUS ALLOGRAFTS FOR THE TREATMENT OF LARGE MENISCUS DEFECTS

In this update we discuss our experience with arthroscopic meniscus allograft transplantation. Whereas scaffolds are mainly used to substitute for partial loss, meniscus allografts are generally used in total or subtotal meniscectomized patients. Meniscus allograft transplantation has gained widespread acceptance throughout Europe as a viable treatment for postmeniscectomy pain in the young patient.[4] Owing to the specific biomechanical characteristics of the lateral compartment, most patients develop early postoperative pain in the lateral compartment after a large meniscectomy, and hence the majority of allograft transplants are performed in the lateral compartment. Of interest also are the differences in surgical techniques between Europe and the United States; although biomechanical data clearly show advantages of bone-block fixation over soft-tissue fixation, a majority of European surgeons prefer all-arthroscopic surgery without bone-block fixation but with transosseous suture fixation.[5,6]

INDICATIONS

Meniscus allograft transplantation represents a potential biologic solution for the symptomatic meniscus-deficient patient who has not yet developed advanced osteoarthritis.[7] The indications for meniscal allograft transplantation have yet to be comprehensively defined. Current recommendations suggest that the procedure is indicated in three clinical scenarios:

1. Young patients with a history of meniscectomy who have pain localized to the meniscus-deficient compartment, a stable knee joint, no malalignment, and articular cartilage with only minor evidence of osteochondral degenerative changes (no more than grade 3 according to the ICRS classification system) are considered ideal candidates for this procedure. Because of the more rapid deterioration in the lateral compartment, a relatively common indication for meniscal transplantation would be a symptomatic, meniscal-deficient lateral compartment.

2. ACL-deficient patients who have had prior medial meniscectomy (who might benefit from the increased stability afforded by a functional medial meniscus) in conjunction with concomitant ACL reconstruction. It is our conviction that an ACL graft is significantly protected by the meniscus allografts as much as the meniscus is protected by an ACL graft.

3. A third context for meniscal transplantation has also been advocated by some. In an effort to avert early joint degeneration, young, athletic patients who have undergone complete meniscectomy might be considered as meniscal transplantation candidates before symptom onset.

CONTRAINDICATIONS

Advanced chondral degeneration is considered a contraindication to meniscal allograft transplantation, although some series suggest that cartilage degeneration is not a significant risk factor for failure. In general, articular cartilage lesions greater than grade 3 according to the ICRS classification system should be of limited surface area and localized. Localized chondral defects may be treated concomitantly—the meniscus transplantation and the cartilage repair or restoration may benefit each other in terms of healing and outcome. Radiographic evidence of significant osteophyte formation or femoral condyle flattening is associated with inferior postoperative results because these structural modifications alter the morphology of the femoral condyle. In general, patients over age 50 have excessive cartilage disease and are suboptimal candidates. Axial malalignment tends to exert abnormal pressure on the allograft, leading to loosening, degeneration, and failure of the graft. A corrective osteotomy should be considered for more than two degrees of deviation toward the involved compartment, as compared with the contralateral limb mechanical axis.

Other contraindications to meniscal transplantation include obesity, skeletal immaturity, instability of the knee joint (which may be addressed in conjunction with transplantation as described earlier), synovial disease, inflammatory arthritis, and previous joint infection.

SURGICAL TECHNIQUE
Specific Steps

The specific steps of the procedure are outlined in Box 59-2.

Allograft Preparation
The allograft is positioned and fixed on a specially designed cork board with three 25-gauge needles. With a scalpel the residual synovial tissue is dissected from the allograft meniscus at the meniscosynovial junction level and discarded.

The upper side of the allograft is marked with a methylene blue skin marker.

Nonresorbable high-strength (FiberWire, Arthrex, Naples, FL) sutures are placed in the anterior and posterior horn of the allograft. In general, three whipstitches are placed on the inner and outer rim of the horn of the allograft (Fig. 59-4). An additional vertical nonresorbable suture (Ethibond 2, Somerville, NJ) is placed at the posteromedial or posterolateral corner of the medial or lateral allograft, respectively. For the

---

BOX 59-2 Steps in the Use of Meniscus Allografts for the Treatment of Large Meniscus Defects

1. Allograft preparation
2. Lateral meniscus allograft transplantation
3. Medial meniscus allograft transplantation

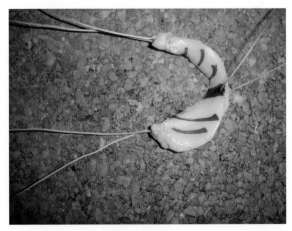

Figure 59-4. Prepared medial meniscal allograft for arthroscopic meniscal transplantation. Whipstitches on the inner and outer rim of the anterior and posterior horn. A vertical nonresorbable suture is placed on the posteromedial corner.

lateral allograft, the posterolateral suture is positioned just anteriorly to the popliteus tendon hiatus; this will serve as a landmark during arthroscopy.

Lateral Meniscus Allograft Transplantation

The classic anteromedial and anterolateral portals are made. An additional anteromedial portal is positioned very medially to gain easy instrumental access for the debridement and resection of the anterior portion of the native lateral meniscus. With a shaver and punch, the remnant meniscus is debrided to the level of the meniscal rim.

A modified ACL aiming device with a low-profile tip is inserted through the medial portal and positioned at the anatomic posterior horn of the lateral meniscus just posterior to the ACL (Fig. 59-5). A guide pin is drilled first and subsequently overdrilled by a 4.5-mm cannulated drill. A double-loop metal wire is introduced through the tunnel from outside in, picked up intra-articularly with an arthroscopic grasper, and pulled out through the lateral portal. Subsequently, a suture passer (Acupass, Smith & Nephew, Memphis, TN) is introduced twice from outside-in just anterior to the lateral collateral ligament and the popliteus tendon into the joint—one suture just below and the second above the native meniscal rim. The looped wires are picked up and pulled out again through the lateral portal. Next, the posterior horn pull suture and the posterolateral pull suture are pulled through using the double looped metal wire and the double-looped suture pass wire. The

prepared lateral allograft is subsequently introduced into the lateral compartment throughout an enlarged lateral portal by pulling progressively on the posterolateral pull suture and the posterior horn pull suture. Care should be taken that the graft does not flip on introduction and that the pull wires do not intertwine. The risk of intertwining wires is greatly reduced by use of a double-loop metal wire for the posterior horn.

The posterior horn is now positioned correctly. Its position can be slightly modified more toward the posterolateral corner or more toward the posterior horn by pulling more on the posterolateral or posterior horn traction wire. One or two all-inside meniscal fixation devices (FasT-Fix, Smith & Nephew) are used to fix the allograft to the meniscal rim. Fixation should be started in the posterolateral corner. Subsequently, inside-out horizontal Ethibond 2/0 sutures are used for fixing the body of the allograft. The anterior horn is fixed using outside-in polydioxanone (PDS) or Ethibond 2/0 sutures.

Before the suture knots are made, the anterior horn is introduced into the knee joint and the anatomic insertion site is identified and prepared in the same manner as for the posterior tunnel. If necessary, its position can be slightly adapted to the graft position. Similar to the procedure for the posterior horn, the anterior tunnel is prepared and the traction suture is pulled through.

First, the meniscal inside-out sutures are knotted (Fig. 59-6). Subsequently, the anterior and posterior horn traction sutures are knotted to each other over a bone bridge on the anteromedial side of the tibia. This procedure reduces the possibly stretched capsule and native meniscal rim tied to the meniscal allograft, by pulling on the anterior and posterior horn by a transosseous suture fixation.

Medial Meniscus Allograft Transplantation

A similar procedure as for the lateral allograft transplantation is performed for the medial allograft transplantation. However, some steps are different and are highlighted in this section.

Additional to the classic anteromedial and anterolateral portal, a posteromedial portal should be used to

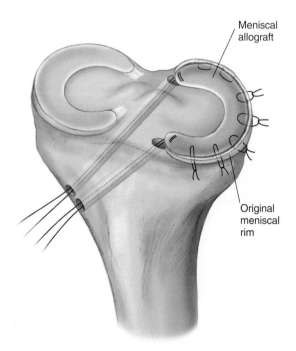

Figure 59-5. The meniscus allograft with two transosseous fixations in combination with all-inside and inside-out sutures. The posteromedial holding suture is also illustrated.

Labels: Meniscal allograft; Original meniscal rim

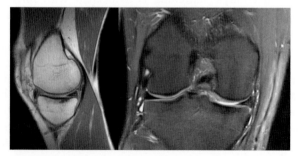

Figure 59-6. Sagittal and coronal magnetic resonance images depicting medial meniscus allograft 1 year after implantation. Note the slightly increased signal compared with the normal lateral meniscus.

identify the original posterior horn attachments of the native meniscus. With use of the same drill guide, the transosseous tunnels can be prepared. These tunnels should be prepared starting on the anterolateral side of the tibia. This direction is more in line with the forces on the traction sutures.

A posteromedial traction suture is used, in accordance with the lateral allograft. On the medial side, however, we lack a clear anatomic landmark such as the popliteal hiatus on the lateral side.

The anterior horn of the native medial meniscus may in some cases be very anterior on the tibial plateau, resulting in a very short transosseous anterior tunnel.

Special Note on Soft Tissue Versus Bone Block Fixation

Biomechanical cadaver studies have shown the superiority of a bony fixation over a soft tissue fixation technique, although a cadaver study showed comparable results.[5,6] Bony fixation, however, has also been shown to be associated with increased risk of cartilage lesions if implantation is incorrect and an increased immunologic reaction owing to the presence of allogeneic bone. In our experience, perfect allograft size matching is essential if bony fixation is to be used. A malpositioned bone block or plugs can inflict damage to the overlying cartilage. Too small a graft will result in a need to overtension the inside-out sutures and possible failure of the soft tissue fixation. Therefore, limited oversizing of the graft is commonly advocated with use of bone plugs or blocks. Separate bone plugs have the potential advantage that the implantation can be somewhat more variable compared with a single bone block. In addition, on the lateral side a straight bone block sometimes induces the need to sacrifice some posterolateral fibers of the ACL.

Today, clinical and/or radiologic differences have not been shown between soft tissue or bone block fixation.

POSTOPERATIVE CONSIDERATIONS

Rehabilitation

Rehabilitation is initially focused on providing mobility to the joint without endangering ingrowth and healing of the graft. Therefore 3 weeks of non–weight-bearing status is prescribed, followed by 3 weeks of partial weight bearing (50% of body weight). Progression to full weight bearing is allowed from week 6 to week 10 postoperatively. The use of a knee brace is not strictly necessary and depends on the morphology and profile of the patient. For the same reasons, range of motion is limited during the first 2 weeks from 0 to 30, to increase by 30 degrees each 2 weeks. Isometric muscle

tonification and cocontraction exercises are prescribed from day 1 postsurgery onward. Straight-leg raises, however, are prohibited during the first 3 weeks. Proprioception training is started after week 3. Swimming is allowed after week 6, and biking after week 12, and running is progressively promoted starting at week 20.

RESULTS

All midterm and long-term studies have shown that medial and lateral meniscal allograft transplantation significantly reduces pain and improves function of the involved knee joint.[4,7]

Previous studies have shown that risk factors for failure and reduced survival time are lower limb malalignment, ACL deficiency, and grade 4 cartilage lesions. Moreover, the additional beneficial effect of a corrective osteotomy in case of a varus malalignment and the importance of a stable knee joint have been clearly demonstrated. The exact position of an associated corrective osteotomy in the valgus knee needs further refinement. More recent studies have not confirmed a significant correlation between the initial cartilage status and clinical failure, challenging the contraindications for arthrosis severity.

Meniscus allograft transplantation represents the biologic solution for the symptomatic, meniscus-deficient patient who has not developed advanced osteoarthritis. A growing body of evidence suggests that pain relief and functional improvement may reliably be achieved at short- and medium-term follow-up, and even in some cases at long-term follow-up (longer than 10 years). Progression of further cartilage degeneration or joint space narrowing is absent in a significant number of patients, indicating a potential chondroprotective effect.

PROSTHETIC POLYCARBONATE-URETHANE MENISCUS IMPLANT FOR THE TREATMENT OF MEDIAL MENISCUS DEFICIENCY

Although in recent years meniscal scaffolds have emerged as a treatment option for younger patients (<45 years of age), the efficacy of such treatment options may decline with age and with the progression of symptoms of osteoarthritis. At a later age—for example, older than 65 years—clinicians often choose to practice more invasive treatment arthroplasty options to treat joint pain by performing unicompartmental or total joint replacement. There is a clear treatment gap, creating a need to accommodate middle-aged patients with a nonbiologic treatment option that can delay more aggressive arthroplasty treatments by relieving pain associated with meniscal dysfunction and the associated joint overload.

A prosthetic medial meniscal implant is proposed as a bridge treatment for middle-aged patients with joint pain associated with a dysfunctional meniscus. A meniscal implant with reliable biomechanical performance that does not rely on regeneration has thus far not been offered in clinical practice. Clinical indications for the use of such an implant must be determined.

METHODS AND MATERIALS

A composite, nonfixed, self-centering, discoid-shaped meniscus implant composed of polycarbonate-urethane, reinforced circumferentially with ultra-high-molecular-weight polyethylene (UHMWPE) fibers, was produced (NUsurface, Active Implants Corporation, Memphis, TN). The concept of a nonanchored device was considered because it allows a simple implantation through a mini-arthrotomy without damaging the bone, cartilage, or ligaments, thus leaving all successive treatment options open. The implant's form was based on extensive magnetic resonance imaging study that included the geometric analysis of more than 100 knee scans; the implant differs from previous interpositional devices by its distinct curb, which runs along the tibial spine and femoral notch to restrict excessive motion and dislocation. Biomechanical optimization of the material properties of the implant was based on in vitro measurements of contact pressure under the implant in cadaver knees and computational finite element (FE) analyses.[8] The last preclinical stage was a sheep study in which an extensive quantitative cartilage evaluation was conducted microscopically, postimplantation.[9] The material properties of the device were tailored to provide it with an optimal pressure distribution ability, to reduce cartilage loads and thus relieve pain. The ability to conform moderately under load without risking the integrity of the device is another important feature that distinguishes it from other interpositional devices.

SURGICAL TECHNIQUE

The specific steps of this procedure are outlined in Box 59-3.

In brief, in a first stage the remaining meniscus tissue is debrided to a stable meniscus rim. The continuity of the meniscus rim and horns is checked, the stability of the cruciate ligaments is documented, and the cartilage degeneration is evaluated. Subsequently a mini-arthrotomy of approximately 5 cm is performed over the medial compartment, the appropriately sized trial implant is introduced into the medial compartment, and the stability and lift-off of the implant are evaluated clinically and with use of fluoroscopy (Fig. 59-7). If

BOX 59-3 Steps in the Use of Prosthetic Polycarbonate-Urethane Meniscus Implant for the Treatment of Medial Meniscus Deficiency

1. The remaining meniscus tissue is debrided to a stable meniscus rim.
2. The continuity of the meniscus rim and horns is checked.
3. The stability of the cruciate ligaments is documented.
4. The cartilage degeneration is evaluated.
5. A mini-arthrotomy is performed over the medial compartment.
6. The appropriately sized trial implant is introduced into the medial compartment.
7. The stability and lift-off of the implant are evaluated clinically and with fluoroscopy.
8. If correct sizing and biomechanical behavior are confirmed, the final implant is introduced.

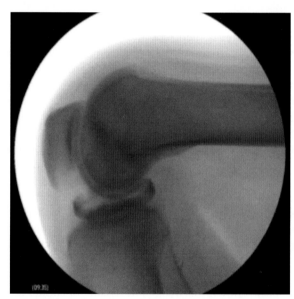

Figure 59-7. Prosthetic trial meniscus implant at 90 degrees of flexion. The implant follows the motion of the femoral condyle during fluoroscopy.

correct sizing and biomechanical behavior are confirmed, the final implant is introduced.

RESULTS

The in vitro evaluation of the final implant in cadaver knees showed that pressure distribution maps under the fiber-reinforced polycarbonate urethane were similar to those attained for the natural meniscus. Important, the contact area was predominantly in the outer third of the tibial plateau surface and was not concentrated in the central region. It was found that the synthetic meniscus performs equally well in distributing joint loads in a 5% range around the "true" size. Additional kinetic

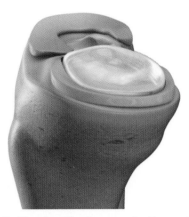

Figure 59-8. The free-floating prosthetic medial meniscus implant surrounded by the native meniscus rim to ensure stability and tracking.

evaluation in cadaver knees with use of fluoroscopy demonstrated good functionality in terms of maintaining contact with the cartilage and smoothness of motion resulting from the self-adjustment ability of the implant. A multicenter European trial is currently being conducted. Although the clinical results should still be considered very preliminary, a clear and significant clinical improvement could be observed in all patients. This benefit was already discernible as soon as 3 months after surgery, unlike with other biologic treatment options.

CONCLUSIONS

The proposed implant is considered a feasible treatment option for patients with medial pain associated with a dysfunctional meniscus resulting from tear or previous meniscectomy in the middle-aged patient (Fig. 59-8). It has been found to reduce cartilage contact pressures to normal levels without relying on tissue regeneration. With its simple implantation and joint-sparing use, this implant has good potential to postpone more aggressive

treatment options to a later age. Currently the device is under clinical investigation for safety and efficacy in a multicenter European study.

REFERENCES

1. Rodkey WG, Steadman JR, Li ST. A clinical study of collagen meniscus implants to restore the injured meniscus. *Clin Orthop Relat Res.* 1999;367(Suppl):S281-S292.
2. Verdonk R, Verdonk P, Huysse W, et al. Tissue ingrowth after implantation of a novel, biodegradable polyurethane scaffold for treatment of partial meniscal lesions. *Am J Sports Med.* 2011;39(4):774-782.
3. Verdonk P, Verdonk R, Huysse W, et al. Successful treatment of painful irreparable partial meniscal defects with a polyurethane scaffold—two year safety and clinical outcomes. *Am J Sports Med.* 2012;40(4):844-853.
4. Elattar M, Dhollander A, Verdonk R, et al. Twenty-six years of meniscal allograft transplantation: is it still experimental? A meta-analysis of 44 trials. *Knee Surg Sports Traumatol Arthrosc.* 2011;19(2):147-157.
5. Huang A, Hull ML, Howell SM. The level of compressive load affects conclusions from statistical analyses to determine whether a lateral meniscal autograft restores tibial contact pressure to normal: a study in human cadaveric knees. *J Orthop Res.* 2003;21:459-464.
6. Paletta GA Jr, Manning T, Snell E, et al. The effect of allograft meniscal replacement on intraarticular contact area and pressures in the human knee. A biomechanical study. *Am J Sports Med.* 1997;25:692-698.
7. Cole BJ, Carter TR, Rodeo SA. Allograft meniscal transplantation: background, techniques, and results. *Instr Course Lect.* 2003;52:383-396.
8. Elsner JJ, Portnoy S, Zur G, et al. Design of a free-floating polycarbonate-urethane meniscal implant using finite element modeling and experimental validation. *J Biomech Eng.* 2010;132(9):095001.
9. Zur G, Linder-Ganz E, Elsner JJ, et al. Chondroprotective effects of a polycarbonate-urethane meniscal implant: histopathological results in a sheep model. *Knee Surg Sports Traumatol Arthrosc.* 2011;19(2):255-263.

Chapter 60

Meniscus Regeneration with Biologic or Synthetic Scaffolds

William G. Rodkey*

Chapter Synopsis

- Efforts should be made to preserve the meniscus, but if this is not possible, meniscus regeneration with biologic or synthetic scaffolds may be an option. Multicenter clinical trials and reports have demonstrated new tissue formation and fewer reoperations after collagen scaffold implantation compared with partial meniscectomy alone for at least 10 years. A synthetic scaffold showed biocompatibility and successful early tissue ingrowth at 1 year. Research continues to develop and refine novel acellular scaffolds to support regeneration and regrowth of lost or damaged meniscus tissue.

Important Points

- Meniscus scaffolds are indicated for partial meniscus loss, whereas meniscus allografts are indicated for total meniscectomy.
- Two meniscus scaffolds, one biologic and one synthetic, are available for human clinical use (not currently in the United States).
- Intact anterior and posterior horn attachments and an intact rim of the involved meniscus are required.
- Knee ligamentous stability and proper axial alignment are necessary before scaffold implantation.
- Meniscus scaffolds are contraindicated in knees with advanced osteoarthritis.
- Successful scaffold implantation is technique specific and dependent.
- Proper postoperative rehabilitation must be followed to avoid early damage to the scaffold.

Clinical and Surgical Pearls

- Preparation of the implant site results in a full-thickness meniscus defect with no residual flaps or loose or degenerative tissue.
- The defect size must be measured accurately, and then the implant should be trimmed by oversizing by about 10%.
- The implant can be delivered into the joint with an atraumatic clamp through an extended portal.
- The scaffold must be sutured to the meniscus rim, preferably with all-inside or inside-out sutures.
- Do not overtighten the sutures; that could damage the implant.
- If the medial compartment is tight, partial release of the medial collateral ligament should be considered.
- If there are comorbidities (e.g., axial malalignment, full-thickness chondral injuries, ligament instability), consider staging the procedures.

Clinical and Surgical Pitfalls

- Inadequate lesion preparation may result in the implant not making uniform contact with the host meniscus rim.
- Improper measuring of the defect or cutting the implant too short leaves the defect incompletely filled.
- Excessive tension on the fixation sutures can damage the scaffold implant.
- Damage to the articular cartilage with the implant delivery device or with the suture devices can occur, especially in a tight knee.
- Placing the implant in a knee with untreated comorbidities can result in excessive biomechanical forces on the scaffold and lead to its damage or prevent adequate cell ingrowth and new tissue formation.

---

*The devices described in this chapter are not currently approved by the U.S. Food and Drug Administration for distribution or use in the United States (as of January 2013).

Contemporary thinking related to the meniscus focuses on preservation, restoration, and reconstruction. The menisci are critical for shock absorption, force transmission, and load distribution across the knee in addition to contributing to stability, joint congruence, articular cartilage nutrition, articular cartilage protection, joint lubrication, and proprioception. Because meniscus injuries often are irreparable, tissue engineering techniques have been used to develop acellular materials to support regrowth of lost meniscus tissue. For an engineered matrix to function as a resorbable meniscus template, of particular importance are the biomechanical properties of the matrix template because the template initially serves the biomechanical function of the meniscus. Thus strength of the engineered template and the subsequent biomechanical properties of the regenerated and remodeled tissue must be adequate for the device to survive initially in the hostile environment of the knee, and then ultimately to function like meniscus tissue. In addition, the scaffold must be conductive for cells as well as permeable to nutrients. Intrinsic biologic signals (e.g., growth factors) and cells must incorporate into the template to enhance the overall regeneration and remodeling process and provide an ideal biologic environment for cellular infiltration and new matrix synthesis.

PREOPERATIVE CONSIDERATIONS

Specific indications and contraindications have been developed for meniscus scaffolds.[1-13]

Indications

- For use in patients with either acute or chronic meniscus injuries
- Prior loss of meniscus tissue with intact anterior and posterior horn attachments and an intact rim over the entire circumference of the involved medial meniscus
- Irreparable meniscus tears requiring partial meniscectomy and requiring greater than 25% removal and with the lesion extending at least into the red-white zone
- Partial meniscus loss in the presence of early osteoarthritis (OA) with Kellgren-Lawrence grade 1 or 2 changes radiographically or Outerbridge grade III or lower changes arthroscopically
- Anterior cruciate ligament (ACL) deficiencies corrected within 12 weeks of the implant surgery
- Patients able and willing to follow postoperative rehabilitation program described later

Contraindications

- Complete meniscus loss or absence of one or both horn attachments.
- Repairable meniscus tear.
- Uncorrected ligamentous instability or insufficiency in the involved knee.
- Uncorrected Outerbridge grade IV (full-thickness) degenerative cartilage lesions and/or advanced OA in the affected joint. Limited clinical observations have suggested that the irregular surfaces of an untreated chondral lesion adjacent to the implant may damage or destroy the implant during the early stages of the regenerative process. No controlled studies have been conducted to confirm these observations, nor have studies been done to evaluate the consequences of having degenerative chondral lesions in other compartments of the involved joint that receives the scaffold.
- Uncorrected malformations or axial malalignment in the lower extremity. Malalignment may excessively overload the involved compartment, possibly resulting in damage to the implant during the early regenerative process. No controlled studies have been conducted to confirm this possibility. Whether or not there is a coexisting OA with the malalignment, consideration should be given to correcting those abnormalities before or at least concurrently with the scaffold implantation.
- Documented allergy to any product of animal or synthetic origin or a history of anaphylactoid reaction.
- Systemic or local infection.
- Medical history that is positive for, but not restricted to, severe degenerative osteoarthrosis, rheumatoid arthritis, relapsing polychondritis, or inflammatory arthritis.

SURGICAL TECHNIQUE

Two different meniscus scaffolds have been used clinically in humans and are in common use in several parts of the world. They are discussed in this chapter. Both the Collagen Meniscus Implant (CMI)[1-8,11-13] (Ivy Sports Medicine, Montvale, NJ) as well as Actifit[9,10] (Orteq Sports Medicine, London, United Kingdom) have comparable surgical implantation techniques. Therefore the techniques and steps described here pertain equally to both.

The patient is prepared and positioned for knee arthroscopy in a standard manner. General anesthesia is preferred. The arthroscopic portals should be the same as those preferred by the surgeon for meniscus repair.

Surgical Steps

Box 60-1 outlines the surgical steps of this procedure.

Preparation of Implant Bed

Preparation of the implant site results in a full-thickness meniscus defect (i.e., no residual flaps, no loose or degenerative tissue). The remaining meniscus rim should be intact over the entire length. The prepared defect site should maintain a uniform width of the meniscus rim and extend into either the red-white or red-red zone of the meniscus (Fig. 60-1). When the rim extends out to the red-white zone, puncture holes are made in the rim with use of a soft tissue microfracture awl or similar instrument to extend the blood supply. The anterior and posterior attachment points are trimmed square to accept the implant (Fig. 60-2).

Measurement of Defect Size

After implant site preparation, the defect is measured with the specifically designed measuring device. Because the implant is designed with fixed widths and curvatures, the arc length of the defect site is needed to size the implant properly. Measurements are taken with the measuring rod, which is loaded into the cannula, starting at the posterior aspect of the lesion and continuing until the correct arc length is noted (Fig. 60-3).

Implant Delivery into the Joint

The implant is sized 10% larger than the measured defect (Fig. 60-4). The sized implant is inserted into the joint through an enlarged medial portal with a curved atraumatic vascular clamp (14- to 16-cm-long Cooley clamp) (Fig. 60-5). With the insertion clamp, the implant is guided into the prepared defect (Fig. 60-6).

Suturing the Implant to the Remaining Meniscus

With the implant positioned properly, it is fixed to the host meniscus rim. The original technique used only an inside-out suture method, but that has mostly been changed to an all-inside technique as described in the next section. With use of an inside-out suturing technique, the implant is sutured to the remaining meniscus with size 2-0 braided polyester sutures. The anterior and posterior aspects of the implant are secured with horizontal mattress sutures, typically starting in the posterior aspect of the implant. Vertical mattress sutures are used throughout the remainder of the implant. The sutures should be placed about 5 mm apart midway between the inner and outer margins of the implant to

---

BOX 60-1 Surgical Steps

1. Complete a thorough arthroscopic diagnostic examination, inspecting all geographic areas of the knee. Perform all other intra-articular procedures before completing the meniscus scaffold implantation.

2. Prepare the implant site to ensure a full-thickness meniscus defect (i.e., no residual flaps, loose or degenerative tissue). The remaining meniscus rim should be intact over the entire length. The prepared defect site should maintain a uniform width of the meniscus rim extending to the red-white or red-red zone.

3. The defect size must be measured accurately; then the implant should be trimmed by oversizing it by about 10%.

4. The appropriately sized implant is inserted into the joint through an enlarged portal with a curved atraumatic vascular clamp (e.g., 14- to 16-cm-long Cooley clamp). With the insertion clamp, the implant is guided into the prepared defect.

5. With the implant positioned properly, it is fixed to the host meniscus rim, preferably with all-inside or inside-out sutures. During tying or tightening, the sutures should be tensioned just enough to allow apposition of the implant to the meniscus rim, but not overtightened, which could damage the scaffold.

6. If the medial compartment is tight, partial release of the medial collateral ligament should be considered.

7. If there are comorbidities (e.g., axial malalignment, full-thickness chondral injuries, ligament instability), consider staging the procedures.

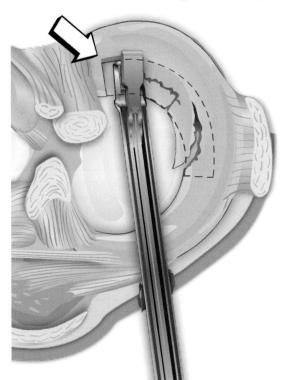

Figure 60-1. Preparation of the implant bed requires meticulous removal of the pathologic tissue to ensure a full-thickness lesion with a stable meniscus rim *(arrow)* as demonstrated in this illustration.

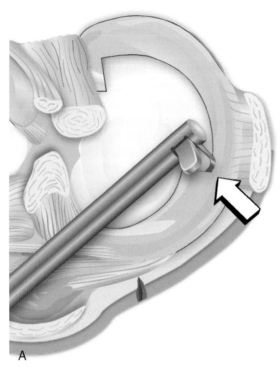

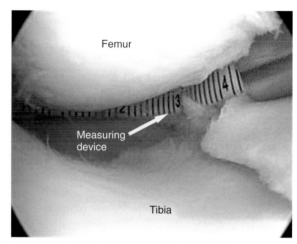

Figure 60-3. A flexible measuring device is used to measure the arc length of the defect to size the meniscus implant properly.

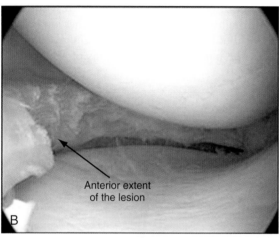

Figure 60-2. Both the anterior and posterior extents of the lesion are made square with radial debridement to better accommodate the implant as noted by the black arrow. (**B,** *Courtesy Dr. Dirk Holsten, Koblenz, Germany.*)

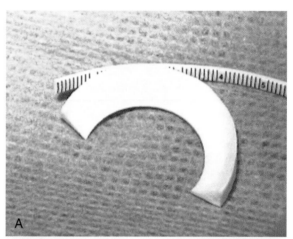

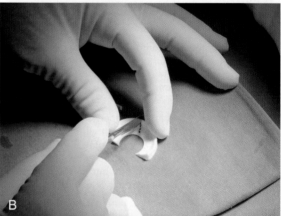

Figure 60-4. The flexible measuring rod is used to measure the length of the implant along its outer rim. The implant length is carefully and accurately measured, then the length is increased by approximately 10% before the implant is cut to ensure adequate length.

provide the greatest resistance to cutting through the implant. When the SharpShooter suturing device (Ivy Sports Medicine) (Fig. 60-7) is used, it is helpful to advance the needle about 2 mm out of the cannula before placement of the stitch so that with slight posterior pressure, proper positioning of the implant is ensured before the needle is advanced. Once both suture arms have been passed, care must be taken to pull the two arms of the sutures together at the same time to avoid any sawing action of the suture on the implant. Care should be taken to protect the surrounding neurovascular structures. After placement of all sutures, they should be tied over the capsule through the

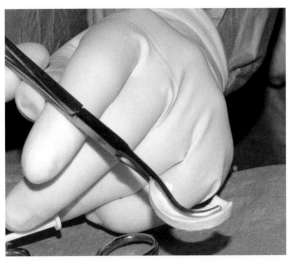

Figure 60-5. The trimmed implant is secured in a curved atraumatic vascular clamp (e.g., 14- to 16-cm-long Cooley clamp) then inserted into the joint through an enlarged portal.

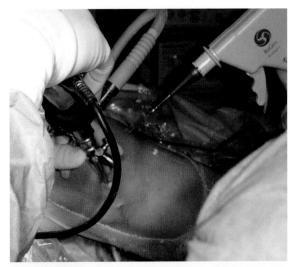

Figure 60-7. An inside-out suturing device is used for arthroscopic placement and advancement of the suture needles. *(Courtesy Dr. Juan Carlos Monllau, Barcelona, Spain.)*

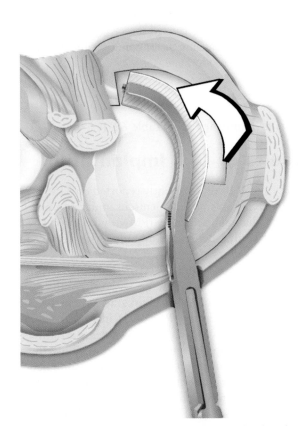

Figure 60-6. With the insertion clamp, the implant is guided into the prepared defect.

posteromedial skin incision while the implant remains under arthroscopic visualization. During tying the sutures should be tensioned just enough to allow apposition of the implant to the meniscus rim, but not over tightened. Direct arthroscopic visualization helps ensure correct suture tension.

Alternative Procedures for Implantation with All-Inside Suturing

The current procedures typically involve fixation with an all-inside suturing device such as the FasT-Fix (Smith & Nephew Endoscopy, Andover, MA). This approach can be more time-efficient and potentially minimize risks inherently associated with an inside-out suture procedure. When an all-inside suture technique is used, the need for an additional posteromedial skin incision and preparation of the joint capsule is eliminated. The all-inside suture system is used to fix the implant with horizontal and vertical mattress sutures as previously described. It is recommended to first place the posterior horizontal suture (Fig. 60-8), then the vertical sutures working anteriorly (Fig. 60-9), and finally the anterior horizontal suture. If the implant extends far anterior, for the most anterior fixation sutures the SharpShooter suturing device with an anterior cannula may be used to place inside-out sutures.

POSTOPERATIVE CONSIDERATIONS

Rehabilitation activities should follow the recommended standard program,[2,8,9,11-13] which is as follows:

- Day 1 until end of week 4:
  - Crutch walking, brace locked at full extension
  - Passive range-of-motion (ROM) exercises from 0 to 60 degrees of flexion
  - Week 1: no weight bearing (WB)
  - Weeks 2 to 4: slow increase of partial WB to 50% WB

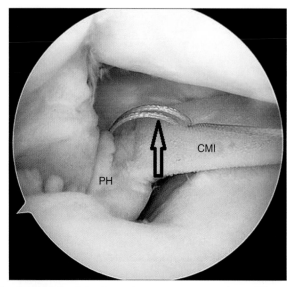

Figure 60-8. A horizontal mattress suture *(arrow)* is placed from the collagen meniscus implant *(CMI)* to the posterior horn *(PH)* attachment as the first suture.

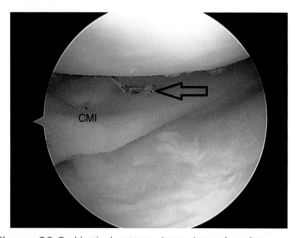

Figure 60-9. Vertical sutures *(arrow)* are placed to secure the collagen meniscus implant *(CMI)* scaffold to the meniscus rim.

- Daily patella mobilization (until week 8), quadriceps strengthening exercises
- Weeks 5 and 6, in addition to existing program:
  - Passive ROM exercises from 0 to 90 degrees of flexion
  - Increase partial WB from 50% to 90%
  - Continue use of brace
- Weeks 7 and 8, in addition to existing program:
  - Unlock brace, but continue its use
  - Active flexion-extension exercises up to full ROM as tolerated
  - Gradually discontinue crutches while increasing to full WB
  - Begin additional strength-training exercises

- Week 9 through 6 months:
  - Discontinue brace and crutches
  - Continue strength-training and agility exercises with gradually increased intensity
- Month 7 and beyond:
  - Return to full unrestricted activities after 6 months or later, depending on intensity of sports activity

Complications

Most of the complications reported with use of meniscus scaffolds have involved the surgical procedure rather than the implants themselves.[2,8-10,13] There exists the possibility of an immune or allergic response to the scaffold materials, but the components of both the biologic and the synthetic scaffolds are in wide medical use for other applications.[3,8,9] As noted earlier, improper fixation of the implant to the host meniscus rim could lead to its dislodgement. Untreated comorbidities might lead to damage to the scaffold or inadequate cellular ingrowth into the implant. Neither type of implant has been reported to have caused direct harm to a joint.[1-13] If the scaffold is causing an ongoing problem, it can be explanted with moderate ease.

RESULTS

Results are summarized in Table 60-1.

Results of CMI Implantation

Rodkey and colleagues recently reported on 311 patients with an irreparable medial meniscus injury or a previous partial medial meniscectomy (PMM) who were enrolled in a CMI study.[8] Patients randomly either received the CMI or served as partial-meniscectomy-only controls. Reoperation rates and survivorship analysis were determined.[5,6,8] Mean follow-up was 59 months (range, 16 to 92). Based on 141 relooks at 1 year, the CMI resulted in significantly ($P = .001$) increased meniscus tissue compared with the original index partial meniscectomy. The implant supported meniscus-like matrix production and integration while it was assimilated and resorbed. Patients who had previously undergone prior partial meniscectomy and received an implant regained significantly more of their lost activity (Tegner index) than did controls ($P = .02$).[7,8] Through five years, the patients who received implants underwent significantly fewer nonprotocol reoperations than controls ($P = .04$).[6,8] The authors concluded that the new meniscus-like tissue is stable and appears safe and biomechanically competent.[8]

Monllau and colleagues evaluated clinical outcomes of CMI after a minimum of 10 years' follow-up in 25 patients.[2] At 10 years the mean Lysholm score improved

TABLE 60-1. Results

Rodkey et al[6,8]	New biomechanically competent meniscus-like tissue forms and is stable for at least 5 years Safe—Complications similar to those of meniscectomy Enhances meniscus function Improved clinical outcomes in patients who had previous meniscectomy Improved survivorship vs. partial meniscectomy (PM) at 5 years
Rodkey et al[7]	Compared results of collagen meniscus implant (CMI) with those of PM alone at 6 years Average 6-year Tegner index (TI) score for CMI patients = 0.47 47% of lost activity regained with scaffold Average 6-year TI score for PM controls = 0.22 22% of lost activity regained with PM alone Clinically and statistically significant (P = .028) TI score for CMI improved from 42% at 2 years to 47% at 6 years (P < .05) TI score for PM controls *decreased* from 29% to 22% from 2 to 6 years (P < .05) Noteworthy that CMI patients continued to *gain* activity from 2 to 6 years, but PM controls *lost* activity over same time
Monllau et al[2]	10-year follow-up in 25 patients after medial CMI Meniscus substitution with CMI provided significant pain relief and functional and activity improvements at minimum 10-year follow-up Safe and low failure rate in the long term No development or progression of DJD
Zaffagnini et al[13]	10-year follow-up in 33 patients after medial CMI compared with medial PM alone All patients clinically evaluated at time 0, at 5 years, and at minimum 10 years after surgery (mean follow-up, 133 months) Significant improvement with use of the CMI at minimum 10-year follow-up compared with partial medial meniscectomy alone based on extensive clinical and imaging findings for pain, activity level, radiographic, and MRI outcomes
Zaffagnini et al[12]	Lateral CMI implanted in professional soccer player after failed partial lateral meniscectomy Returned to competition at 10 months Tegner score improved from 3 preoperatively to 10 at 6 months and 3 years No pain and 100-point Lysholm score at 3 years Has played more than 80 professional games since his return
Verdonk et al[9,10]	52 patients enrolled in a multisite nonrandomized study of Actifit 34 received medial Actifit implant, and 18 received lateral implant No inflammatory reaction observed during 12-month relook MRI findings at 12 months postimplantation showed stable or improved cartilage scores in index compartment compared with baseline Viable tissue with no evidence of necrosis or cell death found in all biopsy samples taken at 12-month relook arthroscopy Tissue ingrowth with meniscus-like cells visible in distinct layers Statistically significant improvements compared with baseline (P < .05) for IKDC and Lysholm scores and for knee pain on VAS at 12 months No longer-term results available as of this writing

DJD, Degenerative joint disease; *IKDC*, International Knee Documentation Committee; *MRI*, magnetic resonance imaging; *VAS*, visual analogue scale.

from 59.9 preoperatively to 87.5 at final follow-up (P = .001). The results were good or excellent in 83% of the population. The mean pain score on a visual analog scale improved by 3.5 points at final follow-up. Patient satisfaction with the procedure was 3.4 of 4 points. Radiographic evaluation showed either minimal or no narrowing of the joint line. Magnetic resonance imaging (MRI) showed nearly normal findings in 64% of patients and normal findings in 21%. There were two failures but no complications related to the device. The authors concluded that the CMI provides significant pain relief

and functional improvement after a minimum of 10 years' follow-up. No significant development or progression of degenerative knee joint disease was observed.[2]

Zaffagnini and colleagues also carried out a 10-year follow-up in 33 nonconsecutive patients who received the CMI or underwent PMM alone and served as controls.[13] All patients were clinically evaluated at time 0 and at 5 years and a minimum of 10 years after surgery (mean follow-up, 133 months). The authors reported on extensive clinical and imaging findings that pain, activity level, and radiographic and MRI outcomes were significantly improved with use of the CMI at a minimum 10-year follow-up compared with PMM alone.[13]

Clinical Results of Actifit Implantation

In a multisite nonrandomized study of the Actifit, 52 patients were enrolled.[9,10] Thirty-four patients received a medial Actifit implant, and 18 received a lateral implant. The mean age of the subjects was 31 years, and the majority were male (75%). Length of the meniscus defects ranged from 30 to 70 mm (mean, 47 mm). No inflammatory reaction to the scaffold implant was observed during arthroscopic examination at 12-month relook. Anatomic MRI findings at 12 months postimplantation showed stable or improved cartilage scores in the index compartment compared with baseline. At 3 months postimplantation, early evidence of tissue ingrowth in the peripheral half of the scaffold was observed on MRI in 86% of patients. Viable tissue with no evidence of necrosis or cell death was observed in all biopsy samples taken at the 12-month relook arthroscopy, consistent with the biocompatibility of the scaffold. Further histologic analyses revealed tissue ingrowth with meniscus-like cells visible in distinct layers with an indication of ongoing regeneration, remodeling, and maturation of tissue. Statistically significant improvements compared with baseline ($P < .05$) were reported for functionality on the International Knee Documentation Committee (IKDC) and Lysholm scores as well as for knee pain on a visual analogue scale (VAS) at 3, 6, and 12 months postimplantation. For the five subcomponents of the Knee injury and Osteoarthritis Outcome Score (KOOS) questionnaire, statistically significant improvements ($P < .05$) were reported in pain, daily living, and quality of life at 3, 6, and 12 months postimplantation, and in sports and recreation and symptoms at 6 and 12 months postimplantation.[9,10]

CONCLUSION

The two devices currently in clinical use are reviewed earlier,[1-13] but other promising techniques for meniscus preservation and replacement may be on the horizon. There is a constant search for new and clinically useful modes of meniscus treatment, but partial meniscus replacement with scaffolds for regeneration and regrowth of lost meniscus tissue seems a reasonable and feasible first step in the right direction.[1-13] *Remember, save the meniscus!*

REFERENCES

1. Bulgheroni P, Murena L, Ratti C, et al. Follow-up of collagen meniscus implant patients: Clinical, radiological, and magnetic resonance imaging results at 5 years. *Knee.* 2010;17:224-229.
2. Monllau JC, Gelber PE, Abat F, et al. Outcome after partial medial meniscus substitution with the collagen meniscal implant at a minimum of 10 years' follow-up. *Arthroscopy.* 2011;27:933-943.
3. Rodkey WG. Menaflex collagen meniscus implants: basic science. In: Beaufils P, Verdonk R, eds. *The Meniscus.* Berlin-Heidelberg, Springer-Verlag; 2010:367-371.
4. Rodkey WG, Briggs KK, Steadman JR. Collagen meniscus implant (CMI)—treated patients have increased activity levels after two years. *Osteoarthritis Cartilage.* 2007; 15(Suppl):B86.
5. Rodkey WG, Briggs KK, Steadman JR. Survivorship analysis confirms that collagen meniscus implants (CMI) decrease reoperation rates in chronic patients. *Osteoarthritis Cartilage.* 2007;15(Suppl):B87.
6. Rodkey WG, Briggs KK, Steadman JR. Collagen meniscus implants (CMI) decrease reoperation rates in chronic knee patients compared to meniscectomy only: A 5-year survivorship analysis. *Knee Surg Sports Traumatol Arthrosc.* 2008;16(Suppl 1):S14.
7. Rodkey WG, Briggs KK, Steadman JR. Function and return to activity outcomes six years after partial meniscectomy vs. collagen meniscus implants assessed with Lysholm scores and Tegner Index. *Knee Surg Sports Traumatol Arthrosc.* 2010;18(Suppl 1):S14-S15.
8. Rodkey WG, DeHaven KE, Montgomery WH, et al. Comparison of the collagen meniscus implant to partial meniscectomy: A prospective randomized trial. *J Bone Joint Surg Am.* 2008;90:1413-1426.
9. Verdonk R, Verdonk P, Heinrichs EL. Polyurethane meniscus implant: technique. In: Beaufils P, Verdonk R, eds. *The Meniscus.* Berlin-Heidelberg, Springer-Verlag; 2010: 389-394.
10. Verdonk R, Verdonk P, Huysse W, et al. Tissue ingrowth after implantation of a novel, biodegradable polyurethane scaffold for treatment of partial meniscal lesions. *Am J Sports Med.* 2011;39:774-782.
11. Zaffagnini S, Marcheggiani Muccioli G, Giordano G, et al. Synthetic meniscal scaffolds. *Tech Knee Surg.* 2009;8: 251-256.
12. Zaffagnini S, Marcheggiani Muccioli GM, Grassi A, et al. Arthroscopic lateral collagen meniscus implant in a professional soccer player. *Knee Surg Sports Traumatol Arthrosc.* 2011.
13. Zaffagnini S, Marcheggiani Muccioli GM, Lopomo N, et al. Prospective long-term outcomes of the medial collagen meniscus implant versus partial medial meniscectomy. A minimum 10-year follow-up study. *Am J Sports Med.* 2011;39:977-985.

Chapter 61

Combined Anterior Cruciate Ligament Reconstruction and Meniscal Allograft Transplantation

M. Mustafa Gomberawalla and Jon K. Sekiya

Chapter Synopsis
- Combined meniscal and anterior cruciate ligament (ACL) deficiency alters knee function and predisposes the patient to accelerated degenerative changes. Combined meniscal allograft transplantation and ACL reconstruction has been advocated to treat this combined deficiency. A size-matched meniscus allograft is transplanted into the appropriate compartment. For revision ACL reconstructions, we prefer to use a double-bundle allograft technique. Clinical results have shown normal to near-normal IKDC scores and return to recreational activities in most patients.

Important Points
- Patients should be under 40 years of age with both meniscal and ACL deficiency.
- Transplantation should be avoided in the presence of advanced chondral changes.
- The meniscal allograft is affixed with use of two bone plugs and bone tunnels (for the medial meniscus) or a bone bridge and trough (for the lateral meniscus).
- Patients may return to recreational activities; however, high-impact sports should be avoided indefinitely.

Clinical and Surgical Pearls
- For the medial meniscus, keep the bone plugs relatively short.

- A traction suture is used in the posterior horn of the transplanted meniscus to guide its intra-articular reduction.
- Intercompartment visualization is significantly improved with the use of a femoral distractor.
- One to 2 mm of the native meniscus rim should be left intact and will be used as a bed for fixation.

Clinical and Surgical Pitfalls
- An appropriately size-matched meniscus allograft should be used.
- The tibial ACL tunnel(s) can encroach on the bony fixation sites of the meniscus.
- The bone plugs (medially) or bone trough (laterally) should be created at the anatomic insertion sites to avoid malpositioning of the meniscal transplant.
- Ensure that full range of motion (including extension) is obtainable at the conclusion of the procedure.

Video
- Video 61-1: Allograft preparation
- Video 61-2: Meniscal site preparation
- Video 61-3: Meniscal allograft fixation
- Video 61-4: ACL tunnel preparation and graft passage

The menisci play a crucial role in maintaining the structure and function of the normal knee. They contribute to shock absorption, joint lubrication, knee stabilization, proprioception, and load sharing.[1-3] These roles are significant in protecting the articular cartilage. For example, the medial meniscus carries up to 50% of the load in the medial compartment when the knee is extended.[4] Fairbank showed significant changes in the knee joint after medial and lateral meniscectomies.[5] Although chondral changes occur more rapidly after lateral meniscectomies, medial meniscectomy more predictably results in degeneration within the knee.[5,6] These findings lead surgeons toward meniscal-preserving treatments whenever possible.[7] Unfortunately, in certain patients meniscal pathology may be severe enough to necessitate subtotal or total meniscectomy to appropriately address a patient's symptoms.

The progression toward degeneration in postmeniscectomy knees is accelerated with an associated injury to the anterior cruciate ligament (ACL).[8,9] In addition, the results of ACL reconstruction in knees with medial meniscal deficiency are usually worse than in knees with an intact medial meniscus.[10] Thus, the menisci and ACL likely play a synergistic role in preserving knee stability. The medial meniscus acts as a secondary stabilizer to anterior tibial translation. Medial meniscectomy in the ACL-deficient knee increases anterior tibial translation by 58% to 90%.[3] With ACL deficiency, forces in the medial meniscus increase from 52% to 197%.[11] In addition, a combined ACL and medial meniscal deficiency results in anteromedial rotatory instability of the knee. For this combined deficiency, performance of meniscal allograft transplantation combined with ACL reconstruction has been advocated to diminish pain, to improve knee stability and function, and to delay degenerative changes in the knee. We present our preferred technique to address this challenging condition as well as our clinical outcomes.

PREOPERATIVE CONSIDERATIONS

History

Before any major reconstructive procedure, it is important to thoroughly evaluate the symptoms the patient may be experiencing, the preinjury and postinjury levels of function, and his or her goals for after treatment. The history should include the initial injury, any treatments (conservative and surgical) for the injury, and what symptoms the patient is experiencing. Typically, the patient has a history of an acute knee injury that may include an episode of "giving way." He or she has likely undergone meniscectomy, and possibly ACL

reconstruction. Despite these treatments, pain in the affected compartment and symptomatic instability may persist. Obtaining previous operative reports as well as arthroscopic images from prior surgeries is important to understand the status of the menisci.

Physical Examination

The physical examination should begin with inspection to document the presence of an effusion or visible swelling, trauma, or skin compromise. Next, the range of motion and strength are documented. The patient's stance, gait pattern, and overall limb alignment should be evaluated and compared with the contralateral side. Joint line tenderness and degree of quadriceps atrophy (if any) should also be noted. Ligamentous stability of the knee should be assessed and compared with uninjured side. Specific attention should be paid to evaluation of the ACL with the Lachman, pivot-shift, and anterior drawer tests. Increased anterior tibial translation during the anterior drawer test that is equal to or greater than translation noted during the Lachman test suggests a loss of secondary stabilizers, most commonly from a deficient posterior horn of the medial meniscus, but also from posteromedial or posterolateral insufficiency.[12,13]

Imaging

Radiographs

Bilateral weight-bearing posteroanterior (PA) views at 45 degrees of flexion, lateral views, and sunrise views are obtained. Long-leg films are used to evaluate mechanical axis alignment and are essential if meniscus replacement surgery is being considered.

Magnetic Resonance Imaging

The integrity of the ACL, subchondral bone, meniscal tissue, and other ligamentous structures is assessed. T1-weighted coronal and sagittal images are specifically used to evaluate the remaining meniscus (Fig. 61-1).

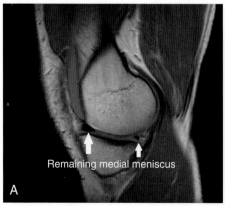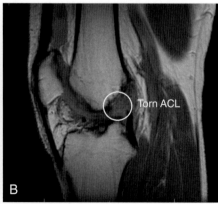

Figure 61-1. Magnetic resonance image (T1-weighted, sagittal view) of the knee demonstrating a deficient medial meniscus **(A)** and a complete anterior cruciate ligament tear **(B)**.

Indications and Contraindications

Candidates for combined ACL reconstruction and meniscal transplantation are patients under 40 years of age with symptomatic instability (despite previous ACL reconstruction) and meniscal deficiency with pain localized to the affected compartment. Ideally, patients should have intact cartilage surfaces with minimal chondral wear (grade I or II changes) and should not have limb malalignment. If the affected limb is malaligned, this should be addressed with an osteotomy to realign the weight-bearing axis before or concomitantly with the reconstruction-transplantation. Large grade IV lesions can be concomitantly reconstructed with fresh osteochondral allograft replacement. Nonoperative treatment including bracing and activity modification will likely have failed. Significant chondral changes (grade III or higher), inflammatory arthritis, history of previous infections, or a body mass index greater than 35 should be considered contraindications to the procedure. Before surgery, the patient's willingness to cooperate with a comprehensive rehabilitation program should be assessed. In addition, given the complexity of this problem, staged diagnostic scope is usually indicated to determine what will need to be done.

SURGICAL TECHNIQUE

Allograft Selection

Appropriate sizing of the meniscal allograft facilitates healing of the graft after transplantation. Thus meniscal grafts should be matched in both size and laterality. Measurements from the PA and lateral radiographs of the knee are used to size the meniscus, as described by Pollard and colleagues—the most common technique used by American Association of Tissue Banks (AATB)–certified tissue banks.[14] This sizing method allows for an accurate estimate (within 3 to 4 mm) of the graft[14] without the need for additional imaging. This size is given to the tissue bank, and an appropriately matched graft is obtained. The meniscal allografts are sterility harvested and fresh-frozen. They should not be irradiated before transplantation.

To reconstruct the ACL concomitantly with meniscal transplantation, we prefer to use a tibialis anterior allograft tendon. In revision procedures we prefer to reconstruct the ACL with a double-bundle technique. Alternatively, bone-patellar tendon-bone allograft may also be used. We prefer allograft in these situations as opposed to autograft, because it hastens postoperative recovery and decreases donor site morbidity in general in knees that have undergone multiple or previous operations. The allograft should be fresh frozen and may be irradiated before use.

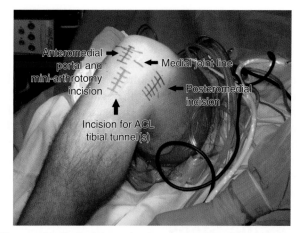

Figure 61-2. Incisions, landmarks, positioning, and the use of a lateral post for the surgical procedure.

Anesthesia and Positioning

We prefer to use general anesthesia for most procedures (unless contraindicated). Often, a femoral and sciatic nerve block will also be used to aid in postoperative pain control. The patient is positioned supine on the operating room table. A sandbag is taped onto the bed under the foot to help support the knee at approximately 70 degrees of flexion. A tourniquet is applied high on the thigh, along with a lateral post at the level of the tourniquet.

Surgical Landmarks, Incisions, and Portals

Figure 61-2 shows the following elements:

- Landmarks: Medial and lateral joint line, borders of the patellar tendon, fibular head, and tibial tubercle.
- Portals: Standard anteromedial and anterolateral arthroscopy portals are marked out. The anteromedial or anterolateral portal will be extended to create a mini-arthrotomy on the side of the meniscal transplant.
- Incisions: A proximal medial tibial incision will be used to create the tibial tunnel(s) for the ACL reconstruction. A posteromedial or posterolateral incision will be used for meniscal fixation, depending on whether a medial or lateral meniscal transplant will be performed.

Examination Under Anesthesia and Diagnostic Arthroscopy

Once appropriate anesthesia has been induced, a thorough examination of the injured knee is performed, and the knee is compared with the contralateral side. Specifically, anterior laxity is assessed with the Lachman, anterior drawer, and pivot-shift tests. With medial meniscal deficiency, anteromedial rotatory instability is evaluated. Diagnostic arthroscopy is performed, and the chondral surfaces of the affected and other compartments are noted. The decision to proceed should be reconsidered, and the transplant possibly abandoned if grade III or higher chondral changes are noted. The amount of remaining meniscus is also noted (Fig. 61-3). This highlights the need for a staged diagnostic scope, because fresh cartilage allografts and even fresh-frozen meniscal allograft must be preordered and size matched before the index procedure is performed.

Specific Steps

The specific steps of this procedure are outlined in Box 61-1.

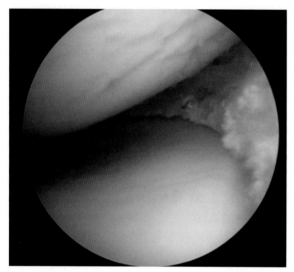

Figure 61-3. Arthroscopic view of the medial compartment demonstrating a near-total meniscectomy.

1. Allograft Preparation

After confirmation of the diagnosis, the allografts are thawed per the vendor's guidelines. The medial meniscus will be fixed with a bone plug technique, and the lateral meniscus will be fixed with a bone bridge and trough (Fig. 61-4).

For the medial meniscus, two 7-mm bone plugs are fashioned from the osseous portion of the meniscal allograft attachment to the donor tibia for the anterior and posterior horns. The bone plugs are secured with No. 2 braided, nonabsorbable suture. In addition, No. 3 braided, nonabsorbable sutures are placed within the posteromedial corner to assist in graft passage and later open fixation. The anterior and posterior horns are labeled with an indelible marker to aid in alignment once the graft is passed into the joint (Fig. 61-5). For the lateral meniscus, a bone bridge measuring 8 to 9 mm is fashioned and maintains the relationship of the attachments of the anterior and posterior horns. The bone bridge is fixed with No. 2 braided, nonabsorbable sutures. In addition, No. 3 braided, nonabsorbable sutures are placed within the posterolateral corner to assist with graft passage and later open fixation (Fig. 61-6).

BOX 61-1 Specific Surgical Steps

1. Allograft preparation
2. Meniscal rim preparation
3. Meniscal insertion site preparation
4. Meniscus allograft passage
5. Meniscus allograft fixation
6. Anterior cruciate ligament tunnel preparation and graft passage
7. Closure

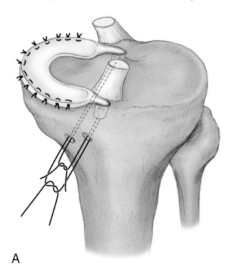
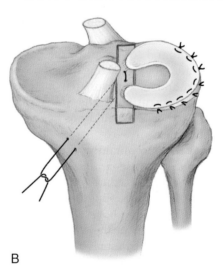

A   B

Figure 61-4. Schematic representation of meniscal allograft fixation showing bone tunnels for the medial meniscus **(A)** and bone bridge and trough for the lateral meniscus **(B)**. The graft is additionally fixed to the native meniscal rim with sutures placed with an inside-out technique.

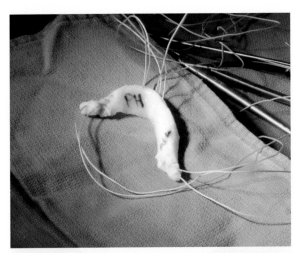

Figure 61-5. Prepared medial meniscus transplant with two bone plugs and traction sutures in the posterior horn.

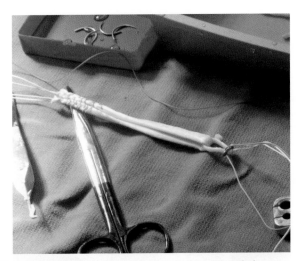

Figure 61-7. Prepared tibialis anterior allograft for complete anterior cruciate ligament reconstruction with a closed-loop EndoButton (Smith & Nephew, London).

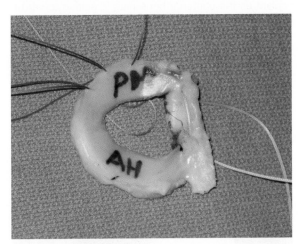

Figure 61-6. Prepared lateral meniscus transplant with a bone bridge and traction sutures in the posterior horn.

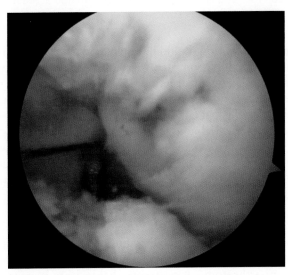

Figure 61-8. Arthroscopic view of the medial compartment. The anterior cruciate ligament guide is positioned over the posterior attachment of the medial meniscus before the guide pin is placed.

For preparation of the ACL graft, two tibialis anterior allografts measuring 6 to 7 mm in diameter are fashioned with No. 2 braided, nonabsorbable sutures on each side, and a 15-mm closed-loop EndoButton (Smith & Nephew, London) is placed in each graft (Fig. 61-7).

2. Meniscal Rim Preparation

The remaining meniscus in the involved compartment is identified and debrided until a 1- to 2-mm rim is remaining. This will serve as a base for suture fixation and enhance healing of the graft to native tissue. Next, the anterior and posterior horn attachments are identified. A femoral distractor is sometimes used to provide varus or valgus stress and improve visualization within the involved compartment.[15]

3. Meniscal Insertion Site Preparation

For the medial meniscus, two transosseous bone tunnels are created at the attachments of the anterior and posterior horns on the tibia, respectively. With the help of a standard ACL guide, a guide pin is placed at the anatomic insertion site of the posterior horn of the meniscus (Fig. 61-8). The pin is subsequently overdrilled with a 7-mm cannulated reamer. The ACL guide is then used to create a similar 7-mm bone tunnel at the attachment of the anterior horn of the medial meniscus.

For the lateral meniscus, a bone trough is fashioned in the lateral tibial plateau incorporating the attachment sites of the anterior and posterior horns. A ¼-inch curved osteotome is brought into the joint. The curve of the osteotome should face medially as it hugs the lateral aspect of the ACL insertion site. A sagittal cut is made with the osteotome in an anterior-to-posterior

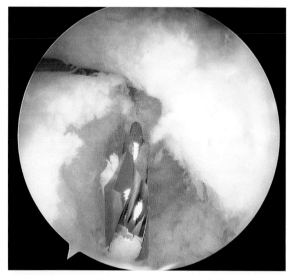

Figure 61-9. Arthroscopic view of the lateral compartment. The bony trough is created with an osteotome, and two suture tunnels are created at least 10 mm apart.

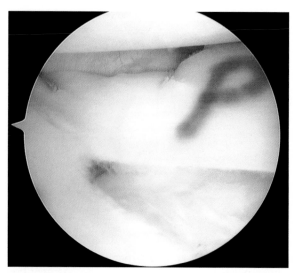

Figure 61-10. Arthroscopic view of the medial meniscal transplant as the posterior bone plug is guided toward the posterior bone tunnel.

direction. Caution should be taken to avoid encroaching on the ACL insertion site, where tunnels will be created for the ACL reconstruction. This step is repeated to create a second cut further lateral on the plateau and parallel to the first cut. The bone bridge is then removed, and prefabricated gouges are used to finish the trough to a diameter of 8 to 9 mm. With an ACL drill, two holes are made in the bone trough, separated by at least 10 mm. These holes will be used for suture passage and meniscal allograft fixation (Fig. 61-9).

4. Meniscus Allograft Passage

For the medial meniscus, the anteromedial arthroscopy portal is enlarged (approximately 3 to 4 cm) to create a mini-arthrotomy. A posteromedial incision is created, centered over the posterior aspect of the medial collateral ligament. The sartorius fascia is incised, and the dissection is carried down to develop the interval between the semimembranosus and the medial gastrocnemius until the posteromedial joint capsule is exposed. The allograft is passed through the mini-arthrotomy and appropriately oriented with use of the previously created anterior and posterior marks. The sutures from the anterior and posterior bone plugs are passed with a suture passer through their respective bone tunnels. Next, the posterior horn of the meniscal allograft is introduced into the joint. The posteromedial traction sutures are passed through the posteromedial incision and used to guide the posterior bone plug into its bone tunnel (Fig. 61-10). The anterior bone plug is guided toward its bone tunnel until the allograft is appropriately reduced into the medial compartment. The sutures in the bone plugs are tensioned until the plugs are sitting tightly in their bone tunnels. The sutures are tightened

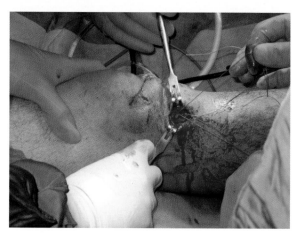

Figure 61-11. Sutures in the medial meniscal bone tunnels being tied over a bony bridge on the lateral tibial metaphysis.

and tied over separate plastic buttons, ensuring good circumferential tension on the allograft (Fig. 61-11).

For the lateral meniscus, the anterolateral arthroscopy portal is enlarged to create a mini-arthrotomy. In addition, a posterolateral incision is made, centered over the posterior aspect of the lateral collateral ligament (LCL). The interval between the Gerdy tubercle and the biceps femoris is developed, and the posterolateral joint capsule is exposed between the LCL and the lateral head of the gastrocnemius. The sutures in the anterior and posterior portions of the bone bridge are threaded through the previously drilled holes in the bone trough with the help of a suture passer. This introduces the meniscus into the joint in the correct orientation. The posterolateral traction sutures are passed through the posterolateral incision to help reduce the allograft into the joint, guiding the bone bridge toward the trough. The sutures in the bone bridge are tightened until the bone bridge is well seated in the bone trough and are tied over a cortical bridge on the tibia.

5. Meniscus Allograft Fixation

The meniscus is then secured to the native meniscal remnant with an arthroscopic inside-out technique. The posteromedial or posterolateral open sutures are secured to the respective posteromedial or posterolateral capsule with a free needle. Then multiple inside-out superior and inferior meniscus sutures are passed through the posterior horn and body of the meniscus (Fig. 61-12). After this, the anterior horn is repaired with an open technique through the arthrotomy with O-braided nonabsorbable sutures to the native anterior horn (Fig. 61-13).

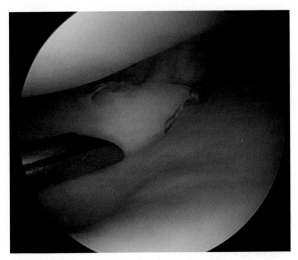

Figure 61-12. Arthroscopic view of inside-out sutures securing the medial meniscal transplant to the native meniscal rim.

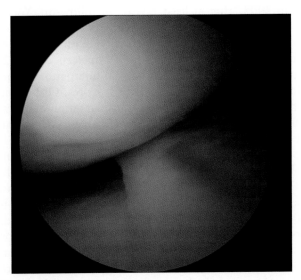

Figure 61-13. Arthroscopic view of the completed medial meniscal transplant.

6. Anterior Cruciate Ligament Tunnel Preparation and Graft Passage

Special care must be taken in performing an ACL reconstruction in conjunction with a meniscal transplant. Specifically, on the tibial side the ACL tunnels can encroach on the bone trough created for the lateral meniscus or on the anterior bone tunnel created for the medial meniscus. Thus we prefer to complete the meniscal transplantation and fixation of the meniscal allograft before starting the ACL reconstruction. Also, especially with double-bundle ACL tunnels, we prefer to use anterolateral tibial tunnels for both medial and lateral meniscus transplants.

Although a single-bundle technique may be used in some situations such as primary reconstructions, we prefer a double-bundle allograft technique in revision reconstructions. With use of a standard ACL guide, a guide pin is placed in the anteromedial and posterolateral bundle insertion sites into the tibia. This is over-reamed with a 7-mm reamer. Careful attention should be paid so that the tibial tunnels do not encroach on the meniscal allograft transplant sites. Next, the knee is hyperflexed, and a guide pin is placed into the anteromedial and posterolateral bundle origins on the femur, through the medial portal. These are over-reamed with a 7-mm cannulated reamer (Fig. 61-14). Next, the EndoButton reamer is used to break through the lateral femoral cortex.

The posterolateral graft is passed first, followed by the anteromedial graft. The EndoButton in each graft is flipped, which is verified with intraoperative fluoroscopy (Fig. 61-15). Next, the posterolateral bundle is tensioned in full extension and affixed in the tibial tunnel with a graft bolt or Intrafix (DePuy Orthopaedics, Warsaw, IN). The anteromedial bundle is tensioned

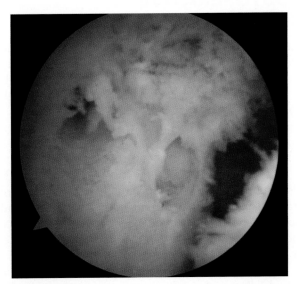

Figure 61-14. Arthroscopic view of the femoral tunnels for a double-bundle anterior cruciate ligament reconstruction.

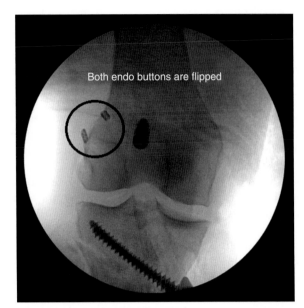

Both endo buttons are flipped

Figure 61-15. Intraoperative fluoroscopy is used to verify that both EndoButtons (Smith & Nephew, London) in each bundle of the anterior cruciate ligament allograft reconstruction are flipped. Previous interference screws in the femur and osteotomy hardware in the tibia are noted.

at 70 degrees of flexion and fixed to the tibia in a similar fashion. Range of motion of the knee is assessed, including the ability to obtain full knee hyperextension.

7. Closure

Arthroscopy portals are closed with simple sutures. We prefer to close larger incisions in a layered fashion.

POSTOPERATIVE REHABILITATION

The patient is immediately placed into a hinged knee brace. Initial rehabilitation focuses on regaining range of motion, with the goals of obtaining full extension by 1 week and 100 degrees of flexion by 4 to 6 weeks postoperatively. Partial weight bearing with crutches is permitted immediately with the brace locked in extension, with gradual advancement to weight bearing as tolerated.

At 4 to 6 weeks postoperatively crutches may be discontinued and the patient should bear weight as tolerated. Isometric strengthening and closed-chain quadriceps exercises are started under a focused physical therapy program. Low-resistance activities are initiated at 8 weeks.

After 3 months, gait balance should be achieved, and closed chain strengthening exercises are further advanced. Low-impact jogging may be initiated at 5 to 6 months postoperatively. Low- and moderate-impact

TABLE 61-1. Results from Combined Meniscal Transplantation and Anterior Cruciate Ligament Reconstruction

Study	No. of Patients	Follow-up	Results
Yoldas et al[16] (2003)	20	2 years	19 of 20 normal to near-normal IKDC score 75% participated in moderate sports
Sekiya et al[17] (2003)	28	2.8 years	86%-90% normal to near-normal IKDC score 90% normal to near-normal Lachman score
Graf et al[18] (2004)	8	8.5 years	7 of 8 normal to near-normal IKDC score 6 of 8 returned to recreational sports

IKDC, International Knee Documentation Committee.

sports may be initiated at 6 to 9 months. However, high-impact activities are discouraged indefinitely.

Complications

- Incomplete healing or recurrent tears of the transplanted meniscus
- Infection
- Arthrofibrosis
- Neurovascular injury (to the saphenous or peroneal nerve)

RESULTS

After combined ACL reconstruction and meniscal transplantation, good results are achieved in approximately 85% of patients (Table 61-1).

In 2003, after at least 2 years of follow-up, Yoldas and colleagues[13] presented 20 patients who had undergone combined ACL reconstruction with (medial or lateral) meniscal transplantation. Nineteen of the 20 patients had normal to near-normal International Knee Documentation Committee (IKDC) scores. Of patients who had undergone meniscal transplantation and revision ACL reconstruction, 75% were able to participate in moderate sports activities without instability.

In 2003, after 2.8 years of follow-up, Sekiya and colleagues[17] reported similar results in 28 patients who had undergone combined ACL reconstruction and meniscal transplantation. Of these patients, 86% to 90% had normal to near-normal IKDC scores. In addition, the physical and mental components of the Short Form 36 (SF-36) score were higher for patients than those of age- and gender-matched populations. Nearly 90% of patients had normal or near-normal Lachman and pivot-shift test scores.

In 2004, Graf and colleagues[18] presented long-term results after 8.5 years of follow-up of patients who had undergone medial meniscal transplantation and ACL reconstruction. Seven of the eight patients had normal to near-normal IKDC scores. Six of the eight patients were extremely pleased with the outcome and had returned to recreational sports. All eight patients stated that they would recommend the procedure to a friend.

REFERENCES

1. Henning C, Lynch M. Current concepts of meniscal function and pathology. *Clin Sport Med.* 1985;4:259-265.
2. Krause W, Pope M, Johnson R, et al. Mechanical changes in the knee after meniscectomy. *J Bone Joint Surg Am.* 1976;58:599-604.
3. Levy I, Torzilli P, Warren R. The effect of medical meniscectomy on anterior-posterior motion of the knee. *J Bone Joint Surg Am.* 1982;64:883-888.
4. Seedhom B, Wright V. Functions of the menisci: a preliminary study. *J Bone Joint Surg Br.* 1974;56:381-382.
5. Fairbank T. Knee joint changes after meniscectomy. *J Bone Joint Surg Br.* 1948;30:664-670.
6. Johnson R, Kettelkamp D, Clark W, et al. Factors affecting late results after meniscectomy. *J Bone Joint Surg Am.* 1974;56:719-729.
7. Morgan C, Wojtys E, Casscells C, et al. Arthroscopic meniscal repair evaluated by second look arthroscopy. *Am J Sports Med.* 1991;19:632-638.
8. Noyes F, Schipplein O, Andriachi T. The anterior cruciate ligament-deficient knee with varus alignment: an analysis of gait adaptations and dynamic joint loadings. *Am J Sports Med.* 1992;20:707-716.
9. Veltri D, Warren R, Wickiewicz TOS. Current status of allograft meniscal transplantation. *Clin Orthop Relat Res.* 1994;303:44-55.
10. Shelbourne K, Gray T. Results of anterior cruciate ligament reconstruction based on meniscus and articular cartilage status at the time of surgery: five-to-fifteen year evaluations. *Am J Sports Med.* 2000;28:446-452.
11. Allen C, Wong E, Livesay G, et al. Importance of the medial meniscus in the anterior cruciate ligament-deficient knee. *J Orthop Res.* 2000;18:109-115.
12. Sekiya JK, Whiddon DR, Zehms CT, et al. A clinically relevant assessment of PCL and posterolateral corner injuries: Evaluation of isolated and combined deficiency. *J Bone Joint Surg Am.* 2008;90(8):1621-1627.
13. Tibor LM, Marchant MH Jr, Taylor DC, et al. Management of medial-sided knee injuries. Part II: posteromedial corner. *Am J Sports Med.* 2011;39(6):1332-1340.
14. Pollard M, Kang Q, Berg E. Radiographic sizing for meniscal transplantation. *Arthroscopy.* 1995;11:684-687.
15. Kurtz C, Bonner K, Sekiya J. Meniscus transplantation utilizing the femoral distractor. *Arthroscopy.* 2006;22:568.e1-568.e3.
16. Yoldas E, Sekiya J, Irrgang J, et al. Arthroscopically assisted meniscal allograft transplantation with and without combined ACL reconstruction. *Knee Surg Sports Traumatol Arthrosc.* 2003;11:173-182.
17. Sekiya J, Giffin R, Irrgang J, et al. Clinical outcomes after combined meniscal allograft transplantation and ACL reconstruction. *Am J Sport Med.* 2003;31:896-906.
18. Graf K, Sekiya J, Wojtys E. Long-term results after combined medial meniscal allograft transplantation and ACL reconstruction: minimum 8.5-year follow-up study. *Arthroscopy.* 2004;20:129-140.

Chapter 62

Combined Anterior Cruciate Ligament Reconstruction and High Tibial Osteotomy

Davide Edoardo Bonasia and Annunziato Amendola

Chapter Synopsis
- This chapter describes the indications, planning, and surgical technique for combined anterior cruciate ligament (ACL) reconstruction and high tibial osteotomy (HTO). Both medial opening wedge and lateral closing wedge HTO have been described.

Important Points
- A preoperative workup to define the degree of varus is essential to correctly plan the surgery and achieve good results. The terms *primary, double,* and *triple varus* simplify the assessment of alignment and ligamentous deficiencies in a varus knee.
- Performance of combined ACL reconstruction and HTO is indicated in the following situations:
  - ACL rupture and severe varus alignment or hyperextension (more than 20 degrees)
  - ACL rupture and double or triple varus
  - ACL rupture, varus alignment, and symptomatic medial knee arthritis
  - ACL rupture, varus alignment, and lateral joint opening
  - ACL rupture, varus alignment, and external tibial rotation
  - ACL rupture and varus thrust
  - ACL rupture, varus alignment, and medial meniscus deficiency or osteochondral defects

Clinical and Surgical Pearls
- The role of the tibial slope in anteroposterior knee stability is very important. The effect of opening and closing wedge HTO as well as the plate positioning on the tibial slope should be known, to precisely correct the tibial slope when necessary.
- During the ACL reconstruction, soft tissue graft is preferred because it allows more freedom in tibial tunnel positioning when the osteotomy is present, compared with the patellar tendon graft.

Clinical and Surgical Pitfalls
- The osteotomy should always be performed before the ACL reconstruction to avoid damages to the graft. In performing the ACL reconstruction, the most anterior screws of the osteotomy plate may prevent a correct tibial tunnel drilling. In this situation the screws need to be removed and repositioned after introduction of the graft into the joint.

In all patients with knee instability associated with joint arthrosis, thorough evaluation of the coronal (varus or valgus) and sagittal (tibial slope) alignment must be performed. In the past, knee instability was a contraindication to osteotomy. More recently, however, indications for high tibial osteotomy (HTO) have expanded to also include knee instability.[1-3] This chapter describes the indications, planning, and surgical technique for combined anterior cruciate ligament (ACL) reconstruction and HTO.

PREOPERATIVE CONSIDERATIONS

Indications

In the varus knee with ACL deficiency it is important to define the degree of varus alignment. The terms *primary, double,* and *triple varus* simplify the assessment of alignment and ligamentous deficiencies in a varus knee. *Primary varus* refers to the overall tibiofemoral varus osseous alignment (including medial meniscus and medial tibiofemoral articular cartilage loss). *Double varus* entails varus osseous alignment combined with separation of the lateral tibiofemoral compartment caused by lateral ligamentous damage (lateral condylar lift-off). The *triple varus knee* refers specifically to varus alignment resulting from (1) tibiofemoral osseous alignment, (2) increased lateral tibiofemoral compartment separation, and (3) varus recurvatum in extension caused by the abnormal increase in external tibial rotation and knee hyperextension, with involvement of the entire posterolateral ligament complex. The selection of an appropriate treatment must take into account the associated ligamentous injuries in addition to the varus malalignment.[4]

The use of combined ACL reconstruction and HTO is indicated in the following situations:

1. ACL rupture and severe varus alignment or hyperextension (more than 20 degrees)
2. ACL rupture and double or triple varus
3. ACL rupture, varus alignment, and symptomatic medial knee arthritis
4. ACL rupture, varus alignment, and lateral joint opening (lateral complex reconstruction or repair can be considered if residual lateral instability is present after combined HTO and ACL reconstruction)
5. ACL rupture, varus alignment, and external tibial rotation

6. ACL rupture and varus thrust
7. ACL rupture, varus alignment, and medial meniscus deficiency or osteochondral defects, when a combined medial meniscus transplant or performance of resurfacing procedures is planned

These conditions are usually encountered in chronic ACL-deficient knees. Use of combined ACL reconstruction and HTO is rarely indicated in the acute setting, even if a primary varus alignment is present.

Planning

We commonly plan the osteotomy as described by Dugdale and colleagues[5] with a mild (3 to 5 degrees) valgus overcorrection (Fig. 62-1). After the correction, the mechanical axis (the line connecting the center of the femoral head with the center of the ankle joint) should pass through a point located at 62.5% of the tibial width, as measured from the tip of the medial edge of the proximal tibia. This point lies slightly lateral to the tip of the lateral tibial spine. In planning for opening wedge HTO, one line is drawn from this point to the center of the femoral head, and another line is drawn from this point to the center of the ankle joint. The angle between the two lines represents the angle of correction (α) (see Fig. 62-1). Next, the osteotomy line is measured from medial (approximately 4 cm below the joint line) to lateral (tip of the articular fibular head). This measurement is transferred to both rays of the α

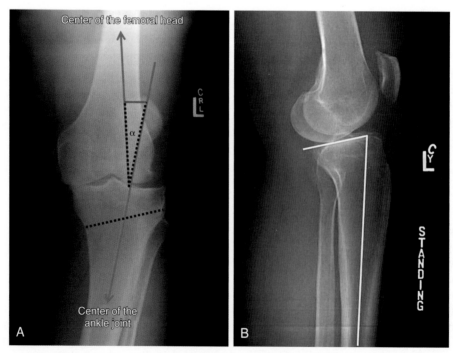

Figure 62-1. Preoperative planning of opening wedge high tibial osteotomy (HTO; see text). **A,** Anteroposterior view of the knee for the coronal planning. **B,** Lateral view of the knee for the sagittal planning.

angle from the vertex. In this fashion the α angle is defined by two identical segments (equal to the osteotomy length), which are then connected by another line. This line serves as the base of an isosceles triangle and corresponds to the opening that should be achieved medially at the osteotomy site (see Fig. 62-1).

In younger patients without medial compartment arthritis, a more neutral alignment is planned after correction (50% of the tibial width, 0 degrees of mechanical axis).

In performing combined ACL reconstruction and HTO, the sagittal planning is very important. The tibial slope can be decreased with a more posterior plate positioning, to protect the graft (see Fig. 62-1).

Hyperextension deformity is more commonly associated with posterior cruciate ligament (PCL) or posterolateral corner (PLC) injury. However, with ACL failure resulting from hyperextension, increasing the tibial slope will correct the hyperextension; but if the slope is severely increased, this will put the ACL reconstruction at risk. Therefore in individuals with deformity of the tibial slope (<6 degrees), a mild correction of the slope is indicated. If the slope is normal (>6 degrees), it should be left as is.

Surgical planning is similar for closing wedge HTO. The α angle is calculated as described for opening wedge HTO, but the osteotomy itself is different and entails two cuts. The proximal osteotomy line is usually horizontal and is placed 2 to 2.5 cm distal to the joint line. The proximal and distal osteotomy should define the angle of correction (α). With closing wedge HTO, it is more difficult to accurately change or correct the tibial slope, which is usually decreased after the procedure.

SURGICAL TECHNIQUE

Both opening wedge and closing wedge HTO can be performed, according to surgeon's preference. Our preferred technique is opening wedge HTO. Also, the choice of the ACL graft and reconstruction technique is a matter of preference of the surgeon.

Surgical Steps

Opening Wedge High Tibial Osteotomy

The surgery is performed with the patient supine on a radiolucent operating table (Box 62-1).[1,3] A lateral post is positioned at the level of the thigh so that the foot can be dropped out of the table and at least 120 degrees of knee flexion can be achieved (Fig. 62-2). Intravenous antibiotic prophylaxis is performed. A tourniquet is placed around the proximal thigh. HTO is performed first. A 5-cm longitudinal incision is made, extending from 1 cm below the medial joint line midway between the medial border of the tubercle and the posteromedial border of the tibia.[1,3] If a hamstring autograft is

---

BOX 62-1 Surgical Steps in Medial Opening Wedge Osteotomy

1. Operative draping and surface anatomy references drawn on skin
2. Exposure of proximal medial tibial cortex with retractor placement
3. Guide pin placement just proximal to proposed osteotomy line
4. Fluoroscopy to ensure integrity of the lateral tibial cortex
5. Two Arthrex (Naples, FL) osteotomes for "stacking" technique to accomplish initial opening of osteotomy
6. Screw jack technique for opening osteotomy
7. Placement of graduated wedge to preoperatively calculated depth
8. Placement of wedged Puddu plate anterior to single stem of the graduated wedge
9. Puddu plate fixation as far posterior as possible to avoid iatrogenic changes in posterior tibial slope
10. Corticocancellous wedge and morselized femoral head allograft
11. Placement of correctly sized wedge anterior to Puddu plate for added stability
12. Femoral tunnel preparation
13. Tibial tunnel preparation
14. Insertion of soft tissue graft into the joint

---

preferred, harvesting of the graft is performed at this point, to avoid damage to the tendons during proximal tibia exposure. The sartorius fascia is exposed by sharp dissection, and the pes anserinus is then retracted distally with a blunt retractor, exposing the superficial fibers of the medial collateral ligament (sMCL). The distal sMCL insertion is partially detached with a Cobb elevator. A blunt Hohmann retractor is then passed deep to the MCL to protect the posterior neurovascular structures. Next, the medial border of the patellar tendon is identified and retracted laterally with a hook or a second blunt lever. A guidewire is then drilled into the proximal tibia.[1,3] The starting point of the wire is the anteromedial (AM) tibia at the level of the superior border of the tibial tubercle (about 4 cm distal from the joint line). The wire must be inserted aiming toward the tip of the fibular head (1 cm below the lateral articular surface). The guidewire positioning is assessed with fluoroscopy (Fig. 62-3). The tibial osteotomy is performed immediately distal to the guide pin, to protect against proximal migration of the osteotomy into the joint. The slope of the osteotomy in the sagittal plane is critical and should mimic the proximal tibial joint slope.[1,3] A small oscillating saw is used to cut the tibial cortex from the tibial tubercle around to the posteromedial corner under direct vision. Thin, flexible osteotomes are then used to advance the osteotomy to within

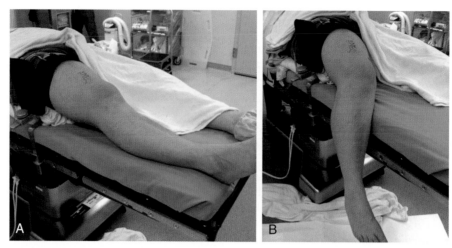

Figure 62-2. Patient positioning. **A,** The patient is supine on a radiolucent operating table, and a tourniquet is placed around the proximal thigh. **B,** A lateral post is positioned at the level of the thigh so that the foot can be dropped from the table and at least 120 degrees of knee flexion can be achieved.

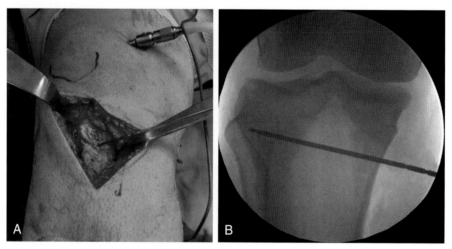

Figure 62-3. A, Exposure of the anteromedial tibia and insertion of the guidewire for the osteotomy. **B,** Fluoroscopic control of wire positioning (anteroposterior view).

1 cm of the lateral tibial cortex (Fig. 62-4). This is achieved with use of intermittent fluoroscopy and graduated osteotomes.[6] The mobility of the osteotomy is checked by gentle manipulation of the leg with a valgus force and encouraged, if needed, by piling up two or three osteotomes.[1,3] Graduated wedges are then engaged into the osteotomy and advanced slowly until the desired opening has been achieved (Fig. 62-5). Once the calculated preoperative correction has been achieved, a long alignment rod is used to check the mechanical axis. The rod is centered over the hip and ankle joints and, according to the preoperative planning, should lie at 62.5% or 50% of the tibial width, as measured from medial to lateral. The sagittal plane correction should also be assessed by fluoroscopy and by looking carefully at the size of the osteotomy opening. Considering the triangular shape of the tibia, if the opening at the level of the AM tibia is half the size of the opening at the level of

the posteromedial tibia, the preexisting slope is maintained (Fig. 62-5B). The wedges (and the plate) can be moved anterior or posterior, according to the correction planned on the sagittal plane.

Once the desired correction has been achieved and the plate positioning determined, the plate is placed and the wedges are removed (see Fig. 62-5). Various plates are available for fixation of the opening wedge osteotomy: conventional, locking, long or short plates, and with or without a spacer.[2] To further decrease the tibial slope, one distal screw is positioned and then the knee is kept in full extension while the first proximal screw is inserted. In this fashion, the osteotomy gap closes anteriorly and the slope decreases. Fluoroscopic control is used to assess proximal and distal positioning of the screws. When a conventional Puddu plate is used, attention should be paid to position the proximal screws more posteriorly than usual, to have enough bone for

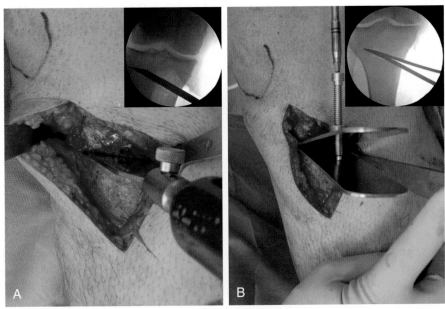

Figure 62-4. A, After the cortex has been cut with an oscillating saw, the osteotomy is performed with graduated osteotomes under fluoroscopic control, with care taken to leave the lateral hinge intact (1 cm from the lateral cortex). **B,** When the bone cut has been completed anteriorly and posteriorly and some degrees of opening are noted with valgus stress, the osteotomy site can be distracted.

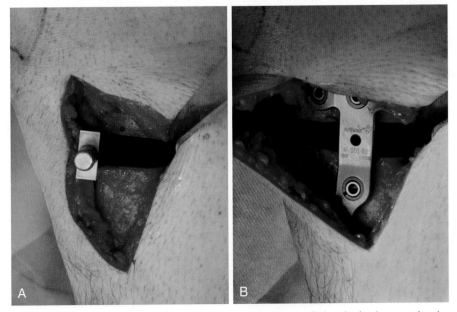

Figure 62-5. A, Graduated wedges are then inserted in the osteotomy until the desired correction is achieved. **B,** Plating is then performed.

the tibial tunnel of the ACL reconstruction. For the same reasons, when a long locking T-plat is used, the most anterior screw should not be inserted proximally.[7] Alternatively, all proximal screws are positioned, and if the tibial tunnel is interfering with one of them, the screw is removed. Then the tibial tunnel is drilled and the screw is positioned in another direction under direct visualization and before the graft is retrieved into the tunnel (see Figs. 62-7B and 62-10). This will avoid damage to the graft during screw insertion.

Closing Wedge High Tibial Osteotomy

Patient positioning and preparation are the same as for opening wedge HTO. A longitudinal midline incision is performed. Dissection is carried out through the lateral aspect of the knee. The fascia of the anterior compartment is incised along the anterolateral (AL) crest of the tibia. A Cobb elevator is used to elevate the tibialis anterior muscle from the tibial surface, and the iliotibial band is elevated from the Gerdy tubercle proximally. The common peroneal nerve is protected throughout the procedure. Many techniques have been described for the proximal tibiofibular joint, including (1) joint excision or disruption, (2) fibular osteotomy (10 cm distal from the fibular head), and (3) excision of the fibular head. The lateral edge of the patellar tendon is identified; the first retractor is placed beneath it, and the second is placed on the posterolateral tibial edge, to protect the neurovascular structures.

With this technique, the proximal tibia is exposed and a laterally based wedge can be removed with an angular cutting guide. To reduce the risk of intra-articular fracture, the outer cortex and large portion of the wedge can be removed with saw cuts, along with the medial half with use of a combination of curettes, rongeurs, and osteotomes, to within 1 cm of the medial cortex. Fluoroscopic control can be used to assess the completeness of wedge removal. Once the osteotomy is closed, position and alignment are checked with the fluoroscope and fixation is then completed, usually with staples or a plate.[1,3]

Once the osteotomy has been plated, the ACL reconstruction can be performed, according to the preferred technique and graft selection, through the same incision as the HTO. Performing the ACL first has two main risks: (1) the graft can be damaged in performance of the tibial bone cut, and (2) the osteotomy can slacken (or overtension) the graft.

Graft Harvesting

When a bone–patellar tendon–bone (BPTB) autograft is used, the incision should be prolonged 3 cm proximally, unless a two-incision technique is preferred for the harvesting. In this situation a 2- to 3-cm horizontal incision is performed at the level of the inferior patellar pole. According to the preferred technique, the central third (around 10 mm) of the patellar tendon is harvested, with trapezoidal patellar and tibial bone plugs (usually around 9×22 mm). Two or three No. 2 nonabsorbable braided traction sutures are inserted in each plug. The lengths of the tendon and the bone plugs are measured. The bone-tendon junction of the femoral plug is marked with a sterile surgical pen.

As previously mentioned, when a hamstring autograft is used, this should be harvested before the HTO, according to the preferred technique. On the back table the graft is doubled after it has been passed through an extracortical flip button fixation device. The distal ends are armed together with No. 2 nonabsorbable braided suture. The graft is then sized, pretensioned at around 15 N, and kept in a moist sponge.

Tibialis anterior of hamstring allograft can be used as well. The allograft is prepared as described for the hamstring autograft. We prefer soft tissue graft, either hamstring autograft or tibialis anterior allograft. These grafts allow for tunnel variability, particularly at the tibial tunnel where the osteotomy is present.

Anterior Cruciate Ligament Reconstruction

A complete diagnostic arthroscopy is performed through standard AM and AL portals. The AM portal is made tangential to the patellar tendon. Any associated pathologies (meniscal or chondral injuries) are identified and treated at this point. The remaining ACL stump is removed with a mechanical shaver until the tibial and femoral footprints are well visualized. A minimal notchplasty is performed with a shaver or an acromioplasty bur (Fig. 62-6).

An arthroscopic over-the-top offset guide is inserted into the joint through the AM portal (see Fig. 62-6). If the medial wall of the lateral femoral condyle is not adequately visualized through the AL portal, an accessory AM portal can be established to introduce the femoral guide. The over-the-top guides are available with different offsets. The appropriate offset should be decided to preserve a 2-mm posterior wall. For example, if a 10-mm diameter (5-mm radius) femoral tunnel is planned, a 7-mm offset guide is used to maintain 2 mm of the posterior wall ($7 - 5 = 2$ mm). With the knee at 120 degrees of flexion, a guide pin is drilled at around the 10 o'clock position (right knee) or the 2 o'clock position (left knee) on the coronal plane. The exit point of the pin through the skin of the lateral thigh should be evaluated. If the pin is exiting too posteriorly with respect to the femoral shaft, the pin should be repositioned to minimize the risk of posterior wall disruption. A cannulated reamer is used to create the femoral tunnel drilling. A No. 2 braided shuttling suture is looped and passed through the eyelet of the guide pin. The guide pin is pulled from the lateral side of the thigh; the two free ends of the suture are retrieved proximally, and the loop is kept outside the AM portal (see Fig. 62-6). The free ends are secured with a Kelly clamp.

Then a tibial ACL guide is inserted into the joint through the AM portal (Figs. 62-7 and 62-8). Landmarks for the correct positioning of the tibial tunnel are the PCL, the anterior horn of the lateral meniscus, and the tibial spines. The ACL guide is positioned about 7 mm anterior to the PCL, posterior to the anterior horn of the lateral meniscus and on the lateral wall of the medial tibial spine. When a BPTB graft is used, the length of the tibial tunnel is important. This is determined by measuring the length of the graft and subtracting the femoral bone plug and the intra-articular portion of the graft (usually 30 mm). A guide pin is drilled into the proximal tibia from a point located halfway between the tibial tubercle and the posteromedial corner of the tibia. The length of the tibial tunnel can then be checked by measuring on the guide pin. A cannulated reamer with the same diameter as the tibial bone plug is used to drill the tibial tunnel on the guide pin. As previously mentioned, if the tibial tunnel is interfering with one of the plate screws, the screw is removed, the tibial tunnel is drilled, and the screw is positioned in another

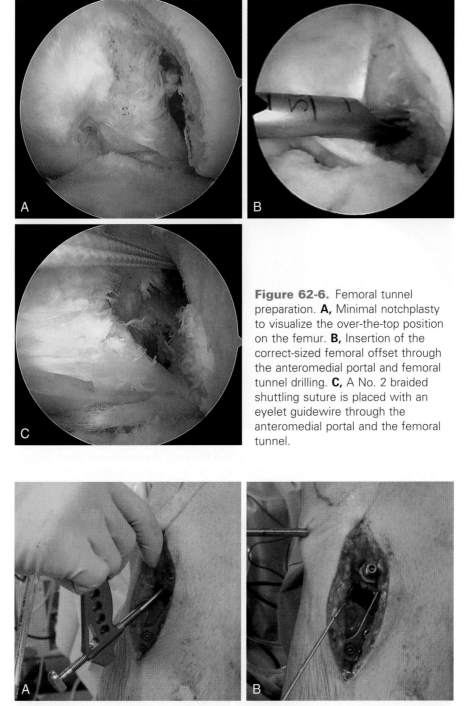

Figure 62-6. Femoral tunnel preparation. **A,** Minimal notchplasty to visualize the over-the-top position on the femur. **B,** Insertion of the correct-sized femoral offset through the anteromedial portal and femoral tunnel drilling. **C,** A No. 2 braided shuttling suture is placed with an eyelet guidewire through the anteromedial portal and the femoral tunnel.

Figure 62-7. A, Tibial tunnel preparation. **B,** Note that sometimes the proximal anterior screw of the plate needs to be removed and repositioned to allow for the tibial tunnel drilling.

direction. This is done under direct visualization and before the graft is retrieved into the tunnel.

An arthroscopic grasper is inserted into the tibial tunnel, and the loop of the suture, previously positioned in the femoral tunnel, is then retrieved out of the tibial tunnel distal aperture (see Fig. 62-8C and D). The graft is then inserted into the joint and fixed (Figs. 62-9 and 62-10).

Fixation of the Graft and Postoperative Rehabilitation

Our preferred fixation for the ACL is as follows. When a BPTB graft is used, fixation is achieved with two interference screws on both the femoral (first) and tibial sides. When a soft tissue autograft or allograft is used, fixation is achieved proximally with an extracortical flip button device and distally with an interference screw.

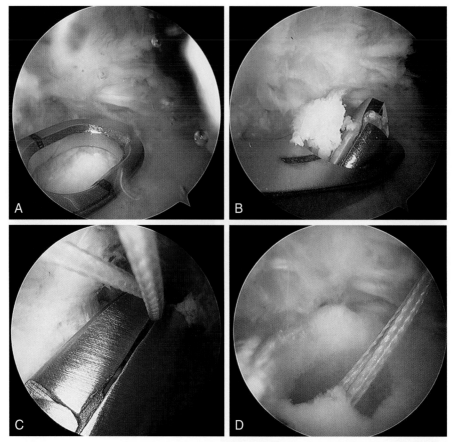

Figure 62-8. Arthroscopic phases of the tibial tunnel preparation. **A,** Positioning of the tibial guide on the distal anterior cruciate ligament footprint. **B,** Positioning of the guidewire. **C** and **D,** Once the tunnel has been drilled over the guidewire, the shuttle suture previously positioned in the femur is retrieved from the tibial tunnel with an arthroscopic grasper.

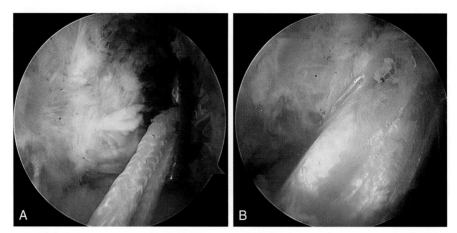

Figure 62-9. Insertion of a soft tissue graft into the joint (arthroscopic images). **A,** The graft is pulled through the tunnels with a previously positioned flip button device on the femoral side. **B,** Graft correctly seated in the tunnels.

In performing an opening wedge HTO, if the osteotomy gap is larger than 10 mm, this is grafted with corticocancellous autograft or allograft. The wounds are closed, and a postoperative hinged knee brace is positioned (Fig. 62-11).

POSTOPERATIVE CONSIDERATIONS

Postoperatively the patient is permitted toe-touch weight bearing in the hinged knee brace (0 to 90 degrees

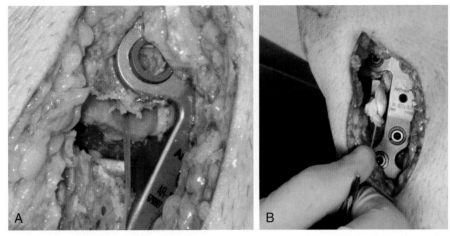

Figure 62-10. Insertion of a soft tissue graft into the joint. If the anterior screw was removed for the tibial tunnel drilling (**A**), it needs to be repositioned in another direction before the graft is inserted (**B**).

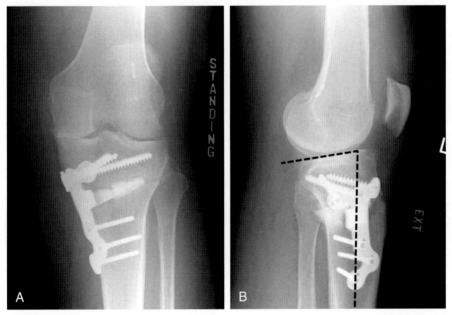

Figure 62-11. Postoperative radiographs after combined high tibial osteotomy and anterior cruciate ligament reconstruction. **A,** Anteroposterior view. **B,** Lateral view showing the decreased tibial slope, compared with preoperative view (see Fig. 62-1).

allowed) for 6 weeks. At 6 weeks, if adequate healing is evident on radiographs, the hinged brace is discontinued, range of motion is no longer restricted, and weight bearing may be increased to 50% of body weight. At 12 weeks new radiographs are obtained, and if consolidation is complete, full weight bearing is allowed. Physical therapy is continued for 3 more months, and return to sports is allowed 6 months after surgery.

RESULTS

In the literature review, the overall results of the osteotomy either alone or combined with ligamentous reconstruction are encouraging.

Fowler and colleagues[8] treated seven ACL-deficient knees with varus alignment or thrust and medial knee arthrosis with HTO alone and reported significant clinical improvement in all patients. Dejour and colleagues,[9] out of 50 ACL-deficient knees with acquired varus treated with HTO and ACL reconstruction, showed a 91% satisfaction rate. In the study by Noyes and colleagues[10] of HTO in ACL-deficient knees, the authors reported reduction of pain in 71%, elimination of giving way in 85%, and resumption of light recreational activities in 66% of patients. Williams and colleagues[11] retrospectively compared closed wedge HTO alone with simultaneous combined ACL reconstruction and closed wedge HTO in patients with chronic ACL deficiency, medial compartment arthritis, and varus deformity. They concluded that the simultaneous procedure had superior short-term outcomes and lower complication rates. Bonin and colleagues found that simultaneous combined ACL reconstruction and closed or open wedge HTO both yielded satisfactory long-term results.[12] Boss and colleagues performed combined BPTB ACL reconstruction, augmented with the Kennedy-ligament device, and HTO (24 lateral closing and three medial opening) in 27 patients. They reported excellent results in 75% of the patients.[13] Imhoff and Agneskirchner performed simultaneous ACL reconstruction and HTO in 58 patients, with improvement in pain, swelling, and giving-way symptoms in all of them.[14]

REFERENCES

1. Amendola A. The role of osteotomy in the multiple ligament injured knee. *Arthroscopy*. 2003;19(1):11-13.
2. Clatworthy M, Amendola A. The anterior cruciate ligament and arthritis. *Clin Sports Med*. 1999;18(1):173-197.
3. Rossi R, Bonasia DE, Amendola A. The role of high tibial osteotomy in the varus knee. *J Am Acad Orthop Surg*. 2011;19(10):590-599.
4. Noyes FR, Barber-Westin SD. High tibial osteotomy in knees with associated chronic ligament deficiencies. In: Jackson DW, ed. *Master Techniques in Orthopaedic Surgery: Reconstructive Knee Surgery*. 3rd ed. Lippincott Williams & Wilkins; 2008:317-360
5. Dugdale TW, Noyes FR, Styer D. Preoperative planning for high tibial osteotomy: the effect of lateral tibiofemoral separation and tibiofemoral length. *Clin Orthop Relat Res*. 1992;(274):248-264.
6. Vasconcellos DA, Griffin JR, Amendola A. Avoiding and managing complications in osteotomies of the knee. In: Meislin RJ, Halbrecht J, eds. *Complications in Knee and Shoulder Surgery: Management and Treatment Options for the Sports Medicine Orthopedist*. London, UK: Springer; 2009;115-132.
7. Amendola A, Bonasia DE. Results of high tibial osteotomy: review of the literature. *Int Orthop*. 2010;34(2):155-160.
8. Fowler P, Kirkley A, Roe J. Osteotomy of the proximal tibia in the treatment of chronic anterior cruciate ligament insufficiency. *J Bone Joint Surg Br*. 1994;76:26.
9. Dejour H, Neyret P, Boileau P, et al. Anterior cruciate reconstruction combined with valgus tibial osteotomy. *Clin Orthop Relat Res*. 1994;299:220-228.
10. Noyes FR, Barber-Westin SD, Hewett TE. High tibial osteotomy and ligament reconstruction for varus angulated anterior cruciate ligament-deficient knees. *Am J Sports Med*. 2000;28:282-296.
11. Williams III RJ, Kelly BT, Wickiewicz TL, et al. The short-term outcome of surgical treatment for painful varus arthritis in association with chronic ACL deficiency. *J Knee Surg*. 2003;16:9-16.
12. Bonin N, Ait Si Selmi T, Donell ST, et al. Anterior cruciate reconstruction combined with valgus upper tibial osteotomy: 12 years follow-up. *Knee*. 2004;11:431-437.
13. Boss A, Stutz G, Oursin C, et al. Anterior cruciate ligament reconstruction combined with valgus tibial osteotomy (combined procedure). *Knee Surg Sports Traumatol Arthrosc*. 1995;3(3):187-191.
14. Imhoff AB, Agneskirchner JD. Simultaneous ACL replacement and high tibial osteotomy: indication, technique, results. *Tech Knee Surg*. 2002;1(2):146-154.

Chapter 63

Osteochondral Allografting in the Knee

Andreas H. Gomoll, Richard Kang, and Brian J. Cole

Chapter Synopsis
- This chapter summarizes the indications for and technique and results of osteochondral allograft transplantation for the treatment of symptomatic cartilage defects of the knee.

Important Points
- Osteochondral transplants are indicated for symptomatic, full-thickness chondral defects. Osteoarthritis, with the exception of very specific circumstances, is a contraindication.
- Two techniques are presented: the dowel (Mega-OATS) technique and the less commonly used shell allograft.

Clinical and Surgical Pearls
- Ensure that the graft has been received in acceptable condition and that the size and side are correct before the patient is anesthetized.
- Adequate exposure is key to ensure perpendicular pin placement.

- Takedown of the meniscus can improve access, especially for posterior defects; this is repaired during closing.
- A positioning device can be helpful to stabilize the extremity in hyperflexion for very posterior lesions.
- Dilate the recipient site and bevel the graft edges to facilitate introduction with little force.
- It is preferable to recess the graft rather than to leave it proud.

Clinical and Surgical Pitfalls
- Do not use excessive force to seat the graft, because this results in chondrocyte death. Ideally, the graft should be seated with use of manual pressure and range of motion.
- Grafts most commonly fail through the bone, not the cartilage; make sure to keep the plug thin (6 to 8 mm) so that only little bone has to be incorporated.
- Avoid excessive impact activities during the first year. The subchondral bone is only slowly substituted and is at its weakest several months after the operation.

Osteochondral allografting in the knee has been used for more than 20 years to reconstruct osteochondral defects resulting from trauma, malignant disease, and developmental disorders.[14] In current practice, osteochondral allografts are most commonly used for the treatment of symptomatic osteochondritis dissecans and other chondral lesions that have failed primary treatment, such as internal fixation of osteochondritis dissecans fragments, marrow stimulation, mosaicplasty, and autologous chondrocyte implantation. Increasingly, allografts are now also being used as the primary treatment in situations in which other restorative procedures have demonstrated limited success, such as in the very large or uncontained defect and in the older population of patients. Although use of the procedure was initially limited by the low number of available grafts, fresh allograft tissue is becoming increasingly available as a result of improved harvesting and storage protocols, but the supply is still outpaced by a rapidly increasing demand.

PREOPERATIVE CONSIDERATIONS
History

Osteochondral allografting is indicated in patients with osteochondral or, less frequently, isolated chondral or osseous defects. Patients with osteochondritis dissecans often report a history of failure of other treatment modalities, such as immobilization, open reduction and fixation of the fragment, and simple excision. The onset of symptoms is mostly insidious, with no distinctive trauma. Conversely, chondral defects often result from athletic injuries that lead to tears of the anterior cruciate ligament or the meniscus, which in turn result in acute or secondary damage to the articular surface. Lastly, young patients with osteonecrosis and secondary articular collapse can be amenable to osteochondral allografting in an attempt to avoid joint replacement surgery.

Typical History

- Prior knee injury or surgery
- Activity-related knee pain and swelling
- Mechanical symptoms, such as locking, catching, and giving way

Physical Examination

- Variable amounts of effusion
- Varus alignment in large medial femoral condyle lesions
- Pain to deep palpation of the affected compartment
- Usually intact range of motion, but can be limited in the presence of loose bodies
- Quadriceps atrophy correlates with duration of symptoms
- Catching or crepitation in the involved compartment

Imaging

Radiography

Figure 63-1 illustrates the following radiographic positions:

- Standing anteroposterior view with knee in full extension
- Standing posteroanterior view with knee in 30 to 60 degrees of flexion (notch, tunnel or Rosenberg view)
- Lateral view
- Patellar sunrise view
- Bilateral long-leg alignment views

Magnetic Resonance Imaging

Magnetic resonance imaging is the "gold standard" for osteochondral lesions. Fluid or edema behind the lesion is suggestive of an unstable fragment.

Evaluate the extent and depth of osseous involvement. Beware of high sensitivity for subchondral edema, which leads to false positives for osseous disease. Computed tomography (CT) scan, especially when combined with arthrography, can provide very high resolution for both cartilage and subchondral bone (Fig. 63-2). This can be particularly helpful to evaluate for subchondral sclerosis and cysts that might have to be addressed by bone grafting.

Indications and Contraindications

The typical candidate for osteochondral allografting has a large full-thickness chondral or osteochondral defect; prior procedures, such as the repair of an unstable osteochondritis dissecans lesion, microfracture, osteochondral autograft transfer, and autologous chondrocyte implantation, have failed. Some lesions preclude the use of other cartilage repair procedures because of their large size, specific location, or associated deep

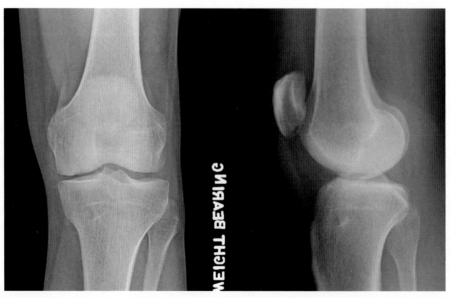

Figure 63-1. Anteroposterior and lateral radiographs of an osteochondral lesion of the medial femoral condyle. The patient had previously been treated with pinning of an osteochondritis dissecans lesion, then underwent bone grafting because of failure of the initial procedure.

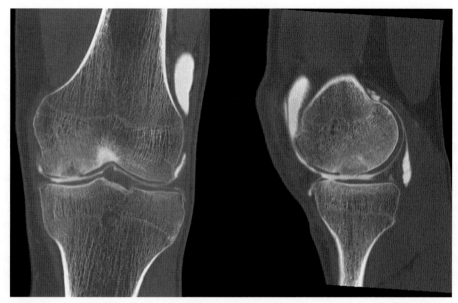

Figure 63-2. Coronal and sagittal computed tomography images show an osteochondral defect of the medial femoral condyle without cartilage cover.

osseous defects. Localized unipolar lesions larger than 2 to 3 cm^2 provide an optimal environment for osteochondral grafting.[1,8,9,12]

Comorbidities that must be addressed either before or at the time of the osteochondral allografting procedure include malalignment, ligament deficiency, and meniscal insufficiency. Bipolar lesions are a relative contraindication and result in less predictable outcomes. Both lesions should be treated concomitantly; the larger and deeper defect is commonly allografted, and the kissing lesion is often amenable to microfracture.

Allograft Preservation and Graft Sizing

Traditionally, grafts were retrieved and reimplanted fresh within 24 to 48 hours. Current standard clinical practice[19] uses prolonged fresh osteochondral allografts that are stored for 2 to 4 weeks at approximately 4° C. The extended storage time allows for bacterial and viral testing before release, and also facilitates scheduling. Grafts are generally size, side, and compartment specific—for example, a left medial femoral condyle defect is treated with use of a left medial femoral hemicondyle graft. Given the popularity of the procedure, wait times for suitable grafts have increased, and the use of contralateral side and compartment grafts has become more common—for example, use of the right lateral hemicondyle to treat aforementioned left medial femoral condyle defect. Graft size is determined on preoperative MRI or CT scans, or AP and lateral radiographs obtained with sizing markers for correction of magnification. In general, size mismatch is more acceptable when the graft is larger rather than smaller than

the recipient condyle. The tissue banks usually require the width of the tibial plateau, as well as the width and length of the hemicondyle. Also, it is helpful to relate the size of the defect and likely required dowel size. Although no consensus exists, we accept grafts that are smaller by 1 to 2 mm or larger by up to 5 mm.

SURGICAL TECHNIQUE

Anesthesia and Positioning

On the basis of the preferences of the surgeon, anesthesiologist, and patient, the procedure can be performed with use of general, spinal, or regional anesthesia or a combination thereof. Before induction of anesthesia, the surgeon must ensure that the fresh graft is size- and side-matched and of sufficient quality. The patient is positioned supine on a standard operating table with a thigh tourniquet. Especially in posterior lesions of the femoral condyle, a leg positioning device is helpful to stabilize the knee in hyperflexion.

Surgical Landmarks, Incisions, and Portals

Landmarks
- Patella
- Patellar tendon
- Tibial tubercle

Incisions
- Anterior midline or paramedian skin incision
- Medial or lateral peripatellar arthrotomy, subvastus or midvastus approach

Structures at Risk

- Infrapatellar branch of the saphenous nerve
- Articular surfaces (at risk during arthrotomy)
- Patellar tendon (risk of avulsion with vigorous retraction)
- Menisci

Examination Under Anesthesia and Diagnostic Arthroscopy

Examination under anesthesia should reveal stable ligaments and full range of motion. Although it is not mandatory, diagnostic arthroscopy as an initial staging procedure is helpful to better assess the extent of the chondral lesion as well as to rule out associated pathologic changes, such as ligamentous or meniscal insufficiency.

Specific Steps

The specific steps of the procedure are outlined in Box 63-1.

1. Exposure

Osteochondral allografting is an open procedure requiring the use of an arthrotomy sized to be consistent with the location and extent of the lesion (Fig. 63-3). Most commonly, an anterior midline incision is made from the proximal pole of the patella to the tibial tubercle, but medial or lateral paramedian incisions can be used as well. The incision is carried down to the capsule; then full-thickness skin flaps are raised to make a mobile window. A medial or lateral peripatellar capsulotomy is performed from the mid-level of the patella to slightly below the joint line. Occasionally, more extensile approaches are required, especially for posterior lesions and those on the lateral femoral condyle. In these situations a formal quadriceps tendon splitting parapatellar

approach with subluxation of the patella can provide adequate exposure. More limited incisions, such as the subvastus and midvastus approaches, have recently gained popularity, and we think that these approaches allow accelerated postoperative quadriceps rehabilitation. The patella is retracted with either a Z or bent Hohmann retractor placed into the notch. We have found it helpful to release the fat pad and to dissect the anterior meniscal horn from the capsule for better exposure, especially with small incisions.

The most commonly used technique is the press-fit plug technique; several proprietary systems have been developed to facilitate graft sizing and preparation (Fig. 63-4). For comprehensiveness, we also discuss the shell graft technique, which is technically more challenging but allows the treatment of very large and irregularly shaped defects not amenable to the plug technique, or

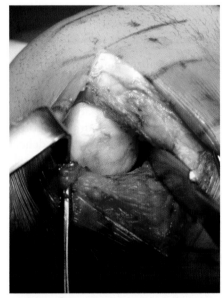

Figure 63-3. Peripatellar arthrotomy exposing a chondral defect on the medial femoral condyle.

BOX 63-1 Surgical Steps

1. Exposure

Press-Fit Plug Technique
2a. Defect preparation
2b. Allograft preparation
2c. Graft insertion and fixation

Shell Technique
2a. Defect preparation
2b. Allograft preparation
2c. Graft insertion and fixation
3. Closure

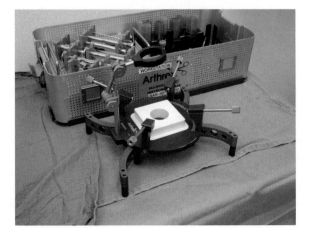

Figure 63-4. Osteochondral allograft instrumentation (Arthrex, Naples, FL).

those so far posterior that perpendicular pin placement is not possible.

Press-Fit Plug Technique

2a. Preparation of the Recipient Site

Once the lesion is exposed, the abnormal cartilage is identified. It is of utmost importance to reconstruct the normal geometry of the articular surface with the donor graft.

1. Place a cylindric sizing guide on the defect to determine the optimal plug diameter (Fig. 63-5).
2. A circumferential mark is made around the guide, followed by a mark at the 12-o'clock position of the recipient cartilage.
3. A guide pin is placed perpendicularly through the cannulated sizer into the center of the defect to a depth of 2 to 3 cm (Fig. 63-6).
4. A reamer is used to create a recipient socket with a depth of 6 to 8 mm (Fig. 63-7). In cases of osteonecrosis, reaming should extend into bleeding bone (release the tourniquet).
5. The depth of the socket is measured in all four quadrants, and the floor is penetrated multiple times to improve vascularization (Fig. 63-8).

2b. Preparation of the Donor Graft

1. Identify and outline the appropriate donor site on the donor hemicondyle. The graft is also marked at the 12-o'clock position to match the orientation of the recipient site (Fig. 63-9).

2. Secure the donor condyle in the allograft workstation.
3. The bushing with the appropriate graft size diameter is placed in the workstation over the marked donor site and set to the appropriate angle to match the contour of the recipient site.

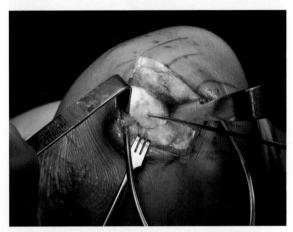

Figure 63-6. The guide pin has been placed perpendicular to the articular surface.

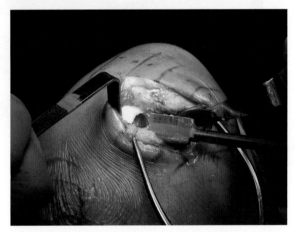

Figure 63-7. Reaming the recipient socket to approximately 6 to 8 mm depth.

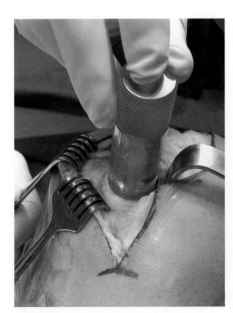

Figure 63-5. Determination of the optimal plug diameter with use of cannulated sizing guides.

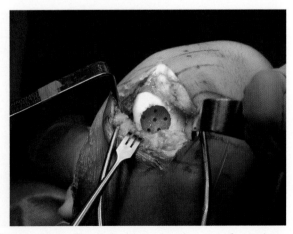

Figure 63-8. The defect base has been perforated to improve vascularization.

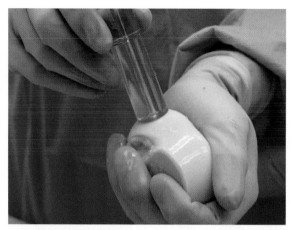

Figure 63-9. Matching the size and location of the donor site.

4. A core reamer is used to harvest an osteochondral cylinder from the donor condyle under constant irrigation (Fig. 63-10).
5. After extraction of the graft from the donor harvester, the depth measurement guide is used to mark out the four quadrants of the graft to match the depths recorded from the recipient site.
6. The allograft is held with the allograft forceps and trimmed down with a saw to match the recipient socket depth (Fig. 63-11).
7. Marrow elements of the subchondral bone, which are more immunogenic than the cartilage or the subchondral bone itself, are irrigated out with pulse lavage.

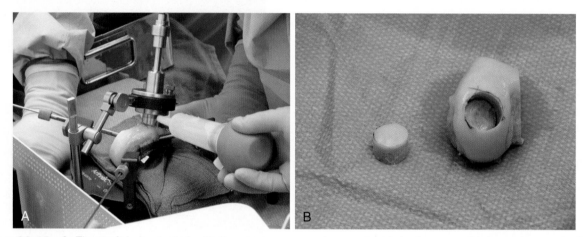

Figure 63-10. A, The graft is harvested with the core reamer under constant irrigation to avoid thermal necrosis. **B,** The graft cylinder after retrieval from the donor condyle.

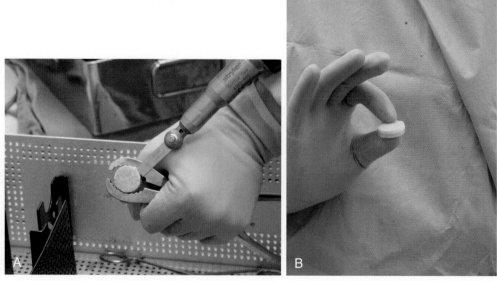

Figure 63-11. A, The graft is cut to the appropriate thickness to correspond to the depth of the recipient socket. **B,** Final appearance of the prepared graft before insertion.

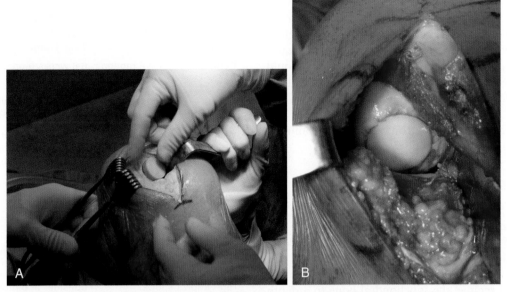

Figure 63-12. **A,** The graft is inserted by hand to avoid injury to the cartilage. **B,** The graft is flush with the recipient articular surface.

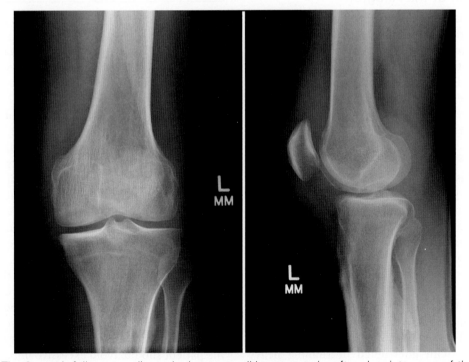

Figure 63-13. The 6-month follow-up radiograph shows a well-incorporated graft and maintenance of the joint space.

2c. Graft Insertion and Fixation

1. An additional 0.5 mm of dilation is achieved by insertion of a calibrated dilator into the recipient site.
2. The graft's corners may be beveled to assist insertion. It is generally preferable to trim the graft slightly rather than require the use of excessive force to seat the graft, which will lead to chondrocyte injury and death.
3. The graft is press-fitted into the recipient defect (Fig. 63-12).
4. The knee is taken through a range of motion with the appropriate varus and valgus stress to load the graft. This both aids in seating of the graft and assessment of any mechanical interaction with the meniscus, which would manifest as catching and popping. It is preferable to recess the graft rather than to leave it proud (see Fig. 63-13).

5. Smaller contained grafts are usually stable with press-fit fixation alone. Larger-diameter grafts (>18 mm in diameter) and those that are not circumferentially contained (peripheral defects—for example, osteochondritis dissecans [OCD] lesions) should be secured with supplemental fixation, ideally a resorbable compression screw. If metal screws are used, the hardware should be removed after a few months, because screws could become prominent and damage the opposing articular surface.

Shell Allograft Technique

2a. Preparation of the Recipient Site

1. The lesion is outlined with a surgical pen.
2. A No. 15 blade is then used to outline the borders of the lesion.
3. A bur, saw, and/or curettes are used to debride the defect and remove the subchondral bone to a depth of 4 to 5 mm.

2b. Preparation of the Allograft

1. The allograft is marked with a surgical pen to match the shape of the recipient site. The allograft should be slightly oversized to allow for trimming during several trial fittings.
2. A shell graft is fashioned with 4 to 5 mm of subchondral bone.
3. Marrow elements are pulse-lavaged out of the subchondral bone.

2c. Graft Placement and Fixation

1. Place graft flush with the articular surface of recipient site. If the graft has been trimmed too thinly and is recessed more than 1 mm, bone graft can be placed behind the graft.
2. Fixation is established with bioabsorbable or metal compression screws.

3. Closure

The knee is taken through a full range of motion to ensure that the graft is stable and does not cause catching or locking. The arthrotomy is closed per the surgeon's preference with interrupted or running heavy suture. Skin closure is performed in several layers with subcuticular resorbable sutures or staples.

POSTOPERATIVE CONSIDERATIONS

Rehabilitation

General rehabilitation guidelines are described in Table 63-1. The benefit of continuous passive motion after osteochondral allografting is less clear than after marrow-stimulating techniques or autologous

TABLE 63-1. Rehabilitation Protocol after Osteochondral Allografting

Modality	Time Frame
Continuous passive motion	6-8 weeks (optional but desirable)
Brace	6-12 weeks (patellofemoral or tibial-femoral grafts)
Weight-bearing status	Toe-touch weight bearing or non–weight bearing for 6-12 weeks (based on size of graft)
Closed chain exercises, straight-leg raises	Immediately postoperatively
Stationary cycling	Beginning at 4-8 weeks postoperatively
Light recreational sports	Consider at 4-6 months postoperatively
High-impact sports	Consider at 6 months postoperatively for smaller lesion; not recommended for larger lesions

chondrocyte implantation because mature cartilage is transplanted. It may be useful, however, to improve range of motion and reduce the risk of postoperative stiffness.

Full range of motion is allowed unless dictated otherwise by concomitant procedures (i.e., meniscus transplantation, osteotomy, ligament repair). After the first postoperative visit at 1 week, patients start supervised physical therapy for range-of-motion exercises along with quad sets and patellar mobilization. During this period, the patients remain on non–weight-bearing status. At 6 weeks, weight-bearing status is gradually advanced to full weight bearing; brace use is discontinued once quad control is reestablished, and closed chain strengthening exercises are added to the rehabilitation protocol. By 3 months, patients are expected to have regained full and pain-free range of motion with nearly normal quadriceps strength, and recreational sports may be resumed at 6 months postoperatively. However, the patient should avoid excessive impact loading of the allograft during the first year.

Complications

- General surgical complications, including infection, stiffness, neurovascular damage and deep vein thrombosis (DVT)
- Osteochondral allograft-related complications, including the following[4,5,17]:
  - Graft nonunion, fragmentation, or collapse (months to years postoperatively)
  - Disease transmission (HIV, hepatitis)

TABLE 63-2. Results of Osteochondral Allografting

Study	No. of Knees and Diagnosis	Mean Age (y)	Location	Mean Follow-up	Results
Meyers et al[16] (1989)	40 FCD	38	F, T, PF	3.6 years	78% success
Garrett & Wyman[10] (1994)	17 OCD	20	F	3.5 years	94% success
Ghazavi et al[11] (1997)	126 OD	35	F, T, PF	7.5 years	85% success
Chu et al[6] (1999)	55 FCD	35	F, T, PF	75 months	76% good to excellent 16% failure
Aubin et al[2] (2001)	60 FCD	27	F	10 years	Kaplan-Meier Survival Rate: 10 years: 85% 15 years: 75%
Shasha et al[18] (2003)	65 OD	43	T	12 years	Kaplan-Meier Survival Rate: 5 years: 95% 10 years: 80% 15 years: 65% 20 years: 46%
Emmerson et al[7] (2007)	66 OCD	29	F	7.7 years	72% good to excellent 15% underwent reoperation
McCulloch et al[15] (2007)	25 FCD	35	F	3 years	88% graft survival 84% patient satisfaction
Görtz et al[13] (2010)	28 AVN	24	F	2 years	89% graft survival

AVN, Avascular necrosis; *F,* femur; *FCD,* focal chondral defect; *OCD,* osteochondritis dissecans; *OD,* osteochondral defect; *PF,* patellofemoral; *T,* tibia.

RESULTS

After osteochondral allograft transplantation, good to excellent results are achieved in nearly 85% of procedures, and patients demonstrate a measurable decrease in pain and increase in activity level (Table 63-2). The degree of graft incorporation can be assessed on follow-up radiographs.

REFERENCES

1. Alford JW, Cole BJ. Cartilage restoration, part 2: techniques, outcomes, and future directions. *Am J Sports Med.* 2005;33:443-460.
2. Aubin PP, Cheah HK, Davis AM, et al. Long-term follow-up of fresh femoral osteochondral allografts for posttraumatic knee defects. *Clin Orthop Relat Res.* 2001; 391:S318-S327.
3. Beaver RJ, Mahomed M, Backstein D, et al. Fresh osteochondral allografts for post-traumatic defects in the knee: a survivorship analysis. *J Bone Joint Surg Br.* 1992;74: 105-110.
4. Bugbee WD, Convery FR. Osteochondral allograft transplantation. *Clin Sports Med.* 1999;18:67-75.
5. Bugbee WD. Fresh osteochondral allografts. *J Knee Surg.* 2002;15:191-195.
6. Chu CR, Convery FR, Akeson WH, et al. Articular cartilage transplantation. Clinical results in the knee. *Clin Orthop Relat Res.* 1999;360:159-168.
7. Emmerson BC, Görtz S, Jamali AA, et al. Fresh osteochondral allografting in the treatment of osteochondritis dissecans of the femoral condyle. *Am J Sports Med.* 2007;35(6):907-914.
8. Fox JA, Freedman KB, Lee SJ, et al. Fresh osteochondral allograft transplantation for articular cartilage defects. *Oper Tech Sports Med* 2002;10:168-173.
9. Garrett J. Fresh osteochondral allografts for treatment of articular defects in osteochondritis dissecans of the lateral femoral condyle in adults. *Clin Orthop Relat Res.* 1994;303:33-37.
10. Garrett J, Wyman J. The operative technique of fresh osteochondral allografting of the knee. *Oper Tech Orthop.* 2001;11:132-137.
11. Ghazavi MT, Pritzker KP, Davis AM, et al. Fresh osteochondral allografts for post-traumatic osteochondral defects of the knee. *J Bone Joint Surg Br.* 1997;79: 1008-1013.
12. Gitelis S, Cole BJ. The use of allografts in orthopaedic surgery. *Instr Course Lect.* 2002;51:507-520.
13. Görtz S, De Young AJ, Bugbee WD. Fresh osteochondral allografting for steroid-associated osteonecrosis of the femoral condyles. *Clin Orthop Relat Res.* 2010;468(5): 1269-1278.
14. Gross AE, Kim W, Las Heras F, et al. Fresh osteochondral allografts for posttraumatic knee defects: long-term followup. *Clin Orthop Relat Res.* 2008;466(8):1863-1870.
15. McCulloch PC, Kang RW, Sobhy MH, et al. Prospective evaluation of prolonged fresh osteochondral allograft transplantation of the femoral condyle: minimum 2-year follow-up. *Am J Sports Med.* 2007;35(3):411-420.

16. Meyers MH, Akeson W, Convery FR. Resurfacing of the knee with fresh osteochondral allograft. *J Bone Joint Surg Am*. 1989;71:704-713.

17. Oakeshott RD, Farine I, Pritzker KP, et al. A clinical and histologic analysis of failed fresh osteochondral allografts. *Clin Orthop Relat Res*. 1988;233:283-294.

18. Shasha N, Krywulak S, Backstein D, et al. Long-term follow-up of fresh tibial osteochondral allografts for failed tibial plateau fractures. *J Bone Joint Surg Am*. 2003;85 (suppl 2):33-39.

19. Williams JM, Virdi AS, Pylawka TK, et al. Prolonged-fresh preservation of intact whole canine femoral condyles for the potential use as osteochondral allografts. *J Orthop Res*. 2005;23:831-837.

Chapter 64

Microfracture Technique in the Knee

Kai Mithoefer

Chapter Synopsis

- Microfracture is a safe, minimally invasive, technically simple, and cost-effective marrow stimulation technique that provides effective short-term functional improvement of small to medium cartilage defects. Appropriate indications, attention to surgical detail, and well-structured rehabilitation help to optimize the outcome from this cartilage repair technique. Shortcomings include limited hyaline repair tissue, variable repair cartilage volume, subchondral bone changes, functional deterioration in some patients, and unclear long-term efficacy. Despite its limitations, microfracture is still the most frequently used cartilage repair technique.

Important Points

- Indication: Symptomatic cartilage lesions of femur, patella, and tibia smaller than 4 cm^2.
- Technical steps: Debridement, calcified cartilage removal, systematic microfracture from periphery with use of a spiral pattern, leaving 3 to 4 mm between individual microfracture holes.
- Individualized rehabilitation addresses unique defect characteristics and associated pathology.

Clinical and Surgical Pearls

- Preoperative patient counseling and close cooperation with well-trained physical therapists improves postoperative rehabilitation.

- Gentle but thorough removal of calcified cartilage improves repair tissue volume and adherence.
- Systematic placement of microfracture holes optimizes clot adherence and mesenchymal stem cell distribution and reduces risk for subchondral bone collapse and bony overgrowth.
- Criteria-based progression during postoperative rehabilitation avoids activity-related pain and swelling.

Clinical and Surgical Pitfalls

- Insufficient debridement to a stable peripheral cartilage margin and failure to remove the calcified cartilage layer limit peripheral and basilar integration.
- Compromised subchondral bone plate integrity can occur with inappropriate microfracture technique.
- Insufficient subchondral bone penetration with limited access to mesenchymal stem cells may reduce the quality and quantity of the repair cartilage tissue.
- Clot displacement or limited integration of repair tissue may occur from premature weight bearing.

Video

- Video 64-1: Anterior cruciate ligament tunnel preparation and graft passage

---

Articular cartilage injuries affect an estimated 900,000 individuals in the United States every year, resulting in considerable morbidity and disability for affected individuals with a substantial associated burden on the healthcare system.[1] Treatment of articular cartilage injury in the knee still presents a great therapeutic challenge owing to the limited regenerative capacity of articular cartilage. Although no validated treatment algorithm exists for treating articular cartilage lesions in the knee, the arthroscopic microfracture technique is commonly used as a first-line option and frequently serves as the standard technique against which other cartilage repair procedures are compared.[2-4] Developed by Steadman in the 1980s, this widely used marrow stimulation procedure is generally regarded as safe and cost-effective.[5] Histologic studies have demonstrated that microfracture results in a fibrocartilage or hybrid fibrohyaline repair tissue with variable proteoglycan and type II collagen content.[3,6] Microfracture is a minimally invasive and technically simple procedure clinically, and current scientific data demonstrate that close adherence to the indications for, technical details of, and postoperative rehabilitation after this technique will help to optimize the outcomes from this cartilage repair procedure in the knee.

PREOPERATIVE CONSIDERATIONS

History

Obtaining a thorough history in patients with knee cartilage defects is a critical first step in the selection of patients who are appropriate candidates for microfracture. Symptoms from cartilage defects are usually nonspecific and can mimic other knee pathology such as meniscal tears. Pain on weight bearing is frequent and is often present during impact activities. Catching and locking sensations can occur from cartilage flaps or larger defects. Joint effusion is frequently reported, particularly after demanding impact activities. Defects of the femoral condyles often produce focal tenderness over the condyle rather than the joint line. Patellar or trochlear lesions usually lead to pain when ambulating up and down stairs, driving a car, or rising from a seated or squatting position. Symptoms of patellar instability may be reported. Articular cartilage defects may manifest acutely, such as after joint trauma including knee ligament tears, or they may be a chronic issue. Any history of previous knee surgeries should be noted, because microfracture is most effective as a first-line treatment.

Physical Examination

Physical examination includes evaluation of gait pattern as well as hip, knee, and ankle range of motion. The knee should be routinely evaluated for ligamentous instability, patellar maltracking or instability, and lower extremity malalignment. Any joint effusion should be noted. Depending on defect location and size, mechanical symptoms may or may not be present and may overlap with meniscal test findings. The patient's body mass index (BMI) should be assessed because it has been shown to correlate with functional outcome after microfracture.[1,7-9]

Preoperative Imaging

Plain radiographs including weight-bearing anteroposterior (AP), lateral, and Merchant views are obtained. In addition, a 45-degree flexion posteroanterior (PA) or Rosenberg view and long-leg films can help to identify the presence of osteochondral lesions, joint space narrowing, patellar maltracking, and overall lower extremity malalignment. Cartilage-sensitive magnetic resonance imaging (MRI) is a sensitive, specific, and accurate tool for noninvasive diagnosis of articular cartilage injury.[8]

It provides useful information about the status of the menisci, ligaments, and subchondral bone, as well as the size and depth of the lesion. Owing to the pathologic changes in the surrounding cartilage the final size of the defect usually is larger than defect size measured on preoperative MRI.[1]

Indications and Contraindications

Microfracture is indicated for symptomatic, high-grade (grade III or IV) chondral defects of the knee in active patients who are physiologically too young for arthroplasty. This technique is most successful as a first-line treatment for isolated chondral lesions up to 4 cm² that involve the femoral condyles, trochlea, and patella. Prerequisites for successful microfracture include adequate range of motion, appropriate axial alignment or patellar tracking, ligamentous stability, and the ability to comply with the postoperative rehabilitation. Adjuvant procedures can be performed simultaneously to address coexisting pathology without negative effects on the postoperative functional outcome and activity level. Detailed indications and contraindications for microfracture are listed below.

Indications

- Symptomatic cartilage lesions of femur, patella, tibia (including incidental defects)
- Defect size less than 4 cm²
- Short preoperative duration of symptoms (optimally <12 months)
- Patient age (optimally <45 years)

Contraindications

Absolute Contraindications

- Generalized degenerative joint changes
- Limited patient compliance
- Uncontained chondral lesions
- Severe axial malalignment of greater than 5 degrees for femoral condyle lesions (surgical realignment required)
- Patellar maltracking or instability for patellofemoral lesions
- High-grade ligamentous instability (surgical stabilization required for translation >10 mm)
- Tumor
- Infection
- Inflammatory arthropathy
- Systemic cartilage disorder

Relative Contraindications

- Preoperative duration of symptoms longer 12 months
- Body mass index greater than 30
- Meniscal deficiency

- Moderate to advanced chondropenia
- Defect size greater than 4 cm²
- Patient age greater than 60 years

Preoperative Planning and Counseling

Based on the history, physical examination findings, and radiologic information, the indication for microfracture or adjuvant procedures is discussed with the patient preoperatively. In-depth preoperative patient counseling is critically important to determine the patient's demands, to assess his or her ability to comply with the postoperative rehabilitation, and to create realistic expectations and goals for postoperative knee function and activity level.

SURGICAL TECHNIQUE

Positioning of the extremity must allow knee motion without limitation. A tourniquet is placed on the proximal thigh but not routinely inflated. Portals are positioned according to the location of the cartilage lesion to provide optimal access to the articular cartilage defect. Standard anterolateral and anteromedial portals can be used for lesions of the central femoral condyles. For defects of the posterior condyles, portals should be placed lower to facilitate access to and visualization of the defects. Far medial or lateral portals can be added if necessary. Superolateral portals can be helpful for patellar and trochlear lesions. Thorough diagnostic arthroscopy is performed to identify any additional intra-articular pathology such as meniscal tears, ligamentous disruption, patellar maltracking, or multiple cartilage defects.

Specific Steps

The specific steps of this procedure are outlined in Box 64-1.

Surgical treatment of meniscal pathology is addressed before microfracture, whereas ligamentous reconstruction is performed after microfracture to allow for better visualization. Simultaneous treatment of concomitant pathology avoids repetitive operative morbidity and associated prolonged rehabilitation.

The cartilage defect is identified, and existing cartilage flaps are debrided back to a stable and healthy peripheral margin with an arthroscopic shaver or ring curette (Fig. 64-1). The size of the articular lesion is measured with a calibrated probe and recorded. If debridement reveals that the lesion is not contained by an intact cartilage margin, microfracture cannot be used because sufficient pooling of the marrow clot cannot be achieved. The arc of motion during which the lesion articulates with the opposing joint surface is carefully

---

BOX 64-1 Surgical Steps

1. Complete arthroscopic joint survey to identify associated pathology and assess joint cartilage status.
2. Debride chondral defect to stable and healthy surrounding cartilage margins, and determine final defect size.
3. Gently but thoroughly remove calcified cartilage layer, avoiding bleeding from subchondral bone.
4. Start microfracture in periphery of defect with perpendicular access of the awl tip to the defect base.
5. Systematically penetrate the subchondral bone plate with use of a spiral pattern, leaving 3 to 4 mm between individual microfracture holes.
6. Ensure appropriate depth of the penetration to subchondral bone marrow by visualization of fat droplets or bleeding from the individual microfracture holes.
7. Close portal incisions tightly and avoid drain placement.

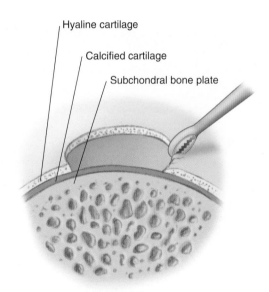

Hyaline cartilage

Calcified cartilage

Subchondral bone plate

Figure 64-1. Debridement of the loose cartilage flaps to create a stable peripheral cartilage margin using an arthroscopic shaver. *(From Mithoefer K, Williams RJ 3rd, Warren RF, et al. Chondral resurfacing of articular cartilage defects in the knee with the microfracture technique. Surgical technique. J Bone Joint Surg Am. 2006;88[Suppl 1 Pt 2]:294-304.)*

---

recorded. Knowledge of this range of contact has important implications for postoperative rehabilitation. A curette is used to carefully remove the calcified cartilage layer from the base of the lesion (Fig. 64-2). The calcified cartilage layer is a thin layer between the deep zone of the cartilage and subchondral bone and can increase in thickness with age. Removal of the calcified cartilage has been shown to improve bonding of the repair tissue to the subchondral bone after microfracture.[6] The calcified cartilage can be difficult to differentiate visually but

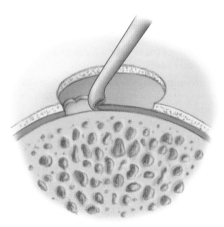

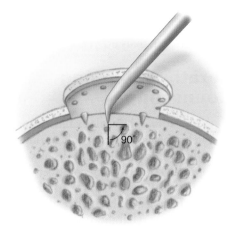

Figure 64-2. Gentle intraoperative debridement of the calcified cartilage with use of a curette for manual feedback control. *(From Mithoefer K, Williams RJ 3rd, Warren RF, et al. Chondral resurfacing of articular cartilage defects in the knee with the microfracture technique. Surgical technique. J Bone Joint Surg Am. 2006;88[Suppl 1 Pt 2]:294-304.)*

Figure 64-4. Initiation of the microfracture penetrations at the periphery of the lesion with perpendicular alignment of the awl for optimal penetration of the subchondral bone plate. *(From Mithoefer K, Williams RJ 3rd, Warren RF, et al. Chondral resurfacing of articular cartilage defects in the knee with the microfracture technique. Surgical technique. J Bone Joint Surg Am. 2006;88[Suppl 1 Pt 2]:294-304.)*

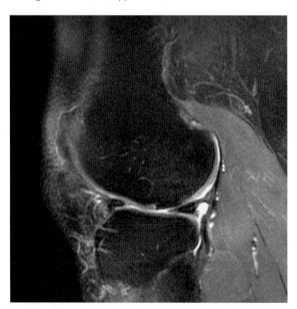

Figure 64-3. Sagittal fast spin echo magnetic resonance image demonstrating marked subchondral overgrowth *(arrow)* with resultant thinning of the overlying repair cartilage

can be distinguished more easily from the hard underlying subchondral bone plate by tactile feedback. Use of a curette provides better manual feedback than use of an arthroscopic shaver and avoids excessive debridement with thinning of the subchondral bone. Excessive removal of the subchondral bone may stimulate subchondral bone overgrowth and should be avoided. This phenomenon is observed in 25% to 49% of patients after microfracture and leads to relative thinning of the overlying repair cartilage layer with resultant biologic and biomechanical implications for the repair tissue quality (Fig. 64-3). After appropriate removal of the

calcified cartilage layer, microfracture holes are created with commercially available awls. The conical shape of the instruments is designed for controlled depth penetration and easy removal of the impacted instrument tip. Penetration of the subchondral bone is performed with the instrument tip perpendicular to the subchondral bone plate. Perpendicular alignment ensures appropriate depth of penetration into the subchondral bone marrow and avoids skiving of the tip during impact with the mallet. Skiving of the instrument can create large longitudinal disruptions of the subchondral bone plate and may affect its biomechanical integrity. Skiving can also be avoided by gently toeing in the tip of the instrument. Microfracture awls are available with tip angulation of 30, 45, 60, and 90 degrees and facilitate access to cartilage lesions in all areas of the knee joint. For femoral condyle or trochlear lesions, the 30- or 45-degree awls readily provide perpendicular alignment of the instrumentation (Fig. 64-4). Knee motion can also help to optimize instrument positioning. The 90-degree awl is frequently used for patellar defects. Perpendicular penetration of the 90-degree awl through the patellar subchondral bone plate is facilitated by impacting the grip of the instrument rather than its end. This technique in combination with manual stabilization and counterpressure on the patella will help to prevent skiving with the instrument (Fig. 64-5).

The microfracture holes are created on the periphery (Fig. 64-6) of the defect first and then continued toward the center of the lesion in a systematic spiral pattern (Fig. 64-7). This systematic approach provides homogeneous distribution of the microfracture holes throughout the entire cartilage defect and maximizes adherence

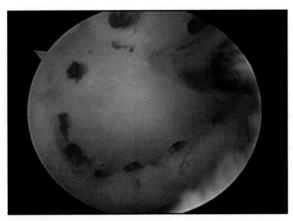

Figure 64-5. Arthroscopic image of the initial microfracture penetrations at the periphery of the cartilage defect.

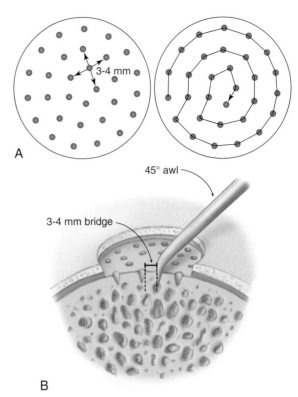

Figure 64-7. The systematic spiral pattern (**A**) of microfracture penetrations to ensure homogeneous distribution of the microfractures while maintaining sufficient subchondral bone bridges between individual penetrations (**B**). *(From Mithoefer K, Williams RJ 3rd, Warren RF, et al. Chondral resurfacing of articular cartilage defects in the knee with the microfracture technique. Surgical technique. J Bone Joint Surg Am. 2006;88[Suppl 1 Pt 2]:294-304.)*

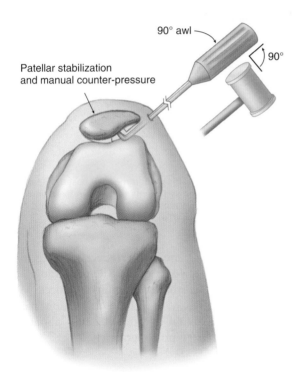

Figure 64-6. The technique for microfracture of patellar lesions. *(From Mithoefer K, Williams RJ 3rd, Warren RF, et al. Chondral resurfacing of articular cartilage defects in the knee with the microfracture technique. Surgical technique. J Bone Joint Surg Am. 2006;88[Suppl 1 Pt 2]:294-304.)*

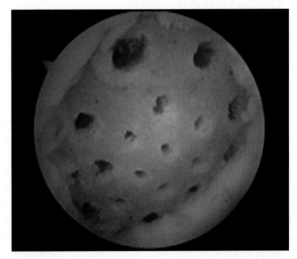

Figure 64-8. Arthroscopic view of the treated defect confirming adequacy of the microfractures by release of fat droplets and blood from the individual holes.

of the mesenchymal clot at the base (Figs. 64-8 and 64-9). Carefully, 3- to 4-mm-wide bone bridges are maintained between the individual holes to preserve subchondral bone plate integrity and function. Release of fatty droplets from the microfracture holes indicates adequate depth of the microfracture. Once the entire defect has been treated, the bony debris on the rim of

the microfracture holes is removed by curettage or arthroscopic shaver. Adequate release of blood and marrow fat droplets from the microfracture holes can be confirmed by eliminating arthroscopic pump pressure. Once adequate access to the subchondral bone

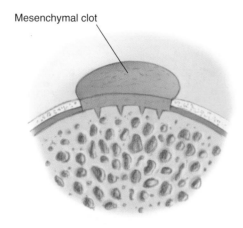

Mesenchymal clot

Figure 64-9. The pooling of the mesenchymal clot in the treated cartilage defect and the anchoring effect of the microfracture penetrations. *(From Mithoefer K, Williams RJ 3rd, Warren RF, et al. Chondral resurfacing of articular cartilage defects in the knee with the microfracture technique. Surgical technique. J Bone Joint Surg Am. 2006;88[Suppl 1 Pt 2]: 294-304.)*

marrow has been ensured, the arthroscope is removed from the joint. No drains are used to avoid removal of the pluripotent mesenchymal clot from the cartilage defect by suction or direct abrasion by the drain during postoperative joint mobilization. A compression dressing is placed and cryotherapy used routinely for control of postoperative swelling.

POSTOPERATIVE CONSIDERATIONS

Rehabilitation

Appropriate rehabilitation after treatment of articular cartilage defects of the knee with microfracture helps mesenchymal stem cell differentiation in the clot while avoiding detrimental compression and shear forces on the developing repair cartilage tissue (Box 64-2). Rehabilitation presents a critical component for successful treatment outcome and follows different guidelines for femorotibial lesions and patellofemoral defects. Although general timelines can be useful, progression through rehabilitation should be achieved individually based on the lesion characteristics, surgical details, and patient symptoms. Concomitant procedures such as ligament reconstruction, meniscal surgery, or osteotomy may alter the postoperative rehabilitation protocol.

Postoperative Imaging

Second-look arthroscopy is not routinely recommended. Postoperative cartilage-sensitive MRI provides reliable information about repair cartilage fill and integration with additional evaluation of the underlying

---

BOX 64-2 Microfracture Rehabilitation Timeline*

Femoral Defects

Touch-down weight bearing for 2 weeks, then progression of 25% per week

CPM 6 to 8 hours per day for 6 weeks

Closed kinetic chain exercises (biking) without resistance at 2 weeks

Start limited-arc open kinetic chain exercises at 6 to 8 weeks

Initiate impact exercises (jogging) at 4 months if no pain or effusion

Start plyometric drills at 5 months

Return to cutting, jumping activities at 5 to 6 months

Sport-specific skill program and functional progression at 6 months

Gradual return to high-impact athletics by 6 to 8 months

Patellar and Trochlear Defects

WBAT for 8 weeks with brace locked at 0 to 20 degrees

CPM 6 hours per week for 6 to 8 weeks at 0 to 45 degrees

Start closed kinetic chain exercises without resistance at 2 to 4 weeks

Limited-arc ROM exercises until 12 weeks

Start open kinetic chain exercises after 12 to 16 weeks

Initiate impact activities at 6 to 7 months

Return to high-impact athletics at 8 to 12 months

*Individualized progression is recommended based on patient's lesion characteristics and symptoms rather than fixed timelines. *CPM,* Continuous passive motion; *ROM,* range of motion; *WBAT,* weight bearing as tolerated.

---

subchondral bone plate with respect to integrity and overgrowth. Newer functional MRI technologies such as T2 mapping, delayed gadolinium-enhanced MRI of cartilage (dGEMRIC), or T1rho relaxation mapping can be used to obtain additional detail about repair cartilage morphology postoperatively.

RESULTS

Results of the procedure are summarized in Table 64-1.

A systematic review described the clinical results of 28 studies including 3122 patients.[1] Microfracture effectively improved knee function in all studies during the first 24 months postoperatively, although several studies reported a decrease in function with higher failure rates occurring after 2 years.[4,8,9,14] However, average functional improvement remained above preoperative levels in all studies beyond 2 years after microfracture.[8-12,17] Several factors were identified that affected clinical outcome after microfracture, including age (better results with age below 40 years), location of the lesion, duration of symptoms (longer than 12 months), lesion size (smaller than 4 cm²), preoperative activity

TABLE 64-1. Clinical Outcome of Microfracture

Study	Type	Surgery	Follow-up	Patient Population	Clinical Results
Blevins et al[10] (1998)	Prospective	MF	3.7 years	Athletes	76% improvement
Steadman et al[11] (2003)	Prospective	MF	11 years	Traumatic, <45 years	80% improvement
Steadman et al[12] (2003)	Prospective	MF	4.5 years	Athletes	76% return to sport
Miller et al[13] (2004)	Prospective	MF	2.6 years	Degenerative	Tegner-Lysholm improvement
Mithoefer et al[8] (2005)	Prospective	MF	41 months	Mixed	67% good-excellent IKDC score decreased >2 years
Gudas et al[2] (2005)	Randomized	MF vs. OAT	37 months	Athletes	Good-excellent 52% (MF) and 96% (OAT)
Gobbi et al[14] (2005)	Prospective	MF	72 months	Athletes	70% improvement Tegner score decreased >2 years
Kreuz et al[15,16] (2006)	Prospective	MF	36 months	Mixed	Better results with age <40 years
Mithoefer et al[9] (2006)	Prospective	MF	41 months	Mixed athletes	44% return to sport (overall) 71% return to sport (competitive athletes)
Knutsen et al[3] (2007)	Randomized	MF vs. ACT	60 months	Mixed	77% improvement
Saris et al[14] (2009)	Randomized	MF vs. CCI	36 months	Mixed	Better KOOS with CCI
Miller et al[17] (2010)	Prospective	MF	48 months	Mixed	Lysholm score decrease after 2 years Results better with age <45 years

ACT, Autologous chondrocyte transplantation; *CCI*, characterized chondrocyte implantation; *IKDC*, International Knee Documentation Committee; *KOOS*, knee injury and osteoarthritis outcome score; *MF*, microfracture; *OAT*, osteochondral autograft transfer.

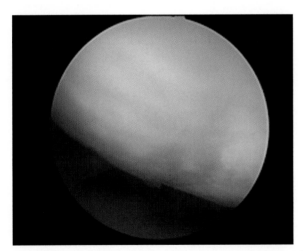

Figure 64-10. Arthroscopic appearance of the defect 23 months after microfracture.

level (Tegner score higher than 4), body mass index (below 30 kg/m²), and level of competition for athletes (better return to sport in competitive athletes).[1,8-10,15,16] Defect fill on MRI can be highly variable and correlates with functional outcome.[8] Macroscopic repair cartilage quality positively affected long-term failure rate, but the influence of histologic repair tissue quality remained inconclusive.[1,3] Randomized comparison of microfracture with autologous chondrocyte transplantation showed no significant difference in clinical function at 5 years.[3] Randomized comparison with characterized chondrocyte implantation and osteochondral autograft transfer demonstrated significantly lower knee function for microfracture at 3 years.[2,4] Overall, microfracture provides effective short-term functional improvement of knee function, but insufficient data are available on its long-term results (Fig. 64-10).

REFERENCES

1. Mithoefer K, McAdams T, Williams RJ, et al. Clinical efficacy of the microfracture technique for articular cartilage repair in the knee: an evidence-based systematic analysis. *Am J Sports Med.* 2009;37:2053-2063.
2. Gudas R, Kalesinskas RJ, Kimtys V, et al. A prospective randomized clinical study of mosaic osteochondral autologous transplantation versus microfracture for the treatment of osteochondral defects in the knee joint in young athletes. *Arthroscopy.* 2005;2:1066-1075.
3. Knutsen G, Drogset JO, Engebretsen L, et al. A randomized trial comparing autologous chondrocyte implantation with microfracture. Findings at five years. *J Bone Joint Surg Am.* 2007;89:2105-2112.
4. Saris DB, Vanlauwe J, Victor J, et al. TIG/ACT/01/2000&EXT Study Group. Treatment of symptomatic cartilage defects of the knee: characterized chondrocyte

implantation results in better clinical outcome at 36 months in a randomized trial compared to microfracture. *Am J Sports Med.* 2009;37(Suppl 1):10S-19S.

5. Steadman JR, Rodkey WG, Singleton SB, et al. Microfracture technique for full-thickness chondral defects: technique and clinical results. *Oper Tech Orthop.* 1997;7: 300-304.

6. Frisbie DD, Morisset S, Ho CP, et al. Effects of calcified cartilage on healing of chondral defects treated with microfracture in horses. *Am J Sports Med.* 2006;34: 1824-1831.

7. Mithoefer K, Williams 3rd RJ, Warren RF, et al. Chondral resurfacing of articular cartilage defects in the knee with the microfracture technique. Surgical technique. *J Bone Joint Surg Am.* 2006;88(Suppl 1 Pt 2):294-304.

8. Mithoefer K, Williams 3rd RJ, Warren RF, et al. The microfracture technique for the treatment of articular cartilage lesions in the knee. A prospective cohort study. *J Bone Joint Surg Am.* 2005;87:1911-1920.

9. Mithoefer K, Williams 3rd RJ, Warren RF, et al. High-impact athletics after knee articular cartilage repair: A prospective evaluation of the microfracture technique. *Am J Sports Med.* 2006;34:1413-1418.

10. Blevins FT, Steadman JR, Rodrigo JJ, et al. Treatment of articular cartilage defects in athletes: an analysis of functional outcome and lesion appearance. *Orthopedics.* 1998;21:761-767.

11. Steadman JR, Briggs KK, Rodrigo JJ, et al. Outcomes of microfracture for traumatic chondral defects of the knee: average 11-year follow-up. *Arthroscopy.* 2003;19: 477-484.

12. Steadman JR, Miller BS, Karas SG, et al. The microfracture technique in the treatment of full-thickness chondral lesions of the knee in national football league players. *J Knee Surg.* 2003;16:83-86.

13. Miller BS, Steadman JR, Briggs KK, et al. Patient satisfaction and outcome after microfracture of the degenerative knee. *J Knee Surg.* 2004;17(1):13-17.

14. Gobbi A, Nunag P, Malinowski K. Treatment of chondral lesions of the knee with microfracture in a group of athletes. *Knee Surg Sports Traumatol Arthrosc.* 2005;13: 213-221.

15. Kreuz PC, Erggelet C, Steinwachs MR, et al. Is microfracture of chondral defects in the knee associated with different results in patients aged 40 years or younger? *Arthroscopy.* 2006;22:1180-1186.

16. Kreuz PC, Steinwachs MR, Erggelet C, et al. Results after microfracture of full-thickness chondral defects in different compartments in the knee. *Osteoarthritis Cartilage.* 2006;14:1119-1125.

17. Miller BS, Briggs KK, Downie B, et al. Clinical outcomes following the microfracture procedure for chondral defects in the knee: A longitudinal data analysis. *Cartilage.* 2010;1:108-112.

Chapter 65

Primary Repair of Osteochondritis Dissecans in the Knee

Jonathan M. Frank, Geoffrey S. Van Thiel, L. Pearce McCarty III, and Brian J. Cole

Chapter Synopsis

- Osteochondritis dissecans (OCD) is a pathologic process that results in the detachment of subchondral bone and its overlying articular cartilage from the underlying bone. Several options are available to treat adult OCD, including debridement, drilling, loose body removal, microfracture, arthroscopic reduction and internal fixation (ARIF), osteochondral autografting and allografting, and autologous chondrocyte implantation (ACI). Primary repair is described in this chapter.

Important Points

- A course of nonoperative treatment should have failed first.
- Can be done via arthroscopic or open technique; it is important to get an accurate reduction.
- Must stimulate healing at the base of the lesion.
- Absorbable or nonabsorbable implants may be used.

Clinical and Surgical Pearls

- It is essential to achieve appropriate visualization of the lesion and the base of the defect. An open approach may be used as needed.
- A larger arthrotomy is required for access to patellofemoral lesion.
- Lesion stability after fixation is essential.
- Excision of a portion of the anterior fat pad can improve visualization of the lesion and greatly facilitate insertion of cannulated implants during arthroscopic treatment.

- Treatment of OCD lesions should be thought of as fracture fixation. Compression should be generated along a vector orthogonal to the fracture site to optimize healing.
- In the arthroscopic treatment of medial femoral condyle lesions, particularly classic lesions that abut the intercondylar notch, it is often easiest to hinge the lesion open along its intercondylar edge.

Clinical and Surgical Pitfalls

- A free fragment with minimal subchondral bone has a very low probability of healing.
- Nonabsorbable implants can be removed at 8 weeks to assess for healing and to prevent screw prominence with fragment settling.
- In removing headless, variable-pitch screws, a noncannulated screwdriver should be used to initiate removal. The torque required to initiate unscrewing of a well-seated screw is sufficient to cause the tip of a cannulated screwdriver to break. After a total of approximately two thirds of the screw has been unscrewed, a guidewire should be inserted and the cannulated screwdriver used to complete the removal.
- Follow a strict postoperative protocol with non–weight-bearing status.

 Video

- Video 65-1: Primary repair of osteochondritis dissecans

Osteochondritis dissecans (OCD) is a pathologic process that results in the detachment of subchondral bone and its overlying articular cartilage from the underlying bone.[1-3] The destabilized area is now vulnerable to fragmentation and shear forces. The end result is degenerative changes and subsequent loss of function of the affected compartment. The cause remains unknown; however, it is likely multifactorial and may be related to repetitive microtrauma or an acute traumatic or ischemic incident, genetic predisposition, endocrine dysfunction, or an ossification abnormality.[4-6]

The prevalence of OCD is estimated at 15 to 30 cases per 1000 patients annually, affecting the medial femoral condyle (lateral aspect most commonly) in 80% of patients, lateral femoral condyle in 15%, and patello-femoral in 5%.[7,8] Very little is known about the natural history of untreated OCD lesions. Studies by Lindén and colleagues[7] and Twyman and colleagues[9] suggest that patients with adult-onset OCD who are left un-treated have a higher risk of developing osteoarthritis and that this likelihood is proportional to the side of the lesion. In effect, symptomatic lesions are always treated for fear of the sequelae of leaving these lesions to progress toward their inevitable osteoarthritic con-clusion. The goal of reparative procedures is to restore the integrity of the native subchondral interface and preserve the overlying articular cartilage.[10] Several options are available to treat adults with OCD, includ-ing debridement, drilling, loose body removal, micro-fracture, arthroscopic reduction and internal fixation (ARIF), osteochondral autografting and allografting, and autologous chondrocyte implantation (ACI). Un-fortunately, no consensus exists as to the best treatment option. The surgeon's clinical expertise, the character of the defect, and the patient's goals dictate the best treat-ment option. It is well established, though, that primary repair by rigid, compressive fixation of unstable lesions offers an attractive and effective means of treatment by preserving the native osteochondral surface.

PREOPERATIVE CONSIDERATIONS

History and Physical Examination

Patients often report several months of stiffness and activity-related swelling and poorly localized pain. They may report catching or locking symptoms exacerbated by increased activity, a result of a stable lesion detaching and effectively acting as a loose body.

Physical examination is often more informative but can also be misleading. Observe for a change in gait, specifically an antalgic gait. There may be an effusion, loss in range of motion, and quadriceps atrophy depend-ing on severity. Because the most common location for an OCD lesion is on the medial femoral condyle by the trochlea, tenderness may be elicited with palpation over this area and can be confused for patellofemoral pain. Observe for the Wilson sign—the patient will ambulate with the affected leg in relative external rotation to decrease contact of the lesion with the medial tibial eminence. Reproduction of pain through internal rota-tion of the tibia between 30 and 90 degrees of flexion and relief with subsequent external rotation is the Wilson test. It has low sensitivity, but if the result is positive initially, it reliably becomes negative with healing of the lesion.[11,12]

Imaging

Plain radiographs should include standard anteroposte-rior, flexion weight-bearing anteroposterior (notch view), lateral, and Merchant views. The notch view is useful for identifying posterior condyle lesions.

OCD lesions commonly appear as an area of osteo-sclerotic bone with a high-intensity line between the defect and the epiphysis (Fig. 65-1).

Magnetic resonance imaging (MRI) is the most informative imaging modality, providing information on the quality of bone edema, subchondral separation, and cartilage condition, as well as lesion size, location, and depth. Meeting one of the following four criteria will provide up to 97% sensitivity and 100% specificity in predicting lesion stability (Fig. 65-2)[13-16]:

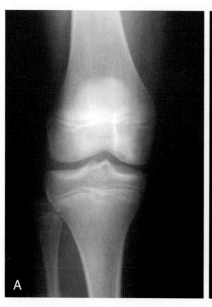 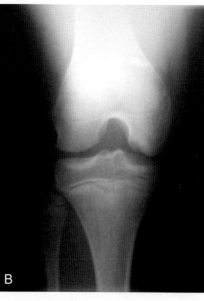

Figure 65-1. A, Weight-bearing anteroposterior radiograph of a right knee in a skeletally immature patient depicting a classic osteochondritis dissecans lesion. **B,** Weight-bearing, 30-degree flexed posteroanterior radiograph, or tunnel view, in the same patient. The osteochondritis dissecans lesion is visualized much more readily with this view.

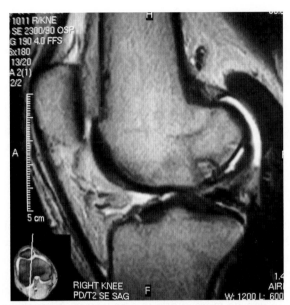

Figure 65-2. Proton density, T2-weighted sagittal magnetic resonance image through the lateral femoral condyle. A high signal intensity interface between the osteochondritis dissecans lesion and underlying bone suggests instability.

1. Thin, ill-defined or well-demarcated line of high signal intensity, measuring 5 mm or more in length at the interface between the OCD lesion and underlying subchondral bone
2. Discrete rounded area of homogeneous high signal intensity, 5 mm or more in diameter beneath the lesion
3. Focal defect with an articular surface of the lesion with a width of 5 mm or more
4. High–signal intensity line traversing the articular cartilage and subchondral bone plate into the lesion

Indications for and Contraindications to Surgery

Surgical planning requires an evaluation of all the different data points that have thus far been gathered from the history, physical examination, and imaging. Putting together a picture that looks at the patient's age, characteristics of the lesion (quality of articular cartilage; size of associated subchondral bone; shape, thickness, and location of the lesion), diagnostic information provided by MRI and arthroscopy, and preference of the operating surgeon will aid in the choice of surgery and the plan of attack.

Initial conservative management is primarily activity modification with a reduction in weight bearing through use of crutches or possibly even casting in noncompliant patients. The goal is to allow time for lesion healing while limiting factors that may promote further degradation and separation. Radiographs are usually taken 3 months after the start of nonsurgical therapy to assess the status of the lesion and the condition of the subchondral bone. In a study by Sales de Gauzy and colleagues that looked at outcomes of OCD lesions in active children after cessation of sports activities, the researchers found an improvement in the lesions and recommended against surgical intervention.[17] However, these results may not translate well to those who are not active sports participants. For these patients, limiting weight bearing and instructing on range-of-motion exercises to prevent stiffness may be viable options. An argument can be made, though, that nonsurgical management should be reserved for only skeletally immature patients because the risk of further degradation and loose body formation is high in adults. Surgical intervention is absolutely indicated if the lesion becomes detached or unstable or if the quality of pain worsens.

The ideal OCD lesion for primary repair is the unstable lesion in situ in an active, symptomatic patient who acknowledges and is willing to comply with postoperative weight-bearing and activity restrictions and who understands the need for a second procedure for implant removal. In addition, patients who fail to demonstrate symptomatic or radiographic improvement after 6 months of appropriate nonoperative therapy should also be considered for surgical treatment. Primary repair is not recommended in the case of grossly unstable lesions that have produced a loose body with less than 3 mm of subchondral bone remaining on the fragment. These lesions may be treated with excision of the loose body and either marrow stimulation or one of a variety of secondary salvage cartilage restoration techniques. A cartilage flap can be fixed with screw or pin fixation, whereas a lesion that is partially lifted from the subchondral bone will require an intervention to improve bloodflow—usually via drilling or microfracture awl—followed by fixation.[18] Furthermore, cancellous autograft is used in cases of subchondral bone loss to replace the lost subchondral support for the chondral surface.

Results after primary repair of appropriately selected OCD lesions in the knee have typically been reported as good to excellent, with fragment union reported in 72% to 100% of patients.[19-28]

SURGICAL TECHNIQUE

With a congruent reduction of the osteochondral flap, primary repair of an OCD lesion may be performed either arthroscopically or with use of a small parapatellar arthrotomy. An incongruent reduction with articular step-off, however, typically requires an open technique to permit autologous bone grafting at the base of the lesion. Reduction and fixation of suitable fragments that are detached and floating loosely inside the joint also generally require an open technique. It has been shown that these fragments continue to grow via nutrition supplied by the synovial fluid. Thus these fragments can be contoured to fit into the defect appropriately and subsequently fixed.

Anesthesia and Positioning

Choice of anesthesia option depends on the preferences of the surgeon, patient, and anesthetist, with consideration of the patient's comorbidities. After appropriate muscle relaxation, a standard examination under anesthesia is performed to document range of motion and ligamentous stability. The patient is positioned supine on a standard operating room table with a padded thigh tourniquet, and the affected extremity is secured in a standard leg holder placed around the proximal thigh to permit broad access to the knee. The contralateral extremity may be positioned in an obstetric-type leg holder. When this type of device is used, care should be taken to provide adequate padding around the fibular head to protect the common peroneal nerve, because the leg has a tendency to externally rotate and thereby place undue pressure on this area. The bed is placed in 15 to 20 degrees of reflex to take the lumbar spine out of extension. The foot of the operating room table is dropped completely. An additional advantage of this type of positioning is ease of access should one wish to confirm the placement of implants by intraoperative fluoroscopy.

Surgical Landmarks, Incisions, and Portals

Begin by marking out the patella, patellar tendon edges, and tibial tubercle; these will serve as the landmarks. If the procedure is performed via an arthroscopic technique, standard lateral and medial portals are made. An accessory instrumentation portal for placement of fixation is also required. This portal should be established by standard spinal needle localization such that fixation can be orthogonal to the plane of the lesion.

An open technique can use a midline utility skin incision (may be adjusted slightly medial or lateral of midline, depending on location of lesion) with a medial or lateral parapatellar arthrotomy. Patellar lesions treated in an open fashion require a larger arthrotomy to permit partial or complete eversion and exposure of the lesion. For standard condylar lesions, a mini-arthrotomy, extending from the joint line to midpatellar level, should be sufficient. Be careful to avoid the meniscus or patellar tendon because these structures are at risk of injury. Unfortunately, though, often the infrapatellar branch of the saphenous nerve is unavoidably sacrificed.

Specific Steps

The key surgical steps for primary repair remain essentially unchanged whether the lesion is approached in an open or arthroscopic fashion (Box 65-1).

1. Diagnostic Arthroscopy

A complete, systematic arthroscopic evaluation of each compartment and its structures is performed to identify any additional sources of intra-articular disease.

2. Identification and Assessment of Lesion Stability

With use of the elbow of a standard arthroscopic probe, the boundaries and stability of the lesion are assessed. In many cases the borders of the lesion are obvious, with fissuring, fibrillation, and even gross gapping in the articular surface (Fig. 65-3). However, definition of the lesion can be more subtle in some cases. Nevertheless, even without obvious visual clues, a distinct transition from firm to soft or the ballottement of a segment of

---

BOX 65-1 Surgical Steps: Primary Repair of Osteochondritis Dissecans in the Knee

1. Diagnostic arthroscopy
2. Identification and assessment of lesion stability
3. Debridement of lesion bed and undersurface of the fragment
4. Microfracture of lesion bed with further debridement as needed and assessment of fragment reduction
5. Fixation of lesion
6. Implant removal (for nonabsorbable implants, 3 to 4 months after fixation)

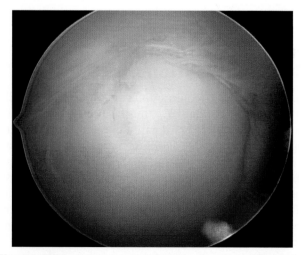

Figure 65-3. Large osteochondritis dissecans lesion of the medial femoral condyle bordering the intercondylar notch. Cartilage fissuring and fibrillation demarcate lesion borders.

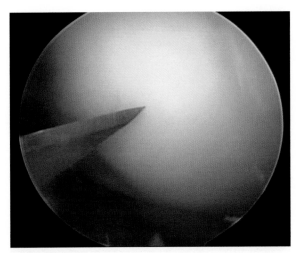

Figure 65-4. With no evident fissuring, a knife can be used to demarcate and access the base of the lesion.

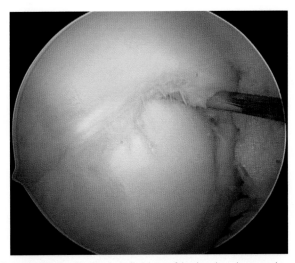

Figure 65-5. Further definition of lesion borders and arthroscopic assessment of lesion stability are carried out with a standard arthroscopic probe.

articular cartilage can typically be appreciated while one moves the elbow of the probe from normal cartilage to that overlying a lesion. The tactile feedback received is that of the elbow of the probe falling into a small crevasse as the lesion boundary is crossed. In the rare situation in which the lesion cannot be identified through visualization and tactile feedback, intraoperative fluoroscopy can confirm the lesion's location. Occasionally a knife is needed to demarcate the lesion and access the base of the defect (Fig. 65-4).

3. Debridement of Lesion Bed and Undersurface of the Fragment

Any disruption in the articular surface or observation of ballottement with palpation confirms instability and indicates a need to expose and to debride the lesion. Careful manipulation of the lesion boundary with a probe will typically reveal a tendency for the lesion flap to hinge open in one particular direction (Fig. 65-5). For lesions bordering on the intercondylar notch, the general tendency is for the lesion to hinge on the intercondylar side (Fig. 65-6). A 15-degree arthroscopic Bankart elevator can be useful in opening the lesion. Once it is fully exposed, use a curette to debride the base of the lesion of fibrinous tissue or sclerotic bone. A shaver or spherical bur (4 to 4.5 mm; an angled instrument may be useful and should be available) is used to clean the undersurface of the osteochondral fragment and further debride the base of the lesion (Fig. 65-7).

4. Microfracture of Lesion Bed with Further Debridement as Needed and Assessment of Fragment Reduction

A standard set of microfracture awls is used to penetrate the base of the lesion at 5-mm intervals. Inflow should be shut off after microfracture to confirm efflux of marrow elements from the base of the lesion (Fig. 65-8).

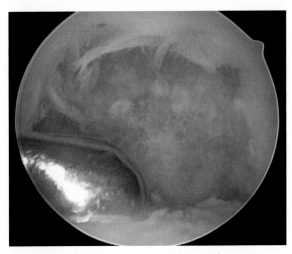

Figure 65-6. The lesion is opened on an intact fibrocartilaginous hinge that borders the intercondylar notch.

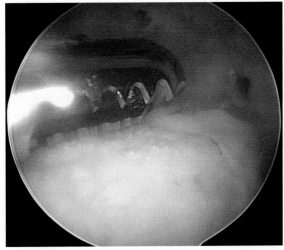

Figure 65-7. A mechanized shaver or bur is used to debride the base of the lesion and undersurface of the fragment.

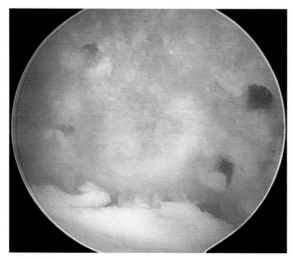

Figure 65-8. Microfracture is performed on the base of the lesion. Appropriate depth of penetration is confirmed by visualization of marrow efflux from perforations.

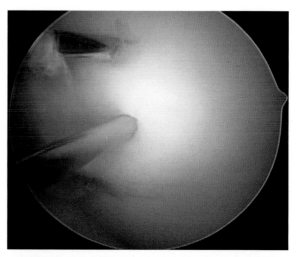

Figure 65-9. Two guidewires are placed to control rotation during fixation with cannulated implants.

If the process of microfracture generates an uneven surface that may impede congruent reduction, a small bur can be used to smooth out the lesion bed. The osteochondral fragment is then reduced and held firmly in place with the elbow of a probe. Attention is given to the congruency of the reduction. Any step-off greater than 1 mm suggests the need for bone autograft to the lesion bed.

5. Fixation of Lesion

With spinal needle localization, a line orthogonal to the plane of the lesion is established and an accessory portal is made. This is an extremely important step; application of compressive force along a nonorthogonal vector can produce shear and nonanatomic reduction of the osteochondral fragment.

A variety of implants can be used for fixation. We currently prefer a nonabsorbable, cannulated, headless, variable-pitch compression screw because of the rigidity of fixation provided and compatibility with an arthroscopic technique. Cannulated implants are also recommended for an open technique, given that implant guidewires are often used to maintain reduction during fixation. Bioabsorbable and metallic screw options are available; however, each has its own drawbacks. Problems with metallic implants include a required second surgery for removal and interference with MRI. With regard to bioabsorbable implants, there are reports of sterile effusions, sterile abscess, production of intra-articular loose bodies from dissociation of the head from the shaft as a result of absorption at the head-neck junction, and screw back-out resulting in damage to the opposing articular surface.[29-34] However, these complications may be more related to the type of biomaterial than to biomaterials in general.[35]

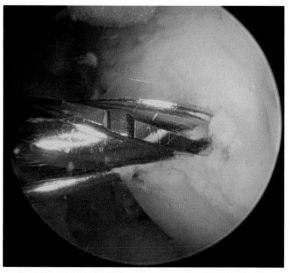

Figure 65-10. A cannulated drill bit is introduced and drilled to the appropriate depth.

With use of an ipsilateral viewing portal, a guidewire is introduced through the accessory instrumentation portal and drilled into the lesion (Fig. 65-9). A second guidewire is then placed to provide counter-torque during drilling and placement of the first screw. Small lesions may permit use of a single screw for adequate fixation, but larger lesions may require two or even three screws, and careful consideration should be given to the spacing of implants to avoid crowding and fracture of the osteochondral flap itself. Because these lesions occur in a younger population with excellent bone quality, implants will typically obtain generous purchase and can easily generate excessive compression at the lesion site, fracturing the osteochondral flap with excessive tightening. Slight overdrilling may help prevent overtightening (Fig. 65-10). When cannulated implants are used, it is helpful to remove the guidewire once the

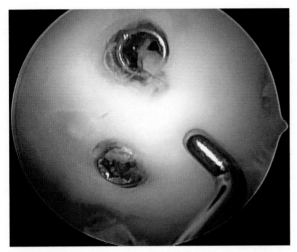

Figure 65-11. After fixation, the lesion is probed for stability.

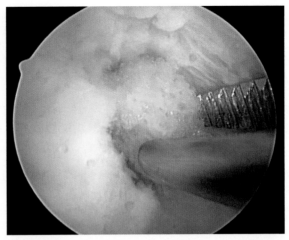

Figure 65-12. Placement of bone graft into the defect.

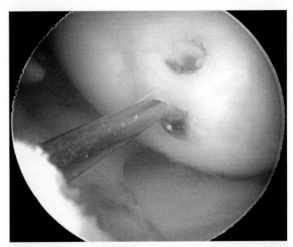

Figure 65-13. The accessory instrumentation portal is reestablished at the appropriate angle for removal of implants.

screw has been seated two thirds of the way and to finish seating the screw with a noncannulated screwdriver. This avoids difficulty in removing the guidewire and eliminates the risk of breakage of a cannulated screwdriver tip by the torque generated by the compression screw. Implants are countersunk to permit range of motion without risk of injury to the opposing articular surface (Fig. 65-11). After fixation, the lesion is probed for stability and observed through several cycles of flexion and extension for flap motion.

For lesions requiring autograft, adequate cancellous graft can be obtained from the Gerdy tubercle with minimal additional morbidity. If it is available, an 8-mm-diameter harvesting trocar for osteochondral autograft transfer can be used to harvest the bone graft in a minimally invasive fashion. A 1-cm vertical incision is made overlying the Gerdy tubercle. A subperiosteal flap is elevated, and the harvesting trocar is introduced with slight distal and medial angulation. Depending on the size of the lesion, one or two plugs will provide sufficient graft. Alternatively, a slightly longer incision can be made over the Gerdy tubercle, a 1-cm cortical window made with an osteotome, and a curette used to remove cancellous autograft. The cortical flap is then replaced, and the incision is irrigated and closed in layers. Cancellous autograft is then tamped into the base of the lesion until a congruent reduction has been obtained (Fig. 65-12). Fixation is then applied as described earlier.

6. Implant Removal (for Nonabsorbable Implants, 3 to 4 Months After Fixation)

Implant removal is typically performed arthroscopically, regardless of initial fixation technique. Diagnostic arthroscopy is performed to reevaluate the joint and to assess healing of the lesion. Spinal needle localization is used to establish the appropriate vector for implant

removal (Fig. 65-13). A noncannulated screwdriver is used to initiate screw removal because a sufficient amount of torque may be applied during this process to fracture the tip of a cannulated screwdriver. Once the screw has been backed out several turns, a guidewire is threaded down the shaft of the screw and a cannulated screwdriver completes removal. Once the tip of the screw has been disengaged from the articular surface, the guidewire is clamped with a hemostat at a point distal to the tip of the screw to prevent loss of the screw in the joint or extra-articular soft tissue. The lesion should then be probed for stability and the knee brought through a cycle of flexion and extension (Fig. 65-14).

POSTOPERATIVE CONSIDERATIONS

Follow-up will typically occur in 7 to 10 days for suture removal and postoperative non–weight-bearing

TABLE 65-1. Summary of Results of Studies of Primary Repair of Osteochondritis Dissecans of the Knee

Study	Mean Follow-up	Lesion Location (No. of Knees)	Implant	Outcome
Tabaddor et al[36] (2010)	39.6 months	MFC (14), LFC (5), P (5)	Poly 96L/4D-lactide copolymer	Healing in 22 of 24 knees
Gomoll et al[22] (2007)	6 years	MFC (12)	Metallic CCS	Healing in 12 of 12 knees
Nakagawa et al[26] (2005)	5 years	MFC (4), LFC (1), T (3)	PLLA (7), bone peg (1)	Healing in 7 of 8 knees
Larsen et al[24] (2005)	2.6 years	MFC (7)	PGA-PLLA copolymer	Healing in 6 of 7 knees
Makino et al[25] (2005)	4.2 years	MFC (14), LFC (1)	Metallic VPCCS	Healing in 14 of 15 knees; 13 of 15 knees "normal" by IKDC score
Dervin et al[21] (1998)	2.75 years	MFC (9)	PLLA	Healing in 8 of 9 knees
Kivistö et al[23] (2002)	4 years	MFC (18), T (10)	Hoffmann dynamic metal staples	Healing in 23 of 28 knees
Rey Zuniga et al[27] (1993)	1.3 years	MFC (11)	Metallic VPCCS	Healing in 8 of 11 knees
Cugat et al[20] (1993)	3.5 years	MFC (14), T (1)	Metallic CCS	Healing in 15 of 15 knees
Anderson et al[19] (1990)	6 years	MFC (17)	Threaded Kirschner wire	Healing in 16 of 17 knees

CCS, Cannulated compression screw; *IKDC*, International Knee Documentation Committee; *LFC*, lateral femoral condyle; *MFC*, medial femoral condyle; *PGA*, polyglycolic acid; *PLLA*, poly-L-lactic acid; *T*, trochlea; *VPCCS*, variable pitch cannulated compression screw.

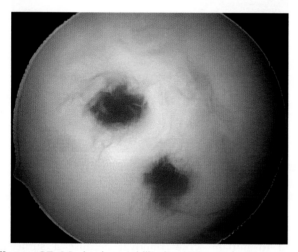

Figure 65-14. Lesion stability is reassessed after removal of fixation.

anteroposterior and lateral radiographs, which are repeated at regular 4- to 6-week intervals until healing of the lesion is observed. Patients with metallic implants are often kept on heel-touch–weight-bearing status until implant removal, whereas those with bioabsorbable implants are advanced after 6 weeks. Passive range of motion is prescribed for 4 to 6 weeks, followed by active range of motion. Heel slides, quadriceps sets, straight-leg raises, and ankle pumps are initiated immediately postoperatively.

Patients treated with nonabsorbable implants are kept on non–weight-bearing status until implant removal, whereas those with bioabsorbable implants are advanced after 6 weeks. Passive range of motion is prescribed for 4 to 6 weeks, followed by active range

of motion. Heel slides, quadriceps sets, straight-leg raises, and ankle pumps are initiated immediately postoperatively.

RESULTS

Results of studies are summarized in Table 65-1.

REFERENCES

1. Cahill BR, Phillips MR, Navarro R. The results of conservative management of juvenile osteochondritis dissecans using joint scintigraphy. A prospective study. *Am J Sports Med*. 1989;17(5):601-605, discussion 605-606.
2. Magnussen RA, Carey JL, Spindler KP. Does operative fixation of an osteochondritis dissecans loose body result in healing and long-term maintenance of knee function? *Am J Sports Med*. 2009;37(4):754-759.
3. Steinhagen J, Bruns J, Deuretzbacher G, et al. Treatment of osteochondritis dissecans of the femoral condyle with autologous bone grafts and matrix-supported autologous chondrocytes. *Int Orthop*. 2010;34(6):819-825.
4. Aichroth P. Osteochondritis dissecans of the knee. A clinical survey. *J Bone Joint Surg Br*. 1971;53(3):440-447.
5. Mackie T, Wilkins RM. Case report: Osteochondritis dissecans in twins: treatment with fresh osteochondral grafts. *Clin Orthop Relat Res*. 2010;468(3):893-897.
6. Schenck RC, Goodnight JM. Osteochondritis dissecans. *J Bone Joint Surg Am*. 1996;78(3):439-456.
7. Lindén B. The incidence of osteochondritis dissecans in the condyles of the femur. *Acta Orthop Scand*. 1976; 47(6):664-667.
8. Hughston JC, Hergenroeder PT, Courtenay BG. Osteochondritis dissecans of the femoral condyles. *J Bone Joint Surg Am*. 1984;6:1340-1348.

9. Twyman RS, Desai K, Aichroth PM. Osteochondritis dissecans of the knee. A long-term study. *J Bone Joint Surg Br.* 1991;73(3):461-464.

10. Mandelbaum BR, Browne JE, Fu F, et al. Articular cartilage lesions of the knee. *Am J Sports Med.* 1998;26(6):853-861.

11. Conrad JM, Stanitski CL. Osteochondritis dissecans: Wilson's sign revisited. *Am J Sports Med.* 2003;31(5):777-778.

12. Wilson JN. A diagnostic sign in osteochondritis dissecans of the knee. *J Bone Joint Surg Am.* 1967;49(3):477-480.

13. De Smet AA, Fisher DR, Graf BK, et al. Osteochondritis dissecans of the knee: value of MR imaging in determining lesion stability and the presence of articular cartilage defects. *AJR Am J Roentgenol.* 1990;155(3):549-553.

14. De Smet AA, Ilahi OA, Graf BK. Untreated osteochondritis dissecans of the femoral condyles: prediction of patient outcome using radiographic and MR findings. *Skeletal Radiol.* 1997;26(8):463-467.

15. Flynn JM, Kocher MS, Ganley TJ. Osteochondritis dissecans of the knee. *J Pediatr Orthop.* 2004;24(4):434-443.

16. Friel NA, Bajaj S, Cole BJ. Articular cartilage injury and adult OCD: treatment options and decision making. In: McCarty L III, ed. *Surgical techniques of the shoulder, elbow, and knee in sports medicine.* Philadelphia: Elsevier; 2008:517-526.

17. Sales de Gauzy J, Mansat C, Darodes PH, et al. Natural course of osteochondritis dissecans in children. *J Pediatr Orthop B.* 1999;8(1):26-28.

18. Morelli M, Poitras P, Grimes V, et al. Comparison of the stability of various internal fixators used in the treatment of osteochondritis dissecans—a mechanical model. *J Orthop Res.* 2007;25(4):495-500.

19. Anderson AF, Lipscomb AB, Coulam C. Antegrade curettement, bone grafting and pinning of osteochondritis dissecans in the skeletally mature knee. *Am J Sports Med.* 1990;18(3):254-261.

20. Cugat R, Garcia M, Cusco X, et al. Osteochondritis dissecans: a historical review and its treatment with cannulated screws. *Arthroscopy.* 1993;9(6):675-684.

21. Dervin GF, Keene GC, Chissell HR. Biodegradable rods in adult osteochondritis dissecans of the knee. *Clin Orthop Relat Res.* 1998;(356):213-221.

22. Gomoll AH, Flik KR, Hayden JK, et al. Internal fixation of the unstable Cahill Type-2C osteochondritis dissecans lesions of the knee in adolescent patients. *Orthopedics.* 2007;20(6):487-490.

23. Kivistö R, Pasanen L, Leppilahti J, et al. Arthroscopic repair of osteochondritis dissecans of the femoral condyles with metal staple fixation: a report of 28 cases. *Knee Surg Sports Traumatol Arthrosc.* 2002;10(5):305-309.

24. Larsen MW, Pietrzak WS, DeLee JC. Fixation of osteochondritis dissecans lesions using poly(L-lactic acid)/poly(glycolic acid) copolymer bioabsorbable screws. *Am J Sports Med.* 2005;33(1):68-76.

25. Makino A, Muscolo DL, Puigdevall M, et al. Arthroscopic fixation of osteochondritis dissecans of the knee: clinical, magnetic resonance imaging, and arthroscopic follow-up. *Am J Sports Med.* 2005;33(10):1499-1504.

26. Nakagawa T, Kurosawa H, Ikeda H, et al. Internal fixation for osteochondritis dissecans of the knee. *Knee Surg Sports Traumatol Arthrosc.* 2005;13(4):317-322.

27. Rey Zuniga JJ, Sagastibelza J, Lopez Blasco JJ, et al. Arthroscopic use of the Herbert screw in osteochondritis dissecans of the knee. *Arthroscopy.* 1993;9(6):668-670.

28. Thomson NL. Osteochondritis dissecans and osteochondral fragments managed by Herbert compression screw fixation. *Clin Orthop Relat Res.* 1987;(224):71-78.

29. Barfod G, Svendsen RN. Synovitis of the knee after intraarticular fracture fixation with Biofix. Report of two cases. *Acta Orthop Scand.* 1992;63(6):680-681.

30. Fridén T, Rydholm U. Severe aseptic synovitis of the knee after biodegradable internal fixation. A case report. *Acta Orthop Scand.* 1992;63(1):94-97.

31. Friederichs MG, Greis PE, Burks RT. Pitfalls associated with fixation of osteochondritis dissecans fragments using bioabsorbable screws. *Arthroscopy.* 2001;17(5):542-545.

32. Scioscia TN, Giffin JR, Allen CR, et al. Potential complication of bioabsorbable screw fixation for osteochondritis dissecans of the knee. *Arthroscopy.* 2001;17(2):E7.

33. Takizawa T, Akizuki S, Horiuchi H, et al. Foreign body gonitis caused by a broken poly-L-lactic acid screw. *Arthroscopy.* 1998;14(3):329-330.

34. Tegnander A, Engebretsen L, Bergh K, et al. Activation of the complement system and adverse effects of biodegradable pins of polylactic acid (Biofix) in osteochondritis dissecans. *Acta Orthop Scand.* 1994;65(4):472-475.

35. Mukherjee DP, Pietrzak WS. Bioabsorbable fixation: scientific, technical, and clinical concepts. *J Craniofac Surg.* 2011;22(2):679-689.

36. Tabaddor RR, Banffy MB, Andersen JS, et al. Fixation of juvenile osteochondritis dissecans lesions of the knee using poly 96L/4D-lactide copolymer bioabsorbable implants. *J Pediatr Orthop.* 2010;30(1):14-20.

Chapter 66

Osteonecrosis of the Knee

Michael B. Boyd, Simon Görtz, and William D. Bugbee

Chapter Synopsis

- Osteonecrosis (ON) of the knee is a challenging condition; its cause is unclear. ON of the knee can be broken down into two categories: primary or spontaneous ON and secondary ON. Nonsurgical treatment can be pursued for lower-grade lesions. Surgical treatment of ON of the knee includes arthroscopy, core decompression, osteochondral grafting, realignment procedures, and prosthetic arthroplasty. This chapter focuses on the presentations of and treatment options for ON of the knee.

Important Points

- Degenerative subchondral bone cysts (usually large, isolated defects about the medial femoral condyle) are commonly misdiagnosed as ON but are rather a variant presentation of early osteoarthritis.
- Defining the stage and lesion size (volume and surface area) are keys to sound application of our treatment algorithm.
- Subchondral fracture or collapse drastically alters prognosis and limits treatment options.

Clinical and Surgical Pearls

- For deep posterior femoral condyle lesions to be accessed, the meniscus may need to be detached and reflected, leaving a cuff of tissue for later repair.
- If mobilization of the patella is necessary, the fat pad can be released while the anterior horn of the opposite meniscus is protected.

Clinical and Surgical Pitfalls

- Concomitant distal femoral osteotomy and juxtaposed femoral condyle osteochondral allografting are not recommended; procedures should be staged to avoid nonunion of the allograft.
- Uncemented total knee arthroplasty (TKA) is not recommended in the treatment of ON.
- When performing TKA for multifocal ON, have stems available.

Osteonecrosis (ON) of the knee is a difficult clinical entity. Although the exact causes of ON are not well understood, there are several theories. However, the diagnosis of ON of the knee can be arduous, and its management remains challenging and controversial. In general, ON of the knee can be classified as (1) primary or spontaneous ON (also known as *Ahlbäck disease*) or (2) secondary ON, commonly associated with known risk factors. Spontaneous ON of the knee is usually unilateral and typically affects just a single femoral condyle. Secondary ON is often multifocal, bilateral, and/or polyarticular. This chapter focuses on the unique presentations of and various treatment options for ON of the knee.

Secondary ON can result from vascular insufficiency or occlusion, direct cell damage, or elevated intraosseous pressures. Radiofrequency or laser use can lead to postarthroscopic ON. In addition, the use of mechanical instruments can alter cartilaginous biomechanics, leading to postarthroscopic ON.

PREOPERATIVE CONSIDERATIONS

History

A thorough history may simplify the diagnosis of ON and help delineate an effective treatment algorithm. For spontaneous ON, antecedent (often minor) trauma should be elucidated. Likewise, the use of arthroscopic instrumentation, including radiofrequency wands, has been implicated in a separate entity recognized as post-arthroscopic ON. Risk factors for secondary ON should be sought, the most common being corticosteroid use, alcohol abuse, and systemic lupus erythematosus, with multiple risk factors potentiating the odds for the development of the disease.

A common error is to misdiagnose degenerative subchondral bone cysts commonly seen in osteoarthritis as spontaneous ON of the knee, which typically affects obese female patients over the age of 55 years. Postarthroscopic ON most often involves the femoral condyles and rarely affects the plateaus and patella. In secondary ON, screening additional joints might be of benefit, even in the absence of current symptoms.

Signs and Symptoms

Spontaneous Osteonecrosis

- Sudden pain usually over the medial aspect of knee (may be initiated by a minor injury or arthroscopy)
- Increased pain at night and with activity (postarthroscopic ON: pain localized to compartment where surgery was performed)

Secondary Osteonecrosis

- Long-standing insidious pain (although some patients may be asymptomatic)
- Diffuse pain that may be difficult to localize

Physical Examination

- Range of motion: may be decreased secondary to pain, muscle spasm, or subchondral collapse
- Swelling, effusion; may or may not be present
- Ligaments: usually stable

Spontaneous Osteonecrosis

- High sensitivity to touch over osteochondral lesion lesion(s) (usually involving the medial femoral condyle)

Secondary Osteonecrosis

- Nonspecific knee pain (especially with multiple lesions); contralateral knee should be scrutinized

Imaging

Radiography

- Weight-bearing anteroposterior (AP) radiograph of knee in full extension with a radiopaque magnification marker (Fig. 66-1A)

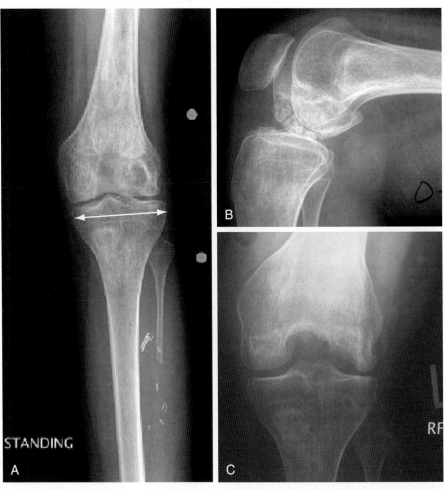

Figure 66-1. A, Anteroposterior standing radiograph of a knee with a radiopaque magnification marker (*arrow* demonstrates the tibial width dimension used for allograft sizing). **B,** Non–weight-bearing 90-degree-flexion lateral view of a knee demonstrating secondary osteonecrosis. **C,** Notch view of a knee depicting secondary osteonecrosis.

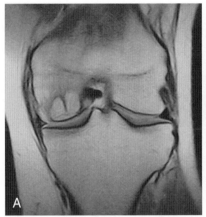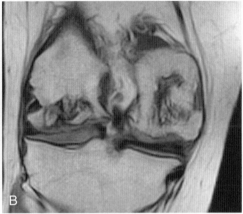

Figure 66-2. A, Magnetic resonance imaging (MRI) scan of a knee exhibiting spontaneous osteonecrosis. **B,** MRI scan of a knee demonstrating secondary osteonecrosis.

- Non–weight-bearing 90-degree-flexion lateral view of knee (Fig. 66-1B)
- Notch (Fig. 66-1C) or Rosenberg view of knee

Optional

- Merchant view of patellofemoral joint
- Long-leg AP mechanical axis view to evaluate for axial malalignment

Other Modalities

- Magnetic resonance imaging (MRI) can help to confirm the diagnosis and the extent of lesion(s) (Fig. 66-2).
- Technetium-99m bone scanning is generally unreliable but may assist in diagnosis when radiographs are negative. Bipolar uptake is more indicative of osteoarthritis, except in the *late* stages of ON. Conversely, simultaneous atraumatic ON of the ipsilateral tibial plateau and femoral condyle is certainly possible during *any* stage and usually causes more intense uptake than osteoarthritis.

Staging

The Aglietti classification for spontaneous ON of the knee (modified Koshino) and the Mont and Hungerford classification for secondary ON of the knee (modified Ficat and Arlet) are described in Boxes 66-1 and 66-2.

Treatment

Nonoperative Treatment (Only in Low-Grade, Low-Symptom, Precollapse Lesions)

- Nonsteroidal antiinflammatory drugs (NSAIDs), if tolerated
- Analgesics
- Pharmacologic treatment based on underlying disease process

---

BOX 66-1 Aglietti Classification for Spontaneous Osteonecrosis of the Knee (Modified Koshino Classification)

Stage I: Normal radiographs, magnetic resonance imaging scans

Stage II: Some flattening of the weight-bearing portion of the condyle

Stage III: Subchondral radiolucency with surrounding sclerosis without sequestration

Stage IV: Increased sclerosis with subchondral collapse and sequestration; visible as a calcium plate

Stage V: Secondary degenerative changes (narrowing of joint space, osteophyte formation, subchondral sclerosis) associated with some erosions

---

BOX 66-2 Mont and Hungerford Classification for Secondary Osteonecrosis of the Knee (Modified Ficat and Arlet Classification)

Stage I: Normal radiographs, magnetic resonance imaging scans

Stage II: Cysts and sclerosis present

Stage III: Subchondral collapse is crescent sign

Stage IV: Secondary degenerative changes (narrowing of joint space, osteophyte formation) on both sides of joint

---

- Activity modifications and protective weight bearing
- Closed-chain quadriceps exercises
- Unloader knee brace

Operative Treatment

- Arthroscopy with or without debridement
- Core decompression by extra-articular drilling with or without bone grafting
- Osteochondral allografting (OCA) for large lesions versus osteochondral autografting (osteochondral autograft transfer [OAT]) for small lesions

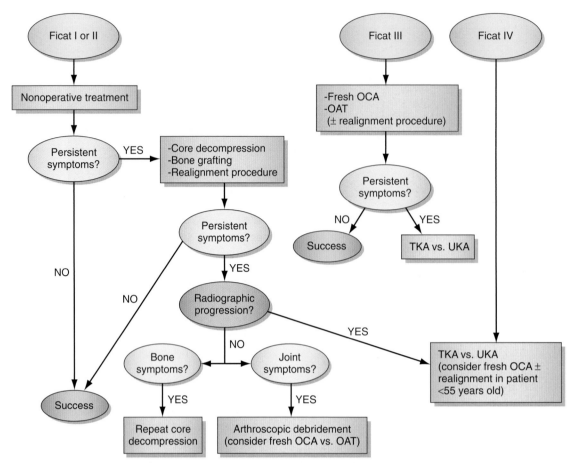

Figure 66-3. Treatment algorithm for osteonecrosis of the knee (modified Mont algorithm). *OCA,* Osteochondral allografting; *OAT,* osteochondral autograft transfer; *TKA,* total knee arthroplasty; *UKA,* unicompartmental knee arthroplasty.

- Realignment procedure—high tibial osteotomy (HTO) for genu varum versus distal femoral osteotomy (DFO) for genu valgum
- Unicompartmental knee arthroplasty (UKA) versus total knee arthroplasty (TKA)

Because of the heterogeneous nature of ON of the knee both in cause and stage, no single technique is always preferred. Treatment should be individualized. Core decompression and use of allograft with or without realignment are our preferred treatments for the younger patient population and are further discussed in this chapter. Our general treatment algorithm (Fig. 66-3) is included.

Core Decompression—Brief Description

Extra-articular drilling is recommended in the treatment of symptomatic ON of the knee in presubchondral collapse stages. Core decompression can be done in conjunction with knee arthroscopy. A small incision is made just proximal to the metaphyseal flare for femoral lesions and just medial to the tubercle for tibial lesions. With fluoroscopic guidance, a 3- to 6-mm trephine

is advanced to within 3 mm of the subchondral bone. The surgeon may elect to lightly pack autologous iliac crest bone graft inside the lesion. Postoperatively, the patient is restricted to 50% partial weight bearing for 4 to 6 weeks.

Fresh Osteochondral Allografting for Osteonecrosis of the Knee

Indications and Contraindications

Fresh OCA may be considered a biologic alternative to arthroplasty in young (younger than 50 years) individuals with ON of the knee. OCA is particularly attractive for this indication, because the allograft procedure can address the osseous and chondral components of juxta-articular necrotic lesions by replacing them with orthotopic tissue to restore joint homeostasis. Typically the lesions should be more than 2 cm (approximately) in diameter. OAT is an acceptable alternative for smaller lesions with compromised articular cartilage.

Relative contraindications to fresh OCA include uncorrected limb malalignment and joint instability. The senior author (W.D.B.) has not found steroid dependency to be a contraindication to fresh OCA, as previously reported in the literature. Allograft use should not be considered an alternative to TKA or UKA in a patient with symptoms, age, and activity level appropriate for prosthetic replacement. Finally, fresh OCA should not be performed in the individual with advanced multicompartmental knee arthrosis.

Surgical Planning

Concomitant Procedures

Significant limb malalignment, ligamentous instability, or meniscal deficiency can be addressed either before or in combination with fresh osteochondral allograft transplantation. Concomitant DFO and use of femoral condyle osteochondral allograft is not recommended owing to the increased risk of nonunion of the juxtaposed allograft. Rather, the procedures should be staged to avoid this potential complication.

Allograft Sizing

A measurement of the width of the tibial diaphysis, a few millimeters inferior and parallel to the plateau, is made via a standing AP knee radiograph with a radiopaque sizing marker (see Fig. 66-1A). After correction for magnification, the measurements are communicated to the tissue bank for a matched donor.

SURGICAL TECHNIQUE— FRESH OSTEOCHONDRAL ALLOGRAFTING

Anesthesia and Positioning

Anesthesia

- General
- Epidural
- Spinal
- With or without regional

Positioning

- Supine on a standard operating room table
- Padded thigh tourniquet
- Leg holder to position knee in 70 to 100 degrees of flexion to access the lesion

Surgical Landmarks, Incisions, and Portals

Useful Surgical Landmarks

- Patella
- Patellar tendon
- Joint line
- Tibial tubercle

Approaches

- Midline incision with medial or lateral parapatellar mini-arthrotomy
- Standard medial parapatellar arthrotomy for bicondylar lesions

Structures at Risk

- Anterior horn of medial or lateral meniscus, patellar tendon

Examination Under Anesthesia and Diagnostic Arthroscopy

Examine the knee range of motion and stability under anesthesia. Perform diagnostic arthroscopy before the allograft procedure if questions regarding the meniscus and/or articular cartilage persist.

Specific Steps

See Box 66-3 for specific steps of this procedure.

1. Exposure

A standard midline incision is made from approximately the center of the patella to the tip of the tibial tubercle (Fig. 66-4). A medial or lateral parapatellar arthrotomy is then made extending from the superomedial or superolateral aspect of the patella down to the distal end of

BOX 66-3 Surgical Steps
1. Exposure
2. Recipient site preparation
3. Fresh osteochondral allograft preparation
4. Graft insertion and fixation
5. Closure

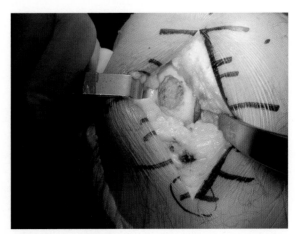

Figure 66-4. Standard midline incision and medial parapatellar approach.

the incision. The incision can be extended for bicondylar lesions. Care is taken to preserve the anterior horn of the meniscus after incision through the infrapatellar fat pad. For access to deep posterior femoral condyle lesions, the meniscus may need to be detached anteriorly and reflected out of the arthrotomy, leaving a cuff of tissue for later repair. Retractors are placed medially and laterally to better expose the condyle. One of these retractors is carefully placed in the notch, retracting the patella and protecting the cruciate ligaments. The knee is then flexed to the appropriate level to visually deliver the lesion to the arthrotomy. If additional mobilization of the patella is necessary, the fat pad can be released further, staying anterior to the anterior horn of the opposite meniscus.

2. Recipient Site Preparation

Two techniques are used for OCA: the dowel and the shell techniques. When possible, use of a dowel or plug (generally 20 mm or larger) is the preferred technique because the instrumentation facilitates the procedure (Fig. 66-5). This is the typical scenario for spontaneous ON of the knee. Often, however, the disease is too extensive for a dowel or multiple dowels, and a free-hand shell technique is performed (typical for secondary ON lesions).

With the dowel technique, the lesion is inspected and probed to assess its margins. A guidewire is then drilled perpendicular to the curvature of the articular surface into the center of the lesion. The graft is sized with cannulated dowels. A cannulated cutting reamer is used to penetrate and score the surrounding articular cartilage. Next, removal of 3 to 4 mm of subchondral bone is performed with the appropriately sized cannulated core reamer. We recommend transplanting as little allograft bone as possible and as much as necessary to ease implantation, minimize bioburden, and optimize incorporation. If indicated, further necrotic bone can be reamed down to bleeding margins, not to exceed 6 to 10 mm. Deeper lesions can be curetted by hand and packed with autologous bone graft as appropriate. The guidewire is then removed (Fig. 66-6). The depth of the lesion is measured in four quadrants (Fig. 66-7). If necessary, multiple small drill holes can be made in the cancellous bone to decompress the lesion. At times, a second graft is necessary to cover the entire lesion. In this situation the dowel technique is repeated as described earlier, overlapping the grafts (Fig. 66-8) and making sure to secure the primary graft to avoid spin out.

Alternatively, the entire condyle might be involved, rendering it difficult to graft with simple dowels (Fig. 66-9A). In this situation the recipient site is prepared with a free-hand technique with a motorized oscillating saw, osteotomes, and/or burs. The goal is to produce a simple, reproducible geometric pattern (Fig. 66-9B). This often incorporates the entire hemicondyle. The dimensions and position of the prepared site are measured and transferred to the allograft.

3. Fresh Osteochondral Allograft Preparation

With the dowel technique, the matching anatomic location on the donor graft is identified. The graft is held

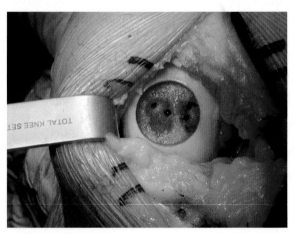

Figure 66-6. Dowel technique. Lesion reamed down to bleeding bone.

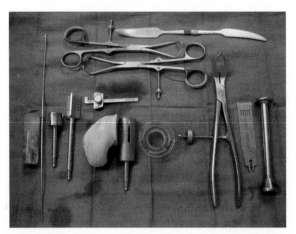

Figure 66-5. Dowel technique instrumentation and fresh hemicondylar femoral allograft.

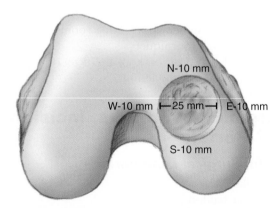

Figure 66-7. Depth measurements of a dowel in four quadrants (N, S, E, and W).

securely with two large tenaculum bone clamps. A saw guide is placed perpendicular to the articular surface. The appropriately sized tube saw is placed over the guide and is used to core the graft (Fig. 66-10) under constant irrigation. The graft is then amputated from the condyle with a perpendicular cut at its base from an oscillating saw. The previously measured recipient site depths are marked at the four corresponding quadrants of the graft. The graft is placed in bone-holding forceps, exposing the subchondral bone, and the oscillating saw is used to make the final cut at the marks. Fine adjustments can be made with a bone rasp, and the edges can be chamfered to ease implantation. To reduce

the immunogenicity of the graft, it is then copiously irrigated with bacitracin solution with the pulsatile lavage system to remove any remaining bone marrow elements (Fig. 66-11).

With the shell technique the cuts are made freehand, creating a geometric match of the recipient site (Fig. 66-12). Repeat trial fittings are performed. The graft is modified accordingly until the articular geometry is restored. The graft is otherwise treated as described earlier.

4. Graft Insertion and Fixation

With the appropriate orientation, the allograft dowel is manually inserted and seated with thumb pressure, or gently tapped in place until flush. If necessary, the recipient site can be expanded with an oversized dilator. Fine adjustments to the allograft are made; a Freer or dental pick is used to remove a seated graft. Typically an excellent press-fit is noted on circumferentially contained grafts (Fig. 66-13); however, the graft can be secured further with bioabsorbable pins. With a shell graft, fixation is obtained with a combination of bioabsorbable pins and small titanium screws. The knee is then put through a range of motion to assess for graft stability and for possible impingement, especially at the notch.

5. Closure

Standard layered closure of the arthrotomy is performed over a ⅛-inch drain.

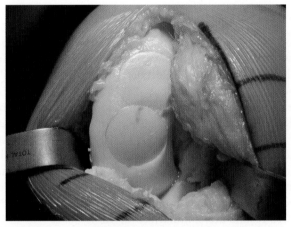
Figure 66-8. Overlapping dowel technique.

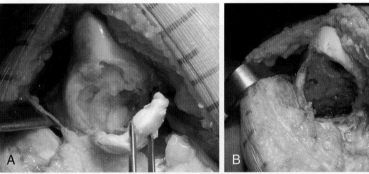
Figure 66-9. A, Severe secondary osteonecrosis lesion affecting the lateral femoral hemicondyle, necessitating a shell technique. **B,** Lesion after debridement into simple geometric configuration.

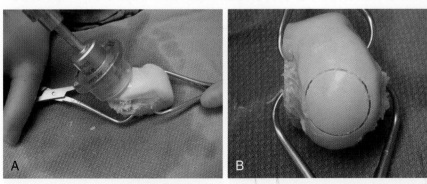
Figure 66-10. A, Preparation of dowel allograft with a reamer. **B,** View of dowel allograft before removal from condyle.

POSTOPERATIVE CONSIDERATIONS

Hospital Course

- Hospital admission for 23 to 48 hours
- Intravenous antibiotics for 24 hours
- Drain removed on postoperative day 1

Rehabilitation

- Immediate touch-down weight-bearing with unlimited range of motion and quadriceps strengthening for 6 to 12 weeks

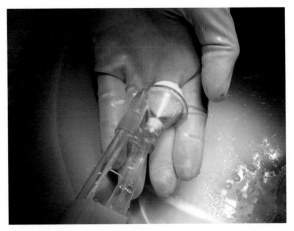

Figure 66-11. The allograft is washed thoroughly with a jet-lavage system to remove bone marrow elements.

- Stationary bicycle at 4 weeks
- With meniscal detachment and repair and large posterior grafts, flexion is limited to 60 degrees for 4 to 6 weeks
- Progressive weight-bearing beginning at 8 to 12 weeks
- Sports and recreation at 6 months

Complications

- Delayed union or nonunion of the allograft
- Infection
- Arthrofibrosis

RESULTS

Core decompression can be an effective way to treat low-grade ON of the knee, before the development of subchondral collapse. Recent data have shown 76% good to excellent clinical results for fresh OCA in steroid-induced ON of the knee in the young patient. UKA has been shown to be successful for the treatment of end-stage spontaneous ON of the knee. TKA is an excellent treatment for all end-stage osteonecroses. The use of cemented stems during TKA improves the long-term results in patients with multifocal ON. Uncemented TKA is no longer recommended in the treatment of ON. These results are summarized in Table 66-1.

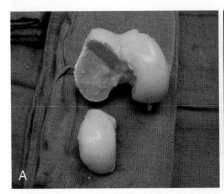
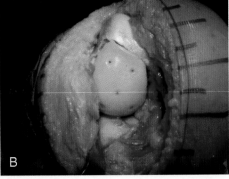

Figure 66-12. A, Example of shell allograft. **B,** Shell allograft implanted in lesion seen in Figure 66-9.

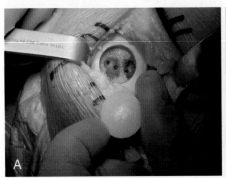
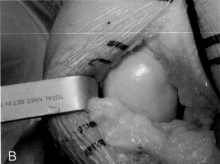

Figure 66-13. A, Example of dowel graft adjacent to recipient site. **B,** Excellent press-fit of dowel graft.

TABLE 66-1. Clinical Results of Various Options for Treatment of Osteonecrosis

Procedure	Type	Author	Mean Follow-up	Miscellaneous Notes	Outcome
Nonoperative treatment	Secondary	Mont et al[1] (1997)	11 years	Mean asymptomatic period—11 months; all but 6 required TKA by 6 years	26 of 32 (81%) unsuccessful
Core decompression	Secondary	Jacobs et al[2] (1989)	4.5 years	16 of 18 patients with steroid-induced ON lesions	7 of 7 (100%) stage I or II successful; 11 of 21 (52%) stage III successful
Core decompression	Spontaneous	Forst et al[3] (1998)	3 years	No late stages	16 of 16 (100%) successful
Core decompression	Secondary	Mont et al[4] (2000)	7 years	No late stages; 15 successfully treated knees needed repeat surgery	72 of 91 (79%) successful
Core decompression	Secondary	Marulanda et al[5] (2006)	3 years	Small-diameter, early stage lesions	56 of 61 (92%) successful
High tibial osteotomy	Spontaneous	Koshino[6] (1982)	5.1 years	23 knees with concomitant core decompression or bone grafting	35 of 37 (95%) successful
High tibial osteotomy	Spontaneous	Takeuchi[7] (2009)	3.3 years	30 knees with concomitant chondral debridement and bone substitute	Mean KSS improved from 51 to 93
UKA, TKA	Spontaneous	Aglietti[8] (1983)	4.4 years	35 TKA, 2 UKA—all stages included	35 of 37 (95%) successful
UKA	Spontaneous	Marmor[9] (1993)	5.5 years	2 of 4 failures from subsequent ON of opposite femoral condyle	30 of 34 (88%) successful
UKA	Spontaneous	Myers et al[10] (2006)	5 years	Part of meta-analysis, 64 patients	90% good to excellent clinical results, 87% survivorship
TKA	Spontaneous, secondary	Bergman and Rand[11] (1991)	4 years	Only a 68% 5-year predicted implant survivorship with use of revision because of use of pain as endpoint	33 of 38 (87%) successful
TKA	Secondary	Seldes et al[12] (1999)	5.3 years	5 patients required revision (3—aseptic loosening; 2—sepsis)	26 of 31 (84%) successful
TKA	Spontaneous, secondary	Mont et al[13] (2002)	9 years	Improved results attributed to use of cement in all patients and stems as warranted	31 of 32 (97%) successful
TKA	Spontaneous	Myers et al[10] (2006)	4 years	Part of meta-analysis, 148 patients	92% good to excellent clinical results, 97% survivorship
TKA	Secondary	Myers et al[10] (2006)	8 years	Part of meta-analysis, 150 patients	74% good to excellent clinical results, 80% survivorship
Fresh OCA, Debridement, HTO, CD	Spontaneous, secondary	Bayne et al[14] (1985)	4.8 years	Failure after 18 months in 3 of 3 patients with steroid-induced ON treated only with fresh OCA	6 of 13 (46%) SONK successful; 4 of 7 (57%) AONK successful
Fresh-Frozen OCA	Spontaneous, secondary	Flynn et al[15] (1994)	4.2 years	Young patient group, 2 patients with steroid-induced ON converted to TKA	12 of 17 (71%) successful
Fresh OCA	Secondary	Görtz et al[16] (2010)	5.6 years	Young patient group with large steroid-induced ON lesions	19 of 25 (76%) good to excellent results; 25 of 28 (89%) graft survival

AONK, secondary (acquired) osteonecrosis of the knee; *CD,* core decompression; *HTO,* high tibial osteotomy; *KSS,* Knee Society Score; *OCA,* osteochondral allografting; *ON,* osteonecrosis; *SONK,* spontaneous osteonecrosis of the knee; *TKA,* total knee arthroplasty; *UKA,* unicompartmental knee arthroplasty.

REFERENCES

1. Mont MA, Tomek IM, Hungerford DS. Core decompression for avascular necrosis of the distal femur—long term followup. *Clin Orthop Relat Res.* 1997;334:124-130.
2. Jacobs MA, Loeb PE, Hungerford DS. Core decompression of the distal femur for avascular necrosis of the knee. *J Bone Joint Surg Br.* 1989;71(4):583-587.
3. Forst J, Forst R, Heller KD, et al. Spontaneous ostenecrosis of the femoral condyle: casual treatment by early core decompression. *Arch Orthop Trauma Surg.* 1998;117:18-22.
4. Mont MA, Baumgarten KM, Rifai A, et al. Atraumatic ostenecrosis of the knee. *J Bone Joint Surg Am.* 2000;82:1279-1290.
5. Marulanda G, Seyler TM, Sheikh NH, et al. Percutaneous drilling for the treatment of secondary osteonecrosis of the knee. *J Bone Joint Surg Br.* 2006;88(6):740-746.
6. Koshino T. The treatment of spontaneous osteonecrosis of the knee by high tibial osteotomy with and without bone-grafting or drilling of the lesion. *J Bone Joint Surg Am.* 1982;64:47-58.
7. Takeuchi R, Aratake M, Bito H, et al. Clinical results and radiographical evaluation of opening wedge high tibial osteotomy for spontaneous osteonecrosis of the knee. *Knee Surg Sports Traumatol Arthrosc.* 2009;17(4):361-368.
8. Aglietti P, Insall JN, Buzzi R. Idiopathic osteonecrosis of the knee. Aetiology, prognosis and treatment. *J Bone Joint Surg Br.* 1983;65(5):588-597.
9. Marmor L. Unicompartmental arthroplasty for osteonecrosis of the knee joint. *Clin Orthop Relat Res.* 1993;294:247-253.
10. Myers TG, Cui Q, Kuskowski M, et al. Outcomes of total and unicompartmental knee arthroplasty for secondary and spontaneous osteonecrosis of the knee. *J Bone Joint Surg Am.* 2006;88(suppl 3):76-82.
11. Bergman NR, Rand JA. Total knee arthroplasty in osteonecrosis. *Clin Orthop Relat Res* 1991;273:77-82.
12. Seldes RM, Tan V, Duffy G, et al. Total knee arthroplasty for steroid-induced osteonecrosis. *J Arthroplasty.* 1999;14(5):533-537.
13. Mont MA, Rifai A, Baumgarten KM, et al. Total knee arthroplasty for osteonecrosis. *J Bone Joint Surg Am.* 2002;84:599-603.
14. Bayne O, Langer F, Pritzker KP, et al. Osteochondral allografts in the treatment of osteonecrosis of the knee. *Orthop Clin North Am.* 1985;16:727-740.
15. Flynn JM, Springfield DS, Mankin HJ. Osteoarticular allografts to treat distal femoral osteonecrosis. *Clin Orthop Relat Res.* 1994;303:38-43.
16. Görtz S, De Young A, Bugbee W. Fresh osteochondral allografting for steroid-associated osteonecrosis of the femoral condyles. *Clin Orthop Relat Res.* 2010;468:1269-1278.

Chapter 67

Osteochondral Autograft for Cartilage Lesions of the Knee

Kenneth G. Swan Jr, R. David Rabalais, and Eric McCarty

Chapter Synopsis
- Osteochondral autograft transplant surgery (OATS) remains an important technique for medium (1 to 3 cm^2) chondral defects. When appropriate indications are met, very good success rates can be expected. Meticulous technique for single-plug or multiple-plug ("mosaicplasty") transplant surgery is imperative to achieve a congruent articulation.

Important Points
- Physical examination findings are often unimpressive. Operative decision making is based more on history, radiographs or magnetic resonance imaging scans, and initial arthroscopic findings.
- Inappropriate indications or overlooking contraindications may lead to early autograft failure.
- *Indications:* Isolated small to medium (1 to 3 cm^2) full thickness chondral lesions
- *Contraindications:* Generalized or inflammatory arthritis, uncorrected malalignment, uncorrected knee instability
- Technique can be performed arthroscopically or via open technique. Larger defects that require multiple plugs are best performed via open technique.

Clinical and Surgical Pearls
Preoperatively
- Thoroughly evaluate need for malalignment correction or ligament stabilization before OATS.

- Ensure patient can comply with prolonged non–weight-bearing status postoperatively.

Intraoperatively
- Make sure graft harvest, recipient site coring, and graft implantation are performed with a trajectory perpendicular to the articular surface.

Postoperatively
- Monitor patient for painful hemarthrosis that may limit range of motion (ROM).
- Aspiration may be required.

Clinical and Surgical Pitfalls
- Postoperative hemarthrosis may occur secondary to donor site defect. Backfilling the donor site with bone and cartilage cored from recipient site may help healing and prevent hemarthrosis.
- Drains are placed intraoperatively and may be removed in the recovery room or the next day.
- If hemarthrosis develops, aspiration may be required in the office on follow-up to alleviate pain and maximize early ROM.

Defects of articular cartilage are a relatively common problem encountered by the sports medicine physician. Isolated cartilage defects can occur secondary to acute trauma or can be atraumatic in nature. The latter often occur in the form of osteochondritis dissecans, the cause of which is not fully understood, and can be found in juveniles and in adults. The distinction is important, because patients with open physes have a much better prognosis with nonoperative treatment.[1]

Patients with symptomatic focal cartilage defects are candidates for operative treatment to relieve symptoms and also to potentially prevent subsequent arthritic changes.[2] Surgical treatment options include arthroscopic debridement, microfracture, autologous chondrocyte implantation (ACI), matrix-induced chondrocyte transplantation, osteochondral autograft transplant surgery (OATS), and osteochondral allograft transplantation. OATS may be the best option in appropriately selected patients. There are several different transplant systems available, but the concept remains the same: the transplantation of full-thickness osteochondral bone plugs from an area of the knee that is non–weight-bearing or has low contact pressures to the osteochondral defect of the ipsilateral knee.

PREOPERATIVE CONSIDERATIONS

History

Patients with focal osteochondral lesions typically have pain and swelling that is intermittent in nature. The history may mimic that of mensical pathology.

Typical History
- Patient age—varies from adolescence to middle age
- Intermittent pain
- Pain elicited by low- or high-impact activities (tibiofemoral disease) or stair climbing and prolonged sitting (patellofemoral disease)
- Recurrent swelling
- Frequently a history of acute or distant trauma, including patellar dislocation
- Mechanical symptoms common
- Symptoms referable to an associated loose body

Physical Examination

Typical Physical Examination Findings
- Effusion
- Relatively preserved range of motion (ROM)
- Possible joint line tenderness
- Possible patellar instability, apprehension

Physical examination findings may be unimpressive; patient history and radiographs or magnetic resonance imaging (MRI) scans are often more telling.

Physical Factors Affecting Surgical Planning
- Limb malalignment (may compromise repair, require realignment procedure)
- Concomitant ligamentous injury (may require prior or concomitant reconstruction)

Imaging

Radiography
- Standard anteroposterior (AP) and lateral knee views.
- Sunrise patellofemoral view to visualize patellar and trochlear lesions.

- Notch view may be best to visualize lateral aspect of medial femoral condyle (typical location of osteochondral defects [OCDs]).[3]
- A mechanical axis view is obtained if malaligment is suspected.

Additional Imaging
- MRI is necessary to best evaluate location and size of articular cartilage lesions. MRI is also important for evaluation of menisci, ligaments, and remainder of articular cartilage.
- Bone scans, computed tomography, and tomograms are not as useful as MRI for evaluation of OCDs and the remainder of the knee.
- Contrast arthrography (intra-articular or intravenous) may prove to be more sensitive than MRI alone, which can have a high false-negative rate.[4]
- Arthroscopy remains the gold standard for evaluation of articular cartilage lesions.

Indications

The indications for OATS are narrow. The patient generally has a small, isolated lesion in an otherwise healthy knee. However, concomitant ligament, meniscus, or alignment pathology may be present and can be addressed simultaneously or with a staged procedure.

Typically during concomitant procedures the surgeon performs autologous osteochondral grafting and anterior cruciate ligament (ACL) reconstruction or hightibial osteotomy. During ACL reconstruction the osteochondral grafting should proceed after meniscal or other cartilage pathology has been addressed and notchplasty has been performed, but before ACL graft fixation. This is to avoid damage to the newly implanted osteochondral plugs. Osteotomy is typically performed after the OATS procedure.

We prefer to perform single-plug autograft transplants on defects 1 cm^2 in diameter or smaller, with allograft transplants used for larger defects. However, some authors perform autograft transplants on defects as large as 4 cm^2, with good results[5] with use of multiple plugs of varying size (aka "mosaicplasty").

Contraindications
- Generalized arthritis
- Inflammatory arthritis
- Lesions smaller than 1 cm^2 for single plugs
- Lesion larger than 3 cm^2 for multiple plugs
- Uncorrected malalignment or knee instability

Surgical Planning

Osteochondral defects are frequently diagnosed in the office after history and physical examination and interpretation of radiographs and MRI scans. The patient and surgeon might then plan for single-stage surgery with arthroscopic examination of the knee to assess the defect. If applicable, an autograft transplant with single or multiple plugs can be performed. The number and size of osteochondral plugs required cannot be determined until the defect has been thoroughly examined via arthroscopy. Defects that are discovered to be excessively large may require allograft transplant, which must be anticipated and planned for. Typically this is performed as a second procedure.

At times, OCDs are not appreciated preoperatively and are discovered during routine knee arthroscopy. The morbidity of the procedure and its rehabilitation process is quite different from that of a standard knee arthroscopy. These patients usually require a second procedure for definitive treatment at a later date unless the surgeon and patient have discussed this possibility preoperatively.

Surgical Steps

See Box 67-1 for a summary of the surgical steps.

Expanded Surgical Technique

Three different systems are commercially available in the United States. All three are very similar and differ in the available graft sizes and minor variations of technique. A comparison is shown in Table 67-1. An example of the necessary equipment is shown in Figure 67-1.

Positioning

The patient is positioned supine with a lateral post, and a sandbag is taped to the bed to facilitate fixed 90-degree flexion of the knee. The surgeon should be able to flex the knee to 120 degrees with ease. A sliding footstep may be used to allow different angles of knee flexion. Alternatively, an arthroscopic leg holder may be used per surgeon preference. We typically do not drop the foot of the bed. A tourniquet is applied but not elevated, and the operative site is prepared and draped. The

---

BOX 67-1 Surgical Steps for Osteochondral Autograft Transfer

1. Diagnostic arthroscopy to debride and measure defect. Plan number, size and placement of specific grafts. Remainder of procedure can be performed as mini-open if desired.
2. Place donor harvester perpendicular to donor site and tamp harvester to required depth. View measurement on outside of harvester.
3. Disengage graft from local bed. Method of disengaging the graft varies with system.
4. Remove graft donor assembly from knee with autograft plug and measure depth of plug.
5. Tamp recipient harvester into defect to desired depth (1 to 2 mm deeper than plug). Keep recipient harvesting tools perpendicular to articular surface.
6. Insert graft under direct visualization through optional clear tube. Be careful to keep tube on articular surface during implantation.
7. Remove clear tube and gently seat graft with plastic tamp until graft is flush with articular surface.

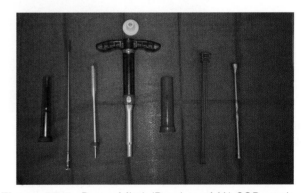

Figure 67-1. Depuy Mitek (Raynham, MA) COR repair system.

TABLE 67-1. Specific Aspects of the Three Different Commercially Available Osteochondral Autograft Systems

System	Graft Sizes (Diameter)	Specific Technical Differences	Comments
Single-use osteochondral autograft transplant surgery (OATS; Osteochondral Autograft Transfer System [Arthrex, Naples, FL])	6-, 8-, 10-mm plugs	Disengaging graft from bed requires 90-degree rotation from starting position	Must lever graft from donor bed
COR repair system (Depuy Mitek, Norwood, MA)	4-, 6-, 8-mm plugs	Disengaging donor grafts from bed requires two complete turns with T-handle	Toothed harvester allows undercutting of donor graft from donor bed
Mosaicplasty systems (Smith & Nephew, Andover, MA)	2.7-, 3.5-, 4.5-, 6.5-, 8.5-mm plugs	Toggle graft to remove from donor bed	Dilator used in recipient site to compact surrounding bone; smaller grafts available

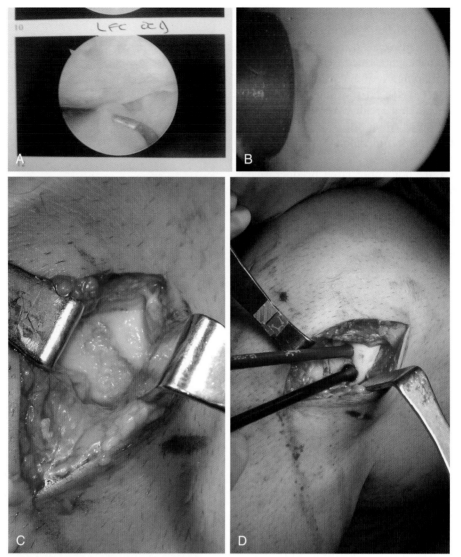

Figure 67-2. A, Femoral condyle defect, arthroscopic view. **B,** The 8-mm defect sizer. **C,** Large condylar defect viewed from mini-open approach. **D,** Open sizing and templating for mosaicplasty.

tourniquet may be inflated if arthroscopic visualization becomes difficult because of intra-articular bleeding.

Arthroscopy

The surgeon performs diagnostic arthroscopy of the knee. Portal sites can be varied to maximize perpendicular access to the donor and recipient sites. This can be performed with spinal needles before the portals are made. A central patellar tendon portal can provide good access to the medial surfaces of the medial and lateral femoral condyles.[6] The defect site is identified, and loose debris, cartilage flaps, and superficial fibrocartilage are removed with a mechanized resector. A thorough evaluation of the patellofemoral joint should be performed with consideration for donor site grafting ramifications. The knee should be carefully inspected for loose bodies, with examination of the lateral and medial gutters and posterior medial and lateral recesses.[7] Examination of

the condyles in full flexion should be performed to identify any other defects of the weight-bearing surface. The defect is measured with measurement probes or size-specific cannulas that vary with the particular system (Fig. 67-2). The surgeon at this time should evaluate the curvature of the surrounding articular cartilage and plan the number and size of grafts to be used. We routinely use an all-arthroscopic technique, but, depending on defect size and surgeon preference, a mini-arthrotomy (2 to 3 cm) may be used for both harvest and implantation. We routinely do not inflate the tourniquet throughout the procedure.

Graft Harvesting

Available donor sites include the lateral femoral condyle above the sulcus terminalis, the peripheral aspect of the medial femoral condyle, and the lateral and superior aspect of the intercondylar notch. The medial aspect of the medial femoral condyle can be easier to access during graft harvest because the intra-articular distention can push the patella laterally.[6] Contact pressures may be lower in donor sites from the distal medial trochlea.[5,8] The central condylar notch is routinely removed during notchplasty and roofplasty during ACL reconstruction, but the curvature is generally concave and has poorer congruity with typical recipient sites on the lateral and medial femoral condyles.[9] We routinely use the superior medial aspect of the medial femoral condyle as a donor site. The largest size amenable to single-plug harvest is 1 cm^2 in diameter, as discussed earlier. Multiple plugs should be harvested for defect sizes of 1 to 3 cm^2 in diameter. We harvest multiple plugs from the same side of the knee as the defect to be filled (medial-medial, lateral-lateral). The knee is ranged from extension to flexion to allow the mini-arthrotomy to accommodate either the donor or the recipient site.

Each system has a T-handle–type system that must be assembled at the back table and varies with the graft diameter that is to be used. This donor harvester is then inserted into the knee perpendicular to the articular surface and held firmly against the cartilage during the extraction. Holding the donor harvester firmly against the surface ensures that a cylindric (not crooked) graft is harvested and helps prevent loss of the graft in the joint during extraction. The donor harvester is impacted with a mallet to the desired depth of penetration, usually 15 mm. The different systems then recommend different techniques to extract the graft from the surrounding bed. The Osteochondral Autograft Transfer System uses a 90-degree rotation both clockwise and counterclockwise from the starting position. The COR system has a "tooth" at the distal aspect of the harvester. When the desired depth has been achieved, the T-handle is rotated two full revolutions to undercut the graft, minimizing leverage against the native bone. The Mosaicplasty system recommends "gentle toggling" to break the deep subchondral bone before graft removal (Fig. 67-3).

Measure the graft length after removal to plan defect drilling. This is performed either through referenced lines on the exterior of a clear sheath holding the graft or by placement of the graft on the back table in a moist sponge, depending on system used. Reinsertion of the plunger into the donor site defect can also assist with measurement of depth.

Recipient Site Preparation

At this point the surgeon should have a clear plan for number of grafts, placement of specific graft plugs, and depth of each plug. The knee can now be further flexed if needed to ensure a perpendicular drilling of the defect. The diameter of the reamer used should correspond to the diameter of the graft taken. The appropriately sized reamer can now be used to drill the recipient hole. Each recipient hole should be separated from adjacent holes

with at least a 1- to 2-mm bridge. The depth of each recipient hole should be 1 to 2 mm deeper than the measured plug. This reduces resultant force during impaction[10] and can minimize intraosseous pressure, although some systems recommend more of a "line-to-line" fit. The Mosaicplasty system recommends dilation of the recipient hole before insertion. All loose cartilage and bone fragments can be safely removed with a small curette (Fig. 67-4).

Graft Implantation

At this time the graft should be in the delivery tube. The delivery tube is seated perpendicular to the reamed hole of matching size and held firmly against the surface. Graft implantation is achieved with gentle tapping of the impactor (plunger) with a mallet. The use of excessive force and large blows should be avoided.[10] Once the graft is almost fully seated and stable in the hole, the delivery tube is removed (Fig. 67-5). Care should be taken not to shear off the cartilage cap of the graft during removal of the insertion tube.[7] Gentle impaction with a plastic rod or impactor is performed until the surface of the graft is flush with the level of the surrounding articular cartilage. The graft should not be left proud. This can result in increased contact pressures[11] or increased gap formation at the graft-tunnel junction with perigraft fissuring, fibroplasia, and subchondral cavitations.[12] If the graft is accidentally impacted deeper than the surrounding surface, the surgeon may drill an adjacent small recipient hole and elevate the graft with an arthroscopic probe to the desired level.[6]

Large Defects

Several pitfalls are encountered in addressing large defects. First, achieving good surface congruity is more difficult. The surgeon should ream recipient sites perpendicular to the surface in the central areas while increasing obliquity 10 to 15 degrees inward toward the periphery.[7] In addition, care must also be taken not to violate adjacent recipient holes when reaming. The sequence of graft harvest, reaming, and implantation should be performed for each individual hole in a step-by-step manner until the defect is covered.[6] The spacing of 1 to 2 mm between grafts in the recipient site should be similar to the spacing of grafts in smaller defects. The surgeon should not obtain all grafts then ream all recipient holes.

An alternative method for treating large defects is to augment the osteochondral autografting procedure with microfracture of the pathologic perimeter. Lane and colleagues studied this technique in a goat model, with histologic, biochemical, and biomechanical follow-up evaluation showing promising results for this hybrid technique.[13]

The donor site can be left as is and usually fills with bone and fibrocartilage.[14] Alternatively, if the bone plug

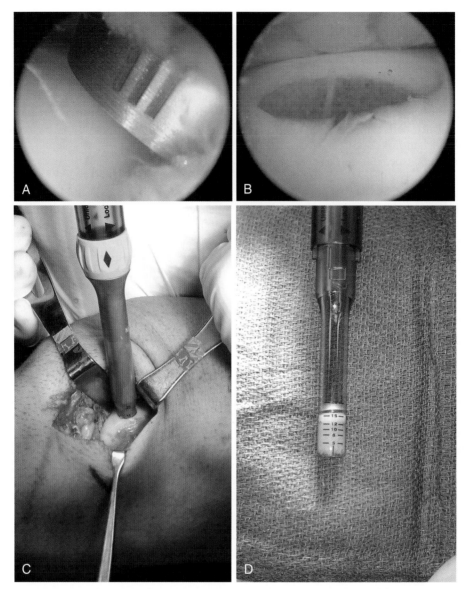

Figure 67-3. A, Arthroscopic graft harvest from the medial aspect of the medial femoral condyle with use of the donor harvester. **B,** Donor site. **C,** Open lateral femoral condyle donor plug harvest. **D,** Harvested osteochondral autograft transplant surgery plug.

removed from the recipient site is whole (depending on the harvester system used), it can be plugged back into the donor defect. This can be sewn into position with chromic suture or fixated with a SmartNail (ConMed, Utica, NY) if it is not stable via press-fit. Another alternative is to backfill the defect with a commercially available bone or cartilage graft substitute. However, some investigators have reported local reactions to these devices,[15] and we do not typically use them. Filling the defect theoretically can decrease donor site morbidity, including postoperative hematoma formation.

Wound Closure

The knee should be cleared of all debris and irrigated. Standard wound closure is performed over suction drains.

POSTOPERATIVE CONSIDERATIONS

- The patient is observed in postoperative recovery.
- Drains are removed before discharge.
- Operative dressing is changed at 48 hours.
- Perioperative antibiotics are instituted at the surgeon's preference.
- Continuous passive motion is begun on the first postoperative day.

Complications

- Infection
- Hematoma formation
- Poor motion

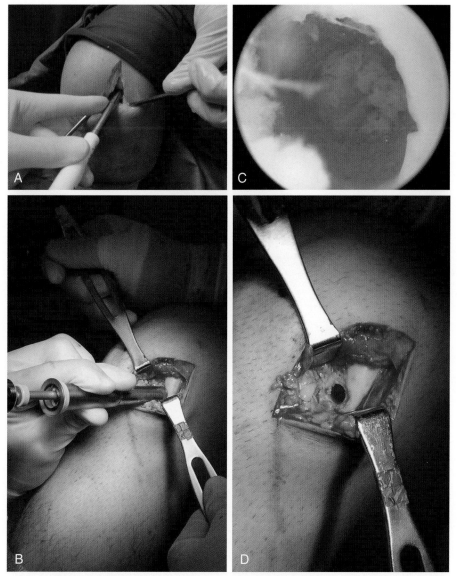

Figure 67-4. The osteochondral recipient site is prepared to appropriate depth with use of the recipient harvester via an arthroscopic or mini-open technique. Recipient site as seen (**A**) arthroscopically and (**B**) open. Recipient site after coring as seen (**C**) arthroscopically and (**D**) open.

- Thromboembolic events
- Reflex sympathetic dystrophy
- Loose body formation
- Dislodging or loosening of the graft
- Donor site morbidity
- Progression of osteoarthritis
- Continued symptoms from the affected region

Rehabilitation

- Non–weight-bearing status for 6 weeks
- Toe-touch weight-bearing until 8 to 12 weeks to ensure full graft maturation

- Consideration of continuous passive motion for 4 to 6 weeks, 4 hours/day
  - Midrange settings for cartilage nutrition rather than for maximization of knee ROM
- Active ROM (AROM) and passive ROM (PROM) to be instituted as the patient can tolerate motion
- Avoid high-impact activities until 16 to 20 weeks

RESULTS

The results in the literature are generally good for patients with small defects but are difficult to interpret because of differences in operative technique, defect

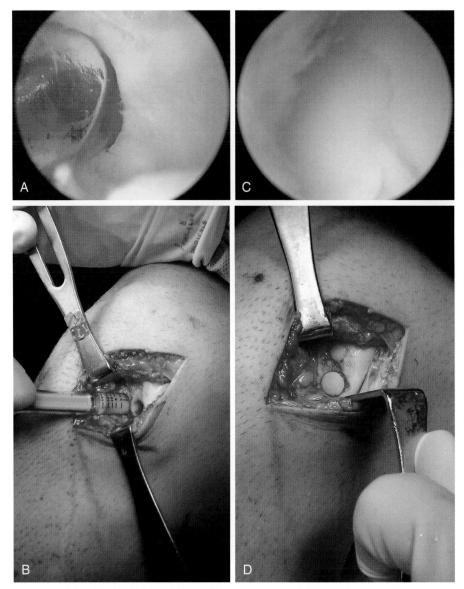

Figure 67-5. Arthroscopic mini-open technique. **A,** Plug insertion as seen arthroscopically. **B,** Open plug insertion site. **C,** Single osteochondral plug as seen arthroscopically. **D,** Open mosaicplasty.

size, and donor site location. Some studies consist of single-plug transfers, whereas in others mosaicplasty was performed. In addition, the majority of published reports are less-than-optimal in that they are of level IV evidence. Results are summarized in Table 67-2. Some of the more significant studies are as follows.

Hangody and colleagues[14] have the most extensive experience in the literature. In a 2010 report they described 383 athletes who were treated with autologous osteochondral transplantation (mosaicplasty) and followed for 2 to 17 years (average 9.6 years). The researchers report 91% good to excellent results for femoral condyle implantations. The results significantly decreased for tibial plateau defects (86%), and patella and trochlea defects (74%); donor site disturbances

were identified in 3% of the patients. Patient age younger than 30 and medium graft size (6.5- and 8.5-mm plugs) were correlated with better results. Larger plugs were likely to cause greater donor site morbidity, whereas smaller plugs were said to be too fragile to incorporate.

Horas and colleagues reported a prospective, randomized study comparing 40 patients who had undergone either ACI (20) or OATS (20) for lesions 3.2 to 5.6 cm^2 at 2 years follow-up. The postoperative Lysholm scores were lower at 6, 12, and 24 months in the ACI group; results of the Meyers and Tegner scoring systems were equal between the two groups at 24 months.[16]

Gudas and colleagues published a prospective randomized study comparing arthroscopic mosaic

TABLE 67-2. Brief Overview of Results of OATS in the Literature

Author	Number	Follow-Up	Results	Scoring System	Type of Study	Level of Evidence
Hangody et al[14] (2010)	354	10 years	91% good to excellent (femoral condyles)	HSS	Case series Mosaicplasty	IV
Horas et al[16] (2003)	40 (20 OATS vs. 20 ACI)	24 months	Lysholm score lower at 6, 12, 24 months for ACI; Tegner score equal at 24 months	Lysholm, Tegner	Prospective, randomized OATS (multiple plugs) vs. ACI	II
Gudas et al[17] (2005)	57 (28 OATS vs. 29 microfracture)	37.1 months	96% good to excellent with OATS 52% good to excellent with microfracture	HSS, ICRS	Prospective, randomized OATS (multiple plugs) vs. microfracture	II
Chow et al[18] (2004)	30	45.1 months	83% good to excellent Lysholm score, 87% "normal knee" on IKDC	Lysholm, IKDC	Case series Multiple plugs	IV
Koulalis et al[19] (2004)	18	27.2 months	12 "normal" 6 "near normal"	ICRS	Case series Mosaicplasty	IV
Andres et al[20] (2003)	19 (22 knees)	24 months	88% of mosaicplasty with OA "improved"	WOMAC, SF-36, VAS	Comparative case series Mosaicplasty in osteoarthritis	III
Outerbridge et al[21] (2000)	16 (18 knees)	7.6 years	83% good	Cincinnati	Case series with patella donor graft, single graft	IV
Laprell et al[22] (2001)	29	8.1 years	26/29 "normal" or "nearly normal"	ICRS	Case series One or two plugs	IV
Ma et al[23] (2004)	18	42 months	89% good to excellent	Lysholm, Tegner	Case series Multiple plugs	IV
Bobic[24] (1996)	10	2 years	"Promising results"		Case series OATS (multiple plugs) + ACI reconstruction	IV
Sharpe et al[25] (2005)	13	3 years	10/13 with "significant improvement"	KSS	Case series OATS (multiple plugs) + ACI	IV
Sanders et al[26] (2001)	21	22 months	Maximum signal intensity of grafts at 4-6 weeks		Case series of MRI results, multiple plugs	IV
Marcacci et al[20] (2007)	30	7 years	77% good to excellent	ICRS	Case series Clinical and MRI follow-up	IV

ACI, Autologous chondrocyte implantation; *HSS,* Hospital for Special Surgery; *ICRS,* International Cartilage Repair Society; *IKDC,* International Knee Documentation Committee; *MRI,* magnetic resonance imaging; *OA,* osteoarthritis; *OATS,* osteochondral autograft transplant surgery; *SF-36,* Short Form 36; *VAS,* visual analogue scale; *WOMAC,* Western Ontario and McMaster Universities Osteoarthritis Index.

osteochondral autologous transplantation (28) with microfracture (29) in 57 femoral condyle lesions smaller than 4 cm² at 37.1 months. The authors reported 96% good to excellent results with the OATS group compared with 52% for the microfracture group with the Hospital for Special Surgery (HSS) and International Cartilage Repair Society (ICRS) scoring systems.[17]

Other studies have shown slightly less successful results. Marcacci reported 77% good or excellent results at 7-year follow-up. Size of lesion and number of plugs

was correlated with outcome. Follow-up MRI showed complete maintenance of filled cartilage defect in 63% of patients; donor sites were covered but still detectable in all patients.[27] Kock and colleagues reported interesting bone scintigraphy results 4 years after osteochondral autograft transplantation. They noted excellent results at the recipient site (changed from abnormal to normal in 11 of 13 patients) but noted persistently increased activity at the donor site in 9 of 11 patients. Many of these patients had retropatellar crepitus at final follow-up 3 to 5 years postoperatively. The authors noted that the size of the plugs harvested (up to 12.9 mm) from the lateral trochlea may explain the negative donor site findings.[28]

Finally, Reddy and colleagues have reported on the morbidity of the donor site (knee) in patients treated with osteochondral transplant surgery for talar lesions. Small to medium plugs (3.5 to 6.5 mm) were harvested from the intercondylar notch or the lateral aspect of the proximal lateral femoral condyle. Patients had asymptomatic knees before surgery, but 4 of 11 had poor knee scores 47 months postoperatively. Despite this, 9 of 11 patients were satisfied or somewhat satisfied with their ankle surgery.[29]

It appears that very good results can be obtained with the OATS procedure, but donor site morbidity is not insignificant and must be explained to the patient.

CONCLUSION

There are several options for the orthopedic surgeon in addressing the patient with a focal cartilage defect of the knee. Osteochondral autografting with either single or multiple plugs provides the surgeon with a viable solution for the defect smaller than 3 cm². Single-plug techniques are appropriate for defects smaller than 1 cm², whereas multiple-plug techniques are appropriate for defects larger than 3 cm². This technique can be used in combination with other knee procedures such as ACL reconstruction and high-tibial osteotomy. The procedure is straightforward and supported by the published literature to be as good as, if not superior to, other techniques such as microfracture or ACI for defects in this size range. Further research is being explored, and techniques are emerging, such as matrix induced chondrocyte transplantation. However, OATS remains a viable and very successful treatment option for appropriately selected patients.

REFERENCES

1. Cahill BR. Osteochondritis dissecans of the knee: treatment of juvenile and adult forms. *J Am Acad Orthop Surg.* 1995;3(4):237-247.
2. Linden B. Osteochondritis dissecans of the femoral condyle: a long term follow-up study. *J Bone Joint Surg Am.* 1977;59(6):769-776.
3. Milgram JW. Radiological and pathological manifestations of osteochondritis dissecans of the distal femur. A study of 50 cases. *Radiology.* 1978;126(2):305-311.
4. Stanitski CL. Correlation of arthroscopic and clinical examinations with magnetic resonance imaging findings of injured knees in children and adolescents. *Am J Sports Med.* 1998;26(1):2-6.
5. Garretson 3rd RB, Katolik LI, Verma N, et al. Contact pressure at osteochondral donor sites in the patellofemoral joint. *Am J Sports Med.* 2004;32(4):967-974.
6. Hangody L, Rathonyi GK, Duska Z, et al. Autologous osteochondral mosaicplasty. Surgical technique. *J Bone Joint Surg Am.* 2004;86(Suppl 1):65-72.
7. Poelstra KA, Neff ES, Miller MD. *Osteochondral Autologous Plug Transfer in the Knee.* Philadelphia: Elsevier; 2004.
8. Ahmad CS, Cohen ZA, Levine WN, et al. Biomechanical and topographic considerations for autologous osteochondral grafting in the knee. *Am J Sports Med.* 2001;29 (2):201-206.
9. Bartz RL, Kamaric E, Noble PC, et al. Topographic matching of selected donor and recipient sites for osteochondral autografting of the articular surface of the femoral condyles. *Am J Sports Med.* 2001;29(2): 207-212.
10. Whiteside RA, Jakob RP, Wyss UP, et al. Impact loading of articular cartilage during transplantation of osteochondral autograft. *J Bone Joint Surg Br.* 2005;87(9): 1285-1291.
11. Wu JZ, Herzog W, Hasler EM. Inadequate placement of osteochondral plugs may induce abnormal stress-strain distributions in articular cartilage—finite element simulations. *Med Eng Phys.* 2002;24(2):85-97.
12. Pearce SG, Hurtig MB, Clarnette R, et al. An investigation of 2 techniques for optimizing joint surface congruency using multiple cylindrical osteochondral autografts. *Arthroscopy.* 2001;17(1):50-55.
13. Lane J, Healey R, Chen A, et al. Can osteochondral grafting be augmented with microfracture in an extended-size lesion of articular cartilage? *Am J Sports Med.* 2010;38(7): 1316-1323.
14. Hangody L, Dobos J, Baló E, et al. Clinical experiences with autologous osteochondral mosaicplasty in an athletic population: a 17-year prospective multicenter study. *Am J Sports Med.* 2010;38(6):1125-1133.
15. Adams M, Gehrmann R, Bibbo C, et al. *In vivo assessment of incorporation of bone graft substitute plugs in osteoarticular autograft transplant surgery. Presented at the AOSSM annual meeting.* Rhode Island: Providence; 2010.
16. Horas U, Pelinkovic D, Herr G, et al. Autologous chondrocyte implantation and osteochondral cylinder transplantation in cartilage repair of the knee joint. A prospective, comparative trial. *J Bone Joint Surg Am.* 2003;85(2):185-192.
17. Gudas R, Kalesinskas RJ, Kimtys V, et al. A prospective randomized clinical study of mosaic osteochondral autologous transplantation versus microfracture for the treatment of osteochondral defects in the knee joint in young athletes. *Arthroscopy.* 2005;21(9):1066-1075.
18. Chow JC, Hantes ME, Houle JB, et al. Arthroscopic autogenous osteochondral transplantation for treating knee cartilage defects: a 2- to 5-year follow-up study. *Arthroscopy.* 2004;20(7):681-690.
19. Koulalis D, Schultz W, Heyden M, et al. Autologous osteochondral grafts in the treatment of cartilage defects of the knee joint. *Knee Surg Sports Traumatol Arthrosc.* 2004;12(4):329-334.
20. Andres BM, Mears SC, Somel DS, et al. Treatment of osteoarthritic cartilage lesions with osteochondral autograft transplantation. *Orthopedics.* 2003;26(11):1121-1126.

21. Outerbridge HK, Outerbridge RE, Smith DE. Osteochondral defects in the knee. A treatment using lateral patella autografts. *Clin Orthop Relat Res.* 2000;(377):145-151.

22. Laprell H, Petersen W. Autologous osteochondral transplantation using the diamond bone-cutting system (DBCS): 6-12 years' follow-up of 35 patients with osteochondral defects at the knee joint. *Arch Orthop Trauma Surg.* 2001;121(5):248-253.

23. Ma HL, Hung SC, Wang ST, et al. Osteochondral autografts transfer for post-traumatic osteochondral defect of the knee: 2 to 5 years follow-up. *Injury.* 2004;35(12):1286-1292.

24. Bobic V. Arthroscopic osteochondral autograft transplantation in anterior cruciate ligament reconstruction: a preliminary clinical study. *Knee Surg Sports Traumatol Arthrosc.* 1996;3(4):262-264.

25. Sharpe JR, Ahmed SU, Fleetcroft JP, et al. The treatment of osteochondral lesions using a combination of autologous chondrocyte implantation and autograft: three-year follow-up. *J Bone Joint Surg Br.* 2005;87(5):730-735.

26. Sanders TG, Mentzer KD, Miller MD, et al. Autogenous osteochondral "plug" transfer for the treatment of focal chondral defects: postoperative MR appearance with clinical correlation. *Skeletal Radiol.* 2001;30(10):570-578.

27. Marcacci M, Kon E, Delcogliano M, et al. Arthroscopic autologous osteochondral grafting of cartilage defects of the knee. *Am J Sports Med.* 2007;35(12):2014-2021.

28. Kock N, van Tankeren E, Oyen W, et al. Bone scintigraphy after osteochondral autograft transplantation in the knee. *Acta Orthop.* 2010;81(2):206-210.

29. Reddy S, Pedowitz D, Parekh S, et al. The morbidity associated with osteochondral harvest from asymptomatic knees for the treatment of osteochondral lesions of the talus. *Am J Sports Med.* 2007;35(1):80-85.

Chapter 68

Complex Problems in Knee Articular Cartilage

Rachel M. Frank, Jaskarndip Chahal, Geoffrey S. Van Thiel, and Brian J. Cole

Chapter Synopsis
- Treatment of combined knee pathology is a challenging problem.
- The inter-relationship among malalignment, meniscus pathology, articular cartilage disease, and instability results in complex clinical scenarios.

Important Points
- For successful operative management of these patients, proper patient selection is critical.
- Determining the cause of symptoms (predominantly pain) can be especially difficult in knees with multiple pathologies, and treatment of incidental lesions must be avoided.

Clinical and Surgical Pearls
- Do not treat incidental defects; stick to predefined pathology.
- Always treat malalignment in the setting of cartilage or meniscal disorders.

Clinical and Surgical Pitfalls
- Do not overcorrect with a high tibial osteotomy into an affected lateral compartment.
- Do not perform meniscal transplant or a cartilage procedure in the setting of malalignment.

Patients with knee pain often have coexisting pathoanatomic conditions at the index clinic visit, which may in turn have multiple causes (Box 68-1). With advancements in surgical techniques, available grafts, and imaging modalities, the ability to successfully perform complex cartilage procedures in even the most challenging patient is improving. However, this aforementioned group of patients with multiple coexisting knee pathologies remains a difficult population, especially with regard to determining which (if any) of the lesions is the cause of symptoms. Cartilage lesions may be simply incidental in nature, and the decision to treat is based on their confirmed contribution to a patient's symptomatology.

The combination of malalignment, ligamentous instability, and chondral and meniscal damage presents multiple challenges.[1] Corrective procedures for each of these problems performed in isolation have historically produced adequate results; however, combined procedures to treat combined pathologies have proven essential for the success of any single procedure.[1,2] Consideration of both patient-specific factors (e.g., age, activity level, expectations) and disease-specific factors is a requisite for treatment planning and optimization of short- and long-term clinical outcomes.

Many surgical options are available for the patient with multiple knee pathologies and are often used in combination. Meniscal deficiency can be treated with debridement, direct repair, or meniscal allograft transplantation. Ligamentous pathology can be addressed with direct repair or reconstruction depending on the region of injury. Articular cartilage pathology can be addressed with a variety of procedures including debridement, microfracture, autologous chondrocyte implantation (ACI), and osteochondral autograft or allograft. Finally, medial compartment disease with varus malalignment can be addressed with a high tibial osteotomy (HTO) that unloads the diseased medial compartment, and lateral compartment disease with valgus malalignment can be treated with a distal femoral osteotomy (DFO) that unloads the lateral compartment. More recently, HTO has been used as a concomitant malalignment corrective procedure in patients undergoing cartilage and/or meniscus surgery in an attempt to offload the compartment in which cartilage surgery is performed.[1-4] A recent systematic review performed by Harris and colleagues[2] analyzed clinical outcomes in patients undergoing combined meniscal allograft transplantation and cartilage repair or restoration. Of the six studies included, 110 patients were identified as having undergone meniscal allograft transplantation and either ACI (n = 73), osteochondral allograft transplantation (n = 20), or osteochondral autograft transplantation (n = 17). In addition, three patients underwent concomitant microfracture. Of note, 33% of patients (36 of 110) underwent other concomitant procedures including HTO or DFO, ligament reconstruction, and/or hardware removal. The authors noted improved outcomes in combined procedures compared with isolated surgery in four of the six studies. Overall, 12% of patients experienced failure of their combined procedure that necessitated revision surgery, and 85% of these failures were noted to be related to the meniscus procedure as opposed to the cartilage procedure.[2]

For all of these procedures, whether performed in isolation or concurrently, proper patient selection and determination of which lesion(s) is responsible for generating symptoms are crucial. As mentioned previously, treating incidental lesions must be avoided.

PATHOPHYSIOLOGY

In a knee with multiple pathologies (meniscal deficiency, chondral defect, malalignment, and ligament instability), each entity must be considered individually with respect to its influence on the overall status of the knee. Meniscectomy is a commonly performed procedure in sports medicine. It is minimally invasive and can produce satisfactory outcomes in a majority of patients, especially those desiring a quick return to activity. However, the procedure is not without risks when it comes to the long-term health of the knee. Subtotal meniscectomy decreases joint contact area[5] and increases peak stress.[5] After subtotal or total meniscectomy, there is a fourteen-fold increased relative risk of developing unicompartmental arthritis.[6-8] Furthermore, multiple studies have demonstrated worse outcomes associated with young age, chondral damage found at time of meniscectomy,[9,10] ligamentous instability,[11-13] and/or tibiofemoral malalignment. In addition, meniscal repair as well as meniscal transplantation have less favorable outcomes when

performed with untreated concomitant instability, malalignment, and/or articular cartilage disease.[1,4,14-16] Thus, although addressing multiple coexisting pathologies in a single patient's knee is certainly challenging, neglecting to correct concomitant comorbidity can compromise overall results and in the worst case scenario lead to a uncorrectable salvage situation.

Damage to the articular cartilage occurs for a variety of reasons, including mechanical overload, developmental defects, genetic failures, and traumatic impact. Articular cartilage injury leads to an increase in degenerative joint disease, especially with bipolar "kissing" lesions. Full-thickness chondral injuries can be extremely problematic, causing knee swelling, pain at night and with rest, and severe activity-related pain.[17,18] Furthermore, it is necessary to determine if a chondral lesion has any underlying subchondral bone changes because this feature would affect decision making in the perioperative period.

Knee malalignment causes excessive loading of articular cartilage, which can lead to degenerative joint disease. The mechanical axis (center of femoral head to intercondylar eminence to center of ankle) of the leg is different from the weight-bearing axis (center of femoral head to center of ankle). Because the anatomic axis of the femur differs from the mechanical axis, the normal anatomic weight-bearing axis of the knee is approximately 5 to 7 degrees of valgus. Furthermore, in a normal knee approximately 60% of the weight-bearing force is transmitted through the medial compartment. Varus malalignment[19] shifts the center of the knee joint lateral to the mechanical axis, leading to medial tibial cartilage volume and thickness loss, as well as increases in tibial and femoral denuded bone.[19] Valgus malalignment shifts the center of the knee medial to the mechanical axis, leading to increased, unbalanced lateral-sided forces. Osteotomy procedures (HTO, DFO) alter the biomechanical axis by shifting load away from the damaged compartment. The pathophysiologic principle of this procedure is to correct the weight-bearing axis if possible to avoid rapid and irreversible progression of unicompartmental degenerative joint disease.[20-22]

PREOPERATIVE CONSIDERATIONS

Patient Presentation

Patients with complex, combined knee pathologies typically report unilateral, single compartment knee pain. Often their symptoms are chronic in nature, because it takes time for any one of these isolated injuries to have an additive effect on another. This goes to the core of the complexity of treating patients with multiple knee pathologies. Diagnosing and treating any injury occurring in isolation is usually rather straightforward;

TABLE 68-1. Common Patient Presentations

Symptom	Condition in Which Symptom Is Common
Intermittent pain ("comes and goes")	Articular cartilage injury, malalignment
Swelling, rest pain	Articular cartilage injury, malalignment
Mechanical symptoms (clicking, locking)	Meniscus injury
Joint line pain and tenderness to palpation	Meniscus, articular cartilage, ligament injury
Sensation of instability	Ligament injury, meniscus injury
Multiligament injury	Ligament injury

however, multiple concurrent injuries tend to expedite the development of degenerative disease. Therefore these patients may also be seen after at least one, if not more, previous (and unsuccessful) surgical intervention. Only occasionally are these types of patients seen acutely after a traumatic event. Other common components of the patient presentation are outlined in Table 68-1.

The history of the patient with combined knee pathologies will not be as straightforward as that of the typical sports medicine patient with a defined traumatic twisting, pivoting, or instability event. Therefore it is vital for the clinician to be suspicious for a knee with combined pathology. Nonetheless, it is important to elicit a certain requisite set of symptoms—specifically, localized pain (retropatellar, medial or lateral), swelling, mechanical symptoms, and/or instability (side-to-side instability, or instability with pivoting and twisting).

Physical Examination

For any patient with combined knee pathology, a standard physical examination of both knees and lower extremities should be performed. Specific physical examination maneuvers can include the following:

- Inspection
  - Alignment in the sagittal, coronal, and transverse planes
  - Muscle bulk
  - Prior surgical incisions
- Palpation
  - Tenderness
  - Crepitus (medial, lateral, patellofemoral)
- Active and passive range of motion
  - Hip
  - Knee
- Strength assessment
  - Core strength
  - Quad strength

- Hamstring flexibility and iliotibial band assessment (Ober test)
- Neurovascular examination
- Patellar examination
  - Tilt
  - Apprehension
  - J sign
  - Static and dynamic Q angle assessment
  - Crepitus
- Tests of stability and special tests
  - Pivot shift, Lachman, anterior drawer
  - Posterior drawer
  - Varus and valgus stress (at full extension and at 30 degrees of flexion)
  - McMurray
  - Anteromedial rotary instability: should be assessed with the knee in 90 degrees of flexion with the patient supine
  - Posterolateral rotary instability: should be assessed with the patient prone while external rotation is applied to both knees in 30 and 90 degrees of flexion for side-to-side comparison

Patients with unilateral joint effusion are likely to have cartilage pathology, although this physical examination finding is not specific. Patients with tenderness to palpation posterior to the midline of joint line are more likely to have meniscal pathology, whereas those with tenderness anterior to the midline of joint line may have patellofemoral, chondral, or meniscal (displaced tears) pathology. Nevertheless, with combined pathology, symptoms can be difficult to differentiate. Most patients have preserved strength and range-of-motion, unless their degenerative disease has progressed far enough to cause weakness and/or stiffness.

Leg length and gait should be assessed in every patient as well, because these findings may have significant implications on surgical planning. Overall alignment and the presence of clinical genu valgum or varum should also be documented.

Imaging

Imaging for patients with combined knee pathologies can include the following:

- Radiographs
  - Standard weight-bearing radiographic series (anteroposterior [AP], lateral, Merchant)
    - Weight-bearing AP views in extension
    - Weight-bearing posteroanterior (PA) views in 45 degrees of flexion
  - Weight-bearing double-stance long-leg axis series
  - Sizing radiographs (for meniscus transplantation and osteochondral allograft transplantation candidates) (Fig. 68-1)

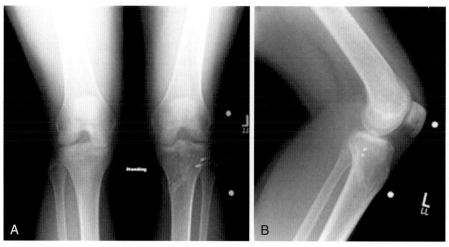

Figure 68-1. Anteroposterior and lateral sizing radiographs.

○ Standing bilateral 45-degree flexion PA view of knee with the x-ray tube directed at 10 degrees caudal. The 10-cm marker should be placed on the lateral aspect of the affected knee at the level of the joint space.

○ Lateral non–weight-bearing knee view. The 10-cm marker should be placed next to the knee cap at the level of the joint space.

- Magnetic resonance imaging (MRI)
- Computed tomography (CT)

MRI is useful for examining soft tissue integrity. Specific sequences can be used to identify articular cartilage, menisci, ligamentous structures, and other intra-articular structures and pathology. In general, a minimum of a 1.5-Tesla MRI is required for adequate resolution to view cartilage abnormalities. Bone marrow edema seen on MRI can be indicative of unicompartmental overload. CT scans can be helpful as adjunctive imaging modalities, especially in the patient with prior surgery (e.g., bone tunnels in previous anterior cruciate ligament [ACL] reconstruction). Other imaging modalities, including bone scans, may provide information regarding degenerative activity in the condyles, plateaus, or patella.

Records of Prior Treatment

Many of the patients with combined pathologies of the knee have a history of previous surgical intervention. In our practice, it is routine to request all operative reports and arthroscopic images to date to help optimize the treatment planning and decision making for the patient. When such information is not available, we recommend performance of a new MRI scan and a diagnostic arthroscopy to survey the knee and assess cartilaginous, ligamentous, and meniscal structures.

TREATMENT OPTIONS

Nonoperative Treatment

Nonoperative approaches include the following:

- Activity modification
- Rest
- Physical therapy
- Nonsteroidal anti-inflammatory drugs (NSAIDs)
- Corticosteroid injections
- Hyaluronic acid injections
- Platelet-rich plasma therapy

Although often effective at symptomatic relief, these modalities typically provide only temporary relief for patients with complex knee injuries.

Operative Treatment

See Figs. 68-2 to 68-5 for details of the operative treatment.

For the surgical management of patients with combined knee pathologies, particular attention must be paid to surgical indications. To reiterate, treatment should be aimed at lesions that are truly responsible for a given patient's symptoms, and not those that are simply incidental in nature. This is especially important during diagnostic arthroscopy procedures, when a previously unknown cartilage injury may be detected but may simply be an incidental finding that is not responsible for any symptoms.

Combined procedures will be effective only in patients with appropriate indications for surgery. Patients who are young and active are ideal candidates for these procedures, whereas older, less active patients may benefit from arthroplasty-based options. Furthermore, only patients who demonstrate an ability to tolerate and comply with rehabilitation protocols should

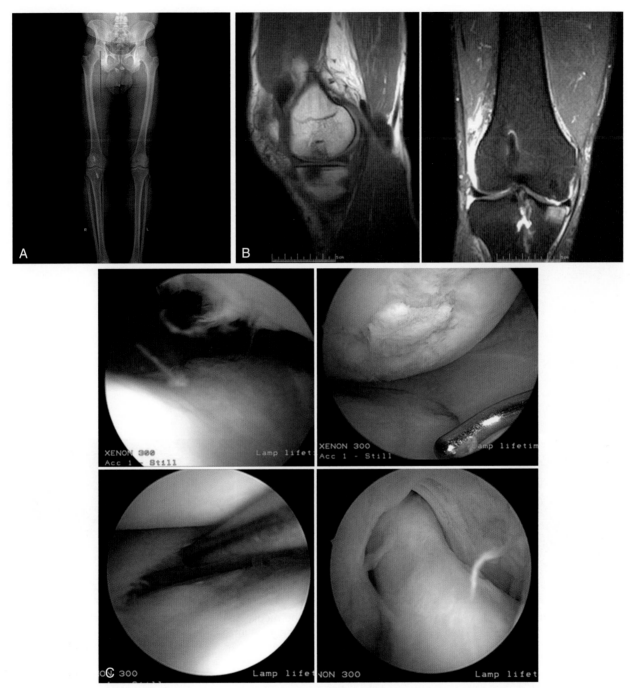

Figure 68-2. Surgical management of a 47-year-old man with a history of prior right anterior cruciate ligament (ACL) reconstruction and right medial femoral condyle (MFC) osteochondral autograft transplant surgery (OATS) now presenting with an acute traumatic knee injury. The patient ultimately underwent medial opening wedge high tibial osteotomy (HTO), medial tibial plateau subchondroplasty, and MFC osteochondral allograft (OA) transplantation. **A,** Standing radiograph showing varus alignment with a plan for a 7.5-degree correction. **B,** Magnetic resonance imaging (MRI) scans showing failed OATS procedure, subchondral edema, and an intact ACL. **C,** Images from the staging arthroscopy showing a grade IV 20- × 20-mm MFC focal chondral defect at the site of the prior OATS failure, grade II patellar changes, and an intact ACL.

Continued

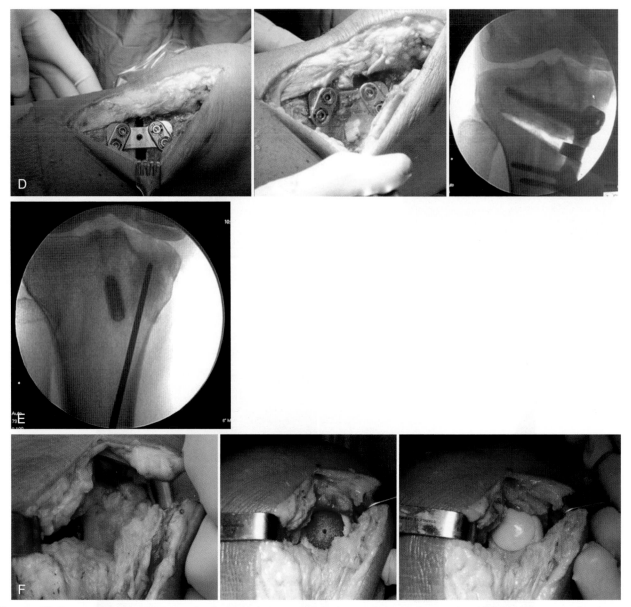

Figure 68-2. cont'd. D, Intraoperative images demonstrating the medial opening wedge HTO. **E,** Intraoperative images demonstrating the medial tibial plateau subchondroplasty. **F,** Intraoperative images demonstrating MFC OA transplantation.

be considered for surgery. Understanding patient expectations is crucial; the patient must understand that the knee will still not be a normal knee and that activity restrictions after several of these procedures may exist. Relative contraindications for such procedures include the following:

- Generalized (tricompartmental) osteoarthritis
- An inability to comply with rehabilitation
- Unrealistic patient expectations
- Obesity with body mass index over 40

Surgical approaches for patients with combined knee pathologies depend on the specific pathologies. Treatments may be performed in one operative setting or may be staged. The various surgical options include

osteotomy (for malalignment); ligamentous repair or reconstruction (for ligamentous instability); articular cartilage debridement; microfracture; ACI and osteochondral autograft or allograft transplantation (for articular cartilage disease); and meniscus debridement, repair, or transplantation (for meniscus pathology). The techniques for each of these procedures performed in isolation are discussed elsewhere in this text; the following treatment sections will focus on the less commonly encountered, clinically complex presentations.

Malalignment with Chondral or Meniscal Defect

HTO procedures[23,24] treat varus malalignment by decreasing the biomechanical load in the medial compartment of the knee. Similarly, DFO procedures treat valgus malalignment by decreasing the biomechanical load in the lateral compartment. There has been a renewed interest in HTO because of the growing number of chronologically and physiologically young patients with medial compartment disease. Arthroplasty is certainly not the ideal option because running and impact activities are not recommended after arthroplasty, but such activities are permitted after HTO. In fact, pending other concomitant knee pathologies and corrective

surgeries, there are no major activity restrictions after HTO. Furthermore, with HTO, newer techniques and instrumentation such as locking plates with variable screw angles have improved fixation, early postoperative results, and patient satisfaction.[25,26] Recent literature suggests that there is no difference in clinical outcomes after total knee arthroplasty in patients with previous HTO compared with those without previous HTO.[27-30] HTO has also been instrumental in treating patients who previously had contraindications for

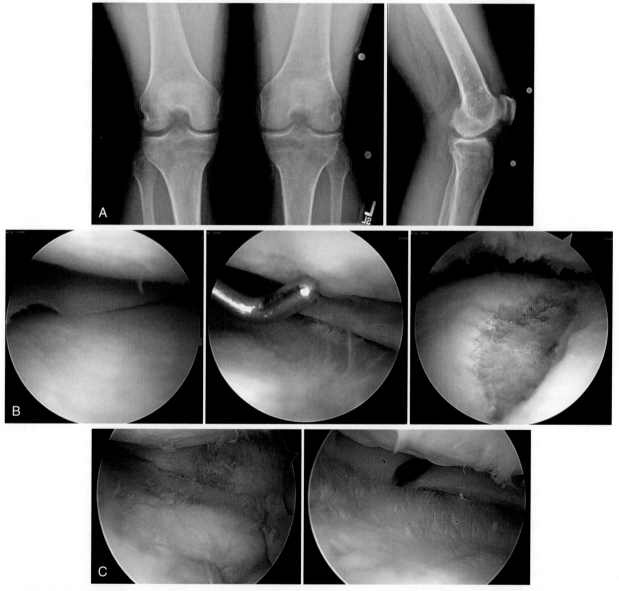

Figure 68-3. Surgical management of a 44-year-old man with a history of prior left knee partial lateral meniscectomy, followed by subsequent lateral meniscus repair with lateral femoral condyle (LFC) microfracture, followed by lateral meniscus allograft transplantation (LMT) with a distal femoral varus osteotomy (DFVO). All procedures were performed because of continued lateral knee pain. The patient ultimately underwent LFC osteochondral allograft, revision LMT, and a DeNovo Natural Tissue (NT) Graft (Zimmer, Inc., Warsaw, IN/ISTO Technologies, Inc., St Louis, MO) procedure to the trochlea. **A,** Posteroanterior (PA) and lateral radiographs demonstrating degeneration of the lateral compartment. **B,** Images from the staging arthroscopy showing a grade IV 4- × 12-mm defect in the trochlea, a grade IV 14- × 14-mm defect in the LFC, and evidence of prior LMT with extrusion of the graft and a posterior horn tear. **C,** Intraoperative images demonstrating the appearance of the lateral meniscus before and after revision LMT.   *Continued*

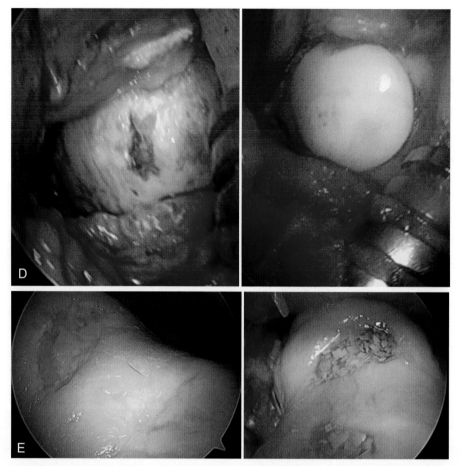

Figure 68-3. cont'd. D, Intraoperative images demonstrating the appearance of the LFC before and after the osteochondral allograft transplantation. **E,** Intraoperative images demonstrating the appearance of the trochlea before and after the DeNovo NT procedure.

meniscal and/or chondral reconstructive procedures secondary to tibiofemoral malalignment.[1]

Concomitant HTO with cartilage and meniscus restoration procedures has been increasing in popularity, because malalignment is a contraindication to performing such procedures in isolation.[1] Recent studies have shown that patients with uncorrected varus malalignment do not achieve optimal outcomes with cartilage restorative procedures,[31,32] and biomechanical and clinical studies have shown the benefits of restoring alignment before or concomitantly with chondral or meniscal restorative procedures.[33-38] For example, HTO performed with a medial meniscus transplant has the potential to both unload the compartment and potentially improve the outcome of a transplant in a varus knee.[1,16,22,39-43] Furthermore, biomechanical evidence from Van Thiel and colleagues[21] has demonstrated the mechanical benefits of performing HTO with meniscus transplantation. These procedures performed in isolation in the presence of tibiofemoral malalignment may have worse outcomes and higher failure rates as a result of mechanical overload of the repaired tissue. Alignment-correcting procedures such as HTO may unload the damaged compartment enough to allow healing and

protect the cartilage and/or meniscal restoration being performed.

The issue of correcting alignment after failed ACL reconstruction has also received a recent increase in attention. One must consider malalignment and thus medial compartment overload as a factor leading to failure of the initial ACL reconstruction. In these patients, correcting the weight-bearing axis with HTO before or during the ACL revision may be appropriate. In patients with ACL deficiency, it may also be beneficial to decrease the tibial slope by placing the plate more posterior along the tibia.[44]

Relative contraindications to HTO include multicompartmental degenerative disease. Even mild lateral compartment disease at the time of HTO can be detrimental to the success of the procedure. Similarly, patellofemoral compartment disease is a relative contraindication, and if the HTO is the procedure of choice, it may be possible to concomitantly perform a Maquet (anterior) or Fulkerson (anteromedial) tibial tubercle osteotomy to treat the patellofemoral disease. Other relative contraindications to HTO include lateral meniscus deficiency, inflammatory arthritis (as this leads to tricompartmental degenerative joint disease), and patients unwilling to comply with the prescribed rehabilitation after HTO.

Good to excellent results with HTO have been reported in the literature, but there are several potential drawbacks. Although the procedure may effectively offload the most diseased compartment, it may also place increased stress on other compartments (e.g., lateral, patellofemoral). Second, reported results of HTO progressively worsen over time, whereas medium- to long-term arthroplasty results are excellent.[45] Coventry and colleagues[46] have reported a 10-year survival rate of 63% in knees with 5 degrees of valgus angulation; of note, improved results were reported in patients with greater degrees of correction (87% with 6 to 7 degrees and 94% with more than 8 degrees). The authors also noted significantly worse survival of the HTO in patients who were substantially overweight. More recently, Efe and colleagues[21] reported on the outcomes of 199 knees that had undergone closing wedge HTO and reported an 84% survival at 9.6 years postoperatively, with knee function outcomes that were good or excellent in 64% of patients. Of note, 36 HTOs were converted to total knee arthroplasties.[47] Reported complications[47-49] after

HTO (with estimated complication rates) include the following:

- Loss of correction
- Intraoperative or postoperative lateral cortex fracture (up to 18.2%)
- Deep venous thrombosis (2.4%)
- Delayed union or nonunion (0.7% to 4.4%)
- Symptomatic hardware (11%)
- Infection (2% to 55%)
- Common peroneal nerve damage (2% to 16%)

Meniscal Defect with Femoral Condylar Cartilage Defect

The biomechanical and functional relationship between the meniscus and femoral articular cartilage is complex. Damage to one of these structures is often associated with damage to the other. As described in detail in the literature, unicompartmental arthritis is a known outcome in up to 70% of patients after near-total meniscectomy, with a relative risk of up to 14 times when compared with matched controls.[5-8] Even partial meniscectomy can significantly increase tibiofemoral contact

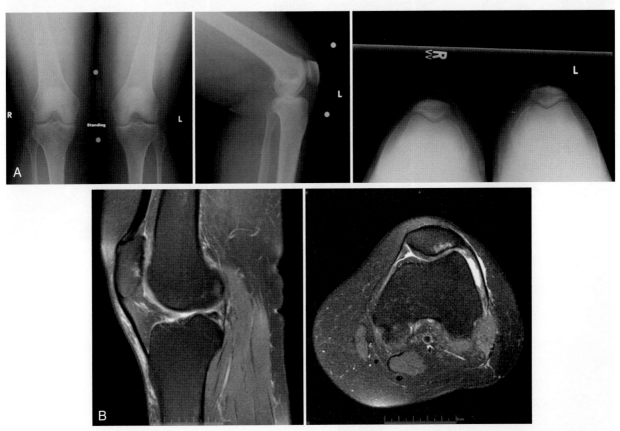

Figure 68-4. Surgical management of a 35-year-old woman with a 5-year history of bilateral knee pain (left greater than right) especially with squatting and stairs. The patient ultimately underwent left knee anteromedialization (AMZ) and augmented microfracture (BioCartilage, Arthrex, Naples, FL). **A,** Preoperative posterolateral, lateral, and sunrise radiographs demonstrating no joint space narrowing or patellar tilt and a normal sulcus. **B,** Preoperative magnetic resonance imaging scan demonstrating a focal chondral defect in the lateral facet of the patella with associated subchondral edema.

Continued

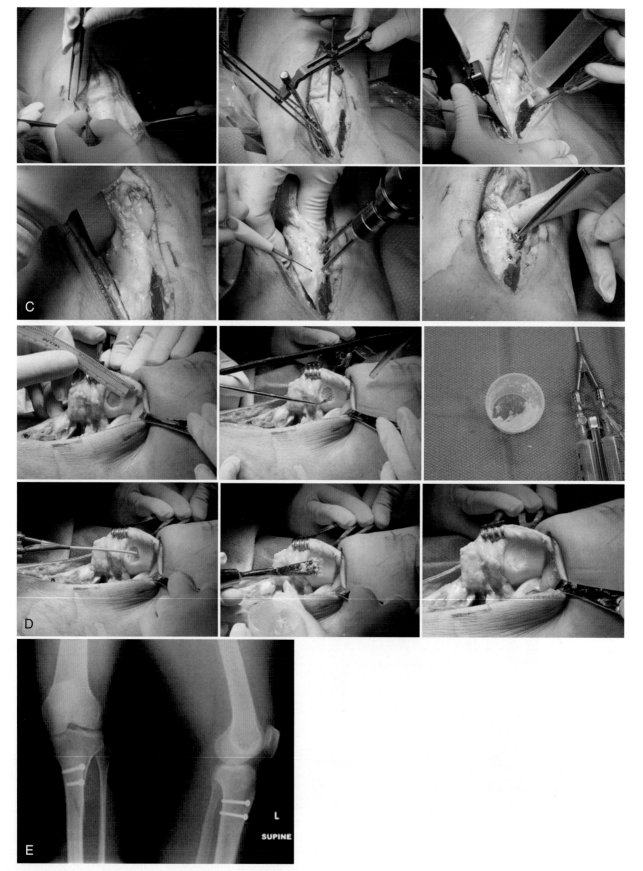

Figure 68-4. cont'd. C, Intraoperative images demonstrating the surgical steps for the AMZ. **D,** Intraoperative images demonstrating the surgical steps for the augmented microfracture. **E,** Postoperative radiographs showing intact hardware.

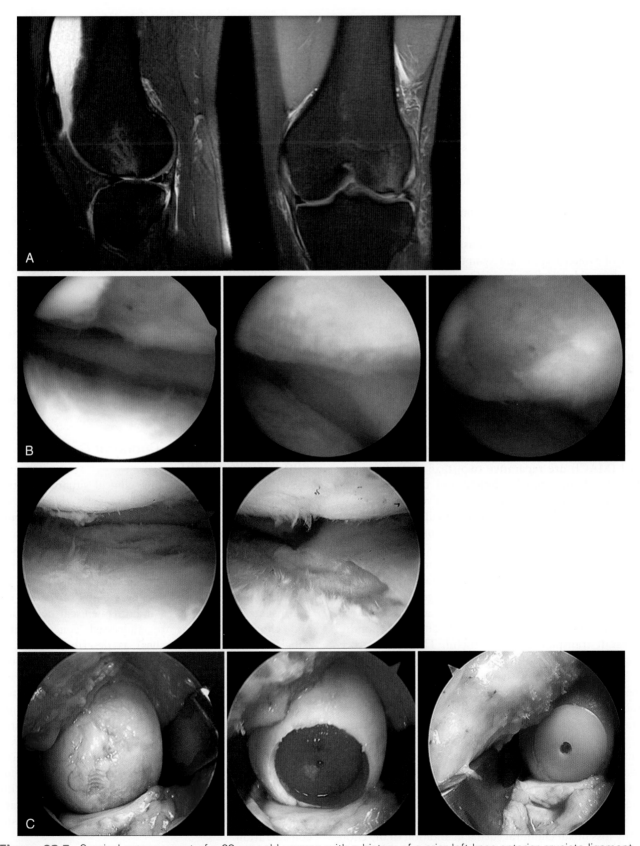

Figure 68-5. Surgical management of a 23-year-old woman with a history of a prior left knee anterior cruciate ligament reconstruction and partial lateral meniscectomy who reported new-onset left knee pain affecting activities of daily living. The patient ultimately underwent left knee meniscus allograft transplantation (LMT) with lateral femoral condyle (LFC) osteochondral allograft (OA). **A,** Preoperative magnetic resonance imaging scan demonstrating LFC subchondral edema and disruption of the lateral meniscus. **B,** Intraoperative images from the diagnostic arthroscopy demonstrating an LFC osteochondral defect and a lateral meniscectomized state. **C,** Intraoperative images demonstrating the definitive treatment of LMT and LFC OA transplantation.

pressures, especially on the lateral side.[50] Treatment options for isolated meniscal pathology include debridement, repair, and transplantation. Repair techniques are useful for tears in the peripheral one third of the meniscus and include outside-in, inside-out, and all-inside techniques. Meniscus allograft transplantation is an invasive technique useful for patients who are symptomatic in the ipsilateral compartment after prior subtotal meniscectomies. Various transplantation techniques have been described, including the bridge-in-slot technique, bone-plug technique, dovetail technique, and free-end technique.[51,52]

With regard to isolated chondral defects, there are several surgical techniques for articular cartilage disease. The single most important consideration is determination of which lesions are symptomatic and which are simply incidental in nature. Operative treatment typically starts with debridement, which is considered a first-line arthroscopic approach that can produce palliative results. Microfracture is a reparative procedure that is best for small (<2 cm^2) unipolar lesions. This marrow-stimulating technique is highly dependent on appropriate technical execution and has over two decades of successful outcomes reported in the literature.[53,54] The key to the success of this procedure is the creation of vertical walls to contain the resultant mesenchymal stem cell clot that attempts to fill in the full-thickness chondral defect with fibrocartilage. ACI and matrix-induced ACI (MACI) are reparative two-stage procedures best used for large condylar lesions (>4 cm^2) or patellar lesions without significant bony involvement. The ACI technique uses the patient's own articular cartilage cells secured down with a periosteal flap or collagen membrane; the goal is to fill in full-thickness cartilage defects with hyaline or fibrocartilage. The procedure can be particularly useful in the patellofemoral joint.

For medium-sized articular cartilage lesions (2 to 4 cm^2), reconstructive procedures such as osteochondral autograft transplant surgery (OATS) and osteochondral allograft transplantation are useful. The OATS procedure is typically used for medium-sized lesions that can be treated with one or two donor site plugs taken from the non–weight-bearing region of the ipsilateral knee and transferred to the damaged area. With osteochondral allograft transplantation, donor plugs from a fresh or prolonged fresh size-matched hemicondyle are used. This can be particularly beneficial during a combined ligament or meniscus procedure, because autograft transfer may add further insult to the knee. This technique is best for medium and large (>4 cm^2) lesions or those that are uncontained or associated with significant bony loss or subchondral edema in addition to the chondral disease.[4,18,55]

Whereas microfracture and osteochondral allograft transplants are most routinely used for condylar lesions in our practice, ACI is our preferred treatment for patellofemoral chondral defects. For patients with failed prior cartilage surgery on the medial and lateral femoral condyles, our preferred treatment is prolonged fresh osteochondral allograft transplantation. In patients with failed ACI for the patellofemoral joint, newer techniques such as DeNovo Natural Tissue (NT) Graft (Zimmer, Inc., Warsaw, IN/ISTO Technologies, Inc., St Louis, MO) are currently under investigation. Although each patient must be evaluated on a case-by-case basis, our general algorithm for osteochondral defects is as follows:

- Osteochondral lesion scoped for first time and noticed without prior awareness: debridement versus microfracture
  - If lesion is debrided only, then patient would be candidate for prolonged fresh osteochondral allograft graft in future if symptoms were to develop.
- Osteochondral lesion with bone marrow edema or failed prior cartilage surgery: osteochondral allograft transplantation
- Patellofemoral lesion: ACI with tibial tubercle osteotomy (realignment procedure)
  - Now also starting to use DeNovo NT for such lesions

Meniscal Deficiency, Chondral Defect, and Malalignment

Perhaps the most challenging clinical situation in the context of articular cartilage surgery is the triad of meniscal deficiency, chondral defect, and malalignment. As described earlier, patients with near-total meniscal deficiency who may benefit substantially from meniscal allograft transplantation have historically been contraindicated for this procedure if they are known to have a concomitant full-thickness chondral defect on the ipsilateral side.[56] Even if both meniscal deficiency and chondral defects are addressed concomitantly (single or staged approaches) as described earlier, a subset of patients will continue to have diminished outcomes because of malalignment and the resulting continuous overload of the involved compartment. Recently, successful outcomes have been reported in patients undergoing concomitant meniscus allograft transplantation, cartilage restoration, and realigning osteotomy.[1,2] Depending on the specific clinical situation, these procedures can be performed in a staged or concurrent fashion, each with potential issues (Table 68-2). With regard to the surgical technique and the appropriate order of procedures, several factors should be taken into consideration.

- For medial and lateral compartment procedures:
  - A diagnostic knee scope is used to confirm need for the planned operation.

TABLE 68-2. Pros and Cons of Concurrent and Staged Procedures

	Pros	Cons
Concurrent	One procedure	Longer surgical time (more complications, more postoperative stiffness)
Staged	Shorter procedures Potentially easier recoveries	Multiple operations (multiple anesthesia risks, multiple recoveries)

- Meniscal transplantation with technique of choice is then performed. An inside-out repair with use of vertical mattress sutures is performed; the sutures are tied in extension.
- Realigning osteotomy should be performed after meniscus allograft transplantation to protect the osteotomy from the abduction and adduction movements required during the meniscus transplantation.
- A midline incision is made and a medial vastus–sparing or lateral parapatellar arthrotomy is performed. Fresh osteochondral allograft transplantation is performed at the conclusion of the surgery.
- For patellofemoral procedures:
  - Longitudinal midline incision.
  - Lateral parapatellar arthrotomy.
  - Tibial tubercle osteotomy is performed first, with fixation with two 4.5 cortical screws.
  - If associated medial patellofemoral ligament reconstruction is performed, two 5-mm patellar holes are drilled to a depth of 20 mm. The hamstring allograft is fixed with two SwiveLock anchors (Arthrex, Naples, FL). The other end of the graft is passed through a 7-mm hole through the MPFL origin in the femur. Fixation is on the femoral side in the final step (after ACI).
  - The patella is everted and the ACI procedure is performed in the standard fashion.
  - Finally, fixation and tensioning of the MPFL graft on the femoral side are performed in the routine fashion.

Meniscal Deficiency or Chondral Defect with Ligamentous Deficiency

With regard to the patient with combined meniscus or cartilage defect and ligamentous deficiency, ligamentous repair or reconstruction is an appropriate and often necessary surgical option. One of the more challenging components of these procedures is determining whether a cartilage lesion found at the time of ligament reconstruction (e.g., a small, isolated, full-thickness medial femoral chondral defect noted arthroscopically during a planned ACL reconstruction) is truly symptomatic or whether it is simply an incidental finding. In the acutely ligamentously injured knee, chondral defects are rarely addressed with more than simple debridement or microfracture. In these patients it is considered appropriate to reconstruct the ligament and observe the newly discovered chondral lesion. It is possible, and even likely, that after appropriate rehabilitation for the ligament reconstruction, the patient may be completely pain and symptom free despite the presence of a known chondral defect. These clinical scenarios become more problematic as the time to ACL reconstruction increases, because both the frequency[57-59] and severity (i.e., pain) of meniscal and chondral injury[58,60,61] increase with increasing time to surgery. In the setting of chronic ACL deficiency and medial meniscus tear, it has been shown biomechanically that meniscus repair improves anterior-posterior tibial translation and overall rotatory stability.[62] Similarly, in the chronically ligament-deficient patient with a concomitant chondral lesion, it is more likely that addressing both the ligament and cartilage defects will improve pain and functional outcomes. In these patients, the order of procedures is important, with several key points as follows:

- If marrow stimulation or OATS is to be performed, a concomitant ligamentous reconstruction and cartilage repair or reconstruction can be performed.
- With combined meniscus transplantation and ACL repair, the ACL tunnels are made in the standard fashion. For medial transplants, the tibial tunnel is made as oblique as possible, with the lateral aspect of the tibial footprint entered to avoid interference with the slot.
- Complete the meniscus allograft transplantation procedure with use of the preferred technique (slot versus bone plugs).
- Pass the ACL graft and fix on the femoral side.
- Perform the osteochondral allograft transplantation procedure through medial or lateral arthrotomy.
- Perform tibial fixation of the ACL graft.

RESULTS

When the following procedures are performed individually for isolated pathology, there are numerous reports of good to excellent outcomes: osteotomies for malalignment,[24,46,63-67] ACL reconstruction for instability,[11,12,68-70] cartilage restoration for chondral disease,[71-73] and meniscus repair or transplantation for meniscal disease (Table 68-3).[14-17,74,76,77] In the setting of treatment for combined pathologies, the reported outcomes are not as consistent. As the number of problems in the knee increases, the outcomes are generally diminished, irrespective of the treatment employed. Central to the complexity of these clinical challenges is that all of these conditions

TABLE 68-3. Results of Knee Articular Complex Procedures

Author	No. of Patients	Procedure	Average Follow-up	Results
Gomoll et al[1] (2009)	7	Meniscus transplant, chondral repair, osteotomy	24 months	7/7 increased function 6/7 return to unrestricted activity
Cameron and Saha[74] (1997)	67	Meniscus transplant in 21 Meniscus transplant and ACL reconstruction in 5 Meniscus transplant and osteotomy in 34 Meniscus transplant, valgus HTO, and ACL reconstruction in 7	31 months	Meniscus transplant 91% good to excellent results Meniscus and ACL reconstruction 80% good to excellent results Meniscus transplant and osteotomy 85% good to excellent results Meniscus transplant, valgus HTO, and ACL reconstruction 86% good to excellent results
Farr et al[3] (2007)	36	Meniscus transplant, ACI	24 months	Four revisions, no difference between subgroups with ACL or osteotomy
Rue et al[4] (2008)	31	Meniscus transplant, cartilage restoration (52% ACI, 43% osteochondral allograft)	37 months	76% (80% ACI, 71% osteochondral allograft) satisfied with result and improved outcomes
Bhosale et al[75] (2007)	8	Meniscus transplant, ACI	38 months	75% improved function at 1 year, 62.5% improved at 3.2 years
Verdonk et al[43] (2006)	27	Meniscus transplant, osteotomy	10 years	83.3% survival at 10 years with osteotomy, 74.2% survival without
Harris et al[2] (2011)	110	Six different studies—meniscus transplant, cartilage restoration	Varied	12% of patients experienced failure; 85% of these were caused by the meniscus Four of the six studies showed improved outcomes with combined techniques. Two of the six studies showed that isolated procedures were better.

ACI, Autologous chondrocyte implantation; *ACL,* anterior cruciate ligament; *HTO,* high tibial osteotomy.

are essentially interrelated.[55] For example, chondral disease can be caused by malalignment, which leads to excessive stress on articular cartilage and meniscal pathology.

Currently, there are a limited number of outcome studies for combined procedures, and it is difficult to draw definitive conclusions based on the short- and long-term studies that are available. Gomoll and colleagues[1] reported on seven patients with concomitant meniscus transplantation, chondral repair, and osteotomy. In this clinical study, six of the seven patients returned to unrestricted activities, and all experienced significant increases in Knee Injury and Osteoarthritis Outcome Score (KOOS), International Knee Documentation Committee (IKDC) score, and Lysholm score at 24 months postoperatively. Cameron and Saha[74] reported on 63 patients (67 knees) undergoing meniscus transplantation with or without concomitant procedures. At 31 months postoperatively, 58 of 67 transplants (87%) knees had good to excellent results. Of note, in 21 knees with isolated meniscal transplantations, 91% had good to excellent outcomes. In five knees that underwent concomitant ACL reconstruction, 80% had good to excellent outcomes. In 34 knees that underwent concurrent osteotomy, 85% had good to

excellent outcomes. Finally, in seven knees that underwent concomitant osteotomy and ACL reconstruction, 86% had good to excellent outcomes. Farr and colleagues[3] reported on 36 patients who underwent concurrent meniscus transplantation and ACI. Of the 29 available for follow-up, 16 had additional concurrent procedures, including tibial tubercle osteotomy, ACL reconstruction, and/or HTO. The authors found significant improvements in outcome surveys, visual analogue pain scale scores, and patient satisfaction, with no differences found among subgroups. Within 2 years postoperatively, the authors reported four failures; the patients went on to undergo revision procedures. Rue and colleagues[4] reported on 31 knees with combined meniscus transplantation and cartilage restoration. Fifty-two percent underwent concomitant ACI, and 48% underwent osteochondral allograft. At 3.1 years postoperatively, 76% (80% ACI, 71% osteochondral allograft) were satisfied with their outcomes and showed statistically significant improvements in Lysholm and IKDC scores. There were no significant differences found between groups. Bhosale and colleagues[75] reported on eight patients who underwent concomitant ACI with meniscus allograft transplantation and reported 75% with improved function and pain relief at 1 year postoperatively and 62.5% with improved functional at 3.2 years postoperatively. Verdonk and colleagues[43] reviewed 27 patients who underwent medial meniscal transplantation and found that patients who also underwent HTO had significantly greater improvements in pain and functional scores than those who underwent isolated transplants. Of note, the 10-year survival rates were 83.3% for the group with a combined transplant and osteotomy versus 74.2% for the medial transplant only group.

Finally, as noted in the recent systematic review by Harris and colleagues,[2] 110 patients in six different studies underwent combined meniscal allograft transplantation and cartilage repair or restoration. All studies reported improvements in clinical outcomes; however, 12% of patients experienced failure of their combined procedure that necessitated revision surgery, and 85% of these failures were noted to be related to the meniscus procedure as opposed to the cartilage procedure.[2] Of note, improved outcomes in combined procedures as compared with isolated surgery were found in four of the six studies, whereas in two of the studies the outcomes of combined surgery were not as good as those of either procedure performed in isolation.

SUMMARY

Treatment of combined knee pathology is a challenging problem. The inter-relationship among malalignment, meniscus pathology, articular cartilage disease, and instability results in complex clinical scenarios. For successful operative management of these patients, proper patient selection is critical. Determining the cause of symptoms (predominantly pain) can be especially difficult in knees with multiple pathologies, and treating incidental lesions must be avoided. Current biomechanical and clinical studies suggest a role for combined surgical procedures (either single or staged), but further long-term studies are needed to determine if these results stand over time. In addition, further investigation into new meniscus replacement alternatives including bioactive scaffolds, synthetic implants, and tissue-engineered menisci as well as advances in cartilage restoration with scaffolds, particulated articular cartilage implantation (autograft or juvenile allograft donor), and stem cells will continue to create nonarthroplasty alternatives for young patients with advanced unicompartmental degenerative joint disease.

REFERENCES

1. Gomoll AH, Kang RW, Chen AL, et al. Triad of cartilage restoration for unicompartmental arthritis treatment in young patients: meniscus allograft transplantation, cartilage repair and osteotomy. *J Knee Surg.* 2009;22(2):137-141.

2. Harris JD, Cavo M, Brophy R, et al. Biological knee reconstruction: a systematic review of combined meniscal allograft transplantation and cartilage repair or restoration. *Arthroscopy.* 2011;27(3):409-418.

3. Farr J, Rawal A, Marberry KM. Concomitant meniscal allograft transplantation and autologous chondrocyte implantation: minimum 2-year follow-up. *Am J Sports Med.* 2007;35(9):1459-1466.

4. Rue JP, Yanke AB, Busam ML, et al. Prospective evaluation of concurrent meniscus transplantation and articular cartilage repair: minimum 2-year follow-up. *Am J Sports Med.* 2008;36(9):1770-1778.

5. Lee SJ, Aadalen KJ, Malaviya P, et al. Tibiofemoral contact mechanics after serial medial meniscectomies in the human cadaveric knee. *Am J Sports Med.* 2006;34(8):1334-1344.

6. McNicholas MJ, Rowley DI, McGurty D, et al. Total meniscectomy in adolescence. A thirty-year follow-up. *J Bone Joint Surg Br.* 2000;82(2):217-221.

7. Roos EM, Ostenberg A, Roos H, et al. Long-term outcome of meniscectomy: symptoms, function, and performance tests in patients with or without radiographic osteoarthritis compared to matched controls. *Osteoarthritis Cartilage.* 2001;9(4):316-324.

8. Roos H, Lauren M, Adalberth T, et al. Knee osteoarthritis after meniscectomy: prevalence of radiographic changes after twenty-one years, compared with matched controls. *Arthritis Rheum.* 1998;41(4):687-693.

9. Burks RT, Metcalf MH, Metcalf RW. Fifteen-year follow-up of arthroscopic partial meniscectomy. *Arthroscopy.* 1997;13(6):673-679.

10. Maletius W, Messner K. The effect of partial meniscectomy on the long-term prognosis of knees with localized, severe chondral damage. A twelve- to fifteen-year followup. *Am J Sports Med.* 1996;24(3):258-262.

11. Hart AJ, Buscombe J, Malone A, et al. Assessment of osteoarthritis after reconstruction of the anterior cruciate ligament: a study using single-photon emission computed tomography at ten years. *J Bone Joint Surg Br.* 2005;87(11):1483-1487.

12. Ruiz AL, Kelly M, Nutton RW. Arthroscopic ACL reconstruction: a 5-9 year follow-up. *Knee.* 2002;9(3):197-200.

13. Shirazi R, Shirazi-Adl A. Analysis of partial meniscectomy and ACL reconstruction in knee joint biomechanics under a combined loading. *Clin Biomech (Bristol, Avon).* 2009;24(9):755-761.

14. Kang RW, Lattermann C, Cole BJ. Allograft meniscus transplantation: background, indications, techniques, and outcomes. *J Knee Surg.* 2006;19(3):220-230.

15. Noyes FR, Barber-Westin SD. Meniscus transplantation: indications, techniques, clinical outcomes. *Instr Course Lect.* 2005;54:341-353.

16. Packer JD, Rodeo SA. Meniscal allograft transplantation. *Clin Sports Med.* 2009;28(2):259-283, viii.

17. Cole BJ, Carter TR, Rodeo SA. Allograft meniscal transplantation: background, techniques, and results. *Instr Course Lect.* 2003;52:383-396.

18. Cole BJ, Pascual-Garrido C, Grumet RC. Surgical management of articular cartilage defects in the knee. *J Bone Joint Surg Am.* 2009;91(7):1778-1790.

19. Sharma L, Eckstein F, Song J, et al. Relationship of meniscal damage, meniscal extrusion, malalignment, and joint laxity to subsequent cartilage loss in osteoarthritic knees. *Arthritis Rheum.* 2008;58(6):1716-1726.

20. Sharma L, Song J, Felson DT, et al. The role of knee alignment in disease progression and functional decline in knee osteoarthritis. *JAMA.* 2001;286(2):188-195.

21. Van Thiel G, Frank R, Gupta A, et al. Biomechanical evaluation of a high tibial ostetomy with a meniscal transplant. *8th World Congress of the International Cartilage Repair Society.* Miami, FL, 2009.

22. Verdonk PC, Demurie A, Almqvist KF, et al. Transplantation of viable meniscal allograft. Survivorship analysis and clinical outcome of one hundred cases. *J Bone Joint Surg Am.* 2005;87(4):715-724.

23. Anbari A. Proximal Tibial and distal femoral osteotomy. In: Cole B, Gomoll A, eds. *Biologic Joint Reconstruction: Alternatives to Arthroplasty.* Thorofare: Slack; 2009.

24. Wright JM, Crockett HC, Slawski DP, et al. High tibial osteotomy. *J Am Acad Orthop Surg.* 2005;13(4):279-289.

25. Brosset T, Pasquier G, Migaud H, et al. Opening wedge high tibial osteotomy performed without filling the defect but with locking plate fixation (TomoFix) and early weight-bearing: prospective evaluation of bone union, precision and maintenance of correction in 51 cases. *Orthop Traumatol Surg Res.* 2011;97(7):705-711.

26. Schroter S, Mueller J, van Heerwaarden R, et al. Return to work and clinical outcome after open wedge HTO. *Knee Surg Sports Traumatol Arthrosc.* 2012.

27. Meding JB, Keating EM, Ritter MA, et al. Total knee arthroplasty after high tibial osteotomy. *Clin Orthop Relat Res.* 2000(375):175-184.

28. Meding JB, Wing JT, Ritter MA. Does high tibial osteotomy affect the success or survival of a total knee replacement? *Clin Orthop Relat Res.* 2011;469(7):1991-1994.

29. van Raaij TM, Bakker W, Reijman M, et al. The effect of high tibial osteotomy on the results of total knee arthroplasty: a matched case control study. *BMC Musculoskelet Disord.* 2007;8:74.

30. van Raaij TM, Reijman M, Furlan AD, et al. Total knee arthroplasty after high tibial osteotomy. A systematic review. *BMC Musculoskelet Disord.* 2009;10:88.

31. Minas T. Autologous chondrocyte implantation in the arthritic knee. *Orthopedics.* 2003;26(9):945-947.

32. Minas T. The role of cartilage repair techniques, including chondrocyte transplantation, in focal chondral knee damage. *Instr Course Lect.* 1999;48:629-643.

33. Gallo RA, Feeley BT. Cartilage defects of the femoral trochlea. *Knee Surg Sports Traumatol Arthrosc.* 2009;17(11):1316-1325.

34. Sterett WI, Steadman JR. Chondral resurfacing and high tibial osteotomy in the varus knee. *Am J Sports Med.* 2004;32(5):1243-1249.

35. Sterett WI, Steadman JR, Huang MJ, et al. Chondral resurfacing and high tibial osteotomy in the varus knee: survivorship analysis. *Am J Sports Med.* 2010;38(7):1420-1424.

36. Van Thiel GS, Frank RM, Gupta A, et al. Biomechanical evaluation of a high tibial osteotomy with a meniscal transplant. *J Knee Surg.* 2011;24(1):45-53.

37. Verma NN, Kolb E, Cole BJ, et al. The effects of medial meniscal transplantation techniques on intra-articular contact pressures. *J Knee Surg.* 2008;21(1):20-26.

38. Willey M, Wolf BR, Kocaglu B, et al. Complications associated with realignment osteotomy of the knee performed simultaneously with additional reconstructive procedures. *Iowa Orthop J.* 2011;30:55-60.

39. Bonasia DE, Amendola A. Combined medial meniscal transplantation and high tibial osteotomy. *Knee Surg Sports Traumatol Arthrosc.* 2010;18(7):870-873.

40. Garrett JC. Meniscal transplantation. *Am J Knee Surg.* 1996;9(1):32-34.

41. Noyes FR, Barber-Westin SD, Hewett TE. High tibial osteotomy and ligament reconstruction for varus angulated anterior cruciate ligament-deficient knees. *Am J Sports Med.* 2000;28(3):282-296.

42. Peters G, Wirth CJ. The current state of meniscal allograft transplantation and replacement. *Knee.* 2003;10(1):19-31.

43. Verdonk PC, Verstraete KL, Almqvist KF, et al. Meniscal allograft transplantation: long-term clinical results with radiological and magnetic resonance imaging correlations. *Knee Surg Sports Traumatol Arthrosc.* 2006;14(8):694-706.

44. Giffin JR, Vogrin TM, Zantop T, et al. Effects of increasing tibial slope on the biomechanics of the knee. *Am J Sports Med.* 2004;32(2):376-382.

45. Morgan MC, Gillespie B, Dedrick D. Survivorship analysis of total knee arthroplasty. Cumulative rates of survival of 9200 total knee arthroplasties. *J Bone Joint Surg Am.* 1992;74(2):308-309.

46. Coventry MB, Ilstrup DM, Wallrichs SL. Proximal tibial osteotomy. A critical long-term study of eighty-seven cases. *J Bone Joint Surg Am.* 1993;75(2):196-201.

47. Efe T, Ahmed G, Heyse TJ, et al. Closing-wedge high tibial osteotomy: survival and risk factor analysis at long-term follow up. *BMC Musculoskelet Disord.* 2011;12:46.

48. Miller BS, Downie B, McDonough EB, et al. Complications after medial opening wedge high tibial osteotomy. *Arthroscopy.* 2009;25(6):639-646.

49. Spahn G. Complications in high tibial (medial opening wedge) osteotomy. *Arch Orthop Trauma Surg.* 2004;124(10):649-653.

50. Alford JW, Lewis P, Kang RW, et al. Rapid progression of chondral disease in the lateral compartment of the knee following meniscectomy. *Arthroscopy.* 2005;21(12):1505-1509.

51. Brophy RH, Matava MJ. Surgical options for meniscal replacement. *J Am Acad Orthop Surg.* 2012;20(5):265-272.

52. Lee AS, Kang RW, Kroin E, et al. Allograft meniscus transplantation. *Sports Med Arthrosc.* 2012;20(2):106-114.

53. Steadman JR, Miller BS, Karas SG, et al. The microfracture technique in the treatment of full-thickness chondral lesions of the knee in National Football League players. *J Knee Surg.* 2003;16(2):83-86.

54. Steadman JR, Rodkey WG, Briggs KK. Microfracture to treat full-thickness chondral defects: surgical technique, rehabilitation, and outcomes. *J Knee Surg.* 2002;15(3):170-176.

55. Cole BJ, Harner CD. Degenerative arthritis of the knee in active patients: evaluation and management. *J Am Acad Orthop Surg.* 1999;7(6):389-402.

56. Alford W, Cole BJ. The indications and technique for meniscal transplant. *Orthop Clin North Am.* 2005;36(4):469-484.

57. Chhadia AM, Inacio MC, Maletis GB, et al. Are meniscus and cartilage injuries related to time to anterior cruciate ligament reconstruction? *Am J Sports Med.* 2011;39(9):1894-1899.

58. Slauterbeck JR, Kousa P, Clifton BC, et al. Geographic mapping of meniscus and cartilage lesions associated with anterior cruciate ligament injuries. *J Bone Joint Surg Am.* 2009;91(9):2094-2103.

59. Tayton E, Verma R, Higgins B, et al. A correlation of time with meniscal tears in anterior cruciate ligament deficiency: stratifying the risk of surgical delay. *Knee Surg Sports Traumatol Arthrosc.* 2009;17(1):30-34.

60. Fok AW, Yau WP. Delay in ACL reconstruction is associated with more severe and painful meniscal and chondral injuries. *Knee Surg Sports Traumatol Arthrosc.* 2012;21:928-933.

61. Maffulli N, Binfield PM, King JB. Articular cartilage lesions in the symptomatic anterior cruciate ligament-deficient knee. *Arthroscopy.* 2003;19(7):685-690.

62. Ahn JH, Bae TS, Kang KS, et al. Longitudinal tear of the medial meniscus posterior horn in the anterior cruciate ligament-deficient knee significantly influences anterior stability. *Am J Sports Med.* 2011;39(10):2187-2193.

63. Coventry MB. Upper tibial osteotomy for osteoarthritis. *J Bone Joint Surg Am.* 1985;67(7):1136-1140.

64. Gardiner A, Gutierrez Sevilla GR, Steiner ME, et al. Osteotomies about the knee for tibiofemoral malalignment in the athletic patient. *Am J Sports Med.* 2010;38(5):1038-1047.

65. Preston CF, Fulkerson EW, Meislin R, et al. Osteotomy about the knee: applications, techniques, and results. *J Knee Surg.* 2005;18(4):258-272.

66. Wolcott M. Osteotomies around the knee for the young athlete with osteoarthritis. *Clin Sports Med.* 2005;24(1):153-161.

67. Wolcott M, Traub S, Efird C. High tibial osteotomies in the young active patient. *Int Orthop.* 2010;34(2):161-166.

68. Asano H, Muneta T, Ikeda H, et al. Arthroscopic evaluation of the articular cartilage after anterior cruciate ligament reconstruction: a short-term prospective study of 105 patients. *Arthroscopy.* 2004;20(5):474-481.

69. Kessler MA, Behrend H, Henz S, et al. Function, osteoarthritis and activity after ACL-rupture: 11 years follow-up results of conservative versus reconstructive treatment. *Knee Surg Sports Traumatol Arthrosc.* 2008;16(5):442-448.

70. Louboutin H, Debarge R, Richou J, et al. Osteoarthritis in patients with anterior cruciate ligament rupture: a review of risk factors. *Knee.* 2009;16(4):239-244.

71. Alford JW, Cole BJ. Cartilage restoration, part 1: basic science, historical perspective, patient evaluation, and treatment options. *Am J Sports Med.* 2005;33(2):295-306.

73. Buckwalter JA, Mankin HJ. Articular cartilage: degeneration and osteoarthritis, repair, regeneration, and transplantation. *Instr Course Lect.* 1998;47:487-504.

72. Alford JW, Cole BJ. Cartilage restoration, part 2: techniques, outcomes, and future directions. *Am J Sports Med.* 2005;33(3):443-460.

74. Cameron JC, Saha S. Meniscal allograft transplantation for unicompartmental arthritis of the knee. *Clin Orthop Relat Res.* 1997(337):164-171.

75. Bhosale AM, Myint P, Roberts S, et al. Combined autologous chondrocyte implantation and allogenic meniscus transplantation: a biological knee replacement. *Knee.* 2007;14(5):361-368.

76. Hergan D, Thut D, Sherman O, et al. Meniscal allograft transplantation. *Arthroscopy.* 2010.

77. Noyes FR, Barber-Westin SD, Rankin M. Meniscal transplantation in symptomatic patients less than fifty years old. *J Bone Joint Surg Am.* 2004;86-A(7):1392-1404.

Autologous Chondrocyte Implantation in the Knee

Scott D. Gillogly and Andrew Gelven

Chapter Synopsis

- Autologous chondrocyte implantation (ACI) is indicated for symptomatic full-thickness chondral defects of the knee in patients 15 to 50 years of age (up to 55 years in some cases). Although diagnostic imaging and examination are important, arthroscopic assessment provides the final confirmation of the appropriateness of this biologic treatment for cartilage repair. A chondral biopsy is performed to obtain patient's healthy cartilage to grow sufficient cells for reimplantation at the second stage of the open cell implantation technique. Postoperative rehabilitation allows for protection and stimulation of the maturing chondrocytes, ensuring the best opportunity for return to improved symptom-free function.

Important Points

Indications

- Symptomatic predominantly full-thickness chondral defects (grade III to IV lesions) and osteochondritis dissecans lesions of the femoral condyles and trochlea
- Medium to large focal lesions, typically larger than 2.5 cm^2

Contraindications

- Advanced or diffuse osteoarthritis
- Bipolar sclerotic bone-on-bone "kissing" cartilage lesions
- Inflammatory arthropathy

Symptoms of Chondral Defects

- Pain with weight bearing or increased loading
- Pain with stairs or getting into and out of a chair for patellofemoral defects
- Complaints of mechanical symptoms such as locking, catching, or giving way; point tenderness in the involved area
- Recurrent swelling

Surgical Technique Highlights

- Chondral biopsy is required initially for the autologous chondrocytes to be cultured and grown.
- ACI is an open procedure requiring adequate exposure.
- The defect(s) is prepared by sharply demarcating the edge of the defect and removing all degenerated cartilage remnants down through the calcified cartilage layer without violating the subchondral plate.
- The defect is sized by making a template and transferring the size and shape to the covering membrane of periosteum or an absorbable type I/III collagen membrane.
- The covering membrane is sutured to the edges of the defect and sealed with fibrin glue to make a watertight seal.
- Autologous cells are then injected under the membrane and the injection site closed and sealed.
- Continuous passive motion is an early key component of an extensive rehabilitation process that maximizes the maturation of the chondrocytes.

Clinical and Surgical Pearls

- Adequate exposure is paramount to consistent defect preparation and cell implantation.
- Defects with uncontained edges may require alternate methods to securely attach the covering membrane, such as micro–suture anchors or drill holes through bone.
- Perform any concomitant procedures before completing the cell implantation, which should be the last portion of the procedure.
- Ensure that the defect is debrided back to a rim of the healthiest-appearing remaining cartilage, allowing a stable firm edge to which to suture the covering membrane.

Continued

Clinical and Surgical Pitfalls

- Paramount to biologic repair of an articular cartilage defect is establishing the most "normal" or balanced intra-articular environment within the knee.
- Requires that mechanical alignment, ligamentous stability, and meniscal function be optimally treated either before or concomitantly with ACI.
- Multiple defects can be treated with ACI at the same implantation.

- Early emphasis on range of motion helps prevent the potential complication of flexion or extension contracture.
- The use of an absorbable type I/III collagen membrane has greatly diminished the complication of graft hypertrophy requiring arthroscopic debridement, seen in about 25% of patients when their periosteum was used as a covering membrane.

Articular cartilage defects are often seen during knee arthroscopy and are noted on magnetic resonance imaging (MRI) with relative frequency in young athletes.[1,2] When the defects are symptomatic, they can cause disability comparable with that associated with advanced knee osteoarthritis.[3] Despite the frequency of articular cartilage injury, methods for treatment of the cartilaginous lesions did not produce good long-term results until the development of the technique by Peterson and colleagues of autologous chondrocyte implantation (ACI), first reported in 1994, which has gained a major role in the treatment of large full-thickness chondral injuries.[4] Results are now available with up to 20 years of follow-up, and more than 75% of the patients have had improvement with relatively minor complications.[4-11] In this technique, a small biopsy specimen of healthy chondral tissue is obtained arthroscopically; this specimen then undergoes in vitro chondrocyte amplification in cell culture, returning autologous chondrocyte cells available for implantation into the defect at the second stage of the repair procedure. The goal with use of autologous chondrocytes is to produce a repair tissue that more closely resembles the morphologic characteristics of the type II hyaline cartilage, thus restoring the durability and natural function of the knee joint.[4,12,13]

PREOPERATIVE CONSIDERATIONS

History (Signs and Symptoms)

An adequate history is the initial step in determining whether ACI is the appropriate treatment for a suspected chondral defect. Patients with femoral condylar lesions commonly have pain with weight bearing or increased loading and mechanical symptoms such as catching, locking, or giving way. Persistent or intermittent swelling is also a common complaint. Often patients are able to localize the area of pain or tenderness. The presence of a patellofemoral defect will produce similar complaints, but with symptoms exacerbated by stairs, getting into and out of a chair or car, and anterior knee pain. Patellar subluxation symptoms are often present as well. It is prudent to match the patient's complaints to the location of the chondral defect to determine that the symptoms are originating from the defect and are not caused by other, coexisting pathology. Finally, individual patient characteristics must be considered in the treatment planning; these include age, body mass index, concomitant knee pathology, smoking, compliance, and expectations. With known chondral defects, additional information is frequently available through previous operative reports and intraoperative images. This will give some indication of the size, location, and number of defects present within the knee. Taking advantage of any available information will help in determining the suitability of the defect for ACI.

Physical Examination

Physical examination is helpful to match the patient's symptoms to the location of the actual defect. Basic observation of gait and gross alignment provide information about the patient's level of function. A thorough evaluation of the knee can quickly establish the presence of an effusion, determine any ligamentous instability or motion deficits, and reveal areas of tenderness with palpation or provocative testing. Should there be questions regarding the examination findings, MRI can provide additional information. Evaluation of the menisci includes provocative meniscal tests and an assessment of radiographs and possibly MRI scans.

Imaging

To adequately evaluate a patient for any cartilage treatment including ACI, it is imperative that weight-bearing anteroposterior (AP) and 45-degree posteroanterior (PA) views be obtained. In addition, patellar alignment radiographs should be obtained with lateral and sunrise views. This allows evaluation of the alignment of the tibiofemoral and patellofemoral portions of the knee and gives an indication of any underlying bone involvement associated with the defect. A long-leg limb alignment radiographic view should be used to assess the mechanical axis and determine the potential need for realignment (Fig. 69-1). The greater availability of office-based digital imaging has made obtaining these long-limb alignment views very practical. As mentioned, MRI can then be used to assess for the presence of both ligamentous injury and damage to the menisci, as well as to define the degree of subchondral bone involvement. Increased signal and edema of a chronic nature in the subchondral bone may indicate persistent overload of the involved compartment and may indicate the need for a realignment procedure in addition to ACI. Bone loss of more than 7 to 8 mm in depth necessitates bone grafting before or at the time of cell implantation. Although MRI is helpful to evaluate subchondral bone loss and the soft tissues of the knee, owing to the wide variations in magnetic resonance field strengths and imaging protocols, at present it does not have consistent sensitivity or specificity to evaluate the full extent of chondral injury or other, more subtle changes to the cartilage.

Indications and Contraindications[4,5,8,14,15]

ACI is indicated for symptomatic, full-thickness chondral lesions and osteochondritis dissecans (OCD) lesions of the femoral condyles and trochlea in physiologically young patients (aged 15 to 55 years) who can be compliant with the rehabilitation protocol (Fig. 69-2). Results of treatment of chondral injuries of the patella with ACI have become much more consistently favorable with realignment and appropriate patellar tracking. ACI is not indicated as a treatment for advanced osteoarthritis or in the presence of bipolar sclerotic bone-on-bone lesions (Fig. 69-3). ACI is also contraindicated in active inflammatory arthritis or infection. In summary, the prerequisites for a successful outcome in treatment of a full-thickness focal chondral defect with ACI include appropriate bony alignment, ligamentous stability, meniscal function, adequate motion and muscle strength, and patient compliance without significant arthritic changes.

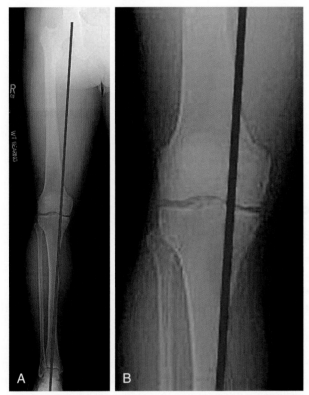

Figure 69-1. A, Long-limb alignment view with mechanical axis in place from center of femoral head to center of ankle. **B,** Note that line passes through the medial compartment on the expanded view, indicating varus malalignment and the need for osteotomy in conjunction with any autologous chondrocyte implantation of the medial femoral condyle.

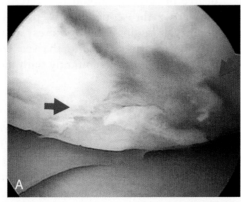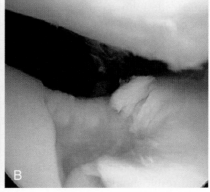

Figure 69-2. Appropriate indications for autologous chondrocyte implantation with traumatic femoral condyle lesion in **A** and a traumatic trochlear lesion in **B.**

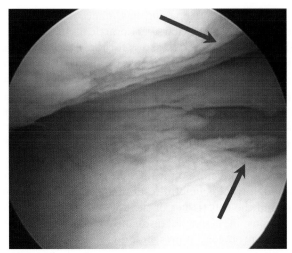

Figure 69-3. Note the bipolar exposed bone and diffusely thinned articular cartilage on the femoral condyle and tibia *(arrows)*. This is *not* an appropriate indication for autologous chondrocyte implantation.

BOX 69-1 Surgical Steps

Stage 1: Arthroscopic Assessment and Chondral Biopsy
- The knee is thoroughly evaluated in all three compartments.
- If a chondral lesion is considered appropriate for autologous chondrocyte implantation (ACI), a biopsy specimen is obtained.

Stage 2: (Open) Autologous Chondrocyte Implantation
- Arthrotomy
- Defect preparation
- Periosteal harvest
- Periosteum or covering membrane fixation
- Watertight sealing of the periosteal or cover membrane graft
- Implantation of chondrocytes
- Wound closure

SURGICAL TECHNIQUE

Anesthesia and Positioning

Typically ACI is performed with general anesthesia augmented by use of peripheral nerve blocks for postoperative pain management. In general, we prefer to have the peripheral block in place before initiation of the procedure. The peripheral block is either a femoral or sciatic block or both. Depending on the complexity of the procedure (multiple lesions or concomitant bony procedures), we have had high patient satisfaction with use of a catheter pain pump for the peripheral block for 2 to 3 days postoperatively.

The patient is placed on the operating table in the supine position. The involved lower extremity is positioned so that the knee may be placed into maximum flexion if necessary, and rests with the foot on a sandbag or other positioning device so that the knee is at 90 degrees of flexion. Prophylactic antibiotics are routinely used. After preparation and draping, a midline incision is generally recommended, followed by a medial or lateral parapatellar arthrotomy, exposing the corresponding chondral injury for condyle defects. For patellar defects and many trochlear defects, the patella is generally reflected superiorly through a tibial tubercle osteotomy that is commonly performed for purposes of patellofemoral realignment. As with any surgical procedure, good exposure is critical for performance of the intended technique and good outcome. The approach must allow the surgeon access to properly suture the covering membrane to the chondral defect with 6-0 Vicryl suture. The end result should never be compromised for the sake of an ill-advised concern for keeping the approach small.

Surgical Landmarks, Incisions, and Portals

- Tibial tubercle
- Inferior, lateral, and medial poles of the patella
- Patellar tendon
- Lateral femoral condyle (LFC) and medial femoral condyle (MFC)
- Tibial plateau

Prior incisions must be taken into account; at least a 5- to 7-cm skin bridge should be left between incisions.

Examination Under Anesthesia and Diagnostic Studies

An examination of the knee with the patient under general anesthesia is beneficial in revealing pathology such as ligamentous laxity in the relaxed patient. This degree of scrutiny should be exercised during the preliminary arthroscopic biopsy procedure so that any abnormal finding that requires surgical intervention may be incorporated into the second-stage operation and performed concomitantly with the ACI procedure.

Specific Steps

Box 69-1 describes the specific steps of this procedure.

ACI is a two-staged procedure. The first stage is intended for the chondral biopsy but also serves as a determination of the suitability of the chondral lesion for ACI. At this time the size, location, and depth of the defect, the status of the surrounding articular cartilage and underlying bone, and the status of the opposing chondral surfaces are all definitively evaluated. Containment of the defect as well as determination of other pathologies that might require treatment for optimal ACI results are assessed. Typically the defects treated by this technique are larger than 2.5 cm²; the average size in our series has been well over 5.6 cm².[4,8,16-18]

Stage 1: Arthroscopic Assessment and Chondral Biopsy

A standard arthroscopic approach to the knee is used. The knee must be thoroughly evaluated in all three compartments. Any coexisting pathology should be noted, and plans are made to address any deficiencies either before or concomitantly with the ACI procedure. Examination under anesthesia again confirms previous clinical assessments.

If a chondral lesion is considered appropriate for ACI, a biopsy is performed. The most common sites are the superomedial edge of the MFC or the superolateral edge of the LFC that is non–weight bearing and nonarticulating with the tibia or patella. Other frequently biopsied areas are the intercondylar notch of the MFC and LFC; the procedure is much like notchplasty for anterior cruciate ligament (ACL) reconstruction, except only the appropriate amount of full-thickness healthy cartilage is removed during the biopsy. An arthroscopic gouge or ring curette is used to obtain several slivers of full-thickness cartilage, each approximately the size of a pencil eraser (i.e., 5 mm by 10 mm)—about 200 to 300 mg of tissue. After the slivers have been removed from the knee, they are placed in the biopsy medium and shipping vial in a sterile fashion. For the final autologous cultured chondrocytes to be obtained, the cartilage is enzymatically digested, and the approximately 200,000 to 300,000 cells contained in the cartilage sample are amplified to approximately 12 million cells per 0.4 mL of culture medium. This takes approximately 6 weeks, but the process can be interrupted after 2 weeks by cryopreservation if necessary. Up to 1.2 mL (48 million cells) can be obtained through standard culture, but additional cells can be obtained with additional cell passage.[14]

Stage 2: (Open) Autologous Chondrocyte Implantation[4,19,18]

Arthrotomy

A standard medial or lateral parapatellar incision and arthrotomy are used for exposure. As with any surgical procedure, exposure is essential. If the lesion is located on the central portion of the condyle, a mini-arthrotomy can be used. For larger or hard-to-reach chondral injuries, a midline incision with a medial or lateral parapatellar arthrotomy and eversion of the patella can be used. This may be especially useful when the lesion is on the posterior portion of the condyles. One can use a subvastus approach rather than cutting the quadriceps tendon when feasible, although it does not seem to alter the postoperative course.

Defect Preparation

During debridement of the defect, all damaged and unhealthy appearing cartilage, calcified cartilage, and fibrocartilage must be removed. Any thinned, fissured, or damaged surrounding cartilage needs to be debrided to an edge, leaving healthy firm articular cartilage (Fig. 69-4). Bleeding may introduce stem cells and fibroblasts into the defect and dilute the chondrocyte population. When minor punctate bleeding is encountered in the base of the defect, it can be controlled with thrombin or epinephrine-soaked Neuro Patties sponges, fibrin glue, or low-wattage electrocautery. The goal of adequate debridement of the defect is to have a dry bed with clean subchondral bone and a healthy, sharply demarcated surrounding cartilage border at the periphery. This is best accomplished by scoring of the periphery of the defect with a No. 15 scalpel blade and use of curettes to remove the damaged tissue. Our method for obtaining the correct size for the periosteal or cover membrane graft is to create a template from sterile paper (glove wrapper) (Fig. 69-5). Alternatively, the foil from a suture pack can be molded to the defect, which also creates an accurate template. The template is cut, oversizing by 1 to 1.5 mm around the circumference because the harvested periosteum tends to contract. When absorbable collagen membrane is used, there is no need to oversize the patch.

Periosteal Harvest

If periosteum is chosen for the covering membrane, the harvest is performed beginning at the proximal medial tibia, two fingerbreadths distal to the pes anserinus and medial collateral ligament insertion on the subcutaneous border. An incision is made just anterior to the posterior border of the tibia. All fat and fascia layers should be removed from the periosteum with both sharp and blunt dissection with a moist sponge. Leaving the thin fascia layer on the periosteum is one of the most common mistakes in harvesting the periosteal graft. The template is then placed over the exposed periosteum, and a scalpel (No. 15 blade) is used to sharply demarcate the periosteal graft. A sharp curved periosteal elevator is used to gently elevate the periosteum off the bone.

Although use of a periosteal patch is the only method currently approved by the U.S. Food and Drug Administration (FDA), use of a periosteal graft for a covering membrane has been abandoned in Europe and the rest of the world because of the propensity of periosteum to produce graft hypertrophy necessitating arthroscopic debridement in more than 25% of patients.[14] An alternative option to periosteum for covering the defect and

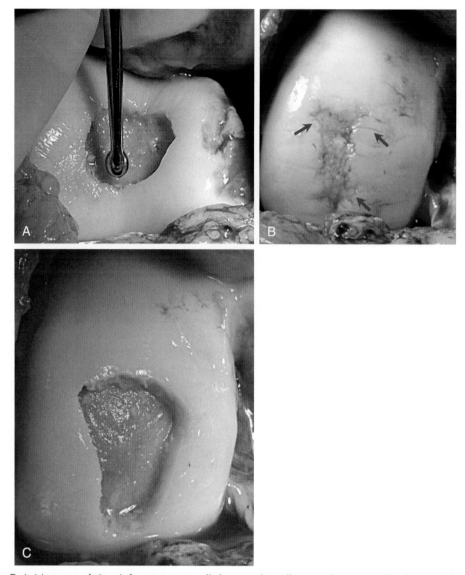

Figure 69-4. A, Debridement of the defect removes all damaged cartilage and exposes the bone without penetration of the subchondral bone. It is easiest to accomplish with small curettes as shown. **B,** Note the fissures and unstable cartilage *(arrows)* extending from edges of obvious full-thickness areas. **C,** All unstable and damaged cartilage needs to be debrided back to a stable rim of healthy articular cartilage for completion of the preparation for cell implantation.

containing the cells is an absorbable "off-the-shelf" collagen membrane. Fortunately, there have been good clinical outcomes with a less than 2% reoperation rate with the collagen membrane covering. The membrane is FDA approved for other indications, but its use is "off label" for ACI at the discretion of the surgeon and patient. We have used the collagen membrane exclusively for the past 3 years with excellent results, a 1% reoperation rate, and easier return to full motion postoperatively.[14]

Periosteum or Covering Membrane Fixation

The covering membrane (periosteum or absorbable collagen membrane patch) is aligned over the defect in the orientation matching the template with the cambium layer or deep layer facing the defect. The membrane is then sutured to the cartilage rim with multiple 6-0 Vicryl interrupted sutures spaced every 2 to 3 mm (Fig. 69-6). If the defect is uncontained—meaning that there is not a circumferential rim of healthy cartilage through which sutures can be passed—suture anchors may be used to attach the periosteal graft on the uncontained side. The knots should be tied on the membrane side, not over the surface of the cartilage, thus minimizing any friction or toggling that could cause loosening of the knots. Redundant membrane graft can be trimmed while the patch is being secured, ensuring that even tension is maintained on the graft. A small opening is maintained on one edge of the graft to allow injection of chondrocyte cells.

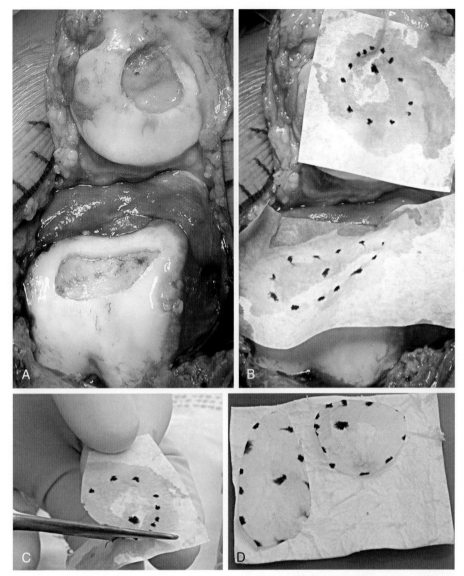

Figure 69-5. A, Defects of the trochlea and patella after debridement. **B** and **C,** Sterile glove paper is used to make a paper template of the exact size of the defect, which can then be cut out on the back table. **D,** Paper templates used as guides to then cut out either periosteal graft or, in this example, the absorbable collagen covering membrane.

Watertight Sealing of the Periosteal or Cover Membrane Graft

The watertight integrity of the secured graft can be tested with an 18-gauge catheter and a saline-filled 1-mL syringe placed deep to the periosteum through the small opening. Additional sutures can be placed as necessary to ensure a watertight seal. The suture line at the periosteal–cover membrane graft edge is then sealed with fibrin glue; one of the commercially available preparations is used.

Implantation of Chondrocytes

The sterile cells are aspirated from the shipping vial into a 1-mL syringe with use of sterile technique. The autologous chondrocytes are then introduced through the syringe with an 18-gauge plastic angiocatheter and injected under the membrane graft (see Fig. 69-6). The injection site is then closed with one or two additional sutures and sealed with fibrin glue. No additional manipulation of the joint should follow the implantation.

Wound Closure

The arthrotomy and wound are then closed in a layered fashion, and a soft sterile dressing and knee immobilizer are applied to the knee. A drain is not typically used so as not to create any suction on the graft. Wound hemostasis should be achieved in routine fashion.

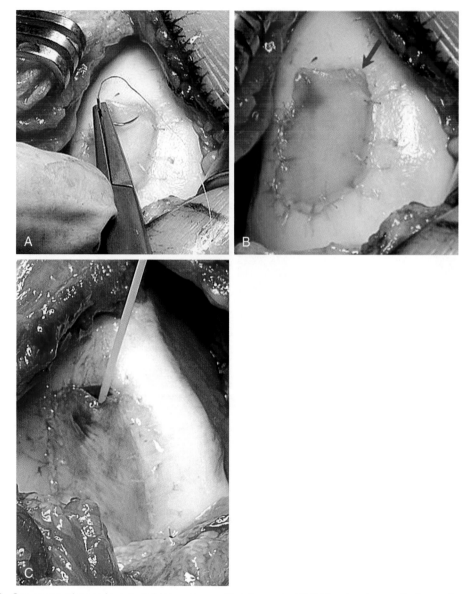

Figure 69-6. **A,** Cover membrane is sutured into place with interrupted 6-0 Vicryl sutures. **B,** A small opening *(arrow)* is left for the cells to be injected. **C,** The cells are injected under the membrane cover with a plastic angiocatheter. The injection site is then closed with an additional suture and fibrin glue, which seals the entire edge (circumference of membrane cover-cartilage interface).

Combined Procedures[12,11,17]

- Tibiofemoral malalignment: osteotomy (Fig. 69-7)
  - Addressed at the time of ACI
  - Overcorrection generally not required; off-loading is generally all that is desired
  - Suturing of the periosteum and implantation of the cells are completed after the osteotomy is fixed
- Ligamentous insufficiency: ligament reconstruction
  Ligament reconstruction should be performed first by the normal method (arthroscopic ACL reconstruction before arthrotomy), then the ACI is performed. This protects the periosteal or membrane cover graft.

The ACI rehabilitation program is the overriding protocol postoperatively.
- Meniscal deficiency: meniscal transplantation
  - Considered in knees that have undergone a total meniscectomy in the same compartment as the chondral injury.
  - Meniscal transplantation in younger patients versus osteotomy in older patients with long-standing meniscectomy.
  - Again, meniscal transplantation should be performed first with the surgeon's preferred technique, and the ACI should follow to prevent disruption of the periosteal graft by any necessary manipulation.

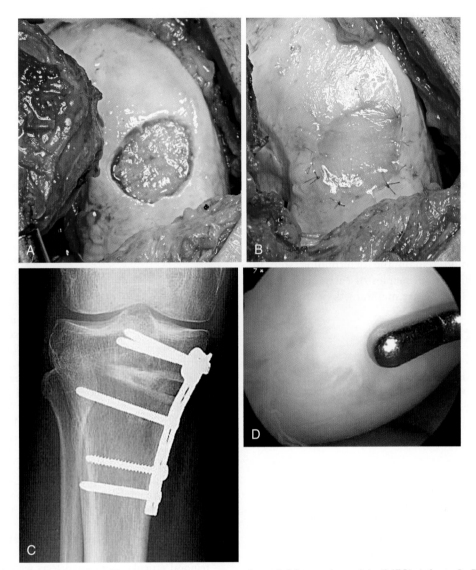

Figure 69-7. A 35-year-old male with varus malalignment and medial femoral condyle (MFC) defect. **A,** Defect in MFC. **B** and **C,** Defect treated with autologous chondrocyte implantation and concomitant medial opening wedge high tibial osteotomy. **D,** Second-look arthroscopy 11 months postoperatively during hardware removal shows defect fully filled with repair tissue with firmness to probing of the surrounding normal articular cartilage.

- Patellofemoral malalignment: anteromedialization of tibial tubercle
  - May perform realignment at initial arthroscopy if ACI is not to be performed in the patellofemoral joint. Otherwise, perform realignment at time of ACI; the defect is more readily approached when the patella and tendon are reflected proximally by detaching the tubercle osteotomy and turning it cranially.
  - After the ACI the tubercle is attached with lag technique in the predetermined position for realignment.
- Bone deficiency: bone grafting
  - Autologous bone graft placed in debrided defect bed

  - ACI 4 to 6 months after bone graft, allowing for bone graft incorporation

POSTOPERATIVE CONSIDERATIONS

Rehabilitation[5,8,20]

- Continuous passive motion (CPM) is started within 24 hours of implantation.
- Initial touch-down weight bearing is usually progressed to full weight bearing after 4 to 6 weeks.
- Early strengthening should include quadriceps, hip abductor, and core muscle exercises performed in non–weight-bearing positions.

- Progress to balance and proprioception exercises as soon as weight-bearing limits allow.
- Impact loading activities start after 6 to 8 months.
- Patellar and trochlear defect repairs are protected from open chain exercises and shear loading for at least the first 3 months.

Rehabilitation after ACI is based on the maturation process of the chondrocytes, the size of the defect, and the location of the defect.[5,19] The concept of a slow gradual maturation of the repair tissue is crucial to understanding the rehabilitation after ACI.[5] The hyaline-like repair tissue must be both protected and stimulated to allow the maturation and remodeling of the tissue in the proper manner. When multiple procedures are performed, ACI should remain the determining step in rehabilitation while the principles of early motion and progressive joint loading are maintained.

Complications[6,18]

- Arthrofibrosis (2%)
- Graft failure or delamination (1.4%)
- Periosteal overgrowth (1.3% to 25%)
- Mechanical symptoms (1%)
- Infection (1%)

RESULTS

Peterson and colleagues recently published findings from long-term follow-up of 10 to 20 years for 224 patients treated with ACI. Seventy-four percent rated their status as better or the same as in the previous years. Overall, 92% were satisfied with their outcome and would undergo ACI again.[10] In a study by Rosenberger and colleagues that looked at 56 patients older than 45 who underwent ACI for full-thickness chondral defects of the knee with an average follow-up of 4.7 years, 72% of patients rated themselves as good or excellent. In addition, 78% felt improved from baseline and 81% would elect ACI again for treatment of their chondral defects.[11]

ACI is also used to treat patellofemoral cartilage defects. Pascual-Garrido and colleagues examined 62 patients treated with ACI of patellofemoral defects with or without a realignment procedure. At 4 years' follow-up, significant improvement was seen in Lysholm, Knee Injury and Osteoarthritis Outcome Scale (KOOS), International Knee Documentation Committee (IKDC), Tegner, Cincinnati, and Short Form 12 physical outcome scores. Association with prior failed cartilage procedures showed no significant difference, but association with anteromedialization procedures did trend toward better outcomes.[7]

These results show strong objective and subjective satisfaction in patients and their treating physicians.

The mechanical durability of ACI cartilage also appears to be significantly greater compared with fibrocartilage regeneration techniques as evaluated by second-look arthroscopy and duration of satisfactory results.[8,9,15,21,22] Overall, ACI is a reliable and consistent treatment option in the armamentarium of the orthopedic surgeon treating cartilage injuries.

REFERENCES

1. Curl WW, Krome J, Gordon ES, et al. Cartilage injuries: a review of 31,516 knee arthroscopies. *Arthroscopy.* 1997;13:456-460.
2. Hirshorn KC, Cates T, Gillogly S. Magnetic resonance imaging documented chondral injuries about the knee in college football players: 3 year National Football League combined data. *Arthroscopy.* 2010;26:1237-1240.
3. Heir S, Nerhus TK, Røtterud JH, et al. Focal cartilage defects in the knee impair quality of life as much as severe osteoarthritis: a comparison of knee injury and osteoarthritis outcome score in 4 patient categories scheduled for knee surgery. *Am J Sports Med.* 2010;38:231-237.
4. Brittberg M, Lindahl A, Nilsson A, et al. Treatment of deep cartilage defects in the knee with autologous chondrocyte transplantation. *N Engl J Med.* 1994;331: 889-895.
5. Gillogly SD, Myers TH, Rienhold MM. Treatment of full-thickness chondral defects in the knee with autologous chondrocyte implantation. *J Orthop Sports Phys Ther.* 2006;36(10):751-764.
6. Micheli LJ, Browne JE, Erggelet C, et al. Autologous chondrocyte implantation of the knee: multicenter experience and minimum 3 year follow-up. *Clin J Sports Med.* 2001;11:223-228.
7. Pascual-Garrido C, Slabaugh MA, L'Heureux DR, et al. Recommendations and treatment outcomes for patellofemoral articular cartilage defects with autologous chondrocyte implantation: prospective evaluation at average 4-year follow up. *Am J Sports Med.* 2009;37:(Suppl 1): 33S-41S.
8. Peterson L, Lindahl A, Brittberg M, et al. Autologous chondrocyte transplantation: biomechanics and long-term durability. *Am J Sports Med.* 2002;30(1):2-12.
9. Peterson L, Minas T, Brittberg M, et al. Two- to 9-year outcome after autologous chondrocyte transplantation of the knee. *Clin Orthop Relat Res.* 2000;374:212-234.
10. Peterson L, Vasiliadis HS, Brittberg M, et al. Autologous chondrocyte implantation: a long-term follow-up. *Am J Sports Med.* 2010;38:1117-1124.
11. Rosenberger RE, Gomoll AH, Bryant T, et al. Repair of large chondral defects of the knee with autologous chondrocyte implantation in patients 45 years or older. *Am J Sports Med.* 2008;36:2336-2344.
12. Brittberg M. Autologous chondrocyte transplantation. *Clin Orthop Relat Res.* 1999;367S:S147-S155.
13. Richardson J, Caterson B, Evans E, et al. Repair of human articular cartilage after implantation of autologous chondrocytes. *J Bone Joint Surg Br.* 1999;81:1064-1068.
14. Gomoll AH, Farr J, Gillogly SD, et al. Surgical management of articular cartilage defects of the knee, an

instructional course lecture 362, American Academy of Orthopaedic Surgeons. *J Bone Joint Surg Am*. 2010;92: 2470-2490.

15. Knutsen G, Engebretsen L, Ludvigsen TC, et al. Autologous chondrocyte implantation compared with microfracture in the knee. *J Bone Joint Surg Am*. 2004:86: 455-464.

16. Cole BJ, D'Amato M. Autologous chondrocyte implantation. *Oper Tech Orthop*. 2001;11:115-131.

17. Gillogly SD. Autologous chondrocyte implantation: complex defects and concomitant procedures. *Oper Tech Sports Med*. 2002;10:120-128.

18. Minas T. Autologous cultured chondrocyte implantation in the repair of focal chondral lesions of the knee: clinical indications and operative technique. *J Sports Traumatol Rel Res*. 1998;20:90-102.

19. Gillogly SD, Voight M, Blackburn T. Treatment of articular cartilage defects of the knee with autologous chondrocyte implantation. *J Orthop Sports Phys Ther*. 1998;28:241-251.

20. Hamby TS, Gillogly SD, Peterson L. Treatment of patellofemoral articular cartilage injuries with autologous chondrocyte implantation. *Oper Tech Sports Med*. 2002;10:129-135.

21. Bentley G, Biant LC, Carrington M, et al. A prospective, randomised comparison of autologous chondrocyte implantation versus mosaicplasty for osteochondral defects in the knee. *J Bone Joint Surg Br*. 2003;85: 223-230.

22. Gillogly, SD, Kendall CB. Cell-based therapy with autologous chondrocyte implantation. In: Cole B, Gomoll A, eds. *Biologic Joint Reconstruction, Alternatives to Arthroplasty*. Thorofare, New Jersey: Slack Inc; 2009:139-145.

Chapter 70

High Tibial Osteotomy

Mark McConkey, Sami Abdulmassih, and Annunziato Amendola

Chapter Synopsis

- High tibial osteotomy (HTO) is a valuable procedure and, when performed with attention to appropriate indications and contraindications, has good outcomes reported in the literature. In this chapter we describe the surgical technique for medial opening wedge HTO.

Important Points

- HTO changes both the coronal and the sagittal plane alignment. Medial opening wedge HTO has a tendency to increase the tibial slope, whereas lateral closing wedge HTO has a tendency to decrease the tibial slope.
- Indications for HTO are varus limb alignment with the following:
  - Unicompartmental medial compartment arthritis in a physiologically young and active person
  - Chronic soft tissue laxity
  - Medial meniscal allograft transplantation procedure
  - Cartilage resurfacing procedure in the medial compartment

Clinical and Surgical Pearls

- The patient with isolated medial-sided degenerative joint disease who is indicated for HTO should be highly active, motivated, and aware that pain relief may not be complete or permanent.

- In the varus knee, slight overcorrection into valgus is encouraged. In most cases the preoperative template should aim to correct the mechanical axis to 62.5% of the width of the plateau.
- Guide pin placement is critical. Do not accept anything less than optimum pin placement.
- The guide pin is inserted from the medial tibial cortex approximately 4 cm distal to the joint line toward the superior aspect of the proximal tibiofibular joint (passing just above the level of the tibial tubercle).

Clinical and Surgical Pitfalls

- The tip of the guide pin should be far enough from the joint line (farther than 1.5 cm).
- Keep the guide pin in place while performing the osteotomy distal to it to prevent propagation of the osteotomy toward the joint line
- The beveled side of the AO osteotome should be away from the joint line
- The osteotomy should be perpendicular to the tibial shaft in the sagittal plane so that the plate would be aligned with and in good apposition to the proximal tibial metaphysis.

High tibial osteotomy (HTO) has been successfully to treat arthritis of the knee in symptomatic patients for many years. Arthritis of the knee joint is commonly localized to one compartment, offering the potential to offload that compartment as a pain-relieving treatment of the disease. Sagittal and coronal alignment directly affects distribution of force across the compartments of the knee; malalignment often accompanies unicompartmental knee arthritis, leading to tissue overload and exacerbation of pain and joint degeneration. Osteotomies are used to redirect weight-bearing forces across the knee joint for a number of reasons. Varus-producing proximal tibial osteotomies are increasingly being employed for indications other than arthritis, including revision anterior cruciate ligament (ACL) reconstruction in a varus limb, chronic posterolateral corner instability, or off-loading of an osteoarticular graft or meniscal allograft.

A proximal tibial osteotomy can take several forms, including valgus-producing opening and closing wedge procedures, varus-producing opening and closing wedge procedures, and procedures designed to primarily affect the sagittal plane. Currently, one of the most commonly employed HTOs is the valgus-producing medial opening wedge osteotomy—the focus of this chapter. Combined proximal tibial osteotomy with ACL reconstruction is covered in a separate chapter.

PREOPERATIVE CONSIDERATIONS

The two most commonly performed valgus-producing HTOs are the medial opening wedge and lateral closing wedge osteotomies. Each has advantages and disadvantages, which are briefly discussed in the following sections.

History

Medial opening wedge HTO has increased in popularity in recent years for a number of reasons. The theoretical advantages of employing an opening wedge osteotomy over a closing wedge procedure include the following:

1. The usual deformity is proximal tibia vara; therefore the osteotomy directly addresses the anatomic deformity.
2. Preservation of bone to the proximal tibia restores anatomy and potentially makes future arthroplasty procedures less technically challenging.
3. Disruption of the proximal tibiofibular joint and anterior compartment of the leg are prevented.
4. The peroneal nerve can be avoided.
5. Only one bone cut is required.
6. The correction can be modified intraoperatively.
7. It is relatively easy to combine the HTO with other procedures (e.g., ACL reconstruction, meniscal allograft).

The disadvantages of the medial-sided procedure include the following:

1. Theoretically higher risk of nonunion as a result of the creation of a bony gap
2. Potential donor site morbidity if autograft is used or infectious disease transmission if allograft is used
3. Longer period of restricted weight bearing

Less common surgical options available to modify the coronal and sagittal alignment of the proximal tibia include the dome osteotomy or gradual correction with an external fixator. These operations both offer the ability to correct large deformities that are not correctable by either opening or closing wedge techniques. These techniques are beyond the scope of this chapter.

Imaging

Radiographic assessment of an HTO candidate varies slightly depending on the indication for surgery. However, regardless of the indication, all patients at our institution undergo a routine knee series including a full-length alignment film. The knee radiographs include bilateral anteroposterior (AP) weight-bearing films in full extension, bilateral posteroanterior weight-bearing films taken at 45 degrees of knee flexion, and lateral and skyline views of the affected knee. In the patient with medial compartment osteoarthritis, the radiographs are needed to assess the extent of the medial compartment osteoarthritis and to rule out extensive degeneration in the patellofemoral and lateral joint compartments. Other findings to note on the preoperative radiographs are the distal femoral and proximal tibial angles for deformity, sagittal tibial slope, lateral tibial subluxation, and joint incongruence. On the full-length radiograph, the weight-bearing axis is drawn from the center of the hip to the center of the ankle, which determines where the load passes through the knee joint.

A number of potential methods can be used to calculate the size of the osteotomy.[1-3] We currently employ the method described by Dugdale and colleagues,[2] which corrects the weight-bearing axis to 62.5% of the width of the plateau, or 3 to 5 degrees of mechanical valgus. An example of the calculation can be seen in Figure 70-1. If there is excess varus malalignment because of soft tissue laxity, the difference in congruence angle on the affected and unaffected legs noted on the bilateral standing full-length AP radiograph is subtracted from the correction.

Indications and Contraindications

Indications for an HTO include clinical and radiographic varus and (1) medial compartment arthrosis with or without mild to moderate asymptomatic radiographic patellofemoral arthrosis; (2) symptomatic ligamentous instability with medial compartment arthrosis; (3) recurrent ACL rupture with significant joint deformity; and (4) medial compartment pain in the setting of previous total medial meniscectomy, osteochondritis dissecans, or significant chondral damage.[4]

Isolated medial-sided degenerative joint disease with varus malalignment remains the most common indication for opening wedge HTO. The patient should be motivated and aware that pain relief may not be complete or permanent. Patients under the age of

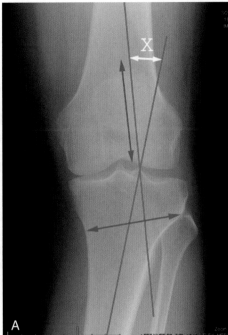

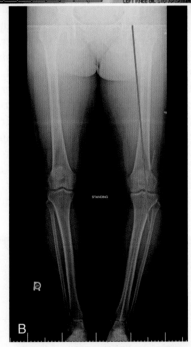

Figure 70-1. A, A long-leg anteroposterior radiograph is used to template the osteotomy. Correction of the weight-bearing axis is achieved to 62.5% of the medial-to-lateral plateau distance. A line is drawn from the center of the femoral head to the point on the plateau corresponding to the new weight-bearing axis. Another line is drawn from the weight-bearing axis to the center of the ankle joint. The angle formed by the intersection of these lines is the angle of the osteotomy. **B,** For the size of the osteotomy in millimeters to be calculated, the length of the osteotomy *(blue arrows)* is measured and overlaid onto the intersection of the weight-bearing axis. The distance between the femoral and tibial weight-bearing lines approximates the size of the osteotomy at the medial metaphysis.

50 and with a body mass index (BMI) of less than 25 are good candidates and demonstrate improved survivorship.[5,6] An HTO in a patient with an unstable knee and malalignment may improve pain and instability symptoms and potentially delay the onset of cartilage degeneration.[7,8]

Absolute contraindications to HTO for medial compartment osteoarthritis include inflammatory arthritis and significant lateral tibiofemoral joint disease. Poorer outcomes after HTO have been correlated with severe articular destruction,[9] significant patellofemoral disease,[10] increased age,[6,9,11] lateral tibial thrust,[6] decreased range of motion,[6] or joint instability.[12] Recent literature presents evidence that ACL deficiency correlates with higher likelihood of long-term survival, suggesting that joint instability may not predict a poorer outcome.[5] The preceding findings should be considered with each patient's clinical picture, serve as a basis to counsel each patient on the potential for a good functional outcome, and should not be thought of as definitive reasons to avoid performing an osteotomy.

SURGICAL TECHNIQUE

In many institutions, HTO is not a commonly performed procedure, so the surgeon is responsible for ensuring that the operating room is set up appropriately and the implants are available. The surgeon must be familiar with the procedure and the instrumentation and must guide the surgery. Fluoroscopy is essential, and a unit must be available and positioned appropriately in the operating room before the operation is started. A discussion should be undertaken with the patient and the anesthesia team regarding the risks and benefits of peripheral nerve blockade. Although some institutions perform HTO as an outpatient procedure, it is significantly painful, so the patient and hospital should be prepared for an overnight stay.

Anesthesia and Positioning

After general or spinal anesthesia has been given, the patient is positioned supine on a radiolucent table. Preoperative antibiotics are given within 1 hour before the start of the procedure. A thigh tourniquet is applied, and all bony prominences are well padded. Next the fluoroscopy unit is positioned in the room. If the surgeon chooses to use the large C-arm, it should be positioned on the contralateral side of the patient to allow the surgical team easy access to the limb at all times during the procedure. We prefer to use the small C-arm during an HTO. The leg can be abducted off the side of the bed and placed over the fluoroscopy unit, which allows the use of a standard, nonradiolucent surgical bed. It also significantly decreases the radiation to which the surgical team is exposed.

Surgical Incisions

A standard sterile preparation is completed, and the leg is draped free. The planned incision and important bony landmarks are marked (Fig. 70-2). A bump is placed under the knee to allow slight flexion, and the tourniquet is inflated. If additional procedures are to be performed before the osteotomy (e.g., arthroscopy, ACL reconstruction, osteochondral allograft), the surgeon should consider waiting to inflate the tourniquet so as not to exhaust tourniquet time before the completion of the HTO. A longitudinal incision is made midway between the tibial tubercle and the posterior tibial metaphysis, beginning 1 cm inferior to the medial joint line and extending 6 cm distally. Electrocautery is used to dissect along the medial border of the patellar tendon. A retractor is placed posterior to the tendon for protection. If needed, the superior 2 to 3 mm of patellar tendon can be elevated from the tibial tubercle. The pes anserinus and superficial medial collateral ligament are raised as a single flap with electrocautery and a Cobb elevator. When the posterior tibial cortex is reached, a retractor is carefully placed directly along the posterior tibial cortex to protect the neurovascular structures (Fig. 70-3).

Specific Steps

Table 70-1 outlines the specific steps of the procedure.

A guide pin is drilled from the medial tibial cortex approximately 4 cm distal to the joint line toward the superior aspect of the proximal tibiofibular joint (Fig. 70-4). Fluoroscopy is used to assess the position of the wire. A corticotomy is then made inferior to the wire with a small oscillating saw (Fig. 70-5). It is important to keep the wire superior to the osteotomy to shield the joint from intra-articular fracture. A thin, flexible AO osteotome is employed to begin the osteotomy and is tapped into place inferior to the wire. The osteotome is then advanced medially, anteromedially, and posteromedially with use of fluoroscopy to assess progress (Fig. 70-6). Once the osteotome has been seated approximately 1 cm from the lateral cortex, it is removed, and the large stackable osteotome is tapped into place. Markings on the osteotomes allow the surgeon to gauge the depth of the osteotomy.

Another osteotome is then stacked inferior to the large osteotome until the medial cortex can be seen to hinge open. The large osteotome is used superiorly to once again protect the lateral joint from intra-articular fracture (Fig. 70-7). The osteotomes are removed, and the calibrated wedges are carefully tapped into place to the depth predetermined on the preoperative template. Again, fluoroscopic images are used to assess the depth and to ensure that no intra-articular fracture has occurred (Fig. 70-8). At this point an alignment guide or cautery cord can be used to assess the correction with the large C-arm. We feel that the accuracy assessment intraoperatively with fluoroscopy and an alignment guide or cautery cord is inherently poor and prefer to

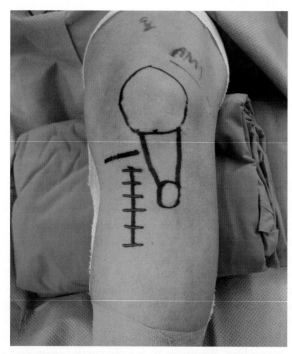

Figure 70-2. The patient is positioned supine with a bump under the knee to allow for knee flexion. Landmarks are drawn, and the incision is taken from the medial joint line down distal to the tibial tubercle. The incision is halfway between the tubercle and the posteromedial tibia.

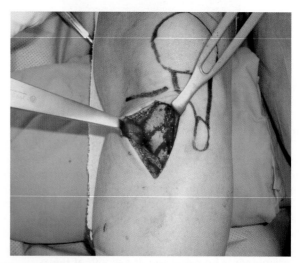

Figure 70-3. The incision is made and the medial soft tissues including pes anserinus and the superficial medial collateral ligament are raised as one full thickness flap. An Army-Navy retractor is placed under the patellar tendon, and a Hohmann retractor along the posterior tibia.

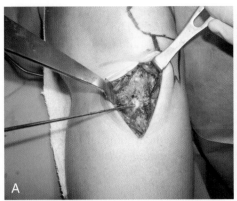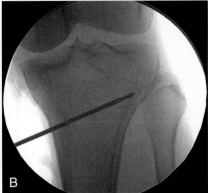

Figure 70-4. A, A guidewire is placed from the medial tibial metaphysis approximately 4-5 cm distal to the joint line directed toward the superior aspect of the proximal tibiofibular joint. Care is taken to ensure the patellar tendon insertion is distal to the osteotomy site. **B,** Fluoroscopy is used to ensure the tip of the wire is 1 cm from the lateral cortex and 1.5 to 2 cm from the lateral tibial plateau.

TABLE 70-1. Surgical Steps for High Tibial Osteotomy

1. Preoperative checklist	Consent, antibiotics, tourniquet, fluoroscopy, radiolucent table, implants, company representative, bone graft or substitute
2. Incision	Incision is 6 cm, midway between tibial crest and posterior cortex Pes anserinus and sMCL elevated as single flap Retractors posterior to patellar tendon and along posterior tibial cortex
3. Osteotomy	Guide pin placed from medial tibial cortex toward superior aspect of tibiofibular joint Small oscillating saw for corticotomy *inferior* to guide pin Flexible osteotome under fluoroscopy guidance Wide Arthrex osteotome tapped into place, and narrower osteotome stacked inferior to it under fluoroscopic guidance, opening the osteotomy
4. Hardware insertion	Graduated wedges inserted to predetermined depth Anterior wedge removed, and plate inserted Shaft screw drilled and placed to attach plate to bone Knee extended to decrease anterior opening to ensure no increase in slope Remainder of screws placed and fluoroscopically checked Bone graft or substitute placed if necessary
5. Closure	Tourniquet deflation Thorough irrigation and hemostasis Reapproximation of pes anserinus over plate Skin closure Hinged knee brace

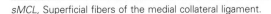
sMCL, Superficial fibers of the medial collateral ligament.

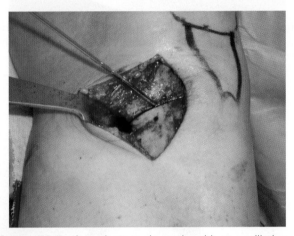

Figure 70-5. A corticotomy is made with an oscillating saw distal to the guidewire, and the osteotomy is started with a flexible osteotome. Attention is paid to ensure that the osteotomy is proximal to the patellar tendon insertion. Fluoroscopy is used to monitor the progression of the osteotomy.

rely on preoperative templating and intraoperative clinical assessment.

The anterior wedge is removed, allowing the plate with the appropriately sized wedge block to be inserted (Fig. 70-9). The plate should be inserted as far posteriorly as possible to reduce the chance of increasing the posterior slope. The bump is now placed under the heel to allow full extension of the knee and extension through the osteotomy. The posterior slope is not significantly changed if the opening anteriorly is half the size of the opening posteriorly.[13]

Screws are sequentially placed, with fluoroscopy used to ensure no hardware complications have occurred. Whether small corrections (<7.5 mm) require bone graft or bone graft substitute is debated. We typically use a bone graft substitute for all corrections (Fig. 70-10). If the osteotomy is done in combination with an allograft procedure (e.g., osteochondral or meniscal

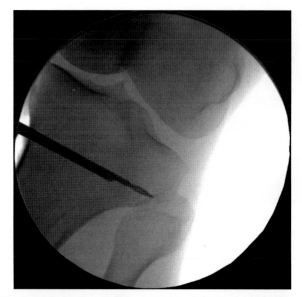

Figure 70-6. The flexible osteotome is used to perform the osteotomy after the corticotomy is completed with the oscillating saw. It is important that the osteotomy be inferior to the wire to protect from intra-articular fracture.

allograft) we use the remaining allograft bone as the graft source. The wound is thoroughly washed and closed in a standard fashion.

POSTOPERATIVE CONSIDERATIONS

Patients undergoing an HTO are kept in the hospital for one night and discharged home the following day. A hinged knee brace is applied in the operating room to be worn full time for the first 6 weeks.

Rehabilitation

The patient is placed on non–weight-bearing status, with the brace allowing motion from 0 to 90 degrees, for the first 6 weeks and progresses to partial weight bearing until 8 weeks if follow-up radiographs demonstrate healing. With smaller corrections (<7.5 mm), earlier weight bearing may be initiated at the discretion of the surgeon. Active-assisted range of motion in the

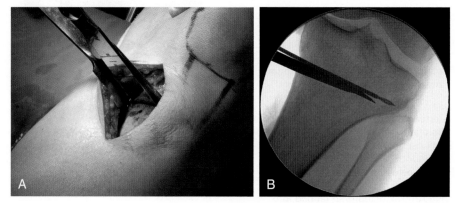

Figure 70-7. The stackable osteotomes are used. First the wide osteotome is buried after ensuring that the cut is complete anteriorly and posteriorly. The narrower osteotome is tapped into place inferior to the wide osteotome until the metaphysis can be hinged open.

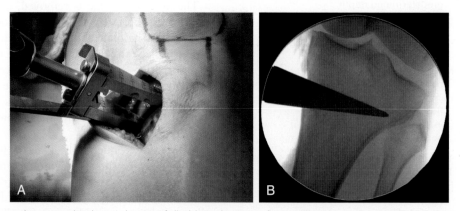

Figure 70-8. Once the metaphysis can be carefully hinged open a few millimeters, the parallel wedges are tapped into place. The size of the opening wedge was determined on the preoperative templating and can be checked with the alignment rod or electrocautery cord as needed.

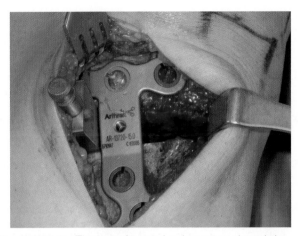

Figure 70-9. The anterior wedge is removed, and the plate with the appropriate-size wedge block is inserted into the osteotomy. Before fixation of the plate, the surgeon should ensure that the osteotomy opens approximately twice as wide posteriorly as anteriorly. This will ensure that the posterior slope of the tibial plateau will remain unchanged.

brace can be performed as tolerated, as can straight-leg raises and calf strengthening. At 8 to 12 weeks, if healing is progressing well, the patient is progressed to full weight bearing and advanced to aggressive strengthening with physical therapy. The patient should expect to walk without crutches within 8 weeks of surgery. Return to work is possible in 2 to 3 weeks if the patient works at a desk. Return to laboring work and sports activities is expected to be at approximately 3 to 4 months.

RESULTS

The vast majority of the articles reporting long-term results of HTO involve lateral closing wedge osteotomies, often treated with cylinder cast immobilization (Table 70-2). Recent literature on long-term results of HTO reports good outcomes up to 20 years postoperatively.[5,9,15,16] In 2005, Tang and Henderson[15] reported a survivorship rate of 74.7% at 10 years and 66.9% at 15 and 20 years in a cohort of patients treated with

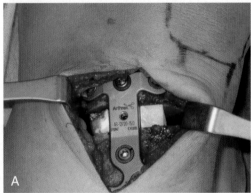
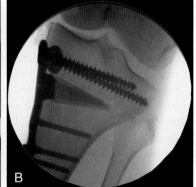

Figure 70-10. The plate is fixed with locking screws; bone graft substitute has been placed. Final fluoroscopic images demonstrating no hardware complications or joint penetration and no intra-articular fracture.

TABLE 70-2. Long-Term Results of High Tibial Osteotomy

Author	Technique	Results
Naudie et al[6] (1999)	Closing wedge, dome	75% at 5 years, 51% at 10 years, 39% at 15 years, 30% at 20 years
Sprenger and Doerzbacher[12] (2003)	Closing wedge	65%-74% at 10 years
Koshino et al[14] (2004)	Closing wedge	97.3% at 7 years, 95.1% at 10 years, 86.9% at 15 years
Tang and Henderson[15] (2005)	Closing wedge	89.5% at 5 years, 74.7% at 10 years, 66.9% at 15 and 20 years
Papachristou et al[16] (2006)	Closing wedge	80% at 10 years, 66% at 15 years, 52.8% at 17 years
Flecher et al[9] (2006)	Closing wedge	85% at 20 years
Gstottner et al[11] (2008)	Closing wedge	94% at 5 years, 79.9% at 10 years, 65.5% at 15 years, 54.1% at 18 years
Akizuki et al[17] (2008)	Closing wedge	97.6% at 10 years, 90.4% at 15 years
DeMeo et al[18] (2010)	Opening wedge	70% at 8 years, Lysholm and HSS scores improved from 54.2 and 75.9 to 89.1 and 92.7 at 2 years
Hui et al[5] (2011)	Closing wedge	95% at 5 years, 79% at 10 years, 56% at 15 years

HSS, Hospital for Special Surgery.

closing wedge HTO fixed with a staple and immobilized in a cast. After a similar procedure, Papachristou and colleagues[16] reported a 66% survival at 15 years and 53% survival rate at 17 years. Flecher and colleagues[9] reported 85% survivorship at 20 years in 301 patients after closing wedge HTO. In 2011, Hui and colleagues[5] reported a retrospective review of 413 patients who had undergone closing wedge HTO. They reported an 85% satisfaction rate and 95%, 79%, and 56% survival at 5, 10, and 15 years, respectively.

Contemporary long-term results of medial opening wedge HTOs in the literature are nonexistent, but some early and midterm results have been reported.[18,19] DeMeo and colleagues[18] reported midterm survivorship of opening wedge HTO. They found Lysholm and Hospital for Special Surgery (HSS) scores improved from 54.2 and 75.9 preoperatively to 89.1 and 92.7 at 2 years postoperatively, respectively. They also reported a survivorship of 70% at 8 years in a total of 20 patients.

Opening wedge HTO is increasingly used in combination with other procedures around the knee for diseases other than unicompartmental joint degeneration (i.e., revision ACL surgery, off-loading of osteoarticular or meniscal allografts, chronic posterolateral soft tissue laxity). For example, Naudie and colleagues[8] performed 17 HTOs on 16 patients with symptomatic hyperextension varus thrust. At an average follow-up of 56 months, all patients had an improvement in their activity level postoperatively, and 15 of 16 were satisfied and would undergo the procedure again. Overall, the results of HTO in these combined procedures are difficult to assess owing to the complexity of the problem, the heterogeneity of the injury pattern, and the combined nature of the surgery.

CONCLUSIONS

HTO is a valuable procedure in the arsenal of the modern knee surgeon. The most common indication is unicompartmental medial-sided arthritis of the knee in a physiologically young person. The long-term results of this procedure are not yet known, but good long-term outcomes at 15 to 20 years have been demonstrated with closing wedge procedures. The use of an HTO should also be considered in situations such as off-loading of meniscal allografts, osteoarticular autografts or allografts, and chronic soft tissue laxity and malalignment. The described surgical technique offers a reproducible procedure with several advantages over the closing wedge technique.

REFERENCES

1. Coventry MB. Upper tibial osteotomy for osteoarthritis. *J Bone Joint Surg Am.* 1985;67:1136-1140.
2. Dugdale TW, Noyes FR, Styer D. Preoperative planning for high tibial osteotomy: The effect of lateral tibiofemoral separation and tibiofemoral length. *Clin Orthop Relat Res.* 1992:248-264.
3. Minaci A, Ballmer FT, Ballmer PM, et al. Proximal tibial osteotomy: A new fixation device. *Clin Orthop Relat Res.* 1989;250-259.
4. Amendola A, Bonasia DE. Results of high tibial osteotomy: Review of the literature. *Int Orthop.* 2010;34:155-160.
5. Hui C, Salmon LJ, Kok A, et al. Long-term survival of high tibial osteotomy for medial compartment osteoarthritis of the knee. *Am J Sports Med.* 2011;39:64-70.
6. Naudie D, Bourne RB, Rorabeck CH, et al. Survivorship of the high tibial valgus osteotomy: A 10- to 22-year followup study. *Clin Orthop Relat Res.* 1999;367:18-27.
7. Badhe NP, Forster IW. High tibial osteotomy in knee instability: The rationale of treatment and early results. *Knee Surg Sports Traumatol Arthrosc.* 2002;10:38-43.
8. Naudie DD, Amendola A, Fowler PJ. Opening wedge high tibial osteotomy for symptomatic hyperextension-varus thrust. *Am J Sports Med.* 2004;32:60-70.
9. Flecher X, Parratte S, Aubaniac JM, et al. A 12-28-year followup study of closing wedge high tibial osteotomy. *Clin Orthop Relat Res.* 2006;452:91-96.
10. Rudan JF, Simurda MA. High tibial osteotomy. A prospective clinical and roentgenographic review. *Clin Orthop Relat Res.* 1990;255:251-256.
11. Gstottner M, Pedross F, Liebensteiner M, et al. Long-term outcome after high tibial osteotomy. *Arch Orthop Trauma Surg.* 2008;128:111-115.
12. Sprenger TR, Doerzbacher JF. Tibial osteotomy for the treatment of varus gonarthrosis. Survival and failure analysis to twenty-two years. *J Bone Joint Surg Am.* 2003;85:469-474.
13. Noyes FR, Goebel SX, West J. Opening wedge tibial osteotomy: The 3-triangle method to correct axial alignment and tibial slope. *Am J Sports Med.* 2005;33:378-387.
14. Koshino T, Yoshida T, Ara Y, et al. Fifteen to twenty-eight years' follow-up results of high tibial valgus osteotomy for osteoarthritic knee. *Knee.* 2004;11:439-444.
15. Tang WC, Henderson IJ. High tibial osteotomy: long term survival analysis and patients' perspective. *Knee.* 2005;12:410-413.
16. Papachristou G, Plessas S, Sourlas J, et al. Deterioration of long-term results following high tibial osteotomy in patients under 60 years of age. *Int Orthop.* 2006;30:403-408.
17. Akizuki S, Shibakawa A, Takizawa T, et al. The long-term outcome of high tibial osteotomy: a ten- to 20-year follow-up. *J Bone Joint Surg Br.* 2008;90:592-596.
18. DeMeo PJ, Johnson EM, Chiang PP, et al. Midterm follow-up of opening-wedge high tibial osteotomy. *Am J Sports Med.* 2010;38:2077-2084.
19. Amendola A, Fowler P, Litchfield R, et al. Opening wedge high tibial osteotomy using a novel technique: Early results and complications. *J Knee Surg.* 2004;17:170-175.

Chapter 71

Distal Femoral Osteotomy

Sami Abdulmassih, Mark McConkey, and Annunziato Amendola

Chapter Synopsis

- Distal femoral osteotomy is a common surgical procedure. It has many indications and contraindications, and has good outcomes in the literature with appropriate indications. In this chapter we describe the step-by-step surgical technique for both lateral opening wedge and medial closing wedge distal femoral osteotomy.

Important Points

- Distal femoral osteotomy changes only the coronal plane alignment and has no effect on the patellar height.
- Indications for distal femoral osteotomy are as follows:
  - Lateral compartment gonarthrosis with valgus limb
  - Lateral femoral condyle osteochondritis dissecans (OCD) lesion with valgus limb alignment in isolation or in addition to cartilage resurfacing
  - Deficient lateral meniscus with valgus limb alignment when lateral meniscal transplantation is considered
  - Valgus deformity with or without valgus thrust in chronic medial collateral ligament (MCL) or MCL and cruciate instabilities
  - Chronic patellar instability with valgus knee alignment

Clinical and Surgical Pearls

- In the varus knee, slight overcorrection into valgus is encouraged, but in the valgus knee, the most common complication is overcorrection into varus, and this must be avoided. Therefore when doing the preoperative planning, shift the mechanical axis to the medial tibial spine but not beyond that.
- Guide pin placement is critical. Do not accept anything less than optimum pin placement, because this guides the surgery in both techniques.

- In lateral closing wedge osteotomy the pin should be inserted 2 cm proximal to the lateral epicondyle, aiming toward the proximal third of the medial epicondyle. It should pass in approximately a 20-degree oblique direction in the coronal plane, in the middle of the lateral femoral cortex in the sagittal plane, and parallel to the floor in the axial plane.
- In medial closing wedge osteotomy the pin should be inserted 2 cm proximal and parallel to the distal femoral articular surface in the coronal plane, in line with long axis of the femur in the sagittal plane (approximately at the junction of the anterior and middle third of the medial condyle), and parallel to the floor in the axial plane.

Clinical and Surgical Pitfalls

- In lateral opening wedge osteotomy:
  - The tip of the guide pin should be far enough from the medial cortex as well as from the joint line (farther than 1.5 cm).
  - Create the osteotomy on the proximal side of the guide pin to prevent shifting of the osteotomy toward the joint line.
  - The beveled side of the AO osteotome should be away from the joint line.
  - The osteotomy should be perpendicular to the femoral shaft in the sagittal plane so that the proximal part of the plate would be aligned with and in good apposition to the shaft.
- In medial closing wedge osteotomy:
  - The chisel should be inserted in line with the long axis of the femur in the sagittal plane so that the plate will align with and be in good apposition to the shaft.

Lower limb alignment is a very important and critical concept in orthopedic surgery. It has many effects on limb function in the short term as well as in the long term. The use of distal femoral osteotomy has increased in recent years; its indications have expanded, improved outcomes have been reported, and surgical technique and fixation methods have improved.

Generally speaking, proximal tibial osteotomy is used to correct a varus limb malalignment, whereas distal femoral osteotomy is used to correct a valgus limb malalignment. The osteotomy can be either a lateral opening wedge or a medial closing wedge. The trend has shifted recently toward performing distal femoral lateral opening wedge osteotomy for many reasons, including the relatively easier surgical exposure, the more accurate degree of correction, and the less complex fixation technique.

In this chapter we describe the step-by-step surgical technique for distal femoral lateral opening wedge and medial closing wedge osteotomies. Patient evaluation and indications and contraindications of these techniques are also discussed, including a summary of reported outcomes from the literature.

Several studies have investigated the association between valgus limb alignment and the development and progression of lateral compartment osteoarthritis (OA). Brouwer and colleagues[1] found that valgus alignment was associated with a borderline significant increase in the development of knee OA (odds ratio [OR] 1.54; 95% confidence interval [95% CI] 0.97–2.44). Other studies have found a strong correlation between valgus alignment and the progression of knee OA.[2,3] A cross-sectional study by Issa and colleagues[4] showed that the presence of cartilage defects in the lateral compartment increased with greater valgus malalignment. Lateral unicompartmental knee arthroplasty (UKA) is performed much less commonly than medial UKA, and therefore the available data on long-term outcomes are limited.

In addition, modern knee procedures such as osteochondral resurfacing and meniscal transplantation have evolved in recent years and gained popularity, often necessitating a concomitant joint unloading procedure to increase the longevity of the reconstruction. Corrective varus-producing osteotomies around the knee to correct valgus alignment are common and a valuable adjunct to other knee surgeries to improve outcomes.

PREOPERATIVE CONSIDERATIONS

History

In general, proximal tibial osteotomy is used to correct varus limb malalignment, and distal femoral osteotomy is used to correct valgus limb malalignment. A proximal

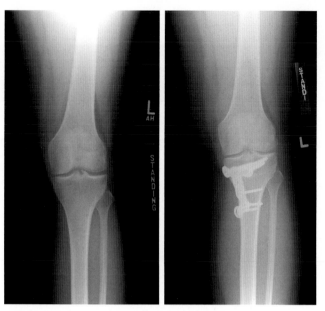

Figure 71-1. A valgus-producing high tibial osteotomy results in obliquity of the tibiofemoral joint line.

tibial osteotomy can be used to correct valgus malalignment, but this usually leads to a change in the joint line orientation (Fig. 71-1).[5] Perhaps, small corrections can be tolerated in the proximal tibia.

The main differences between proximal tibial and distal femoral osteotomies are their effect on the tibial slope and the patellar height.

It is well known that proximal tibial osteotomy alters the tibial slope, with opening wedge having the tendency to increase the slope[6] and closing wedge having the tendency to decrease the slope. This change in the slope has an effect on knee kinematics and stability. In addition, the tibial osteotomy will alter the contact mechanics through a full range of motion, whereas the femoral osteotomy will change the contact forces mainly near extension.[5]

Although there are complications that may accompany any osteotomy including femoral osteotomy, the alignment changes with distal femoral osteotomy involve only the coronal plane. In the varus knee, slight overcorrection into valgus is encouraged, but in the valgus knee the most common complication is overcorrection into varus, and this must be avoided. Patellar height changes after distal femoral osteotomy are also minimal and largely ignored[7] compared with proximal tibial osteotomy.

Physical Examination

Patient evaluation begins by taking a good history and performing an appropriate physical examination to determine if the patient is an appropriate candidate for realignment surgery.

Imaging

Radiographic evaluation should include weight-bearing anteroposterior (AP) and 45-degree flexion posteroanterior (PA; Rosenberg) views, lateral, and skyline or merchant views of both knees for comparison. If assessment of limb alignment is considered, bilateral long-leg views (hips to ankles) should be performed. Magnetic resonance imaging (MRI) may be indicated depending on the differential diagnosis—that is, meniscal or cartilage status.

Sometimes a single standing long-leg view reveals an obscure deformity if clinical findings do not correlate with the initial long-leg view (Figs. 71-2), especially if there is a valgus thrust.

The mechanical axis, which is a line drawn from the center of the femoral head to the center of the talus (Fig. 71-3), should normally pass through the center of the knee joint between the two tibial spines or just lateral to the medial spine.

When a distal femoral osteotomy is indicated, the degree of correction is calculated by use of the long-leg view to make the mechanical axis pass through the medial tibial spine and not beyond that point to prevent overcorrection and medial compartment overload.

A line is drawn from the center of the femoral head to the medial tibial spine. Another line is drawn from the center of the talus to the same point (medial tibial spine), and the angle between these two lines is the angle of correction (Fig. 71-4).

Rather than calculating the correction angle in degrees, calculating the actual correction in millimeters is more practical and avoids an extra step. This conversion is made by drawing the planned osteotomy wedge or triangle (planned level, length, angle of inclination, and angle of correction) on the distal femur and measuring the width of the base of this wedge at the lateral femoral cortex (Figs. 71-5 to 71-7).

Indications

- Lateral compartment gonarthrosis with valgus limb alignment (mechanical axis passes through the lateral compartment)
- Lateral femoral condyle osteochondritis dissecans (OCD) lesion with valgus limb alignment in isolation or in addition to other surgical procedures such as autograft or allograft osteochondral resurfacing
- Deficient lateral meniscus with valgus limb alignment when lateral meniscal transplantation is considered (mechanical axis passes through or beyond the lateral tibial spine)
- Valgus deformity with or without valgus thrust in chronic medial collateral ligament (MCL) or MCL

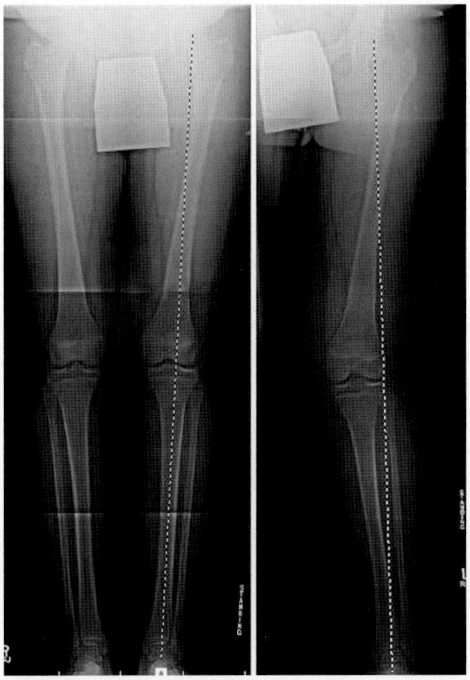

Figure 71-2. A 16-year-old boy who was indicated for lateral meniscal transplantation. Long-leg view initially did not reveal a big valgus deformity, although clinically he was in valgus; a standing one-leg view was ordered and showed the increase in the valgus deformity.

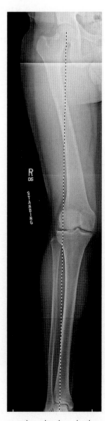

Figure 71-3. The mechanical axis is a line drawn from the center of the femoral head to the center of the talus on a standing long-leg view.

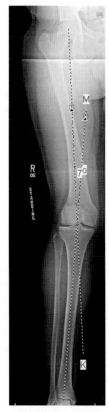

Figure 71-4. The angle of correction between a line, *K,* drawn from the center of the femoral head to the desired level on the tibial articular surface (usually between the two tibial spines) and another line, *M,* drawn from the center of the talus to the same point on the tibial articular surface.

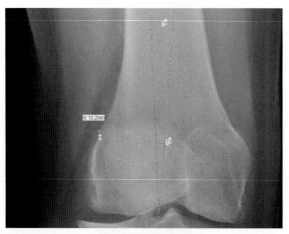

Figure 71-5. The first method of converting the angle of correction into millimeters. A wedge representing the planned osteotomy with the planned level, length, angle of inclination, and angle of correction is drawn, and the width of the base of this wedge at the lateral femoral cortex is the millimeters of correction (here 10.2 mm).

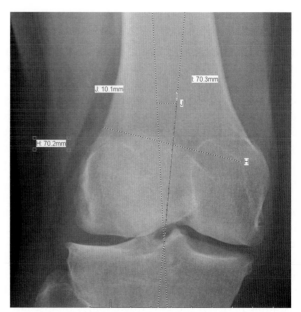

Figure 71-6. The second method of converting the angle of correction into millimeters. A line representing the osteotomy cut with the planned level and angle of inclination is drawn. The length of this line is measured (here 70.2 mm). Another line with the same measured length is drawn over one of the limbs of the angle of correction starting from the tip (the desired point of correction on the tibial articular surface). The width of the base of the triangle formed is the millimeters of correction.

and cruciate instabilities (mechanical axis passes beyond the lateral tibial spine)

- Chronic patellar instability with valgus knee alignment

Indications for medial closing wedge distal femoral osteotomy are as follows:

- Angle of correction greater than 17.5 degrees
- Limb length discrepancy in favor of the operated limb
- Presence of risk factors that delay healing—for example, smoking, neuropathy, poor bone quality, obesity

Contraindications

Absolute Contraindications

- Extreme valgus deformity associated with a subluxation of the tibia
- Tricompartmental arthritis
- Flexion contracture greater than 15 degrees

Relative Contraindications

- Osteonecrosis of the lateral femoral condyle
- Severe patellofemoral OA

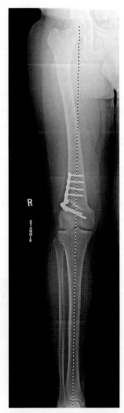

Figure 71-7. Follow-up long-leg radiograph of the patient shown in Figs. 71-3 to 71-6 3 months after the distal femoral lateral opening wedge osteotomy with a 10-mm plate showing the mechanical axis passing between the two tibial spines as planned before surgery.

- High body mass index
- Rheumatoid arthritis[8]

SURGICAL TECHNIQUES

Lateral Opening Wedge Distal Femoral Osteotomy Technique

Positioning

We use the toothed T-shaped plate for fixation. The patient is put in the supine position with a sandbag or bolster under the buttock of the operative side. A nonsterile tourniquet is applied except in very short extremities, in which case we use a sterile tourniquet. We use the mini–C-arm for fluoroscopy during the procedure; it is positioned on the ipsilateral side in the operating room.

A lateral knee post is used at the level of the tourniquet if a knee scope is indicated before the osteotomy, and it is removed after the arthroscopy to allow abduction of the leg toward the mini–C-arm (Fig. 71-8). After preparation and sterile draping of the entire extremity, the tourniquet is inflated to 300 mm Hg. The hip is

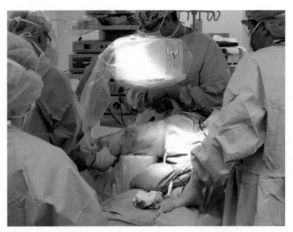

Figure 71-8. The mini–C-arm is used from the ipsilateral side for intraoperative assessment. The lateral knee post that is used during knee arthroscopy has been removed to allow extremity motion toward the mini–C-arm.

flexed and adducted, and a sterile bump is put underneath the thigh with the knee flexed to around 90 degrees.

Surgical Incisions

A 12- to 15-cm longitudinal lateral skin incision is made on the distal third of the thigh starting 2 cm distal to the lateral femoral epicondyle.

The soft tissues are dissected down to the iliotibial band, which is incised along the skin incision. The vastus lateralis muscle is elevated off the intermuscular septum with use of electrocautery and a periosteal elevator. Cauterization of the perforating vessels is very important. Cautery is used to cut the periosteum down to the bone at the metaphyseal level and retract it anteriorly and posteriorly to expose the lateral cortex with the joint capsule left intact. Curved blunt retractors are applied anteriorly and posteriorly. Care is taken to protect the posterior neurovascular structures throughout the procedure.

Specific Steps

Box 71-1 describes the specific steps of this procedure.

The knee is extended and a guidewire is inserted under fluoroscopic guidance starting 2 cm proximal to the lateral epicondyle and aiming toward the proximal third of the medial epicondyle. The wire should be advanced at approximately a 20-degree angle in the coronal plane while being centered in the middle of the lateral femoral cortex in the sagittal plane and parallel to the floor in the axial plane (Fig. 71-9).

The guidewire is kept in place during the osteotomy to prevent intra-articular fracture.

A thin microsagittal saw is used to cut the lateral, anterior, and posterior cortices parallel to and along the proximal aspect of the guidewire and perpendicular to the long axis of the femur in the sagittal plane so that the T-shaped plate fits the femoral cortex proximally. Sharp and thin AO osteotomes are used to complete the osteotomy under fluoroscopic guidance (Fig. 71-10). The osteotomy is continued medially to within 1 cm of the medial cortex. At this point the wide osteotomy blade is inserted and a narrower blade is stacked proximal to it to open the osteotomy site. The blades are removed and gentle manual varus stress is applied to check that the osteotomy will open (Fig. 71-11). The wedge opener is inserted with a mallet, slowly and carefully, to the depth that will allow for the desired amount of correction (in millimeters of opening) (Fig. 71-12).

Fluoroscopy is used to assess the osteotomy opening and can be used to assess limb alignment with an alignment rod or electrocautery cord in addition to clinical inspection for the limb correction. The distal femoral osteotomy plate with the desired depth of the tooth is inserted and fixed with two or three unicortical 6.5-mm cancellous screws distally (inserted parallel to the osteotomy) and four 4.5-mm bicortical screws proximally (inserted perpendicular to the long axis of the femur) (Figs. 71-13 to 71-15). Autograft or allograft bone or tricalcium phosphate wedges are inserted anterior and posterior to the plate (if correction is more than 7.5 mm). Fixation and alignment are again confirmed with fluoroscopy. The tourniquet is released, and homeostasis is obtained. The wound is closed in layers without a drain.

BOX 71-1 Surgical Steps: Lateral Opening Wedge Distal Femoral Osteotomy Technique

- Under fluoroscopic guidance, the guide pin is inserted from lateral to medial 2 cm proximal to the lateral epicondyle in a 20-degree oblique direction, aiming toward the proximal third of the medial epicondyle.
- The osteotomy is made proximal to the guide pin with the guide pin in place and is completed using the AO osteotome.
- The distal femur is exposed and retractors are applied.
- The guide pin is removed.
- The wide osteotomy blade and another narrower blade proximal to it are used to open the osteotomy site.
- Fluoroscopy might be used to check the length and position of the distal drill bit, which should be almost parallel to the osteotomy.
- The wedge opener is inserted to the desired amount of correction in millimeters (or 2 mm more to facilitate plate insertion). The toothed plate is then put in place and fixed using the proximal cortical and the distal cancellous screws.
- The toothed plate in place before bone graft application.
- The plate is fixed and bone graft is applied.

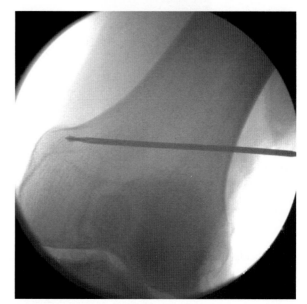

Figure 71-9. Under fluoroscopic guidance, the guide pin is inserted from lateral to medial 2 cm proximal to the lateral epicondyle in a 20-degree oblique direction aiming toward the proximal third of the medial epicondyle.

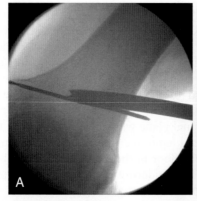
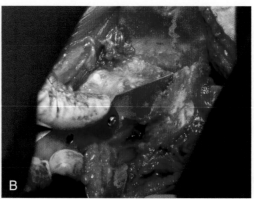

Figure 71-10. A, The osteotomy has been made proximal to the guide pin, and it is completed using the AO osteotome. **B,** The distal femur is exposed and retractors are applied. The guide pin is in place. The osteotomy is completed with the AO osteotome proximal to the guide pin.

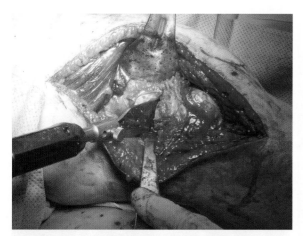

Figure 71-11. The guide pin is removed.

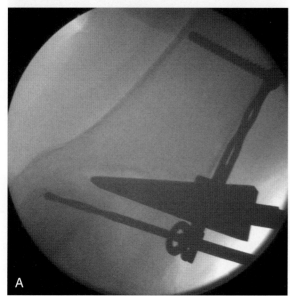

A

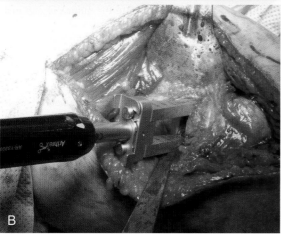

B

Figure 71-12. **A,** The wedge opener is used to open the osteotomy to the planned level, then the toothed plate is put in place and fixed. Fluoroscopy might be used to check the length and position of the distal drill bit, which should be almost parallel to the osteotomy. **B,** The wedge opener is inserted to the desired amount of correction in millimeters (or 2 mm more to facilitate plate insertion).

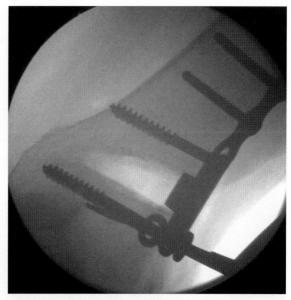

Figure 71-13. The toothed plate in place before bone graft application.

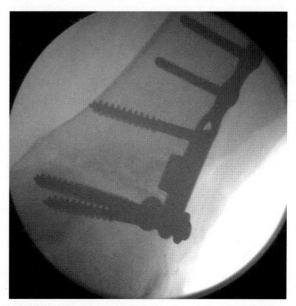

Figure 71-14. The plate has been fixed, and the bone graft has been applied.

Postoperative Considerations

Postoperatively the osteotomy is protected in a hinged knee brace (0 to 90 degrees) for 6 weeks. The patient is kept on non–weight-bearing status for 6 weeks postoperatively. If there is radiographic evidence of union at 6 weeks, the patient is gradually advanced to partial weight bearing. Full weight bearing may commence at 12 weeks, with appropriate evidence of radiographic healing. Physiotherapy is used for range-of-motion exercises in the brace until the osteotomy is healed.

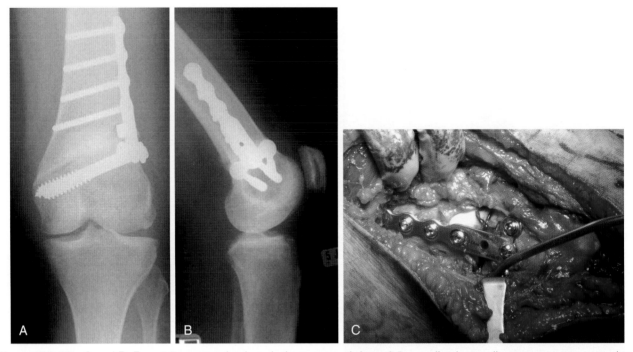

Figure 71-15. A and **B,** Four 4.5-mm proximal cortical screws and three 6.5-mm distal cancellous screws were used to fix the plate. Note that the osteotomy is perpendicular to the femoral shaft to allow good position of the T-plate in the middle of the femoral shaft on the lateral radiograph. **C,** The plate is applied and fixed with the proximal cortical and the distal cancellous screws.

Medial Closing Wedge Distal Femoral Osteotomy Technique

Surgical Incisions

The setup is similar to that for the lateral opening wedge technique. The procedure starts with a 12- to 15-cm medial longitudinal skin incision starting from the level of the joint line and going proximally. The subcutaneous tissue is dissected down to the fascia of the vastus medialis proximally and the joint capsule distally. The fascia is divided along the skin incision. The vastus medialis is elevated off the medial intermuscular septum and is reflected laterally to expose the medial femoral condyle and the femoral cortex. Care is taken to protect the femoral vessels in the adductor canal by elevating them through subperiosteal dissection off the medial femoral cortex throughout the procedure.

Specific Steps

Box 71-2 outlines the steps of this procedure.

Subperiosteal blunt Hohmann retractors are used to maintain exposure of the femoral shaft. Posterior perforating arteries should be cauterized. Most of the dissection is performed with the extremity in a figure-of-four position (the hip is flexed and externally rotated; the knee is flexed). Then a guide pin is inserted in the medial femoral condyle 2 cm proximal and parallel to the distal femoral articular surface in the coronal plane, in line with the long axis of the femur in the sagittal plane

> **BOX 71-2** Surgical Steps: Medial Closing Wedge Distal Femoral Osteotomy Technique
>
> 1. Under fluoroscopic guidance, the guide pin is inserted parallel and 2 cm proximal to the joint line.
> 2. The guide pin is checked on the lateral view to determine at what level in the sagittal plane (anterior to posterior) the chisel should be inserted.
> 3. The chisel is inserted parallel to the guide pin and just proximal to it.
> 4. The chisel is checked on the lateral view; it should be centered along the long axis of the femur.
> 5. The blade of the 90-degree blade plate is inserted parallel to the joint line.
> 6. A wedge of bone (5- to 10-mm base) has been removed proximal to the blade.
> 7. The arm of the plate is pushed toward the femoral cortex, and 4.5-mm cortical screws are inserted.
> 8. Four 4.5-mm bicortical screws are inserted.
> 9. An additional 6.5-mm lag screw is inserted in oblique fashion if the osteotomy is too close to the blade of the plate for additional fixation.

(approximately at the junction of the anterior and middle third of the medial condyle) and parallel to the floor in the axial plane (Fig. 71-16).

Fluoroscopy in the AP and lateral projections is used to confirm the desired placement of the guide pin with

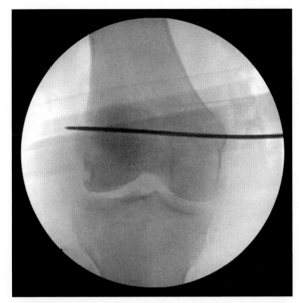

Figure 71-16. Under fluoroscopic guidance, the guide pin is inserted parallel and 2 cm proximal to the joint line.

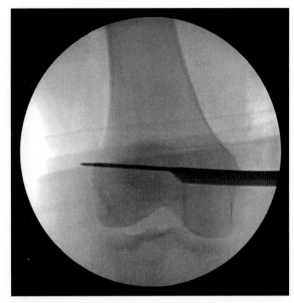

Figure 71-18. The chisel is inserted parallel to the guide pin and just proximal to it.

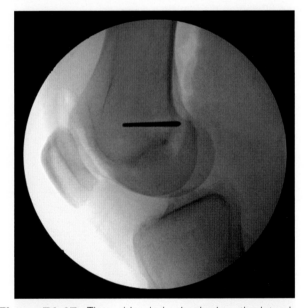

Figure 71-17. The guide pin is checked on the lateral view to determine at what level in the sagittal plane (anterior to posterior) the chisel should be inserted.

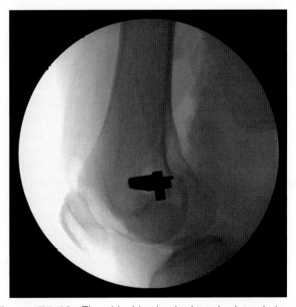

Figure 71-19. The chisel is checked on the lateral view; it should be centered along the long axis of the femur.

respect to the joint (Fig. 71-17). This is the most important part of the procedure because the realignment will end up at 90 degrees to the position of this guidewire (a 90-degree blade plate is used with the blade parallel to this pin). A longitudinal line is marked on the medial part of the femoral cortex parallel to the long axis of the femur proximal and distal to the osteotomy site to ensure that correct rotational alignment is restored after insertion of the blade chisel.

Three 4.5-mm drill holes are made in the medial femoral cortex just proximal to the guide pin (the central hole is in line with the guide pin and the other two holes are anterior and posterior to the central hole). These drill holes are for the entrance of the blade plate chisel and for prevention of uncontrolled fracture of the femur. The chisel is then inserted to a depth of 50 to 70 mm, depending on the size of the distal femur (Fig. 71-18). The plate holder is used to guide the chisel and to obtain optimal apposition of the plate to the long axis of the femur. Fluoroscopy is used to guide the insertion of the chisel. After insertion of the chisel, AP and lateral images are obtained to confirm its alignment (Fig. 71-19). A closing wedge osteotomy with a 5- to 10-mm-based wedge is made 1 cm proximal to the chisel (Fig. 71-20).

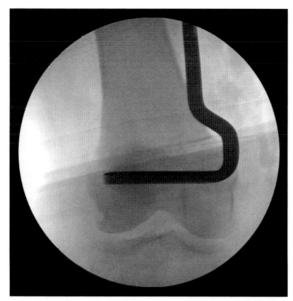

Figure 71-20. The blade of the 90-degree blade plate is inserted parallel to the joint line. A wedge of bone (5- to 10-mm base) has been removed proximal to the blade.

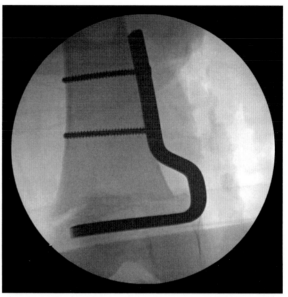

Figure 71-21. The arm of the plate is pushed toward the femoral cortex, and 4.5-mm cortical screws are inserted. Note the automatic correction of the deformity according to the 90-degree blade plate.

Because the proximal cortical fragment has a smaller diameter, it can be easily inserted into the cancellous bone of the distal fragment. This allows an increase in the magnitude of the angular correction if desired. It also provides additional stability and bony apposition and promotes more rapid healing of the osteotomy site.

Rotational alignment is maintained, and the 90-degree offset dynamic compression plate is inserted. If the plate cannot be brought into contact with the medial femoral diaphyseal cortex after insertion of the blade, a slot can be created to better accommodate the shoulder of the blade plate until satisfactory contact has been achieved. The osteotomized bony wedge is morcellized and used as an autograft along the medial aspect of the osteotomy. With the 90-degree blade plate positioned properly along the medial part of the femoral cortex, screws are inserted into the plate with use of compression techniques. The medial part of the femoral cortex and the transepicondylar femoral line are now at 90 degrees to each other (Figs. 71-21 to 71-25). This results in a desired anatomic tibiofemoral angle of approximately 0 degrees. The vastus medialis is then tacked back to the medial septum with interrupted sutures, and the skin and subcutaneous tissues are closed in a routine fashion.

Postoperative Considerations

Postoperatively the osteotomy is protected in a hinged knee brace for 6 weeks. The patient is kept on non–weight-bearing status for 6 weeks postoperatively. If there is radiographic evidence of union at 6 weeks, the patient is gradually advanced to partial weight bearing. Full weight bearing may commence at 12 weeks, with

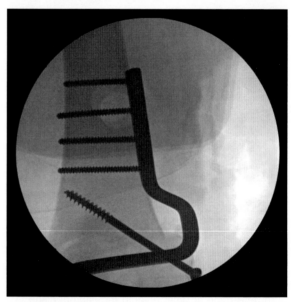

Figure 71-22. Four 4.5-mm bicortical screws are inserted. An additional 6.5-mm lag screw is inserted in an oblique fashion if the osteotomy is too close to the blade of the plate for additional fixation.

appropriate evidence of radiographic healing. Physiotherapy is used for a range-of-motion exercises in the brace until the osteotomy is healed.

Complications

Complications of distal femoral osteotomy in general are similar to the complications seen in other lower extremity surgery.

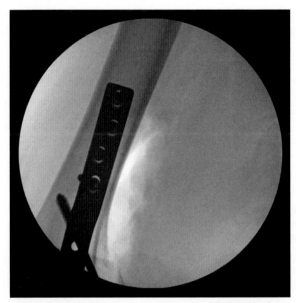

Figure 71-23. Lateral view showing good position of the plate.

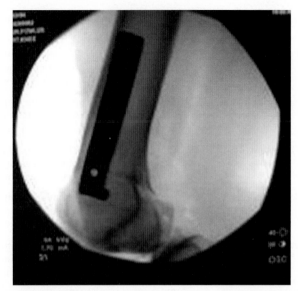

Figure 71-25. Lateral view showing the optimal position of the plate along the femoral shaft approximately at the level of the junction of the anterior and middle third of the medial femoral condyle.

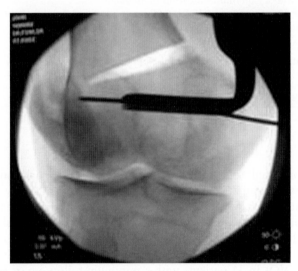

Figure 71-24. Anteroposterior view showing the best position of the osteotomy wedge (not too close to the blade of the plate). There is no need for additional fixation in this instance.

The specific complications related to the distal femoral opening wedge osteotomy are as follows:

- Undercorrection or overcorrection of the deformity
- Intra-articular fracture—when the guide pin is positioned too close to the joint, leaving too little metaphyseal cancellous bone between the osteotomy and the joint surface, or when opening of the osteotomy is attempted before all the osteotomy cuts have been completely made[9]
- Displacement or subluxation at the osteotomy site—when the medial hinge is unstable because of

propagation of the osteotomy through the opposite cortex or when the degree of correction is too big
- Malunion and nonunion of the osteotomy—when the patient has risk factors or when the patient starts bearing weight too early
- Delayed healing, which was found to be frequent by Jacobi and colleagues[10]
- Frequent troublesome irritation caused by the plate being on the iliotibial band[10]

RESULTS

The results of distal femoral osteotomy for the treatment of lateral compartment gonarthrosis in the literature are generally good (Table 71-1). Puddu and colleagues[11] reported their experience with 4 to 14 years of follow-up with a series of 21 patients who underwent open wedge distal femoral osteotomy. All patients showed improvement in the International Knee Documentation Committee (IKDC) and Hospital for Special Surgery (HSS) scores, with excellent results for the last six patients. The remainder of the studies we reviewed used the closing wedge technique. Healy and colleagues[8] reported a series of 23 distal femoral osteotomies in patients with a median age of 56 years and a mean follow-up of 4 years; 83% of the knees were rated as good or excellent according to the HSS knee score, which had improved from an average of 65 points preoperatively to 86 points postoperatively. Finkelstein and colleagues[12] did a survivorship analysis of 21 knees with distal femoral closing wedge osteotomy in 20 patients. At an average of 133 months, 13 osteotomies were still

TABLE 71-1. Long-Term Results of Distal Femoral Osteotomy

Authors	Technique	Results
Puddu et al[11] (2007)	Opening wedge	21 patients with 4 to 14 years of follow-up All patients showed improvement in the IKDC and HSS scores, with excellent results for the last six patients.
Healy et al[8] (1988)	Closing wedge	23 patients with a mean follow-up of 4 years A total of 83% rated as good or excellent HSS scores; an average improvement of 65 points preoperatively to 86 points postoperatively.
Finkelstein et al[12] (1996)	Closing wedge	21 knees in 20 patients After an average of 133 months, 13 procedures were still successful, seven had failed, and one patient had died.
Aglietti and Menchetti[13] (2000)	Closing wedge	18 patients with an average follow-up of 9 years A total of 77% were rated as good or excellent by the Knee Society rating system. Scores improved for pain and function.
Wang and Hsu[14] (2005)	Closing wedge	30 patients with a mean follow-up of 99 months Twenty-five patients had a satisfactory result, and two had a fair result. The remaining three patients underwent total knee arthroplasty.
Backstein et al[15] (2007)	Closing wedge	40 patients with a mean follow-up of 123 months In 60%, good or excellent results; 20% had been converted to total knee arthroplasty, 7.5% had fair results and 7.5% had poor results.
Kosashvili et al[16] (2010)	Closing wedge	33 knees in 30 patients with a minimum follow-up of 10 years Overall failure rate of 48.5% at a mean of 15.6 years; mean modified Knee Society scores improved from 36.8 preoperatively to 77.5 at 1 year after DFVO.
Cameron et al[17] (1994)	Closing wedge	35 patients with chronic MCL instability Improvement in gait pattern was achieved in 34 of 35 patients.
Paley et al[18] (1994)	Closing wedge	Excellent results in 19 out of 23 patients with MCL laxity corrected by osteotomy and distraction osteogenesis.

DFVO, Distal femoral varus osteotomy; *HSS,* Hospital for Special Surgery; *IKDC,* International Knee Documentation Committee; *MCL,* medial collateral ligament.

successful, seven had failed, and one patient had died. The researchers concluded that the probability of survival at 10 years was 64% (95% CI 48% to 80%).

Aglietti and Menchetti[13] reported the results of 18 knees in 18 patients with an average age of 54 years and average follow-up of 9 years. Seventy-seven percent were rated as good or excellent by the Knee Society rating system. The knee and functional scores improved from 54 points to 89 points and from 65 points to 86 points, respectively. One knee required a subsequent total knee arthroplasty 5 years after osteotomy because of severe and persistent pain. Wang and Hsu[14] reported the results of 30 knees in 30 patients with a mean follow-up of 99 months using the HSS knee-rating system and physical examination. Twenty-five patients (83%) had a satisfactory result, and two had a fair result. The remaining three patients had a conversion to a total knee arthroplasty. The cumulative 10-year survival rate for all patients was 87% (95% CI 69% to 100%).

Backstein and colleagues[15] reported on 40 distal femoral varus osteotomies (DFVOs) with a mean follow-up of 123 months. Sixty-percent of the procedures had good or excellent results, 20% had been

converted to total knee arthroplasty, 7.5% had fair results, and 7.5% had poor results. The 10-year survival rate was 82% (95% CI 75% to 89%), and the 15-year survival rate was 45% (95% CI 33% to 57%). Kosashvili and colleagues[16] found an overall failure rate of 48.5% at a mean of 15.6 years on 33 consecutive DFVOs in 31 patients with a minimum follow-up of 10 years. Mean modified Knee Society scores improved from 36.8 preoperatively to 77.5 at 1 year after DFVO.

The reported results of distal femoral osteotomy for other indications are rare. Cameron and Saha[17] treated 35 patients with chronic MCL instability with a distal femoral osteotomy. Improvement in gait pattern was achieved in 34 of 35 patients, but the MCL usually remained lax even after the osteotomy. This, however, is not usually a functional problem with daily activity. Paley and colleagues[18] reported excellent results in 19 of 23 patients with MCL laxity corrected by osteotomy and distraction osteogenesis.

CONCLUSIONS

In short, lower limb alignment is a very important and critical concept in orthopedic surgery. Distal femoral osteotomy is a common surgical procedure used to correct a valgus limb malalignment. It has many indications and has been shown to be effective for a number of patients. However, for the best long-term outcome, one should be mindful of the contraindications as well as the potential pitfalls of this procedure.

REFERENCES

1. Brouwer GM, van Tol AW, Bergink AP, et al. Association between valgus and varus alignment and the development and progression of radiographic osteoarthritis of the knee. *Arthritis Rheum.* 2007;56(4):1204-1211.
2. Cerejo R, Dunlop DD, Cahue S, et al. The influence of alignment on risk of knee osteoarthritis progression according to baseline stage of disease. *Arthritis Rheum.* 2002;46(10):2632-2636.
3. Sharma L, Song J, Felson DT, et al. The role of knee alignment in disease progression and functional decline in knee osteoarthritis. *JAMA.* 2001;286(2):188-195.
4. Issa SN, Dunlop D, Chang A, et al. Full-limb and knee radiography assessments of varus-valgus alignment and their relationship to osteoarthritis disease features by magnetic resonance imaging. *Arthritis Rheum.* 2007;57(3): 398-406.
5. Chambat P, Si Selmi TA, Dejour D, et al. Varus tibial osteotomy. *Oper Tech Sports Med.* 2000;8(1):44-47.
6. Marti CB, Gautier E, Wachtl SW, et al. Accuracy of frontal and sagittal plane correction in open-wedge high tibial osteotomy. *Arthroscopy.* 2004;20(4):366-372.
7. Closkey RF, Windsor RE. Alterations in the patella after a high tibial or distal femoral osteotomy. *Clin Orthop Relat Res.* 2001;(389):51-56.
8. Healy WL, Anglen JO, Wasilewski SA, et al. Distal femoral varus osteotomy. *J Bone Joint Surg Am.* 1988;70(1): 102-109.
9. Vasconcellos DA, Giffin JR, Amendola A. Avoiding and managing complications in osteotomies of the knee. In: Meislin RJ, Halbrecht J, eds. *Complications in Knee and Shoulder Surgery: Management and Treatment Options for the Sports Medicine Orthopedist.* London: Springer; 2009:115-132.
10. Jacobi M, Wahl P, Bouaicha S, et al. Distal femoral varus osteotomy: Problems associated with the lateral open-wedge technique. *Arch Orthop Trauma Surg.* 2011;131(6):725-728.
11. Puddu G, Cipolla M, Cerullo G, et al. Osteotomies: The surgical treatment of the valgus knee. *Sports Med Arthrosc.* 2007;15(1):15-22.
12. Finkelstein JA, Gross AE, Davis A. Varus osteotomy of the distal part of the femur. A survivorship analysis. *J Bone Joint Surg Am.* 1996;78(9):1348-1352.
13. Aglietti P, Menchetti PP. Distal femoral varus osteotomy in the valgus osteoarthritic knee. *Am J Knee Surg.* 2000; 13(2):89-95.
14. Wang JW, Hsu CC. Distal femoral varus osteotomy for osteoarthritis of the knee. *J Bone Joint Surg Am.* 2005; 87(1):127-133.
15. Backstein D, Morag G, Hanna S, et al. Long-term follow-up of distal femoral varus osteotomy of the knee. *J Arthroplasty.* 2007;22(4), Suppl 1, 2-6.
16. Kosashvili Y, Safir O, Gross A, et al. Distal femoral varus osteotomy for lateral osteoarthritis of the knee: A minimum ten-year follow-up. *Int Orthop.* 2010;34(2): 249-254.
17. Cameron JC, Saha S. Management of medial collateral ligament laxity. *Orthop Clin North Am.* 1994;25(3): 527-532.
18. Paley D, Bhatnagar J, Herzenberg JE, et al. New procedures for tightening knee collateral ligaments in conjunction with knee realignment osteotomy. *Orthop Clin North Am.* 1994;25(3):533-555.

Chapter 72

Patellar Tendon Autograft for Anterior Cruciate Ligament Reconstruction

Aman Dhawan and Charles A. Bush-Joseph

Chapter Synopsis

- The bone–patellar tendon–bone autograft is the most commonly used graft during the last 15 years and the graft of choice of physicians treating National Collegiate Athletic Association (NCAA) Division 1A and professional athletes. This is because of the graft's ready accessibility, mechanical strength, and bone healing. In this chapter we highlight the harvest procedure as well as transtibial and medial portal femoral independent surgical techniques for anatomic anterior cruciate ligament (ACL) reconstruction using bone–patellar tendon–bone autograft.

Important Points

- Surgical steps
  1. Graft harvest
  2. Graft preparation
  3. Notch preparation
  4. Femoral tunnel placement
  5. Tibial tunnel placement
  6. Graft placement and fixation
  7. Closure

Clinical and Surgical Pearls and Pitfalls

- Harvest the tendinous and tibial plug portions of the bone–patellar tendon–bone autograft with the leg in flexion.
- Harvest of the patellar plug in extension with the foot on a sterile Mayo stand will allow the superior skin flaps to be more easily mobilized.
- Changing hands while the saw is used during graft harvest enhances visualization of the bone cuts.

- Make a triangular cut for the tibial bone plug and a trapezoidal cut for the patellar bone plug. The latter avoids penetration into the patellar articular surface.
- A shorter femoral bone plug (10 × 20 mm) should be fashioned if a femoral independent drilling technique is used. This will facilitate the turn the graft has to make within the notch after exiting the tibial tunnel.
- Notch preparation should be carried out with a motorized shaver and arthroscopic electrocautery device. Do not use a burr to perform osteoplasty, because this may obliterate the landmarks used to facilitate anatomic femoral tunnel placement.
- The use of a curved femoral aimer, flexible guide pin, and reamers will facilitate visualization without the resource challenges with maintaining a hyperflexed position and the change in orientation hyperflexion induces in the landmarks for femoral ACL tunnel placement.
- While the bone–patellar tendon–bone ACL graft is pulled through the tibial tunnel, a probe or looped arthroscopic suture retriever should be used to help lever the pulling suture at the intra-articular entrance of the tibial tunnel. This will keep the pulling vector in line with the tibial tunnel, as well as keeping the sutures from abrading on the intra-articular tunnel entrance.
- Graft-tunnel mismatch is a concern with the medial portal femoral independent technique, because the femoral tunnel, femoral bone plug, and intra-articular length of the ACL will likely be shorter than when a transtibial technique is used. Therefore we recommend creating a long tibial tunnel to help manage this.

Anterior cruciate ligament (ACL) rupture commonly occurs among both professional and amateur athletes. Because the ACL is the primary restraint to anterior displacement of the tibia on the femur and a secondary stabilizer to tibial rotation, an ACL-deficient knee can lead to meniscal injury, functional instability, and early-onset osteoarthritis.[1] These are potentially devastating consequences in certain populations of patients, especially in athletes who participate in cutting or pivoting activities. The ACL is the most frequently torn knee ligament requiring surgical repair, and more than 100,000 ACL reconstructions are performed each year in the United States.[2]

A variety of decisions must be made when performing ACL reconstruction, including surgical technique, graft source, and graft fixation. Graft options may include autograft (bone–patellar tendon–bone, hamstring, and quadriceps tendon) or allograft (bone–patellar tendon–bone, Achilles tendon, and anterior tibialis tendon) tissue. The bone–patellar tendon–bone autograft has been the most commonly used graft during the last 15 years and is the graft of choice of physicians treating National Collegiate Athletic Association (NCAA) Division 1A and professional athletes.[3-7] This is because of the graft's ready accessibility, good mechanical strength, bone healing, and interference screw fixation. One of our primary goals in ACL reconstruction is to reapproximate the native ACL anatomy with respect to tibial and femoral tunnel placement. This anatomy has been well described in the literature. Several surgical techniques for drilling the femoral and tibial ACL tunnels can be used to accomplish this, including transtibial drilling, medial portal femoral independent drilling, outside-in femoral independent drilling, and two-incision ACL reconstruction. This chapter details the surgical technique for anatomic transtibial and medial portal femoral independent endoscopic ACL reconstruction with a bone–patellar tendon–bone autograft.

PREOPERATIVE CONSIDERATIONS

History

The diagnosis of ACL injury is often apparent from the characteristic history that is provided by the patient. Typical descriptions of the injury mechanism include the following:

- A noncontact injury that occurred during a change-of-direction maneuver, such as pivoting, cutting, or decelerating.
- The patient may have noted knee hyperextension during an awkward landing.

- A "pop" was heard or felt during the event.
- Acute onset of significant swelling that often developed in minutes to hours.
- A sensation of instability limits the ability to return to play.
- The patient reports catching or locking (signifies meniscal disease, stump impingement, or loose bodies).
- The patient's age, history of anterior knee pain or patellar instability and other previous knee injury, and contralateral knee instability are critical to decision making.

Physical Examination

The physical examination is essential in the diagnosis of ACL injury and the evaluation of associated pathologic changes, such as meniscal or chondral damage and associated ligamentous injury.

Assessment of the injured knee includes evaluation of gait, limb alignment, presence of an effusion, knee range of motion, patellar instability, anterior knee or joint line tenderness, and varus or valgus laxity. The Lachman and pivot-shift tests remain the most specific examinations for the evaluation of ACL injury. A positive result of the posterior drawer test, posterior sag, or increased tibial external rotation at 30 or 90 degrees signals the presence of associated posterior cruciate ligament (PCL) or posterolateral corner injury. Instrumented knee arthrometry with anterior drawer testing at 30 degrees can be helpful in confirming ACL injury when the side-to-side difference is greater than 3 mm.

Imaging

Radiography

Despite recent trends, plain radiographic imaging remains critical in the initial evaluation of patients with suspected ACL injuries. Weight-bearing radiographs are essential to visualize joint space, notch architecture, and bone alignment. Lateral radiographs may reveal an avulsion of the tibial eminence or lateral capsule (Segond fracture). Radiographic views commonly used in evaluating patients with knee ligament injuries include the following:

- Weight-bearing anteroposterior radiograph in full extension
- Weight-bearing posteroanterior 45-degree flexion radiograph
- Non–weight-bearing 45-degree flexion lateral view
- Axial view of the patellofemoral joint (Merchant view)

Magnetic Resonance Imaging

Magnetic resonance imaging is performed to evaluate the ACL, PCL, medial collateral ligament, lateral collateral ligament, menisci, and associated articular cartilage injury.

Indications and Contraindications

The ideal candidate for an ACL reconstruction with bone–patellar tendon–bone autograft is a young, active patient with no effusion, full range of motion, and no patellar tendon disease. In addition, patients with symptomatic intra-articular disease, such as meniscal injury or loose bodies, may benefit from earlier surgical intervention. Of note, it is vital to educate the patient concerning the risks and benefits of the various graft options for the patient to make the final informed decision. For example, patients in certain professions, such as roofers and carpet layers, should be counseled about the increased incidence of discomfort with kneeling.

ACL reconstruction with a bone–patellar tendon–bone autograft is relatively contraindicated in patients with degenerative joint disease, in patients with a history of patellar tendon disease, and in those patients who are sedentary, inactive, or elderly. In addition, patients who have limited motion preoperatively or who are unable to comply with a rigorous postoperative protocol are poor candidates as well. Patients with a history of anterior knee pain or pain with kneeling should be advised to choose a different graft option. Last, ACL reconstruction in the skeletally immature patient remains a challenge and requires extensive discussion of the risks and benefits involved. In patients with significant growth remaining, soft tissue grafts such as hamstring, rather than bone–patellar tendon–bone grafts, are thought to pose less risk of premature physeal closure.

Surgical Planning

Preoperative rehabilitation is essential to successful surgical outcomes. Before surgery, all patients undergo extensive physical therapy, focusing on closed-chain hamstring and quadriceps stretching and strengthening to regain full range of motion and a normal gait pattern.

SURGICAL TECHNIQUE

Anesthesia and Positioning

After induction of general, spinal, or regional anesthesia, the patient is placed in the supine position on a standard operating room table. A thorough examination under anesthesia is performed.

Examination under anesthesia includes the Lachman test, anterior and posterior drawer tests, varus and valgus stress testing, and pivot shift test. Evaluation of external rotation at 30 and 90 degrees of flexion is important to assess the stability of the posterolateral corner. Comparison examination of the contralateral knee is done as well. If pivot shift testing demonstrates clear ACL insufficiency, the bone–patellar tendon–bone graft can be harvested before diagnostic arthroscopy.

At this time a tourniquet is placed and the thigh is secured in a leg holder for added stability. The contralateral leg is positioned in a well-padded foot holder with the knee and hip flexed to protect the peroneal nerve. The foot of the operating room table is then dropped, and the waist is flexed to diminish the amount of lumbar extension (Fig. 72-1). The leg is prepared and

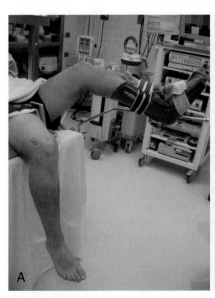
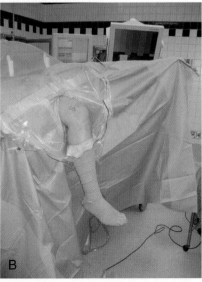

Figure 72-1. Positioning of the patient before **(A)** and after **(B)** draping.

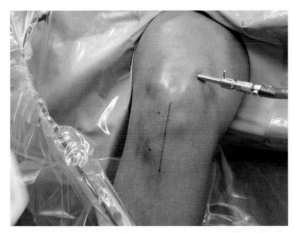

Figure 72-2. Surgical landmarks and skin incision.

draped in sterile fashion while preoperative antibiotics are administered.

Incision

The longitudinal incision for the bone–patellar tendon–bone harvest starts at the most distal aspect of the patella, just medial to the midline, coursing distally to 2 cm below the tibial tubercle (Fig. 72-2). Alternatively, the use of transverse skin incisions over the lower pole of the patella and tibial tubercle may provide a more cosmetic skin scar and potentially avoid injury to the infrapatellar branch of the saphenous nerve.

Portals

- Superolateral (outflow) portal
- Anterolateral portal
- Anteromedial portal
- Far medial inferomedial portal (for medial portal drilling technique)
- Inferomedial portal placed through the patellar tendon defect from harvest (for transtibial technique)

Examination Under Anesthesia and Diagnostic Arthroscopy

Examination under anesthesia is completed as previously described. Of note, if the examination under anesthesia is unclear regarding ACL rupture, diagnostic arthroscopy is performed before harvesting of the bone–patellar tendon–bone graft.[5]

With diagnostic arthroscopy the surgeon evaluates the patellofemoral joint, medial and lateral gutters, suprapatellar pouch, and medial and lateral compartments to assess for any meniscal disease, loose bodies, and articular cartilage injury. The intercondylar notch is visualized as well to evaluate the PCL and ACL for injury.

> **BOX 72-1** Surgical Steps
>
> - Graft harvest
> - Graft preparation
> - Notch preparation
> - Femoral tunnel placement
> - Tibial tunnel placement
> - Graft placement and fixation
> - Closure

Specific Steps

Box 72-1 outlines the surgical steps of this procedure.

1. Bone–Patellar Tendon–Bone Graft Harvest

After the anatomic landmarks have been appropriately marked and the knee is flexed, a longitudinal incision, just medial to midline, is made from the distal tip of the patella to 2 cm distal to the tibial tubercle. This incision allows graft harvest and placement of the tibial tunnel through the same operative approach. This incision is carried directly down to the transverse fibers of the peritenon of the patellar tendon. After skin flaps are raised both medially and laterally, a No. 15 blade is used to incise the peritenon longitudinally at its midline. Metzenbaum scissors extend this cut proximally and distally and undermine the peritenon medially and laterally to fully expose the entire patellar tendon.

The patellar tendon's width is measured proximally and distally and marked with a marking pen. The bone–patellar tendon–bone autograft ideally is 10 mm wide with 10- × 25-mm bone plugs (10- × 20-mm femoral plug for medial portal femoral independent technique). Parallel longitudinal incisions spaced 10 mm apart are made in the patellar tendon, then the periosteum and soft tissues overlying the tibial and patellar bone cuts are outlined with the blade. The tendon incisions are performed with the knee flexed, thus keeping the patellar tendon on tension. Extension of the knee aids in skin flap mobilization and thus visualization for the transverse crosscuts at the patellar and tibial bone block edges.

At this point, an oscillating saw is used to make first the tibial then the patellar bone plug. With use of the nondominant thumb to stabilize the saw and the index finger to protect the graft between the inner and outer portion of the graft (Fig. 72-3), the tibial cortex is scored longitudinally on profile to remove an equilateral triangle of bone. This leaves a maximal amount of bone around the tibial tubercle and remaining patellar tendon to minimize the risk of postoperative complications, such as patellar tendon avulsion or tubercle

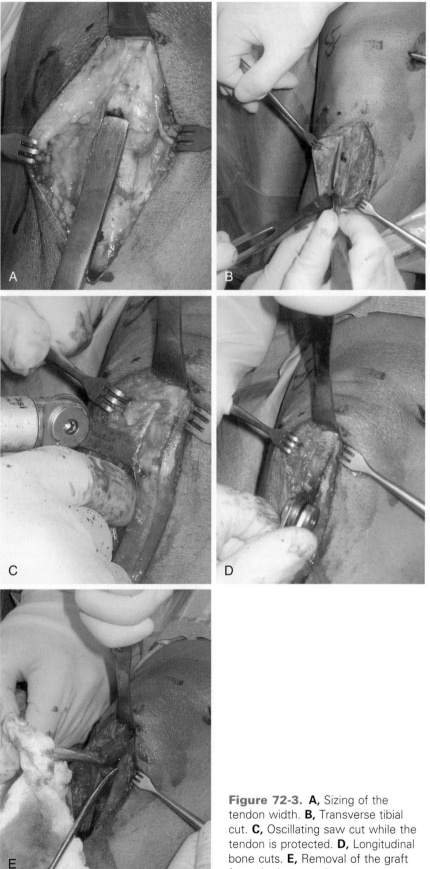

Figure 72-3. A, Sizing of the tendon width. **B,** Transverse tibial cut. **C,** Oscillating saw cut while the tendon is protected. **D,** Longitudinal bone cuts. **E,** Removal of the graft from the harvest site.

fracture. The distal transverse tibial crosscut is made with the saw held at a 45-degree oblique angle to the cortex by use of the corner of the blade on each side of the plug, but the tibial bone plug is left in place at this time. The patellar tendon bone plug is then made in a trapezoidal shape, with a depth not exceeding 6 to 7 mm to avoid damage to the articular surface. Once again, the proximal transverse crosscut is made at a 45-degree oblique angle to the cortex. The saw is then placed parallel to the medial and lateral edges to complete the patellar bone plug crosscuts. Half-inch and quarter-inch curved osteotomes are now used to carefully mobilize the bone plugs without levering. A lap sponge can be placed around the freed tibial plug to improve traction, and Metzenbaum scissors are used to carefully remove any remaining fat or soft tissues. Once it is freed, the graft is wrapped in a moist sponge and walked to the back table by the operative surgeon, where it is placed in a safe location known to all members of the surgical team.

2. Graft Preparation

Ten-millimeter by 25-mm bone plugs are sized for a transtibial technique. If a medial portal technique is used for femoral drilling, we recommend that the length of the femoral bone plug be sized to 20 mm. This shorter length will assist with navigating the proximal bone plug through the notch and docking of the graft into the femoral tunnel after exit through the aperture of the tibial tunnel. The first step involves measurement and documentation of the overall graft length, the length of the bone plugs, and the length of the tendinous portion of the graft. At this time the bone plugs are sized with a small rongeur to remove excess bone and to contour the bone appropriately to fit the desired tunnel diameter, frequently 10 mm. Excess bone should be saved for grafting of the harvest sites. If one bone plug is wider, we prefer to use it on the tibial side, where we usually drill an 11-mm tunnel.

Next, drill holes are made in the tibial and femoral bone blocks. Various configurations have been described. We prefer two holes in the tibial and one hole in the femoral bone block for heavy nonresorbable sutures (Fig. 72-4). These holes can be placed either through the cortex or parallel to it; the latter decreases the risk of cutting the sutures during interference screw placement but also decreases pull-out strength from the bone block. A sterile pen is used to mark the cortical surface of the tibial bone plug to assist in graft orientation; the femoral bone plug is marked at the bone-tendon junction to better assess correct seating of the plug within the tunnel.

3. Notch Preparation

Visualization of the native anatomy of the ACL and surgical anatomic landmarks on the femur and tibia is

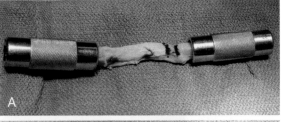
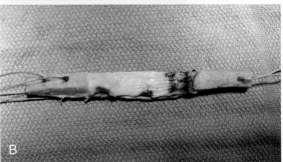

Figure 72-4. Graft preparation. **A,** The graft is sized to fit through a 10-mm tunnel. **B,** The finally prepared patellar tendon autograft with sutures passed through the femoral and tibial bone plugs.

critical to accurate placement of the tunnels for reconstruction. After the diagnostic arthroscopic evaluation of the knee and all intra-articular work have been completed (e.g., meniscal repair), preparation of the notch should commence. With a combination of arthroscopic meniscal punch, motorized shaver, and electrocautery, the residual ACL tissue should be removed from the lateral femoral intercondylar notch. Preserving a small amount of fibers on the ACL tibial footprint will aid in placement of the tibial aiming device for guide pin placement. Care should be taken to preserve the osseous landmarks on the lateral femoral condyle as best as possible to help guide femoral tunnel placement. To this end, electrocautery should be used, as opposed to a shaver, bone cutter, or bur on the lateral femoral condyle proper. To aid in visualization of the native ACL footprint, a 70-degree scope is used through the anterolateral portal. This provides an en face view of the wall of the lateral femoral condyle similar to use of the 30-degree scope placed through the anteromedial portal, while eliminating the "sword fighting" inherent with visualizing and working from two medial portals (Fig. 72-5).[8,9] The 70-degree scope also provides a bird's-eye view of the native tibial ACL footprint and landmarks, which may help aid placement.

4. Femoral Tunnel Placement: Medial Portal, Femoral Independent Technique

The femoral tunnel is drilled first, using the medial portal femoral independent technique. This will help minimize fluid extravasation. We prefer to use a separate far inferomedial accessory portal for guidewire

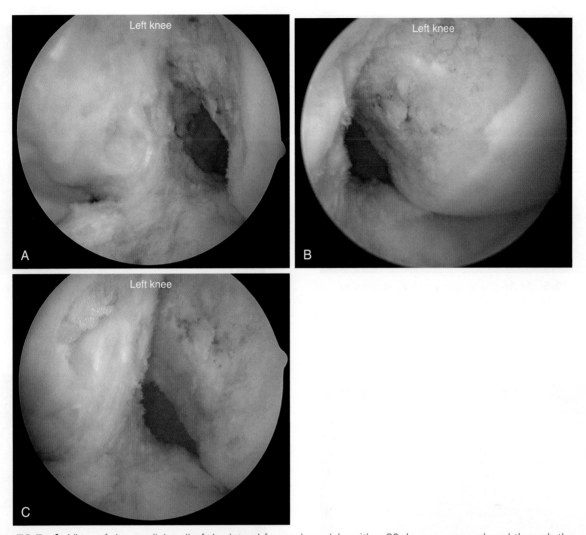

Figure 72-5. A, View of the medial wall of the lateral femoral condyle with a 30-degree scope placed through the anterolateral portal. **B,** View with a 30-degree scope placed through the anteromedial portal. **C,** View with a 70-degree scope placed through the anterolateral portal.

placement and drilling because this position will aid in placement of the drilled femoral tunnel in the anatomic ACL femoral footprint. A standard anteromedial portal can be created early in the procedure to perform meniscal and chondral work in the standard fashion as well as access the posterior aspect of the wall of the lateral femoral condyle for notch preparation. This far inferomedial accessory portal should be placed under direct arthroscopic visualization approximately 3 to 4 cm medial to the patellar tendon and just superior to the meniscus (Fig. 72-6). With an 18-gauge spinal needle, check that the femoral footprint of the native ACL is easily accessed while ensuring that the medial femoral condyle is at a safe distance from the ensuing reamers.

We prefer using curved aiming devices with flexible guide pins and reamers (Stryker, Kalamazoo, MI). This circumvents the challenges with obtaining and

maintaining hyperflexion during femoral tunnel placement, enhances visualization through better fluid egress within the notch, and aids in visualization of the notch in the standard orientation versus hyperflexion, which may be disorienting to surgeons, especially when new to this technique (Fig. 72-7).[8] The guide pin is flexible and makes the turn through the confines of the curved aimer. When it leaves the aimer and enters the lateral femoral condyle, it takes a straight path into and through the lateral femoral condyle. The femoral bone plug therefore docks into a straight tunnel, not a curved one. We have not encountered any problems docking the femoral bone plug as a result of the shape of the femoral tunnel. For single tunnel ACL reconstruction, and with the notch visualized at 90 degrees of knee flexion, the flexible guide pin should be placed posterior and inferior to the well-visualized lateral intercondylar ridge, directly onto the bifurcate ridge, approximately 7 mm

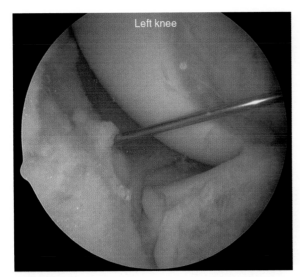

Figure 72-6. An 18-gauge spinal needle is used to localize the far inferomedial accessory portal for femoral independent drilling. This portal should be approximately 3 to 4 cm medial to the patellar tendon and just superior to the meniscus.

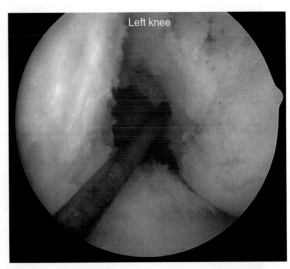

Figure 72-8. The flexible femoral guide pin is placed posterior and inferior to the well-visualized lateral intercondylar ridge, directly onto the bifurcate ridge, approximately 7 mm from the "back wall."

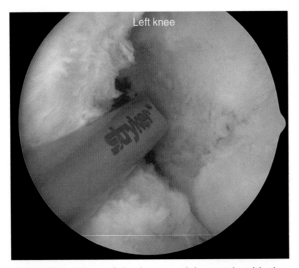

Figure 72-7. View of the intercondylar notch with the knee at 90 degrees of flexion and a curved femoral aiming device.

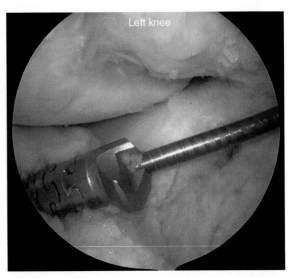

Figure 72-9. The reamer must be visualized as it enters the joint over the guide pin through the inferomedial accessory portal. This is to ensure that no chondral scuffing of the medial femoral condyle occurs during its passage from portal entrance to the lateral femoral condyle.

from the "back wall" (Fig. 72-8).[10] This will yield a 2-mm back wall once reaming has been completed with a 10-mm flexible reamer. The reamer must be visualized as it enters the joint over the guide pin through the inferomedial accessory portal. This is to ensure that no chondral scuffing of the medial femoral condyle occurs during its passage from portal entrance to lateral femoral condyle (Fig. 72-9).

With use of the flexible guide pin and reamers, the tunnel will tend to "posteriorize." Be wary of this, and reexamine the entrance to the femoral tunnel after reaming 2 to 3 mm to ensure an adequate back wall.

This tunnel should be reamed to a depth of no more than 25 mm; any further depth risks blowing out the lateral cortex of the femur. After reaming, the two free ends of a passing suture are threaded through the eyelet of the flexible guide pin and passed out the lateral thigh. A clamp is placed on the looped end and two free ends (looped end through the medial portal and free ends through the lateral thigh) of this looped passing suture and will be used later for graft passage (passing suture-in-waiting).

Femoral Tunnel Placement for Transtibial Technique

The retrograde femoral tunnel offset guide is placed through the tibial tunnel. This guide courses through the joint and hooks the posterior aspect of the notch in the over-the-top position. Ideally, the tunnel originates at the 11-o'clock position in the right knee and the 1-o'clock position in the left knee. The guide assists in avoiding posterior cortical wall blowout if it is positioned appropriately. A 10-mm–diameter tunnel is usually drilled in the posterior cortex with a 7-mm offset guide, resulting in a 2-mm posterior wall. On occasion, when the orientation of the tibial tunnel interferes with correct placement of the femoral tunnel, the femoral offset guide can be placed (with the knee hyperflexed) through an accessory inferomedial portal. The arthroscopic pump is turned off, the femoral guide is placed in the over-the-top position, and a probe is placed into the joint through the inferomedial portal to retract and protect the PCL.

A guide pin is drilled approximately 3 cm into the femur; in the pull-through technique, a Beath pin is used in place of the shorter guide pin and drilled through the femur and out the skin. A 10-mm reamer is placed over the guide pin, and the tunnel is reamed initially only to a depth of 1 cm. The reamer is then retracted, allowing verification of posterior wall integrity. Reaming is resumed to a depth of 5 to 7 mm more than the length of the femoral bone plug to eliminate graft mismatch. As the reamer is removed, the pump inflow is turned on, and loose bone can once again be collected with Owens gauze.[5,6] Final tunnel integrity can be assessed by removal of the reamer and guide pin and placement of the arthroscopic camera through the tibial tunnel and directly into the femoral tunnel.

5. Tibial Tunnel Placement

Medial Portal Femoral Independent Technique

The tibial tunnel is placed after completion of femoral tunnel placement. The tibial tunnel is placed through the same incision that was used for the graft harvest. The ideal placement of the guide pin is in the native ACL tibial, in the sagittal plane midway between the anterior and posterior edges of the anterior horn of the lateral meniscus and between the tibial spines in the coronal plane (Fig. 72-10). A small amount of residual ACL tibial stump can be left attached after notch preparation to help aid guide pin placement. Any residual tissue can be removed after reaming of the tibial tunnel. Graft-tunnel mismatch is a concern with the medial portal femoral independent technique because the femoral tunnel, femoral bone plug, and intra-articular length of the ACL will likely be shorter than when a transtibial technique is used.[11] Therefore we recommend

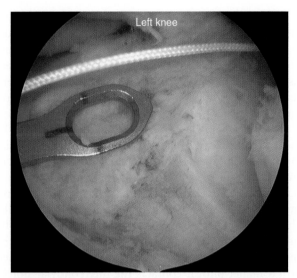

Figure 72-10. Placement of the tibial guide pin is in the native anterior cruciate ligament tibial footprint. In the sagittal plane it is located midway between the anterior and posterior edges of the anterior horn of the lateral meniscus and between the tibial spines in the coronal plane.

creating a long tibial tunnel to help manage this. The guide should be introduced intra-articularly through the standard anteromedial portal and should be set at 60 degrees; this will create a long tibial tunnel. The superior arm of the guide should be parallel to the floor to prevent inadvertent creation of a more steeply angled, and thus shorter, tibial tunnel.

Transtibial Technique

The tibial tunnel is placed through the same incision that was used for the graft harvest. The entrance for the tibial tunnel is approximately 1.5 cm medial to the tibial tubercle and 1 cm proximal to the pes anserine tendons. A 1-cm longitudinal periosteal incision is made parallel and just proximal to the hamstrings, and a medially based rectangular periosteal flap is elevated to expose cortical bone. Care is taken to avoid injury to the medial aspect of the patellar tendon, the superficial medial collateral ligament, and the pes anserine tendons. Orientation of the tibial tunnel is crucial with transtibial technique, because it determines the position of the femoral tunnel.

A tibial guide aids in drilling and proper placement of the tibial tunnel. In general, the "N + 10" rule helps determine the tibial guide angle. The rule adds 10 degrees to the length of the graft (e.g., 45-mm tendon plus 10 yields a 55-degree angle); in a majority of procedures, a 55-degree angle can be used. The guide is then introduced through an accessory inferomedial portal created through the patellar tendon defect from the harvest.

Placement of the guide pin is at the level of the posterior edge of the anterior horn of the lateral meniscus, or approximately 7 mm anterior to the PCL, and just lateral to the medial tibial spine. This placement is necessary to allow for correct localization and placement of the femoral tunnel on the wall of the lateral femoral condyle.

The stylet is appropriately positioned intra-articularly, and the cannulated guide aimer is placed on the tibial cortex 1.5 cm medial to the tibial cortex and 1 cm proximal to the pes anserinus tendons. The guide pin is placed through the guide arm and drilled into the joint, and proper pin position is confirmed arthroscopically. The leg is then extended slowly to make certain that the pin is not impinging on the superior notch. After the knee is returned to a flexed position, the pin is advanced with a mallet until it contacts the intercondylar notch, thus stabilizing the pin during reaming.

The arthroscopy pump is turned off, the appropriately sized cannulated reamer (usually 10 or 11 mm) is placed over the guide pin, and the tibial tunnel is reamed. Bone chips can be collected with Owens gauze as the reamer is removed. At this time, the inflow pump is turned on; the ledge at the posterior aspect of the tibial tunnel is removed with a chamfer reamer and smoothed down with an arthroscopic hand rasp.

6. Graft Passage and Fixation

For both transtibial and femoral independent techniques, care should be exercised to clean out both entrances to the tibial tunnel and the intra-articular entrance to the femoral tunnel. All residual soft tissue and loose bone should be removed from these locations to prevent the graft from getting hung up there. For the medial portal femoral independent technique, the passing suture-in-waiting is unclamped and the looped end is retrieved intra-articularly and in a retrograde manner through the tibial tunnel.

The femoral bone plug suture is threaded through the looped passing suture (or Beath pin slot for transtibial technique) and retrieved proximally by pulling the suture from its exit site on the lateral thigh. The sutures of the femoral bone plug and the tibial bone plug are held taught as the graft is pulled through the knee. We recommend use of a probe or looped arthroscopic suture retriever to help lever the pulling suture at the intra-articular entrance of the tibial tunnel. This will keep the pulling vector in line with the tibial tunnel, as well as keeping the sutures from abrading on the intra-articular tunnel entrance.

A probe can be used to ensure proper orientation and seating of the femoral bone plug with the tendinous portion posteriorly, and the cancellous bone anteriorly, as it enters the femoral tunnel. Once the femoral bone plug is completely seated in the femoral tunnel, a nitinol guide pin (Linvatec, Largo, FL) is placed into the femoral

tunnel at the 11-o'clock position of the graft. The knee can be flexed to 110 to 120 degrees, which may allow easier passage of the guide pin within the femoral tunnel. The pin should be introduced without resistance; otherwise pin divergence should be suspected. A satellite pusher can be used to seat the femoral bone plug as needed. The tibial bone plug should be evaluated at this time for graft-tunnel mismatch.

Before fixation of the graft, graft position should be evaluated by direct visualization to ensure proper position without notch or PCL impingement. Femoral graft fixation is performed with an interference screw placed over the nitinol guidewire. The knee may be hyperflexed to assist with obtaining the correct angle. The screw should be placed against the cancellous surface of the bone plug, away from the tendon insertion, to diminish the risk of graft injury or laceration. At this time the tibial bone plug is externally rotated 180 degrees (toward the lateral side). This maneuver allows the tibial screw to be placed along the cortical surface and anterior. This screw placement avoids possible damage to the graft by a posteriorly placed screw with the knee in flexion as well as limiting impingement that may occur with an anteriorized graft and a posteriorly placed screw.

The knee is placed in full extension with an axial load to the extremity; tension is then held firmly on the tibial sutures, and a nitinol wire is placed anterior to the tibial plug. If a femoral independent drilling technique is used, we do not recommend fixation of the graft in any flexion, to prevent capturing the knee and preventing full extension. The interference screw is advanced and seated just below the cortical surface of the tibia. At this time, the arthroscope is placed into the knee, the ACL is visualized and probed to ensure proper tension, and a Lachman test and pivot shift test are performed (Fig. 72-11).

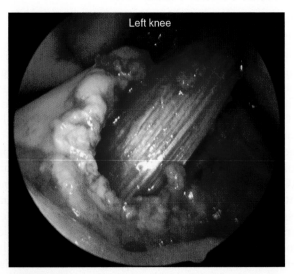

Figure 72-11. Final appearance of the anterior cruciate ligament reconstruction.

7. Closure

After irrigation with sterile saline, the knee is flexed to avoid excessive shortening. The patellar tendon defect is approximated with three or four simple interrupted No. 1 Vicryl sutures. The periosteal flap raised to drill the tibial tunnel is closed with No. 1 Vicryl as well. Bone graft from the reamings is placed in the patellar and tibial bone defects. The peritenon is closed with a running 2-0 Vicryl suture, and the incision is closed with interrupted 2-0 Vicryl for the subcutaneous tissues and a running 3-0 Prolene pullout stitch for the skin. The arthroscopy portals are closed with simple 3-0 Prolene stitches.

The wound and portals are injected with 0.5% bupivacaine (Marcaine) for postoperative analgesia. Steri-Strips and a sterile dressing are applied, followed by Kerlix, an ice cryotherapy device, and an elastic wrap. Finally, the leg is placed in a knee immobilizer or hinged knee brace locked in extension.

POSTOPERATIVE CONSIDERATIONS

Rehabilitation

Rehabilitation focuses on accelerated, closed chain exercises with a goal of achieving full range of motion while maintaining stability and avoiding patellofemoral symptoms.

Postoperative Protocol

Immediate full weight bearing is permitted locked in extension.

- Week 1: Quad sets, straight-leg raises, and patellar mobilizations are initiated with the knee in extension.
- Weeks 2 to 4: Start closed chain extension exercises, hamstring curls, and stationary biking.
- Weeks 4 to 6: Start use of stair climbing machines. Goal range of motion: 120 degrees of flexion to full extension.
- Weeks 6 to 12: Begin advanced closed chain exercises, light jogging, and outdoor biking.
- Months 4 to 6: Start sports-specific exercises and plyometrics; initiate agility drills and gradual return to sports. The patient is discharged from supervised physical therapy to a home or health club program.

Complications

The reoperation rate after patellar tendon reconstruction with bone–patellar tendon–bone autograft ranges from 4% to 31%.[7] In a comprehensive literature review of arthroscopic ACL reconstruction with bone–patellar tendon–bone autografts, Nedeff detailed the mean rates of reoperation as 13%, arthrofibrosis as 7% (1% to 12%), and infection as 0.4% (0% to 4%).[7] Other complications include the following:

- Graft fracture
- Graft contamination
- Femoral tunnel posterior wall blowout
- Graft impingement
- Graft-tunnel mismatch
- Persistent instability secondary to graft malposition
- Failure of graft incorporation
- Patellar tendon rupture, patellar fracture, patellofemoral symptoms, kneeling pain
- Compartment syndrome, complex regional pain syndrome, deep venous thrombosis

RESULTS

The clinical results of ACL reconstruction with bone–patellar tendon–bone autograft are shown in Table 72-1.

TABLE 72-1. Clinical Results of Anterior Cruciate Ligament Reconstruction with Bone–Patellar Tendon–Bone Autograft

Author	Follow-Up	Outcome
Buss et al[12] (1993)	2-year minimum	59/68 (87%) excellent or good
Bach et al[3] (1998)	2-year minimum	96/103 (93%) mostly or completely satisfied
Kleipool et al[13] (1998)	4-year minimum	26/32 (81%) normal or nearly normal
Otto et al[14] (1998)	9-year minimum	52/68 (77%) normal or nearly normal
Webb et al[15] (1998)	2-year minimum	71/82 (87%) normal or nearly normal
Jomha et al[16] (1999)	7-year minimum	55/59 (93%) normal or nearly normal
Ao et al[17] (2000)	1-year minimum	18/20 (90%) excellent or good
Deehan et al[4] (2000)	5-year minimum	81/90 (90%) normal or nearly normal
Jäger et al[18] (2003)	10-year minimum	62/74 (84%) normal
Chaudhary et al[19] (2005)	1-year minimum	68/78 (87%) excellent or good
Salmon et al[20] (2006)	13-year minimum	65/67 (97%) normal or nearly normal

REFERENCES

1. Beynnon BD, Johnson RJ, Abate JA, et al. Treatment of anterior cruciate ligament injuries, part 1. *Am J Sports Med.* 2005;33:1579-1602.
2. Owings MF, Kozak LJ. Ambulatory and inpatient procedures in the United States 1996. *Vital Health Stat 13.* 1998;139:1-119.
3. Bach Jr BR, Levy ME, Bojchuk J, et al. Single-incision endoscopic anterior cruciate ligament reconstruction using patellar tendon autograft. Minimum two-year follow-up evaluation. *Am J Sports Med.* 1998;26:30-40.
4. Deehan DJ, Salmon LJ, Webb VJ, et al. Endoscopic reconstruction of the anterior cruciate ligament with an ipsilateral patellar tendon autograft. A prospective longitudinal five-year study. *J Bone Joint Surg Br.* 2000;82:984-991.
5. Ferrari J, Bush-Joseph C, Bach Jr BR. Endoscopic anterior cruciate ligament reconstruction with patellar tendon autograft: surgical technique. *Tech Orthop.* 1998;13: 262-274.
6. Flik K, Bach Jr BR. Anterior cruciate ligament reconstruction using an endoscopic technique with patellar tendon autograft. *Tech Orthop.* 2005;20:361-371.
7. Nedeff DD, Bach Jr BR. Arthroscopic anterior cruciate ligament reconstruction using patellar tendon autografts: a comprehensive review of contemporary literature. *Am J Knee Surg.* 2001;14:243-258.
8. Bedi A, Altchek DW. The "footprint" anterior cruciate ligament technique: an anatomic approach to anterior cruciate ligament reconstruction. *Arthroscopy.* 2009;25 (10):1128-1138.
9. Bedi A, Dines J, Dines DM, et al. Use of the 70° arthroscope for improved visualization with common arthroscopic procedures. *Arthroscopy.* 2010;26(12):1684-1696.
10. Zantop T, Diermann N, Schumacher T, et al. Anatomical and non-anatomical double-bundle anterior cruciate ligament reconstruction: Importance of femoral tunnel location on knee kinematics. *Am J Sports Med.* 2008;36: 678-685.
11. Bedi A, Raphael B, Maderazo A, et al. Transtibial versus anteromedial portal drilling for anterior cruciate ligament reconstruction: a cadaveric study of femoral tunnel length and obliquity. *Arthroscopy.* 2010;26(3):342-350.
12. Buss DD, Warren RF, Wickiewicz TL, et al. Arthroscopically assisted reconstruction of the anterior cruciate ligament with use of autogenous patellar-ligament grafts. Results after twenty-four to forty-two months. *J Bone Joint Surg Am.* 1993;75:1346-1355.
13. Kleipool AE, Zijl JA, Willems WJ. Arthroscopic anterior cruciate ligament reconstruction with bone–patellar tendon–bone allograft or autograft. A prospective study with an average follow up of 4 years. *Knee Surg Sports Traumatol Arthrosc.* 1998;6:224-230.
14. Otto D, Pinczewski LA, Clingeleffer A, et al. Five-year results of single-incision arthroscopic anterior cruciate ligament reconstruction with patellar tendon autograft. *Am J Sports Med.* 1998;26:181-188.
15. Webb JM, Corry IS, Clingeleffer AJ, et al. Endoscopic reconstruction for isolated anterior cruciate ligament rupture. *J Bone Joint Surg Br.* 1998;80:288-294.
16. Jomha NM, Pinczewski LA, Clingeleffer A, et al. Arthroscopic reconstruction of the anterior cruciate ligament with patellar-tendon autograft and interference screw fixation. The results at seven years. *J Bone Joint Surg Br.* 1999;81:775-779.
17. Ao Y, Wang J, Yu J, et al. [Arthroscopically assisted anterior cruciate ligament reconstruction using patellar tendon autograft fixed with interference screw]. *Zhonghua Wai Ke Za Zhi.* 2000;38:250-252.
18. Jäger A, Welsch F, Braune C, et al. [Ten year follow-up after single incision anterior cruciate ligament reconstruction using patellar tendon autograft]. *Z Orthop Ihre Grenzgeb.* 2003;141:42-47.
19. Chaudhary D, Monga P, Joshi D, et al. Arthroscopic reconstruction of the anterior cruciate ligament using bone–patellar tendon–bone autograft: experience of the first 100 cases. *J Orthop Surg (Hong Kong).* 2005;13: 147-152.
20. Salmon LJ, Russell VJ, Refshauge K, et al. Long-term outcome of endoscopic anterior cruciate ligament reconstruction with patellar tendon autograft: minimum 13-year review. *Am J Sports Med.* 2006;34:721-732.

Chapter 73

Allografts for Anterior Cruciate Ligament Reconstruction

Michael Walsh and Asheesh Bedi

Chapter Synopsis

- The use of allograft tissue in anterior cruciate ligament (ACL) reconstruction continues to gain popularity; with a reported 1.5 million allografts used per year, the number has more than doubled over the past decade. This is likely secondary to improved sterilization procedures, better collection practices, and increased confidence in the overall stability. In addition, current literature indicates that there is no difference in clinical outcome between allograft and autograft use in a number of populations of patients. Consequently there is increasing importance placed on the surgeon's understanding of allograft tissue options, collection and sterilization procedures, indications for use, and surgical techniques used with allograft tissue.

Important Points

- Potential advantages of use of allograft tissue compared with autograft include the following:
  - Decreased donor site morbidity
  - Pain,[1,2] patellar fracture,[3] patellar tendon rupture,[4,5] saphenous nerve injury[6]
  - Decreased operating room time
  - Improved cosmesis
- Potential disadvantages of allograft use include the following:
  - Cost
  - Availability
  - Reliability of vendors
  - Slower graft incorporation
  - Possibility of disease transmission and/or immunologic response[7]
  - Potentially increased risk of failure among younger athletes[8]
- In ACL reconstruction, graft selection should be done on an individual basis; however, in certain populations of patients, allograft may be preferable over autograft,

whereas in others the opposite may be true.[7-9] Patients in whom allograft may be preferred include the following:
  - Patients 40 years of age and older
  - Patients with decreased functional demands or expectations
  - Skeletally immature athletes
  - Patients with history of patellofemoral pain
  - Patients with history of previous patellar surgery
  - Laborers or athletes who frequently kneel
  - Patients undergoing revision ACL reconstruction
  - Patients undergoing multiligament reconstructive surgery
- Those patients in whom allograft is less desirable include the following:
  - High-level athletes younger than 40 years old
  - Elite-level athletes
  - Sprinters or hurdlers who require full terminal flexion strength
  - Patients with concern for disease transmission and immunocompromised patients

Clinical and Surgical Pearls

- Patients should be allowed to make informed decisions on graft choice after a full discussion of risks and benefits with the treating surgeon.
- Have informed consent from the patient to use an allograft.
- Know your allograft supplier's track record and tissue-processing techniques, including use of irradiation and proprietary cleansing techniques.
- Have a second allograft available should something go wrong with the original graft (label error, tissue quality, technical error, contamination), or discuss use of the patient's own tissue if something is wrong with the allograft.

Continued

- Prepare anatomic sockets with an independent drilling technique. Use of the described footprint method ensures an anatomic reconstruction that is not vulnerable to variable patient anatomy or errant referencing of other intra-articular landmarks. Nonanatomic ACL reconstructions are at increased risk for failure independent of autograft or allograft selection.
- Oscillating saws and rongeurs are best for removal of excess bone and sizing of the bone plug.
- Achilles allograft may be favorable owing to bone-to-bone fixation and a large cross-sectional area and favorable time-zero biomechanical properties.
- Allografts may be reasonable options for ACL reconstruction in patients age 40 years and older, particularly those with existing patellofemoral pain and/or extensor mechanism disorders.

Clinical and Surgical Pitfalls
- It is critical to recognize and treat associated malalignment and ligamentous injury, including

medial collateral ligament (MCL), lateral collateral ligament (LCL), and posterior cruciate ligament (PCL) injury. Failure to recognize and treat these conditions will predispose the allograft ACL reconstruction to failure.
- Both Achilles and BTB allografts require careful preparation of the bone plug to avoid fracture; bone crimpers should not be used.
- With bone–patellar tendon–bone allografts, length and graft-tunnel mismatch can be an issue, and tibial tunnel length should be adjusted accordingly.
- Allograft tissue incorporates more slowly than autograft, and bone plug nonunion has been reported.[10,11] A delayed return to play may help minimize the risk of graft failure secondary to inadequate host incorporation.

The use of allografts has enjoyed considerable clinical success in many soft tissue reconstructive procedures, including anterior cruciate ligament (ACL) reconstruction, one of the most common orthopedic procedures performed today. With more than 250,000 new ACL ruptures reportedly each year,[12,13] estimates indicate that 300,000 ACL reconstructions are performed annually, with approximately 240,000 (80%) performed with autograft tissue and 60,000 (20%) with allograft tissue.[7] Rationales for increased use of allograft tissue include more effective sterilization procedures,[14] organized collection and distribution of tissue, and increased confidence in the overall stability of allografts.[15-17]

The orthopedic surgeon has a number of graft options for reconstructive surgery of the ACL. Bone–patellar tendon–bone (BPTB) and hamstring autografts have historically been used for ACL reconstructive surgery, with numerous peer-reviewed studies reporting favorable clinical outcomes.[18-21] However, the use of allograft tissue for ACL reconstruction has increased.[18-20] These grafts avoid potential donor site morbidity associated with hamstring or patellar tendon graft harvest, including donor site pain,[1,2] patellar fracture,[3] patellar tendon rupture,[4,5] saphenous nerve injury,[6] and residual extensor mechanism or hamstring weakness.[1,22-24] Currently available allograft tissue includes BPTB; Achilles, hamstring, or tibialis tendon; and tensor fascia lata (Fig. 73-1). The increasing demand for allograft tissue in ACL reconstruction is attributed to potentially decreased

donor site morbidity and postoperative pain, decreased operating room time, increasing availability from tissue banks, and improved cosmesis. However, potential disadvantages include cost,[25,26] availability, reliability of vendors, slower graft incorporation, the possibility of disease transmission and/or immunologic response,[7] and a potentially increased risk of failure among younger athletes.[8]

Ideal ACL grafts have the following characteristics[27]:

- Structural properties similar to native ACL
  – Before implantation
  – After implantation
- Should allow secure fixation
- Should permit rapid biologic incorporation and ligamentization
- Should limit donor site morbidity

PREOPERATIVE CONSIDERATIONS

Contributing Mechanisms to Anterior Cruciate Ligament Injuries

Extrinsic Factors
- Ground or playing field (uneven field, wet or muddy conditions)

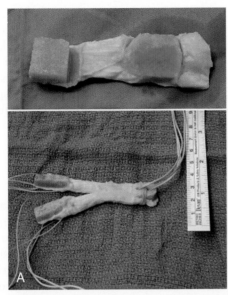
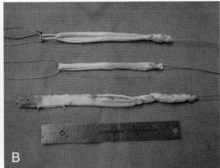

Figure 73-1. Assorted graft options. **A,** Bone–patellar tendon–bone allograft. Note the dual bone blocks, which improve incorporation time and fixation strength. **B,** Assorted allograft tissues: semitendinosus tendon *(top),* gracilis *(middle),* and Achilles tendon *(bottom).* (*A, Courtesy Jon K. Sekiya, MD, and Elsevier. B, Courtesy Jon K. Sekiya, MD.*)

- Level of competition (higher level)
- Playing style (more aggressive)
- Shoe surface (cleats versus noncleats)
- Weather (rain, extreme cold)

Intrinsic Factors

- Body size and limb girth
- Flexibility, strength, reaction time
- Hamstring weakness, quadriceps dominance
- Hormonal fluctuation (suspicion of increased laxity at ovulatory and postovulatory phase)
- Increased Q angle (greater than 14 degrees in men and greater than 17 degrees in women)
- Ligamentous laxity
- Notch width
- Jump landing technique
- Pelvic width

History

As always, a thorough history should be obtained. This should include age, prior activity level, mechanism of injury, symptoms of preinjury or postinjury instability and pain, and history of previous or concomitant knee injuries. Patient expectations, including desired activity level, are critical in helping to guide selection of autograft or allograft reconstruction. A history of immunocompromise or previous graft failure is also important and may influence graft selection.

Typical History

- A majority of injuries (70%) are noncontact, involving deceleration and a dynamic valgus or adduction moment, with the quadriceps contracted against an extended knee.
- A minority of injuries (30%) are contact, with fixed lower leg and internal rotation, valgus stress, or hyperextension injury.
- The classic description is of a popping sensation followed by immediate pain and swelling of the knee.
- The patient reports a feeling of instability or giving-way episodes with cutting or pivoting activity.

Physical Examination

General Examination

- Assessment of standing alignment is critical for every patient. Significant varus alignment increases the risk of failure after ACL reconstruction and may warrant realignment with associated osteotomy.
- Gait should be examined to assess for associated varus thrust. The presence of a thrust often indicates associated lateral collateral and posterolateral (PL) corner complex insufficiency, and a failure to recognize this will increase the risk of failure of the ACL reconstruction.
- Effusion and hemarthrosis may be present.
- Preexisting scars may provide insight into previous surgical procedures and/or graft source.
- Range of motion. It is critical to achieve resolution of effusion and restoration of motion before ACL reconstructive surgery to minimize risk of postoperative stiffness and arthrofibrosis. A mechanical block to full extension or flexion despite resolution of an effusion is often indicative of an associated bucket-handle meniscal tear.[28]

- Joint line tenderness is often indicative of an associated meniscal injury, or secondary to the typical bone contusion pattern of a pivot-shift event.

Specific Tests

- All tests should be performed on the involved and the contralateral limbs, because side-to-side differences are most important in the detection of subtle differences in stability and ligamentous integrity.
- Anterior drawer and Lachman tests are critical for assessment of anterior translational instability. Relative differences between limbs are more important than absolute measurements of translation to indicate ACL insufficiency.
- Anteromedial (AM) rotatory stability to assess the integrity of the medial collateral and posterior oblique ligaments. Occult posteromedial corner injury can increase the risk of ACL reconstruction failure.[29-31]
- Anterolateral rotatory instability and "dial" testing to assess integrity of the lateral collateral and PL corner complex. Missed PL corner injury is a well-recognized cause of failure after ACL reconstruction.[29-31]
- Varus and valgus examination of the knee in full extension and 30 degrees of flexion to assess collateral ligament integrity. Associated collateral ligament injury may warrant delayed surgical intervention or operative repair and must be addressed with ACL injury to avoid failure of the reconstruction.
- Pivot-shift testing with axial load and valgus stress is critical to assess functional instability and rotational instability secondary to ACL insufficiency. Note that the pivot-shift test result may be negative in the setting of an associated bucket-handle tear of the meniscus or medial collateral ligament (MCL) insufficiency that prevents valgus loading of the knee. Presence of fat lobules in aspirated fluid may be confirmatory of associated fracture or osteochondral trauma.

Imaging

Radiographs (Fig. 73-2)

- Standing, long-leg radiographs are essential for assessment of mechanical alignment of the extremities. Asymmetric varus alignment must be addressed to avoid failure of the ACL reconstruction.
- Anteroposterior, lateral, and sunrise views of the knee should be obtained. Loose bodies, spine avulsion fractures, and occult plateau fractures may be identified. Segond fractures with lateral capsular avulsion fragments are pathognomonic of ACL injury but are not universally present with ACL injury. The presence of patella alta, patella baja, or tibial tubercle apophysitis may be a relative contraindication to autogenous patellar tendon graft selection.
- A flexion weight-bearing (Rosenberg) view should be obtained to assess for significant tibiofemoral joint space narrowing. The presence of significant osteoarthritic changes may be a relative contraindication to ACL reconstruction.

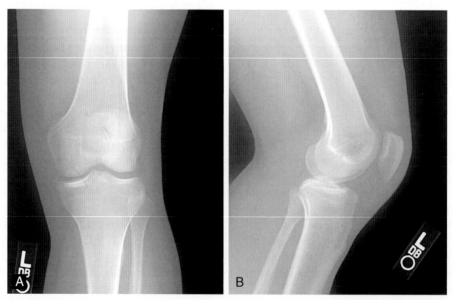

Figure 73-2. Weight-bearing long-leg alignment anteroposterior (**A**) and lateral (**B**) radiographs and dedicated knee radiographs are important for assessment and preoperative planning. Loose bodies, spine avulsion fractures, and occult plateau fractures may be identified. In addition, the presence of Segond fractures, patella alta, patella baja, or tibial tubercle apophysitis may be recognized.

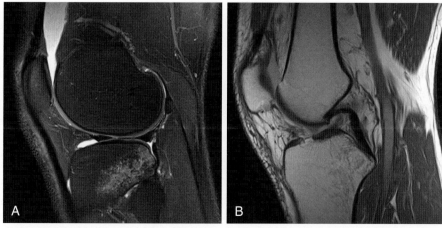

Figure 73-3. Sagittal magnetic resonance images demonstrating (**A**) the discontinuity of anterior cruciate ligament fibers and (**B**) edema in the lateral tibial plateau and lateral femoral condyle.

Magnetic Resonance Imaging

Magnetic resonance imaging has a high sensitivity (94.4%) and specificity (94.3%) for full-thickness tear[9] (Fig. 73-3).

Direct Signs of Anterior Cruciate Ligament Tear[32]

- Focal or diffuse discontinuity of the ACL. The fibers must be assessed in at least two planes to confirm discontinuity.
- Abnormal ACL signal (increased signal intensity).
- Decreased slope of residual ACL fibers or wavy configuration.

Indirect Signs of Anterior Cruciate Ligament Tear[32]

- Deep lateral femoral notch sign—deep depression of lateral condylopatellar sulcus
- Abnormal posterior cruciate ligament (PCL) orientation
- Typical contusion in lateral femoral condyle and PL tibial plateau
- Uncovering of posterior horn of lateral meniscus
- Segond fracture
- Associated medial or lateral meniscal injury

Indications and Contraindications

The approach to graft election for ACL reconstruction must be determined on an individual basis after a thorough review of the risks and benefits of autograft and allograft sources. Patients should make an informed decision about graft type used for ACL reconstruction. However, there are populations of patients in whom allograft may be preferable over autograft[7,9]:

- Patients 40 years of age and older may have an equivalent rate of failure with autograft or allograft ACL reconstruction.[8]
- Patients with decreased functional demands or expectations, including a return to low-intensity, recreational sports
- Skeletally immature athletes, to avoid physeal or apophyseal injury associated with autogenous graft harvest.
- Patients with history of patellofemoral pain or previous patellar surgery (realignment, tendon repair, fracture).
- Laborers or athletes who frequently kneel, such as roofers, masons, firefighters, wrestlers, baseball catchers, and football linemen.
- Patients undergoing revision ACL or multiligament reconstructive surgery.

Patients in whom allograft is less desirable include the following:

- High-level athletes younger than 40 years of age
- Sprinters and hurdlers or elite-level athletes who require full terminal flexion strength
- Patients with concern for disease transmission or immunocompromised patients

SURGICAL TECHNIQUE

Allograft Selection

The surgeon has multiple options when it comes to choosing allograft tissue, including patellar tendon, hamstring, Achilles tendon, tibialis anterior tendon, and tensor fascia lata. These may be procured from one of the many tissue banks currently in practice. It has been reported that there are more than 80 tissue banks that are current members of the AATB, with at least 60 more banks that are not currently members.[22] It is prudent for the surgeon to be knowledgeable about the soft tissue bank's methods of procurement, sterilization, and preparation before using its allografts, because these factors can significantly affect a patient's outcome.

Although the number of infections is likely underreported, allograft transplantation infection rates are very low; the reported incidence is less than 1% (0.0004% to 0.014%).[33,34] Despite this low incidence, many surgeons continue to be concerned with the risk of allograft disease transmission.[33] This phenomenon has been well documented[35,36] with regard to transmission of human immunodeficiency virus (HIV), hepatitis B virus (HBV), and hepatitis C virus (HCV), group A streptococcus, *Clostridium* species, and prions. In addition, many surgeons have concerns about regulatory practices and the biomechanical properties of tissue after sterilization.

Currently, all human cells or tissues intended for transplantation into a human recipient are regulated as HCT/P, or "human cell, tissue, and cellular and tissue-based product."[34,37] Any institution that recovers, processes, stores, or handles allograft tissue consequently not only must register with the Center for Biologics Evaluation and Research[33] of the U.S. Food and Drug Administration (FDA), but also is strongly encouraged to seek certification from the AATB's voluntary accreditation program, which ensures that tissue banks that seek its certification follow strict guidelines for tissue processing. Because of past disease transmission, the FDA now mandates that all donor tissue be screened for HIV types 1 and 2, HBV, HCV, *Treponema pallidum*, and human transmissible spongiform encephalopathies with use of advanced nucleic acid testing (NAT) techniques.[34] NAT sharply reduces the diagnostic window and excludes donors with high viremia.[38] In addition, the AATB requires members to conduct NAT testing and provide negative *Clostridium* and *Streptococcus pyogenes* tissue culture results.[34,37] Although accreditation by the AATB is not required, tissue banks are urged to seek certification. Lack of accreditation can be a warning to the surgeon about the quality of the allografts provided by the tissue bank.

After appropriate donor screening, including exhaustive reviews of medical and social histories for risk factors for infectious disease, allograft tissue must undergo processing to ensure that pathogens are not concomitantly transferred. It should be noted that the Current Good Tissue Practice does not necessarily mandate aseptic handling or sterilization before transplantation of donor tissue; however, tissue recovery is typically performed with use of aseptic technique, in a standard operating room setting.[34,37] Tissue procured under these conditions is not necessarily sterile—contamination may still be introduced by health care workers or the donor's endogenous flora.[34]

After procurement, specimens are sterilized. There is currently no single preferred sterilization process; however, the two main processes for sterilization are irradiation and proprietary chemical processing. The FDA maintains that biologic medical devices are acceptable if a sterility assurance level (SAL) of 10^{-3} (1 in 1000 chance that a living microbe exists) is attained. Human tissues may be considered sterile only if these specimens have an SAL of 10^{-6}. However, allografts that have not been treated with gamma or electron-beam irradiation or ethylene oxide are not likely to be sterile.[39] Irradiation of soft tissue allografts is a delicate balancing act. Gamma radiation sterilization is an effective technique[33,40] that works by inducing excitation of molecules and ions for radical-induced chemical reactions, which subsequently leads to demise of pathogens. Although irradiation of 25 to 40 kGy can inactivate HIV and eliminate spores, the free-radical formation resulting from these doses has been shown to significantly alter the biomechanics of soft tissue grafts. Generation of free radicals distorts the integrity of the allograft tissue, which has been demonstrated in a number of studies showing decreasing allograft biomechanical integrity and enzyme resistance in irradiated tendons[41,42] with increasing doses of irradiation (Table 73-1).[43-45] The underlying reasons for this poor biomechanical integrity are not yet well understood. Gamma irradiation above 20 to 25 kGy is now seldom used because of this concern.[22]

Another sterilization technique, no longer employed, is ethylene oxide gas. This technique was shown to have excellent external sterilization properties, but it demonstrated poorer tissue penetration and its byproducts have been shown to inhibit tissue remodeling. Ethylene oxide gas was also shown to cause host tissue reactions and synovial inflammation and subsequently has not been used in the past 10 years.[33,34,37]

Chemical sterilization entails a series of staged cleansing, disinfection, and rinsing in an effort to remove lipids and cells from tissue. Some commonly used proprietary tissue sterilization processes include the Clearant Process (Clearant, Los Angeles, CA); Allowash XG (LifeNet, Virginia Beach, VA); BioCleanse (RTI Biologics, Alachua, FL); and Tutoplast (Tutogen Medical, Alachua, FL). Although each formulation is used with slightly different methods, proprietary sterilization typically includes bathing of the graft in the solution, followed by spinning of the graft with or without hydrogen peroxide, a possible second rinse, and then irradiation.

Tissues are then deep frozen and stored at −70° to −80° C until surgery. Deep freezing has not been shown to alter the biomechanics of the graft. It does not destroy

TABLE 73-1. Biomechanical Properties of Various Anterior Cruciate Ligament (ACL) Allograft and Autografts

Graft Type	Time Zero Ultimate Strength (N)	Time Zero Stiffness (N/mm)	Advantages	Disadvantages
Achilles tendon allograft[27]	4617	685	Large size (67 mm² cross-sectional area) Bone block for femoral fixation	Only one bone block Risk of insertional tendinopathy Difficulty contouring calcaneal bone block
Bone–patellar tendon–bone (BTB) allograft[27]	2977	620	Two bone blocks for early incorporation Ability to use aperture interference screws	Smaller cross-sectional area (35 mm²) Increased chance for graft-tunnel mismatch
Quadrupled hamstring allograft[27]	4090	776	Three times normal ACL stiffness, two times BTB stiffness	Smaller cross-sectional area (53 mm²) Longer incorporation time Soft tissue fixation
Quadriceps tendon allograft[27]	2352	463	Robust size (62 mm² cross-sectional area) Bone block for improved femoral fixation and incorporation	Only one bone block compared with BTB Longer tibial-sided incorporation time
Tensor fascia lata[53]	3266	414	Lower likelihood of graft-tunnel mismatch Relatively comparable strength and stiffness compared with other grafts	Soft tissue fixation Longer incorporation time
Looped tibialis anterior allograft[27]	4122	460	Lower likelihood of graft-tunnel mismatch	Small size (37 mm² cross-sectional area) Soft tissue fixation Longer incorporation time
Quadrupled hamstring autograft[27]	4090	776	Same as hamstring allograft but with lower immunogenicity, faster incorporation than allograft	Same as hamstring allograft Potential donor site morbidity
BTB autograft[27]	2977	620	Same as BTB allograft but without risk of immunogenic reaction, faster incorporation than allograft	Donor site morbidity Patella fracture risk Anterior knee pain Risk of graft-tunnel mismatch
Intact ACL[27]	2160	242		

viruses such as HIV or HCV, but does decrease antigenicity to some extent.

Anesthesia and Positioning

Choice of anesthesia is typically determined based on discussion among the surgeon, the anesthetist, and the patient, but surgery may be performed with use of regional, spinal, or general anesthesia. A preoperative or postoperative femoral nerve block may also aid in postoperative pain control but is typically not required with allograft ACL reconstructive surgery. The patient is placed in the supine position on the operating table, and a thorough examination under anesthesia (EUA) is performed. A tourniquet is applied to the proximal thigh, and a circumferential leg holder is applied just distal to the tourniquet. The contralateral leg is well padded and allowed to rest on the table. A seat belt is applied to the chest to fasten the patient to the table.

The leg is then prepared and draped with use of meticulous sterile technique.

Surgical Landmarks, Incisions, and Portals

Landmarks
- Inferior pole of the patella
- Patellar tendon
- Tibial tubercle
- Tibial plateau
- Medial and lateral femoral condyles

Portals and Incisions
- The lateral portal is typically placed lateral to the inferior pole of the patella and 1 to 2 mm lateral to the patellar tendon. This location is critical to allow for avoidance of the fat pad and unencumbered

visualization of the lateral wall and ACL femoral footprint.

- The medial portal is placed under direct visualization by spinal needle guidance after diagnostic arthroscopy. The needle should be placed directly above the anterior horn of the medial meniscus and achieve a low-to-high trajectory toward the center of the ACL femoral footprint. This position allows appropriate access and trajectory for an AM portal and an independent drilling technique for femoral socket preparation. The needle must also be placed to ensure sufficient clearance from the medial femoral condyle for subsequent reaming. If a dual medial portal technique is used, a "viewing" medial portal may be placed high and central just adjacent to the patellar tendon at the level of the inferior pole of the patella. The "working," accessory medial portal for reaming is placed more medial and inferior, just above the anterior horn of the medial meniscus.
- The pretibial incision is placed on the proximal medial tibial metaphysis just superior to the pes tendon sheath and anterior to the inserting fibers of the MCL. For bone-tendon-bone allograft reconstruction, this location may need adjustment to

change the tibial tunnel length to minimize the risk of graft tunnel mismatch. For soft tissue or Achilles allograft reconstruction, graft tunnel mismatch is typically not a concern because the excess graft may be trimmed after tibial fixation.

Examination Under Anesthesia and Diagnostic Arthroscopy

Before draping, a thorough (EUA should be completed, including Lachman, anterior and posterior drawer, varus and valgus stress, pivot-shift, and dial testing. The results should be compared with those of the contralateral leg. External rotation and thigh-foot angles at 30 and 90 degrees should be evaluated for PL instability. If the examination is equivocal for complete ACL injury or functional instability, diagnostic arthroscopy should be completed before graft harvest and preparation.

After a thorough EUA, the surgical procedure should begin with arthroscopic evaluation of the knee. The medial and lateral compartments should be carefully inspected for meniscal or chondral pathology (Fig. 73-4). In the favorable healing environment of an associated ACL reconstruction, meniscal tears should be

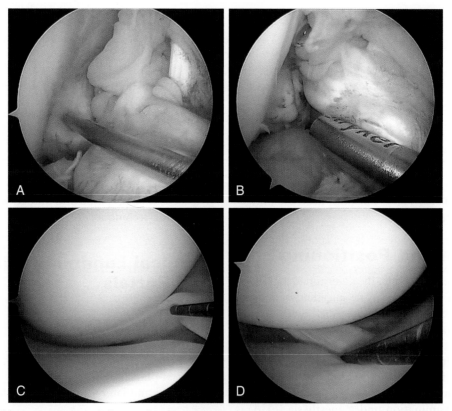

Figure 73-4. A, After completion of diagnostic arthroscopy, a spinal needle is introduced into the medial compartment under direct visualization. The spinal needle is inserted directly above the anterior horn of the medial meniscus. The spinal needle must be positioned sufficiently distant from the medial femoral condyle to avoid iatrogenic injury with reamer passage (see earlier) but sufficiently medial to provide unencumbered access to the lateral wall and femoral footprint in as perpendicular an orientation as possible. **B,** Demonstrating easy clearance of the femoral condyle with a shaving device. **C,** Inspection of the meniscus and chondral surfaces. **D,** Inspection of the popliteal hiatus.

aggressively repaired if the tear pattern is amenable in the red-white and red-red zones. Full-thickness chondral defects should be addressed as well, often with microfracture for small, full-thickness defects on the weight-bearing condylar surfaces. Significant patellofemoral chondromalacia or arthrosis is also important to document and may provide further support for use of an allograft or hamstring autograft over an autogenous patellar tendon ACL reconstruction. Arthroscopic drive-through signs in the medial and lateral compartment should also be noted and may be important signifiers of occult collateral ligament insufficiency that was not appreciated on the EUA.

Specific Steps: The Footprint Anterior Cruciate Ligament Technique[46]

Box 73-1 describes the specific steps in this procedure.

1. Footprint Preparation

Footprint preparation is critical to the success of this procedure, because footprints are the primary references used in tunnel placement. With use of a radiofrequency device, the tibial ACL footprint is detached approximately 2 mm above its bony insertion, allowing for clear definition of the oval footprint and its margins. Then the radiofrequency probe is used to clearly demarcate the center of the tibial footprint bisecting the AM and PL bundles (Fig. 73-5). The remaining distal ligament stump may then be resected with a shaver device.

Attention is then directed toward the femoral footprint. As with the tibia, the femoral attachment is gently debrided, leaving only the residual 2 mm of the femoral footprint on the lateral wall of the femur to precisely define its margins (Fig. 73-6). A notchplasty is not

---

BOX 73-1 Surgical Steps

1. Footprint preparation
2. Graft preparation
3. Tibial tunnel preparation
4. Femoral tunnel preparation
5. Graft insertion and fixation
6. Closure

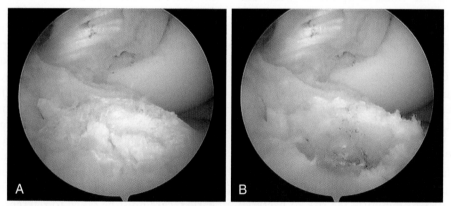

Figure 73-5. A, Tibial footprint. A radiofrequency probe can be used to demarcate the center of the footprint. The remaining ligament stump can be debrided with a shaver (**B**).

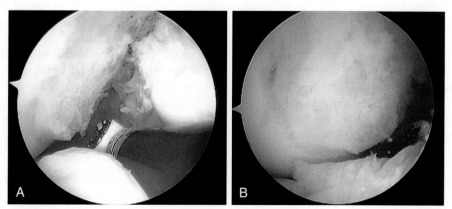

Figure 73-6. A, As with the tibia, the femoral footprint can be prepared by isolating the center of the footprint with a radiofrequency probe, followed by debridement of remaining ligament stump tissue. A 70-degree arthroscope may be helpful for improved visualization of the femoral wall from the lateral portal. **B,** A demarcated femoral footprint.

required for anatomic ACL reconstruction. However, in certain cases of a stenotic, A-frame notch, a gentle anterior margin notchplasty is performed to improve visualization of the femoral footprint and to avoid graft-wall impingement and attenuation. A 70-degree arthroscope may be helpful in certain procedures to provide a panoramic view of the lateral wall and femoral ACL footprint. Use of the 70-degree arthroscope with this footprint technique allows femoral tunnel preparation, graft passage, and fixation to all be performed with excellent visualization and without repositioning of the camera, creation of accessory medial portals, or knee hyperflexion.

The center of the tibial and femoral footprint is marked with a microfracture awl device for later guide-wire placement and socket reaming. Preservation of the margins of the footprints allows for direct measurement of the footprint dimensions and placement in the center of the native ligament attachment, bisecting the AM and PL bundles. The intercondylar and bifurcate ridge can be useful references on the femoral side to confirm central placement. The direct measurement confirms preservation of a posterior back wall when interference fixation will be used. Care should be taken to ensure central marking in the tibial footprint as well. The native footprint extends as anteriorly as the intermeniscal ligament, and historical referencing from the PCL or tibial spines has resulted in relatively posterior placement of the tibial socket primarily within the PL bundle of the footprint. Capture of the AM bundle fibers on the tibial footprint is as critical as anatomic femoral socket position to achieving a biomechanically optimal, single-bundle ACL reconstruction.[47]

2. Graft Preparation

The allograft is thawed by soaking it in normal saline at room temperature. We have typically augmented the saline with antibiotics to minimize the risk of bacterial colonization with graft preparation. It has been our preference to use an Achilles tendon with a bone block for allograft ACL reconstruction. This graft offers several advantages, including bone-to-bone fixation and a large soft tissue cross-sectional area similar to quadriceps tendon autograft that is particularly useful for tunnel fill in the setting of revision surgery. Also, the time-zero load-to-failure is approximately 4000 N, comparable to quadrupled hamstring autograft.[48] Although these grafts may be purchased presized, we have typically prepared them by trimming the calcaneal bone plug to 9 to 11 mm by approximately 25 mm in length based on the size of the femoral footprint. The soft tissue is folded to maximize cross-sectional area and prepared with a locking, nonabsorbable suture.

A mark should be made on the nontendinous side of the prepared bone plug to confirm complete seating into the prepared femoral socket and to facilitate interference screw placement with minimal risk of injury to the graft tendon fibers. Three 1.6-mm holes are drilled through the plug perpendicular to the cortical surfaces, and a No. 5 braided polyester suture is passed through each hole to facilitate shuttling and seating of the bone plug into the femoral socket.

If a soft tissue allograft is used, graft preparation is minimal and requires only locking sutures to be placed in each end. However, care must be taken to ensure that the femoral socket is prepared with sufficient depth to allow for seating of at least 20 mm of graft. This is a potential concern with use of suspensory femoral fixation devices and a short femoral socket that can result from independent, medial portal drilling techniques. If a bone-tendon-bone allograft is used, care must be taken to adjust tibial tunnel length to avoid graft-tunnel mismatch. This is a potentially greater concern with patellar tendon allograft than with autograft, because the graft may not be proportionate to the size or height of the patient.

3. Tibial Tunnel Preparation

Tibial tunnel preparation is performed in a routine fashion. An external starting point is identified along the anterior fibers of the MCL and just superior to the pes tendon sheath to provide sufficient coronal obliquity. Although graft-tunnel mismatch is rarely a concern with allograft reconstruction, this starting point may be adjusted proximally or distally to adjust tibial tunnel length for bone-tendon-bone allograft. A 2-cm skin incision is made at this point, and skin flaps are elevated. The sartorial fascia and proximal margin of the pes tendon sheath are identified and retracted inferiorly. A periosteal window is created just proximal to the pes tendon sheath and anterior to the inserting MCL fibers. A commercial ACL tunnel guide is then targeted toward the true center of the defined footprint. As discussed earlier, care must be taken to reference the center of the tibial footprint and not surrogate measurements from the PCL or tibial spines, which can result in errant posterior placement of the tibial tunnel into the PL bundle fibers only (Fig. 73-7). The guide angle is typically set at approximately 52 to 55 degrees but is adjusted to target the previously determined location of the tibial aperture on the proximal tibial metaphysis. The guide pin is drilled through the guide, and it is arthroscopically verified that the pin breaches the previously defined center of the ACL footprint between the AM and PL bundles. The pin is then reamed with the appropriately sized reamer based on the size of the prepared graft.

4. Femoral Tunnel Preparation

The femoral tunnel is prepared with use of an independent drilling technique. Although a transtibial technique can be used, multiple studies have demonstrated risk for nonanatomic femoral socket position, iatrogenic

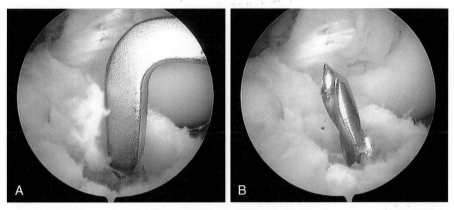

Figure 73-7. A, Targeting the center of the tibial anterior cruciate ligament footprint with the tibial guide under direct visualization. **B,** A guide pin through the center of the tibial footprint.

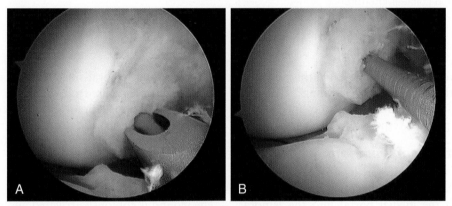

Figure 73-8. Femoral socket reaming. **A,** Demonstrating a flexible guide pin in position at center of the femoral footprint. Note the perpendicular orientation to the lateral wall and superolateral trajectory of the pin. This trajectory is critical to maximize the length of the femoral socket while simultaneously achieving an anatomic tunnel position. **B,** After pin placement, a flexible reamer is placed over the pin to prepare the femoral socket.

rereaming of the tibial tunnel, and a PL-to-AM graft mismatch configuration.[49-52] We have used an AM portal drilling technique with a flexible guidewire and reaming system. With the lateral wall of the notch and femoral footprint in clear view with the 70-degree arthroscope in the lateral portal, the cannulated guide is introduced through the AM portal and positioned at the previously marked center of the femoral ACL footprint. Care should be taken to orient the guide to achieve a supero-lateral trajectory of the guidewire. The flexible system affords the advantage of allowing socket preparation and reaming in modest hyperflexion. A straight guide pin and reaming system can be used effectively but requires greater hyperflexion and has the potential for blind reaming secondary to limited visualization from the fat pad (Fig. 73-8A).

With the guide in position, the flexible guide pin is positioned into the previously created awl hole at the center of the femoral ACL footprint. The knee is then flexed to 115 degrees before drilling of the pin to improve superolateral trajectory and achieve safe clearance from the medial femoral condyle. The pin is passed out of the lateral skin of the distal thigh. An exit point in the region of the distal vastus lateralis is typically confirmatory of an appropriate, oblique trajectory of the femoral socket. Once the guidewire has been passed, the appropriately sized flexible reamer is advanced over the wire and can be directly visualized while reaming is performed in modest hyperflexion (Fig. 73-8B). For an Achilles allograft, a femoral socket of length 25 mm is adequate for seating and fixation of the bone plug. However, for soft tissue allografts, a longer socket may be desirable and necessary for sufficient tendon-bone interface for healing with use of suspensory fixation devices. The presence of a back wall can be confirmed after reaming a short distance. The reamer and pin are removed and bony debris cleared with a shaver device. The tunnel position, depth, and walls can be directly visualized and evaluated with the 70-degree arthroscope in the lateral portal without adjustment or repositioning

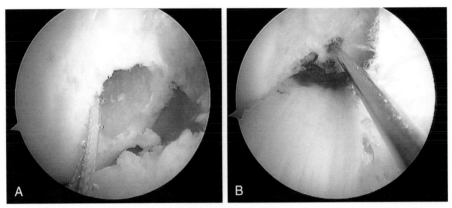

Figure 73-9. Graft insertion. **A,** Prepared femoral socket with shuttle suture in place. **B,** The graft is shuttled into the femoral socket. To facilitate graft passage, the leg is brought into relative extension as the graft is pulled through the tibial tunnel and the femoral bone plug is pulled completely within the notch. The knee is then flexed to a resting position of 90 degrees, and the plug is oriented and seated into the femoral socket without difficulty. The graft is then fixed in the femoral socket with a colinear interference screw.

to the medial or accessory portal. We find this advantageous to avoid the instrument "crowding" that can occur with visualization and reaming from medial and accessory medial portals, respectively.

5. Graft Insertion and Fixation

The free ends of a looped, nonabsorbable suture are placed in the eyelet of the guidewire. The wire is then advanced through the medial portal into the femoral tunnel and out the superolateral thigh. After clamping of the free ends, the suture loop is visualized within the notch and retrieved through the tibial tunnel with a probe or claw grasper (Fig. 73-9A). The shuttle sutures of the graft bone plug are then brought into the tunnels by use of the looped passing suture.

In comparison to a conventional transtibial technique, independent drilling techniques result in nonparallel tibial and femoral tunnels. To facilitate graft passage, the leg is brought into relative extension as the graft is pulled through the tibial tunnel, thus aligning the vector of pull with the tibial tunnel. Once the femoral bone plug has been pulled completely into the notch, the knee is allowed to flex to a resting position of 90 degrees and the bone plug is oriented and subsequently seated into the femoral socket (Fig. 73-9B). Care is taken to rotate the bone plug before seating in the femoral socket in the most favorable orientation for safe interference fixation on the nontendinous side of the graft. Graft fixation is performed in a standard fashion, typically by use of interference screw fixation on the femoral side. Care must be taken to hyperflex the knee to ensure colinearity of the bone plug and interference screw. If soft tissue allograft such as hamstring or tibialis anterior tendon is used, metallic screws typically should be avoided because they may damage

the graft. After femoral-sided fixation, the graft is cycled, tensioned, and secured on the tibial side in 10 to 15 degrees of flexion with an interference device. Suspensory fixation also may be used for augmentation of fixation, particularly in the setting of osteopenic proximal tibial bone.

6. Closure

The wound is copiously irrigated and the periosteal flap over the tibial tunnel external aperture is approximated and closed with absorbable sutures. The deep dermal layer is closed with absorbable sutures and the subcutaneous layer is closed with a running, nonabsorbable Prolene suture. The portals are closed with simple, nonabsorbable sutures. A well-padded, sterile dressing is applied. A cryotherapy device is also placed and fastened with an elastic bandage.

POSTOPERATIVE CONSIDERATIONS
Follow-up

The patient is seen in the clinic within the first postoperative week and again 2 weeks postoperatively for wound check and suture removal (Fig. 73-10).

The patient is instructed postoperatively to initiate knee flexion exercises, straight-leg raises, isometric quadriceps exercises, and patellar mobilization. In the absence of associated meniscal repair, full range of motion, resolution of effusion, and significant return of quadriceps function is desirable by 4 weeks postoperatively. In the setting of associated meniscal repair, range of motion of only 0 to 90 degrees is permitted, to minimize shear forces on the repair.

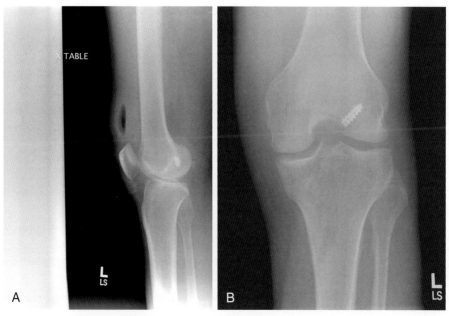

Figure 73-10. Postoperative radiographs demonstrating anatomic socket position and colinear interference screw fixation on the femoral side. Soft tissue interference fixation was used on the tibial side.

Rehabilitation

- Patients may bear weight as tolerated with a knee brace locked in extension after a return of reasonable quadriceps strength and control. This typically occurs by 2 weeks postoperatively. Immediate cryotherapy, effusion control, range of motion, and straight-leg raise exercises are initiated postoperatively.
- Physical therapy is initiated in the second postoperative week, with emphasis on achieving full range of motion, particularly terminal extension and beginning flexion exercises.
- Patients may begin bicycling, leg-press exercises, and balanced quadriceps and hamstring strengthening by 3 to 4 weeks postoperatively. As long as full range of motion and resolution of the effusion are achieved, with stable and symmetrical Lachman examination findings, light in-line jogging is permitted at 12 weeks postoperatively. If symmetrical quadriceps strength is documented in the involved and contralateral limb by leg-press examination at 5 months postoperatively, an agility program is initiated. These exercises focus on return of proprioception, balance, and proper techniques for jumping and landing. For an uncomplicated recovery, return to sports is permitted at 6 to 8 months postoperatively. Allograft reconstruction may be delayed relative to autograft reconstruction in this regard, because the incorporation and ligamentization of the graft are known to be slower and ongoing for 9 to 12 months postoperatively.

Complications

Intraoperative Complications

- Graft laceration
- Inadequate fixation and pull-out
- Posterior femoral wall blowout
- Graft-tunnel mismatch for bone-tendon-bone allografts
- Nonanatomic socket preparation
- Neurovascular injury

Postoperative Complications

- Traumatic graft failure
- Failure of biologic incorporation
- Disease transmission (HIV or HCV risk approximately 1 in 1,600,000)[31]
- Infection
- Arthrofibrosis

RESULTS

Recent systematic reviews of the literature suggest that in evaluating the general population undergoing ACL reconstruction with either allograft or autograft, clinical outcomes with respect to laxity, functional testing, and failure rate are equivalent. In addition, allograft use has been shown to have the benefit of significantly decreased postoperative pain and smaller incisions. However, in the young athlete it has been reported that both allograft and high activity level are risk factors for graft failure, and when matched together have a multiplicative effect on likelihood of ACL graft failure (Table 73-2).[8]

TABLE 73-2. Outcome Studies Comparing Laxity After Allograft and Autograft Anterior Cruciate Ligament (ACL) Reconstruction

Author	Follow-up	Outcome
Saddemi et al[54] (1993)	1-4 years	No significant difference in KT1000 laxity >5 mm (6% vs. 0%) comparing BTB allograft with autograft.
Lephart et al[55] (1993)	1, 2 years	No significant difference in quadriceps index (92% ± 6.2% vs. 95% ± 4.2%) comparing BTB allograft with autograft No difference in torque acceleration energy at 240 deg/sec (N-m) (31.5 ± 9.2 vs. 31.1 ± 11.0).
Harner et al[19] (1996)	3-5 years	No significant difference in KT1000 testing (autograft laxity of 1.9 mm vs. 1.8 mm in allograft).
Stringham et al[56] (1996)	3 years	No significant difference in KT1000 side-to-side laxity (<3 mm) comparison (80% in autograft group, 70% in allograft group).
Shelton et al[57] (1997)	2 years	No significant difference in KT1000 side-to-side laxity (<3 mm) comparison between BTB allografts (73%) and autografts (70%) ($P > .05$).
Peterson et al[58] (2001)	5 years	No significant difference in KT1000 measured side-to-side laxity (<3 mm), comparing BTB allograft (73%) and autograft (67%) ($P > .05$).
Chang et al[59] (2003)	2-year minimum	No significant difference in KT1000 laxity >5 mm (9% vs. 9%) comparing BTB allograft with autograft ($P = 0.7$).
Kustos et al[60] (2004)	3 years	No KT1000 testing done. Authors state Lachman test results slightly more positive in autograft group, but this was deemed not clinically significant. No significant difference in average Lysholm scores (allograft, 84.1; autograft, 89.9).
Barrett et al[61] (2005)	3 year autograft, 4 year allograft	No significant difference between allograft and autograft, respectively, in (1) mean maximum KT1000 arthrometer side-to-side distance (1.46 mm vs. 0.104 mm, $P = .398$), (2) side-to-side difference ≤3 mm (86% vs. 96%, $P = .226$). or (3) >5 mm side-to-side difference (7% vs. 0%, $P = .150$).
Poehling et al[20] (2005)	5 years	Increased laxity by KT1000 in allograft (2.8 in autografts vs. 3.0 mm in allografts, but insignificant P value. ($P = .0520$). No difference noted in side-to-side KT1000 testing.
Bach et al[15] (2005)	2-year minimum	Measured side-to-side laxity with KT1000 preoperatively and postoperatively. *Preop* mean maximum manual translations of the affected knees were 14 mm and 7.5 mm for the unaffected knee ($P < .001$). *Postop* values decreased to 7.6 mm and 6.9 mm, respectively ($P < .001$).
Prodromos et al[62] (2007)	2-year minimum	Meta-analysis measuring KT1000 stability of autograft vs. allograft reconstructions. Normal stability (<2 mm side-to-side difference) was 72% vs. 59%, respectively ($P < .01$), whereas abnormal stability (>5 mm side-to-side difference) was 5% vs. 14%, respectively ($P < .01$). BTB autograft normal stability was 66% vs. 57% for allografts ($P < .01$). Hamstring autograft normal and abnormal stability rates were 77% and 4% and were compared with soft tissue allografts as a group, which had values of 64% and 12% ($P < .01$).
Krych et al[63] (2008)	2-year minimum	Meta-analysis of outcomes. Higher failure rate (OR, 5.03; $P = .01$) and more likely to have a hop test result less than 90% of the nonoperative side (OR, 5.66; $P < .01$) in allograft group. No KT1000 results available; authors report no difference in Lachman or IKDC scores. No significant difference when irradiated specimens thrown out of study.
Sun et al[64] (2009)	4-9 years	No significant difference in KT2000 measured maximum laxity between autograft (2.4 ± 0.7 mm) and allograft groups (2.5 ± 0.9 mm) ($P = .369$). No significant difference between either group in side-to-side difference <3 mm or >5 mm ($P = .465$).
Sun et al[65] (2009)	2-5 years	Measured side-to-side laxity with KT2000, 87.8% of patients in autograft group vs. 31.3% in the irradiated-allograft group had a side-to-side difference <3 mm ($P = .011$).
Tibor et al[66] (2010)	2-year minimum	No difference in positive Lachman test result, pivot-shift test result, IKDC grade, or graft failure. Significant increase in KT1000 laxity >3 mm (31.1% vs. 16.0%).
Kaeding et al[8] (2010)	2 years	Patient age and ACL graft type both significant predictors of graft rupture. Fourfold increase in ACL graft rupture with allograft with respect to age ($P < .01$). Patients aged 10-19 showed highest failure rate ($P < .01$). For each 10-year decrease in age, odds of graft rupture increased 2.3 times.
Mascarenhas et al[67] (2010)	3-14 years	No significant difference on KT1000 side-to-side testing between autograft (1.11 ± 2.56) and allograft groups (1.78 ± 3.11) ($P = .466$).

TABLE 73-2. Outcome Studies Comparing Laxity After Allograft and Autograft Anterior Cruciate Ligament (ACL) Reconstruction—cont'd

Author	Follow-up	Outcome
Tian et al[68] (2010)	2-year minimum	Significant difference on KT2000 side-to-side testing between autograft (2.4 ± 0.6 mm) and irradiated allograft (5.5 ± 3.6 mm) in group B ($P < 0.05$).
Foster et al[69] (2010)	Unknown	Systematic review. After substitution of missing standard deviation values, KT1000 testing showed significant difference in side-to-side comparison: allograft 1.4 ± 0.02 mm vs. autograft 1.9 ± 0.01 mm ($P < .02$). No statistical difference in <3 or >5 mm side-to-side difference ($P > .1$ and $P > .5$ respectively).
Sun et al[70] (2011)	2.5-year minimum	Significantly increased laxity >5 mm in allograft group; $P = .00021$. No difference in IKDC score, functional and subjective evaluations, or activity level.
Sun et al[71] (2011)	5-9 years	No difference in maximal displacement with KT2000 between autograft (5.3 ± 3.1 mm) and allograft (5.6 ± 2.5 mm) ($P = .416$). No statistical difference in <3 mm (83.5% vs. 78%) or >5 mm (7.7% vs. 8.4%) side-to-side difference ($P = .968$).

BTB, Bone–patellar tendon–bone; *IKDC*, International Knee Documentation Committee; *OR*, odds ratio.

REFERENCES

1. Aglietti P, Buzzi R, D'Andria S, et al. Patellofemoral problems after intraarticular anterior cruciate ligament reconstruction. *Clin Orthop Relat Res.* 1993;(288): 195-204.

2. Rubinstein Jr RA, Shelbourne KD, VanMeter CD, et al. Isolated autogenous bone-patellar tendon-bone graft site morbidity. *Am J Sports Med.* 1994;22(3):324-327.

3. Christen B, Jakob RP. Fractures associated with patellar ligament grafts in cruciate ligament surgery. *J Bone Joint Surg Br.* 1992;74(4):617-619.

4. Bonamo JJ, Krinick RM, Sporn AA. Rupture of the patellar ligament after use of its central third for anterior cruciate reconstruction. A report of two cases. *J Bone Joint Surg Am.* 1984;66(8):1294-1297.

5. Marumoto JM, Mitsunaga MM, Richardson AB, et al. Late patellar tendon ruptures after removal of the central third for anterior cruciate ligament reconstruction. A report of two cases. *Am J Sports Med.* 1996;24(5): 698-701.

6. Figueroa D, Calvo R, Vaisman A, et al. Injury to the infrapatellar branch of the saphenous nerve in ACL reconstruction with the hamstrings technique: clinical and electrophysiological study. *Knee.* 2008;15(5):360-363.

7. Cohen SB, Sekiya JK. Allograft safety in anterior cruciate ligament reconstruction. *Clin Sports Med.* 2007;26: 597-605.

8. Kaeding CC, Aros B, Pedroza A, et al. Allograft versus autograft anterior cruciate ligament reconstruction: predictors of failure from a MOON prospective longitudinal cohort. *Sports Health.* 2011;3(1):73-81.

9. Strickland S, MacGillivray J, Warren R. Anterior cruciate ligament reconstruction with allograft tendons. *Orthop Clin North Am.* 2003;34:41-47.

10. Berg EE. Tibial bone plug nonunion: a cause of anterior cruciate ligament reconstructive failure. *Arthroscopy.* 1992;8(3):380-384.

11. Jackson DW, Corsetti J, Simon TM. Biologic incorporation of allograft anterior cruciate ligament replacements. *Clin Orthop Relat Res.* 1996;(324):126-133.

12. Marrale J, Morrissey MC, Haddad FS. A literature review of autograft and allograft anterior cruciate ligament reconstruction. *Knee Surg Sports Traumatol Arthrosc.* 2007;15:690-704.

13. Miller AC. A review of open and closed kinetic chain exercises following ACL reconstruction. Available at http://www.brianmac.demon.co.uk/kneeinj.htm. Accessed March 13, 2012.

14. Greenberg DD, Robertson M, Vallurupalli S, et al. Allograft compared with autograft infection rates in primary anterior cruciate ligament reconstruction. *J Bone Joint Surg Am.* 2010;92(14):2402-2408.

15. Bach Jr BR, Aadalen KJ, Dennis MG, et al. Primary anterior cruciate ligament reconstruction using fresh-frozen, nonirradiated patellar tendon allograft. *Am J Sports Med.* 2005;33:284-292.

16. Bedi A, Feeley BT, Williams RJ III. Management of articular cartilage defects of the knee. *J Bone Joint Surg Am.* 2010;92:994-1009.

17. Tom JA, Rodeo SA. Soft tissue allografts for knee reconstruction in sports medicine. *Clin Orthop Relat Res.* 2002;402:135-156.

18. Carey JL, Dunn WR, Dahm DL, et al. A systematic review of anterior cruciate ligament reconstruction with autograft compared with allograft. *J Bone Joint Surg Am.* 2009;91:2242-2250.

19. Harner CD, Olson E, Irrgang JJ, et al. Allograft versus autograft anterior cruciate ligament reconstruction; 3- to 5-year outcome. *Clin Orthop Relat Res.* 1996;324: 134-144.

20. Poehling GG, Curl WW, Lee CA, et al. Analysis of outcomes of anterior cruciate ligament repair with 5-year follow-up: Allograft versus autograft. *Arthroscopy.* 2005; 21:774-785.

21. Shelbourne KD, Nitz P. Accelerated rehabilitation after anterior cruciate ligament reconstruction. *Am J Sports Med.* 1990;18:292-299.

22. Aglietti P, Buzzi R, Zaccherotti G, et al. Patellar tendon versus doubled semitendinosus and gracilis tendons for anterior cruciate ligament reconstruction. *Am J Sports Med.* 1994;22(2):211-217; discussion 217-218.

23. Kleipool AE, van Loon T, Marti RK. Pain after use of the central third of the patellar tendon for cruciate ligament reconstruction. 33 patients followed 2-3 years. *Acta Orthop Scand*. 1994;65(1):62-66.

24. Sachs RA, Daniel DM, Stone ML, et al. Patellofemoral problems after anterior cruciate ligament reconstruction. *Am J Sports Med*. 1989;17(6):760-765.

25. Cooper MT, Kaeding C. Comparison of the hospital cost of autograft versus allograft soft-tissue anterior cruciate ligament reconstructions. *Arthroscopy*. 2010;26(11):1478-1482.

26. Oro FB, Sikka RS, Wolters B, et al. Autograft versus allograft: an economic cost comparison of anterior cruciate ligament reconstruction. *Arthroscopy*. 2011;27(9):1219-1225.

27. Baer GS, Harner CD. Clinical outcomes of allograft versus autograft in anterior cruciate ligament reconstruction. *Clin Sports Med*. 2007;26(4):661-681.

28. Noyes FR, Wojtys EM, Marshall MT. The early diagnosis and treatment of developmental patella infera syndrome. *Clin Orthop Relat Res*. 1991;(265):241-252.

29. LaPrade RF, Resig S, Wentorf F, et al. The effects of grade III posterolateral knee complex injuries on anterior cruciate ligament graft force: A biomechanical analysis. *Am J Sports Med*. 1999;27:469-475.

30. Noyes FR, Barber-Westin SD, Roberts CS. Use of allografts after failed treatment of rupture of the anterior cruciate ligament. *J Bone Joint Surg Am*. 1994;76:1019-1031.

31. O'Brien SJ, Warren RF, Pavlov H, et al. Reconstruction of the chronically insufficient anterior cruciate ligament with the central third of the patellar ligament. *J Bone Joint Surg Am*. 1991;73:278-286.

32. Bining J, Andrews G, Forster B. The ABCs of the anterior cruciate ligament: a primer for magnetic resonance imaging assessment of the normal, injured, and surgically repaired anterior cruciate ligament. *Br J Sports Med*. 2009;43:856-862.

33. McAllister DR, Joyce MJ, Mann BJ, et al. Allograft update. The current status of tissue regulation, procurement, processing, and sterilization. *Am J Sports Med*. 2007;35:2148-2158.

34. Vaishnav S, Vangsness Jr CT. New techniques in allograft tissue processing. *Clin Sports Med*. 2009;28:127-141.

35. Kainer MA, Linden JV, Whaley DN, et al. Clostridium infections associated with musculoskeletal-tissue allografts. *N Eng J Med*. 2004;350:2564-2571.

36. Mroz TE, Joyce MJ, Steinmetz MP, et al. Musculoskeletal allograft risks and recalls in the United States. *J Am Acad Orthop Surg*. 2008;16:559-565.

37. Vangsness Jr CT, Dellamaggiora RD. Current safety sterilization and tissue banking issues for soft tissue allografts. *Clin Sports Med*. 2009;28:183-189.

38. Pruss A, Monig HJ. Current standards in tissue banking. *ISBT Science Series*. 2010;5:148-154.

39. Joyce MJ. Safety and FDA regulations for musculoskeletal allografts: perspective of an orthopaedic surgeon. *Clin Orthop Relat Res*. 2005;435:22-30.

40. Kaminski A, Gut G, Marowska J, et al. Mechanical properties of radiation-sterilised human bone-tendon-bone grafts preserved by different methods. *Cell Tissue Bank*. 2009;10:215-219.

41. Gorschewsky O, Klakow A, Riechert K, et al. Clinical comparison of the Tutoplast allograft and autologous patellar tendon (bone- patellar tendon-bone) for the reconstruction of the anterior cruciate ligament. *Am J Sports Med*. 2005;33:1202-1209.

42. Seto A, Gatt Jr CJ, Dunn MG. Radioprotection of tendon tissue via crosslinking and free radical scavenging. *Clin Orthop Relat Res*. 2008;466:1788-1795.

43. Hoburg AT, Keshlaf S, Schmidt T, et al. Effect of electron beam irradiation on biomechanical properties of patellar tendon allografts in anterior cruciate ligament reconstruction. *Am J Sports Med*. 2010;38:1134-1140.

44. Mehta VM, Mandala C, Foster D, et al. Comparison of revision rates in bone-patella tendon-bone autograft and allograft anterior cruciate ligament reconstruction. *Orthopedics*. 2010;33(1):12.

45. Seto A, Gatt Jr CJ, Dunn MG. Improved tendon radioprotection by combined cross-linking and free radical scavenging. *Clin Orthop Relat Res*. 2009;467:2994-3001.

46. Bedi A, Altchek DW. The "footprint" anterior cruciate ligament technique: An anatomic approach to anterior cruciate ligament reconstruction. *Arthroscopy*. 2009;25(10):1128-1138.

47. Bedi A, Musahl V, O'Loughlin P, et al. A comparison of the effect of central anatomical single-bundle anterior cruciate ligament reconstruction and double-bundle anterior cruciate ligament reconstruction on pivot-shift kinematics. *Am J Sports Med*. 2010;38(9):1788-1794.

48. West RV, Harner CD. Graft selection in anterior cruciate ligament reconstruction. *J Am Acad Orthop Surg*. 2005;13(3):197-207.

49. Bedi A, Musahl V, Steuber V, et al. Transtibial versus anteromedial portal reaming in anterior cruciate ligament reconstruction: an anatomic and biomechanical evaluation of surgical technique. *Arthroscopy*. 2011;27(3):380-390.

50. Bedi A, Raphael B, Maderazo A, et al. Transtibial versus anteromedial portal drilling for anterior cruciate ligament reconstruction: a cadaveric study of femoral tunnel length and obliquity. *Arthroscopy*. 2010;26(3):342-350.

51. Musahl V, Voos JE, O'Loughlin PF, et al. Comparing stability of different single- and double-bundle anterior cruciate ligament reconstruction techniques: a cadaveric study using navigation. *Arthroscopy*. 2010;26(9 Suppl):S41-S48.

52. Steiner ME, Battaglia TC, Heming JF, et al. Independent drilling outperforms conventional transtibial drilling in anterior cruciate ligament reconstruction. *Am J Sports Med*. 2009;37(10):1912-1919.

53. Chan DB, Temple HT, Latta LL, et al. A biomechanical comparison of fan-folded, single-looped fascia lata with other graft tissues as a suitable substitute for anterior cruciate ligament reconstruction. *Arthroscopy*. 2010;(12):1641-1647.

54. Saddemi SR, Frogameni AD, Fenton PJ, et al. Comparison of perioperative morbidity of anterior cruciate ligament autografts versus allografts. *Arthroscopy*. 1993;9(5):519-524.

55. Lephart SM, Kocher MS, Harner CD, et al. Quadriceps strength and functional capacity after anterior cruciate

ligament reconstruction. Patellar tendon autograft versus allograft. *Am J Sports Med.* 1993;21(5):738-743.

56. Stringham DR, Pelmas CJ, Burks RT, et al. Comparison of anterior cruciate ligament reconstructions using patellar tendon autograft or allograft. *Arthroscopy.* 1996;12(4):414-421.

57. Shelton WR, Papendick L, Dukes AD. Autograft versus allograft anterior cruciate ligament reconstruction. *Arthroscopy.* 1997;13(4):446-449.

58. Peterson R, Shelton W, Bomboy A. Allograft versus autograft patellar tendon anterior cruciate ligament reconstruction: a 5-year followup. *Arthroscopy.* 2001;17:9-13.

59. Chang SK, Egami DK, Shaieb MD, et al. Anterior cruciate ligament reconstruction: allograft versus autograft. *Arthroscopy.* 2003;19:453-462.

60. Kustos T, Bálint L, Than P, et al. Comparative study of autograft or allograft in primary anterior cruciate ligament reconstruction. *Int Orthop.* 2004;28(5):290-293.

61. Barrett G, Stokes D, White M. Anterior cruciate ligament reconstruction in patients older than 40 years: allograft versus autograft patellar tendon. *Am J Sports Med.* 2005;33(10):1505-1512.

62. Prodromos C, Joyce B, Shi K. A meta-analysis of stability of autografts compared to allografts after anterior cruciate ligament reconstruction. *Knee Surg Sports Traumatol Arthrosc.* 2007;15(7):851-856.

63. Krych AJ, Jackson JD, Hoskin TL, et al. A meta-analysis of patellar tendon autograft versus patellar tendon allograft in anterior cruciate ligament reconstruction. *Arthroscopy.* 2008;24(3):292-298.

64. Sun K, Tian SQ, Zhang JH, et al. Anterior cruciate ligament reconstruction with bone-patellar tendon-bone autograft versus allograft. *Arthroscopy.* 2009;25(7):750-759.

65. Sun K, Tian S, Zhang J, et al. Anterior cruciate ligament reconstruction with BPTB autograft, irradiated versus non-irradiated allograft: a prospective randomized clinical study. *Knee Surg Sports Traumatol Arthrosc.* 2009;17(5):464-474.

66. Tibor LM, Long JL, Schilling PL, et al. Clinical outcomes after anterior cruciate ligament reconstruction: A meta-analysis of autograft versus allograft tissue. *Sports Health: A Multidisciplinary Approach.* 2010;2(1):56-72.

67. Mascarenhas R, Tranovich M, Karpie JC, et al. Patellar tendon anterior cruciate ligament reconstruction in the high-demand patient: evaluation of autograft versus allograft reconstruction. *Arthroscopy.* 2010;26(9 Suppl):S58-S66.

68. Tian S, Zhang J, Wang Y, et al. A prospective study on anterior cruciate ligament reconstruction with patellar tendon autograft versus gamma irradiated allograft. *Zhongguo Xiu Fu Chong Jian Wai Ke Za Zhi.* 2010;24(3):282-286.

69. Foster TE, Wolfe BL, Ryan S, et al. Does the graft source really matter in the outcome of patients undergoing anterior cruciate ligament reconstruction? An evaluation of autograft versus allograft reconstruction results: a systematic review. *Am J Sports Med.* 2010;38(1):189-199.

70. Sun K, Zhang J, Wang Y, et al. Arthroscopic anterior cruciate ligament reconstruction with at least 2.5 years' follow-up comparing hamstring tendon autograft and irradiated allograft. *Arthroscopy.* 2011;27(9):1195-1202.

71. Sun K, Zhang J, Wang Y, et al. Arthroscopic reconstruction of the anterior cruciate ligament with hamstring tendon autograft and fresh-frozen allograft: a prospective, randomized controlled study. *Am J Sports Med.* 2011;39(7):1430-1486.

Chapter 74

Hamstring Tendon Autograft for Anterior Cruciate Ligament Reconstruction

Keith Lawhorn and Stephen M. Howell

Chapter Synopsis

- This chapter presents a proven transtibial tunnel anterior cruciate ligament (ACL) technique that uses a three-dimensional tibial guide to place the tunnels without posterior cruciate ligament (PCL) and roof impingement. The featured graft construct is a double-looped hamstring graft with slippage-resistant, high-stiffness, strong fixation. The rationale and clinical outcome of brace-free aggressive rehabilitation with this tunnel placement technique and graft construct are supported by peer-reviewed studies that are discussed.

Important Points

- Customized coronal and sagittal placement of the tibial tunnel is critical for positioning the femoral tunnel via a transtibial tunnel technique.

- In the coronal plane, widen the notch, center the tibial tunnel between the tibial spines, and angle the tunnel at 60 to 65 degrees off the medial joint line to minimize loss of flexion and instability from PCL impingement.

- In the sagittal plane, center the tibial tunnel 4 to 5 mm posterior and parallel to the intercondylar roof with the knee in full extension to minimize loss of extension and instability from roof impingement.

- Consider the use of slippage-resistant, high-stiffness, strong fixation; a double-looped hamstring graft;

aggressive brace-free rehabilitation; and a return to sport at 4 months based on in vivo analysis of graft lengthening.

Clinical and Surgical Pearls

- Perform a lateral wallplasty until the space between the lateral femoral condyle and PCL is wide enough for the ACL graft.

- Drill the tibial guide pin with the knee in terminal extension.

- Rotate the femoral aimer down the sidewall of the lateral condyle.

- Angle the WasherLoc tibial fixation screw toward the fibular head.

- Tension the graft bundles equally with the knee in full extension.

Clinical and Surgical Pitfalls

- Position the anteromedial portal adjacent to the medial border of the patellar tendon so the tibial guide centers in the notch.

- Almost always perform a lateral wallplasty to make room for the graft.

- Perform a roofplasty only when the roof overhangs the notch.

The use of autogenous hamstring tendons for anterior cruciate ligament (ACL) reconstruction continues to grow in popularity. The superb biomechanical properties of these looped tendons coupled with the low morbidity of graft harvest make this tissue an ideal graft for ACL reconstruction. Furthermore, autogenous hamstring grafts are an excellent graft source for skeletally immature patients. Improved tunnel placement techniques along with improved graft fixation devices also add to the appeal of hamstring grafts for ACL surgery. The use of two smaller-diameter tendon grafts affords the surgeon the ability to use hamstring grafts when performing either single or double-bundle ACL reconstruction techniques. This chapter focuses on the use of a single-tunnel ACL reconstruction technique that uses a scientifically proven transtibial tunnel technique and double-looped hamstring grafts fixed with high-strength slippage-resistant tibial and femoral devices.

PREOPERATIVE CONSIDERATIONS

ACL injury most commonly occurs during a noncontact deceleration change of direction maneuver. Patients typically feel and possibly hear a "pop" at the time of injury. Patients experience acute pain and are unable to continue their sport or activity. Comprehensive provocative examination testing and physical examination findings in the acute and chronic settings are outlined in Box 74-1 and Table 74-1. Anteroposterior (AP), lateral, and oblique radiographs are obtained to assess for fractures in the acute setting. A fracture along the lateral rim of the tibial plateau is a Segond fracture or lateral capsular sign and is pathognomonic for ACL tear. In most cases, no fracture is seen. Magnetic resonance imaging (MRI) may be useful in the acute setting to confirm a suspected ACL tear and to detect any additional ligamentous, meniscal or chondral injuries at the time of injury. In the chronic setting, MRI is seldom needed to identify ACL injury because provocative Lachman and pivot-shift testing results are positive.

Patients who experience an ACL tear and subsequent instability will benefit from surgical reconstruction. Young patients, particularly skeletally immature patients, should undergo early ACL reconstruction to restore rotational knee stability and minimize the risk of meniscal tears.[1,2] Potential growth disturbances in skeletally immature patients is a concern; however, the incidence of growth disturbance with a hamstring graft is very low, and the deformity can be better salvaged than with the meniscal-deficient knee. A table of indications and relative contraindications for surgery is presented in Box 74-2.

SURGICAL TECHNIQUE
Patient Positioning

Position the patient supine on the operating table and place a tourniquet around the proximal thigh of the

TABLE 74-1. Provocative Examination Tests

Examination	Significance
Lachman and pivot-shift test	ACL injury
Straight-leg raise	Extensor mechanism injury
Patella apprehension	Patella instability
MPFL tenderness	Patella instability
Varus or valgus laxity at 30 degrees	Collateral ligament injury
Varus or valgus laxity at 0 degrees	Capsular injury
Tibial external rotation at 30 degrees	PLC injury
Tibial external rotation at 90 degrees	PCL injury
Posterior drawer at 90 degrees	PCL injury
Quadriceps active test	PCL injury
Joint line tenderness	Meniscal tear, chondral injury, capsular avulsion
Lateral tibial plateau tenderness	Bone bruise, fracture
Extension recurvatum test	PCL and PLC combined injury
Reverse pivot shift test	PCL combined injury

ACL, Anterior cruciate ligament; *MPFL,* medial patellofemoral ligament; *PCL,* posterior cruciate ligament; *PLC,* posterolateral corner.

BOX 74-1 Examination Findings in the Acute Versus the Chronic Anterior Cruciate Ligament (ACL)–Deficient Knee

Acute ACL Injury
- Swelling, hemarthrosis
- Pain
- Decreased range of motion
- Lachman test result—positive
- Pivot shift limited by pain

Chronic ACL Injury
- Minimal or no swelling
- Lack of pain (if pain is present, suspect meniscal tear, bone bruise, chondral injury)
- Normal motion
- Lachman test result—positive
- Pivot shift—positive

BOX 74-2 Indications and Contraindications for Anterior Cruciate Ligament Reconstruction

Indications
- High-demand athlete
- Skeletally immature patient
- Repairable meniscal tear
- Symptomatic instability
- Instability with activities of daily living
- Refusal of patient to change lifestyle

Relative Contraindications
- Older sedentary patient
- No symptomatic instability
- Willingness to alter lifestyle
- Advanced arthritis

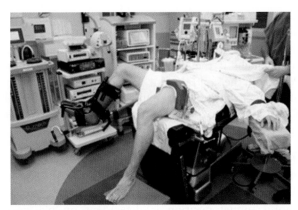

Figure 74-1. Our preferred patient setup.

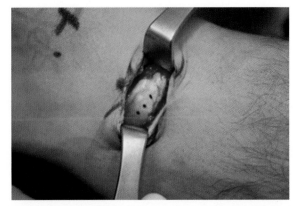

Figure 74-2. The dotted line at the inferior border of the gracilis tendon represents the transverse incision in the sartorius fascia used to expose the gracilis and semitendinosus tendons.

BOX 74-3 Surgical Steps
• Tendon harvest
• Portal placement
• Tibial tunnel placement
• Femoral tunnel placement
• Prepare WasherLoc
• EZLoc sizing and insertion
• WasherLoc tibial fixation
• Bone graft tibial tunnel

WasherLoc and EZLoc, Biomet Sports Medicine, Warsaw, IN.

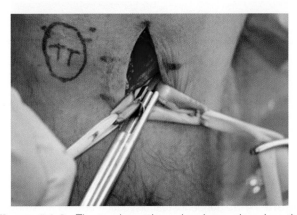

Figure 74-3. The tendon stripper has been placed on the gracilis tendon. Penrose drains isolate each tendon and allow for counterforce during tendon stripping.

operative leg. Position the operative leg in a standard knee arthroscopy leg holder with the foot of the operating table flexed completely. The leg holder can be adjusted and rotated proximally to allow for greater knee flexion. Position the contralateral leg in an Allen stirrup with the hip flexed and abducted with mild external rotation. Ensure that there is no pressure on the peroneal nerve and calf (Fig. 74-1). Alternatively, the surgeon can position the operative leg flexed over the side of the table using a lateral post and maintain the contralateral leg extended on the operating table. Prepare, drape, and exsanguinate the leg and inflate the tourniquet.

Preferred Surgical Technique

Box 74-3 provides the steps of this procedure.

Tendon Harvest

Make a 2- to 3-cm vertical incision along the posteromedial crest of the tibia, centered three fingerbreadths below the medial joint line. A vertical incision allows the surgeon a more extensile incision should it be necessary to lengthen the incision for ease of hamstring harvest. Making the incision obliquely or transversely might decrease the risk of sensory nerve injury, but these incisions are not extensile and need to be optimally placed. Incise the skin and subcutaneous fat down to

the sartorius fascia. Palpate the hamstring tendons and incise the sartorius fascia horizontal and parallel inferior to the gracilis tendon and proximal to the semitendinosus tendon (Fig. 74-2). Flex the knee to 90 degrees and develop a plane by sweeping a finger in the proximal and posterior direction deep to the sartorius fascia along the gracilis tendon. Flex the finger to capture the gracilis tendon. Loop a Penrose drain around the tendon. Release any fascial slips from the inferior border of the gracilis. Strip the gracilis tendon from its musculotendinous junction with a blunt tendon stripper. Pull back on the gracilis tendon insertion site and identify the semitendinosus tendon along the inferior border of the gracilis. Loop a Penrose drain around the semitendinosus tendon (Fig. 74-3). Identify and cut any fascial slips to the medial gastrocnemius originating from the inferior border of the semitendinosus tendon. Strip the tendon with a blunt tendon stripper (see Fig. 74-3). Prepare the tendons by stripping the muscle from the tendon with scissors or a broad periosteal elevator (Fig. 74-4). Place an absorbable No. 1 stitch in the end of each tendon for tensioning. Double-loop and size the tendons with sizing sleeves. Select the diameter of the tendons by

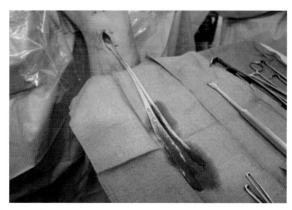

Figure 74-4. Proximal tendon ends are first cleaned of muscle with a broad periosteal elevator and stitched before removal from the tibial insertion site.

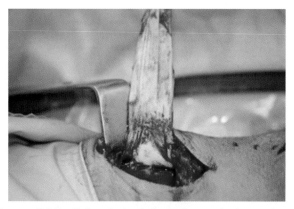

Figure 74-5. Subperiosteal dissection at the hamstring insertion site allows for additional 5 to 10 mm of length.

choosing the smallest-diameter sleeve that freely slides over the looped tendons. Subperiosteally remove the tendons from the anterior tibial crest at their common tendinous insertion, including 5 to 10 mm of periosteum (Fig. 74-5). Suture the common tendinous insertion with a single suture. Store the tendons in the sizing sleeve and a damp sponge in a kidney basin on the back table. Cover the kidney basin with an occlusive Ioban sheet to ensure the safety of the graft on the back table.

Portal Placement

Establish inferolateral and inferomedial portals adjacent to the edges of the patella tendon starting 5 to 10 mm distal to the inferior pole of the patella. The medial portal must touch the edge of the patella tendon because if it is placed more medial the tibial guide may not stay seated in the intercondylar notch with the knee in full extension. An optional outflow portal can be established superiorly.

Perform diagnostic arthroscopy. Treat any meniscal or articular cartilage injuries. Identify and remove the torn remnant ACL stump. It is not necessary to completely denude the tibial insertion of the native ACL

tissue. In fact, retaining a portion of the insertion of the native ACL helps seal the edges of the ACL graft at the joint line and does not result in a cyclops lesion and roof impingement if the tibial tunnel has been positioned properly in the sagittal plane. Remove the synovium and soft tissue in the notch to expose the lateral edge of the PCL. Remove any of the ACL origin from the over-the-top position with an angled curette and shaver.

Tibial Tunnel Placement

When a transtibial tunnel technique is used, the key step is correct placement of the tibial tunnel because the femoral tunnel position is dependent on placement, especially in the coronal plane. Most failures regarding tunnel placement are the result of aberrant tibial tunnel placement. Consider the use of a three-dimensional guide (Howell 65° Tibial Guide, Biomet Sports Medicine, Warsaw, IN) that is designed specifically to correctly position the tibial tunnel in the coronal and sagittal planes to avoid graft impingement on the PCL and roof and to properly restore the tension pattern in the graft similar to the intact ACL. This tibial guide customizes the sagittal and coronal placement of the tunnel for individual differences in knee anatomy including the width of the notch, the slope of the intercondylar roof, and the hyperextension of the knee.

Insert the 65° Tibial Guide through the medial portal. Advance the guide into the intercondylar notch. The tip of the guide is 9.5 mm wide, which mimics the width of an 8- or 9-mm wide ACL graft. Typically the guide contacts the lateral femoral condyle and deforms the PCL because the space is narrower than the width of the graft. Perform a lateral wallplasty to the apex of the notch by removing bone from the lateral wall until the tip of the guide passes into the notch without deforming the PCL. Performing a wallplasty moves the tibial tunnel laterally away from the PCL and minimizes PCL impingement. Do not remove bone from the intercondylar roof unless overhanging osteophytes are present because the 65° Tibial Guide references the intercondylar roof when setting the sagittal position of the tibial tunnel.

Insert the 65° Tibial Guide through the anteromedial portal into the intercondylar notch, and fully extend the knee (Fig. 74-6). While extending the knee visualize that the tip of the guide is inside the notch and the arm of the guide contacts the trochlea groove. Place the heel of the patient on a Mayo stand to maintain the knee in maximum hyperextension. Stand on the lateral side of the leg and insert the coronal alignment rod through the proximal hole in the guide. Rotate the 65° Tibial Guide in the coronal plane until the coronal alignment rod is parallel to the joint and perpendicular to the long axis of the tibia (see Fig. 74-6). Insert the combination bullet guide–hole changer into the 65° Tibial Guide, and advance the bullet until it is seated against the

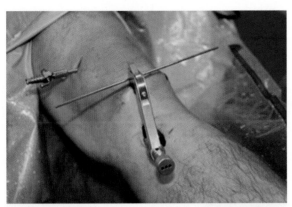

Figure 74-6. The tibial guide is positioned through the medial portal with the coronal alignment rod parallel to the joint line or perpendicular to the long axis of tibia. The knee is in full extension and remains in this position during guide pin placement.

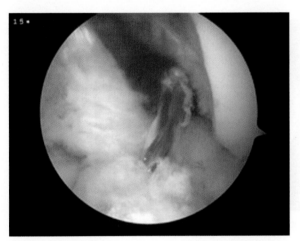

Figure 74-7. Customized tibial guide pin placement viewed from lateral portal.

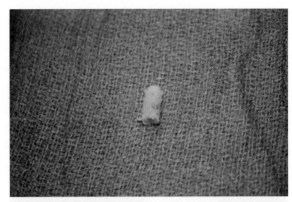

Figure 74-8. Cancellous bone plug harvested from tibia during tunnel preparation will be reinserted into the tibial tunnel once reconstruction has been completed.

anteromedial cortex of the tibia. Drill the tibial guide pin through the lateral hole in the bullet until it strikes the guide intra-articularly with the knee in terminal extension. If you want to check the position of the guide pin, use a C-arm to confirm the position with the tibial guide and guide pin in the knee. Remove the bullet from the tibial guide and remove the guide from the notch. Tap the guide pin into the notch and assess its position.

The tibial guide pin is properly positioned medially and laterally in the coronal plane when it enters the notch midway between the lateral edge of the PCL and the lateral femoral condyle. The guide pin should not touch the PCL and should be directed toward the native ACL femoral footprint (Fig. 74-7). The tibial guide pin is properly positioned rotationally in the coronal plane when the projection of the tibia of the guide pin touches the lateral femoral condyle halfway between the apex and the bottom of the notch. The tibial guide pin is properly positioned anteriorly and posteriorly in the

sagittal plane when there is a 2- to 3-mm space between the guide pin and intercondylar roof with the knee in full extension (see Fig. 74-7). The space can be assessed by manipulating a 2-mm-wide nerve hook probe between the between the guide pin and intercondylar roof in the fully extended knee.

Prepare the tibial tunnel by breaking through the tibial cortex with a drill with the same diameter as the prepared ACL graft. Harvest a bone dowel from the tibial tunnel by inserting a centering rod over the guide pin and then impacting an 8-mm-diameter bone dowel harvester over the tibial guide pin to the subchondral bone. Remove the dowel harvester with cancellous bone dowel (Fig. 74-8). If the tibial guide pin is removed with the bone dowel, replace it by inserting it through a 7- or 8-mm-diameter reamer that has been reinserted into the tunnel. Drill the remainder of the tibial tunnel.

Check for PCL impingement by placing the knee in 90 degrees of flexion and inserting the impingement rod into the notch. A triangular space at the apex of the notch and no contact at the base of the notch between the PCL and impingement rod confirm the absence of PCL impingement (Fig. 74-9). Check for roof impingement by placing the knee in full extension and inserting an impingement rod of the same diameter as the tibial tunnel into the intercondylar notch. The impingement rod should disappear into the intercondylar notch (Fig. 74-10). Free movement of the impingement rod in and out of the notch with the knee in full extension also confirms the absence of roof impingement.

Femoral Tunnel Placement

Place the femoral tunnel via the transtibial technique. Insert the size-specific femoral aimer through the tibial tunnel with the knee in flexion. The size of the offset of the femoral aimer is based on the diameter of the ACL graft and is designed to create a femoral tunnel with a 1-mm back wall. Extend the knee, and hook the tip of the femoral aimer in the over-the-top position. Allow

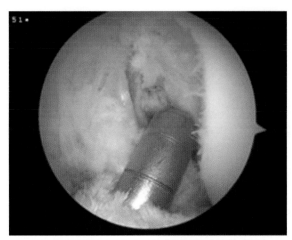

Figure 74-9. Impingement rod angles away from posterior cruciate ligament and toward the native femoral footprint.

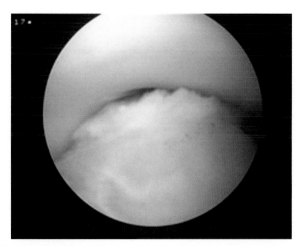

Figure 74-10. With the knee in full extension, the impingement rod should disappear into the intercondylar notch.

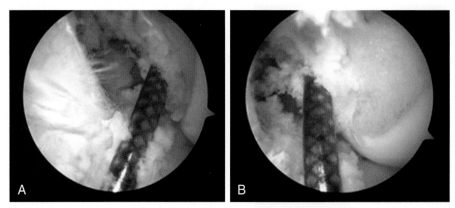

Figure 74-11. Position of the femoral guide pin in the native anterior cruciate ligament footprint.

gravity to flex the knee until the femoral guide seats on the femur. Rotate the femoral aimer a quarter turn lateral away from the PCL, which positions the femoral guide pin farther down the lateral wall of the notch, minimizing PCL impingement. Drill a pilot hole in the femur through the aimer and remove both the guide pin and femoral aimer.

Redirect the femoral guide pin to shorten the femoral tunnel from 35 through 50 mm in length with use of the following technique. Reinsert the femoral guide pin into the pilot hole, and flex the knee to 90 to 100 degrees. Drill the guide pin through the lateral femoral cortex. The guide pin should be located within the native ACL femoral footprint (Fig. 74-11). Pass a cannulated 1-inch reamer the same diameter as the ACL graft over the guide pin. Ream the femoral tunnel. Confirm that the back wall of the femoral aimer is only 1 mm thick. Confirm that the center of the femoral tunnel is midway between the apex and base of the lateral half of the notch (Fig. 74-12). A femoral tunnel placed correctly down the sidewall does not allow room for a second posterolateral tunnel (see Fig. 74-12). Last,

measure the length of the femoral tunnel with the transtibial tunnel depth gauge.

Prepare WasherLoc

Expose the distal aspect of the tibial tunnel by removing a thumbnail portion of the surrounding soft tissue and periosteum. Insert the counterbore aimer into the tibial tunnel. Rotate the guide to aim toward the fibular head. Impact the counterbore awl to create a pilot hole in the tibial tunnel (Fig. 74-13). Drill the anterior tibial tunnel with the counterbore reamer seated in the pilot hole and aimed toward the fibular head. Ream the anterior distal tibial tunnel until it is flush with the posterior wall of the tibial tunnel. Do not ream deeper than the posterior wall into the tibia. Save the bone from the flutes of the reamer.

EZLoc Sizing and Insertion

The EZLoc femoral fixation device is available in two diameters and three lengths to maximize fixation on the cortical bone and optimize bone tunnel surface area and graft length. For femoral tunnel diameters of 7 or 8 mm,

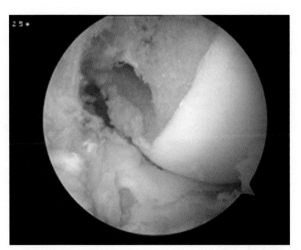

Figure 74-12. Femoral tunnel position in native anterior cruciate ligament footprint with this backwall. Virtually all of the footprint will be filled with graft tissue.

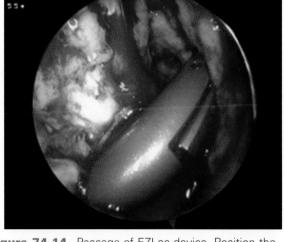

Figure 74-14. Passage of EZLoc device. Position the gold deployment lever laterally.

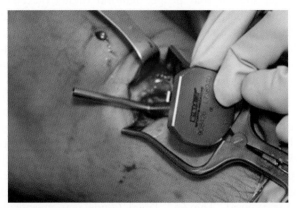

Figure 74-13. Counterbore awl guide being positioned to angle counterbore reamer and screw toward the fibular head.

choose the 7/8 EZLoc device; and for femoral tunnel diameters of 9 or 10 mm, choose the 9/10 EZLoc device. For femoral tunnel lengths of 35 to 50 mm determined by depth gauge measurement, choose a standard-length implant. For femoral tunnel lengths less than 35 mm, choose a short implant, and for femoral tunnel lengths greater than 50 mm, choose a long implant.

With the appropriate-size EZLoc device chosen, insert the passing pin connected to the EZLoc into the tibial tunnel and out of the femoral tunnel under arthroscopic visualization (Fig. 74-14). Pull the passing pin out the lateral thigh until the EZLoc implant is just outside of the tibial incision and tibial tunnel entrance. Pass the graft through the loop of the EZLoc device. Even the ends of the graft and tie the sutures from the ends of the tendons together. With a ruler, measure from the distal aspect of the gold lever arm of the EZLoc, and with a marking pen mark the graft according to the length of the femoral tunnel. This mark will ensure that

the EZLoc has passed lateral and proximal to the proximal-most aspect of the femoral tunnel. Once the marked portion of the graft enters the femoral tunnel, the suture on the EZLoc and passing pin is cut. The passing pin is removed, and tension is pulled on the EZLoc suture deploying the lever arm. Pull tension on the graft strands and rock the graft–EZLoc device back and forth to ensure that the EZLOC is seated on the cortical bone of the lateral femur. Cycle the knee 20 to 30 times, maintaining tension on the graft.

WasherLoc Tibial Fixation

After cycling the knee, position it in full extension. Tie all graft sutures together, and pass an impingement rod through the suture loops. Assemble the WasherLoc to the inserter and drill guide. Place the WasherLoc inserter awl through the pilot hole and capture the strands of the graft within the long tines of the WasherLoc. Have an assistant pull tension on all graft strands equally by pulling on the impingement rod. With all graft strands isolated between the long tines of the WasherLoc, impact the WasherLoc into the graft and bone with a mallet. Remove the inserter awl and drill the far cortex with a 3.2-mm drill through the drill guide. Remove the drill guide and measure the length of the drill hole. Place the measured length 6.0-mm cancellous screw through the WasherLoc, compressing the WasherLoc and graft against the posterior wall of the tibial tunnel (Fig. 74-15).

Bone Graft Tibial Tunnel

Insert the tibial tunnel dilator into the distal aspect of the tibial tunnel. The dilator often can be advanced up the tunnel by hand. Alternatively, gently impact the dilator up the tibial tunnel by tapping lightly with a mallet. Place the plastic sleeve over the tip of the bone

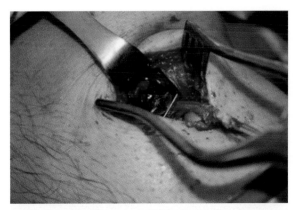

Figure 74-15. WasherLoc fixation of graft with bone graft impacted in tibial tunnel.

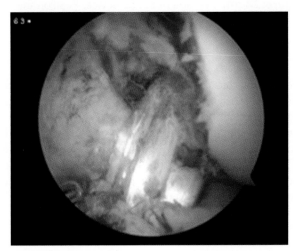

Figure 74-16. Completed anterior cruciate ligament reconstruction.

dowel harvest tube. Position the plastic sleeve at the tip of the harvest tube against the dilated opening of the tibial tunnel. Impact the inner plunger rod to deliver the cancellous bone dowel from the harvest tube into the tibial tunnel. Insert the scope into the joint and inspect the graft (Fig. 74-16). Flex and extend the knee to ensure that no roof or PCL impingement is present. Connect the outer sheath of the arthroscopy handpiece shaver blade to a syringe filled with bupivacaine (Marcaine), advance the sheath under the sartorius fascia along the hamstring tendon sheaths, and inject to provide local anesthesia to the proximal medial thigh. Close the hamstring harvest site in layers, and close the portal sites. Place a sterile dressing and deflate the tourniquet.

POSTOPERATIVE REHABILITATION

The postoperative goals in rehabilitation are given in Table 74-2.

TABLE 74-2. Goals in Rehabilitation

Time	Activity
0-2 weeks	Brace-free, weight bearing as tolerated
2-4 weeks	Stationary bike, quadriceps and hamstring strengthening
8-12 weeks	Jogging, leg press, open and closed chain exercises
12-16 weeks	Add weights and agility exercises
After 16 weeks	Return to sport if single-leg hop distance is greater than 85% of normal side

RESULTS

Several recently published articles question the effectiveness of the transtibial tunnel technique to properly position the femoral tunnel for ACL reconstruction.[3,4] These articles suggest that proper femoral tunnel placement within the native ACL footprint can be inconsistent and difficult to achieve with a transtibial tunnel technique. One criticism of these studies is there is no planar control for tibial tunnel placement. Simply identifying an exit point for the tibial tunnel within the native ACL tibial footprint appears to be inadequate to allow for consistent transtibial placement of the femoral tunnel within the native ACL femoral footprint. Both the sagittal and coronal plane positions of the tibial tunnel are critical, because the tibial tunnel will determine in large part the position of the femoral tunnel and ultimately the ACL graft position when a transtibial tunnel technique is used. The 65° Tibial Guide was specifically developed to position the tibial tunnel in the appropriate sagittal and coronal planes rather than simply choosing a point in the native tibial footprint to prepare the tibia tunnel. Appropriate planar position of the tibial tunnel with use of this guide consistently positions the tibial tunnel in the native ACL tibial footprint for all patients.[5] Coronal plane angulation of 60 to 65 degrees prevents PCL impingement and lateralizes the position of the femoral tunnel more obliquely down the sidewall of the lateral condyle.[6,7] Based on MRI studies, the native ACL position is consistently posterior and parallel to the intercondylar roof when the knee is in full extension.[8,9] Thus the native ACL position is influenced by knee extension and the intercondylar roof angle for any given patient.[10] Use of a coronal alignment rod along with the use of the intercondylar roof anatomy of the knee while the knee is in full extension as described earlier enables the surgeon to consistently and accurately position the tibial tunnel in the correct planes for any given patient.[11] Whereas use of intraoperative fluoroscopy may be helpful in preventing roof impingement, a recent study demonstrated difficulty in solely relying on fluoroscopy to establish proper tibial tunnel placement for all patients because of normal anatomic variability among them.[12] Correct planar position of the tibial tunnel leads to correct femoral tunnel position, resulting in ACL graft tension behavior similar to that of the native ACL.[13,14] Furthermore, complications of roof and PCL impingement are avoided because the 65° Tibial Guide improves the accuracy of ACL graft position, taking into account the anatomic differences between our graft sources and the native ACL.

Second, use of strong, stiff, and slippage-resistant fixation devices further ensures successful outcomes regardless of the use of autogenous hamstring or allograft tissues. In a recently submitted prospective randomized controlled trial comparing autogenous hamstring grafts with anterior tibialis allografts with use of the previously described surgical technique, no differences in subjective or functional outcomes were determined between groups in this appropriately powered study.[15] In addition, a recently published study that used the described surgical technique with fresh-frozen tibialis allograft demonstrated only a 1- to 2-mm overall graft length change in the first 2 months after surgery, with no additional graft length change after 2 months as detected by roentgen stereophotogrammetric analysis.[16] This in vivo study clearly demonstrated the importance of the use of strong and stiff fixation devices coupled with proper tunnel placement via a transtibial tunnel technique to achieve graft isometry, knee stability, and an early return to sport and activity.

REFERENCES

1. Mizuta H, Kubota K, Shiraishi M, et al. The conservative treatment of complete tears of the anterior cruciate ligament in skeletally immature patients. *J Bone Joint Surg Br*. 1995;77:890-894.
2. Shelbourne KD, Patel DV, McCarroll JR. Management of anterior cruciate ligament injuries in skeletally immature adolescents. *Knee Surg Sports Traumatol Arthrosc*. 1996; 4:68-74.
3. Abebe ES, Moorman CT 3rd, Dziedzic TS, et al. Femoral tunnel placement during anterior cruciate ligament reconstruction: an in vivo imaging analysis comparing transtibial and 2-incision tibial tunnel-independent techniques. *Am J Sports Med*. 2009;37:1904-1911.
4. Strauss EJ, Barker JU, McGill K, et al. Can anatomic femoral tunnel placement be achieved using a transtibial technique for hamstring anterior cruciate ligament reconstruction? *Am J Sports Med*. 2011;39:1263-1269.
5. Cuomo P, Edwards A, Giron F, et al. Validation of the 65 degrees Howell guide for anterior cruciate ligament reconstruction. *Arthroscopy*. 2006;22:70-75.
6. Rue JP, Ghodadra N, Bach Jr BR. Femoral tunnel placement in single-bundle anterior cruciate ligament reconstruction: a cadaveric study relating transtibial lateralized femoral tunnel position to the anteromedial and posterolateral bundle femoral origins of the anterior cruciate ligament. *Am J Sports Med*. 2008;36:73-79.
7. Simmons R, Howell SM, Hull ML. Effect of the angle of the femoral and tibial tunnels in the coronal plane and incremental excision of the posterior cruciate ligament on tension of an anterior cruciate ligament graft: an in vitro study. *J Bone Joint Surg Am*. 2003;85:1018-1029.
8. Howell SM, Berns GS, Farley TE. Unimpinged and impinged anterior cruciate ligament grafts: MR signal intensity measurements. *Radiology*. 1991;179:639-643.
9. Howell SM, Clark JA, Blasier RD. Serial magnetic resonance imaging of hamstring anterior cruciate ligament autografts during the first year of implantation. A preliminary study. *Am J Sports Med*. 1991;19:42-47.
10. Howell SM, Barad SJ. Knee extension and its relationship to the slope of the intercondylar roof. Implications for positioning the tibial tunnel in anterior cruciate ligament reconstructions. *Am J Sports Med*. 1995;23:288-294.
11. Howell SM, Gittins ME, Gottlieb JE, et al. The relationship between the angle of the tibial tunnel in the coronal plane and loss of flexion and anterior laxity after anterior cruciate ligament reconstruction. *Am J Sports Med*. 2001; 29:567-574.
12. Kasten P, Szczodry M, Irrgang J, et al. What is the role of intra-operative fluoroscopic measurements to determine tibial tunnel placement in anatomical anterior cruciate ligament reconstruction? *Knee Surg Sports Traumatol Arthrosc*. 2010;18:1169-1175.
13. Howell SM, Hull ML. Checkpoints for judging tunnel and anterior cruciate ligament graft placement. *J Knee Surg*. 2009;22:161-170.
14. Wallace MP, Howell SM, Hull ML. In vivo tensile behavior of a four-bundle hamstring graft as a replacement for the anterior cruciate ligament. *J Orthop Res*. 1997;15: 539-545.
15. Lawhorn K, Howell SM, Traina SM, et al. The effect of graft tissue on anterior cruciate ligament outcomes: a multicenter, prospective, randomized controlled trial comparing autograft hamstrings with fresh-frozen anterior tibialis allograft. *Arthoscopy*. 2012;28:1079-1086.
16. Smith CK, Howell SM, Hull ML. Anterior laxity, slippage, and recovery of function in the first year after tibialis allograft anterior cruciate ligament reconstruction. *Am J Sports Med*. 2011;39:78-88.

Chapter 75

Central Quadriceps Free Tendon Harvest for Anterior Cruciate Ligament Reconstruction

John P. Fulkerson

Chapter Synopsis
- The central quadriceps tendon provides an important anterior cruciate ligament (ACL) reconstruction graft alternative. It may be used as a free tendon graft with predictable success and less pain than other autograft alternatives.

Important Points
- Understanding that the quadriceps tendon is twice as thick as patellar tendon, the surgeon may harvest a 7-mm-thick graft by carefully defining this desired thickness at the time of tendon graft harvest.

Clinical and Surgical Pearls
- Use a hemostat to define the posterior graft thickness by careful spreading.
- Obtain both rectus and intermedius components of the quadriceps tendon to ensure adequate graft bulk.
- Keep the knee flexed for graft harvest to ensure adequate tension in the quad tendon. This facilitates harvest of the graft.
- Stay just medial to the central aspect of the quad tendon where the tendon is thickest.

Clinical and Surgical Pitfalls
- Penetration into the suprapatellar pouch at the time of graft harvest may be remedied easily with a few sutures after turning off inflow into the joint.
- If an inadequate graft is harvested, the surgeon may harvest additional quadriceps tendon and suture to the initial graft.

Central quadriceps free tendon (CQFT) graft reconstruction of the anterior cruciate ligament (ACL) has been refined from earlier descriptions of the procedure using a bone block from the proximal patella in quadriceps tendon for ACL reconstruction. Quadriceps free tendon (without bone) reduces the morbidity of graft harvest and provides a substantial free tendon autograft for ACL reconstruction, saving both time and morbidity.[1,4] The CQFT is an important and desirable autograft alternative for ACL reconstruction. It is harvested from a large tendon donor site without neurovascular complication risk and without risk of patellar fracture.

PREOPERATIVE CONSIDERATIONS

I use central quadriceps tendon for reconstruction in virtually all patients—male and female, competitive athletes and working people. My criteria for surgery, elicited in the history, include recurrent instability related to ACL deficiency that limits daily function or participation in desired athletic activity and an active athletic lifestyle requiring quick turning, pivoting, and cutting such that problems might be predictable without ACL reconstruction. I establish a loss of ACL function by clinical examination to detect positive Lachman and pivot shift test results. I routinely use magnetic resonance imaging for confirmation.

Contraindications include gross obesity, sedentary lifestyle in which ACL reconstruction may not be necessary, immunosuppressive therapy, and smoking on a regular basis. I find that most smokers are willing to give up smoking during the preoperative and postoperative period to allow graft healing. Small women (under 5 feet tall) may have a short quadriceps tendon. Even in such patients, an adequate graft can be harvested. No quadriceps tendon rupture has occurred in any of my patients.

SURGICAL TECHNIQUE

Box 75-1 outlines the specific steps of this procedure.

A (CQFT) graft is readily obtained through a short longitudinal incision at the center of the proximal patella extended approximately 3 to 4 cm (or more as needed) toward the apex of the central quadriceps tendon. With proximal retraction and well-directed lighting, the surgeon will define a 9- to 10-mm-wide central quadriceps graft with a No. 10 scalpel blade. The graft is best harvested with its center 2 to 3 mm medial to the apex of the central quadriceps tendon.[4] After the medial and lateral borders of the graft have been defined, a hemostat is used to define the posterior portion of the graft leaving the back wall of the intermedius portion of quadriceps tendon (Fig. 75-1). A 7-mm-deep graft is relatively easy to harvest and define by use of the hemostat to spread within the intermedius tendon posteriorly to obtain the desired thickness of the quadriceps tendon graft. After ample spreading of the posterior aspect of the intended graft, the graft is released from the proximal patella (distal end of the graft) with a No. 15 scalpel blade (Fig. 75-2). Once the distal end is free, I recommend a uterine T-clamp to hold the released end of the quadriceps tendon graft such that whipstitches of Ultrabraid (Smith & Nephew, Andover, MA) or a similar No. 5–strength suture may be placed in the free end of the graft. I recommend two sets of

whipstitches, front and back, such as four strands of No. 5–strength suture (I prefer Ultrabraid), to hold the graft during the remainder of the harvest.

With whipstitches in the end of the free tendon graft, the more proximal aspect of the quadriceps free tendon graft may be readily harvested via a combination of blunt dissection and use of Metzenbaum scissors. It is important to preserve the integrity of the graft as it is dissected proximally. Once the graft has been defined for a length of 7 to 8 cm, the knee is extended; with the retractor pulling proximally, a 7- to 8-cm-long quadriceps free tendon graft is released proximally, leaving the entire remaining quadriceps tendon intact (Fig. 75-3). Usually, some vastus medialis muscle will be on the graft; this is trimmed off.

With the chosen device used to hold the graft, the sutured end of the graft is secured and whipstitches are

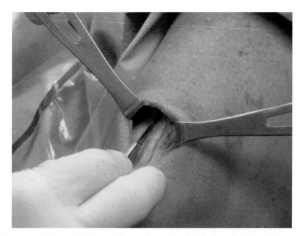

Figure 75-1. With a No. 10 scalpel blade, define a 9- to 10-mm-wide graft, 7 mm in depth (the quad tendon is about 9 mm in thickness). *(Courtesy Julie Lippe, MD.)*

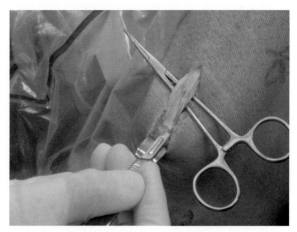

Figure 75-2. A hemostat defines the posterior aspect of the graft. Use a No. 15 scalpel blade to release the quadriceps free tendon graft from the patella, then place whipstitches in the distal end before releasing it proximally. *(Courtesy Julie Lippe, MD.)*

BOX 75-1 Surgical Steps

1. Make incision.
2. Define and make incision for medial and lateral borders of graft to 7 mm thickness.
3. Define posterior portion of graft by spreading with a hemostat.
4. Release graft from the proximal patella.
5. Grasp distal end of graft with uterine T clamp and whipstitch end.
6. Release quadriceps free tendon graft proximally to obtain a 7- to 8-cm-long, 7-mm-thick free tendon graft for anterior cruciate ligament reconstruction.
7. Prepare the quadriceps free tendon graft on a suitable holding platform; make double whipstitches in both ends.
8. Use EndoButton on the proximal end of the graft for femoral fixation, placing one front and one back suture of graft through central holes of the EndoButton. Tie knot adjacent to graft to meeting ends of sutures.
9. Secure the tibial side with a biointerference screw or a button tied at the tibial exit site.

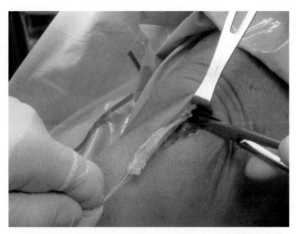

Figure 75-3. The quadriceps free tendon graft is released proximally to provide a 7- to 8-cm-long, 7-mm-thick free tendon graft for anterior cruciate ligament reconstruction. *(Courtesy Julie Lippe, MD.)*

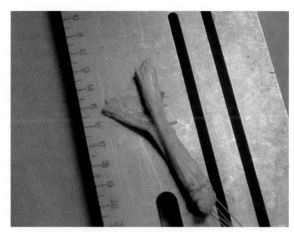

Figure 75-5. The intermedius and rectus components of the quadriceps tendon also make it ideal for double-bundle anterior cruciate ligament reconstruction. *(Courtesy Julie Lippe, MD.)*

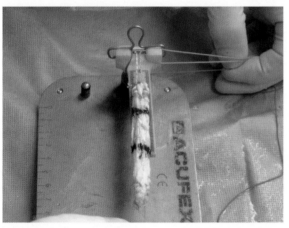

Figure 75-4. The quadriceps free tendon graft is easily prepared on a suitable holding platform, with whipstitches placed in both ends. *(Courtesy Julie Lippe, MD.)*

placed in the distal end as well. My preference is to use an EndoButton (Smith & Nephew) on the proximal end of the graft for femoral fixation. After the socket for the femoral end of the graft has been drilled at the anatomic location, the depth of the socket and EndoButton tunnel are measured with the EndoButton measuring stick. The sutures from one side of the quadriceps free tendon graft are then placed through the central eyes of the Endo-Button, brought down, and tied just adjacent to the tendon graft itself; the length is adjusted to allow for 2 cm of graft in the femoral socket once the EndoButton has been deployed. In this manner the knot may be tied precisely to allow the proper amount of tendon in the femoral socket with the knot tied adjacent to the graft (Fig. 75-4). A double-bundle graft is readily available because of distinct rectus and intermedius components (Fig. 75-5).

Once the graft is locked in place on the femoral side, the tibial side may be secured with a biointerference screw, or a button tied at the tibial exit site.

POSTOPERATIVE CONSIDERATIONS

Patients are placed in a knee immobilizer after surgery but encouraged to bear full weight and to start immediate range of motion. A home program of closed-chain exercises has worked well, and loss of range of motion is extremely uncommon. Most patients achieve motion quickly because pain is less than with other autografts. Closed chain physical therapy may be started after 10 days to 2 weeks (I generally use subcuticular closure). Most patients are off crutches with supportive quadriceps function by 2 weeks from the time of surgery. Patients do closed chain exercises for 3 months and then progress to running.

RESULTS

Short-term pain has been less than with alternative autografts, and satisfaction of patients has been consistently high. In a short-term follow-up study by Joseph and colleagues,[1] patients who had undergone CQFT ACL reconstruction reported pain medication use for 6 days, versus 19 days in a matched group of patients who had received hamstring autografts and 22 days in a comparable group of patients with bone-tendon-bone ACL reconstruction. The patients who had undergone CQFT reconstruction also reached rehabilitation landmarks sooner.

In a long-term follow-up study (all patients more than 2 years after surgery; average, 66 months) of the CQFT for ACL reconstruction,[2] the median International Knee Documentation Committee score at follow-up was 90, the average side-to-side KT1000 difference (20-pound pull) was 1.2 mm, and the single-leg hop quotient was 0.96. There were five graft failures in the group of 124 patients. No patient had anterior knee pain or loss of knee range of motion.

Geib and Shelton[4] have also noted similar favorable longer term results with CQFT for ACL reconstruction. Stability results with central quadriceps free tendon ACL reconstruction are comparable with those of other graft types, but morbidity appears to be less.

Adams and colleagues[5] have demonstrated by mechanical testing that the quadriceps tendon is stronger, in general, after graft harvest than the patellar tendon is before a bone-tendon-bone graft is harvested. Lippe et al[6] have provided a detailed anatomic study of the quadriceps tendon that may be helpful to surgeons wanting to use this autograft alternative in cruciate ligament reconstruction.

REFERENCES

1. Joseph M, Fulkerson J, Nissen C, et al. Short-term recovery after anterior cruciate ligament reconstruction: a prospective comparison of three autografts. *Orthopedics*. 2006;29: 243-248.
2. DeAngelis JP, Fulkerson JP. Quadriceps tendon a reliable alternative for reconstruction of the anterior cruciate ligament. *Clin Sports Med*. 2007;26:587-596.
3. Fulkerson JP. Central quadriceps free tendon for anterior cruciate ligament reconstruction. *Oper Tech Sports Med*. 1999;7:195-200.
4. Geib TM, Shelton WR, Phelps RA, et al. Anterior cruciate ligament reconstruction using quadriceps tendon autograft: intermediate term outcome. *Arthroscopy*. 2009;25(12): 1408-1414.
5. Adams D, Mazzocca A, Fulkerson J. Residual strength of the quadriceps versus patellar tendon after harvesting a central free tendon graft. *Arthroscopy*. 2006;22:76-79.
6. Lippe J, Armstrong A, Fulkerson J. Anatomic guidelines for harvesting a quadriceps free tendon autograft for anterior cruciate ligament reconstruction. *Arthroscopy*. 2012;28(7): 980-984.

Chapter 76

Revision Anterior Cruciate Ligament Reconstruction

Geoffrey S. Van Thiel, Brian Forsythe, Adam B. Yanke, and Bernard R. Bach Jr

Chapter Synopsis

- Acute failure of an anterior cruciate ligament (ACL) reconstruction is most likely a result of a technical error, whereas failure at over 1 year is more commonly the result of a traumatic event. Regardless, a thorough evaluation of tunnel position, hardware and fixation, and concomitant pathology must be completed before any revision procedure.

Important Points

- After failure of an ACL reconstruction:
  - If tunnel position is good, use the same tunnels.
  - If tunnels are malpositioned but not overlapping, proceed with standard ACL reconstruction.
  - If malpositioned tunnels will overlap new tunnels, fill the overlapping tunnel with graft or screw.
  - If concern exists that tunnel expansion will compromise fixation, consider a two-stage procedure with bone grafting as the first step.

Clinical and Surgical Pearls

- In the setting of tunnel expansion or overlapping tunnels, options include the following:

  - Stacking screws
  - Allograft dowels or bone chips placed through a cannula
  - Large bone plugs attached to the graft
- Ensure that all required equipment for hardware removal is present.
- Address malalignment, other ligament insufficiency, meniscal pathology, and articular cartilage defects with a concomitant or staged procedure.
- Fully evaluate tunnel position preoperatively, and begin the procedure with a definitive plan.

Clinical and Surgical Pitfalls

- Defer graft preparation until the tunnels are made. This optimizes the potential of making custom-sized bone plugs if needed in situations in which there may be tunnel expansion or overlap.
- If there is any question about the integrity of tibial fixation, one should consider backup fixation.

Reconstruction of the anterior cruciate ligament (ACL) is one of the most common surgical procedures performed by orthopedic surgeons. However, despite its overwhelming success, 3% to 25% of patients may experience a failure of their reconstruction. Large multicenter studies have suggested that allografts result in higher failure rates in younger athletic patients,[1] but failure can occur with any graft type or patient demographic if the appropriate principles are not followed in the primary reconstruction. In the majority of failures, technical errors can be identified and must be corrected at the revision procedure for knee stability to be restored. This chapter discusses the surgical planning and techniques for revision ACL reconstruction.

PREOPERATIVE CONSIDERATIONS

Classification of Anterior Cruciate Ligament Failures

There are a multitude of contributing factors to the rupture of an ACL graft. However, a general rule of thumb is that if the failure occurs in the first 6 months, it is most likely a result of a technical error, although failure of graft incorporation (especially with allografts), excessive rehabilitation, and premature return to full activities can also play a role. If the failure occurs after 1 year postoperatively, it is most likely a result of a traumatic event.

The most common cause of failure in primary ACL reconstruction is technical error in tunnel placement, typically involving vertical placement of the femoral tunnel (Fig. 76-1). Historically, concern for ACL-roof impingement in extension led some surgeons to place their tibial tunnels too posteriorly. If the femoral tunnel is then drilled transtibially through the posterior tibial tunnel, a subsequent high (anteromedial [AM]) graft position will result from the orientation of the drill guide. The ACL graft is then malpositioned between a posterior tibial tunnel and a high or vertical femoral position. It should also be noted that even with an independent femoral tunnel in an "anatomic" position on the femoral wall, a posterior tibial tunnel will create a vertical graft in the sagittal plane and may not adequately address rotational stability.

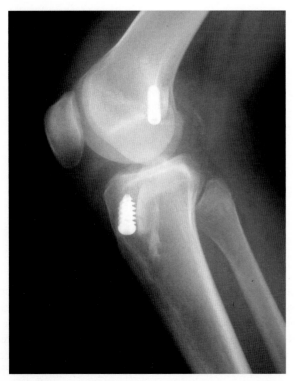

Figure 76-1. Vertical femoral tunnel and posteriorized tibial tunnel.

This mismatched graft position may diminish impingement and improve anteroposterior (AP) stability; however, it fails to restore normal rotational stability of the knee. Abnormal biomechanics are observed, and patients may report subjective instability even though they have a normal Lachman test result and minimal KT1000 side-to-side difference.[5,21] Their rotational instability, however, manifests with a positive pivot glide or 1+ pivot shift even though the Lachman and anterior drawer test results may remain normal. It is important to keep in mind that range of motion may provide important clues regarding the presence of notch impingement and, most important, accurate tunnel placement.[2] Regardless, to restore more normal knee kinematics, patients may require a revision ACL reconstruction.

History

Patients who experience recurrent instability may benefit from a revision reconstruction to stabilize the knee and restore function. Preoperative data collection and planning are important to ensure success of the reconstruction. If available, previous operative notes, arthroscopic images, and imaging are reviewed to determine previous surgical tunnels, graft location, meniscal status, and cartilage defects. In the setting of a previous significant meniscectomy, staged or concomitant meniscal transplantation may be required.

Physical Examination

A thorough physical examination is performed to assess knee stability not only anteriorly but also posteriorly, medially, and laterally. It is critical to exclude a subtle posterolateral or posteromedial laxity that may be contributing to graft attenuation. All test results should be compared with those of the opposite knee. The affected knee's range of motion should be recorded, with particular attention to subtle knee flexion contractures. Patellofemoral crepitation and mobility should be assessed. If it is available, a KT1000 measurement should be performed on both knees to provide objective anterior-posterior translation parameters.

Imaging

If no previous radiographs are available, we recommend obtaining at least four views to determine tunnel orientation and to help decide whether hardware will need to be removed during revision surgery (AP in extension, posteroanterior [PA] Rosenberg, lateral, and skyline). The radiographs will also help assess the slope of the tibial plateau because this can contribute to a failure mechanism. Magnetic resonance imaging can help evaluate concomitant pathologic changes, such as meniscal tears and posterior cruciate ligament (PCL) or posterolateral corner injuries. If there is any suggestion of tunnel widening on conventional radiographs, we routinely obtain a computed tomographic scan to better delineate tunnel expansion.

Graft Choice

Several graft options are available for revision ACL reconstruction. Autografts include hamstring tendon, quadriceps tendon, and patellar tendon from the ipsilateral or contralateral knee. Allograft options include Achilles, patellar, hamstring, quadriceps, and tibialis anterior tendons. Our preference is to use allograft tissue if a patellar tendon autograft has been harvested previously. Although some surgeons prefer the use of a contralateral patellar tendon graft, we have noted that most patients do not want to have their "normal" knee surgically violated. Although biomechanical characteristics of quadrupled hamstring grafts are more than adequate for revision reconstruction, secure fixation in the expanded tunnels can be difficult, especially when soft tissue grafts had been used primarily. Patellar tendon allograft provides bone for supplemental grafting, and extra-large bone blocks can be customized to provide improved tunnel fill for primary interference fixation. In our institution we have historically used nonirradiated patellar tendon allograft for revision procedures, with excellent results.[3]

Indications and Contraindications

Revision ACL reconstruction is indicated after a failed primary reconstruction, defined as a symptomatic, unstable knee that interferes with the activity level desired by the individual patient. Contraindications include significant medical comorbidities and current or recent infection. Uncorrected malalignment, decreased range of motion, and degenerative changes are relative contraindications that can frequently be addressed in staged or concomitant procedures.

Furthermore, a staged procedure should be considered in the following circumstances:

- Tunnel expansion of more than 1.5 cm
- Loss of extension of more than 5 degrees
- Loss of flexion of more than 20 degrees
- Significant varus or valgus malalignment necessitating an osteotomy

SURGICAL TECHNIQUE

Anesthesia and Positioning

Most patients undergo general anesthesia. A femoral nerve block can be useful in controlling postoperative pain, although we rarely use nerve blocks or regional anesthesia. Patients are positioned supine on the operating room table. The foot of the bed is flexed; a tourniquet is applied to the operative thigh, which is then secured in a leg holder. The contralateral leg rests in a gynecologic leg holder with both the hip and the knee flexed no more than approximately 60 degrees to prevent traction on the femoral or peroneal nerves. To prevent lumbar spine extension and traction on the femoral nerve, we reflex the operating bed slightly and place it in Trendelenburg position. It is important to be able to flex the operative knee to approximately 110 degrees of flexion to allow proper placement of the femoral tunnel and screw if a single-incision endoscopic technique is to be used.

Examination Under Anesthesia and Diagnostic Arthroscopy

A thorough examination under anesthesia is performed before the thigh is secured in the leg holder, to reassess ACL incompetency as well as to rule out any other injuries to the PCL, medial collateral ligament, and posterolateral corner complex. Diagnostic arthroscopy is performed to evaluate all potential concomitant pathology. All necessary repairs or debridement are performed before the ACL revision. One should be particularly attentive of partial-thickness meniscal tears, which appear more commonly on the undersurface medially and on the superior surface laterally. Any arthritic changes or articular surface wear should be well documented.

Specific Steps

Box 76-1 outlines the specific steps of this procedure.

1. Notch Preparation

The general principles of ACL reconstruction apply to revision surgery. Before removal of the ACL remnant, inspect the footprints of the torn ACL on both the tibia and femur and mark their location via arthroscopic electrocautery. With use of a combination

---

BOX 76-1 Surgical Steps for Revision Anterior Cruciate Ligament Reconstruction

1. Notch preparation
2. Notchplasty
3. Removal of old hardware
4. Tibial tunnel
5. Femoral tunnel
6. Bone grafting procedures for tunnel widening
7. Graft preparation and placement
8. Femoral fixation
9. Tibial fixation

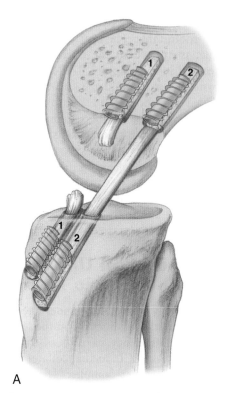
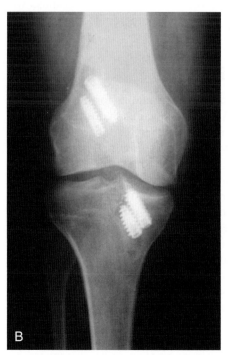

A   B

Figure 76-2. Graft 1 represents a nonanatomic tunnel with a revision procedure completed without removal of any old hardware.

of electrocautery, an arthroscopic curette, and a full-radius shaver, the remnant of the ACL is removed from the lateral wall of the notch all the way back to the "over-the-top" position and from the tibial insertion.

2. Notchplasty

Intercondylar notch impingement and roof impingement are two common causes of ACL failure. A notch width of at least 20 mm is necessary in the midtunnel region to avoid graft impingement. If a notchplasty is necessary, it can be performed with either a quarter-inch osteotome or a spherical bur. The notchplasty is performed from anterior to posterior and from apex to inferior. One should avoid elevating the apex of the notch (unless there are apical notch osteophytes) because the patella contacts this region in the extremes of flexion. A rasp or shaver can be used to smooth the wall of the intercondylar notch. After the notchplasty has been performed, a probe is placed to palpate the "over-the-top" position. One should be able to hook this area easily with a probe; if the probe slides off the back edge, it is advisable to reevaluate and to debride this area further.

3. Removal of Old Hardware

It is critical to consider whether former hardware will require removal or whether it may be bypassed at revision surgery. Various interference screws are commercially available with differing morphologic appearances radiographically. Most can be removed with a standard 3.5-mm screwdriver, but every effort should be made to determine the specific brand of the screw to prepare necessary specialized equipment. This is the first decision point; if previous tunnels are nonanatomic and nonoverlapping, the hardware can generally be left in place (Figs. 76-2 and 76-3). If the tunnels will overlap, the hardware may require initial removal for the new tunnel to be made, but it may have to be subsequently reinserted to provide construct fixation stability. In our experience, bioabsorbable screws are generally not resorbed at the time of revision surgery and frequently fracture on attempted removal secondary to softening. The surgeon may therefore have to ream through these screws to properly position the new tunnel.

If a screw does require removal, a flexible nitinol pin is placed through the screw, and an appropriate screwdriver is used to remove the old screw. This "technical pearl" may facilitate alignment of the screwdriver more easily within the femoral screw hexagonal recess and reduce the possibility of stripping the screw. If the screw is stripped, commercially available screw extractors may need to be used. Alternatively, when the femoral tunnel is placed too vertically, the screw can be advanced forward and not removed, which creates a medial wall support for the new graft.

If the tibial tunnel is in an acceptable position and a metallic screw was used, it needs to be removed as well. On the other hand, the old screw can be left in place if it is bioabsorbable or if it does not interfere with the

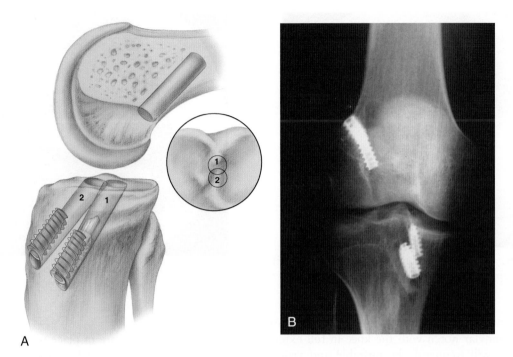

Figure 76-3. Tunnel 1 represents a nonoverlapping malpositioned tibial tunnel with hardware that does not need to be removed at the revision reconstruction.

new tunnel. It is critical to identify the location of the screw before a cortical window is made. If the screw edge is not easily detectable, the surgeon should consider use of intraoperative radiographic imaging to minimize cortical violation, which could subsequently compromise tibial bone plug fixation. One technical pearl that we routinely use during primary ACL reconstruction is to cut the tibial bone plug sutures long, leaving a tail that facilitates location of the screw for later removal if it is needed.

4. Tibial Tunnel

The senior author (B.R.B.) uses an accessory inferomedial or transpatellar portal for placement of the tibial aiming device with the angle set at 55 degrees or slightly higher. The higher the angle, the longer the tibial tunnel. The entry point of the guide pin should be at least 25 mm below the joint line. The establishment of an accessory inferomedial portal or transpatellar portal facilitates proper oblique orientation of the tibial aiming device. In the endoscopic technique, the position of the femoral tunnel is affected by the orientation of the tibial tunnel if it is drilled in a transtibial fashion. If the tibial tunnel is not angled appropriately in the sagittal plane, the resultant femoral tunnel is likely to be positioned too vertically. An entrance point on the tibial cortex midway between the tibial tubercle and the posteromedial border of the tibia will allow proper tunnel orientation (Fig. 76-4).

Intra-articularly, tibial tunnel orientation aims to avoid intercondylar notch impingement. As a general

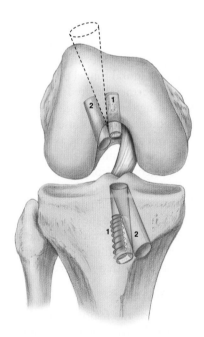

Figure 76-4. The position of the femoral tunnel is affected by the orientation of the tibial tunnel. Tunnel 2 represents the appropriate orientation for a tibial tunnel.

reference point, the pin entry should be at the level of the posterior edge of the anterior horn of the lateral meniscus. Alternatively, some surgeons advocate an entrance point 7 mm anterior to the PCL. In the coronal plane, the device is placed in a central location to allow clearance of the graft between the PCL and notch wall. The knee should be extended to visualize the placement

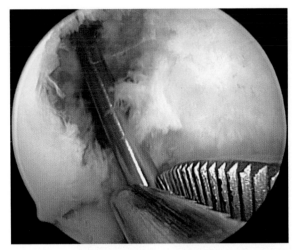

Figure 76-5. The guide pin is tapped into the femur and further stabilized with a Kocher clamp during reaming.

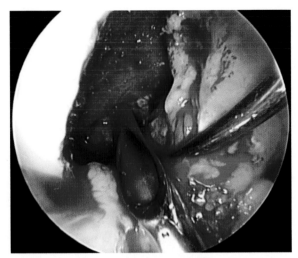

Figure 76-6. A 7-mm offset guide placed through the tibial tunnel. A probe is used to protect the posterior cruciate ligament.

of the tibial pin, which should not impinge on the apex of the intercondylar notch with the knee in full extension. The pin will frequently be unstable and visibly mobile within the previous tibial tunnel and will therefore need to be stabilized before over-reaming. After correct pin placement has been verified, the guide pin is tapped into the femoral wall to improve stability during reaming. It is advisable to perform intraoperative radiographic imaging if there are any concerns regarding either the tibial or femoral tunnel placement. The guidewire can also be further secured with a hemostat or Kocher clamp during reaming (Fig. 76-5). A cannulated acorn or solid fluted reamer is used to make the new tibial tunnel. Sequential reaming is done with a final reamer size of 10 or 11 mm. If tunnel widening is suspected, some surgeons recommend use of a smaller reamer first, then placement of the arthroscope through the tunnel to examine the quality of the tunnel before it is sequentially enlarged to the desired width. Once the tunnel has been made, the arthroscope can be passed up the tibial tunnel to assess for residual soft tissue, which can then be debrided with a shaver or rasp.

5. Femoral Tunnel

The ideal location for the femoral tunnel is in the 1:30 (left knee) or 10:30 (right knee) position with 1 to 2 mm of intact posterior wall. Our goal is to place a femoral tunnel that fills portions of both the AM and posterolateral bundle footprints. Anatomic studies have demonstrated that a transtibial technique with use of an accessory transpatellar portal creates an oblique tibial tunnel orientation whereby the femoral tunnel fills approximately 50% of each bundle footprint.[4,5] Careful inspection of the previous tunnel is performed; if it is in the correct location, it can be reused. However, if it is positioned too anteriorly, a new tunnel is drilled behind it (see Fig. 76-3). In this situation we recommend

keeping the old hardware in place to act as an anterior buttress. On occasion, a deficient posterior wall precludes interference screw fixation with the endoscopic technique, in which case a two-incision technique can be used to secure the ACL on the anterior femur instead.

We generally use a 7-mm offset guide, which is placed transtibially and therefore is sensitive to correct tibial tunnel orientation (Fig. 76-6). If an ideal femoral starting point cannot be achieved with this technique, the femoral tunnel should instead be drilled by use of an accessory inferomedial portal and hyperflexion of the knee to 130 degrees. A provisional guide pin is then drilled to a depth of approximately 3 to 4 cm. The surgeon may feel more resistance while this pin is drilled if it contacts the cortical bone plug from the previous reconstruction.

With a probe used to retract and to protect the PCL, reaming is performed initially to a depth of 6 to 8 mm to make the footprint. The reamer is withdrawn to allow visualization of the preliminary starting point, and a probe is used to verify the integrity of the posterior wall. A 10-mm reamer is routinely used, although one could begin with a smaller-diameter reamer and then convert to the 10-mm reamer. The reamer is usually advanced to a 35-mm depth; a 25-mm bone plug is generally prepared on the graft. This allows for some space for the graft to be potentially recessed if there is a graft-tunnel mismatch. While the reamer is advanced, the surgeon may feel more resistance than in a primary procedure from a previously placed cortical bone plug. Once reaming is completed, cancellous bone debris is removed with the shaver. A rasp or a shaver is used to smooth the anterior edge of the femoral tunnel. The arthroscope is placed transtibially to inspect the femoral tunnel and to rule out posterior wall insufficiency or intratunnel "blowout." An intratunnel blowout could occur if the knee is extended too much during femoral reaming. In general, the knee should be in 80 to 90 degrees of knee flexion to position the femoral aimer. If the knee has to be extended farther to position the femoral aimer, the tibial tunnel may have been placed too far anteriorly, or a posterior ledge at the tibial tunnel entrance may be deflecting the aimer anteriorly.

6. Bone Grafting Procedures for Tunnel Widening

After preparation of both tibial and femoral tunnels, bone grafting may be performed in either a concomitant or staged fashion to address overlapping or widened tunnels (Fig. 76-7). Graft choices include autograft and allograft to avoid the morbidity associated with iliac crest graft harvesting. Allograft bone chips or dowels and bone left over from preparation of the tendon graft are commonly used.[6] In the case of overlapping tunnels, either bone graft or a larger bone plug can be used to fill the defect and still allow interference screw fixation. To minimize extravasation of bone graft material into the joint, we found it helpful to use a clear shoulder-arthroscopy cannula or, alternatively, a 3-mL syringe with the tip cut off. The syringe is filled with morcellized bone graft, introduced through a slightly enlarged arthroscopy portal, and directed into the defect, and the bone graft is delivered by advancement of the plunger. Other options include placing cortical allograft dowels (Fig. 76-8) into the defect or stacking screws to enhance bone plug fixation in overlapping or widened tunnels. Supplemental fixation (EndoButton [Smith & Nephew, Andover, MA], staples, post, suture button) on both the femoral and tibial sides should be considered whenever secure graft fixation may be compromised by enlarged or bone-grafted tunnels.

If bone stock is severely compromised because of extensive tunnel widening, primary bone grafting is advisable. All hardware is removed, and both tibial and femoral tunnels are filled with morcellized bone graft. After 4 months, the patient returns for staged ligament reconstruction.

7. Graft Preparation and Placement

For revision procedures it may be advisable to defer graft preparation until the tunnels have been made. This optimizes the potential of making custom-sized bone plugs if needed in situations in which there may be tunnel expansion or overlap. However, if one makes tunnels without knowing the length of the soft tissue construct, the likelihood of graft-construct mismatch may be increased. As a generalization, if the osseous tunnels do not appear expanded, we will make our tunnels while the graft is being prepared.

In general, the bone plugs are shaped, contoured, and sized to fit 10-mm sizing tubes. Two or three 2-mm holes are drilled through the tibial plug, and No. 5

braided sutures are placed through them. Some surgeons prefer to do the same for the femoral plug; however, we prefer the push-in technique instead.[15] With this method the femoral bone plug is initially oriented with the cancellous bone facing anteriorly and the tendon facing posteriorly. The plug is then pushed through the tibial tunnel by a two-pronged pusher (Fig. 76-9). Before seating of the bone plug is completed, a 14-inch hyperflex nitinol pin is inserted at the 11- to 12-o'clock position of the femoral tunnel, the knee is further flexed, and the pin is advanced until it meets resistance within the depth of the socket. At this point, the bone plug can be advanced until it is flush with the articular margin, and the construct is assessed again for mismatch. If the tibial bone plug resides within the tibial tunnel, one can continue with standard femoral and tibial fixation.

However, if the graft protrudes significantly because of graft-tunnel mismatch, potentially compromising tibial fixation, several treatment options exist: further recessing of the graft into the femoral tunnel; use of staple fixation or screw-post fixation on the tibial side; rotation of the graft up to 540 degrees, which can shorten the graft by up to 6 mm; performance of a free bone block modification (Fig. 76-10); and combination of these modifications (e.g., recession of the femoral bone plug and rotation of the graft[3]). The disadvantage of recessing the graft is that there is an increased chance of tendon laceration during femoral bone plug fixation; staple or screw-post fixation has a lower strength of fixation and increased likelihood of painful hardware. Graft rotation is controversial; although the ultimate failure strength in vitro is similar to that of a nonrotated graft, cyclic loading studies suggest that the graft may be negatively affected with hyper-rotation.[8-11] Our general preference with more than 50% bone plug extrusion on the tibia is to remove the graft, to excise the tibial bone plug (thus making a "pseudo–quadriceps tendon" graft), and to reinsert the graft with standard femoral fixation followed by tibial fixation by insertion of the free bone block into the tibial tunnel and sandwiching of the plug with an interference screw.[7,13] This can be supplemented by a whipstitch through the tendinous portion of the graft, which is then tied over a tibial staple or post.

8. Femoral Fixation

Once the femoral bone plug has been positioned and the hyperflex nitinol pin inserted, a 7- × 25-mm metallic cannulated interference screw is placed over the wire and advanced into the femoral tunnel. It is critical to flex the knee at least 100 degrees to ensure parallel screw placement. One should carefully inspect the graft as the screw is inserted to avoid graft laceration. Ideally, we attempt to place the screw anteriorly on the plug; the plug can effectively function as a skid, allowing

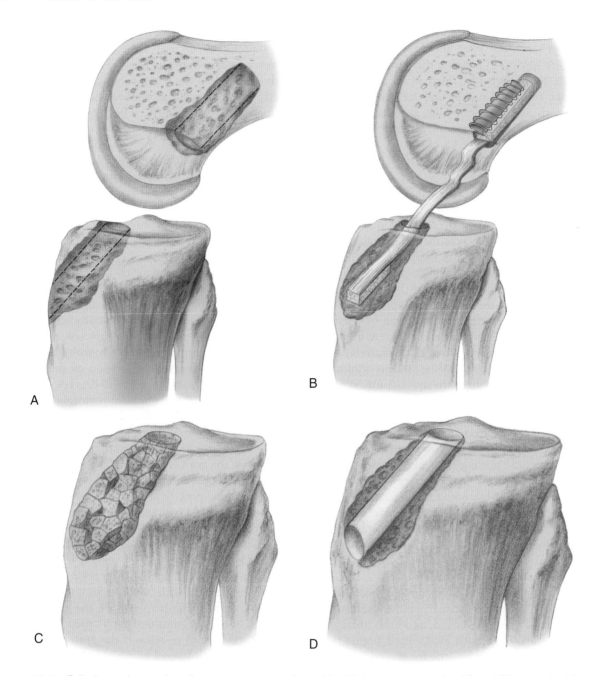

Figure 76-7. Failed anterior cruciate ligament reconstruction with tibial tunnel expansion (**A** and **B**) treated with a staged bone grafting procedure (**C** and **D**).

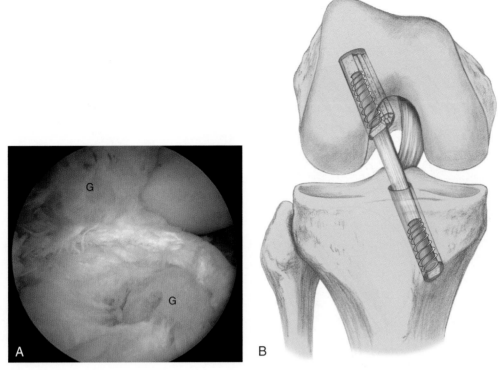

Figure 76-8. A, Allograft dowels have been inserted as bone graft into the previous tunnels. **B,** Multiple allograft dowels can be placed to improve fixation. *G,* Bone graft.

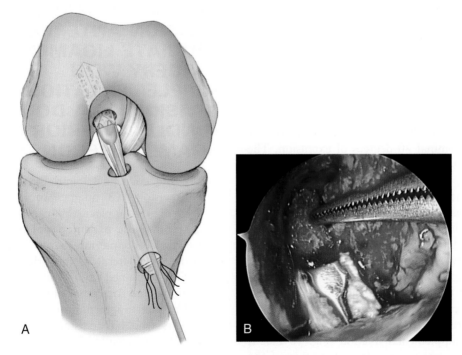

Figure 76-9. Push-in technique. The graft is advanced by a two-pronged pusher.

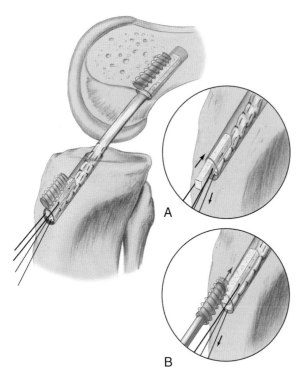

Figure 76-10. Free bone block technique. The bone plug is removed from the tibial portion of the graft and reinserted to improve mismatch and fixation.

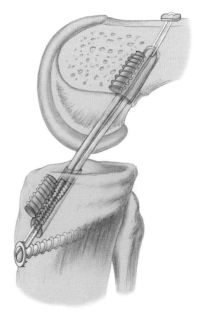

Figure 76-11. Back-up fixation of the graft. A post and washer are used on the tibial side, whereas the femoral side is backed up with a suture button construct.

parallel placement of the screw. If the screw is placed on the side of the plug, the likelihood of screw divergence is increased.

9. Tibial Fixation

The knee is cycled several times, and "gross isometry" is inspected. In general, the graft should shorten only 1 to 2 mm in the terminal 30 degrees of extension. The graft is rotated 180 degrees, and the cannulated metallic interference screw (9 × 20 mm) is placed anteriorly on the cortical surface of the graft. The anterior screw placement also pushes the graft farther posterior so that it is less likely to impinge in extension and prevents the screw from "wandering" if placed posterior to the graft. Finally, if the screw is placed anteriorly, one can extend beyond the tendino-osseous junction without the screw's violating the soft tissue aspect of the graft, whereas if the screw is placed posteriorly, the screw tip could abrade the soft tissue. If the bone is osteopenic, one should consider supplemental fixation (Fig. 76-11). If any excess bone is protruding after placement of the tibial screw, it is cut flush with the tibia by use of a bur or a saw.

Once the graft is secured, it is critical to confirm the integrity of the construct fixation. The knee is multiply cycled and serially examined to confirm that Lachman and pivot-shift test results are normal.

SPECIAL CONSIDERATIONS— REVISION ANTERIOR CRUCIATE LIGAMENT SURGERY WITH SUPPLEMENTATION AND REVISION OF A DOUBLE-BUNDLE ANTERIOR CRUCIATE LIGAMENT RECONSTRUCTION

Brophy and colleagues[14] initially described a double-bundle revision ACL augmentation technique, leaving the original graft in place, that can be applied to a vertical graft in select patient populations. A new tibial tunnel is placed anterior to the original, and a new femoral tunnel lateral to the original on the femoral wall. The combined ACL construct provides robust translational and rotational stability to the tibiofemoral joint. The same augmentation concept may be applied to patients who have sustained partial tears of their native ACL (typically the posterolateral bundle) or partial tears of their anatomically placed ACL reconstruction.[15]

An example of supplementation is illustrated in Figure 76-12 (partial tear of an ACL with intact AM fibers). A new anteriorly placed femoral tunnel is

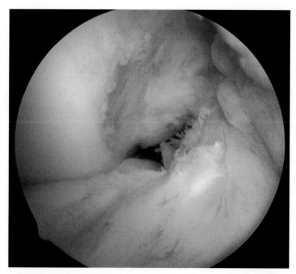

Figure 76-12. Partial tear of an anterior cruciate ligament with intact anteromedial fibers.

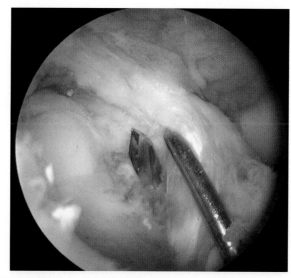

Figure 76-14. Placement of a new tunnel in a posterolateral position while the intact anterior cruciate ligament fibers are protected.

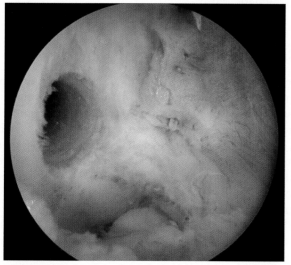

Figure 76-13. Tunnel placed anterior to intact anterior cruciate ligament fibers.

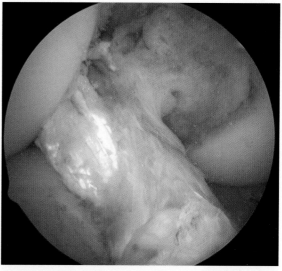

Figure 76-15. Final augmentation with hamstring autograft, secured with cortical, EndoButton (Smith & Nephew, Andover, MA) fixation on the femoral side and interference screw fixation on the tibial side.

depicted in Figure 76-13, with the knee in 90 degrees of flexion. On the tibial side, Figure 76-14 illustrates placement of a new tunnel in a posterolateral position while the intact ACL fibers are protected. Figure 76-15 shows the final augmentation with hamstring autograft, secured with cortical, EndoButton fixation on the femoral side and interference screw fixation on the tibial side.

Failed double-bundle ACL reconstruction may result in compounded technical errors, given that two tunnels have the potential for malposition on both the tibial and femoral sides. Figure 76-16 illustrates a failed a double-bundle ACL reconstruction with hamstring autograft, with a vertically placed AM tunnel. In the setting of a

failed double-bundle procedure, structural support is often needed to fill the large defect created by the two tunnels (Fig. 76-17; the biocomposite screw was placed in the AM tunnel to provide structural support). A new single femoral tunnel can then be drilled in the appropriate anatomic position (see Fig. 76-17). Tibial tunnel coalescence can be managed with allograft dowels in a single-stage fashion, as was done in the failed double-bundle ACL reconstruction shown in Figure 76-8. Overall, revision of a double-bundle procedure can be technically challenging owing to the defect that is created

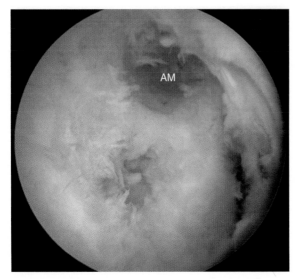

Figure 76-16. Failed double-bundle reconstruction with a vertical anteromedial (AM) tunnel.

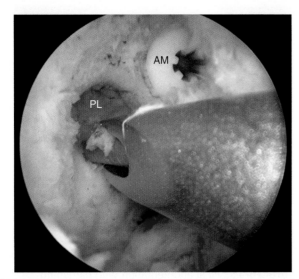

Figure 76-17. Biocomposite screw placed in the anteromedial (AM) tunnel to provide structural support. A new femoral tunnel was drilled through the existing posterolateral (PL) tunnel.

from two femoral tunnels. Appropriate preoperative planning is required.

POSTOPERATIVE CONSIDERATIONS

Rehabilitation

Most patients are allowed to progress to full weight bearing with the knee locked in extension in the brace.

If secure fixation is achieved on both sides of the graft, rehabilitation follows the same protocol as for a primary ACL reconstruction.

Straight-leg raises and quadriceps sets are initiated immediately after surgery. Crutches are generally used for the first 2 weeks, and physical therapy initially concentrates on achievement of full extension and progressive flexion. Full flexion should be reached within 6 weeks. Bicycling (stationary) can be started 1 week after surgery, StairMaster-type exercises at 4 to 6 weeks, and light jogging without cutting or pivoting in 12 weeks. Gradual return to full activities is achieved 6 months after surgery.

Complications

Complications of revision ACL surgery are similar to those seen in primary ACL reconstruction. They include infection, arthrofibrosis, neurovascular injury, and failure of the revision graft to be incorporated or macrotraumatic retear.

RESULTS

Revision ACL reconstruction occurs most commonly for either a traumatic retear or tunnel malposition. In comparing results for revision ACL reconstruction, one should pay close attention to the metrics used.[16-22] This is especially true for tunnel malposition because many studies use their own methodology—there is no universally accepted system for tibial and/or femoral malpositioning. Similarly, cartilage assessment can be either through arthroscopic or radiographic classification. For subjective analysis, the International Knee Documentation Committee (IKDC), Lysholm, and Tegner scores are most commonly used. The results from Table 76-1 demonstrate significant score improvements with ACL revision reconstruction: for IKDC from category C-D to A-B, Lysholm scores from 86 to 93, and Tegner values (the least improved) from 4 to 6.7 at follow-up. These results are similar to outcomes in primary ACL reconstruction; however, fewer patients return to competitive sports, and they are at increased risk for osteoarthritis.

Results of revision ACL reconstruction are less predictable and do not approach the results of primary ACL reconstruction.[4] Patients need to be educated preoperatively that in the setting of a revision ACL reconstruction there are frequently meniscal or chondral abnormalities and the results will not approach those of a primary reconstruction. Overall, an ACL revision after a macrotraumatic failure with good tunnel position will achieve better results that a revised ACL revision required after an aberrant tunnel position.

TABLE 76-1. Summary of Studies and Results

Authors	Study Design	No. of Patients	Age	Technique/ Notes	Reason for Failure	Follow-Up (years)	KT1000	Radiographic OA	IKDC Score	Tegner Score	Lysholm Score
Lind et al[20] (2011)	Case series (4)	128	31 (16-58)	BTB 28%, SemiT/G 41%, allograft 30%, 11% staged	Trauma (30%), unknown (24%), malposition (20%)	6 (2-9)	6.2 to 2.5 mm	N/A	—	4 (1-8)	—
Niki et al[21] (2010)	Therapeutic case-control (3)	29	29 ± 8	BTB recon for synthetic ACL failures	Malposition (75%)	2.8 ± 0.9	1.4 mm at follow-up	Increased OA compared with primary	100% C-D to 70% A-B	5.5 to 4.9	63.8 to 89.4
Denti et al[16] (2008)	Case series (4)	60	31 (16-55)	SemiT/G 56%, BTB 41%, Achilles 3%	Malposition (52%), trauma (35%), biologic (3%)	3.5 (2-6)	56% <3 mm, 34% 3-5 mm, 10% 6-10 mm	N/A	82% A-B	6.7 (0-10)	90.5 (54-100)
Diamantopoulos[17] (2008)	Case series (4)	107	38 ± 9.3	SemiT/G 42%, BTB 38%, quad 20%	Malposition (64%), trauma (24%)	6	None	Increased OA	65.4% A-B	2.8 to 6.3	51.5 to 88.5
Weiler et al[22] (2007)	Cohort study (2)	50	31 ± 8	SemiT/G 46%, SemiT 54%	Malposition (40%-55%)	2.5	2.1 mm at follow-up	N/A	100% C-D to 88% A-B (same as primary)	—	65 to 90 (worse than primary)
Garofalo et al[18] (2006)	Case series (4)	28	27 (18-41)	Quad	Trauma in history (100%), malposition (79%)	4.2 (3.3-5.6)	97% <5 mm maximum manual	N/A	86% C-D to 93% A-B	4.2 to 6.1	68 to 93
Grossman et al[19] (2005)	Case series (4)	29	30.2	BTB allograft 76%, BTB autograft 21%, Achilles 3%	Trauma (40%), malposition (29%), biologic (14%)	5.6	2.78 mm (better with autograft)	OA (34%)	86% A-B	5.2	86.6

ACL, anterior cruciate ligament; *BTB,* bone–patellar tendon–bone; *IKDC,* International Knee Documentation Committee; *N/A,* not applicable; *OA,* osteoarthritis; *quad,* quadriceps; *recon,* reconstruction; *SemiT,* semitendinosus; *G,* gracilis.

REFERENCES

1. Kamath GV, Redfern JC, Greis PE, et al. Revision anterior cruciate ligament reconstruction. *Am J Sports Med.* 2011;39(1):199-217.

2. Shelbourne KD, Klotz C. What I have learned about the ACL: utilizing a progressive rehabilitation scheme to achieve total knee symmetry after anterior cruciate ligament reconstruction. *J Orthop Sci.* 2006;11(3):318-325.

3. Fox JA, Pierce M, Bojchuk J, et al. Revision anterior cruciate ligament reconstruction with nonirradiated fresh-frozen patellar tendon allograft. *Arthroscopy.* 2004;20(8):787-794.

4. Bach Jr BR. ACL reconstruction: revisited, revised, reviewed. *J Knee Surg.* 2004;17(3):125-126.

5. Piasecki DP, Bach Jr BR, Espinoza Orias AA, et al. Anterior cruciate ligament reconstruction: can anatomic femoral placement be achieved with a transtibial technique? *Am J Sports Med.* 2011;39(6):1306-1315.

6. Battaglia TC, Miller MD. Management of bony deficiency in revision anterior cruciate ligament reconstruction using allograft bone dowels: surgical technique. *Arthroscopy.* 2005;21(6):767.

7. Rue JP, Lewis PB, Parameswaran AD, et al. Single-bundle anterior cruciate ligament reconstruction: technique overview and comprehensive review of results. *J Bone Joint Surg Am.* 2008;90(suppl 4):67-74.

8. Berkson E, Lee GH, Kumar A, et al. The effect of cyclic loading on rotated bone-tendon-bone anterior cruciate ligament graft constructs. *Am J Sports Med.* 2006;34(9):1442-1449.

9. Elmans L, Wymenga A, van Kampen A, et al. Effects of twisting of the graft in anterior cruciate ligament reconstruction. *Clin Orthop Relat Res.* 2003;409:278-284.

10. Hame SL, Markolf KL, Gabayan AJ, et al. The effect of anterior cruciate ligament graft rotation on knee laxity and graft tension: An in vitro biomechanical analysis. *Arthroscopy.* 2002;18(1):55-60.

11. Verma N, Noerdlinger MA, Hallab N, et al. Effects of graft rotation on initial biomechanical failure characteristics of bone-patellar tendon-bone constructs. *Am J Sports Med.* 2003;31(5):708-713.

12. Verma NN, Dennis MG, Carreira DS, et al. Preliminary clinical results of two techniques for addressing graft tunnel mismatch in endoscopic anterior cruciate ligament reconstruction. *J Knee Surg.* 2005;18(3):183-191.

13. Brophy RH, Selby RM, Altchek DW. Anterior cruciate ligament revision: double-bundle augmentation of primary vertical graft. *Arthroscopy.* 2006;22(6):683 e681-685.

14. Shen W, Forsythe B, Ingham SM, et al. Application of the anatomic double-bundle reconstruction concept to revision and augmentation anterior cruciate ligament surgeries. *J Bone Joint Surg Am.* 2008;90 Suppl 4:20-34.

15. Denti M, Lo Vetere D, Bait C, et al. Revision anterior cruciate ligament reconstruction: causes of failure, surgical technique, and clinical results. *Am J Sports Med.* 2008;36(10):1896-1902.

16. Diamantopoulos AP, Lorbach O, Paessler HH. Anterior cruciate ligament revision reconstruction: results in 107 patients. *Am J Sports Med.* 2008;36(5):851-860.

17. Garofalo R, Djahangiri A, Siegrist O. Revision anterior cruciate ligament reconstruction with quadriceps tendon-patellar bone autograft. *Arthroscopy.* 2006;22(2):205-214.

18. Grossman MG, ElAttrache NS, Shields CL, et al. Revision anterior cruciate ligament reconstruction: three- to nine-year follow-up. *Arthroscopy.* 2005;21(4):418-423.

19. Lind M, Lund B, Fauno P, et al. Medium to long-term follow-up after ACL revision. *Knee Surg Sports Traumatol Arthrosc.* 2011.

20. Niki Y, Matsumoto H, Enomoto H, et al. Single-stage anterior cruciate ligament revision with bone-patellar tendon-bone: a case-control series of revision of failed synthetic anterior cruciate ligament reconstructions. *Arthroscopy.* 2010;26(8):1058-1065.

21. Weiler A, Schmeling A, Stohr I, et al. Primary versus single-stage revision anterior cruciate ligament reconstruction using autologous hamstring tendon grafts: a prospective matched-group analysis. *Am J Sports Med.* 2007;35(10):1643-1652.

Chapter 77

Anatomic Anterior Cruciate Ligament Concept: Single- and Double-Bundle Anterior Cruciate Ligament Reconstruction

Paulo H. Araujo, Kellie K. Middleton, Gof Tantisricharoenkun, and Freddie H. Fu

Chapter Synopsis

- *Anatomic reconstruction of the anterior cruciate ligament* (ACL) is defined as the functional restoration of the ACL to its native dimensions, collagen orientation, and insertion sites. The aim of anatomic ACL reconstruction is to provide the patient with the greatest potential for a successful outcome.

Important Points

- Four fundamental principles should be observed for anatomic ACL reconstruction to be achieved:
  - Note the patient's native anatomy.
  - Individualize each surgery with respect to the patient's anatomy.
  - Place the tunnels and grafts in the center of the patient's native footprints.
  - Reestablish knee biomechanics by tensioning the grafts to mimic the native ACL as closely as possible.

Clinical and Surgical Pearls

- Tibial insertion site, ACL length, inclination angle, and quadriceps tendon and patellar tendon measurements on magnetic resonance imaging (MRI) are fundamental for good preoperative planning. They provide valuable information that helps to individualize the surgery according to patient's anatomy.
- Proper placement of portals ensures an optimum arthroscopic visualization. The high anterolateral portal must be above the fat pad. Central and accessory medial portals should be created under arthroscopic visualization with a spinal needle used as a guide. The portal placement follows the patient's anatomy.

- Intraoperative measurements with an arthroscopic ruler complement the preoperative MRI measurements and dictate the technique to be used as well as graft source and size, according to individual anatomic characteristics.

Clinical and Surgical Pitfalls

- Careful intraoperative dissection should be performed to correctly identify bony landmarks and soft tissue remnants.
- The torn ligament remnants should be cautiously examined to help recognize the anatomic tibial and femoral insertion sites for the anteromedial (AM) and posterolateral (PL) bundles, which should be marked with use of a thermal device for later tunnel drilling.
- For PL femoral tunnel drilling, at least 120 degrees of knee flexion should be achieved to allow an adequate tunnel length and avoid damage to the posterior wall. The same rule is valid for femoral AM tunnel drilling through the accessory medial portal and for single-bundle technique.
- When the femoral AM tunnel is drilled through the accessory medial portal, care should be taken to ensure that it will not communicate with the PL tunnel; they will be parallel to each other.
- Graft fixation should be done independently for the double-bundle reconstruction. The PL graft is tensioned first and fixed with the knee in full extension, followed by tensioning of the AM graft at 45 degrees of knee flexion.

Over the last two decades, single-bundle anterior cruciate ligament (ACL) reconstruction has largely been a successful operation.[1] Many patients over the short term have been able to return to sports with an improvement in subjective instability of their knee. However, recent studies have also found that a subset of patients experience persistent subjective knee instability and therefore are not able to return to prior activity.[2] Furthermore, long-term evaluation of patients suggests that osteoarthritic changes occur at the same rate as in knees that have not undergone surgery.[3,4] For example, a recent randomized controlled trial found radiographic degenerative changes in 84% of the subjects 11 years after ACL reconstruction.[5] Results such as this, presented in many other papers,[3,4,6] have pushed the focus of ACL reconstruction toward an anatomic approach to more closely restore normal knee function and avoid long-term osteoarthritic changes.

Anatomic reconstruction of the ACL is defined as the functional restoration of the ACL to its native dimensions, collagen orientation, and insertion sites.[7] The aim of anatomic ACL reconstruction is to provide the patient with the greatest potential for a successful outcome. Four fundamental principles should be observed for achievement of this goal. The first is to carefully note the patient's native anatomy. The second is to individualize each surgery with respect to the patient's anatomy. The third is to place the tunnels and grafts in the center of the patient's native footprints. The fourth is to reestablish knee biomechanics by tensioning the grafts to mimic the native ACL as closely as possible.[8]

The traditional anteromedial (AM)-based single-bundle ACL reconstruction was shown to successfully resist anteroposterior (AP) translation forces, but failed to correct rotational instability of the injured knee leading to abnormal knee kinematics.[9,10] It is presumed that with this condition there is an altered wear pattern and subsequent premature evidence of osteoarthritis. Therefore, increasing efforts have been made during the past decade to restore normal knee kinematics. The "forgotten" posterolateral (PL) bundle, which plays an important role in both knee stability in extension and knee rotation in flexion, was found to be indispensable. Several studies have shown the clinical superiority of double-bundle (DB) reconstruction in restoring AP and rotational stability compared with the traditional single-bundle (SB) procedure.[11-17]

The anatomic ACL DB concept views the ACL as two functionally different bundles that work synergistically. Hence the goal of the anatomic ACL reconstruction, which can be accomplished with an SB or a DB technique, is to restore the ACL anatomy as closely as possible and consequently to approximate normal knee kinematics. This chapter discusses the indications, contraindications, and surgical technique of anatomic SB and DB ACL reconstruction.

PREOPERATIVE CONSIDERATIONS

Patient Evaluation

A detailed history and careful physical examination are fundamental to diagnosis of an ACL injury. The mechanism of injury can support the diagnosis and also help discern if there are associated injuries. Certain symptoms are typically related to an ACL injury: an immediate knee effusion and pain along with initial difficulty in bearing weight. These symptoms tend to diminish over the weeks, and eventually the patient will be able to regain a complete range of motion. Sporadic pain and subjective instability of the knee are consistent with a more chronic lesion of the ACL. Clicking and popping in the knee associated with joint line tenderness indicate a simultaneous meniscal injury.

A physical examination should always be conducted on both legs for comparison. The examination includes observation of knee alignment while the patient is seated, standing, and walking and close examination for a joint effusion, muscular atrophy, and ecchymoses. Next, range of motion is assessed, followed by careful palpation of the knee joint to identify tender areas that may indicate concomitant injuries. In the acute setting it can be difficult to perform specific tests including the anterior drawer, posterior drawer, Lachman, pivot shift, reverse pivot shift, McMurray, dial, and varus and valgus stress tests. However, these tests are necessary for a complete knee evaluation and should be performed as soon as possible. In addition to standard physical examination tests, the KT1000 (MEDmetric, San Diego, CA) can quantify the degree of anterior laxity. A 3-mm or greater side-to-side difference suggests an ACL injury.

Imaging

A complete radiographic series including Merchant view for patellar evaluation, weight-bearing posteroanterior (PA) view in 45 degrees of flexion, lateral radiographs in 45 degrees of knee flexion, and full-extension AP radiographs is fundamental to the initial assessment of the injured knee. These films allow evaluation of degenerative changes, previous deformities, and associated fractures or avulsions.

High-quality magnetic resonance imaging (MRI) is used to help identify the rupture pattern of the ACL and associated injuries. Special sequences such as oblique coronal and oblique sagittal views enhance ACL visualization (Fig. 77-1A and B) by cutting MRI sections in the same anatomic alignment as the ACL. MRI also plays a definitive role in preoperative planning for individualized surgery. Measurements of the tibial insertion site, ACL length, ACL inclination angle, and quadriceps and patellar tendon thickness on sagittal view are

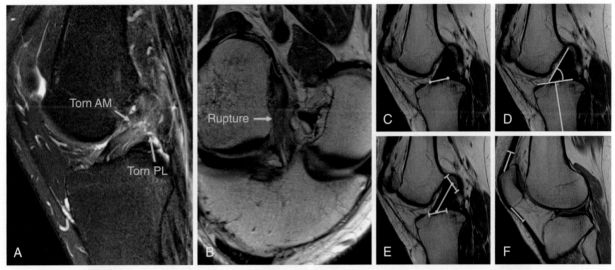

Figure 77-1. Knee magnetic resonance imaging (MRI) scans showing special cuts and MRI measurements. **A,** T2 oblique sagittal view showing a complete anterior cruciate ligament (ACL) tear. **B,** Proton density oblique coronal view showing ACL rupture. **C,** Tibial insertion site measurement. **D,** Sagittal inclination angle of the ACL. **E,** ACL length. **F,** Quadriceps tendon and patellar tendon thickness. *AM,* anteromedial bundle; *PL,* posterolateral bundle.

routinely employed to help determine reconstruction technique and graft choice (Fig. 77-1C to F). For example, DB reconstruction is indicated if the tibial insertion site measures more than 18 mm. An insertion site size less than 14 mm does not easily permit the drilling of two separate tunnels while a 2-mm bone bridge is maintained between them. In this scenario, an SB reconstruction would be the better option.[18-20] In insertion sites between 14 and 18 mm, either an SB or a DB procedure can be performed.

In revision surgeries, three-dimensional computed tomography (CT) scans prove invaluable in identifying previous tunnel placement and bony erosions in relation to the normal ACL insertion sites. Visualization of tunnel placement and anatomic changes aides in surgical planning—determining whether a new tunnel can be drilled, whether the old tunnels can be reused, or whether a two-stage procedure involving bone grafting should be performed instead[8] (Fig. 77-2).

Indications and Contraindications

A surgical approach to an ACL injury is indicated for active patients who participate in cutting, pivoting, jumping, or quick deceleration sports. In addition, patients with physically demanding professions or with subjective knee instability are candidates for surgical reconstruction.

As mentioned in the section on imaging, preoperative MRI insertion site measurements can guide the surgeon's decision to perform an SB or a DB reconstruction. Intraoperative measurements of the tibial insertion site are performed to verify preoperative MRI measurements. The femoral insertion site and notch height and width are also measured intraoperatively to guide the surgeon's technique decision. Tibial and femoral insertion sites smaller than 14 mm and notch widths smaller than 12 mm make the DB reconstruction a technically difficult and more challenging procedure. In such situations an SB reconstruction is preferred. SB reconstruction is also a better option in patients with open physes or multiligamentous injuries.

Patients with a sedentary lifestyle, particularly older adults who experience no symptoms after initial knee rehabilitation, may be eligible for nonoperative management. Contraindications to ACL reconstruction include severe arthritis, infection, and poor patient compliance with a lengthy rehabilitation program.

SURGICAL TECHNIQUE

Once the patient is under anesthesia, a thorough physical examination is conducted and the findings are compared with those of the contralateral extremity. Range of motion, results of Lachman, pivot shift, anterior and posterior drawer, and valgus and varus stress tests, and external and internal rotation at 30 and 90 degrees of knee flexion are documented. The patient is positioned supine on the operating table with the affected knee secured in a leg holder and bent over the end of the table in 90 degrees of flexion. The patient setup should allow at least 120 degrees of knee flexion and full extension (Fig. 77-3), as well as valgus and varus stress. A pneumatic cuff is positioned on the upper thigh of the injured limb and inflated to 250 to 350 mm Hg depending on the size of the patient's limb and his or her mean arterial pressure. The contralateral limb is positioned in the high

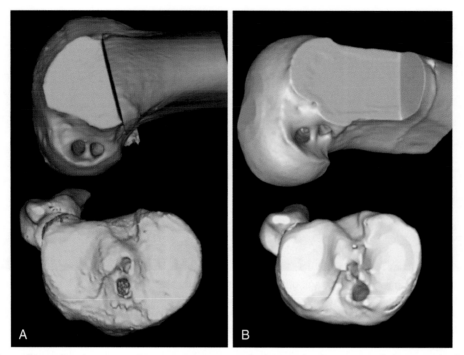

Figure 77-2. Three-dimensional computed tomography scans. **A,** Anatomic placement of the tunnels. **B,** Nonanatomic placement of the tunnels.

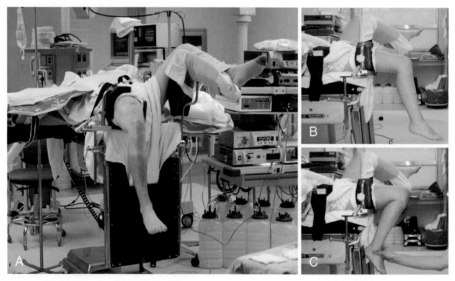

Figure 77-3. Patient setup. **A,** Supine position with the injured limb in a leg holder. **B,** Injured knee resting in 90 degrees of flexion. **C,** Knee flexion of 120 degrees.

lithotomy position away from the surgical field. Care is taken to pad the nonoperative leg to avoid complications such as tourniquet effect or neurologic palsy.

Surgical Steps

Box 77-1 outlines the specific steps of this procedure.

A three-portal technique is used to optimize visualization (Fig. 77-4).[21] First, the high anterolateral (AL) portal is created. The most distal point of this portal is placed at the line of the inferior pole of the patella just lateral to the lateral border of the patellar tendon. This portal avoids the fat pad and provides a broad view of the tibial insertion site. Diagnostic arthroscopy is performed at this point to evaluate chondral and meniscal condition. Next, with use of a spinal needle under direct visualization, a central medial portal (CP) is created where the needle perforates the skin toward the central portion of the intercondylar notch in its lower third. The accessory medial portal (AMP) is created approximately 2 cm medial to the medial border of the patellar tendon and just above the anterior horn of the medial

---

BOX 77-1 Surgical Steps

Single-Bundle Technique	**Double-Bundle Technique**
Preoperative evaluation with use of MRI measurements	Preoperative evaluation with use of MRI measurements
Patient positioning	Patient positioning
Graft harvesting* and preparation	Graft harvesting* and preparation
High anterolateral portal placement	High anterolateral portal placement
Diagnostic scope	Diagnostic scope
Central and accessory portal placement	Central and accessory portal placement
Measurement of insertion sites and notch	Measurement of insertion sites and notch
Marking of insertion sites	Marking of insertion sites
Femoral tunnel placement and drilling	Femoral PL tunnel placement and drilling
Tibial guidewire placement and tunnel drilling	Tibial PL and AM guidewire placement and tunnel drilling
Graft passage	Femoral AM tunnel placement and drilling
Femoral fixation	PL graft passage
Tibial fixation	Femoral and tibial fixation
Closure	AM graft passage and femoral fixation
	Fibrin clot positioning
	AM tibial fixation
	Closure

*For autograft.

AM, Anteromedial; *MRI,* magnetic resonance imaging; *PL,* posterolateral.

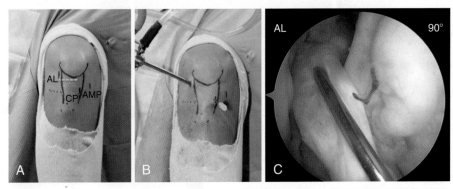

Figure 77-4. Three-portal technique. **A,** High anterolateral portal *(AL)*, central portal *(CP)*, and accessory medial portal *(AMP)*. The distal extremity of AL is on the same level as the inferior pole of the patella just lateral to the lateral border of the patellar tendon. **B,** Spinal needle confirming optimum positioning of the central portal. **C,** Arthroscopic view of the spinal needle showing a good position for the central portal. Spinal needle in the center of the notch following anterior cruciate ligament fibers.

meniscus where the spinal needle crosses the skin to freely reach the femoral insertion site. There should be approximately 2 mm between the spinal needle and the femoral medial condyle to ensure safe drilling. The CP provides a straightforward view of the lateral wall of the intercondylar notch, which obviates the need for notchplasty, thus leaving in place bony and soft tissue landmarks to guide the anatomic placement of femoral tunnels. The AMP is mostly used as a working portal to drill the femoral tunnels.

After assessment of potential meniscal and/or chondral lesions, attention is given to the ACL. With the AL portal used as a viewing portal, the rupture pattern and tibial insertion site are evaluated. The ACL remnants are carefully dissected to identify the AM and PL bundles. A cautery device is used to mark the center of the AM and PL insertion sites (Fig. 77-5). The length of the total insertion site is measured, as well as the size of the individual bundles, with an arthroscopic ruler (Fig. 77-6). The femoral notch width is then measured

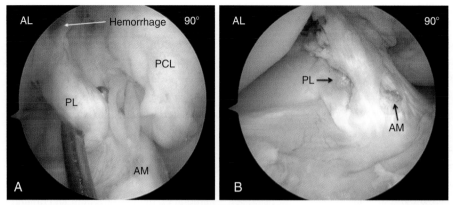

Figure 77-5. Rupture pattern and tibial insertion site marking. **A,** Posterolateral *(PL)* probing showing rupture pattern with laxity and hemorrhage. **B,** Center of anteromedial *(AM)* and PL insertion sites marked with a thermal device. *AL,* Anterolateral; *PCL,* posterior cruciate ligament.

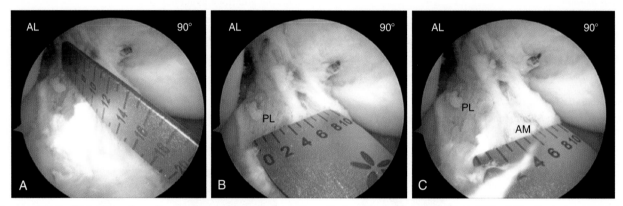

Figure 77-6. Tibial insertion site measurements. **A,** Insertion site length. **B,** Posterolateral *(PL)* width. **C,** Anteromedial *(AM)* width. *AL,* Anterolateral.

with an arthroscopic ruler (Fig. 77-7) with either the CP or AL used as the viewing portal. Notch height is also recorded.

Next, with the scope through the CP, the lateral wall of the intercondylar notch is directly visualized. The femoral insertion site is carefully dissected with a cautery device through the AMP. Both the AM and PL bundle femoral insertion sites are visualized and marked (Fig. 77-8). In the operating position with the knee flexed to 90 degrees, the intercondylar ridge is the upper limit of the ACL femoral insertion site. Another bony landmark, the bifurcate ridge, runs anterior to posterior in the anatomic position and is seen as a vertical ridge with the knee flexed at 90 degrees (Fig. 77-9). This ridge separates the femoral AM and PL insertion sites. Total length of the femoral insertion site as well as AM and PL femoral insertion site widths are obtained (Fig. 77-10). Preoperative and intraoperative measurements reflect the variation of individual anatomy and determine the procedure to be performed—either a DB or an SB reconstruction technique (Table 77-1). Such measurements also help determine graft choice and

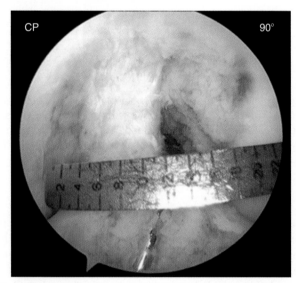

Figure 77-7. Femoral notch width measurement. *CP,* central portal.

TABLE 77-1. Indications

Intraoperative measurements	Tibial or femoral insertion site <14 mm	Tibial or femoral insertion site 14-18 mm	Tibial or femoral insertion site >14 mm	Notch width <12 mm	Notch width >12 mm
Preferred technique	Single bundle	Single bundle or double bundle	Double bundle	Single bundle	Single or double bundle

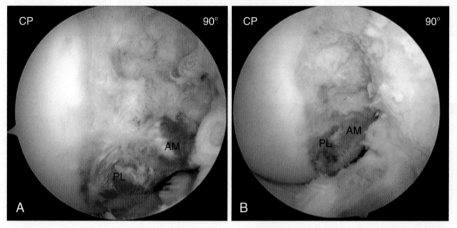

Figure 77-8. Femoral insertion site. **A,** Posterolateral *(PL)* and anteromedial *(AM)* stumps. **B,** PL and AM insertion sites marked with thermal device. *CP,* central portal.

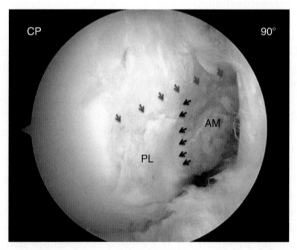

Figure 77-9. Intercondylar ridge *(green arrows)*. Bifurcate ridge *(black arrows)*. *AM,* Anteromedial; *CP,* central portal; *PL,* posterolateral.

size—a soft tissue autograft (preferable), an allograft, or a hybrid graft containing autograft and allograft, which is prepared on the back table during surgery.

A pointed awl is then used to create the initial hole in the center PL insertion site or in the center of the ACL footprint (Fig. 77-11) for a DB or SB reconstruction, respectively. Thereafter the femoral PL tunnel is drilled over a guide pin through the AMP. This tunnel is drilled during maximum knee flexion (at least 120 degrees) to avoid damage to the posterior wall of the lateral condyle,

allow for maximum tunnel length, and permit the tunnel to exit anterior to the peroneal nerve. This drill angle also avoids injury to other lateral knee structures such as the lateral collateral ligament and the PL corner. The femoral tunnel is drilled 20 mm in depth with a power acorn reamer with a drill bit 1 mm smaller than the desired tunnel diameter. The tunnel is then drilled by hand to the appropriate depth required for suspensory femoral fixation. Thereafter a hand dilator is used to establish a tunnel diameter of choice. The same steps apply for SB femoral tunnel drilling. At this point, attention is turned to the tibial side.

A 3- to 4-cm vertical AM incision is made over the proximal tibia centered between the anterior tibial crest and the posterior border of the tibia at the level of the tibial tubercle. This incision is used for drilling both the AM and the PL tibial tunnels. The AL portal is used to place the scope while a tibial tip-to-tip aiming guide set to 45 degrees is positioned through either the CP or the AMP. The guide pin is aimed at the center of the PL bundle footprint previously marked with the thermal device. It is necessary to visualize the posterior root of the lateral meniscus, which is just posterior to the PL footprint, to avoid iatrogenic injury while the tunnel is drilled. A guide pin is advanced into the knee joint starting from a more medial position on the AM tibia. Care must be taken to avoid injury to the medial collateral ligament. After the PL guide pin is advanced, the guide is reset to 55 degrees and the tip of the guide is placed

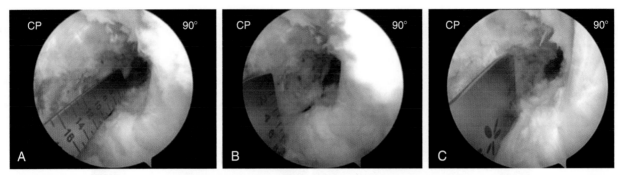

Figure 77-10. Femoral insertion site measurements. **A,** Femoral insertion site length. **B,** Femoral posterolateral *(PL)* width measurement. **C,** Femoral anteromedial *(AM)* width measurement. *CP,* central portal.

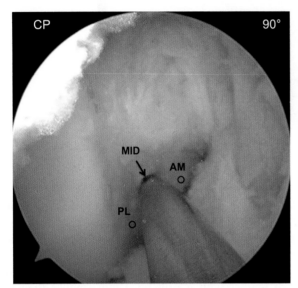

Figure 77-11. Pointed awl for femoral single or double bundle tunnel *(s)* positioning. *PL,* Posterolateral insertion site; *MID,* middle of single-bundle insertion site; *AM,* anteromedial insertion site; *CP,* central portal view.

in the center of the AM bundle footprint (Fig. 77-12). The second guide pin is then advanced starting from a more lateral position on the AM tibial surface. The pins entrances on the tibial surface should be separated to allow for at least 1 cm between the two tunnels (Fig. 77-13). Next, the PL tunnel is drilled to a diameter 1 mm less than the desired size as determined by the patient's insertion site dimensions. Further dilation is carried out by hand. The same steps are then used to drill the tibial AM tunnel.

For the SB procedure, the tibial tunnel is created with the aiming guide at 55 degrees in the center of the ACL footprint, between the AM and PL insertion sites (see Fig. 77-12).

In a DB technique, after drilling of the tibial tunnels, the arthroscope is placed through the CP and focused on the femoral AM tunnel site. The femoral AM tunnel can be drilled with use of three different approaches: through the tibial PL tunnel, through the tibial AM tunnel, or through the AMP. The tibial PL tunnel approach is successful over 60% of the time, whereas the tibial AM tunnel approach is successful only approximately 10% of the time.[22] The transtibial femoral AM tunnel drilling has the advantage of placing the AM tunnel more divergent from the PL tunnel compared with AMP drilling. However, this necessitates the use of a half-moon drill bit when the tibial PL tunnel diameter is smaller than the planned AM femoral tunnel diameter (Fig. 77-14). The AMP approach to the femoral AM footprint is always an option and should be used when the transtibial approach is not feasible.

The femoral tunnel is drilled to a depth of 20 mm with a drill bit 1 mm smaller than the desired diameter. Hand drilling is used to achieve the desired depth as per suspensory femoral fixation specifications. Finally, the tunnel is dilated by hand to the diameter of choice.

When the graft is passed, the PL bundle graft is first advanced from the tibial through the femoral PL tunnels. It is then secured on the femoral side with a suspensory fixation device. Next, the AM graft is advanced following the same steps applied to the PL bundle (Fig. 77-15). The grafts are then tensioned and checked under arthroscopic visualization for full range of motion without impingement on both the notch and the posterior cruciate ligament. In an anatomic ACL reconstruction, no impingement is expected because the native anatomy has been reproduced. The knee is then cycled several times—from full extension to maximum flexion—which applies tension to both the AM and PL grafts. Next, the PL bundle is fixed in full extension and the AM bundle is fixed in 45 degrees of flexion. Both grafts are fixed in the tibial tunnel with interference bioabsorbable screws. For the SB procedure the graft is fixed with use of the same devices as for the DB technique, but with 15 degrees of knee flexion (Fig. 77-15).

An alternative to the most widely used ACL DB reconstruction with four tunnels (two femoral and two tibial) and soft tissue grafts is the anatomic reconstruction with three tunnels (one femoral and two tibial) with a quadriceps tendon. In this technique, the quadriceps tendon graft is harvested with a patellar bone plug,

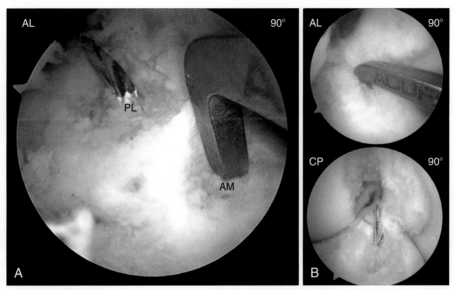

Figure 77-12. Tibial tunnel placement. **A,** Tibial aiming guide set to 55 degrees in the center of anteromedial *(AM)* footprint and posterolateral *(PL)* guidewire in correct position. **B,** Tibial aiming guide in the center of anterior cruciate ligament footprint, between AM and PL insertion sites in the top. Guidewire correctly positioned for SB tibial tunnel in the bottom. *AL,* Anterolateral; *CP,* central portal.

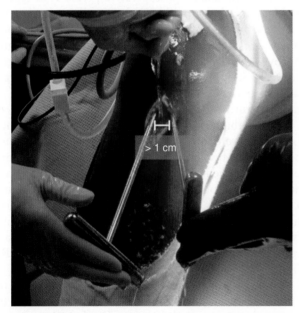

Figure 77-13. Tibial tunnel entrances more than 1 cm apart in the proximal tibial surface.

which can also be used in an SB procedure (Fig. 77-16). For the DB technique, the soft tissue graft end is split in the sagittal plane. The final graft should be at least 6 cm in length in both arms and include a bone block that is 10 × 20 mm. The thickness of the PL and AM bundle grafts can be tailored according to the measurements obtained via MRI before surgery and from intraoperative measurements with an arthroscopic ruler.

A single tunnel is drilled in the center of the femoral insertion site to accommodate the quadriceps graft bone plug. The PL and AM tibial tunnels are then drilled anatomically. The graft is passed through the AMP to the femoral tunnel. Correct positioning of the bone plug should be verified to ensure femoral restoration of PL and AM bundle insertion sites. Femoral fixation is performed with a suspensory device. The two arms of the graft are then placed within the joint and pulled inside out through the tibial tunnels. The PL graft is passed first and fixed at full extension, followed by the AM at 45 degrees of knee flexion. For an SB procedure, the graft is fixed at 15 degrees of knee flexion.

Fibrin Clot

In an attempt to enhance biologic healing of the graft, fibrin clot is added to the ACL reconstruction. During the operation, 50 to 60 mL of blood are collected from the patient and slowly hand stirred in a beaker for approximately 5 minutes until clot formation. A portion of the clot is sutured within the proximal and distal ends of each soft tissue graft to enhance graft incorporation into the tunnel (Fig. 77-17). Finally, part of the clot is also placed between the two individually reconstructed bundles. Both bundle grafts should be secured in the femoral side; the PL bundle graft is then fixed in the tibial side, leaving the AM graft loose. With a suture around its waist, the AM bundle graft is pulled apart from posterolaterally. A cannula containing the clot is introduced through the AMP, and the clot is deposited between the bundle grafts (Fig. 77-17). Next, the AM bundle is released from the suture and fixed in the tibial side, sandwiching the fibrin clot between the two bundles.

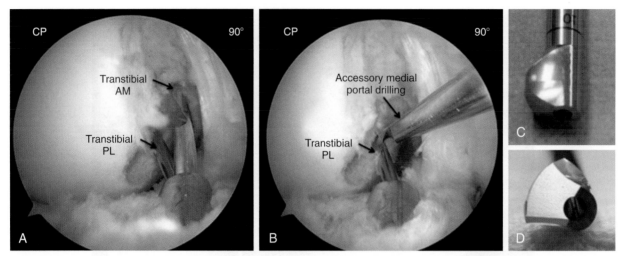

Figure 77-14. Anteromedial *(AM)* femoral tunnel placement. **A,** Through tibial AM tunnel and through posterolateral *(PL)* tibial tunnel. **B,** Femoral AM placement comparison between accessory medial portal (AMP) and PL tibial tunnel. The positioning through PL tibial tunnel allows a more divergent tunnel than through the AMP. **C,** Half-moon drill bit. **D,** Detail of a half-moon drill bit. *CP,* central portal.

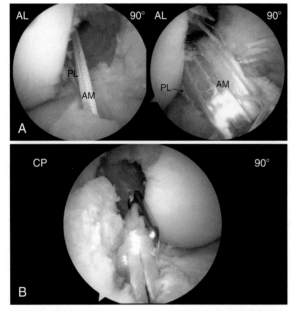

Figure 77-15. Graft passage. **A,** Sutures placed before graft passage for double-bundle reconstruction and both grafts in place in a left knee. **B,** Single-bundle graft passage in a right knee. *AL,* Anterolateral; *AM,* anteromedial; *CP,* central portal; *PL,* posterolateral.

POSTOPERATIVE CONSIDERATIONS

Rehabilitation

After the surgery, the patient's knee is immobilized with the brace locked in full extension for 1 week. Thereafter the brace may be unlocked for assisted exercises. The goal of the immediate postoperative period is to regain motion. Ambulation with crutches is allowed after the first week and use of the crutches can be slowly discontinued as the patient's range of motion and strength improve. Usually after 6 weeks the brace is no longer necessary. Strengthening exercises are slowly integrated into the patient's rehabilitation routine as part of a gradual return to activity.

The rehabilitation after anatomic ACL reconstruction should be carefully followed by physical therapist and surgeon because grafts placed in an anatomic position experience more forces than those placed with a nonanatomic technique. A decision on return to sports should be made cautiously by considering physical examination findings, muscle strength, recovery of normal knee function and, most important, graft healing and maturation, which can be assessed via MRI (Fig. 77-18).

Although inline activities are authorized at 3 to 6 months, cutting activities are allowed only at 9 to 12 months. A prophylactic functional ACL brace is indicated when the patient first returns to sports.

Complications

The DB ACL reconstruction has the same general complications as the SB procedure, including hemarthrosis, effusions, neurovascular injury, arthrofibrosis, wound infection, tibial or femoral fractures, tunnel widening, and deep vein thrombosis.

Overall, DB reconstruction is a more challenging surgery than the SB procedure. The concept of anatomic reconstruction should be first solidified with the SB technique before the DB approach is attempted.

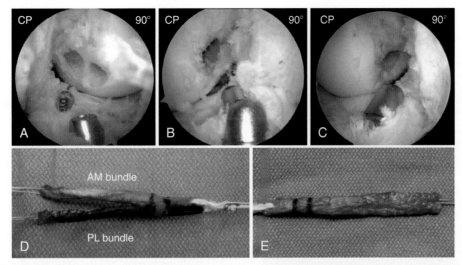

Figure 77-16. Anatomic anterior cruciate ligament reconstruction with use of quadriceps tendon. **A,** Double-bundle four-tunnel technique in a left knee. **B,** Double-bundle three-tunnel technique in a right knee. **C,** Single-bundle technique in a right knee. **D,** Quadriceps tendon split for double-bundle reconstruction. **E,** Quadriceps tendon prepared for single-bundle reconstruction. *AM,* anteromedial; *CP,* central portal; *PL,* posterolateral.

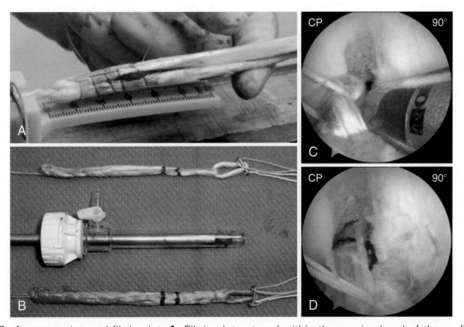

Figure 77-17. Graft preparation and fibrin clot. **A,** Fibrin clot sutured within the proximal end of the graft. **B,** Grafts ready to be passed. Fibrin clot in the tip of the cannula. **C,** Anteromedial *(AM)* bundle pulled apart from posterolateral *(PL)* bundle and the cannula with the fibrin clot properly positioned. **D,** Fibrin clot sandwiched between the AM and PL bundles. *CP,* central portal.

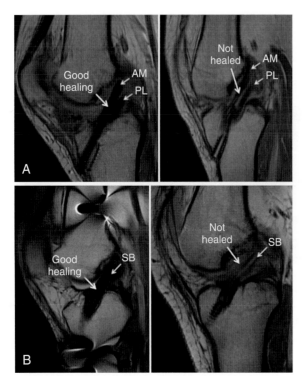

Figure 77-18. Magnetic resonance imaging (MRI) assessment to graft healing. **A,** Double-bundle reconstruction. Mature grafts *(dark)* and good healing response (no gap between grafts) on the left, and an immature graft *(gray)* and bad healing response (gap between grafts) on the right. Both MRI scans taken 8 months postoperatively. **B,** Single-bundle reconstruction showing good graft maturation *(dark)* on the left and an immature graft on the right. Both MRI scans taken at 6 months postoperatively. *AM,* Anteromedial; *PL,* posterolateral; *SB,* single-bundle.

SUMMARY

The anatomic DB concept views the ACL as two functionally different bundles that work synergistically. With an SB technique, the tunnels should be drilled in the center of the ACL footprints, whereas the DB procedure should anatomically replace the AM and PL bundles.

The primary aim of the anatomic reconstruction of the ACL is to closely restore patient's native and individual anatomy. Anatomic ACL reconstruction performed with either an SB or a DB technique better achieves this goal.

REFERENCES

1. Freedman KB, D'Amato MJ, Nedeff DD, et al. Arthroscopic anterior cruciate ligament reconstruction: a metaanalysis comparing patellar tendon and hamstring tendon autografts. *Am J Sports Med.* 2003;31(1):2-11.

2. Biau DJ, Tournoux C, Katsahian S, et al. ACL reconstruction: a meta-analysis of functional scores. *Clin Orthop Relat Res.* 2007;458:180-187.

3. Daniel DM, Stone ML, Dobson BE, et al. Fate of the ACL-injured patient: a prospective outcome study. *Am J Sports Med.* 1994;22(5):632-644.

4. Gillquist J, Messner K. Anterior cruciate ligament reconstruction and the long-term incidence of gonarthrosis. *Sports Med.* 1999;27(3):143-156.

5. Sajovic M, Strahovnik A, Dernovsek MZ, et al. Quality of life and clinical outcome comparison of semitendinosus and gracilis tendon versus patellar tendon autografts for anterior cruciate ligament reconstruction: an 11-year follow-up of a randomized controlled trial. *Am J Sports Med.* 2011;39(10):2161-2169.

6. Pinczewski LA, Lyman J, Salmon LJ, et al. A 10-year comparison of anterior cruciate ligament reconstructions with hamstring tendon and patellar tendon autograft: a controlled, prospective trial. *Am J Sports Med.* 2007; 35(4):564-574.

7. van Eck CF, Schreiber VM, Mejia HA, et al. "Anatomic" anterior cruciate ligament reconstruction: a systematic review of surgical techniques and reporting of surgical data. *Arthroscopy.* 2010;26(9):S2-S12.

8. Van Eck CF, Schreiber VM, Liu TT, et al. The anatomic approach to primary, revision and augmentation anterior cruciate ligament reconstruction. *Knee Surg Sports Traumatol Arthrosc.* 2010;18(9):1154-1163.

9. Woo SL, Kanamori A, Zeminski J, et al. The effectiveness of reconstruction of the anterior cruciate ligament with hamstrings and patellar tendon. A cadaveric study comparing anterior tibial and rotational loads. *J Bone Joint Surg Am.* 2002;84(6):907-914.

10. Yagi M, Wong EK, Kanamori A, et al. Biomechanical analysis of an anatomic anterior cruciate ligament reconstruction. *Am J Sports Med.* 2002;30(5):660-666.

11. Aglietti P, Giron F, Cuomo P, et al. Single- and double-incision double-bundle ACL reconstruction. *Clin Orthop Relat Res.* 2007;454:108-113.

12. Kondo E, Yasuda K, Azuma H, et al. Prospective clinical comparisons of anatomic double-bundle versus single-bundle anterior cruciate ligament reconstruction procedures in 328 consecutive patients. *Am J Sports Med.* 2008;36(9):1675-1687.

13. Muneta T, Koga H, Mochizuki T, et al. A prospective randomized study of 4-strand semitendinosus tendon anterior cruciate ligament reconstruction comparing single-bundle and double-bundle techniques. *Arthroscopy.* 2007;23(6):618-628.

14. Siebold R, Dehler C, Ellert T. Prospective randomized comparison of double-bundle versus single-bundle anterior cruciate ligament reconstruction. *Arthroscopy.* 2008; 24(2):137-145.

15. Yagi M, Kuroda R, Nagamune K, et al. Double-bundle ACL reconstruction can improve rotational stability. *Clin Orthop Relat Res.* 2007;454:100-107.

16. Yasuda K, Kondo E, Ichiyama H, et al. Clinical evaluation of anatomic double-bundle anterior cruciate ligament reconstruction procedure using hamstring tendon grafts: comparisons among 3 different procedures. *Arthroscopy.* 2006;22(3):240-251.

17. Järvelä T. Double-bundle versus single-bundle anterior cruciate ligament reconstruction: a prospective, randomize clinical study. *Knee Surg Sports Traumatol Arthrosc.* 2007;15(5):500-507.

18. Pombo MW, Shen W, Fu FH. Anatomic double-bundle anterior cruciate ligament reconstruction: where are we today? *Arthroscopy.* 2008;24(10):1168-1177.

19. Shen W, Forsythe B, Ingham SM, et al. Application of the anatomic double-bundle reconstruction concept to revision and augmentation anterior cruciate ligament surgeries. *J Bone Joint Surg Am.* 2008;90(Supplement 4): 20-34.

20. van Eck CF, Lesniak BP, Schreiber VM, et al. Anatomic single- and double-bundle anterior cruciate ligament reconstruction flowchart. *Arthroscopy.* 2010;26(2): 258-268.

21. Araujo PH, van Eck CF, Macalena JA, et al. Advances in the three-portal technique for anatomical single- or double-bundle ACL reconstruction. *Knee Surg Sports Traumatol Arthrosc.* 2011.

22. Kopf S, Pombo MW, Shen W, et al. The ability of 3 different approaches to restore the anatomic anteromedial bundle femoral insertion site during anatomic anterior cruciate ligament reconstruction. *Arthroscopy.* 2011; 27(2):200-206.

Chapter 78

Double-Bundle Anterior Cruciate Ligament Reconstruction

Patrick A. Smith

Chapter Synopsis

- Anterior cruciate ligament (ACL) reconstruction is a common surgical procedure, yet there is no single universally accepted reconstructive technique.

- Single-bundle reconstruction is most commonly done, but debate is ongoing as to whether it should be done with the traditional transtibial approach for drilling the femur, or via an independent drilling technique on the femur either through the anteromedial (AM) portal or via a lateral two-incision type of approach.

- More recently, with recognition of the tendency for a vertical nonanatomic graft if the reconstruction is done transtibially, attention has focused on an anatomic single-bundle reconstruction through independent drilling.

- An alternative to an anatomic technique in ACL reconstruction is to perform a double-bundle ACL reconstruction.

- As with single-bundle ACL reconstruction, there are different ways to perform a double- bundle ACL reconstruction.

- This chapter focuses on the all-inside procedure, which is the most minimally invasive technique for double-bundle ACL reconstruction.

Important Points

- A hallmark surgical indication for ACL reconstruction is the subjective sensation of giving way, correlated with objective pivot-shift test results on examination.

- The normal ACL has two primary bundles—anteromedial (AM) and posterolateral (PL).

- Experimental studies have shown benefit to the addition of a PL bundle for rotational stability.

- Two grafts provide potential for better isometry with some portion of graft material tight through full range of motion.

- The all-inside technique is conceptually different via creation of a retrograde tibial socket from inside the joint—not a full tunnel—thereby being innately less invasive; clinically, the procedure seems less painful.

- No transtibial drilling; the procedure involves independent drilling of femoral and tibial sockets with the femur drilled either through the AM portal or "outside-in" as in a two-incision approach.

- An all-inside technique is versatile relative to graft choice; choices include patellar or quadriceps tendon, hamstring autograft or allograft, or a combination thereof.

Clinical and Surgical Pearls

- Issue of graft length in PL socket: Owing to bony anatomy relative to the width of the lateral femoral condyle, the intraosseous distance for the PL bundle is shorter. The goal is to have at least 20 mm of graft in the PL socket for optimal healing. It is preferable not to use an accessory medial portal because that would create an angle of approach to the femur that is too perpendicular and thus further shorten the intraosseous distance. With use of a low AM portal, it is possible to orient the guide pin more obliquely from the femoral starting point to make for a longer intraosseous distance, which is the key to maximal graft in the femoral socket.

- The proprietary RetroCutter (Arthrex, Naples, FL) provides optimal circular cuts for tibial sockets to minimize aperture fragmentation and also maximize space available for two separate tibial sockets to avoid the risk of coalescence. In addition, this device make visualization of the socket position technically easier.

- PL bundle tibial socket creation: It is critical to initiate the starting point on the tibia with the RetroCutter guide pin close to the midline; this greatly facilitates later passage of the RetroScrew (Arthrex) from inside the joint for graft fixation. Otherwise, it is difficult to place the RetroScrew on the driver if not centered in notch.

- A helpful step for RetroScrew fixation of both bundles on the tibia is dilating over a tibial guide wire with the

Continued

RetroScrewdriver (Arthrex) *before* placing the RetroScrew. This provides more room for the RetroScrew to fixate anterior to the graft filling the socket.

- Use a cannula through the AM portal when passing grafts to avoid getting sutures caught in the soft tissue (i.e., fat pad), which can be very frustrating.
- Fix the PL bundle in full extension because the biomechanics of knee motion involves tightening of the PL bundle by 2 to 3 mm as the knee is extended. If the PL bundle is not fixed in full extension, either the joint will be overconstrained and extension will be limited, or the PL graft will stretch and fail.

Clinical and Surgical Pitfalls

- Measurement of graft length is critical with the all-inside technique because femoral and tibial sockets are fixed lengths, along with intra-articular distance; otherwise, grafts could "bottom out" and be lax.
- AM portal drilling for femoral socket creation: Drill the PL socket first to make sure it is not positioned too distally toward the weight-bearing surface of the lateral femoral condyle; if the AM bundle is drilled first, the surgeon risks not leaving enough room for the PL. If the injury is chronic and there are no remaining native PL and AM fibers for orientation for the sockets, the

approach is to be sure that both sockets are positioned posterior to the lateral intercondylar ridge ("resident's ridge") with 2 mm between the sockets and 3 to 4 mm intact from the distal lateral femoral condyle articular surface for the PL bundle.

- If the surgeon is uncomfortable with AM portal drilling, another option is to use an outside-in approach with the FlipCutter (Arthrex). This is a proprietary guide pin that easily converts to a reamer for creation of the femoral sockets from a lateral drilling position.
- If a patient has a small tibial footprint, double-bundle ACL reconstruction may not be feasible. An intra-articular measuring device is used, and if the distance from the front of the posterior cruciate ligament (PCL) to the anterior margin of the ACL footprint is at least 18 mm, all-inside double-bundle ACL reconstruction is possible. The RetroCutter greatly facilitates the double-bundle procedure because it achieves true circular sockets on the tibia, which take up less room than transtibial tunnels; transtibial tunnels create a wider more oval aperture upon entering the knee joint, with a higher propensity for aperture microfracturing.

 Video

- Video 78-1 : All-inside double-bundle allograft anterior cruciate ligament reconstruction

PREOPERATIVE CONSIDERATIONS

An acute anterior cruciate ligament (ACL) tear is typically related to a "giving way" episode, and a noncontact rotational injury is quite common, particularly in football and soccer. Deceleration and landing from a jump are classic mechanisms of injury in basketball players. Patients usually have early swelling with an acute tear consistent with hemarthrosis, and resultant limited motion—especially extension. One should have a high level of suspicion with young female basketball or soccer players who hurt the knee and have diffuse pain and swelling with a difficult examination; an ACL tear should be presumed until proven otherwise. In the chronic setting, patients relate instability with twisting and pivoting, and may also note catching or locking if they have an associated meniscus tear.

Physical examination for an ACL tear is predicated on determination of both pathologic anterior and rotational joint laxity compared with the normal knee. The Lachman test at 30 degrees of flexion is easily done even in the acute setting and is very sensitive for anterior laxity. The pivot-shift maneuver is really the key test, however, because it is diagnostic for rotational instability, which is the disabling feature of an ACL tear—that is, the mechanism that puts the knee at risk for giving way. Joint line tenderness should raise suspicion for a meniscus tear, especially if pain and/or a pop is present

with provocative knee flexion and rotation testing. In the acute setting, lateral joint tenderness may be more related to the common associated bone contusion injury pattern to the lateral femoral condyle anteriorly and the lateral tibial plateau posteriorly.

Standard imaging for an ACL injury includes weight-bearing radiographs, especially important in patients with chronic ACL deficiency to assess for degenerative change or malalignment. Magnetic resonance imaging (MRI) is helpful in acute injury to quantify the extent of lateral compartment bone contusion, which is important relative to consideration of a period of non–weight-bearing time to protect the lateral compartment articular surfaces, particularly if there is associated chondral injury. In the chronic setting, subtle degenerative chondral changes may be seen. MRI is also very useful to assess the status of the collateral ligaments if there is any question of the need for repair or reconstruction of the medial or lateral-PL ligament complex at the time of ACL reconstruction. MRI, of course, also provides valuable information relative to the status of the menisci. Certainly, accurate knowledge about the state of the secondary stabilizers relative to the collateral ligaments and the menisci, along with the condition of the articular surfaces, is helpful for surgical planning.

Options for ACL reconstruction include single-bundle versus double-bundle procedures. In the realm of single-bundle procedures, recent experimental and clinical work has highlighted the potential for vertical graft placement with traditional transtibial drilling of the femur, which in turn can lead to residual instability. This has spawned the term "anatomic" single-bundle reconstruction done with independent drilling of the femur and tibia. The femoral socket can be drilled either through the anteromedial (AM) portal or outside-in, either with a two-incision technique for guide pin placement from the lateral femur into the joint for reaming, or less invasively with a FlipCutter (Arthrex, Naples, FL), which is a guide pin that converts easily to a reamer. Given the fact that the native ACL has at least two major bundles—AM and posterolateral (PL)—an alternative approach would be double-bundle reconstruction, which would conceptually result in an even more anatomic reconstruction.

Certainly, there are numerous ways to perform a double-bundle ACL reconstruction. The overall goal regardless of the chosen technique is to achieve anatomic placement of graft tissue to recreate both the AM and the PL bundles. In its purest sense, double-bundle reconstruction is done with two separate tunnels in the femur and tibia. However, there are described "double-bundle ACL" techniques that use one tibial tunnel with two femoral tunnels, as well as techniques that use one tibial tunnel and one femoral tunnel with splitting of the graft into "bundles" with the fixation used. For a true double-bundle reconstruction, full tibial tunnels are usually created with guides by drilling into the joint from the proximal tibia. The femoral tunnels are then created transtibially, from the AM portal, or via a lateral two-incision type of approach. This chapter outlines the all-inside procedure, which is the most minimally invasive way to perform a double-bundle reconstruction. In the procedure to be detailed, two separate femoral sockets are drilled through the AM portal, and two separate tibial sockets are created in a retrograde manner from within the joint. Fixation is dependent on graft choice but generally consists of suspensory fixation on the femur with retrograde aperture screw fixation on the tibial side.

All-inside ACL reconstruction is based on the principle of creating a tibial socket by reaming from within the joint, as opposed to a traditional full tibial tunnel reamed from outside in. In addition, graft fixation on the tibial side is also done in retrograde fashion with placement of a fixation screw from within the joint. This was originally described in 2006 for single-bundle ACL reconstruction and was termed "no-tunnel" reconstruction"[1] and subsequently was first reported for double-bundle reconstruction in 2008.[2] The driving force for the all-inside technique is its innate minimal invasiveness; the tibial socket is created through a small incision with a 3.0-mm-diameter pin, leading to less overall tibial soft tissue dissection. The key technologic advance is use of the RetroCutter (Arthrex) device. The other major difference from a traditional ACL reconstruction

done through a full tibial tunnel is use of the RetroScrew (Arthrex) placed also from inside the joint for aperture fixation. Anecdotally, it was appreciated early on that patients seemed to have less pain postoperatively with the all-inside technique. Currently, a level I study comparing standard endoscopic single-bundle soft tissue allograft ACL reconstruction with an all-inside approach is being completed with 2-year follow-up data collection. Preliminary results confirm significantly less pain with visual analogue scale (VAS) scoring with the all-inside technique at all follow-up timeframes up to 2 years. It is important to note that no difference in outcome scores with International Knee Documentation Committee (IKDC) and Knee Society Score (KSS) scales has been seen (Smith and colleagues, unpublished data).

Potential indications for double-bundle reconstruction include athletes for whom rotational stability is paramount, particularly in position-dependent situations—for example, running backs, wide receivers, linebackers, and defensive backs in football. Patients who demonstrate inherent physiologic laxity with excessive knee hyperextension also may be appropriate candidates. Finally, for certain revision procedures the double-bundle approach may be most suitable.

A relative shortcoming of double-bundle reconstruction includes the need for harvesting two grafts when one wants to use autograft tissue. Certainly, the procedure is easily performed with two allografts—as illustrated in the surgical case presented in this chapter—but in young athletes, autograft tissue is generally preferable. Initially the all-inside double-bundle procedure with autograft tissue in young athletes was done with use of a doubled semitendinosus graft for the AM bundle and a doubled gracilis for the PL bundle, but a rerupture rate of approximately 7% (Smith, unpublished data) for that group on return to play was considered to be unacceptable. It was speculated that the doubled gracilis tendon was not strong enough for the stresses placed on the PL bundle, especially with joint loading in extension with athletic activity. This led to use of a patellar tendon autograft for the AM bundle and a doubled semitendinosus for the PL bundle in athletes, which has resulted in an acceptable rerupture rate of only 1.5% (Smith, unpublished data). However, this procedure requires use of both the patellar tendon and the semitendinosus, which prevents their use later if failure should occur. In that setting, I have found that an autograft quadriceps tendon single-bundle revision procedure has worked well.

A potential contraindication relates to the difficulty of a revision ACL reconstruction after a double-bundle procedure. The all-inside technique has an advantage in that regard, because creation of tibial sockets—not full bone tunnels—is inherently bone saving. Therefore a single-stage revision reconstruction has not been a problem, and I have even performed revision all-inside double-bundle reconstruction after a failed all-inside double-bundle construction.

SURGICAL TECHNIQUE

The all-inside double-bundle ACL reconstruction discussed here is a case study of a left knee repaired with use of two semitendinosus soft tissue allografts. The PL bundle graft is 7.5 mm in diameter, and the AM bundle graft is 8.0 mm in diameter. The following is an overview of the procedure: Both the PL and AM femoral sockets are first created through the AM portal in hyperflexion for optimal anatomic positioning. Next, the PL tibial socket is created with the RetroCutter from a midline approach. The PL graft is passed and fixated on the femoral side with the suspensory TightRope device (Arthrex), and on the tibial side with a RetroScrew in full extension. The AM tibial socket is then created with the RetroCutter, and this graft is passed and fixed on the femur with the TightRope and on the tibial side with another RetroScrew at 30 degrees of knee flexion. A key point with all-inside surgery is accurate determination of graft length to ensure that a graft does not "bottom out," which would make it lax at time zero. This is easily accomplished by knowing the depth of each graft in the femoral and tibial sockets in addition to measuring the intra-articular length of both grafts. Then, 5 to 10 mm is added to the reamed depth of each tibial socket to accommodate tensioning of each bundle and to ensure that neither graft will be too long.

Specific Steps

Box 78-1 outlines the specific steps of this procedure.

1: Operating Room Setup

It is best to use a foot holder that can easily adjust the angle of knee flexion, especially to facilitate drilling though the AM portal, which is my preference for the femoral sockets. Also, the addition of a simple lateral knee support to stabilize the thigh leads to a hands-free situation so that positioning of the knee at any angle of desired flexion is easily accomplished, making the procedure less labor intensive (Fig. 78-1).

2: Offset Guide to Create Posterolateral Femoral Socket

A 5-mm AM portal offset guide (Arthrex) is passed through the AM portal under the articular surface of the lateral femoral condyle at the 3-o'clock position. In hyperflexion of approximately 120 degrees, a special measuring guide pin (Arthrex) is drilled to create a pilot hole for the PL bundle. This will position the PL femoral socket posteriorly 2 mm from the articular surface of the lateral femoral condyle, and 3 to 4 mm from the distal lateral femoral condyle articular surface. The intraosseous distance is measured to determine depth of the socket to be reamed. In general, a minimum of 20 mm of graft in the PL femoral socket is possible with use of TightRope femoral suspensory fixation in this situation, so this depth is reamed over the pin with a low-profile reamer to protect the medial femoral condyle. The pin is used to pull a passing suture through this PL femoral socket. Notably, a notchplasty is rarely done (Fig. 78-2).

BOX 78-1 Surgical Steps

- Operating room setup—leg holder and thigh support
- Creation of PL femoral socket with offset guide
- Creation of AM femoral socket with low-profile reamer, ensuring 2-mm bone bridge from PL socket
- Creation of PL tibial socket—midline approach
- All-inside shuttle-wire to suture loop
- Intra-articular PL measurement
- Dilation step for PL tibial socket
- PL bundle passage with ACL TightRope fixation
- PL RetroScrew placement
- Final PL bundle inspection
- Creation of AM tibial socket
- AM bundle TightRope passage
- Tibial RetroScrew AM bundle
- Final all-inside double-bundle construct

ACL, Anterior cruciate ligament; *AM,* anteromedial; *PL,* posterolateral.

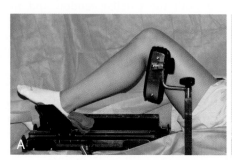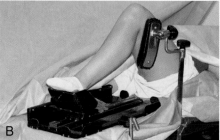

Figure 78-1. A, Lateral view of foot holder with lateral thigh support, which facilitates medial portal femoral drilling. **B,** Front view of operative setup with leg holder and thigh support.

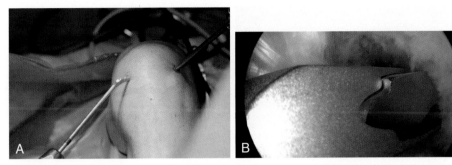

Figure 78-2. A, Anteromedial offset guide passing through the low anteromedial portal. **B,** Offset guide with pin at 3-o'clock position for posterolateral femoral socket with knee hyperflexed.

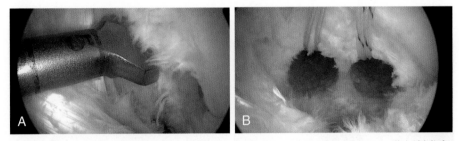

Figure 78-3. A, An 8-mm low-profile reamer over guide pin at 1:30 position for anteromedial (AM) femoral socket, ensuring 2-mm bone bridge from posterolateral (PL) socket. **B,** Ideal position of PL and AM femoral sockets within 2 mm of the posterior lateral femoral articular surface with 2-mm bone bridge with passing sutures.

3: Creation of Anteromedial Femoral Socket Bone Bridge

The AM femoral socket is drilled after the PL socket, leaving a 2-mm bone bridge on the joint side—appreciating that given the different position on the femur that is drilled, there will actually be further divergence of this AM femoral socket compared with the PL socket deeper in the bone. A 6-mm AM portal offset guide (Arthrex) is positioned at the 1:30 position in hyperflexion to allow for 2 mm of bone intact from the PL femoral condyle articular surface, and I check by bringing the 8-mm reamer over the special measuring pin (Arthrex) to ensure the presence of 2 mm of intact bone from the PL femoral socket. Usually reaming is done to a depth of 25 to 30 mm for the AM femoral socket to allow that much graft in that socket with use of the TightRope suspensory femoral fixation. Again, a passing suture is pulled through to the aperture of the AM femoral socket (Fig. 78-3).

Step 4: Creation of Posterolateral Tibial Socket—Midline Approach

A critical pearl is the angle of approach for the PL tibial socket. Specifically, for the all-inside technique a RetroScrew is placed for tibial fixation; but for this to be done for the PL bundle, the PL tibial socket must have an angle that is more midline for later passage of the special RetroScrewdriver (Arthrex) so that the RetroScrew can be flipped up in the notch to be placed on the

RetroScrewdriver. Otherwise, the RetroScrew cannot be easily placed on the RetroScrewdriver. Therefore a small incision is made over the proximal tibial just distal and medial to the tibial tubercle for the starting point for the guide sleeve. The RetroCutter itself is positioned in the joint just lateral to midline in front of the lateral tibial eminence where there is a natural sulcus. In this procedure a 7.5-mm RetroCutter was used. A special 3.0-mm cannulated RetroCutter guide pin (Arthrex) is drilled into the joint on forward and "captures" the RetroCutter, which is reverse threaded on the guide, and then the PL tibial socket is retroreamed to the desired depth—usually 40 mm to account for 30 mm of graft in the PL tibial socket and to accommodate room for graft tensioning. The RetroCutter is delivered back in the joint; once the pin has gone through the guide, which has been left in the joint, the drill is reversed to put the RetroCutter back on the guide so it can then be removed from the joint (Fig. 78-4).

Step 5: All-inside Shuttle-Wire to Suture Loop

Another key pearl is the "how-to" of passing first the graft, and then the intra-articular RetroScrew for later aperture graft fixation on the joint side for the all-inside technique. This is accomplished by creating a suture shuttle with the special RetroCutter guide pin, which is cannulated. This allows passage of a wire that has a loop on one end; this wire is passed through the guide pin right after the tibial socket has been reamed with

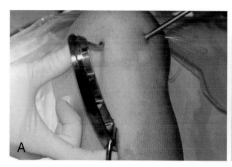
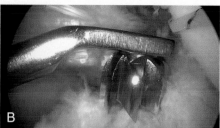

Figure 78-4. A, Important angle of RetroCutter (Arthrex, Naples, FL) guide toward midline to drill posterolateral (PL) tibial socket to facilitate later RetroScrew placement. **B,** The 7.5-mm RetroCutter is placed in front of the posterior cruciate ligament lateral to midline in sulcus, buttressing the lateral tibial eminence to create the PL tibial socket.

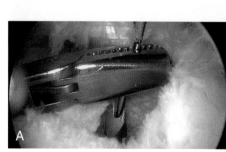
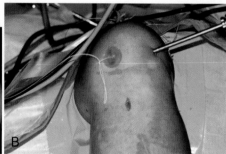

Figure 78-5. A, Wire with loop end is passed through the cannulated RetroCutter (Arthrex, Naples, FL) guide pin after reaming and retrieved through the anteromedial portal, where the PassPort cannula has been placed. **B,** No. 2 FiberStick suture with loop tied in midportion is passed by wire loop back through the posterolateral tibial socket to serve as a shuttle, first for the graft and then for the wire to place the RetroScrew.

the RetroCutter. Do not pull this pin out after reaming, because the 3.0-mm hole through the small tibial incision can be hard to find. The wire is pulled out through the AM portal, where a PassPort (Arthrex) cannula has been placed; this is extremely helpful to avoid catching sutures in the soft tissue of the fat pad, which blocks graft passage and therefore can be can be very frustrating. Next a No. 2 FiberStick (Arthrex) suture with a loop tied in its midportion is passed back through the tibial socket with the wire. The loop of this suture will be used to pull the graft in the tibial socket; then the free end remaining outside the AM portal is tied to the same wire through its loop so that later the wire can be pulled anterior to the graft after it has been passed. In this way the RetroScrewdriver can be passed back over the wire into the joint to allow for RetroScrew aperture fixation (Fig. 78-5).

Step 6: Intra-articular Posterolateral Measurement

It is essential with all-inside surgery to accurately determine graft length because there are blind femoral and tibial sockets; the graft can bottom out and be lax if the graft is too long. Socket depth in the femur and tibia is easily determined at the time of reaming. A special intra-articular measuring device (Arthrex) is used to separately measure the intra-articular distance—in

Figure 78-6, from the center of the PL tibial socket to the aperture at the femoral socket.

Step 7: Dilation Step for Posterolateral Tibial Socket

Another critical pearl is what I term the "dilation step." This is necessary because to fix a graft all-inside with a RetroScrew, the RetroScrewdriver must be placed from below in the socket anterior to the graft *after* the graft has been pulled into the socket. The challenge is that the initial RetroCutter guide pin hole is in the center of this socket, which makes it tight to pass the RetroScrewdriver with the graft already in place. For this process to be facilitated, when the socket is open the RetroScrewdriver is passed over the wire that is initially placed through the cannulated RetroCutter guide pin to be a shuttle for the No. 2 FiberWire suture loop. The RetroScrewdriver is then free to dilate the centering hole more anteriorly, making it easy to pass the RetroScrewdriver for the fixation step anterior to the graft after it has been pulled into the socket (Fig. 78-7).

Step 8: Posterolateral Bundle Passage with Anterior Cruciate Ligament TightRope Fixation

Fixation on the femur is via the TightRope suspensory device. The graft is pulled through the AM portal

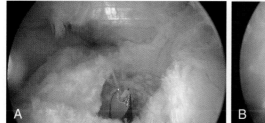
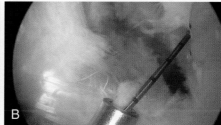

Figure 78-6. A, Ideal posterolateral tibial socket in front of the posterior cruciate ligament lateral to midline with the RetroCutter (Arthrex, Naples, FL) guide pin in place after reaming. **B,** Intra-articular measuring device necessary to determine graft length to ensure the graft is not too long and does not "bottom out" with blind femoral and tibial sockets.

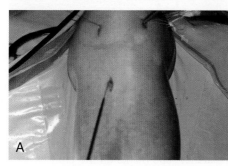
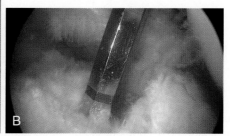

Figure 78-7. A, Outside look of passage of the RetroScrewdriver (Arthrex, Naples, FL) over the guide wire passed after reaming of the posterolateral (PL) tibial socket; advance in the same orientation as socket was reamed. **B,** RetroScrewdriver advanced over guidewire as dilation step into joint. RetroScrewdriver is manipulated to the anterior aspect of the PL tibial socket to make passage of the RetroScrewdriver later, once the graft is in place, much easier.

through the PassPort cannula in place to avoid soft tissue interposition. The blue No. 2 FiberWire passing sutures are pulled out the femur, flipping the button on the cortex. This is facilitated by marking on the white loop the intraosseous distance from the distal end of the button to indicate when it should flip. Next the two shortening sutures are pulled in an alternating fashion to "hoist" the graft to the expected depth (usually 20 mm) in the femoral socket, marked with methylene blue on the graft (Fig. 78-8). The shortening sutures are then cut.

Step 9: Posterolateral RetroScrew Placement

The tibial end of the PL bundle is first shuttled into the tibial socket though the PassPort cannula via the loop of the No. 2 FiberStick suture. Next, the wire attached to the end of the No. 2 FiberStick suture is pulled back through the tibial socket from the AM portal by this suture so it is anterior to the graft. The RetroScrewdriver is then passed over the wire—again, facilitated by the previous dilation step. Next, another No. 2 FiberStick suture is passed through the Retro-Screwdriver and out the PassPort cannula and through a RetroScrew. For this procedure it is a 7-mm-diameter, 20-mm-long poly-L–lactic acid (PLLA) absorbable RetroScrew. A closed mulberry-type knot is tied to secure the RetroScrew to the suture. The RetroScrew is

then pulled back into the joint by the other end of the same suture; once the RetroScrew has been placed on the RetroScrewdriver (and fully seated, as noted by a black laser mark), this suture is cleated securely to the RetroScrewdriver. A tamp is used by an assistant to push down on the RetroScrew, which is tightened by counterclockwise turning of the RetroScrewdriver, by the surgeon while simultaneously bringing the knee right away to absolute full extension (Fig. 78-9).

Step 10: Final Posterolateral Bundle Inspection

Again, the PL bundle is fixed at the tibial aperture with the RetroScrew in absolute full extension. This is critical because the PL bundle lengthens 2 to 3 mm going from flexion into extension, and if it is not fixed at full extension, either the joint could be over-constrained and the patient will lose motion or the PL graft bundle will stretch out and fail. At 90 degrees of flexion, the PL bundle will be slightly lax to probing but will be completely taut to probing in full extension (Fig. 78-10).

Step 11: Creation of Anteromedial Tibial Socket

The same size RetroCutter (7.5 mm in this case) is positioned in the AM footprint 2 mm from the PL tibial RetroScrew to ensure a bone bridge there. The small

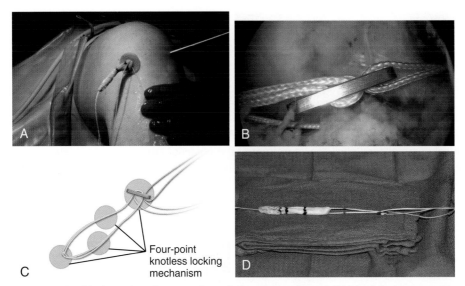

Figure 78-8. A, A 7.5-mm doubled semitendinosus allograft for posterolateral (PL) bundle is passed into the femur with a suture loop from the PL femoral socket through the PassPort cannula (Arthrex, Naples, FL) in the anteromedial portal. **B,** TightRope button is pulled across the joint for PL graft fixation on the femur with a blue passing suture. **C,** Schematic of anterior cruciate ligament TightRope locking points for graft—each side of spliced suture and then from base of suture loop against the button. **D,** Prepared 7.5-mm PL graft before passage with a mark on the suture loop where the button should flip on the lateral femoral cortex based on intraosseous distance, and marks on the graft for expected graft in the femoral socket and intra-articular measurement.

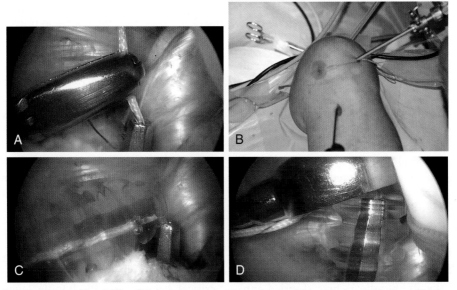

Figure 78-9. A, Retrieving the No. 2 FiberStick through the RetroScrewdriver (Arthrex, Naples, FL) from the anteromedial portal to pass through the RetroScrew. **B,** RetroScrewdriver in place in the posterolateral (PL) tibial socket with the RetroScrew tied to a No. 2 FiberStick and prepared to be passed through the PassPort cannula in the anteromedial portal. **C,** A 7.0-mm RetroScrew in position to be flipped onto the RetroScrewdriver, done by application of tension to the No. 2 FiberStick and use of a hemostat to position the RetroScrew over the end of the RetroScrewdriver; the RetroScrewdriver is then passed into the RetroScrew. **D,** Tamp pushing down on the RetroScrew while the RetroScrewdriver is turned and the knee is brought into full extension to fixate the PL bundle at the tibial aperture.

AM medial tibial incision is always proximal and medial to the small PL tibial incision. The same steps are followed as with the PL bundle, with passage of a wire and dilation with the RetroScrewdriver after retroreaming, and passage of the special No. 2 FiberStick suture with the loop (Fig. 78-11).

Step 12: Anteromedial Bundle TightRope Passage

Just as for the PL bundle previously, the AM bundle is passed through the AM portal via the PassPort cannula with the ACL TightRope button flipped on the lateral

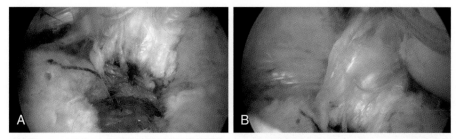

Figure 78-10. A, A 7.0-mm RetroScrew (Arthrex, Naples, FL) in position at the posterolateral (PL) tibial socket aperture with knee in flexed position where the PL bundle is slightly lax. **B,** PL bundle as knee is extended where it tightens by 2 to 3 mm in full extension.

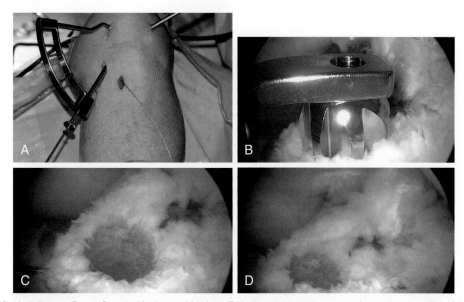

Figure 78-11. A, A 7.5-mm RetroCutter (Arthrex, Naples, FL) in position to create the anteromedial (AM) tibial socket with the posterolateral (PL) tibial incision noted with a suture from the PL bundle. **B,** RetroCutter in place anterior and medial to PL tibial RetroScrew still in the footprint of anterior cruciate ligament, with native fibers noted. **C,** Completed 7.5-mm AM tibial socket with 2-mm bone bridge from the PL tibial RetroScrew. D, Position of AM tibial socket in relation to the PL graft is appreciated.

femoral cortex for secure suspensory fixation. The graft is then hoisted into the femoral socket, usually for a distance of 25 to 30 mm, by the TightRope shortening sutures. The intraosseous distance for the AM femoral socket is always longer than the PL intraosseous distance, which allows for more graft to be placed in the AM femoral socket (Fig. 78-12).

Step 13: Tibial RetroScrew Anteromedial Bundle

After the AM bundle has been shuttled into its tibial socket with the No. 2 FiberStick loop suture, and the wire has been brought anterior to the graft, the AM tibial RetroScrew is placed in the same way as was done for the PL bundle. This RetroScrew is a BioComposite screw; hence the beige color, as opposed to the clear PLLA RetroScrew used for the PL bundle. The Retro-Screw is inserted to the appropriate depth on the RetroScrewdriver, as marked by the laser mark on the

driver. Again, the tamp is used to minimize torque on the RetroScrewdriver during insertion. The AM bundle is fixated at 30 degrees of flexion (Fig. 78-13).

Step 14: Final All-Inside Double-Bundle Construct

On completion, the AM bundle is anterior to the PL bundle and generally is most isometric, being tight both in full extension and particularly in flexion. The PL bundle is minimally lax in flexion and tightens in full extension, becoming parallel to the AM bundle (Fig. 78-14).

POSTOPERATIVE CONSIDERATIONS

Relative to postoperative rehabilitation with all-inside double-bundle ACL reconstruction, standard protocol

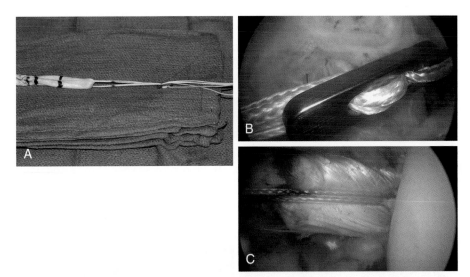

Figure 78-12. **A,** A 7.5-mm allograft for the anteromedial (AM) bundle prepared on anterior cruciate ligament (ACL) TightRope with the first mark on the suture indicating where the button should flip on the lateral femoral cortex with the next mark on the tendon graft for the determined length of graft in the femoral socket. The next mark on the graft represents intra-articular distance for the AM bundle. **B,** ACL Tightrope button passing into the femoral socket. **C,** Shortening sutures for ACL Tightrope noted after the graft has been hoisted in femoral socket.

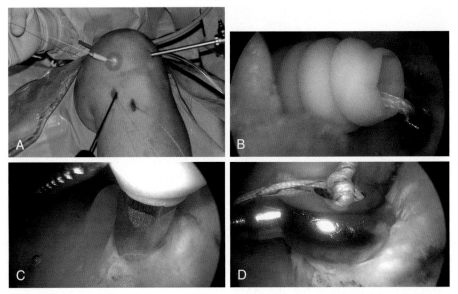

Figure 78-13. **A,** RetroScrewdriver (Arthrex, Naples, FL) in place for anteromedial (AM) bundle tibial fixation with 7-mm BioComposite RetroScrew to pass through the PassPort cannula. **B,** A 7-mm BioComposite RetroScrew coming through the PassPort cannula to be placed on the RetroScrewdriver. **C,** A black laser mark on the RetroScrewdriver confirms the RetroScrew is fully inserted on the RetroScrewdriver. **D,** Tamp facilitates securing of 7-mm RetroScrew for aperture fixation of the AM bundle at 30 degrees of flexion.

includes use of a continuous passive motion machine for the first 2 weeks, with flexion increased as tolerated. Emphasis is on early and aggressive quadriceps strengthening for full extension with the goal of performing straight-leg raises with no lag. Patellar mobilization is encouraged to avoid anterior scarring. Full weight bearing is encouraged, with weaning from crutches once the patient demonstrates good quadriceps function and leg control with a smooth gait pattern. The bike is started usually at 2 weeks. Closed chain strengthening with the leg press is started at 4 weeks, along with minisquats and hamstring curls. Hip and core strengthening is also emphasized at that time. Jogging usually is allowed at 3 months with progression to agility and proprioceptive exercises at 4 months. Sport-specific training begins at 5 months, including jump and landing exercises. Return to sport is usually at 6 months if the patient is ready, based on results of functional

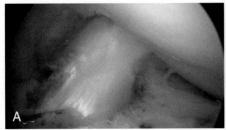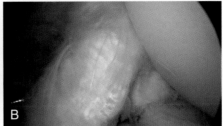

Figure 78-14. A, Final appearance of the anteromedial (AM) bundle after RetroScrew (Arthrex, Naples, FL) aperture tibial fixation. **B,** Final construct with the AM bundle anterior to posterolateral (PL) bundle heading toward 1:30 position on the femur with the PL bundle underneath it attaching toward 3-o'clock position.

assessment testing by the physical therapist and the findings of the orthopedic clinical evaluation in the office at that time.

The all-inside double-bundle procedure is a minimally invasive option for double-bundle ACL reconstruction. It is a flexible procedure, particularly from the standpoint of graft choice. It can be done with gracilis and semitendinosus autografts, or with hamstring allografts as demonstrated in this chapter. Another approach previously mentioned is use of an autogenous patellar tendon graft harvested with bone only from the tibia for the AM bundle, and a doubled semitendinosus autograft for the PL bundle, which is the construct I prefer in contact athletes. A hybrid reconstruction with use of combined autograft and allograft tendon is also feasible. In my personal case series of all-inside double-bundle ACL reconstructions since 2007 with different graft combinations, primarily done in young athletic patients, there are 174 patients with greater than 1 year of follow-up. In that group, there was only one reoperation for a minimal loss of extension caused by anterior scar tissue that was easily corrected with arthroscopic debridement. I have a total of 10 reruptures, all in young athletes under the age of 21, for an overall retear rate of 5.7%. This compares with a recently published report of a systematic review of level I and II single-bundle ACL reconstruction studies with greater than 5 years' follow-up of 2026 patients with a pooled graft retear rate of 5.8%.[3] Again, with sockets rather than full tunnels in the tibia, there is good bone stock remaining; and in my experience, revision after all-inside double-bundle reconstruction has not posed any major technical challenges. Although graft retears still occur with double-bundle ACL reconstruction—similar to single-bundle procedures—the real long-term question is whether a successful double-bundle procedure leads to less late osteoarthritis development than does single-bundle reconstruction, which has shown a concerning high incidence of this late complication.[4,5]

FINAL RESULTS (Box 78-2)

It is well accepted that the normal ACL comprises at least two distinct bundles: the AM and PL bundles.

BOX 78-2 Summary of Studies

- Chhabra and colleagues evaluated characteristics of the two ACL bundles with the posterolateral bundle tighter in extension and the anteromedial bundle tighter in flexion.[7]
- Yagi and colleagues showed in a cadaver study that the double-bundle construct demonstrates better stability than use of a single bundle.[8]
- Zantop and colleagues showed experimentally that the posterolateral bundle achieves better rotational stability.[9]
- Kondo and colleagues and Siebold and colleagues found better stability via the clinical pivot-shift test with double-bundle versus single-bundle techniques, but comparable objective KT1000 results for stability testing.[10]
- Hemmerich and colleagues analyzed three-dimensional knee kinematics and found that double-bundle reconstruction restores better rotation than the single-bundle method.[14]
- Tsai and colleagues found in a cadaver study with simulated pivot shift that all-inside double-bundle reconstruction permits normal restoration of anterior translation, with all-inside single-bundle reconstruction being more lax.[16]
- Walsh and colleagues compared experimentally all-inside double-bundle tibial drilling order and fixation and found the technique of drilling and fixing the PL bundle first provided better ultimate failure load and had less risk of bone bridge fracture.[17]

ACL, Anterior cruciate ligament; *PL,* posterolateral.

They have distinct origins on the tibia and are named respectively on that basis, and have distinct attachment sites on the femur as well.[6] Relative to isometric behavior, they have different patterns of tightening, with the PL bundle tighter in extension and the AM bundle tighter in flexion.[7]

It is simplistic to think that a single-bundle ACL reconstruction would truly be isometric, because the biomechanics of the native ACL are complicated. ACL kinematics has been well tested in cadaver models, and the double-bundle construct has consistently demonstrated better stability than a single bundle.[8] This has been attributable to adding the PL bundle for better rotational stability.[9]

The basic question is whether a double-bundle ACL reconstruction is "more isometric" and therefor ultimately better in the clinical setting. One concern is that the current long-term follow-up studies of single-bundle ACL reconstruction have shown a high rate of osteoarthritis development, which could relate to less-than-optimal restoration of knee kinematics, but it is not known if double-bundle ACL reconstruction will decrease the development of late-onset osteoarthritis. So far, clinical comparison follow-up studies of single-versus double-bundle ACL reconstruction have shown better stability by way of the clinical pivot-shift test, which may have examiner variability, but comparable objective results on KT1000 stability testing of anterior laxity.[10,11] Notably, outcome measures such as the IKDC scores are similar for both procedures.[12] It certainly would be helpful if a consistent rotational testing device became available that could be used in the office to easily and reliably compare rotational knee stability to objectively document whether there is truly enhanced rotational stability with a double-bundle reconstruction. A recent study used MRI to demonstrate that double-bundle constructs are rotationally more stable than single-bundle reconstructions, although this type of testing is both expensive and cumbersome.[13] Another recent clinical study measured three-dimensional knee kinematics and showed that double-bundle reconstruction more closely restored rotational knee kinematics than single-bundle reconstruction when results were compared with a normal control group.[14]

There is literature support for the principles of the all-inside technique, including the double-bundle procedure highlighted in this chapter. Walsh and colleagues first showed, in porcine tibias, that the RetroScrew placed intra-articularly for aperture fixation with the all-inside technique provided 678 ± 109 newtons for ultimate failure load.[15] Tsai and colleagues compared single- versus double-bundle all-inside ACL reconstructions in cadavers, and showed normal restoration of anterior translation during a simulated pivot-shift for the double-bundle construct, with the single-bundle reconstruction significantly more lax than the intact state.[16] Another important cadaver study relates directly to the specific technique for all-inside double-bundle ACL reconstruction described in this chapter. Walsh and colleagues[17] performed a biomechanical analysis in porcine tibias, comparing two sequences for tibial drilling and fixation for all-inside double-bundle ACL reconstruction. They created both tibial sockets first; passed the PL bundle graft, fixing it with a RetroScrew; then repeated this process for the AM bundle graft (2:2 method). This was compared with the creation of the PL tibial socket only with the passage and RetroScrew fixation of this bundle, followed by creation of the AM tibial socket, and then passing and fixing of the graft with the aperture RetroScrew (1:1 method). They found

that creating the PL socket only and fixing that graft separately had higher initial and ultimate failure loads and a result that was stiffer with less susceptibility to bone bridge fracture as compared with the 2:2 technique. They postulated that the superior biomechanical outcomes with the 1:1 method are a result of strain relief of the bone when the AM socket is created after the PL socket has been reamed and the PL graft fixated. Use of the RetroCutter, which has shown less aperture microfracturing than traditional outside-in tibial drilling, also likely plays an important role to further minimize the risk of tibial bone bridge fractures with the all-inside double-bundle construct.[18]

REFERENCES

1. Lubowitz J. No-tunnel anterior cruciate ligament reconstruction: The transtibial all-inside technique. *Arthroscopy.* 2006;22:900e1-900e11.
2. Smith P, Schwartzberg R, Lubowitz J. All-inside, double-bundle, anterior cruciate ligament reconstruction: A no-tunnel, 2-socket, retroconstruction technique. *Arthroscopy.* 2008;24:1184-1189.
3. Wright R, Magnussen R, Dunn W, et al. Ipsilateral graft and contralateral ACL rupture at five years or more following ACL reconstruction: A systematic review. *J Bone Joint Surg Am.* 2011;93(12):1159-1165.
4. Hui C, Salmon L, Kok A, et al. Fifteen-year outcome of endoscopic anterior cruciate ligament reconstruction with patellar tendon autograft for "isolated" anterior cruciate ligament tear. *Am J Sports Med.* 2011;39(1):89-98.
5. Ruiz AL, Kelly M, Nutton RW. Arthroscopic ACL reconstruction: a 5-9 year follow-up. *Knee.* 2002;9:197-200.
6. Girgis F, Marshall J, Monajem A. The cruciate ligaments of the knee joint. Anatomical, functional and experimental analysis. *Clin Orthop Relat Res.* 1975;106:216-231.
7. Chhabra A, Starman J, Ferretti M, et al. Anatomic, radiographic, biomechanical, and kinematic evaluation of the anterior cruciate ligament and its two functional bundles. *J Bone Joint Surg Am.* 2006;88(Supplement 4.):1-4.
8. Yagi M, Wong E, Kanamori A, et al. Biomechanical analysis of an anatomic anterior cruciate ligament reconstruction. *Am J Sports Med.* 2002;30;5:660-666.
9. Zantop T, Herbort M, Raschke M, et al. The role of the anteromedial and posterolateral bundles of the anterior cruciate ligament in anterior tibial translation and internal rotation. *Am J Sports Med.* 2007;35(2):223-227.
10. Kondo E, Yasuda K, Azuma H, et al. Prospective clinical comparisons of anatomic double-bundle versus single-bundle anterior cruciate ligament reconstruction procedures in 328 consecutive patients. *Am J Sports Med.* 2008;36:1675-1687.
11. Siebold R, Dehler C, Ellert T. Prospective randomized comparison of double-bundle versus single-bundle anterior cruciate ligament reconstruction. *Arthroscopy.* 2008;24(2):137-145.
12. Jarvela T, Moisala A, Sihvonen R, et al. Double-bundle anterior cruciate ligament reconstruction using hamstring autografts and bioabsorbable interference screw fixation. *Am J Sports Med.* 2008;36(2):290-297.

13. Izawa T, Okazaki K, Tashiro Y, et al. Comparison of rotary stability after anterior cruciate ligament reconstruction between single-bundle and double-bundle techniques. *Am J Sports Med.* 2011;39;7:1470-1477.

14. Hemmerich A, van der Merwe W, Batterham M, et al. Double-bundle ACL surgery demonstrates superior rotational kinematics to single-bundle technique during dynamic task. *Clin Biomech (Bristol, Avon).* 2011; 26(10):998-1004.

15. Walsh MP, Wijdicks CA, Parker JB, et al. A comparison between a retrograde interference screw, suture button, and combined fixation on the tibial side in an all-inside anterior cruciate ligament reconstruction. *Am J Sports Med.* 2009;37(1):160-167.

16. Tsai AG, Wijdicks CA, Walsh MP, et al. Comparative kinematic evaluation of all-inside single-bundle and double-bundle anterior cruciate ligament reconstruction: A biomechanical study. *Am J Sports Med.* 2010;38(2): 263-272.

17. Walsh MP, Wijdicks CA, Armitage BM, et al. The 1:1 versus the 2:2 tunnel-drilling technique: Optimization of fixation strength and stiffness in an all-inside double-bundle anterior cruciate ligament reconstruction-a biomechanical study. *Am J Sports Med.* 2009;37(8): 1539-1547.

18. McAdams TR, Biswal S, Stevens KJ, et al. Tibial aperture bone disruption after retrograde versus antegrade tibial tunnel drilling: A cadaveric study. *Knee Surg Sports Traumatol Arthrosc.* 2008;16:818-822.

Chapter 79

All-Inside Anterior Cruciate Ligament GraftLink Technique: Second-Generation, No-Incision Anterior Cruciate Ligament Reconstruction

James H. Lubowitz, Christopher S. Ahmad, and Kyle Anderson

Chapter Synopsis
- We describe the anatomic single-bundle, all-inside anterior cruciate ligament (ACL) GraftLink technique with use of second-generation FlipCutter guide pins that become RetroDrills, and second-generation adjustable graft loop length cortical suspensory fixation devices: femoral TightRope and tibial ACL TightRope–Reverse Tension (Arthrex, Naples, FL). The technique is minimally invasive, using only four 4-mm stab incisions. Graft choice is a no-incision allograft or a gracilis sparing, posterior semitendinosus harvest. The graft is sutured four times through each strand in a loop and linked, like a chain, to femoral and tibial adjustable TightRope graft loops. Using this method, graft tension can be increased even after graft fixation. The technique may be modified for double-bundle ACL reconstruction.[1]

Important Points

Indications
- ACL primary or revision procedure, single bundle or double bundle

Contraindications
- Failed ACL with large bone loss

Clinical and Surgical Pearls
- Graft length less than sockets plus intra-articular distance allow all-inside tensioning.
- Meticulous graft preparation is required.
- Anteromedial portal graft passage is used.
- Keep FlipCutter cannula in place after drill pin removal. Insert graft-passing suture and then remove cannula.
- Anatomic tunnel placement is used.

Clinical and Surgical Pitfalls
- Undersized sockets are not permitted because TightRope fixation flips before graft tensioning.

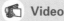 Video
- Video 79-1: All-inside anterior cruciate ligament GraftLink technique: second-generation, no-incision ACL reconstruction

An old orthopedic adage states, "The techniques that I use in the operating room now are different from the techniques I learned during my training."[1]

When it comes to modern anterior cruciate ligament (ACL) surgery, the techniques we use in the operating room today may be different from the techniques we used only 5 years ago.

Five years ago, all-inside ACL reconstruction using the no-incision technique involved use of transtibial drilling of the ACL femoral socket.[2] Unfortunately, the transtibial technique for creating the ACL femoral socket is known to be a risk factor for anatomically mismatched posterior tibial tunnel placement and high anteromedial (AM) femoral tunnel placement.[3-7] As a result, over the last 5 years some surgeons have transitioned to the AM portal technique for creating the ACL femoral tunnel.[4,6,8,9-18] This technique, however, is not without associated potential pitfalls.[4,8,9,12,13,15,16,19,20] In response to these concerns, in 2011 we recommended creating the ACL femoral socket with use of an outside-in

841

technique as an alternative to the anatomic AM portal technique.[3,5,14,15,21-23]

Historically, the outside-in technique for creating the ACL femoral socket fell out of favor because of the requirement for two-incision technique involving a lateral muscle-splitting dissection at the distal femur.[3,4,21,23] Recently, however, new technology including narrow-diameter guide pins that are transformed into retrograde drills[14,15] allows for a "no-incision" outside-in technique to create the ACL femoral socket. The advantages of an outside-in technique for creating the femoral socket include the ability of the surgeon to operate in the comfortable and familiar position of 90 degrees of knee flexion (unlike the AM portal technique), independent placement the femoral socket in an anatomic position unconstrained from drilling through the tibial tunnel, and drilling of a longer socket than with the AM portal technique.[15] In addition, outside-in drilling allows for measurement of the femoral interosseous distance before socket creation with use of standard, outside-in femoral guides and guide pin sleeves. Premeasurement of the socket depth is a safety feature of the outside-in technique because a short tunnel may necessitate that less graft tissue be contained within the femoral socket.[24]

In addition to the use of retrograde drilling pins, two additional technical developments simplify all-inside ACL reconstruction. The first development represents an evolution of cortical suspensory fixation button devices. First-generation cortical suspensory fixation buttons have fixed length graft loops, whereas second-generation cortical suspensory fixation buttons have graft loops that are adjustable in length, such that after the button flips on the cortex, the graft loop may be tightened. This pulls the graft into the socket to completely fill the socket with graft substance. Whereas the first-generation cortical suspensory fixation buttons were designed for femoral fixation, the second-generation adjustable graft loop buttons are also effective for tibial fixation. In addition, the second-generation adjustable graft loop buttons allow for an increase in graft tension while the loop is tightened, allowing the ACL surgeon for the first time to adjust graft tension even after the graft has been fixed in place.

The second important technical development that simplifies all-inside ACL reconstruction is the use of cannulas. Arthroscopic shoulder and hip surgeons have long understood the importance of cannulas for maintaining portals and preventing soft tissue from becoming intertwined in sutures. As a result, we recommend the use of a cannula in the AM arthroscopic instrumentation portal to prevent soft tissue interposition. Furthermore, we introduced a unique guide pin sleeve that transforms into a cannula to maintain access to the narrow-diameter guide pin tracks used to create all-inside sockets, allowing for suture passage and for later graft passage after ACL socket retroconstruction.[1]

PREOPERATIVE CONSIDERATIONS

Indications

- ACL primary or revision procedure: single bundle or double bundle

Contraindications

- Failed ACL with large bone loss

SURGICAL TECHNIQUE

No-tunnel, all-inside socket ACL reconstruction via GraftLink requires learning new techniques for graft preparation, socket creation, and graft fixation. In terms of graft preparation, several important factors must be considered, including incisional cosmesis in selection of a graft source, creation of a graft with a length that is less than the sum of the socket lengths plus the intra-articular graft distance to ensure that the graft does not bottom out in the sockets during final graft tensioning, and learning the GraftLink preparation technique. Femoral and tibial socket creation is performed with second-generation retrodrilling guide pins, and femoral and tibial fixation is completed with second-generation cortical suspensory fixation devices that allow for tensioning with an adjustable graft loop. Our preferred technique is illustrated in Video 79-1.

Special Equipment

- *Graft preparation station and high-strength suture.* High-strength sutures (FiberWire, Arthrex, Naples, FL) secure the graft in a loop. The loop is sewn in linkage with an ACL femoral TightRope adjustable graft loop (Arthrex) and with an ACL tibial reverse TightRope adjustable graft loop (Arthrex; Figs. 79-1 and 79-2). A graft preparation station facilitates

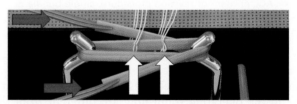

Figure 79-1. The graft is first loaded in linkage with anterior cruciate ligament (ACL) femoral and tibial tightropes *(white arrows)*. Graft free ends are held by hemostats *(red arrows)* and then wrapped around the hooks *(silver)* on a graft preparation station set to graft length (before tensioning) of approximately 65 mm. *(From Lubowitz JH, Ahmad C, Anderson K. All-inside anterior cruciate ligament graft-link technique: Second-generation, no-incision anterior cruciate ligament reconstruction. Arthroscopy. 2011;27:717-727.)*

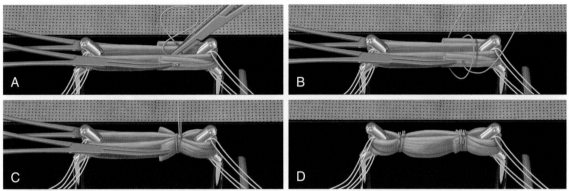

Figure 79-2. GraftLink suture technique. **A,** The graft is loaded in linkage with anterior cruciate ligament (ACL) femoral and tibial tightropes (white suture loops at far left and far right of graft loop). Graft ends are held by hemostats, and wrapped around hooks (silver) of graft preparation station. High-strength suture (No. 2) is passed through the center of each strand of the looped graft. **B,** Suture free ends are crossed and wrapped around the graft. **C,** First wrapped suture is tied in a wrapped cinch. **D,** A second suture is tied in a similar manner immediately next to the first suture (both shown tied and cut). Two additional sutures are placed, cinching the other side of the graft (graft far left). The final construct shown is a graft linked with ACL femoral tightrope on the left, and ACL tibial tightrope-reverse tension on the right. *(From Lubowitz JH, Ahmad C, Anderson K. All-inside anterior cruciate ligament graft-link technique: Second-generation, no-incision anterior cruciate ligament reconstruction. Arthroscopy. 2011;27:717-727.)*

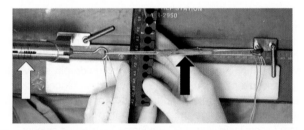

Figure 79-3. The final construct is attached to a spring-loaded tensioning device *(white arrow).* The tension is set to approximately 40 N *(white arrow).* The typical ultimate length of the graft *(black arrow)* is 75 mm after tensioning. The construct shown is a graft linked with an anterior cruciate ligament (ACL) femoral tightrope on the hook of the tensioning device *(left)* and with an ACL tibial tightrope reverse tension on fixed hook of the graft preparation station *(right).* The surgeon holds the graft diameter sizing block and measures in 0.5-mm sizing increments. *(From Lubowitz JH, Ahmad C, Anderson K. All-inside anterior cruciate ligament graft-link technique: Second-generation, no-incision anterior cruciate ligament reconstruction. Arthroscopy. 2011;27:717-727.)*

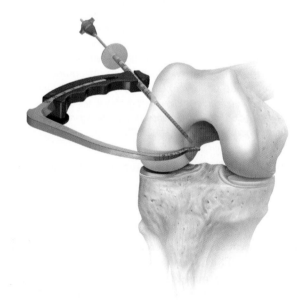

Figure 79-4. Right knee. Second-generation retrograde drill (FlipCutter), and anterior cruciate ligament femoral guide with marking hook. Guide illustrated in anterolateral portal position. Note that the guide pin sleeve has a 7-mm step-off tip that is impacted over the pin into the bony cortex. Flipping a switch on the handle (top) of the FlipCutter will change the guide pin into a retrograde drill. *(From Lubowitz JH, Ahmad C, Anderson K. All-inside anterior cruciate ligament graft-link technique: Second-generation, no-incision anterior cruciate ligament reconstruction. Arthroscopy. 2011;27:717-727.)*

suturing of the graft at a specific length (approximately 65 mm). After suturing, pretensioning of the graft construct results in an ultimate graft length of approximately 75 mm (Fig. 79-3).

• *FlipCutter.* The FlipCutter (Arthrex) is a second-generation retrograde drill. The FlipCutter guide pin becomes a retrograde drill when a switch on the pin handle is flipped. The socket is created with clockwise drilling and retrograde pressure. After use, the FlipCutter retrograde drill is switched back into a guide pin and removed. The FlipCutter is 3.5 mm in diameter to allow for creation of the femoral (Figs. 79-4 and 79-5) and tibial socket (Figs. 79-6 and

79-7) through portal-sized stab incisions for a cosmetic all-inside technique.

• *FlipCutter guide pin sleeve.* The FlipCutter is drilled through a unique graduated-tip guide pin sleeve. The tip of the drill sleeve is stepped with a 7-mm-long

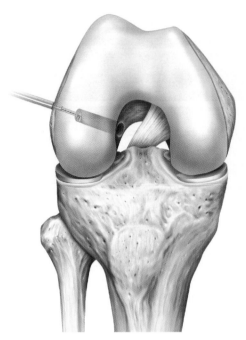

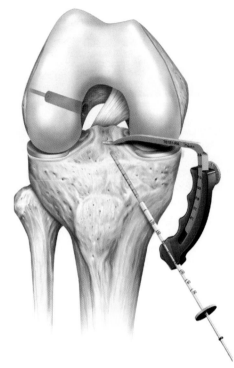

Figure 79-5. Right knee. Second-generation retrograde drill (FlipCutter) creates anterior cruciate ligament femoral socket. Note that the guide pin sleeve has a 7-mm step-off tip impacted over the pin into the bony cortex. Once socket creation is complete, flipping a switch on the handle of the FlipCutter will change the retrograde drill back into a guide pin. *(From Lubowitz JH, Ahmad C, Anderson K. All-inside anterior cruciate ligament graft-link technique: Second-generation, no-incision anterior cruciate ligament reconstruction. Arthroscopy. 2011;27:717-727.)*

Figure 79-6. Right knee. Second-generation retrograde drill (FlipCutter) and anterior cruciate ligament tibial guide with marking hook. Guide illustrated in anteromedial portal position. Cannulated 7-mm step-off tip guide pin sleeve is impacted over the pin into the bony cortex. Once socket creation is complete, flipping a switch on the handle of the FlipCutter will change the guide pin into a retrograde drill. *(From Lubowitz JH, Ahmad C, Anderson K. All-inside anterior cruciate ligament graft-link technique: Second-generation, no-incision anterior cruciate ligament reconstruction. Arthroscopy. 2011;27:717-727.)*

narrow tip. The tip of the cannula is tapped into the distal lateral femoral cortex over the FlipCutter and subsequently into the proximal AM tibial metaphysis. When the tip is advanced to the 7 mm mark, it reaches palpable resistance to further tip advancement because during creation of the retrograde socket the FlipCutter is withdrawn until it stops at the tip of the metal guide pin sleeve. In addition, laser marks on the guide pin sleeve allow for observation of the 7-mm tap-in distance. The 7-mm sleeve protects and preserves a 7-mm cortical bridge and results in the creation of sockets, not full tunnels, on both the femoral and tibial graft sites. Cortical preservation is required for cortical suspensory fixation with a second-generation adjustable graft loop (see Figs. 79-4 to 79-7). After the FlipCutter has been removed, the sleeve is left in place to serve as a cannula and to facilitate simple and reproducible passage of graft-passing sutures and for the graft itself (Fig. 79-8).

- *Passport cannula.* The use of a flexible, silicone cannula (Passport, Arthrex) in the AM arthroscopic portal facilitates all-inside ACL reconstruction by preventing soft tissue interposition. Inner and outer flanges with dams maintain cannula position and minimize fluid leakage from the larger-than-usual portal required for all-inside ACL graft passage with graft passage through the AM portal (Fig. 79-9).

- *Femoral fixation with ACL TightRope.* The ACL TightRope is a second-generation adjustable graft loop suspensory fixation device. The adjustable graft loop has a four-point, knotless locking mechanism that relies on multiple points of friction to create self-reinforcing resistance to slippage under tensioning. The adjustable graft loop decreases in size under tensioning of the free ends or "pull sutures," in effect tensioning the graft into the sockets. Because the TightRope loop is adjustable and "one size fits all," this leads to an overall reduction in inventory and makes first-generation loop calculations required to select the proper length obsolete. The second-generation adjustable loop length technique allows optimal potential for graft-to-socket healing because graft collagen is pulled fully into the socket while the graft loop is tightened.

- *ACL Tightrope–Reverse Tension (ACL TR-RT).* ACL TR-RT is a second-generation adjustable graft

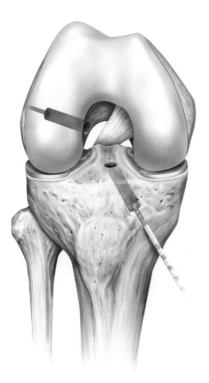

Figure 79-7. Right knee. Second-generation retrograde drill (FlipCutter) creates anterior cruciate ligament tibial socket. Note that the guide pin sleeve has a 7-mm step-off tip impacted over the pin into the bony cortex. Once socket creation is complete, flipping a switch in the handle of the FlipCutter will change the retrograde drill back into a guide pin. *(From Lubowitz JH, Ahmad C, Anderson K. All-inside anterior cruciate ligament graft-link technique: Second-generation, no-incision anterior cruciate ligament reconstruction. Arthroscopy. 2011;27:717-727.)*

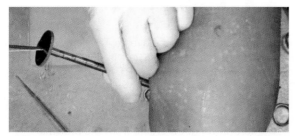

Figure 79-8. Right knee. The femoral socket has been retrodrilled, and the FlipCutter has been removed. Note that the FlipCutter guide pin sleeve has been impacted into the femoral cortex and is held in place (surgeon's gloved and hand). FiberStick suture is loaded into the cannula *(left)*. The FiberStick suture is passed into the joint and retrieved via the anteromedial arthroscopic portal. The femoral graft-passing FiberStick suture is docked and then later retrieved for final anterior cruciate ligament femoral graft passage. *(From Lubowitz JH, Ahmad C, Anderson K. All-inside anterior cruciate ligament graft-link technique: Second-generation, no-incision anterior cruciate ligament reconstruction. Arthroscopy. 2011;27:717-727.)*

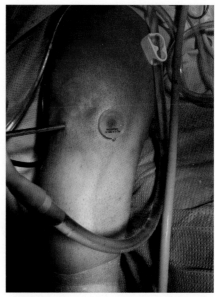

Figure 79-9. Right knee. Flexible, silicone cannula (Passport; *blue*) in the anteromedial arthroscopic portal prevents soft tissue interposition. Inner (not visible) and outer (illustrated) flanges with dams maintain cannula position and minimize fluid leakage from the larger than usual portal required for all-inside anterior cruciate ligament graft passage via the anteromedial portal. The arthroscope *(silver)* is in the anterolateral portal. *(From Lubowitz JH, Ahmad C, Anderson K. All-inside anterior cruciate ligament graft-link technique: Second-generation, no-incision anterior cruciate ligament reconstruction. Arthroscopy. 2011;27:717-727.)*

loop suspensory fixation device. The tibial Tight-Rope is identical to the femoral TightRope with the exception of reversed pull sutures. After the tibial TightRope has been reverse-tensioned with use of the respective free ends of the pull sutures, these free ends are tied over the tibial button with an arthroscopic knot-pushing device for backup fixation and protection of the implant when the pull sutures are cut. Figure 79-10 illustrates the ACL TightRope and ACL TR-RT techniques.

Specific Steps

Box 79-1 outlines the specific steps of this procedure.

Graft Length

All-inside ACL reconstruction results in bone sockets but not full bone tunnels. For the graft to be properly tensioned, it must not bottom out in the sockets, so the graft length must be less than the sum of femoral socket length plus the intra-articular graft distance plus the tibia socket length.[2] As a general guideline, the graft length should be no more than 75 mm after tensioning, with subsequent adjustments in length based on patient size (see Fig. 79-3).

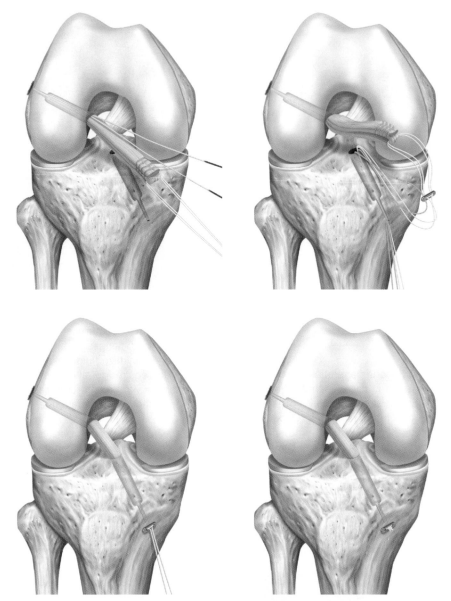

Figure 79-10. Right knee. Anterior cruciate ligament (ACL) tightrope and ACL TightRope–Reverse Tension (TR-RT). In all four illustrations, the lateral femoral cortical suspensory button is flipped. Upper left drawing: Graft is illustrated entering the joint via the anteromedial portal position. Tibial side of graft loop is shown linked to ACL TR-RT *(right, white sutures)*. Emerging superior to the graft from the femoral socket are the ACL femoral tightrope pull sutures *(white with dark blue ends)*. The pull sutures remove the slack from the TightRope's adjustable graft loop, fully seating the graft in the femoral socket. Upper right drawing: Graft is illustrated entering the joint via the anteromedial portal position. Tibial ACL TR-RT passing sutures and pull sutures are passed into the tibial socket. Lower left drawing: Emerging from the proximal anteromedial tibial metaphysis *(bottom right)* are the ACL TR-RT pull sutures *(white)*. The pull sutures remove the slack from the ACL TR-RT's adjustable graft loop, tensioning the graft in the tibial socket over the cortical button *(silver)* which is shown flipped on the metaphysis. Lower right drawing: All-inside, GraftLink, double-TightRope ACL. The tibial ACL TR-RT pull sutures have been tied and cut. *(From Lubowitz JH, Ahmad C, Anderson K. All-inside anterior cruciate ligament graft-link technique: Second-generation, no-incision anterior cruciate ligament reconstruction. Arthroscopy. 2011;27:717-727.)*

Graft Selection

Single Semitendinosus

We recommend a posterior hamstring harvest technique for semitendinosus autografts.[25] This technique is cosmetic and follows the no-incision philosophy. We recommend sparing of the gracilis tendon because if the earlier-stated recommendations for graft length are followed, in most cases the graft may be folded and tripled on itself. If the semitendinosus is short or if the graft

- Determine graft length
- Select the graft
- Prepare the graft
- Create a GraftLink construction
- Determine socket diameter
- Create the femoral socket
- Create the tibial socket
- Mark the graft
- Pass the graft
- Fix the graft
- Tension the graft
- Close the incisions

has an inadequate diameter after being tripled (less than approximately 7.5 mm), the gracilis can then be secondarily harvested.

Allograft

Indications for allograft continue to evolve. If desired and for the proper indications, a soft tissue allograft may be prepared for the GraftLink, following the no-incision cosmetic principle without harvest site morbidity.

Graft Preparation

Graft selection and graft length determination are performed as described earlier.

The two posts of an ACL graft preparation stand are positioned so that the graft length equals the planned graft length when the graft is tripled in loops around the posts and clamped. The posts should be set apart at a distance of 65 mm (see Figs. 79-1 and 79-2) to obtain an ultimate graft length of 75 mm after pretensioning (see Fig. 79-3).

The graft is baseball-stitched into loops with use of a traditional strand of No. 2 high-strength suture (see Fig. 79-2). Two sutures are placed on the tibial side of the graft, and two on the femoral side. Each stitch must pass through each strand of graft collagen, and the suture limbs are crossed and wrapped once around the collagen bundles, creating a self-reinforcing suture noose when tied.

Graft Linkage

Before the graft loop is clamped and sewn, it must be loaded to create links, like a chain (see Fig. 79-1).

We create a GraftLink construct, similar to the links in a chain, in which a femoral ACL TightRope and tibial ACL TR-RT are linked within each end of the loop (see Figs. 79-1 to 79-3).

Socket Diameter

Socket diameter should allow a snug fit with the graft to ensure biologic incorporation.

If the graft is too large, however, or the socket diameter is drilled too small, the graft can get stuck at the socket orifice after the button is flipped, representing a significant intra-operative dilemma. Potential bail-out solutions include the use of tunnel dilators or curettes to enlarge the tunnel. Alternatively, if the adjustable loop is visible, it can be cut arthroscopically to allow the button to be pulled out of the thigh with passing sutures. As a last resort, the distal lateral stab incision can be extended and the button removed through an open approach. Once the button is removed, the graft can then be retrieved and trimmed, or the socket can be redrilled to a larger size. A socket diameter sizing block that measures in 0.5-mm increments is illustrated in Figure 79-3).

Femoral Socket Creation

A soft tissue notchplasty is performed. We perform a minimal bony notchplasty if the notch orifice is stenotic.

It is essential to precisely identify the anatomic ACL footprint centrum on both the femoral and tibial sides.[3-7,10,11,13,15,19,23,26-33] We use radiofrequency through the AM instrumentation portal to mark the femoral and tibial ACL footprints so that they can be identified through both portals.

We then switch the arthroscope to the AM portal. AM portal viewing provides an improved perspective for analyzing the ACL femoral footprint anatomy. At this time we assess and adjust our previous mark to ensure precise placement of the center of the footprint.

The FlipCutter ACL femoral marking hook is then locked into the FlipCutter guide ring at an angle of approximately 100 to 110 degrees. The FlipCutter guide pin sleeve is advanced to the level of the skin to a point approximately 1 cm anterior to the posterior border of the iliotibial band and 2.5 cm proximal to the lateral femoral condyle. A stab incision is made through the skin and iliotibial band, and the cannulated guide pin sleeve for the FlipCutter is pushed down hard to bone with a blunt trocar. A laser mark indicates the femoral intraosseous distance. The guide is adjusted to optimize interosseous distance (a 32-mm distance results in a 25-mm femoral socket with a 7-mm cortical bone bridge). The FlipCutter is advanced with forward drilling into the knee. The FlipCutter handle is then loosened, and a handle switch flips the guide pin tip into RetroDrill position.

Next, the FlipCutter cannulated guide pin sleeve with the graduated 7-mm stepped tip is tapped with a mallet and advanced until resistance is felt. This indicates that the stepped tip is at the distal lateral femoral cortex and can be confirmed by viewing the 5-mm laser marks on the FlipCutter.

The guide pin sleeve is held firmly in place at the proper angle and is not removed until femoral preparation is complete.

With continued forward drilling but with retrograde force, the femoral socket is retrodrilled until the drill blade stops advancing when it contacts the guide pin sleeve tip. The FlipCutter is pushed back into the knee, flipped back into guide pin mode, and removed.

The cannulated guide pin sleeve is not removed.

A FiberStick suture (Arthrex, Naples, FL) is advanced through the cannulated guide pin sleeve, and the arthroscope is placed back through the anterolateral portal. The FiberStick suture is then retrieved through the AM portal, and the femoral graft-passing FiberStick suture is docked with a small clamp during tibial surgery. This femoral graft-passing suture is later undocked for graft passage, after the tibia has been prepared.

Femoral socket creation is illustrated in Figures 79-4, 79-5, and 79-8.

Tibial Socket Creation

With the arthroscope in the anterolateral portal, the FlipCutter ACL tibial marking hook is locked on the FlipCutter guide ring at an angle of approximately 55 to 60 degrees. Guide position and angle are optimized to maximize tibial interosseous distance so the graft does not bottom out during tensioning. A distance of at least 37 mm will result in a 30-mm socket depth with a 7-mm cortical bone bridge. Distance may be read before drilling with use of laser marks on the FlipCutter guide pin sleeve. As a preventative measure, if the distance is short, readjust the guide before drilling.

Tibial socket creation is completed with the FlipCutter by following the steps described earlier for femoral socket creation.

Tibial socket creation is illustrated in Figures 79-6 and 79-7.

Marking the Graft

The first distance that should be measured and marked on the GraftLink construct is the femoral interosseous distance. This distance is marked on the adjustable graft loop, measuring from the tip of the cortical suspensory button while the surgeon holds the button in a "pre-flipped" position. When the mark on the adjustable graft loop reaches the femoral socket orifice during graft passage, this indicates to the surgeon that the button is in the proper position to flip.

The second distance that should be measured and marked on the GraftLink construct is the length of collagen within the femoral socket, with the goal of maximizing the amount of collagen in the socket while ensuring that the graft does not bottom out during tensioning. A typical amount of collagen in the femoral socket is around 25 mm. This distance is marked on the graft itself as measured from the femoral end of the

graft. When the mark on the graft reaches the femoral socket orifice during graft passage, this indicates to the surgeon that femoral graft tensioning is complete.

These steps are then repeated for the tibial side of the graft.

Graft Passage

A cannula (Passport; see Fig. 79-9) prevents soft tissue interposition and is essential because of graft passage through the AM arthroscopic portal. Femoral and tibial graft-passing sutures are retrieved. One technical pearl is to retrieve the femoral and tibial graft-passing sutures from the AM arthroscopic portal at the same time to avoid suture tangling or soft tissue interposition. To further ensure that the sutures are not tangled, the sliding open loop suture retriever (CrabClaw, Arthrex) is used to run the length of the femoral and tibial sutures independently beginning from an intra-articular position and moving extra-articularly through the cannula (Fig. 79-11). Once the surgeon confirms that the sutures are not tangled, femoral tightrope sutures are shuttled via the AM portal to pass the graft through the AM portal and allow fixation of the graft first on the femoral side. Then the tibial sutures are shuttled and the graft is fixed on the tibial side (see Fig. 79-10).

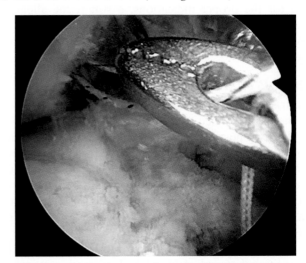

Figure 79-11. Right knee. Anterolateral portal arthroscopic view shows open loop suture retriever (CrabClaw; *silver*) grasping tibial FiberStick graft-passing suture loop *(blue)*, and the femoral graft-passing suture loop *(white with dark stripe;* TigerWire). The technical pearl is that the surgeon must retrieve the femoral and tibial graft-passing sutures from the anteromedial arthroscopic portal at the same time, as illustrated, to avoid soft tissue interposition during subsequent graft passage. Next, the open loop suture retriever runs the length of the femoral and tibial graft-passing sutures, independently, from intra-articular to extra-articular. This doubly ensures that the sutures are not tangled. *(From Lubowitz JH, Ahmad C, Anderson K. All-inside anterior cruciate ligament graft-link technique: second-generation, no-incision anterior cruciate ligament reconstruction.* Arthroscopy *2011;27:717-727.)*

Grafts up to 9.5 mm in diameter can be passed through the AM portal using a 10-mm-diameter Passport cannula. For larger-diameter grafts, the cannula should be removed before graft passage.

Graft Fixation

First we flip, then we fill.

We first shuttle the femoral graft-passing suture via the distal lateral femoral stab incision and pull the adjustable femoral graft loop into the femoral socket through the AM portal until the mark on the graft loop reaches the socket orifice under direct arthroscopic visualization. This indicates that the button has exited the femoral cortex proximally and is ready to flip.

Once the button flips, we pull hard on the graft to ensure solid femoral fixation. Next, tension is applied back and forth on each free end of the suture and on the femoral "pull suture" to seat the graft into the socket.

An advanced technique is to partially seat the femoral side of the graft and to then pass the tibial side such that the graft depth in sockets can be fine-tuned during tensioning.

The flip-then-fill technique is then repeated on the tibia side.

Remember that the tibia ACL TR-RT pull suture free ends are tied over the tibia button at the end of the procedure.

These steps are illustrated in Figure 79-10.

Graft Tensioning

The femoral and tibial pull sutures are used to tension the graft as long as the graft is prepared properly to prevent it from bottoming out in the socket; an overly long graft that bottoms out on the socket floor is not acceptable.

The knee is then taken through a range of motion, and additional tension is applied by pulling the femoral or tibial pull sutures either by hand or by use of a tensioning device on the tibial side. A reverse Lachman maneuver is performed while tension is applied.

Cosmesis

With this technique, the two 4-mm arthroscopic portals and the two 4-mm FlipCutter stab incisions are closed with 3-0 nylon. If autograft is used, the posterior hamstring harvest incision is 1 cm in length and hidden on the posterior aspect of the knee; it is closed with 3-0 nylon.

POSTOPERATIVE CONSIDERATIONS

Rehabilitation

Rehabilitation is the same as for standard ACL rehabilitation with any other technique.

Single-Bundle Versus Double-Bundle Reconstruction

The all-inside ACL GraftLink technique is versatile. The technique described earlier is for an anatomic single-bundle ACL reconstruction and can be modified for double-bundle reconstruction. We hypothesize that fixation with use of four buttons may be simpler than a first-generation all-inside × 2 reconstruction technique with use of cannulated interference screws.[18] An all-inside technique is bone sparing, and the four-button, GraftLink technique even more so; the GraftLink may be an optimal, simple, and reproducible ACL double-bundle technique modification with the advantages described earlier.[1]

Complications

In our series, one patient had a wound infection after a revision procedure that required irrigation and debridement in the second postoperative week. At the time of surgery there was purulence around the tibial button that was subsequently removed with the exposed suture material. The button was noted to have been pushed into the old tibial tunnel, likely because the FlipCutter was drilled either into or directly adjacent to an old tunnel during the revision procedure. The graft was retained and there was no evidence of septic arthritis. The patient was treated with a 6-week course of antibiotics, and the postoperative rehabilitation regimen was modified such that no open chain resisted knee extension was permitted until 12 weeks after the primary surgery. A knee immobilizer was prescribed 2 weeks after irrigation and debridement and was removed for continuous passive motion (CPM) and gentle closed chain stationary cycling (80 rpm). The patient was permitted to bear weight as tolerated.

Another complication involved a 17-year-old patient who was noncompliant with the postoperative rehabilitation protocol and developed knee laxity in the anteroposterior plane after performing squats of more than 400 pounds during the second through sixth postoperative weeks.

RESULTS

Of approximately 75 primary and revision ACL GraftLink procedures with 6-month follow-up, there were two complications, including one wound infection and one knee with increased laxity. In the opinion of the author (Level V evidence), the outcomes of the technique with regard to stability thus far seem superior to those of any other technique practiced during his first 15½ years of practice.

SUMMARY

We describe anatomic single-bundle, all-inside ACL GraftLink technique with use of second-generation Flip-Cutter guide pins that become RetroDrills, and second-generation ACL adjustable graft loop length cortical suspensory fixation devices: the femoral TightRope and the tibial ACL TR-RT. The technique is minimally invasive, using only four 4-mm stab incisions. Graft choice is either no-incision allograft or a gracilis sparing, posterior semitendinosus harvest. The graft is linked to femoral and tibial adjustable TightRope graft loops and sutured four times through each strand with a wrapped stitch to an ultimate graft length of 75 mm after pretensioning. The technique may be modified for double-bundle ACL reconstruction."[1]

REFERENCES

1. Lubowitz JH, Ahmad C, Anderson K. All-Inside Anterior Cruciate Ligament Graft-Link Technique: Second-Generation, No-Incision Anterior Cruciate Ligament Reconstruction. *Arthroscopy.* 2011;27:717-727.
2. Lubowitz JH. No-tunnel anterior cruciate ligament reconstruction: the transtibial all-inside technique. *Arthroscopy.* 2006;22:900i.e1-900.e11.
3. Abebe ES, Moorman CT 3rd, Dziedzic TS, et al. Femoral tunnel placement during anterior cruciate ligament reconstruction: an in vivo imaging analysis comparing transtibial and 2-incision tibial tunnel-independent techniques. *Am J Sports Med.* 2009;37(10):1904-1911.
4. Bedi A, Musahl V, Steuber V, et al. Transtibial Versus Anteromedial Portal Reaming in Anterior Cruciate Ligament Reconstruction: An Anatomic and Biomechanical Evaluation of Surgical Technique. *Arthroscopy.* 2010.
5. Marchant BG, Noyes FR, Barber-Westin SD, et al. Prevalence of nonanatomical graft placement in a series of failed anterior cruciate ligament reconstructions. *Am J Sports Med.* 2010;38(10):1987-1996.
6. Steiner M. Independent drilling of tibial and femoral tunnels in anterior cruciate ligament reconstruction. *J Knee Surg.* 2009;22:171-176.
7. Zantop T, Kubo S, Petersen W, et al. Current techniques in anatomic anterior cruciate ligament reconstruction. *Arthroscopy.* 2007;23:938-947.
8. Baer G, Fu F, Shen W, et al. Effect of Knee Flexion Angle on Tunnel Length and Articular Cartilage Damage During Anatomic Double-Bundle Anterior Cruciate Ligament Reconstruction. *Arthroscopy.* 2008;24S:e31.
9. Basdekis G, Abisafi C, Christel P. Influence of Knee Flexion Angle on Femoral Tunnel Characteristics When Drilled Through the Anteromedial Portal During Anterior Cruciate Ligament Reconstruction. *Arthroscopy.* 2008;24: 459-464.
10. Bottoni CR. Anterior Cruciate Ligament Femoral Tunnel Creation by Use of Anteromedial Portal. *Arthroscopy.* 2008;24:1319.
11. Bottoni CR, Rooney CR, Harpstrite JK, et al. Ensuring accurate femoral guide pin placement in anterior cruciate ligament reconstruction. *Am J Orthop.* 1998;28: 764-766.
12. Golish S, Baumfeld J, Schoderbek R, et al. The Effect of Femoral Tunnel Starting Position on Tunnel Length in Anterior Cruciate Ligament Reconstruction: A Cadaveric Study. *Arthroscopy.* 2007;23:1187-1192.
13. Harner C, Honkamp N, Ranawat A. Anteromedial Portal Technique for Creating the Anterior Cruciate Ligament Femoral Tunnel. *Arthroscopy.* 2008;24:113-115.
14. Kim S, Kurosawa H, Sakuraba K, et al. Development and Application of an Inside-to-Out Drill Bit for Anterior Cruciate Ligament Reconstruction. *Arthroscopy.* 2005;21: 1012.e1-1012.e4.
15. Lubowitz JH, Konicek J. Anterior cruciate ligament femoral tunnel length: cadaveric analysis comparing anteromedial portal versus outside-in technique. *Arthroscopy.* 2010;26(10):1357-1362.
16. Neven E, D'Hooghe P, Bellemans J. Double-Bundle Anterior Cruciate Ligament Reconstruction: A Cadaveric Study on the Posterolateral Tunnel Position and Safety of the Lateral Structures. *Arthroscopy.* 2008;24: 436-440.
17. Smith P. An alternative method for "All-inside" anterior cruciate ligament reconstruction. *Arthroscopy.* 2006;22: 451.
18. Smith P, Schwartzberg R, Lubowitz J. All-inside, double-bundle, anterior cruciate ligament reconstruction: a no tunnel, 2-socket, Retroconstruction technique. *Arthroscopy.* 2008;24:1184-1189.
19. Lubowitz J. Anteromedial Portal Technique for the Anterior Cruciate Ligament Femoral Socket: Pitfalls and Solutions. *Arthroscopy.* 2009;25:95-101.
20. Nakamura M, Deie M, Shibuya H, et al. Potential Risks of Femoral Tunnel Drilling Through the Far Anteromedial Portal: A Cadaveric Study. *Arthroscopy.* 2009;25: 481-487.
21. Harner C, Marks P, Fu F, et al. Anterior cruciate ligament reconstruction: endoscopic versus two- incision technique. *Arthroscopy.* 1994;10:502-512.
22. Puddu G, Cerullo G. My technique in femoral tunnel preparation: the "Retro-Drill" technique. *Tech Orthop.* 2005;20:224-227.
23. Yu J, Garrett W. Femoral Tunnel Placement in Anterior Cruciate Ligament Reconstruction. *Oper Tech Sports Med.* 2009;14:45-49.
24. Zantop T, Ferretti M, Bell K, et al. Effect of Tunnel-Graft Length on the Biomechanics of Anterior Cruciate Ligament-Reconstructed Knees Intra-articular Study in a Goat Model. *Am J Sports Med.* 2008;36:2158-2166.
25. Prodromos CC, Han YS, Keller BL, et al. Posterior mini-incision technique for hamstring anterior cruciate ligament reconstruction graft harvest. *Arthroscopy.* 2005;21: 130-137.
26. Colombet P, Robinson J, Christel P, et al. Morphology of Anterior Cruciate Ligament Attachments for Anatomic Reconstruction: A Cadaveric Dissection and Radiographic Study. *Arthroscopy.* 2006;22:984-992.
27. Ho J, Gardiner A, Shah V, et al. Equal Kinematics Between Central Anatomic Single-Bundle and Double-Bundle Anterior Cruciate Ligament Reconstructions. *Arthroscopy.* 2009;25:464-472.

28. Kaz R, Starman JS, Fu FH. Anatomic double-bundle anterior cruciate ligament reconstruction revision surgery. *Arthroscopy.* 2007;23:1250.e1-1250.e3.

29. Lubowitz J, Poehling G. Watch your footprint: anatomic ACL reconstruction. *Arthroscopy.* 2009;25:1059-1060.

30. Petersen W, Zantop T. Anatomy of the anterior cruciate ligament with regard to its two bundles. *Clin Orthop Relat Res.* 2007;454:35-47.

31. Pombo M, Shen W, Fu F. Anatomic Double-Bundle Anterior Cruciate Ligament Reconstruction: Where Are We Today? *Arthroscopy.* 2008;24:1168-1177.

32. Siebold R, Ellert T, Metz S, et al. Tibial insertions of the anteromedial and posterolateral bundles of the anterior cruciate ligament: morphometry, arthroscopic landmarks, and orientation model for bone tunnel placement. *Arthroscopy.* 2008;24:154-161.

33. Siebold R, Ellert T, Metz S, et al. Femoral insertions of the anteromedial and posterolateral bundles of the anterior cruciate ligament: Morphometry and arthroscopic orientation models for double-bundle bone tunnel placement-A cadaver study. *Arthroscopy.* 2008;24:585-592.

Chapter 80

Transtibial Tunnel Posterior Cruciate Ligament Reconstruction

Gregory C. Fanelli

Chapter Synopsis

- The keys to successful posterior cruciate ligament (PCL) reconstruction are to identify and treat all pathology, use strong graft material, accurately place tunnels in anatomic insertion sites, minimize graft bending, use a mechanical graft tensioning device, use primary and backup graft fixation, and employ the appropriate postoperative rehabilitation program. Adherence to these technical principles results in successful single- and double-bundle arthroscopic transtibial tunnel PCL reconstruction based on stress radiography, arthrometer readings, knee ligament rating scales, and patient satisfaction measurements.

Important Points

- PCL surgical reconstructions may be unsuccessful because of failure to recognize and treat associated ligament instabilities (posterolateral instability and posteromedial instability), failure to treat varus osseous malalignment, and incorrect tunnel placement. The double-bundle double–femoral-tunnel transtibial tunnel PCL reconstruction approximates the anatomy of the PCL by reconstructing the anterolateral and the posteromedial bundles of the PCL. This double-bundle reconstruction more closely approximates the broad femoral insertion of the PCL, enhancing the biomechanics of the PCL reconstruction. Although the double-bundle double–femoral-tunnel transtibial tunnel PCL reconstruction does not perfectly reproduce the normal PCL, there are certain factors that lead to success with this surgical technique:
  - Identification and treatment of all pathology (especially posterolateral and posteromedial instability)
  - Accurate tunnel placement
  - Anatomic graft insertion sites
  - Strong graft material
  - Minimization of graft bending
  - Final tensioning at 70 to 90 degrees of knee flexion

- Graft tensioning with a mechanical tensioning device
- Primary and backup fixation
- Appropriate rehabilitation program

Surgical Pearls

Surgical Steps

- Creation of the posteromedial safety incision
- Elevation of the posterior capsule
- Tibial tunnel drill guide positioning
- Tibial tunnel drilling
- Inside to outside femoral tunnel double-bundle aimer positioning
- Inside to outside femoral tunnel drilling
- Graft passage
- Mechanical graft tensioning and fixation
- Additional surgery (anterior cruciate ligament [ACL] reconstruction, posterolateral reconstruction, posteromedial reconstruction)

Clinical and Surgical Pitfalls

- PCL surgical reconstructions may be unsuccessful because of the following:
  - Failure to recognize and treat associated ligament instabilities (posterolateral instability and posteromedial instability).
  - Failure to treat varus osseous malalignment.
  - Incorrect tunnel placement.
- Neurovascular injury may occur during transtibial tunnel drilling. This is avoided by use of the posteromedial safety incision. The posteromedial safety incision enables the surgeon to do the following:
  - Protect the neurovascular structures.
  - Confirm the accuracy of the tibial tunnel placement.
  - Facilitate the flow of the surgical procedure.

Posterior cruciate ligament (PCL) surgical reconstructions may be unsuccessful because of failure to recognize and treat associated ligament instabilities (posterolateral instability and posteromedial instability), failure to treat varus osseous malalignment, and incorrect tunnel placement.[1-3] The keys to successful PCL reconstruction are to identify and treat all pathology, use strong graft material, accurately place tunnels in anatomic insertion sites, minimize graft bending, use a mechanical graft tensioning device, use primary and backup graft fixation, and employ the appropriate postoperative rehabilitation program. Adherence to these technical points results in successful single- and double-bundle arthroscopic transtibial tunnel PCL reconstruction documented with stress radiography, arthrometer readings, knee ligament rating scales, and patient satisfaction measurements.[4-10] This chapter illustrates my surgical technique of the arthroscopic double-bundle double–femoral tunnel transtibial tunnel PCL reconstruction surgical procedure.

PREOPERATIVE CONSIDERATIONS

History and Physical Examination

The typical history of a patient with a PCL injury includes a direct blow to the proximal tibia with the knee in 90 degrees of flexion. Hyperflexion, hyperextension, and a direct blow to the proximal medial or lateral tibia in varying degrees of knee flexion as well as a varus or valgus force will induce PCL-based multiple-ligament knee injuries. Physical examination of the injured knee compared with the noninjured knee reveals a decreased tibial step-off and a positive result of the posterior drawer test. Because concomitant collateral ligament injury is common (posterolateral and posteromedial corner injuries), posterolateral and posteromedial drawer tests, dial tests, and external rotation recurvatum tests may elicit abnormal results; varus and valgus laxity and even anterior laxity may be present.[11,12] Diagnostic features of different types and combinations of PCL injuries are as follows.

Isolated Posterior Cruciate Ligament Injury
- Abnormal posterior laxity of less than 5 mm
- Abnormal posterior laxity that decreases with tibial internal rotation
- No abnormal varus
- Abnormal external rotation of the tibia on the femur of less than 5 degrees compared with the uninvolved side, tested with the knee at 30 degrees and 90 degrees of knee flexion

Posterior Cruciate Ligament Injury and Posterolateral Corner Injury
- Abnormal posterior laxity of more than 10 mm with a negative tibial step-off
- Abnormal varus rotation at 30 degrees of knee flexion—variable and depends on the posterolateral instability grade
- Abnormal external rotation thigh-foot angle of more than 10 degrees compared with the normal lower extremity, tested at 30 degrees and 90 degrees of knee flexion—If the examiner can see the difference, then posterolateral ligament injury exists.
- Posterolateral drawer test result positive

Combined Anterior Cruciate Ligament and Posterior Cruciate Ligament Injuries
- Grossly abnormal anterior-posterior tibial-femoral laxity at both 25 degrees and 90 degrees of knee flexion
- Positive Lachman and pseudo-Lachman test results
- Positive pivot-shifting phenomenon
- Negative tibial step-off (posterior sag)
- Increased varus-valgus laxity in full extension

Imaging Studies

Radiography

Plain radiographs to evaluate PCL injuries include the following views:

- Anteroposterior weight-bearing view of both knees
- 30-degree flexion lateral view
- Intercondylar notch view
- 30-degree axial view of the patella
- Stress views at 90 degrees of knee flexion of both knees

Other Modalities

Magnetic resonance imaging is helpful in acute injuries, but we have found it to be less beneficial in chronic PCL injuries. Bone scan is used in patients with chronic PCL instability with pain to define early degenerative joint disease.

Indications and Contraindications

My indications for surgical treatment of acute PCL injuries include insertion site avulsions, a decrease in tibial step-off of 8 mm or greater, and PCL tears combined with other structural injuries. My indications for surgical treatment of chronic PCL injuries are when an isolated PCL tear becomes symptomatic and when progressive functional instability develops. Contraindications include poor skin condition, uncorrected bony malalignment, severe degenerative joint disease, and medical conditions that prevent surgical intervention.

SURGICAL TECHNIQUE
Graft Selection

My preferred graft source for PCL reconstruction is allograft tissue. The anterolateral bundle of the PCL is reconstructed with Achilles tendon allograft, and the posteromedial bundle of the PCL is reconstructed with tibialis anterior allograft tissue.

Specific Steps

Box 80-1 outlines the specific steps of this procedure.

The patient is positioned on the operating table in the supine position, and the surgical and nonsurgical knees are examined with the patient under general or regional anesthesia. A tourniquet is applied to the operative extremity, and the surgical leg is prepared and draped in a sterile fashion. Allograft tissue is prepared before the surgical procedure is begun. Standard arthroscopic knee portals are used. The joint is thoroughly evaluated arthroscopically, and the PCL is evaluated via the three-zone arthroscopic technique.[11] The PCL tear is identified, and the residual stump of the PCL is debrided with hand tools and the synovial shaver.

An extracapsular posteromedial safety incision approximately 1.5 to 2.0 cm long is created.[4-10,13,14] The crural fascia is incised longitudinally, with precautions taken to protect the neurovascular structures. The interval is developed between the medial head of the gastrocnemius muscle and the posterior capsule of the knee joint, which is anterior. The surgeon's gloved finger is positioned so that the neurovascular structures are posterior to the finger and the posterior aspect of the joint capsule is anterior to the surgeon's finger. This technique enables the surgeon to monitor surgical instruments

such as the over-the-top PCL instruments and the PCL–anterior cruciate ligament (ACL) drill guide as they are positioned in the posterior aspect of the knee. The surgeon's finger in the posteromedial safety incision also confirms accurate placement of the guidewire before tibial tunnel drilling in the medial-lateral and proximal-distal directions (Fig. 80-1). This is the same anatomic surgical interval that is used in the tibial inlay posterior approach.

The curved over-the-top PCL instruments (Biomet Sports Medicine, Warsaw, IN) are used to elevate the posterior knee joint capsule away from the tibial ridge on the posterior aspect of the tibia. This capsular elevation enhances correct drill guide and tibial tunnel placement (Fig. 80-2).

The arm of the PCL-ACL Drill Guide (Biomet Sports Medicine) is inserted into the knee through the inferior medial patellar portal and positioned in the PCL fossa on the posterior tibia (Fig. 80-3). The bullet portion of the drill guide contacts the anterior medial aspect of the proximal tibia approximately 1 cm below the tibial tubercle, at a point midway between the tibial crest anteriorly and the posterior medial border of the tibia. This drill guide positioning creates a tibial tunnel that is relatively vertically oriented and has its posterior exit point in the inferior and lateral aspect of the PCL tibial anatomic insertion site. This positioning creates an angle of graft orientation such that the graft will turn two very smooth 45-degree angles on the posterior aspect of the tibia (Fig. 80-4).

The tip of the guide in the posterior aspect of the tibia is confirmed with the surgeon's finger through the

---

BOX 80-1 Surgical Steps

- Creation of the posteromedial safety incision
- Elevation of the posterior capsule
- Tibial tunnel drill guide positioning
- Tibial tunnel drilling
- Inside to outside femoral tunnel double-bundle aimer positioning
- Inside to outside femoral tunnel drilling
- Graft passage
- Mechanical graft tensioning and fixation
- Additional surgery (anterior cruciate ligament reconstruction, posterolateral reconstruction, posteromedial reconstruction)

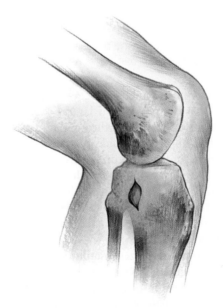

Figure 80-1. Posteromedial safety incision is used to protect the neurovascular structures, confirm the accuracy of the tibial tunnel placement, and facilitate the flow of the surgery. *(Courtesy Biomet Sports Medicine, Warsaw, IN.)*

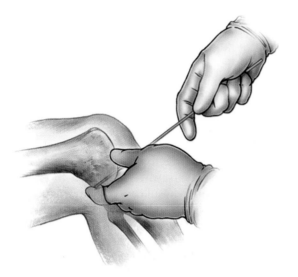

Figure 80-2. Posterior capsule elevation from the proximal tibia with use of curved posterior cruciate ligament instruments to prepare for tibial tunnel creation. *(Courtesy Biomet Sports Medicine, Warsaw, IN.)*

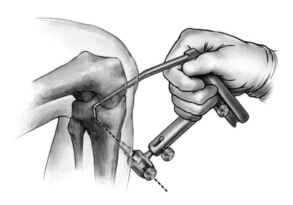

Figure 80-3. Posterior cruciate ligament drill guide positioned for creation of the posterior cruciate ligament tibial tunnel. *(Courtesy Biomet Sports Medicine, Warsaw, IN.)*

extracapsular posteromedial safety incision. Intraoperative anteroposterior (AP) and lateral radiographs may also be used, as well as arthroscopic visualization to confirm drill guide and guide pin placement. A blunt spade-tipped guidewire is drilled from anterior to posterior and can be visualized with the arthroscope, in addition to being palpated with the finger in the posteromedial safety incision. I consider the finger in the posteromedial safety incision the most important step for accuracy and safety.

The appropriately sized standard cannulated reamer is used to create the tibial tunnel. The closed curved PCL curette may be positioned to cup the tip of the guidewire. The arthroscope, when positioned in the posteromedial portal, may visualize the guidewire being captured by the curette and may help in protecting the neurovascular structures. This, in addition to the surgeon's finger in the posteromedial safety incision, helps

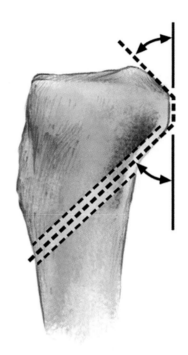

Figure 80-4. Tibial tunnel orientation to eliminate acute graft angle turns around the posterior tibia. *(Courtesy Biomet Sports Medicine, Warsaw, IN.)*

to protect the neurovascular structures. The surgeon's finger in the posteromedial safety incision is monitoring the position of the guidewire. The standard cannulated drill is advanced to the posterior cortex of the tibia. The drill chuck is then disengaged from the drill, and completion of the tibial tunnel reaming is performed by hand. This gives an additional margin of safety for completion of the tibial tunnel. The tunnel edges are chamfered and rasped with the PCL-ACL system rasp.

My preferred method is to perform a double-bundle PCL reconstruction, making the PCL femoral tunnels from inside out. The PCL single-bundle or double-bundle femoral tunnels are made from inside out with the double-bundle aimers (Biomet Sports Medicine). Insertion of the appropriately sized double-bundle aimers through a low anterior lateral patellar arthroscopic portal creates the PCL anterior lateral bundle femoral tunnel. The double-bundle aimer is positioned directly on the footprint of the femoral anterior lateral bundle PCL insertion site. The appropriately sized guidewire is drilled through the aimer, through the bone, and out a small skin incision. Care is taken to ensure there is no compromise of the articular surface. The double-bundle aimer is removed and an acorn reamer is used to endoscopically drill from inside out the anterior lateral PCL femoral tunnel. The tunnel edges are chamfered and rasped. The reaming debris is evacuated with a synovial shaver to minimize fat pad inflammatory response with subsequent risk of arthrofibrosis. The same process is repeated for the posterior medial bundle of the PCL. Care must be taken to ensure that there will be an

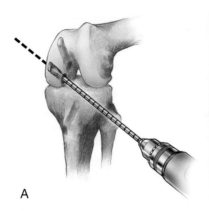
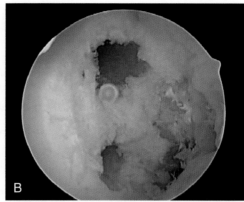

A

B

Figure 80-5. A, Creation of posterior cruciate ligament femoral tunnels from inside out through a low anterolateral arthroscopic portal. **B,** A 5-mm bone bridge is maintained between the anterolateral and posteromedial tunnels. (**A,** *Courtesy Biomet Sports Medicine, Warsaw, IN.*)

adequate bone bridge (approximately 5 mm) between the two femoral tunnels before drilling. This is accomplished with use of the calibrated probe and direct arthroscopic visualization (Fig. 80-5).

The Magellan suture-passing device, the double-bundle aimer (Biomet Sports Medicine), is introduced through the tibial tunnel and into the knee joint and is retrieved through the femoral tunnel with an arthroscopic grasping tool. The traction sutures of the graft material are attached to the loop of the Magellan suture-passing device, and the PCL graft material is pulled into position.

Fixation of the PCL graft is accomplished with primary and backup fixation on both the femoral and tibial sides. Femoral fixation is accomplished with cortical suspensory backup fixation with polyethylene ligament fixation buttons, and aperture opening fixation with the Bio-Core bioabsorbable interference screws (Biomet Sports Medicine). The mechanical graft tensioning boot (Biomet Sports Medicine) is applied to the traction sutures of the graft material on its distal end and tensioned to restore the anatomic tibial step-off. The knee is cycled through several sets of 25 full flexion-extension cycles for graft pretensioning and settling (Fig. 80-6). The PCL reconstruction graft is tensioned in physiologic knee flexion ranges. Graft fixation is achieved with primary aperture opening fixation with use of the Bio-Core bioabsorbable interference screw (Biomet Sports Medicine), and backup fixation with a ligament fixation button, screw and post, or screw and spiked ligament washer assembly (Figs. 80-7 and 80-8).

POSTOPERATIVE CONSIDERATIONS

Rehabilitation

The knee is maintained in full extension for 5 weeks of non–weight-bearing status. Progressive range of motion

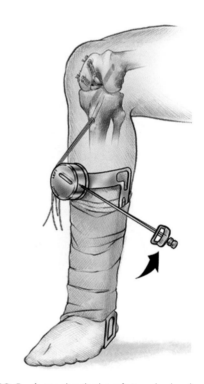

Figure 80-6. A mechanical graft tensioning boot is used for reduction of the tibia on the femur, tensioning of the posterior cruciate ligament (PCL) graft, and maintenance of reduction during PCL tibial fixation. *(Courtesy Biomet Sports Medicine, Warsaw, IN.)*

occurs during weeks 5 through 10. Progressive weight bearing occurs at the beginning of postoperative week 6, progressing at a rate of 20% body weight per week during postoperative weeks 6 through 10. Progressive closed kinetic chain strength training, proprioceptive training, and continued motion exercises are initiated very slowly beginning at postoperative week 11. The long-leg range-of-motion brace is discontinued after the tenth week, and the patient wears a PCL functional brace for all activities. Return to sports and heavy labor

TABLE 80-1. Fanelli Results

Author	Follow-up	Outcome
Fanelli and Edson[4] (2002)	2-10 years	46.0% normal posterior drawer test results and tibial step-offs, and 54.0% grade 1 posterior drawer test results and tibial step-offs in combined PCL and ACL reconstructions No Biomet graft tensioning boot was used (Biomet Sports Medicine, Warsaw, IN).
Fanelli and Edson[5] (2004)	2-10 years	70% normal posterior drawer test results and tibial step-offs for the overall study group, and 91.7% normal posterior drawer test results and tibial step-offs in the subgroup with the Biomet graft tensioning boot in combined PCL posterolateral reconstructions
Fanelli et al[8] (2005)	2 years	86.6% normal posterior drawer test results and tibial step-offs in combined PCL and ACL reconstructions in which the Biomet graft tensioning boot was used
Fanelli et al[10] (2012)	2-6 years	Both the single-bundle and the double-bundle arthroscopic transtibial tunnel PCL reconstruction surgical techniques that included use of allograft tissue and the Biomet mechanical graft tensioning boot provided successful results in PCL reconstructions in the multiple-ligament-injured knee when evaluated with stress radiography, arthrometer measurements, and knee ligament rating scales.

ACL, Anterior cruciate ligament; *PCL,* posterior cruciate ligament.

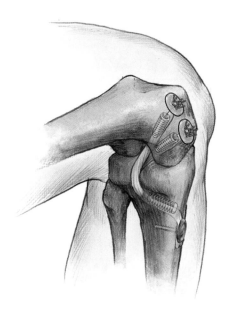

Figure 80-7. The posterior cruciate ligament graft has double fixation on each end of the graft to minimize the risk of fixation failure. *(Courtesy Biomet Sports Medicine, Warsaw, IN.)*

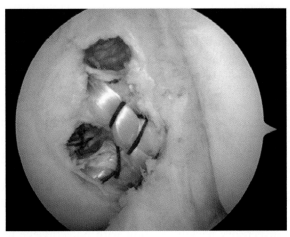

Figure 80-8. Arthroscopic view of double-bundle posterior cruciate ligament reconstruction.

occurs after the ninth postoperative month when sufficient strength, range of motion, and proprioceptive skills have returned.[15]

Complications

PCL reconstruction is technically demanding surgery. Complications encountered with this surgical procedure include failure to recognize associated ligament injuries, neurovascular complications, persistent posterior sag, osteonecrosis, loss of knee motion, anterior knee pain, and fractures. A comprehensive preoperative evaluation, including an accurate diagnosis, a well-planned and carefully executed surgical procedure, and a supervised postoperative rehabilitation program, will help reduce the incidence of these complications.

RESULTS

Both single-bundle and double-bundle PCL reconstruction surgical techniques that use allograft tissue and mechanical graft tensioning provide successful results in PCL reconstruction when evaluated with stress radiography, arthrometer measurements, and knee ligament rating scales (Table 80-1). Mechanical graft tensioning provides better static stability of the PCL reconstruction than manual graft tensioning in my experience.[4,5,8-10]

SUMMARY AND CONCLUSIONS

PCL surgical reconstructions may be unsuccessful because of failure to recognize and treat associated ligament instabilities (posterolateral instability and posteromedial instability), failure to treat varus osseous malalignment, and incorrect tunnel placement. The keys to successful PCL reconstruction are identification and treatment of all pathology, use of strong graft material, accurate placement of tunnels in anatomic insertion sites, minimization of graft bending, use of a mechanical graft tensioning device, use of primary and backup graft fixation, and employment of the appropriate postoperative rehabilitation program. Adherence to these technical details results in successful single-and double-bundle arthroscopic transtibial tunnel PCL reconstruction documented with stress radiography, arthrometer measurements, knee ligament rating scales, and patient satisfaction scores.

REFERENCES

1. Noyes FR, Barber-Westin SD. Posterior cruciate ligament revision reconstruction, part 1. *Am J Sports Med.* 2005;33 (5):646-654.
2. Robinson JR, Bull AMJ, Thomas RR, et al. The Role of the medial collateral ligament and posteromedial capsule in controlling knee laxity. *Am J Sports Med.* 2006;34(11): 1815-1823.
3. Sekiya JK, Haemmerle MJ, Stabile KJ, et al. Biomechanical analysis of a combined double bundle posterior cruciate ligament and posterolateral corner reconstruction. *Am J Sports Med.* 2005;33(3):360-369.
4. Fanelli GC, Edson CJ. Arthroscopically assisted combined ACL/PCL reconstruction. 2-10 year follow-up. *Arthroscopy.* 2002;18(7):703-714.
5. Fanelli GC, Edson CJ. Combined posterior cruciate ligament -posterolateral reconstruction with Achilles tendon allograft and biceps femoris tendon tenodesis: 2-10 year follow-up. *Arthroscopy.* 2004;20 (4):339-345.
6. Fanelli GC, Giannotti BF, Edson CJ: Arthroscopically assisted combined anterior and posterior cruciate ligament reconstruction. *Arthroscopy.* 1996;12(1):5-14.
7. Fanelli GC, Giannotti BF, Edson CJ. Arthroscopically assisted combined posterior cruciate ligament/posterior lateral complex reconstruction. *Arthroscopy.* 1996, 12(5): 521-530.
8. Fanelli GC, Edson CJ, Orcutt DR, et al. Treatment of combined ACL PCL medial lateral side injuries of the knee. *J Knee Surg.* 2005;28(3):240-248.
9. Fanelli GC, Beck JD, Edson CJ. Double bundle posterior cruciate ligament reconstruction: surgical technique and results. *Sports Med Arthrosc.* 2010, 18(4):242-248.
10. Fanelli GC, Beck JD, Edson CJ. Single compared to double bundle PCL reconstruction using allograft tissue. *J Knee Surg.* 2012;25(1):59-64.
11. Fanelli GC, Giannotti BF, Edson CJ. Current Concepts Review. The posterior cruciate ligament: arthroscopic evaluation and treatment. *Arthroscopy.* 1994;10(6): 673-688.
12. Fanelli GC, Feldmann DD. Management of combined ACL/PCL/posterolateral complex injuries of the knee. *Oper Tech Sports Med.* 1999;7(3):143-149.
13. Fanelli GC. *Rationale and surgical technique for PCL and multiple knee ligament reconstruction. Surgical technique guide.* Warsaw, IN: Biomet Sports Medicine; 2008.
14. Fanelli GC, Edson CJ, Reinheimer KN. Posterior cruciate ligament reconstruction: transtibial tunnel surgical technique. *Orthop Today.* 2007;27(2):40-46.
15. Edson CJ, Fanelli GC, Beck JD. Postoperative rehabilitation of the posterior cruciate ligament. *Sports Med Arthrosc.* 2010;18 (4):275-279.

SUGGESTED READINGS

Fanelli GC, ed. *Posterior Cruciate Ligament Injuries: A Practical Guide To Management.* New York: Springer-Verlag; 2001.

Fanelli GC, ed. *The Multiple Ligament Injured Knee. A Practical Guide to Management.* New York: Springer-Verlag; 2004.

Fanelli GC, Beck JD, Edson CJ. Current concepts review: the posterior cruciate ligament. *J Knee Surg.* 2010;23 (2):61-72.

Fanelli GC, Beck JD, Edson CJ. Arthroscopic double bundle posterior cruciate ligament reconstruction surgical technique. *J Knee Surg.* 2010;23(2):89-94.

Fanelli GC, Boyd J. How I manage PCL injuries. *Oper Tech Sports Med.* 2009;17(3):175-193.

Chapter 81

Arthroscopic Double-Bundle Tibial Inlay Posterior Cruciate Ligament Reconstruction

Alexander E. Weber and Jon K. Sekiya

Chapter Synopsis

- Multiple surgical techniques exist for the reconstruction of the posterior cruciate ligament (PCL). The purpose of this chapter is to present the double-bundle all-arthroscopic inlay technique for PCL reconstruction. Furthermore, after a literature-based review we advocate for this surgical technique as the optimal approach to restoring normal knee function after injury to the PCL.

Important Points

- Acute PCL injury results from direct knee trauma.
- In 95% of acute PCL tears there is an associated ligamentous injury (60% of these are posterolateral corner [PLC] injuries).
- A magnetic resonance imaging (MRI) study is important for confirmation of PCL injury as well as a necessity to evaluate the integrity of the PLC.

Surgical Pearls

- The anteromedial portal is placed closer to the patellar tendon than a standard portal and extended into a 2-cm arthrotomy to aid in graft passage.
- Achilles tendon allograft is the graft of choice; tendon length must be greater than 7 cm.
- Always be cognizant of the posterior neurovascular bundle; work with the knee flexed, and drill the guide pin for the tibial socket under fluoroscopic guidance.
- An advantage of the arthroscopic tibial inlay procedure is the retrograde reaming of the tibial socket, which minimizes the risk of injury to the neurovascular bundle.

- Use of the tibial inlay technique eliminates the "killer turn" phenomenon of graft attenuation in the tibial tunnel.
- The femoral tunnels are drilled via an outside-in technique that eliminates the "critical corner" and decreases graft strain.
- The anteromedial portal is converted into a mini-arthrotomy (2 cm), and a cannula is used to prevent incarceration of the graft in the fat pad during graft passage.
- The anterolateral and posteromedial bundles are fixed in 90 degrees of knee flexion.

Surgical Pitfalls

- Ensure adequate bone stock between femoral tunnels to prevent bone tunnel collapse and loss of the advantages of an anatomic double-bundle graft.
- Avascular necrosis of the medial femoral condyle can occur as a result of entry or exit of femoral tunnels within the subchondral bone.
- Loss of motion can result from errors in tunnel placement or excessive graft tensioning.
- Routine palpation of the thigh and calf is necessary to ensure that a compartment syndrome is not developing secondary to fluid extravasation.
- After graft fixation, check for full range of motion to ensure that the knee is not overconstrained.

Video

- Video 81-1: Arthroscopic double-bundle tibial inlay posterior cruciate ligament reconstruction

Posterior cruciate ligament (PCL) injuries are infrequent; however, their treatment remains a difficult clinical problem for the treating orthopedic surgeon. Although clinical outcomes of PCL deficiency are not uniformly poor, recent studies suggest that the kinematics of the PCL-deficient knee are significantly altered from the intact state.[1,2] In similar fashion to that in the anterior cruciate ligament–deficient knee, PCL deficiency redirects the forces across the knee joint.[1,2] The resultant increase in pressure in the medial and patellofemoral compartments may lead to premature and severe arthrosis.[3] In an attempt to restore normal stability to the symptomatic knee, most authors advocate reconstruction of the PCL. There are multiple surgical options for PCL reconstruction, with no gold standard technique. The purpose of this chapter is to present the clinical presentation of, diagnostic approach to, and surgical treatment for injury to the PCL. Furthermore, the technical aspect is focused on the double-bundle arthroscopic inlay surgical technique, because this surgical technique is currently the senior author's (J.K.S.) preferred technique for PCL reconstruction. After discussion of the technical aspects, by way of a review of the current literature we will discuss the advantages of the double-bundle arthroscopic inlay PCL reconstruction and provide evidence as to why this is our advocated and chosen surgical technique for reconstruction of the PCL.

PREOPERATIVE CONSIDERATIONS

History

In the acute setting there is often a history of a direct blow to the pretibial aspect of the lower extremity or a hyperextension injury to the affected knee. An effusion or swelling is often present with an acute PCL injury. A knee dislocation often results in injury to the PCL, which is likely associated with concomitant ligamentous or soft tissue injuries. In the case of severe knee trauma, 95% of patients with a PCL injury have associated ligamentous injuries. The most common associated injury is disruption of the posterolateral knee structures (approximately 60%).[4] In the case of chronic PCL injuries, patients may report pain and instability with activity.

Physical Examination

It is crucial to fully evaluate and appreciate the extent of the injury to the knee in the preoperative setting, and a thorough physical examination may accomplish this objective. Remember to address the presumably intact structures, and do not hesitate to compare the injured knee with the contralateral knee.

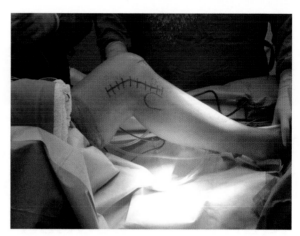

Figure 81-1. Intra-operative physical examination finding of the posterior cruciate ligament–deficient knee; a posterior sag of the right tibia in 90 degrees of flexion.

On physical examination it is crucial to assess the neurovascular status of the affected limb. This is of particular importance if there is suspicion for or history of knee dislocation. Once the neurovascular competence of the injured limb has been confirmed, inspection and palpation of the knee for effusion are performed. Next, the knee should be passively taken through a range of motion, and, if the patient is capable, passive range of motion should be compared with active range of motion. The relationship of the tibial plateau and femoral condyles as well as the natural tibial step-off can be assessed with the knee in a flexed position. The Godfrey test is used to assess for a posterior sag and is performed with the lower leg elevated and the knee flexed to 90 degrees (Fig. 81-1). A posterior drawer test is also performed in 90 degrees of flexion and can evaluate the amount of posterior tibial translation. Often with traumatic PCL injury a concomitant posterolateral corner (PLC) injury is present as well. This injury pattern can be evaluated with a reverse pivot test, dial test, posterolateral drawer test, and varus stress testing at both 30 and 90 degrees of flexion.

Radiography

Plain radiographs (anteroposterior and lateral) of the knee are helpful in that they can rule out fracture in the acute setting and medial or patellofemoral compartment arthrosis in the chronic setting. Long-leg standing films should be obtained if any fixed or dynamic instability is suspected. Posterior tibial subluxation can be evaluated on standard lateral radiographs; however, if there is any doubt, bilateral stress radiographs should be obtained (Fig. 81-2).

Other Imaging Modalities

In the setting of a chronically PCL-deficient knee, a bone scan may be useful to identify the extent of degenerative

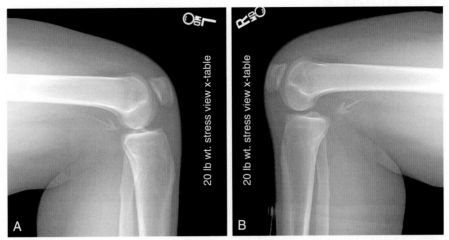

Figure 81-2. Stress radiographs of the bilateral knees. **A,** The normal anatomic position of the tibia in relation to the femur *(arrow)* in a ligamentously intact knee. **B,** Posterior tibial subluxation in relation to the femur *(arrow)* is present in a posterior cruciate ligament–deficient knee.

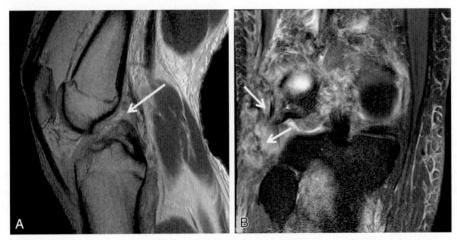

Figure 81-3. Magnetic resonance images of a patient who sustained an acute complete tear of the posterior cruciate ligament (PCL) off the femur (**A**) and a patient with a concomitant posterolateral corner injury in the presence of an acute PCL tear (**B**). Arrows demarcate the aforementioned pathology.

changes that may not be detected on plain radiographs. A magnetic resonance imaging (MRI) study is an essential part of the workup of a PCL injury, not only for confirmation of PCL injury but, more important, for the assessment of associated ligamentous injuries such as those to the PLC that will affect the operative plan and ultimately the clinical outcome (Fig. 81-3).

Indications and Contraindications

Acute isolated grade I or II PCL injuries may be treated with nonoperative, protected weight bearing and rehabilitation. Grade I or II injuries that go on to cause persistent and recurrent instability may be treated surgically. Surgically reconstructing an acute, isolated PCL tear is indicated for a grade III injury, or in the presence of a bone avulsion injury, although not all authors agree

on the existence of an isolated grade III PCL injury.[5-7] The majority of acute PCL injuries occur in conjunction with a knee dislocation or a multiligamentous injury necessitating surgical intervention. The timing of intervention remains controversial; however, an acute reconstruction is generally recommended in the presence of a bone avulsion injury or a combined ligamentous injury (especially a PLC injury).

Acute PCL reconstruction is contraindicated in the setting of a traumatic open knee injury or in the presence of a neurovascular injury requiring repair or reconstruction. Reconstruction of the PCL is contraindicated in a PCL-deficient knee with a chronic, fixed posteriorly subluxed deformity of the tibia or in the PCL-deficient knee in which significant arthrosis is present. In both of the aforementioned circumstances, the senior author recommends a biplane osteotomy rather than a soft tissue reconstruction.

SURGICAL TECHNIQUE

Overview

There are a number of surgical variables to consider before PCL reconstruction, including graft material, number of bundles, and surgical technique (transtibial versus open inlay versus arthroscopic inlay). A recent systematic review addressed the variable of number of bundles and found that although there are no clinical studies to suggest an advantage of double-bundle grafts, there are distinct biomechanical advantages to the double-bundle PCL reconstruction.[8] Most recently, the evolution of the arthroscopic inlay technique has melded the advantages of both the transtibial and open inlay techniques while negating the disadvantages of each technique. For these reasons the double-bundle arthroscopic inlay technique is the PCL reconstruction of choice for the senior author of this chapter (J.K.S.) and is presented here.

Anesthesia and Positioning

In the preoperative holding area the anesthesia team places both femoral and sciatic peripheral nerve catheters for postoperative pain management. The catheters are not to be dosed with anesthetic medication until the postoperative period because a complete postoperative neurovascular assessment is a crucial part of the procedure. The patient is then transported to the operating room and placed supine on a radiolucent table. Fluoroscopy is implemented throughout the procedure, and thus a radiolucent table is a necessity. The patient then undergoes general anesthesia and endotracheal intubation, but no long-acting paralytics are given, to ensure that all neurologic stimulation induces a response. Once the patient has been anesthetized and intubated, a thorough examination under anesthesia is performed to assess the integrity of all ligamentous and soft tissue structures of the knee (Video 81-1). The majority of the procedure is performed at 45 to 90 degrees of flexion; to facilitate these flexion angles, a sandbag is taped to the ipsilateral side of the table at the level of the contralateral heel cord (Fig. 81-4). In addition, flexing the knee, with the use of the sandbag, ensures that the contents of the popliteal fossa fall away from the posterior tibia to allow for safe arthroscopic dissection of the tibial footprint. A well-padded tourniquet is applied to the proximal thigh, although this is infrequently inflated. An advantage to working without the tourniquet is the early detection of a vascular injury if one should occur. Last, a flip-down lateral post is placed at the level of the tourniquet and set in a high position to act as a buttress for the leg.

Specific Steps

Box 81-1 outlines the specific steps of this procedure.

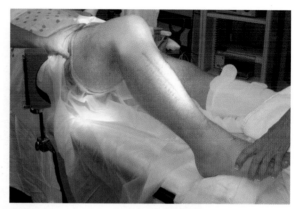

Figure 81-4. Surgical positioning for the arthroscopic inlay procedure. A sandbag or bump is secured to the radiolucent table to allow the operative knee to be ranged in the flexion arc of 45 to 90 degrees.

BOX 81-1 Surgical Steps

- Portal placement
- Creation of the tibial socket
- Graft preparation
- Femoral tunnel
- Graft passage and tibial fixation
- Femoral fixation

Portal Placement

Slight adjustments are made to the standard portal locations for this technique. A standard anterolateral (AL) portal is made, but the anteromedial (AM) portal is established in closer proximity to the patellar tendon for increased access to the posteromedial (PM) joint space. In preparation for graft passage, the AM portal is extended to a 2-cm parapatellar arthrotomy. Next the PM working portal is created. Under direct arthroscopic visualization an 18-gauge spinal needle is used to access the PM aspect of the joint on a line between the PM edge of the tibia and the femoral condyle. To maximize the portal's utility in clearing the tibial footprint, the placement should be approximately 1 cm proximal to the PM joint line.

Once the portals have been created, a thorough diagnostic arthroscopic examination is conducted. The integrity of all ligaments, menisci, and chondral surfaces is thoroughly evaluated. Most important, attention is paid to medial and or lateral compartment opening with valgus or varus stresses, which may be indicative of a PM or PLC injury. In either case a missed corner injury will jeopardize the surgical reconstruction and negatively affect clinical outcome.

Tibial Socket

With the assistance of fluoroscopy and under direct arthroscopic visualization, a PCL guide (Arthrex,

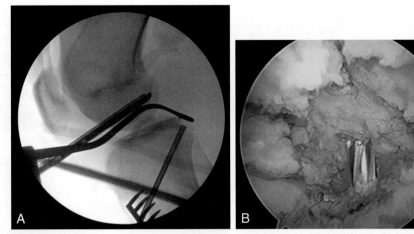

Figure 81-5. Creation of the tibial socket. **A,** Fluoroscopic image demonstrating the posterior cruciate ligament guide and the cannulated drilling of the tibial socket. **B,** Arthroscopic view confirming guide pin and drill at the targeted location 7 mm distal to the proximal edge of the footprint.

Naples, FL) is used to place a guide pin for the tibial socket. The target for insertion of the guide pin is 7 mm distal to the proximal pole of the tibial footprint. A 3.5-mm cannulated drill is used to ream over the guide pin, and the position is confirmed arthroscopically (Fig. 81-5). Care is taken to avoid plunging into the posterior structures of the knee. Two safety mechanisms are employed; the first is the reaming position, which can be confirmed fluoroscopically or with direct arthroscopic visualization, and the second is the protection afforded by the 13-mm footplate built into the drill guide. Once the tunnel has been reamed, the drill and guide pin are removed and replaced by the FlipCutter (Arthrex). The FlipCutter is advanced through the tibial tunnel until it is visualized intra-articularly with the arthroscope. Once the working end is within the joint, the blade is engaged by flipping it into a perpendicular position. A 13-mm diameter tibial socket to a depth of 10 to 12 mm is then drilled in a retrograde fashion (Fig. 81-6). The FlipCutter blade is flipped back into the upright position, and the device is withdrawn.

Graft Preparation

The current graft of choice is the Achilles tendon allograft with a minimum length of 7 cm. There is no literature to suggest a superiority of allograft or autograft either biomechanically or clinically for this surgical technique; however, the Achilles tendon natural raphe between the superficial and deep fibers facilitates the creation of two bundles (Fig. 81-7A). A No. 10 blade is used to sharply develop this interval in line with the longitudinal fibers of the graft to a distance of approximately 1 cm from the calcaneal bone block. The bundles are oriented in the anterior-to-posterior orientation with the larger bundle (8 to 11 mm) for the AL bundle and the smaller bundle (6 to 9 mm) for the PM bundle. Each bundle of the bifid graft is

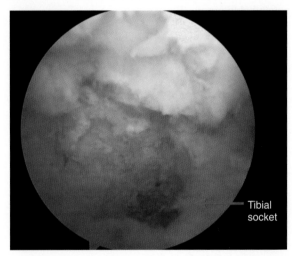

Figure 81-6. Arthroscopic image of the completed tibial socket reamed by the FlipCutter; diameter 13 mm, depth 10 to 12 mm.

whipstitched with a No. 2 braided nonabsorbable suture (Fig. 81-7B).

Attention is then turned to shaping the calcaneal bone plug. Ensuring a proper press-fit of the bone plug into the tibial socket is the key to graft stability.[9] The proper press-fit for a 13-mm socket is a cylindric 12-mm bone plug, which is created with the aid of a coring reamer or hand-whittled with a rongeur. A central tunnel is created within the bone plug and over-reamed to a diameter of 3.5 mm with a cannulated drill system (Fig. 81-8). The 1 cm of tendon left in continuity is then whipstitched with a No. 2 braided nonabsorbable suture. The free ends of this stitch are then passed through the center tunnel of the bone plug from the cortical to the cancellous side of the bone plug (Fig. 81-9). These free limbs will aid in guiding the bone plug into position before they are tied over a post or button to augment tibial fixation. Recently we have employed

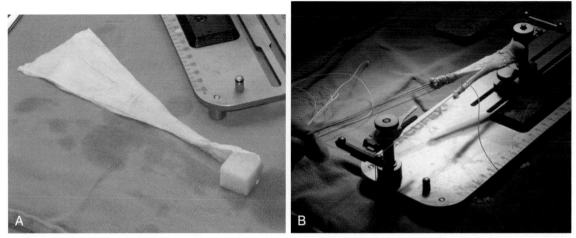

Figure 81-7. Preparation of the soft tissue segment of the tendon-bone graft. **A,** The natural raphe of the Achilles tendon allograft is appreciated before sharp dissection of the graft into two limbs. An approximately 1-cm segment of tendon is left intact at the bone edge of the graft. Each limb is whipstitched and tubularized with a No. 2 braided, nonabsorbable suture (**B**).

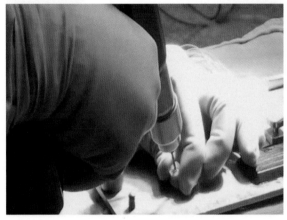

Figure 81-8. Preparation of the bone segment of the tendon-bone graft. After the cubed bone block has been sculpted into a cylinder, the central calcaneal aperture is created with the use of a 3.5-mm drill system.

the use of TightRope fixation (Arthrex, Naples, FL), which we have tested biomechanically in the laboratory. This has equivalent strength and stiffness to previous methods, with easier use and improved visualization for seating of the bone plug fluoroscopically.

Femoral Tunnel

The femoral tunnels are created with an outside-in technique. A skin incision is made anteromedially over the vastus medialis obliquus (VMO) at the level of the medial epicondyle extending in line and anterior to the intermuscular septum. The VMO is elevated and retracted with a Cobb elevator, and an S-shaped retractor is positioned over the anterior femur. Once the periosteum is exposed, the proper starting points are identified to ensure anatomic positioning of the tunnels. The ideal tunnel position for the anterior edge of the AL bundle is 1 to 2 mm off the articular margin of the

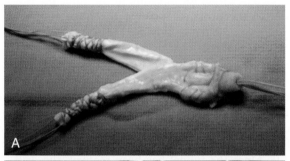

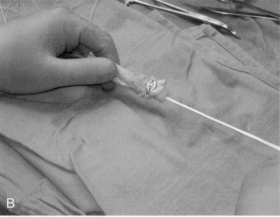

Figure 81-9. The graft is finalized by passage of a No. 2 braided, nonabsorbable suture through the remaining 1 cm of intact tendon at the bone plug end of the graft. **A,** The free limbs are then shuttled through the bone plug to aid in guiding the bone plug into the tibial socket and ultimately assisting with fixation. **B,** A new technique of tibial fixation with use of a TightRope (Arthrex).

medial femoral condyle at the 11:30 (left) or 12:30 (right) clock position. For creation of this tunnel, the guide pin is placed approximately 5 mm posterior to the articular margin (Fig. 81-10). For the PM bundle the guide pin is placed 7 mm off the articular margin at

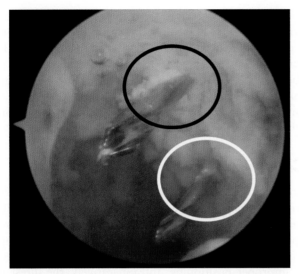

Figure 81-10. Arthroscopic confirmation of anatomic position of the femoral tunnels. The respective guide pins located in the center of the anterolateral *(black circle)* and posteromedial *(white circle)* footprints.

the 9-o'clock (left) or 3-o'clock (right) position. The edge of the drilled tunnel should lie approximately 3 mm away from the articular margin (see Fig. 81-10). Failure to maintain adequate spacing between the tunnels as a result of tunnel convergence will result in bone bridge collapse and loss of the potential benefits of a double-bundle reconstruction.

Graft Passage and Tibial Fixation

As mentioned previously, to ease the passage of the graft, the AM portal is routinely extended into a 2-cm arthrotomy. Care is taken to pass the graft and sutures cleanly through the arthrotomy and fat pad, avoiding incarceration of the graft in the fat pad. We have found that a metal cannula may be useful to guide the graft into the tibial socket. The seating of the bone plug into the tibial socket is confirmed fluoroscopically (Fig. 81-11). Once the tibial pone plug is seated, the tibial side is fixed with a post or button. More recent techniques have used the TightRope.

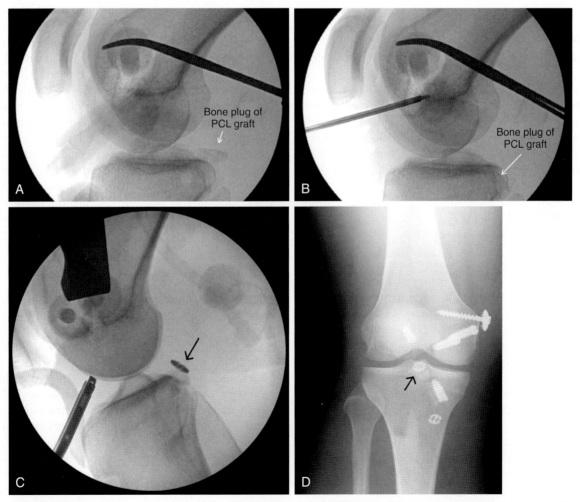

Figure 81-11. Fluoroscopic confirmation of a well-positioned tibial bone plug **(A)**. Once tension has been placed on the suture limbs, the seating of the bone plug in the tibial socket is confirmed **(B)**. When a TightRope is used, the metal button *(arrows)* can be used for confirmation of bone plug location **(C** and **D)**. *PCL,* Posterior cruciate ligament.

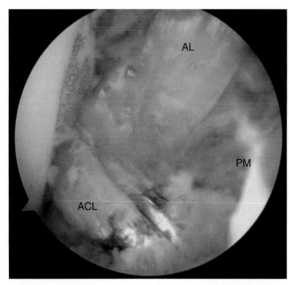

Figure 81-12. The arthroscopic appearance of a completed double-bundle arthroscopic tibial inlay posterior cruciate ligament reconstruction with a concomitant anterior cruciate ligament *(ACL)* reconstruction. *AL,* anterolateral; *PM,* posteromedial.

Femoral Fixation

After the tibial side has been secured, the femoral-sided suture limbs are retrieved through their respective bone tunnels with a looped 18-gauge wire. Before fixation of the AL and PM bundles, the knee and graft are cycled to eliminate laxity in the construct. The bundles are then tensioned at 90 degrees of flexion and fixed with bioabsorbable interference screws. The AL bundle and PM bundles are then backup fixed over a post (Fig. 81-12).

POSTOPERATIVE CONSIDERATIONS

Rehabilitation

Cryotherapy and a hinged knee brace locked in full extension are placed on the operative limb at the conclusion of the procedure. Controlled range-of-motion exercises and partial weight bearing with the operative extremity locked in extension are permissible in the immediate postoperative period. Prone passive knee flexion, quadriceps strengthening sets, and patellar mobilization exercises are expected in the first postoperative month. The stationary bike becomes part of the exercise regimen in the second postoperative month, and in the third postoperative month full flexion is achieved. Closed chain exercises are added in the fourth postoperative month, and athletes are returned to running without cutting motion at 6 months. Gradual return to sport-specific training is incorporated in the 9- to 12-month postoperative period. The current criteria used for return to sport include absence of effusion; satisfactory clinical examination findings; quadriceps and hamstring strength at or above 90% of the contralateral leg; one-leg hop and vertical jump at or above 90% of the contralateral leg; full-speed run, shuttle run, and figure-of-eight running without a limp; and ability to perform squat and rise without difficulty.[7,10]

Complications

Complications associated with PCL reconstruction are rare events but do unfortunately occur. Broadly, complications may be divided into preoperative, intraoperative, and postoperative events. The major preoperative complication is neurapraxia secondary to poor or improper positioning. Intraoperatively, the direst of complications is injury to the popliteal vessels or nerves during drilling. As mentioned previously, with the arthroscopic inlay technique protection from this complication is afforded by the drill guide as well as retrograde reaming with the FlipCutter. Likewise, the arthroscopic inlay technique affords arthroscopic visualization and fluoroscopic confirmation of drill position at all times. Loss of knee motion secondary to excessive graft tensioning or poor graft position is an acknowledged complication that must be avoided. Conversely, undertensioning of the graft leading to residual laxity must also be avoided. Intermittent checks of thigh and calf tone are important to ensure that compartment syndrome does not develop in response to fluid extravasation into the soft tissue. Avascular necrosis of the medial femoral condyle can be avoided by placing the starting and exiting points for the femoral tunnels clear of the subchondral bone. In the postoperative period, overaggressive or overly cautious rehabilitation may lead to graft failure or knee stiffness, respectively.

RESULTS

Although there is a paucity of clinical data regarding the success of the double-bundle arthroscopic inlay PCL reconstruction, this technique is a natural progression in the evolution of the treatment of PCL injury and is grounded in sound biomechanical evidence. In the results section we elaborate on the biomechanical advantages of both double-bundle versus single-bundle reconstruction and tibial inlay versus transtibial reconstructions. The biomechanical advantages are supported with clinical outcomes where available.

A number of in vitro biomechanical studies have found the double-bundle PCL reconstruction to more closely reproduce normal knee biomechanics and kinematics.[11-13] A recent systematic review found that there may be no definitive advantage to double-bundle PCL with regard to anteroposterior stability; however,

TABLE 81-1. Clinical Results of Double-Bundle Arthroscopic Tibial Inlay Posterior Cruciate Ligament Reconstruction

Authors	No. of Patients	Follow-up	Graft Type	Postoperative Objective Measures	Functional Outcome
Kim and Park[19] (2005)	7	Short-term (n = 2 with longer than 1 year)	Achilles tendon allograft	Arthrometric: <3-mm side-side (average)	N/A
Mariani and Margheritini[20] (2006)	9	12-20 months 15 months (average)	Quadriceps tendon autograft	Arthrometric: 3.2-mm side-side (average) Radiographic: 4.6-mm side-side (average)	IKDC score: 5 A, 3 B, 1 C
Kim et al[21] (2009)	10 DBI* vs 11 SBI vs. 8 SBTT	>24 months	Achilles tendon allograft	Arthrometric: DBI 3.6-mm side-side (average) vs SBI 4.7-mm side-side (average) vs SBTT 5.6-mm side-side (average)	Lysholm score: DBI 84.3 (average) vs SBI 79.7 (average) vs SBTT 86.8 (average)

*DBI, Double-bundle arthroscopic inlay technique; IKDC, International Knee Documentation Committee; N/A, not applicable; SBI, single-bundle arthroscopic inlay technique; SBTT, single-bundle transtibial technique.

there is a distinct advantage of double-bundle PCL reconstruction with regard to rotational stability in the setting of unrecognized or untreated PLC injury.[8] There are currently no high-level clinical studies that support the use of double-bundle reconstruction over single-bundle reconstruction or vice versa.[8]

Although there is no gold standard surgical technique for reconstruction of the PCL, the biomechanical advantages of the tibial inlay technique (either open or arthroscopic) in avoiding the "killer turn" and subsequent graft elongation or failure have been documented in cadaveric studies.[14,15] The arthroscopic inlay approach is biomechanically comparable to the open inlay approach at time zero and avoids the morbidity associated with a posterior approach to the knee and violation of the PM joint capsule.[16-18] There are currently three clinical or functional outcome studies involving the double-bundle arthroscopic inlay technique, all with promising results (Table 81-1). Kim and colleagues compared cohorts of single-bundle transtibial reconstructions, single-bundle arthroscopic inlay reconstructions, and double-bundle arthroscopic inlay reconstructions and found that mean Lysholm and range-of-motion at final follow-up were equivalent among all groups; however, the single-bundle transtibial reconstructions had significant increased laxity compared with the double-bundle arthroscopic inlay group.[21]

REFERENCES

1. Logan M, Williams A, Lavelle J, et al. The effect of posterior cruciate ligament deficiency on knee kinematics. *Am J Sports Med.* 2004;32(8):1915-1922.
2. Van de Velde SK, Bingham JT, Gill TJ, et al. Analysis of tibiofemoral cartilage deformation in the posterior cruciate ligament-deficient knee. *J Bone Joint Surg Am.* 2009;91(1):167-175.
3. Boynton MD, Tietjens BR. Long-term follow-up of the untreated isolated posterior cruciate ligament-deficient knee. *Am J Sports Med.* 1996;24(3):306-310.
4. Fanelli GC, Edson CJ. Posterior cruciate ligament injuries in trauma patients. Part II. *Arthroscopy.* 1995;11: 526-529.
5. Fanelli GC, Giannotti BF, Edson CJ. The posterior cruciate ligament arthroscopic evaluation and treatment. *Arthroscopy.* 1994;10(6):673-688.
6. Sekiya JK, Haemmerle MJ, Stabile KJ, et al. Biomechanical analysis of a combined double-bundle posterior cruciate ligament and posterolateral corner knee reconstruction. *Am J Sports Med.* 2005;33:360-369.
7. Sekiya JK, West RV, Ong BC, et al. Clinical outcomes after isolated arthroscopic single-bundle posterior cruciate ligament reconstruction. *Arthroscopy.* 2005;21:1042-1050.
8. Kohen R, Sekiya JK. Single-bundle versus double-bundle posterior cruciate ligament reconstruction. *Arthroscopy.* 2009;25(12):1470-1477.
9. Ruberte Thiele RA, Campbell RB, Amendola A, et al. Biomechanical comparison of figure-of-8 versus cylindrical tibial inlay constructs for arthroscopic posterior cruciate ligament reconstruction. *Arthroscopy.* 2010;26(7): 977-983.
10. Chu BI, Martin RL, Carcia CR, et al. Surgical techniques and postoperative rehabilitation for isolated posterior cruciate ligament injuries. *Orthop Phys Ther Pract.* 2007;19(4):185-189.
11. Harner CD, Janaushek MA, Kanamori A, et al. Biomechanical analysis of a double-bundle posterior cruciate ligament reconstruction. *Am J Sports Med.* 2000;28: 144-151.
12. Race A, Amis AA. PCL reconstruction: in vitro biomechanical comparison of "isometric" versus single and double-bundle "anatomic" grafts. *J Bone Joint Surg Br.* 1998;80:173-179.
13. Whiddon DR, Zehms CT, Miller MD, et al. Double compared with single-bundle open inlay posterior cruciate ligament reconstruction in a cadaver model. *J Bone Joint Surg Am.* 2008;90(9):1820-1829.

14. Bergfeld JA, McAllister DR, Parker RD, et al. A biomechanical comparison of posterior cruciate ligament reconstruction techniques. *Am J Sports Med.* 2001;29:129-136.

15. Markolf KL, Zemanovic JR, McAllister DR. Cyclic loading of posterior cruciate ligament replacements fixed with tibial tunnel and tibial inlay methods. *J Bone Joint Surg Am.* 2002;84:518-524.

16. Campbell RB, Jordan SS, Sekiya JK. Arthroscopic tibial inlay for posterior cruciate ligament reconstruction. *Arthroscopy.* 2007;23(12):1351-1354.

17. Campbell RB, Torrie A, Hecker A, et al. Comparison of tibial graft fixation between simulated arthroscopic and open inlay techniques for posterior cruciate ligament reconstruction. *Am J Sports Med.* 2007;35(10):1731-1738.

18. Zehms CT, Whiddon DR, Miller MD, et al. Comparison of a double-bundle arthroscopic inlay and open inlay posterior cruciate ligament reconstruction using clinically relevant tools: a cadaveric study. *Arthroscopy.* 2008;24(4):472-480.

19. Kim SJ, Park IS. Arthroscopic reconstruction of the posterior cruciate ligament using tibial-inlay and double-bundle technique. *Arthroscopy.* 2005;21:1271.

20. Mariani PP, Margheritini F. Full arthroscopic inlay reconstruction of posterior cruciate ligament. *Knee Surg Sports Traumatol Arthrosc.* 2006;14:1038-1044.

21. Kim SJ, Kim TE, Jo SB, et al. Comparison of the clinical results of three posterior cruciate ligament reconstruction techniques. *J Bone Joint Surg Am.* 2009;91:2543-2549.

Chapter 82

Posterior Cruciate Ligament Tibial Inlay

Anjan P. Kaushik and Mark D. Miller

Chapter Synopsis

- Rupture of the posterior cruciate ligament (PCL) may be seen as an isolated injury or as a part of a more complex multiligamentous knee injury. The PCL tibial inlay is a technique for reconstruction of the PCL that has the advantage of avoiding the "killer turn" that is seen in the transtibial PCL reconstruction. This chapter details the operative treatment of the PCL with a single-bundle tibial inlay technique with bone–patellar tendon–bone (BPTB) autograft. Several studies have described favorable outcomes with this reconstruction.

Important Points

- Ruptures of the PCL occur more commonly in multiligamentous knee trauma than as isolated injuries.
- Posterior tibial translation exceeding 10 mm on stress radiography indicates complete PCL rupture, and translation exceeding 12 mm suggests combined PCL and posterolateral corner injury.
- Surgical indications include grade III PCL injuries, persistently symptomatic grade II PCL injuries, bony avulsion injuries, and multiligamentous knee injury involving the PCL.
- A significant advantage of the posterior approach and PCL tibial inlay technique is the avoidance of the killer turn, which is the acute angulation of the PCL graft that is seen in transtibial PCL reconstructions.
- Rehabilitation of the reconstructed PCL focuses on recovery of full range of motion and strengthening with use of prone extension modalities.

Clinical and Surgical Pearls

- Fully mobilize the medial head of the gastrocnemius with aggressive blunt dissection.
- Use a long retractor that is "toed in" to hold the gastrocnemius while you are drilling the Steinmann pins that will be used for retraction.
- Palpate the posterior prominences. Stay lateral to the more prominent medial prominence.
- Make a generous vertical arthrotomy by extending the initial incision for the trough proximally.
- Make sure that the graft does not spin or get wrapped up during fixation.
- If the graft does not go right up into the femoral tunnel, pass it anteriorly and then up the tunnel. This is performed in two separate steps.
- Cycle the knee and palpate the graft to ensure that there is good tension before final fixation.
- Look down the femoral tunnel during and after interference screw placement with the arthroscope.

Clinical and Surgical Pitfalls

- Do not forget to fix the posterolateral corner if there is a combined injury.
- Do not use a tourniquet or leg holder for more than 120 minutes. This requires a well-planned operation, particularly if a multiple-ligament reconstruction is performed.
- Vigilantly protect the neurovascular bundle at all times, and release the tourniquet before closure to rule out injury to the popliteal vessels.
- Pad the extremities and opposite leg well to prevent pressure injuries.
- Failure to make a generous posterior arthrotomy can make graft passage difficult.
- Do not hesitate to back up graft fixation.
- Do not leave the operating room unhappy.

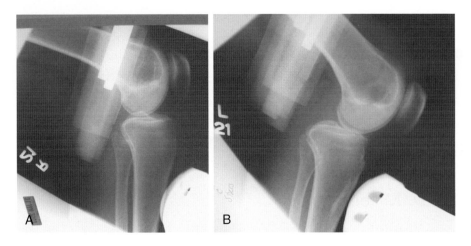

Figure 82-1. A, Normal knee examination finding with Telos testing. **B,** Abnormal Telos test result.

Ruptures of the posterior cruciate ligament (PCL) occur more commonly in multiligamentous knee trauma than as isolated injuries. Because this ligament is damaged much less frequently than its counterpart, the anterior cruciate ligament (ACL), knowledge of and experience in evaluation and management of the PCL still lag behind those of the ACL. Left untreated, the PCL-deficient knee encounters altered kinematics during weight-bearing activities relative to the uninjured knee, because the PCL is the primary restraint to posterior tibial translation at 90 degrees of knee flexion.[1] Accurate, early diagnosis leads to appropriate treatment of PCL injuries.

Clinical examination emphasizes the posterior drawer test for evaluation of PCL stability; however, further assessment of posterior tibial subluxation with Telos stress radiography offers more objective evidence of PCL laxity, particularly when compared with the contralateral knee[2] (Fig. 82-1). Posterior tibial translation exceeding 10 mm on stress radiography indicates complete PCL rupture, and translation exceeding 12 mm suggests combined PCL and posterolateral corner (PLC) injury. Other physical examination maneuvers include the reverse pivot shift, quadriceps sag, and quadriceps active test. Magnetic resonance imaging (MRI) plays a significant role in confirmation of PCL injury and can certainly detect other ligamentous and soft tissue injuries (Fig. 82-2). The optimal method for PCL reconstruction (i.e., transtibial versus tibial inlay; single-bundle versus double-bundle; tunnel positioning) continues to be hotly debated. The goal of this chapter is to detail the operative technique of single-bundle PCL tibial inlay reconstruction, paying close attention to the anatomy and biomechanics of this method.

PREOPERATIVE CONSIDERATIONS

Anatomy and Biomechanics

The PCL is an intra-articular ligament that is divided into two bundles based on function in flexion and

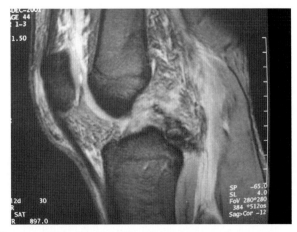

Figure 82-2. Sagittal T2-weighted magnetic resonance imaging scan demonstrating rupture of the posterior cruciate ligament. *(From Gill SS, Cohen SB, Miller MD. PCL tibial inlay and posterolateral corner reconstruction. In: Miller MD, Cole BJ, eds.* Textbook of Arthroscopy. *Philadelphia: Saunders Elsevier; 2004.)*

extension: anterolateral (AL) and posteromedial (PM) (Fig. 82-3). The AL bundle is taut in 90 degrees of flexion and more lax in extension. Conversely, the PM bundle is taut in extension and lax in flexion. Studies show that they appear to have a synergistic relationship for maintaining knee stability.[1] The PCL is 32 to 38 mm long and has an average width of 11 to 13 mm.[1,3]

The proximal and distal bony insertions have two to three times the width of the midportion of the ligament. The PCL attaches to the posterolateral aspect of the medial femoral condyle approximately 10 mm from the articular cartilage, as referenced from a line parallel to the Blumensaat line, and passes in a posterior and lateral direction to attach into a depression on the posterior aspect of the tibia known as the posterior intercondylar facet.[1] The attachment on the posterior tibia is bordered by a medial and lateral prominence and is 1.0 to 1.5 cm distal to the joint line.[3] The meniscofemoral ligaments of Humphrey and Wrisberg run anterior and posterior

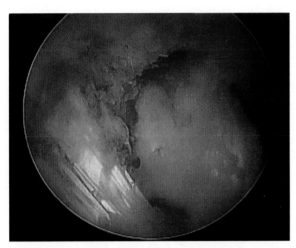

Figure 82-3. Arthroscopic image of the two bundles of the posterior cruciate ligament. The reconstructed anterolateral bundle *(right)* and the intact native posteromedial bundle *(left)* are shown.

BOX 82-1 Surgical Steps of Posterior Cruciate Ligament Reconstruction with a Single-Bundle Tibial Inlay Technique with Bone–Patellar Tendon–Bone Autograft

- Examination under anesthesia and diagnostic arthroscopy
- Graft harvest
- Femoral tunnel placement
- Posterior approach and distal fixation
- Graft passage and proximal fixation

---

to the PCL, respectively, and are secondary stabilizers to posterior tibial translation.[1]

History, Examination, and Indications

Injuries to the PCL occur commonly from dashboard injuries, in which a posteriorly directed blow to the proximal tibia occurs. Hyperextension injuries to the knee can also result in PCL injury. Severe trauma to the knee resulting in knee dislocations can cause multiligamentous knee injuries in which the PCL is ruptured. When the mechanism of injury involves a direct blow to the anterior tibia, the position of the foot often determines the injury pattern; ankle plantarflexion is associated with PCL injuries, whereas ankle dorsiflexion is associated with patellofemoral injury.

The presentation is much less dramatic than that of ACL injuries, and large hemarthroses are less common in PCL injuries. Isolated PCL injuries are frequently grade I or grade II and can be treated nonoperatively. The emphasis for physical therapy in nonoperative management is to obtain full range of motion and to rehabilitate the quadriceps mechanism to counteract posterior tibial subluxation. Quadriceps strengthening is often done with exercises in the prone position. These lower-grade PCL injuries may actually demonstrate "healing" on MRI, with collagen remodeling within the ligament. Because the strength of this "healed" PCL is less than that of a native PCL, persistent ligamentous laxity is common.[4,5] Nonetheless, isolated low-grade PCL injuries can be treated without surgery.

Surgical indications include grade III PCL injuries, persistently symptomatic grade II PCL injuries, bony avulsion injuries, and multiligamentous injury (MLI) of the knee involving the PCL. Isolated grade III PCL injury is rare, and disruption of other soft tissue structures, particularly the PLC, is common. It is essential to identify PCL injuries with associated lateral-sided injuries, because identification of this concomitant injury will affect the treatment approach to reconstruction.

SURGICAL TECHNIQUE

There are several conventional techniques for PCL reconstruction, and newer methods such as computer-assisted ligament reconstruction demonstrate similar outcomes to these conventional approaches.[6] This chapter focuses on the operative treatment of the PCL with a single-bundle tibial inlay technique with bone–patellar tendon–bone (BPTB) autograft.

This technique is called the *inlay* because the bone from the BPTB graft is placed into a trough in the posterior aspect of the tibia at the PCL footprint. A significant advantage of the posterior approach and PCL tibial inlay technique is the avoidance of the "killer turn," which is the acute angulation of the PCL graft that is seen in transtibial PCL reconstructions. This reduces the stress placed across the graft and decreases the potential risk of abrasion and rupture of the graft.[7,8] The single-bundle technique detailed in the next section reliably reconstructs the AL bundle of the PCL in its anatomic insertion site (Fig. 82-4).

It is our preference to use BPTB autograft because it allows a robust bone-to-bone fixation and avoids the problems with allograft, which include delayed incorporation, infection risk, late laxity, and cost. If autograft is unavailable, an allograft with a bone block is a viable option (e.g., Achilles tendon, BPTB, or quadriceps tendon).

Specific Steps

Box 82-1 outlines the specific steps of this procedure.

1. Examination Under Anesthesia, Positioning, and Diagnostic Arthroscopy

The procedure commences with a thorough examination of the knee under anesthesia to confirm the

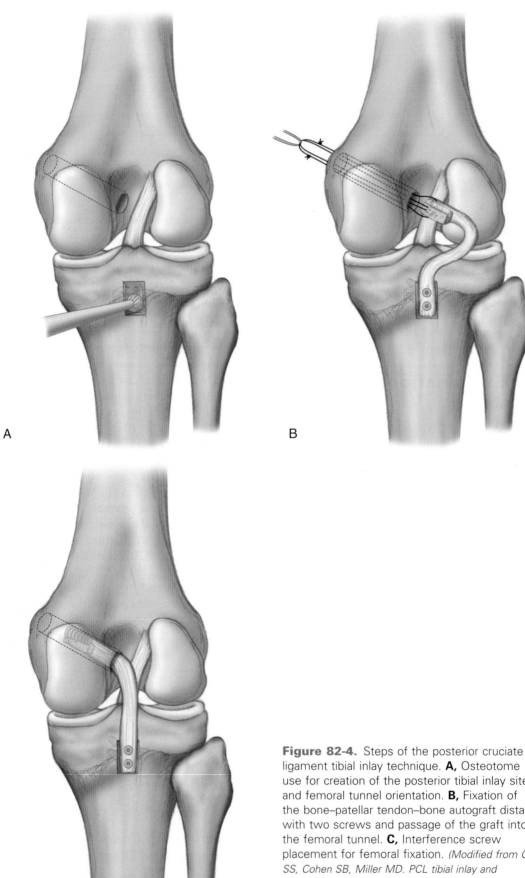

A

B

C

Figure 82-4. Steps of the posterior cruciate ligament tibial inlay technique. **A,** Osteotome use for creation of the posterior tibial inlay site, and femoral tunnel orientation. **B,** Fixation of the bone–patellar tendon–bone autograft distally with two screws and passage of the graft into the femoral tunnel. **C,** Interference screw placement for femoral fixation. *(Modified from Gill SS, Cohen SB, Miller MD. PCL tibial inlay and posterolateral corner reconstruction. In: Miller MD, Cole BJ, eds. Textbook of Arthroscopy. Philadelphia: Saunders Elsevier; 2004.)*

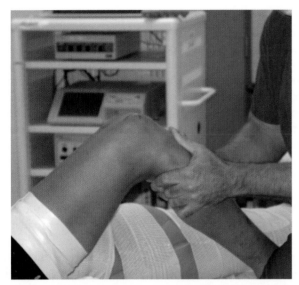

Figure 82-5. Examination of the posterior cruciate ligament under anesthesia with the posterior drawer test. The examiner stabilizes the knee in 90 degrees of flexion and directs a posterior force onto the anterior aspect of the tibia.

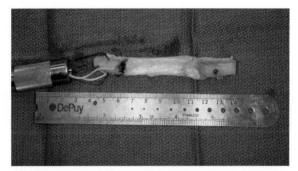

Figure 82-6. The bone–patellar tendon–bone autograft before passage. Note the bullet-shaped bone plug for the femoral side to facilitate passage.

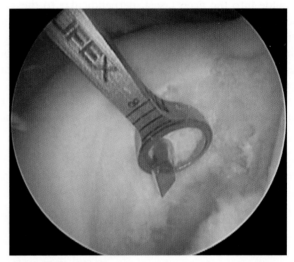

Figure 82-7. Arthroscopic view of the posterior cruciate ligament (PCL) guide in place for single-bundle PCL reconstruction. The guide pin is drilled from outside in.

preoperative examination findings (Fig. 82-5). Demonstration of a positive posterior drawer and posterior sag sign can be confirmed, and testing of the PLC and lateral complex can be more accurately performed with the patient asleep.

A tourniquet is applied high on the thigh and should be deflated before wound closure to ensure that there is no injury to the popliteal vessels. The patient can be positioned supine or in the lateral decubitus position. Arthroscopy can be performed with the patient in the lateral decubitus position, obviating the need for intraoperative repositioning for the posterior approach, or the patient can be repositioned after supine arthroscopy. Our preference is to use a lateral decubitus position for both arthroscopy and PCL reconstruction. The contralateral leg must be adequately padded to avoid pressure necrosis. The operative extremity can be abducted and externally rotated to facilitate the arthroscopy.[9]

A diagnostic arthroscopic examination is then performed to evaluate all intra-articular pathology, including chondral and meniscal damage. The torn PCL may be difficult to recognize until it is viewed completely. An indication of a PCL tear is the "sloppy ACL sign" or ACL pseudolaxity.[10] The torn ends of the PCL are identified, and the stumps are debrided with a shaver while any fibers in continuity are preserved.

2. Graft Harvest

With the operative extremity in the abducted and externally rotated position, the BPTB autograft is harvested from the ipsilateral knee in standard fashion. The bony ends of the graft are prepared in a rectangular shape on the tibial inlay side and in a bullet shape on the femoral

side to allow smooth passage into the femoral tunnel (Fig. 82-6).

3. Femoral Tunnel Placement

The incision for femoral tunnel placement is made at the medial knee anterior and superior to the medial femoral epicondyle. Dissection is carried down in line with vastus medialis to the level of the femoral condyle. The bone should be visualized to protect soft tissue structures during drilling and to later easily identify the tunnel for femoral fixation. The PCL guide is placed with arthroscopic guidance at the 1-o'clock position (right knee) or 11-o'clock position (left knee), 8 mm deep in the medial femoral notch and away from the articular surface (Fig. 82-7). The guide pin is drilled from outside in with use of the PCL guide, and the position is confirmed arthroscopically. The starting point of the guide pin should be proximal (farther from subchondral bone) enough to avoid subchondral collapse or avascular necrosis of the condyle as a complication of drilling the femoral tunnel.[11] The tunnel (approximately 11 to 12 mm in diameter, 30 to 35 mm in depth) is then drilled over the guidewire, and the tunnel edges are debrided with a shaver to facilitate later graft passage. A looped smooth 18-gauge wire is placed through the tunnel into the joint to be used later for passage of the autograft from the posterior knee into the femoral tunnel.

4. Posterior Approach and Distal Fixation

The operative extremity is returned to the lateral decubitus position, and the posterior knee is visualized. A transverse skin incision is made in line with the flexion crease of the knee, providing for excellent exposure and cosmesis (Fig. 82-8A). A hockey stick–shaped incision is made into the deep fascia, perpendicular to the skin incision (Fig. 82-8B). The medial head of the gastrocnemius is a key landmark to identify. Blunt dissection is carried down between the medial head of the gastrocnemius and semimembranosus proximally. The gastrocnemius muscle is mobilized and retracted laterally.

At this point it is useful to place a series of two to four smooth Steinmann pins from the posterior knee

in an anterior direction (Fig. 82-9). These pins are then bent to serve as self-retaining retractors.[12] The gastrocnemius-semimembranosus interval protects the popliteal vessels and tibial nerve, and it is not necessary to directly visualize these posterior neurovascular structures with this technique. After the medial gastrocnemius and neurovascular bundle have been retracted, the posterior capsule of the knee and posterior tibia are identified. The popliteus muscle is commonly encountered in this interval, and the upper portion of the popliteus muscle belly can be reflected to expose the posterior cortex of the tibia (see Fig. 82-9). The medial and lateral prominences bordering the posterior intercondylar facet (the PCL footprint) are identified 1.0 to 1.5 cm distal to the joint line. The lateral prominence is smaller and often more difficult to palpate; however, the medial prominence should be readily apparent.[9]

A generous, vertical posterior capsulotomy is made for deeper dissection to prepare the proximal aspect of the bone trough, and for later passage of the BPTB graft. The medial and lateral prominences are then dissected

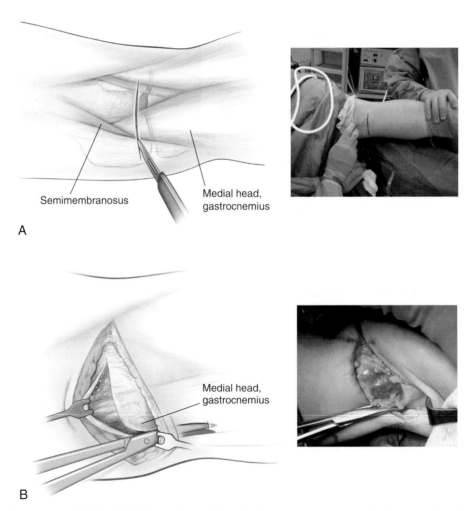

Semimembranosus   Medial head, gastrocnemius

A

Medial head, gastrocnemius

B

Figure 82-8. A, Skin incision. **B,** Fascial incision. *(From Miller MD. Knee and lower leg: Posterior approach to the knee. In: Miller MD, Chhabra AB, Hurwitz S, et al, eds.* Orthopaedic Surgical Approaches. *Philadelphia: Saunders; 2008.)*

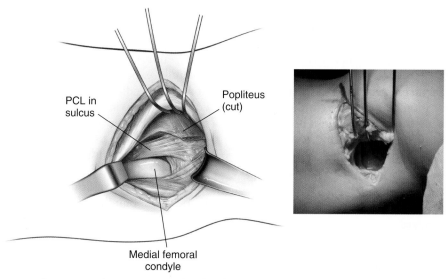

PCL in sulcus

Popliteus (cut)

Medial femoral condyle

Figure 82-9. Steinmann pins retract the gastrocnemius for deep dissection. Vertical capsulotomy and partial reflection of the popliteus muscle exposes the posterior tibia and femoral condyles. *PCL,* Posterior cruciate ligament. *(From Miller MD. Knee and lower leg: Posterior approach to the knee. In: Miller MD, Chhabra AB, Hurwitz S, et al, eds. Orthopaedic Surgical Approaches. Philadelphia: Saunders; 2008.)*

subperiosteally to prepare the trough just lateral to the medial prominence. Preparation of the bone trough for the inlay is fashioned by hand as a vertically oriented rectangular slot, either with osteotomes or with a high-speed bur (see Fig. 82-4A). This trough should be closely matched to the size of the bone plug from the BPTB graft, because this is an inlay graft. After proximal tibial trough preparation is completed near the capsulotomy site, the prepared BPTB graft is then retrieved and inlayed into the trough (see Fig. 82-4B). The graft is secured with two pins from a cannulated screw set, preferentially for a screw diameter of 4.5 mm.

The graft is then passed into the joint with the previously placed looped smooth 18-gauge wire. Screw fixation is then achieved with two bicortical screws securing the bone plug into the posterior trough. Other fixation methods include a single 6.5-mm cancellous screw or a staple. It is our practice to fix the distal graft site with two bicortical 4.5-mm screws, with a washer in the proximal of the two screws (see Fig. 82-4B).

5. Graft Passage and Proximal Fixation

The remainder of the BPTB graft is passed through the posterior capsulotomy into the joint. The bullet-shaped bone plug is passed into the previously drilled and prepared femoral tunnel with the knee at 90 degrees of flexion. After the graft is appropriately positioned in the femoral tunnel, a guide pin is placed on the anterior side of the graft from outside in. While maximum manual tension is applied to the graft, it is important to cycle the knee repeatedly to remove any kinks in the graft. While graft tension is maintained, an anterior drawer force is applied, with the knee at 90 degrees of flexion. An interference screw is then inserted over the guide pin

(see Fig. 82-4C), which should be removed when the interference screw is approximately halfway seated. This avoids binding of the guide pin in the fixation. The screw is then seated fully and the graft is visualized arthroscopically to ensure that the screw is not proud at the joint level. It is essential to maintain constant tension on the BPTB graft until the interference screw is fully seated. Other fixation options, based on the stability of the reconstruction, include double fixation with a post and a washer, medial staples, or over a button on the medial femoral cortex.

The tourniquet should be released before closure of the posterior incision, to rule out potential vascular injury to the popliteal artery or vein. A Hemovac drain may be placed in the wound if there is any concern of postoperative hematoma. The medial and posterior incisions and arthroscopy sites are also closed, and routine dressings applied. The operative leg can be kept in a knee immobilizer or hinged knee brace locked in extension, and neurovascular status should be monitored closely.

POSTOPERATIVE CONSIDERATIONS

Follow-up and Rehabilitation

Immobilization of the knee in extension for the first 2 to 4 postsurgical weeks helps prevent tibial subluxation. Patients should be counseled preoperatively and postoperatively that PCL rehabilitation is more difficult and slower than ACL rehabilitation, and full recovery can take 1 year or longer. Early weight bearing while walking can be deleterious to the graft incorporation; therefore patients are generally kept on non–weight-bearing status for 4 to 6 weeks postoperatively.[13] Alternatively, limited weight bearing with the brace in full extension may be allowed, based on surgeon preference. Rehabilitation of the reconstructed PCL focuses on recovery of full range of motion and strengthening via prone extension modalities. The prone position allows gravity to help achieve full extension and also protects against posterior sag and tibial translation. Active quadriceps activity is encouraged early, with no active hamstring motion or strengthening. Hamstring exercises are generally started actively only after 3 to 4 months.

Complications

PCL reconstructions are technically demanding and can be lengthier than other surgical procedures in sports medicine, particularly if associated injuries of other ligaments must also be addressed. Therefore certain precautions must be taken. Careful positioning and padding of the contralateral extremity must be performed preoperatively to prevent neurapraxia and pressure sores. The most common adverse outcome after PCL reconstruction is loss of motion. This can be related to excessive graft tension, tensioning in extension, and inadequate postoperative rehabilitation.

Although rare, neurovascular injuries may occur with the posterior approach, which places the popliteal artery and tibial nerve at risk. The surgical exposure protects these structures without directly visualizing them, but injuries can still occur.[14] Any concern for popliteal artery damage should prompt consultation with a vascular surgeon, and prophylactic fasciotomies are warranted to avoid reperfusion injury if arterial repair or bypass is needed.

Ligamentous laxity may be persistent postoperatively, evidenced by objective instrumented measures. Fortunately, this laxity is rarely associated with functional instability and may result from stretching of graft fibers or remodeling. Patients are usually unaware of this subtle asymmetry in PCL laxity. Accurate tunnel placement and proper graft tensioning reduce the incidence of laxity after PCL reconstruction.

Other, less common complications include compartment syndrome, osteonecrosis, femoral or tibial fracture, anterior knee pain, and heterotopic ossification.[14]

RESULTS

Long-term follow-up of patients with chronic PCL insufficiency demonstrated that they have higher rates of knee pain, effusion, and chondral damage in the medial and patellofemoral compartments,[15] as well as meniscal damage. However, clinical long-term outcomes are variable, and the majority of patients do well without any surgical intervention.

Several studies of single-bundle tibial inlay PCL reconstruction with minimum follow-up of 2 years have demonstrated favorable outcomes, as measured objectively and with stress radiography.[16-20] Patients can generally expect to return to grade I laxity or better; however, residual laxity after reconstruction has been commonly seen in follow-up. Despite this laxity, patients progress well and have minimal to no symptoms. The functional results of PCL reconstruction are not necessarily correlated with the objective laxity observed.

As the controversy over optimal reconstruction of the PCL persists, multiple investigators have compared PCL single-bundle tibial inlay with double-bundle tibial inlay and transtibial PCL reconstruction. All techniques demonstrate favorable clinical and functional results,[18,19,21] but higher-quality, prospective, randomized controlled trials are still needed to determine the best reconstruction strategy.

REFERENCES

1. Voos JE, Mauro CS, Wente T, et al. Posterior cruciate ligament: anatomy, biomechanics, and outcomes. *Am J Sports Med.* 2012;40(1):222-231.
2. Margheritini F, Mancini L, Mauro CS, et al. Stress radiography for quantifying posterior cruciate ligament deficiency. *Arthroscopy.* 2003;19(7):706-711.
3. Harner CD, Livesay GA, Kashiwaguchi S. Comparative study of the size and shape of human anterior and posterior cruciate ligaments. *J Orthop Res.* 1995;13:429-434.
4. Shelbourne KD, Davis TJ, Patel DV. The natural history of acute, isolated, nonoperatively treated posterior cruciate ligament injuries. *Am J Sports Med.* 1999;27:276-283.
5. Shelbourne KD, Muthukaruppan Y. Subjective results of nonoperatively treated, acute, isolated posterior cruciate ligament injuries. *Arthroscopy.* 2005;21:457-461.
6. Meuffels DE, Reijman M, Scholten RJPM, et al. Computer assisted surgery for knee ligament reconstruction. *Cochrane Database Syst Rev.* 2011;6:CD007601.
7. Berg EE. Posterior cruciate ligament tibial inlay reconstruction. *Arthroscopy.* 1995;11:69-76.
8. Papalia R, Osti L, Del Buono A, et al. Tibial inlay for posterior cruciate ligament reconstruction: a systematic review. *Knee.* 2010;17(4):264-269.
9. Gill SS, Cohen SB, Miller MD. PCL tibial inlay and posterolateral corner reconstruction. In Miller MD, Cole BJ, eds. *Textbook of Arthroscopy.* 1st ed. Philadelphia PA: Saunders Elsevier; 2004:717-728.
10. Fanelli GC, Giannotti BF, Edson CJ. The posterior cruciate ligament: arthroscopic evaluation and treatment. *Arthroscopy.* 1994;10:673-688.
11. Athanasian EA, Wickiewicz TL, Warren RF. Osteonecrosis of the femoral condyle after arthroscopic reconstruction of a cruciate ligament; report of two cases. *J Bone Joint Surg Am.* 1995;77:1418-1422.
12. Miller MD, Olszewski AD. Posterior cruciate ligament injuries. New treatment options. *Am J Knee Surg.* 1995;8:145-154.

13. Edson CT, Fanelli GC, Beck JD. Postoperative rehabilitation of the posterior cruciate ligament. *Sports Med Arthrosc.* 2010;18(4):275-279.

14. Zawodny SR, Miller MD. Complications of posterior cruciate ligament surgery. *Sports Med Arthrosc.* 2010;18(4):269-274.

15. Boynton MD, Tietjens MB. Long-term followup of the untreated isolated posterior cruciate ligament-deficient knee. *Am J Sports Med.* 1996;24:306-310.

16. Cooper DE, Stewart D. Posterior cruciate ligament reconstruction using single-bundle patella tendon graft with tibial inlay fixation: 2- to 10-year follow-up. *Am J Sports Med.* 2004;32:346-360.

17. Jung YB, Tae SK, Jung HJ, et al. Replacement of the torn posterior cruciate ligament with a mid-third patellar tendon graft with use of a modified tibial inlay method. *J Bone Joint Surg Am.* 2004;86:1878-1883.

18. Kim SJ, Kim SH, Kim SG, et al. Comparison of the clinical results of three posterior cruciate ligament reconstruction techniques: surgical technique. *J Bone Joint Surg Am.* 2010;92(Suppl 1 Pt 2):145-157.

19. Panchal HB, Sekiya JK. Open tibial inlay versus arthroscopic transtibial posterior cruciate ligament reconstructions. *Arthroscopy.* 2011;27(9):1289-1295.

20. Seon JK, Song EK. Reconstruction of isolated posterior cruciate ligament injuries: a clinical comparison of the transtibial and tibial inlay techniques. *Arthroscopy.* 2006;22:27-32.

21. May JH, Gillette BP, Morgan JA, et al. Transtibial versus inlay posterior cruciate ligament reconstruction: an evidence-based systematic review. *J Knee Surg.* 2010;23(2):73-79.

Chapter 83

Arthroscopic Posterior Cruciate Ligament Inlay

Fabrizio Margheritini and Pier Paolo Mariani

Chapter Synopsis

- The clinical outcomes of posterior cruciate ligament reconstruction are less satisfactory than those of anterior cruciate ligament reconstruction. Several authors have reported that the graft can be stretched when a traditional Clancy arthroscopic technique is used, and therefore inlay open reconstruction has been suggested as a viable option. The need to combine an arthroscopic procedure with an inlay procedure has been filled by development of a full arthroscopic inlay reconstruction.

Important Points

- *Indications:* Chronic isolated and combined posterior cruciate ligament instability, revision surgery
- *Contraindications:* Acute injuries, dislocation
- *Classification:* Grade I, II (isolated), grade III (combined)
- *Symptom:* Persistent symptomatic complaints, posterior isolated and combined instability
- *Surgical technique:* Arthroscopic posterior cruciate ligament inlay reconstruction

Clinical and Surgical Pearls

- *Clinical:* Stress radiographs are taken to define the amount of posterior subluxation.

- *Graft selection:* Bone block grafts are mandatory. Quadriceps tendon is the graft of choice owing to the mechanical property and easy fit within the knee joint.
- *Portals and setup:* Working position is 90 degrees of knee flexion; posteromedial and posterolateral portals and trans-septal technique are used.
- Use of the tourniquet is not mandatory. Do not inflate it (until necessary), to check intraoperative bleeding.
- Use the radiofrequency as well the shaver with the working area facing the bone, not vice versa, to prevent damage to the neurovascular structures.
- Trim the bone block to the desired size.

Clinical and Surgical Pitfalls

- Neurovascular complications
- Compartment-like syndrome caused by extensive use of pump
- Failure to restore peripheral stability
- Persistent posterior sag

Injuries to the posterior cruciate ligament (PCL) occur more frequently than previously thought, not only among patients who sustain severe trauma of the lower extremity, but also among athletes. Surgical reconstruction of the PCL is recommended for acute injuries that result in severe posterior tibial subluxation and instability, objective criteria that are often met in patients with combined ligamentous injuries. Surgical treatment of the chronic PCL-deficient knee is recommended for patients with persistent symptomatic complaints, such as pain or discomfort that fails to improve with an appropriate physiotherapeutic program. The rationale for performing a reconstruction is to restore normal joint kinematics and forces, thus minimizing the deleterious effects, such early cartilage degeneration, that PCL deficiency has been shown to have on the knee. With these premises in mind, we developed a technique of arthroscopic tibial inlay reconstruction[1] to minimize the graft stresses and allowing a more anatomic reconstruction. This concept has more recently also been applied at the femoral side.[2]

PREOPERATIVE CONSIDERATIONS

Anatomy

The PCL has been considered by some the strongest knee ligament. Synovial tissue reflected from the posterior capsule covers the ligament on its medial, lateral, and anterior surfaces, whereas distally the posterior portion of the PCL blends with the posterior capsule and periosteum. The PCL is 32 to 38 mm long, with a cross-sectional area of 11 mm at its midpoint. The midsubstance of the ligament is approximately one third the diameter of both the femoral and tibial insertion sites. The PCL can be functionally divided into two components: a larger anterolateral (AL) bundle and a smaller posteromedial (PM) bundle. In general, the PCL has a broad, relatively vertical femoral footprint at the AL aspect of the medial femoral condyle, with a midpoint approximately 1 cm proximal to the articular surface. The tibial insertion of the PCL is more consistent than the femoral insertion. The two PCL fiber bundles insert without anatomic separation in a centrally located fovea, or facet, on the posterior aspect of the tibia approximately 1.0 to 1.5 cm distal to the joint line, with the posterior horn of the medial meniscus being the anterior-most extent. The center of the two fiber bundles is located, medially to laterally, at 48% of the mediolateral width of the tibial plateau from the medial tibial edge. The fiber regions should not be confused with the meniscofemoral ligaments, which are distinct and separate structures that need to be preserved in case PCL reconstruction will be performed. The majority of blood supply to the PCL stems from the middle geniculate artery, a branch of the popliteal artery. This vessel also supplies the synovial sheath, which contributes to PCL nourishment as well. Capsular vessels also supply the base of the PCL via branches from the popliteal artery and inferior geniculate arteries.

History

Numerous PCL reconstruction techniques have been described in the literature. Since its first description by Clancy and colleagues[3] in 1983, single-bundle PCL reconstruction has become a popular surgical option. Its focus is on the reconstruction of the larger, stiffer AL bundle via arthroscopic assistance. It has been reported that the grafted substances can be stretched owing to the concentration of stress caused by the acute angle between the graft and the intra-articular apertures of the tunnels. Therefore tibial inlay reconstruction has been proposed as an alternative technique to the transtibial tunnel single-bundle technique since early 1990s.[4] Rather than using a tunnel for tibial attachment, the tibial inlay technique uses a bone trough at the tibial site of PCL insertion to which the bone block of the graft is directly fixed. This type of reconstruction has the specific aim of restoring normal knee kinematics by achieving a more anatomic tibial fixation and by avoiding what has been described as the "killer turn."[5] However, no clear evidence of biomechanical superiority has been demonstrated from either a biomechanical or a clinical standpoint.[6,7] Furthermore, the need for an open approach and the specific setup for performance of a tibial inlay reconstruction have decreased its appeal for some orthopedic surgeons.

SURGICAL TECHNIQUE

Positioning, Examination Under Anesthesia, and Portals

The patient is positioned on the operating room table in the decubitus position with the knee flexed to 70 to 90 degrees, with the foot on the table. A standard arthroscopic inspection is carried out with the usual AL and anteromedial (AM) standard approaches. The key point in this technique is the use of two additional portals—the PM and the posterolateral (PL)—which allows the surgeon to perform the transseptal technique (Fig. 83-1).

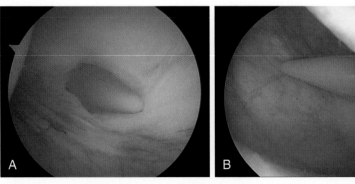

Figure 83-1. A, Posteromedial and **B,** posterolateral portal creation.

BOX 83-1 Surgical Steps in Arthroscopic Posterior Cruciate Ligament (PCL) Inlay

Tibial Inlay

- Quadriceps tendon harvesting and preparation of the graft
- Transseptal approach creation
- Preparation of the tibial slot
- Preparation of the femoral tunnel
- Graft passage and fixation via FiberWire tying on the anterior tibial cortex

Femoral PCL Inlay

- Quadriceps tendon harvesting and preparation of the graft
- Preparation of the femoral slot
- Graft passage and fixation via FiberWire tying on the medial femoral cortex

Specific Steps

Box 83-1 outlines the specific steps of this procedure.

Tibial Posterior Cruciate Ligament Inlay

The quadriceps tendon is the graft of choice owing to the superior biomechanical and anatomic features: it is larger and stronger and has lower harvest morbidity than the patellar tendon graft. It also has a soft tissue end that makes passage through the joint easier. Graft harvesting is accomplished through a short midline incision made approximately 6 cm from the midpatella, extending proximally to provide adequate exposure. Next, the fascial and multiple aponeurotic layers in front of the anterior surface of the patella are incised longitudinally. The osseotendinous junction of the quadriceps tendon at the upper patellar pole is recognized and a bone plug is harvested. Subsequently, the quadriceps tendon comprising the full thickness of the rectus femoris and a partial thickness of the vastus intermedius is incised longitudinally and proximally with a width of 10 mm, a depth of 6 mm, and a length of 8 cm from the top of the patella. The most inferior tendinous part of the vastus intermedius is best left intact to prevent rupture into the suprapatellar pouch. The proximal portion of the patella is prepared with a bone plug with a width of 10 mm, length of 10 mm, and depth of 9 to 10 mm and fashioned into a corticocancellous rectangle to fit the tibial trough. Two corticocancellous 2-mm drill holes are placed so that two FiberWire (Arthrex, Naples, FL) sutures are positioned through the holes.

The arthroscope is then shifted from AL to the PL portal and a motorized shaver is introduced from the contralateral portal. The posterior septum is removed with use of the technique described by Ahn and Ha.[8] The insertion site of the PCL stump on the tibia can then easily be identified (Fig. 83-2); the PCL tibial stump

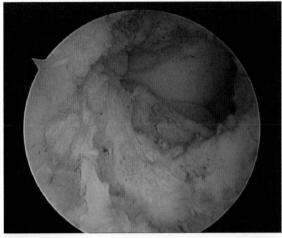

Figure 83-2. Posterior compartment transseptal view. The scope is placed via posterolateral portal looking at the posterior cruciate ligament tibial insertion and the posteromedial compartment.

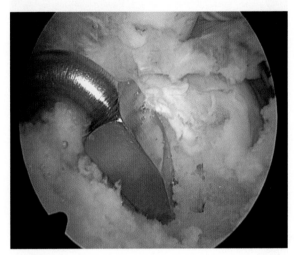

Figure 83-3. Preparation of the tibial slot. The scope is placed via posterolateral portal, and the rasp is inserted through the anteromedial access.

is debrided while the meniscofemoral ligaments are preserved.

When the posterior tibial sulcus has been identified, the periosteum is debrided and the posterior capsule is elevated from the tibial ridge. With curved rasps from the AM portal or with a motorized bur from the PM portal, the posterior sulcus is deepened under direct visualization to fit with the bone block (Fig. 83-3). After the creation of the inlay trough, two small tunnels are drilled within the slot to allow the passage of the sutures fixing the bone block to the slot (Figs. 83-4 and 83-5).

At this time the femoral tunnel is created with a technique that is more surgeon-friendly. Our preference is to perform an arthroscopically assisted outside-in technique. A PCL femoral drill guide is passed through the AM portal. Locating the proper position on the notch is critical; the femoral tunnel should be high in the notch, resembling the position of the AL bundle,

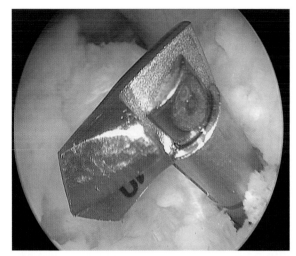

Figure 83-4. Retrograde drill system in situ.

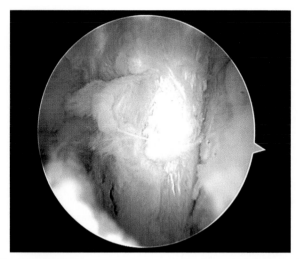

Figure 83-6. Transseptal view of the bone block placed in the tibial slot.

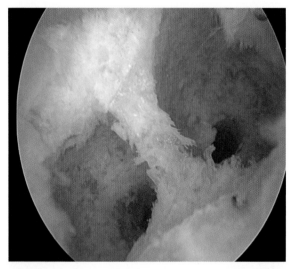

Figure 83-5. Final view of the tibial slot with the two tunnels.

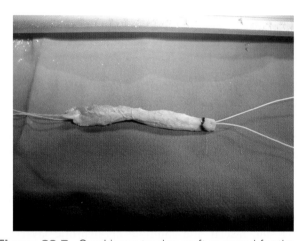

Figure 83-7. Quadriceps tendon graft prepared for the femoral inlay technique. The bone plug is rounder to fit in the circular femoral slot.

approximately 3 to 5 mm behind the articular surface. Ideally, the tunnel's direction is from distal to proximal and it is created via a skin incision, focused on the medial femoral condyle and a subcutaneous dissection to avoid the penetration of the vastus medialis. After completion of the femoral tunnels the graft is ready for passage of the posterior cannula. The bone block is placed on the tibial slot (Fig. 83-6), with the two sutures retrieved anteriorly and secured over the tibial cortex with use of a button to get a stronger tie. The soft tissue end of the graft is then placed in the femoral tunnel and fixed with a bioabsorbable screw at approximately 90 degrees of knee flexion with a maximum anterior drawer applied.

Femoral Posterior Cruciate Ligament Inlay

The first part of the surgery is performed as previously described until the preparation of the graft. The quadriceps tendon–patella construct is trimmed to a round bone plug with a diameter of 10 mm and a thickness of

10 mm (Fig. 83-7). Then a 2.0-mm-diameter hole is drilled at the center of the bone plug perpendicular to the cortex, and one or two FiberWire sutures are passed through this hole and through the tendon at the tendon-bone junction.

First the tibial tunnel is drilled with a transtibial technique. The arthroscopic PCL drill guide is set at 50 to 55 degrees and introduced through the AM portal under direct visualization. The scope is placed via either PM or PL access. Because the large posterior camera aids removal of the posterior septum, a K-wire can be safely placed and the tunnel can be drilled without radiographic control. Specifically, we try to seat the tip of the PCL guide proximally and laterally to preserve the highest possible number of PM fibers. Then the scope is placed through the AL portal, and the PCL femoral stump is debrided. Because the goal of the surgery is to reproduce the AL bundle, we strive to preserve the posteromedial bundle and the menisco-femoral ligament insertion. An inlay graft trough is

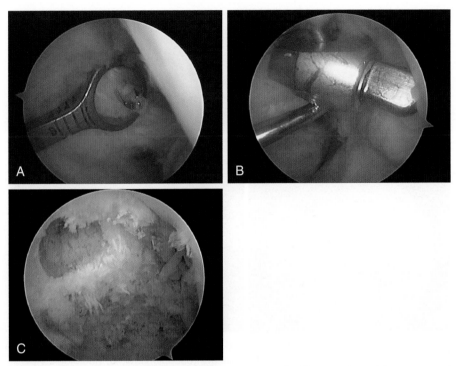

Figure 83-8. Femoral slot preparation. **A,** Outside-in wire placement. **B,** Slot creation with a retrograde drill system. **C,** Arthroscopic view.

created with a retrograde drill system after placement of a K-wire with an outside-in drill guide. The depth of the trough should fit the size of the bone plug (Fig. 83-8).

The graft is passed into the knee joint through the AL portal with the soft tissue pulled through the tibial tunnel with a leading suture. When the bone block is at the desired position, in front of the femoral trough, the bone block is gently seated with the help of a small hammer inserted through the AM portal. The FiberWire suture is retrieved through the femoral tunnel and pulled out of the skin. Usually the bone plug is slightly oversized to achieve a press-fit placement. At this time a skin incision is made on the medial femoral side and the sutures are tightened over an EndoButton (Smith & Nephew Endoscopy, Andover, MA) on the femoral cortex (Fig. 83-9). Distal fixation is achieved with use of a single oversized screw placed anatomically or a screw plus a washer according to both the bone quality and the surgeon's preference. For combined peripheral reconstruction, the distal fixation can be postponed until after the reconstruction of the PL or PM compartment.

POSTOPERATIVE CONSIDERATIONS

Follow-up and Rehabilitation

Full weight bearing usually is avoided for approximately 3 weeks for isolated reconstruction or up to 5 weeks for combined reconstruction to minimize the stresses on the graft. The restoration of motion with passive exercise is encouraged from the second week postoperatively while the knee is protected against gravity with specific brace. Return to sports activity is not allowed any earlier than 7 months postoperatively.

Complications

PCL reconstruction is an uncommon surgery, and a full arthroscopic inlay reconstruction is even more rare. Therefore even if specific complications have not been associated with this technique, certain precautions need to be taken. Risk of neurovascular injuries should be taken into account because of the close proximity of the popliteal artery and tibial nerve. The transseptal portal, if properly created, allows the surgeon to create a big posterior room, not allowing the posterior capsule to spread away from the posterior tibial cortex by use of the fluid pressure. On the other hand, too aggressive a removal of the posterior septum in the distal tibial area can cause fluid to leak within the posterior calf, which can mimic a compartmental-like syndrome. Persistent posterior sag after PCL surgery produces a suboptimal result of PCL reconstruction. Factors contributing to persistent posterior sag include failure to address peripheral instability, early weight bearing in flexion, improper graft placement, and inadequate graft fixation.

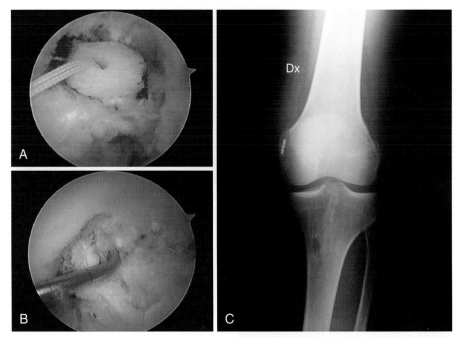

Figure 83-9. The graft is inserted via anterolateral portal and pulled through the tibial tunnel. The bone block is flipped (**A**) with the cancellous part facing the slot and inlayed. **B,** Final arthroscopic view. **C,** Radiologic view.

RESULTS

Clinical and basic scientific research continues to focus on how to best reconstruct the PCL. The concept of inlay reconstruction was first used at the tibial side to reduce the graft stresses showed by some authors in the early 2000s.[5] Subsequently, other studies[9,10] proposed that the true "killer turn" is found on the femoral side rather than on the tibial side, and this was our impetus to develop a femoral PCL inlay technique.

We believe that both tibial and femoral arthroscopic inlay techniques allow the surgeon to take advantage of the superior fixation and graft healing at the insertion site, which typically occurs within the first 4 to 6 weeks after surgery, the same period during which caution is taken to prevent early stresses on the graft.

Biomechanically, the posterior inlay technique has proven to be safe, with the suture providing similar initial and early fixation to that of a standardized, open PCL inlay technique with screw fixation.[11] In conclusion, arthroscopic inlay reconstruction appears to be a secure technique, although clinical studies are needed to see if these methods offer improvements over existing traditional methods.

REFERENCES

1. Mariani PP, Margheritini F. Full arthroscopic inlay reconstruction of posterior cruciate ligament. *Knee Surg Sports Traumatol Arthrosc.* 2006;14(11):1038-1044.
2. Margheritini F, Frascari Diotallevi F, Mariani PP. Posterior cruciate ligament reconstruction using an arthroscopic femoral inlay technique. *Knee Surg Sports Traumatol Arthrosc.* 2011;19(12):2033-2035.
3. Clancy Jr WG, Shelbourne KD, Zoellner GB, et al. Treatment of knee joint instability secondary to rupture of the posterior cruciate ligament. Report of a new procedure. *J Bone Joint Surg Am.* 1983;65(3):310-322.
4. Thomann YR, Gaechter A. Dorsal approach for reconstruction of the posterior cruciate ligament. *Arch Orthop Trauma Surg.* 1994;113(3):142-148.
5. Bergfeld JA, McAllister DR, Parker RD, et al. A biomechanical comparison of posterior cruciate ligament reconstruction techniques. *Am J Sports Med.* 2001;29(2): 129-136.
6. MacGillivray JD, Stein BE, Park M, et al. Comparison of tibial inlay versus transtibial techniques for isolated posterior cruciate ligament reconstruction: minimum 2-year follow-up. *Arthroscopy.* 2006;22(3):320-328.
7. Margheritini F, Mauro CS, Rihn JA, et al. Biomechanical comparison of tibial inlay versus transtibial techniques for posterior cruciate ligament reconstruction: analysis of knee kinematics and graft in situ forces. *Am J Sports Med.* 2004;32(3):587-593.
8. Ahn JH, Ha CW. Posterior trans-septal portal for arthroscopic surgery of the knee joint. *Arthroscopy.* 2000; 16(7):774-779.
9. Handy MH, Blessey PB, Kline AJ, et al. The graft/tunnel angles in posterior cruciate ligament reconstruction: a cadaveric comparison of two techniques for femoral tunnel placement. *Arthroscopy.* 2005;21(6):711-714.
10. Mariani PP, Margheritini F, Camillieri G, et al. Serial magnetic resonance imaging evaluation of the patellar tendon after posterior cruciate ligament reconstruction. *Arthroscopy.* 2002;18(1):38-45.
11. Campbell RB, Torrie A, Hecker A, et al. Comparison of tibial graft fixation between simulated arthroscopic and open inlay techniques for posterior cruciate ligament reconstruction. *Am J Sports Med.* 2007;35(10): 1731-1738.

Chapter 84

Posterolateral Corner Reconstruction

Bryan A. Warme and Warren R. Kadrmas

Chapter Synopsis
- Posterolateral corner (PLC) injuries of the knee can result in chronic instability and contribute to the development of knee arthritis if left untreated. Patients with a PLC injury should have the other knee ligaments evaluated to exclude a multiligamentous injury or knee dislocation. Various reconstruction techniques of the PLC structures have been reported to improve knee stability. Associated injuries and degree of instability can help surgical decision making.

Important Points
- Unstable PLC injuries are amenable to reconstruction and, in certain circumstances, repair. Furthermore, attempted repair can be augmented with reconstruction.
- Chronicity of the injury and associated injuries can assist surgical decision making.
- With multiligamentous knee injury, consideration should be given to use of allograft rather than autograft for reconstruction.

Clinical and Surgical Pearls
- Identify, release, and protect the common peroneal nerve throughout the procedure.

- Make a window through the iliotibial band to access the lateral collateral ligament and popliteal femoral insertions.
- The fibula tunnel trajectory should be angled laterally to medially as you drill anteriorly to posteriorly.
- If a knee dislocation is suspected, vascular injury should be ruled out.

Clinical and Surgical Pitfalls
- Postoperative peroneal palsy is possible even if the nerve is found to be intact. Warn the patient about this risk, and be sure to identify, release, and protect the nerve throughout the procedure.
- Fibula tunnel drilling can cause fracture. Do not attempt to drill too large a tunnel. Tunnels that are 7 to 8 mm in diameter are usually sufficient for adequate reconstruction.
- Failure to identify and address concomitant ligament injuries in the knee can compromise the PLC reconstruction outcome.

Injury to the posterolateral corner of the knee is a rare but often debilitating entity. Posterolateral corner injury is usually associated with additional ligament injury and can be missed on initial physical examination.[1-4] If it is identified early (within 3 weeks), many authors recommend acute repair of the posterolateral corner. However, recent data suggest that the results of reconstruction may be better than those of acute repair.[5]

Reconstruction of the posterolateral corner is indicated for those who are seen 3 weeks after injury or who have inadequate soft tissue for successful repair. Biomechanical data have shown that reconstruction of the posterolateral corner must restore function of the lateral collateral ligament and popliteofibular ligament to resist posterior translation, varus opening, and external rotation of the tibia on the femur.[5-8]

PREOPERATIVE CONSIDERATIONS

History

It is essential to obtain a complete history of the injury at the time of the initial evaluation. Injuries to the posterolateral corner of the knee are rarely isolated and are usually associated with significant trauma to the knee. A detailed account of previous treatments, as well as operative reports, if they are available, should be obtained before consideration of additional surgical intervention.

Typical History

- Acute, traumatic knee injury
- Activity-related instability
- Previous ligament reconstruction (anterior or posterior cruciate ligament) may have failed

Physical Examination

Examination of the cruciate and collateral ligaments as well as of the neurovascular status of the patient should be well documented. A significant percentage of posterolateral corner injuries occur in the setting of knee dislocation. Examination of the acute injury may be limited by pain.

Acute Injury

- Tenderness over posterolateral aspect of the knee with ecchymosis (Fig. 84-1)
- Positive varus instability at 30 degrees (and 0 degrees with combined injury)
- Possible associated ligamentous instability (anterior cruciate ligament, posterior cruciate ligament)
- Positive result of posterolateral drawer test
- Positive result of external rotation (dial) test: increased only at 30 degrees, isolated posterolateral corner injury; increased at 30 degrees and 90 degrees, posterior cruciate ligament and posterolateral corner injuries
- Positive result of external rotation recurvatum test (with combined injury) (Fig. 84-2)
- Positive result of reverse pivot shift test
- Examination findings possibly consistent with peroneal nerve injury

Chronic Injury

- Similar to acute injury, although a varus thrust during gait may develop
- Lateral joint line pain

Imaging

Radiography

- Weight-bearing anteroposterior radiograph in full extension
- Weight-bearing posteroanterior 45-degree flexion radiograph
- Non–weight-bearing 45-degree flexion lateral radiograph
- Patella Merchant radiograph
- Hip-to-ankle alignment film to evaluate position of weight-bearing axis in the knee

Other Modalities

Magnetic resonance imaging is performed to assess meniscus and ligamentous structures. Magnetic resonance arteriography may be considered, in conjunction with magnetic resonance imaging, for evaluation of acute or subacute posterolateral corner injuries in the setting of suspected knee dislocation.

Electromyelography is performed at 3 weeks if peroneal nerve injury is present.

Indications and Contraindications

Reconstruction of the posterolateral corner of the knee is generally indicated for complete disruptions (grade

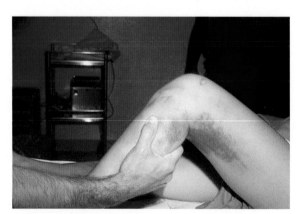

Figure 84-1. Clinical appearance of the knee after posterolateral corner injury.

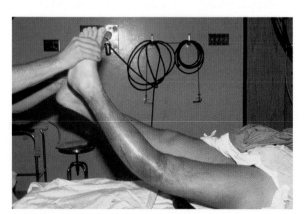

Figure 84-2. Positive result of external rotation recurvatum test.

III) or grade II injuries with symptomatic instability. Associated ligamentous injuries may need to be addressed at the time of posterolateral corner reconstruction. A relative contraindication for posterolateral corner reconstruction is varus knee alignment. High tibial osteotomy, before or in conjunction with the posterolateral corner reconstruction, should be considered in chronic injury.

Surgical Planning

Concomitant Procedures

Significant limb malalignment, chondral injury, or associated ligament injuries may need to be addressed before or in conjunction with the posterolateral corner reconstruction in chronic injury. Our standard technique uses a single graft passed through the fibula head and fixed to the anatomic insertions of the popliteal tendon and lateral collateral ligament on the femur (Figs. 84-3 and 84-4).[9] If there is extreme instability of the posterolateral corner, consideration can be given to adding a tibial tunnel to the construct.[10]

Graft Selection

Graft selection should be discussed with the patient at the preoperative visit. Graft options include hamstring autograft, Achilles tendon allograft, and anterior tibial tendon allograft tissue.

SURGICAL TECHNIQUE

Anesthesia and Positioning

Reconstruction of the posterolateral corner of the knee can be performed under general, combined spinal and epidural, or regional anesthesia on the basis of the patient's, anesthesiologist's, and surgeon's preferences. The patient is placed supine on a standard operating room table, and a tourniquet is applied to the upper thigh. The knee is flexed 20 to 30 degrees over a bump.

Surgical Landmarks

- Fibular head
- Gerdy tubercle
- Lateral epicondyle of the femur

Examination Under Anesthesia and Diagnostic Arthroscopy

Examination under anesthesia is performed to test the ligamentous structures of the knee. Diagnostic arthroscopy may be performed to further evaluate the lateral compartment and intra-articular structures. If combined ligamentous reconstruction, cartilage restoration procedures, and tibial osteotomy are to be considered, they

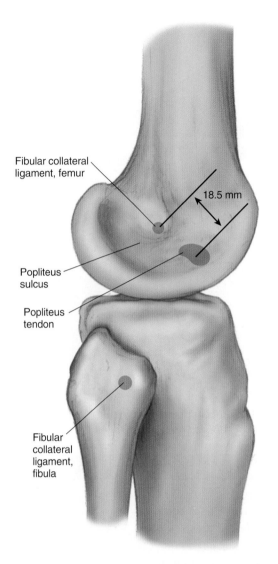

Figure 84-3. Posterolateral corner anatomy and tunnel landmarks. *(Modified from McCarthy M, Camarda L, Wijdicks CA, et al. Anatomic posterolateral knee reconstructions require a popliteofibular ligament reconstruction through a tibial tunnel. Am J Sports Med. 2010;38:1674-1681.)*

may be performed under arthroscopic assistance before the posterolateral corner is addressed.

Specific Steps

Box 84-1 outlines the specific steps of this procedure.

1. Exposure

An incision is made in the skin from a point just proximal and posterior to the lateral epicondyle and extended in line with the iliotibial band to a point just distal to Gerdy tubercle, midway between the Gerdy tubercle and the fibular head (Fig. 84-5A). The incision is carried sharply down to the level of the iliotibial band with a scalpel or electrocautery. Anterior and posterior soft

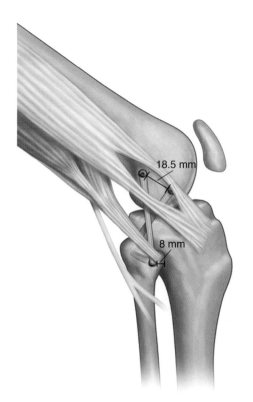

Figure 84-4. Reconstruction technique. *(Copyright 2011 Matthew Bollier, MD, and Aaron Szeto, MFA.)*

BOX 84-1 Surgical Steps

1. Exposure
2. Fibular tunnel preparation
3. Preparation of femoral tunnels
4. Graft preparation
5. Graft passage and fixation
6. Compartment release
7. Closure

---

tissue flaps are raised to expose the lateral epicondyle, the Gerdy tubercle, and the fibular head (Fig. 84-5B).

2. Fibular Tunnel Preparation

The posterior border of the long head of the biceps femoris is identified and incised sharply. The peroneal nerve is identified at the posterior border of the muscle belly and dissected from proximal to distal as it passes across the fibular head. The fascia overlying the peroneal muscles should be released to allow adequate decompression of the nerve. A vessel loop is placed around the nerve for identification and protection throughout the remainder of the procedure. After identification and protection of the peroneal nerve, anterior and posterior subperiosteal dissection of the fibular head is performed. A guidewire is placed from anterior to posterior, aiming slightly medially, approximately

2 cm from the tip of the fibula, and the guidewire over-reamed with a 7-mm reamer (Fig. 84-5D).[9,11] A No. 5 Ethibond (Ethicon, Somerville, NJ) suture is placed through the fibular hole and tagged for later graft passage.

3. Preparation of Femoral Tunnels

Attention is turned to the lateral epicondyle of the femur, which is easily palpated. A 3- to 4-cm incision is made in the iliotibial band at the level of the lateral epicondyle and extended distally. Blunt dissection is performed deep to the iliotibial band, and the lateral collateral ligament remnant and popliteus insertion are visualized. The lateral collateral ligament insertion lies proximal and posterior to the popliteal insertion, separated by an average distance of 18.5 mm (see Figs. 84-3 and 84-5C).[10] Subperiosteal dissection is performed at the popliteal insertion, and a guide pin is drilled into the lateral femoral condyle, with care taken not to penetrate into the joint or intercondylar notch. Accurate placement of the guide pin is confirmed with fluoroscopy. The pin then is overdrilled with a 7-mm reamer to a depth of 20 mm. Next, a slotted guide pin is drilled across the femur, starting at the lateral collateral insertion. Placement of the guide pin is made parallel to the joint line and confirmed with fluoroscopy. This pin is overdrilled with a size 7-mm reamer to a depth of 30 mm. Two No. 2 FiberWire (Arthrex, Naples, FL) sutures are placed in the slot of the guide pin, and the free ends are brought out the medial side of the knee.

4. Graft Preparation

The selected graft is subsequently prepared. A No. 2 FiberWire suture is placed in one end of the graft in a Krakow-type fashion; the other end is left free for future measurement and division.

5. Graft Passage and Fixation

The graft is brought through the fibular tunnel by the previously placed No. 5 Ethibond passing suture. Dissection under the iliotibial band is performed with a large clamp, and both ends of the graft are passed beneath it. The end of the graft with the Krakow suture is docked into the popliteal tunnel with an interference screw. The knee is subsequently reduced and taken through a full range of motion with the tibia held in internal rotation and a valgus stress applied. The free end of the graft is tensioned and brought to the aperture of the lateral collateral femoral tunnel for measurement. A No. 2 FiberWire suture is placed in a Krakow-type fashion from the point marked at the lateral collateral tunnel aperture and extended 20 mm distally. The free end of the graft is then divided immediately distal to the Krakow-type stitch. The suture ends in the graft are then shuttled into the tunnel and brought out the medial side of the knee with the remaining passing suture. With

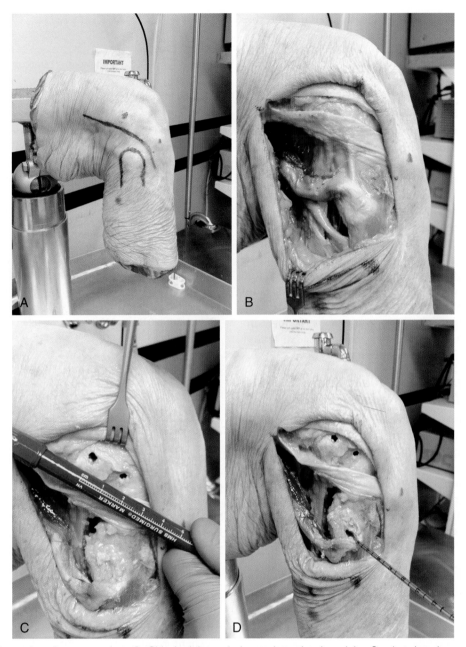

Figure 84-5. Dissection demonstration. **A,** Skin incision relative to lateral epicondyle, Gerdy tubercle, and fibular head. **B,** Normal posterolateral corner anatomy showing peroneal nerve, biceps tendon, and iliotibial band (split as in the reconstruction technique to expose the lateral femoral condyle. **C,** Femoral tunnels at the insertions of popliteal tendon and lateral collateral ligament. **D,** Guide pin demonstrating position and trajectory of fibular tunnel.

the knee held in its reduced position and tension applied to the graft at the free end, the knee is taken through a gentle range of motion to eliminate creep within the graft. The knee is brought to 20 degrees of flexion, and the tibia is maintained in internal rotation with a valgus stress. A soft tissue interference screw is placed from anterior to posterior (and lateral to medial) in the fibular tunnel to secure the graft distally. The lateral collateral limb of the graft is then secured with an interference screw (see Fig. 84-4). In the setting of osteoporotic bone or poor primary fixation, supplemental fixation with a

soft tissue button may be performed on the medial cortex of the femur through a separate small incision.

6. Compartment Release

The anterior and lateral compartments of the leg are released distally with long-handled Metzenbaum scissors before wound closure.

7. Closure

The incisions are closed in layers, and a drain is placed within the wound. Care should be taken to ensure that the peroneal nerve is not under tension during the closure.

Combined Procedures

Tibial Osteotomy and Posterolateral Corner Reconstruction

- High tibial osteotomy should be performed before or in conjunction with the posterolateral corner reconstruction.
- If the procedures are performed in conjunction, the tibial osteotomy should be done before the posterolateral corner reconstruction.
- The medial opening wedge osteotomy is indicated for patients with medial laxity and varus deformity.
- Consider medial opening wedge osteotomy for patients with varus deformity and grade I or grade II varus instability.
- Lateral closing wedge osteotomy is performed in patients with varus deformity without medial laxity or with grade III varus instability.

Combined Cruciate Ligament and Posterolateral Corner Reconstruction

Posterior and anterior cruciate ligaments should be secured within the tibial and femoral tunnels, respectively, before completion of posterolateral corner reconstruction. The knee is held in a reduced position during subsequent fixation of the posterolateral corner. The final posterior or anterior cruciate ligament fixation should be performed after completion of the posterolateral corner reconstruction.

POSTOPERATIVE CONSIDERATIONS

Follow-up

- At 7 to 10 days for suture removal and postoperative radiographs

Rehabilitation

- The patient is initially maintained in non–weight-bearing status in a hinged knee brace; range of motion is limited to 0 to 90 degrees of flexion (continuous passive motion may be used).
- Gentle strengthening exercises are initiated at 4 weeks.
- Progression of weight bearing to full begins 6 to 8 weeks postoperatively.
- In-line running is permitted after 16 weeks.
- Return to full activities is allowed after 6 months (if strength is within 80% of contralateral side).

TABLE 84-1. Results of Posterolateral Corner Reconstruction

Author	Follow-up	Outcome
Noyes and Barber-Westin[12] (1996)	42 months	16/21 (76%) good-excellent
Albright and Brown[13] (1998)	4 years	26/30 (87%) clinical improvement
Latimer et al[14] (1998)	28 months	10/10 (100%) resolution of subjective instability
Stannard et al[5] (2005)	2 years	20/22 (91%) successful
Yoon et al[15] (2006)	Minimum 1 year	Anatomic reconstruction: 20/21 (95%) good-excellent Posterolateral corner sling: 21/25 (84%) good-excellent
Rios et al[9] (2010)	Minimum 2 year	24/24 (100%) Lysholm score 83, Tegner score 6
LaPrade et al[16] (2011)	51 months	54/54 (100%) Cincinnati score 65.7, significant improvement in IKDC score

IKDC, International Knee Documentation Committee.

Complications

- Peroneal nerve injury
- Infection
- Arthrofibrosis
- Recurrent instability

RESULTS

After posterolateral corner reconstruction, good to excellent results can be expected in 85% to 90% of patients (Table 84-1). Patients will generally have resolution of instability but may continue to have some degree of pain, depending on the cartilage injury at the time of the initial trauma. Recent data suggest that the results of anatomic reconstructions may be better than those of procedures that do not attempt to restore the normal anatomy.[15]

REFERENCES

1. Baker Jr CL, Norwood LA, Hughston JC. Acute posterolateral rotatory instability of the knee. *J Bone Joint Surg Am.* 1983;65:614-618.
2. DeLee JC, Riley MB, Rockwood Jr CA. Acute posterolateral rotatory instability of the knee. *Am J Sports Med.* 1983;11:199-207.

3. Hughston JC, Andrews JR, Cross MJ, et al. Classification of knee ligament instabilities. Part II. The lateral compartment. *J Bone Joint Surg Am.* 1976;58:173-179.

4. Hughston JC, Jacobson KE. Chronic posterolateral rotatory instability of the knee. *J Bone Joint Surg Am.* 1985;67:351-359.

5. Stannard JP, Brown SL, Farris RC, et al. The posterolateral corner of the knee: repair versus reconstruction. *Am J Sports Med.* 2005;33:881-888.

6. Gollehon DL, Torzilli PA, Warren RF. The role of the posterolateral and cruciate ligaments in the stability of the human knee: a biomechanical study. *J Bone Joint Surg Am.* 1987;69:233-242.

7. Grood ES, Stowers SF, Noyes FR. Limits of movement in the human knee: effect of sectioning the posterior cruciate ligament and posterolateral structures. *J Bone Joint Surg Am.* 1988;70:88-97.

8. Veltri DM, Warren RF. Anatomy, biomechanics, and physical findings in posterolateral knee instability. *Clin Sports Med* 1994;13:599-614.

9. Rios CG, Leger RR, Cote MP, et al. Posterolateral corner reconstruction of the knee: evaluation of a technique with clinical outcomes and stress radiography. *Am J Sports Med.* 2010;38(8):1564-1574.

10. McCarthy M, Camarda L, Wijdicks CA, et al. Anatomic posterolateral knee reconstructions require a popliteofibular ligament reconstruction through a tibial tunnel. *Am J Sports Med.* 2010;38(8):1674-1681.

11. Arciero RA. Anatomic posterolateral corner knee reconstruction. *Arthroscopy.* 2005;21(9):1147.

12. Noyes FR, Barber-Westin SD. Surgical restoration to treat chronic deficiency of the posterolateral complex and cruciate ligaments of the knee joint. *Am J Sports Med.* 1996;24:415-426.

13. Albright JP, Brown AW. Management of chronic posterolateral rotatory instability of the knee: surgical technique for the posterolateral corner sling procedure. *Instr Course Lect.* 1998;47:369-378.

14. Latimer HA, Tibone JE, ElAttrache NS, et al. Reconstruction of the lateral collateral ligament of the knee with patellar tendon allograft: report of a new technique in combined ligament injuries. *Am J Sports Med.* 1998;26:656-662.

15. Yoon KH, Bae DK, Ha JH, et al. Anatomic reconstructive surgery for posterolateral instability of the knee. *Arthroscopy.* 2006;22:159-165.

16. LaPrade RF, Johansen S, Engebretsen L. Outcomes of an anatomic posterolateral knee reconstruction: surgical technique. *J Bone Joint Surg Am.* 2011;93(suppl 1):10-20.

   Noyes FR, Stowers SF, Grood ES, et al. Posterior subluxations of the medial and lateral tibiofemoral compartments: an in vitro ligament sectioning study in cadaveric knees. *Am J Sports Med.* 1993;21:407-414.

Chapter 85

Medial Collateral Ligament and Posteromedial Corner Repair and Reconstruction

John E. McDonald and Robert F. LaPrade

Chapter Synopsis

- Medial knee injuries can usually be treated nonoperatively. An operative intervention is warranted in certain acute, subacute, and chronic settings. The choice of the repair, augmentation, or reconstruction technique of the medial knee structures should be based on the ability of the technique to recreate the native anatomy and provide for immediate range of motion to prevent complications.

Important Points

- Gapping to valgus stress in full extension at time zero results in an increased chance of failure of nonoperative treatment.
- Tibial MCL lesions have a decreased chance of healing (especially in the setting of a Stener-type lesion), and consideration should be given to direct repair or augmentation.
- Allograft can be used in lieu of autograft for a medial reconstruction in the setting of a multiligament knee injury or if a prior hamstring harvest has been performed.

Clinical and Surgical Pearls

- Range of motion must be tested intraoperatively. It is imperative that the knee can be moved 0 to 90 degrees without significant tension on the repair or reconstruction construct. A very low rate of

arthrofibrosis can be achieved if the knee is moved from 0 to 90 degrees immediately postoperatively.
- It is important to place the distal tibial reconstruction tunnel for the superficial fibers of the medial collateral ligament (sMCL) along the posterior aspect of the attachment site, because tunnels placed too anteriorly were shown to fail when early range of motion was started in cadaver biomechanical testing.
- It is very helpful to find the adductor magnus tendon, which is rarely injured in medial knee injuries, at its attachment to the adductor tubercle to accurately find the sMCL and posterior oblique ligament (POL) femoral attachment sites.

Clinical and Surgical Pitfalls

- We cannot stress enough the importance of testing the safe zone of range of motion intraoperatively to prevent early motion in physical therapy from stretching the grafts and repair.
- It is helpful to notch the distal aspect of the distal sMCL reamed tunnel before placing the interference screw to prevent screw breakage or cutting of the graft.
- Do not ream the proximal sMCL or POL tunnels before placing both eyelet pins and measuring the distance between them to determine that they are anatomically placed. This prevents creation of a tunnel that one later finds is misplaced.

Injury to the medial aspect of the knee has traditionally been thought of as simply a medial collateral ligament (MCL) injury, but more recent research has concluded that the main medial knee structures have a complex relationship and provide both static and dynamic stability. The majority of acute isolated medial knee injuries can be treated nonoperatively, and a full return of function should be expected. The treatment of injuries to the medial knee had undergone a shift from aggressive operative treatment to almost exclusively nonoperative treatment; however, with the advent of new reconstructive techniques and acute augmentation techniques, the pendulum has swung back toward operative treatment in select patients.[1] The surgical reconstruction of choice should recreate the native anatomy and be justified by both biomechanical and clinical research.

PREOPERATIVE CONSIDERATIONS

History

The patient with a medial-sided knee injury can usually recall the injury mechanism. This typically is a valgus load to the knee and can occur when the foot is planted or from a direct lateral blow.[2] The recollection of hearing a "pop" can hint at the presence of a cruciate ligament injury or bone bruise. In the chronic setting, patients will describe the feeling of a side-to-side instability.

Physical Examination

Localized swelling and induration are present around the medial femoral condyle and/or proximal tibia. Deep medial joint line tenderness specifically is usually found only in the setting of a concomitant meniscal injury. The presence of a large hemarthrosis should alert the examiner to a potential combined cruciate ligament injury. The medial structures should be tested by the application of a valgus load at both full extension and 20 degrees of flexion. Isolated medial knee injuries will gap in 20 degrees of flexion, but the presence of gapping at full extension should heighten the suspicion for a concurrent cruciate ligament injury.[3] Of note, in our experience the presence of gapping in full extension at time zero (acute injury) is associated with an increased risk of failure of nonoperative treatment and chronic valgus laxity despite cruciate ligament reconstruction. The medial knee injury can be classified into three grades. Grade I injuries indicate a partial tear of the MCL and, on valgus stress, subjectively gap less than 5 mm. A grade II injury subjectively gaps 5 to 9 mm with valgus stress at 20 degrees of flexion and does not gap in extension.[4] Both of these injuries have firm endpoints with a valgus load. A grade III injury indicates a complete tear of the MCL. This injury subjectively gaps more than 10 mm at 20 degrees of flexion and often gaps at full extension as well. The examiner will typically find a soft or no endpoint.

A thorough ligamentous examination should be performed, including an anterior drawer, posterior drawer, Lachman, pivot-shift, reverse pivot-shift, dial, and posteromedial, anteromedial, and posterolateral drawer tests. It is very important to note that a positive dial test does not always indicate a posterolateral corner injury. Complete injury to the medial structures significantly increases external rotation at 30 and 90 degrees of flexion, resulting in a positive dial test.[5] It often occurs that a chronic medial knee injury will be misdiagnosed as a posterolateral corner injury owing to the presence of a positive dial test.

Imaging

Radiography

The injured and uninjured knees should be imaged with standard anteroposterior, lateral, patellofemoral, Rosenberg, and standing long-leg radiographs. Specifically, films should be evaluated for fractures, loose bodies, and capsular or ligamentous avulsions. In the chronic setting, valgus stress radiographs should be obtained to quantify the amount of medial compartment opening and should be compared with radiographs of the uninjured knee. If there is confusion regarding the exact diagnosis (positive dial test result), varus stress radiographs can be obtained as well. Gapping of more than 3.2 mm at 20 degrees of flexion is indicative of a grade III superficial MCL injury, whereas gapping of 6.5 mm at 0 degrees and 9.8 mm at 20 degrees of flexion is consistent with a complete medial-sided knee injury with rupture of the superficial fibers of the medial collateral ligament (sMCL), deep MCL, and posterior oblique ligament (POL).[6]

Magnetic Resonance Imaging

Magnetic resonance imaging (MRI) should be performed to evaluate for meniscal, cartilaginous, or other ligamentous injury and the presence of a distal meniscotibial Stener lesion, which might indicate the need for operative intervention.[7] The presence of lateral femoral condyle and lateral tibial plateau bone bruises should alert the physician to the possibility of a medial-sided injury. These lesions have been reported in 45% of medial knee injuries and typically resolve within 4 months from the time of injury.[8]

Anatomy

Three main structures provide stability to the medial knee—the sMCL, the deep MCL, and the POL. These structures provide restraint to valgus, external rotation, and internal rotation forces. The sMCL is the primary restraint to valgus load on the knee. It averages 9.5 cm in length and has one femoral and two tibial attachments. The femoral attachment site is not to the medial epicondyle, but is 3.2 mm proximal and 4.8 mm posterior to the medial epicondyle.[9] The proximal tibial attachment is 1.2 cm distal to the joint line and is primarily to soft tissues (anterior arm of the semimembranosus). The distal tibial attachment is reproducibly 6 cm distal to the joint line regardless of the patient's size. The proximal division of the sMCL is important for valgus stability, whereas the distal division is more important in stabilizing external rotation.

The second structure, the deep MCL, is primarily a thickening of the medial joint capsule with a femoral attachment 12.6 mm distal to the sMCL attachment and a tibial attachment 3.2 mm distal to the joint line. In addition, there is a very strong attachment to the medial meniscus.

Last, the POL has several attachments at the knee. This ligament is a thickening of the posteromedial joint capsule and is located posterior to the sMCL. The femoral attachment is 7.7 mm distal and 2.9 mm anterior to the gastrocnemius tubercle, and the tibial attachment of the central arm of the POL is 1 cm posterior to the anterior arm of the semimembranosus bony attachment on the tibia. The POL serves to limit internal rotation and valgus with the knee in full extension.

Indications

Indications for an acute operative repair of the MCL include the presence of a Stener lesion, a complete rupture of the sMCL from the distal insertion on the tibia, and the complete rupture of the medial knee structures from their femoral origin in the setting of a cruciate injury. If immediate postoperative range of motion cannot be started because of the tenuous nature of the repair, an sMCL augmentation should be performed with use of a semitendinosus autograft. A medial reconstruction should be undertaken to correct chronic side-to-side instability with documented medial gapping on stress radiography.

SURGICAL TECHNIQUE

Anesthesia and Positioning

The patient is placed supine on the operating table, and general anesthesia is induced. A preoperative femoral nerve indwelling catheter is placed by the anesthesiologist under ultrasound guidance, and 0.25% bupivacaine is administered for approximately 48 hours postoperatively to assist in postoperative pain control. The nonoperative leg is placed into a well-leg holder, and the fibular head is well padded. A thorough examination under anesthesia is performed, including evaluation of range of motion and the ligamentous examination described earlier. A nonsterile tourniquet is applied to the operative extremity, and the limb is placed into an arthroscopic leg holder after the foot of the bed has been completely lowered (Fig. 85-1). A surgical time-out to verify the operative extremity is performed, and prophylactic antibiotics are administered. The limb is prepared with chlorhexidine and draped in the standard fashion.

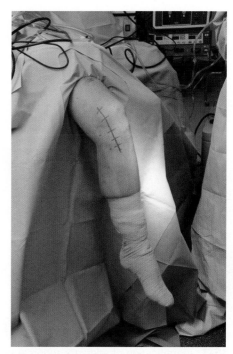

Figure 85-1. Left knee planned medial augmentation repair and reconstruction setup with arthroscopic leg holder.

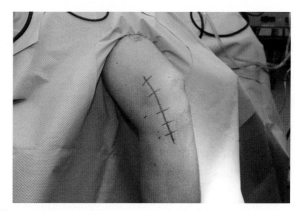

Figure 85-2. Left knee planned medial augmentation repair and reconstruction incision.

Surgical Landmarks, Incisions, and Portals

The incision for a repair of the femoral or tibial attachments of the sMCL should be centered over the attachment sites and be approximately 5 cm long. The incision for a reconstruction or augmentation is an anteromedial incision made 4 cm medial to the patella and extending distally over the midportion of the tibia, approximately 7 to 8 cm distal to the joint line (Fig. 85-2). If an arthroscopy is planned, the anteromedial portal can be made through this incision. It is recommended to perform the medial dissection and identify all of the pertinent landmarks, including the sMCL and POL femoral and tibial attachment sites, before beginning the

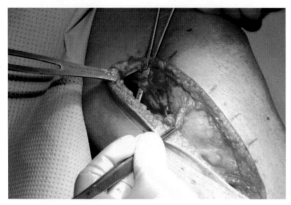

Figure 85-3. Identification of adductor tubercle with a clamp aids in determining the anatomic femoral attachments of the posterior oblique ligament and superficial fibers of the medial collateral ligament.

arthroscopy. The dissection is significantly more challenging once the tissue planes are distorted and the knee is distended from the arthroscopy fluid.

Specific Steps

Box 85-1 outlines the specific steps of the procedure.

1. Repair of Femoral Rupture

The leg is first exsanguinated with an Esmarch bandage, and the tourniquet is inflated to 250 mm Hg. The incision is made centered between the medial epicondyle and the medial border of the patella, and dissection is carried down to the sartorius fascia, with the saphenous nerve and vein identified and protected. The fascia is incised and retracted. The native sMCL and POL and the femoral attachment sites as described earlier should be identified. To best identify these structures, we recommend first identifying the distal attachment of the adductor magnus tendon (Fig. 85-3). The bony prominence slightly distal to its attachment is the adductor tubercle. The medial epicondyle is then distal to this and essentially parallel to the shaft of the femur, averaging 12.6 mm distal and 8.3 mm anterior to the adductor tubercle.[9] In contrast to prior reports, the attachment of the sMCL is actually slightly anterior and proximal to the medial epicondyle. The POL attachment site is next determined by first finding the medial gastrocnemius tendon and following it to the gastrocnemius tubercle. The gastrocnemius tubercle is 2.6 mm distal and 3.1 mm

anterior to the femoral origin of the medial gastrocnemius tendon.[9] The POL attachment is 7.7 mm distal and 2.9 mm anterior to this bony prominence.[9] If the posteromedial capsule is still intact, a vertical incision can be made posterior to the remnants of the sMCL into the joint, and a probe can be used to identify the femoral POL attachment site. A direct repair to bone can usually be accomplished with suture anchors. It is important to tension the sMCL in 20 degrees of flexion, neutral rotation, and slight varus. The POL should be sutured in full extension and in neutral rotation. If the POL is sutured in any degree of flexion, the repair has a very high likelihood of failing when early motion is begun on postoperative day 1. Of note, in contrast to historical literature, the femoral attachment sites for the sMCL and POL are not the medial epicondyle and adductor tubercle, and these structures should not be repaired to these locations. Great care should be taken to identify the anatomic attachments described earlier to recreate the native anatomy and allow for immediate range of motion. If the rupture is midsubstance, a direct suture repair of the two ends can be achieved, but consideration must be given to a concurrent augmentation repair.

2. Repair of Tibial Ruptures

For distally based ruptures, the dissection is carried down to the sartorius fascia, and the fascia is incised. If a Stener lesion is present, the sMCL should be passed posterior to the pes anserinus tendons before repair. The distal tibial sMCL attachment is consistently 6 cm distal to the joint line, and repair to bone can be achieved with suture anchors. It is important to use a position slightly posterior in the footprint to best recreate the anatomic location. When reconstructions methods were biomechanically tested, there was consistent failure when immediate range of motion was undertaken and the distal attachment was positioned slightly anterior in the footprint.

If the repaired tissues are of poor quality or the repair seems tenuous on range-of-motion testing intraoperatively, the surgeon should have a low threshold to perform an augmentation repair with a semitendinosus autograft.

3. Augmentation Repair

If an augmentation repair is planned, the dissection is carried down to the sartorius fascia, and the fascia is carefully dissected. The native sMCL and POL are identified, and the femoral and tibial attachment sites are marked with cautery. The semitendinosus is identified and harvested with an open hamstring harvester; the tendon is left attached to the tibial insertion (Fig. 85-4). The muscle remnants are debrided from the tendon with Metzenbaum scissors (Fig. 85-5). Two double-loaded suture anchors are placed at the sMCL distal attachment

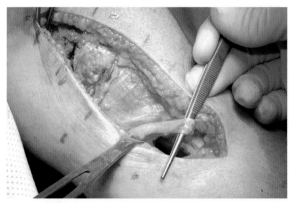

Figure 85-4. Identification of the semitendinosus tendon before harvest.

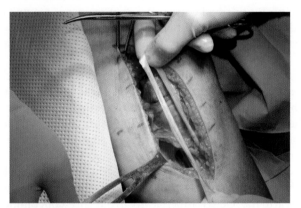

Figure 85-5. After harvesting of the semitendinosus tendon, it is stripped of all muscle.

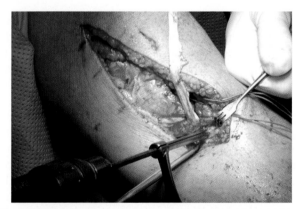

Figure 85-6. Drilling for placement of a double-loaded suture anchor at the distal attachment of the superficial fibers of the medial collateral ligament. Care is taken to achieve a position posterior in the footprint of the attachment site.

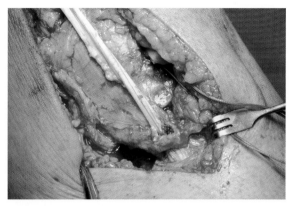

Figure 85-7. While posting the semitendinosus to the distal attachment site of the superficial fibers of the medial collateral ligament (sMCL), it is important to incorporate native sMCL to aid in healing of the augmentation repair.

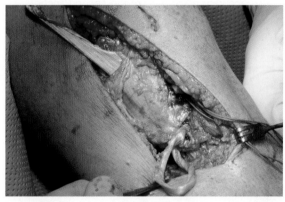

Figure 85-8. The semitendinosus graft has been passed deep to the sartorius fascia but superficial to the joint capsule.

site, 6 cm distal to the joint line and posterior in the footprint. The semitendinosus is "posted" to this attachment site by suturing to the anchors (Fig. 85-6). It is important to incorporate the native sMCL into this construct to facilitate healing and to strengthen the repair (Fig. 85-7). The semitendinosus is then passed deep to the sartorius fascia but superficial to the medial joint capsule along the course of the sMCL (Fig. 85-8). One single-loaded suture anchor is placed 1 cm distal to the joint line to secure the semitendinosus to the tibia at its proximal tibial attachment site. This recreates the proximal tibial attachment of the sMCL. Two double-loaded suture anchors are placed at the femoral attachment site (Fig. 85-9). The semitendinosus is secured to the femur, incorporating native sMCL tissue into the augmentation, while the knee is held in 20 degrees of flexion, neutral rotation, and slight varus (Fig. 85-10). There typically is a significant amount of semitendinosus remaining. It is looped back distally along the course of the augmentation, deep to the sartorius fascia, and secured to itself with No. 1 absorbable sutures while incorporation of the native sMCL tissue is continued (Fig. 85-11). If there is any remaining tendon, it is cut off at the end and disposed of. The knee should be taken through a range of motion to verify that the augmentation is secure from 0 to 90 degrees of flexion, because early range of motion is imperative if an optimal result is to be obtained and for the risk of arthrofibrosis to be decreased.

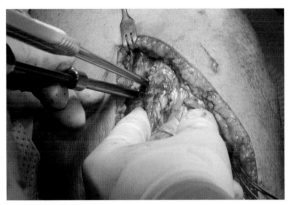

Figure 85-9. Preparing the second tunnel for a double-loaded suture anchor at the femoral attachment site of the superficial fibers of the medial collateral ligament and posterior oblique ligament. The first anchor can be seen still attached to its handle. Leaving this handle in place facilitates accurate placement of the second anchor.

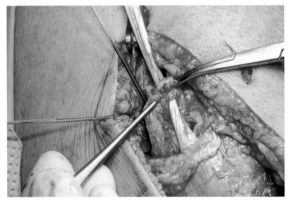

Figure 85-10. Incorporation of native superficial fibers of the medial collateral ligament into the semitendinosus graft aids in healing of the graft.

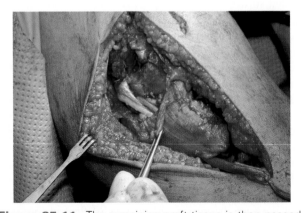

Figure 85-11. The remaining graft tissue is then passed deep to the sartorius fascia again and secured to itself and the native tissue of the superficial fibers of the medial collateral ligament.

4. Medial Knee Reconstruction

The approach for the reconstruction is identical to that for the augmentation. The semitendinosus is harvested for use in the reconstruction. In most patients, at least the remnant of the distal tibial sMCL attachment can be identified deep within the pes anserine bursa and is located 6 cm distal to the joint line. As mentioned earlier, it is critical to place the reconstruction tunnel posterior at the attachment site, not at the anterior portion. During biomechanical testing of this technique, all the reconstruction grafts failed when placed anteriorly.[10]

First, an eyelet pin is passed through the posterior aspect of the distal tibial attachment site transversely across the tibia, with care taken to avoid drilling through the posterior tibial cortex. A 7-mm reamer is reamed to a depth of 25 mm. In smaller patients, the use of a 6-mm reamer may be necessary. Cold irrigation should be used to prevent overheating while reaming.

Second, the identification of the POL tibial attachment is undertaken. This is found at the posteromedial tibia, slightly anterior to the direct arm attachment of the semimembranosus tendon. Exposure can be obtained via an incision along the posterior edge of the anterior arm of the semimembranosus tendon. Similarly to the procedure used for the distal tibia attachment, an eyelet pin is placed across the tibia and should be aimed toward the Gerdy tubercle to avoid any concomitant anterior and posterior cruciate ligament reconstruction tunnels. A 7-mm reamer is used to drill a tunnel 25 mm deep.

The proximal attachment sites of the sMCL and POL are then identified as described earlier. In the chronic setting, these structures can be very difficult to identify, and a detailed dissection is recommended. Occasionally, intraoperative fluoroscopy can be used to identify the correct anatomic femoral attachment sites.[11] Once the site has been correctly identified, an eyelet pin is placed transversely across the femur and aimed anteriorly and proximally to avoid any posterolateral corner reconstruction tunnels and to avoid the common peroneal nerve. The POL site is then addressed before the sMCL tunnel is reamed. This step is to avoid having the tunnels placed in an incorrect location before the distance between the attachment sites has been fully assessed and the relationship to the bony prominences has been reverified. One should always look for native remnant tissue to confirm that the sites are anatomic and to incorporate into the repair. Once both sites have been correctly identified, two 7-mm tunnels are reamed to a depth of 25 mm.

The grafts should be prepared on the back table, with the sMCL reconstruction graft measuring 16 cm and the POL graft measuring 12 cm (Fig. 85-12). The semitendinosus graft should be cut to achieve these lengths. Once the grafts have been prepared, the eyelet pins are repositioned back into the femoral tunnels. Both ends of each graft should be tubularized and are then passed into the femoral tunnels via the eyelet pins. A cannulated bioabsorbable screw is then placed anteriorly in each tunnel to secure each graft.

Both grafts are then passed distally—the POL within the substance of the native POL, and the sMCL under the sartorius fascia and any sMCL native remnants. These are then passed into their respective tunnels with the eyelet pin, and the knee is cycled several times to

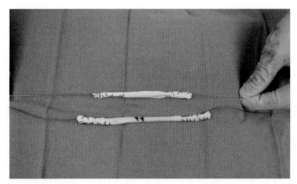

Figure 85-12. Graft preparation of semitendinosus autograft.

eliminate any slack while traction is placed on the grafts. This step is performed to ensure there is no impingement on the grafts by soft tissue or scarring. Once any concomitant cruciate ligament reconstruction grafts have been secured, the medial reconstruction grafts are secured in their tunnels.

The POL graft is secured first in full extension, because the primary function of the POL is to resist internal rotation near full extension.[12] The surgeon should then flex the knee to 90 degrees to ensure that this graft becomes slack. The sMCL graft is then secured in 20 degrees of knee flexion, neutral rotation, and slight varus. Next, the proximal tibial attachment site of the sMCL is addressed. This is located 1.2 cm distal to the medial joint line and is directly medial to the anterior arm of the semimembranosus tendon attachment. A suture anchor is placed at this location, and the graft is secured (Fig. 85-13). This fixation has been shown to replicate that of the native proximal tibial attachment site.[13] Last, the knee is flexed to the point where any repaired tissue appears to be weakening; this determines the safe zone of range of motion that can be started on postoperative day 1. The goal should be to obtain at least 90 degrees of flexion for the safe zone of range of motion.

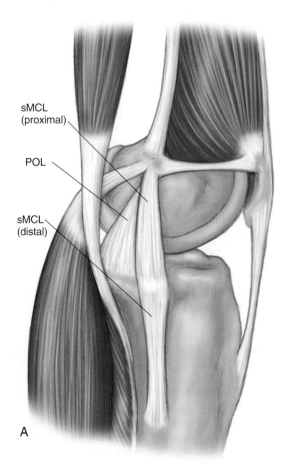

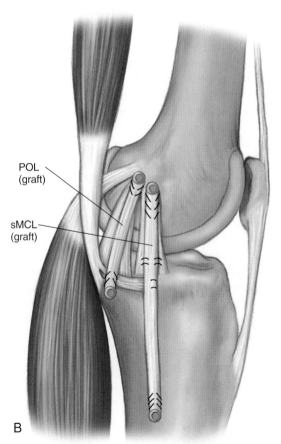

Figure 85-13. The native anatomy (**A**) and the final medial knee reconstruction (**B**) of the superficial fibers of the medial collateral ligament and posterior oblique ligament.

POSTOPERATIVE CONSIDERATIONS

Rehabilitation

Early range of motion is stressed for an anatomic medial knee reconstruction. This rehabilitation focus aims to prevent quadriceps atrophy and intra-articular adhesion formation. The patient begins physical therapy on postoperative day 1 and moves the knee within the safe zone determined intraoperatively for the first 2 weeks. An emphasis is placed on patella mobilization and quadriceps setting exercises. Regardless of the treatment for the medial knee injury, the patient is kept on non–weight-bearing status for 6 weeks. A hinged knee brace is used for 6 weeks throughout the day and night, and it is used for an additional 6 weeks when the patient is outside of the house. The brace is limited 0 to 90 degrees for the first 6 weeks, and then the patient is allowed full range of motion. The initial 6 weeks are focused on range of motion, patellar mobility, quadriceps reactivation, and edema control. Double-leg strengthening begins at 6 weeks if the patient has no effusion and 0 to 90 degrees of knee motion without difficulty. Closed kinetic chain exercises are initiated, and, to limit joint translation, leg presses are limited to 70 degrees of knee flexion. Once weight bearing is initiated, it is imperative to instruct the patient to avoid pivoting motions of the foot, which could stress the reconstruction or repair. Single-leg strengthening begins at approximately 16 to 20 weeks, once a patient can walk without a limp. A full return to activities and sport occurs once the patient is able to pass a sport-specific barrage of functional testing and has objective evidence of healing on valgus stress radiographs.

Complications

Several complications can theoretically occur with repair, augmentation, or reconstruction of the medial knee structures and most commonly include saphenous nerve injury, infection, graft failure, and stretching of the graft or repair with resultant continued side-to-side instability. Arthrofibrosis has typically been considered a relatively common complication when these procedures are performed. However, with use of the augmentation and reconstruction techniques in conjunction with the postoperative rehabilitation protocol described, the senior author (R.F.L.) has not seen one case of arthrofibrosis.

RESULTS

The senior author (R.F.L.) has prospectively evaluated 28 patients with an average age of 32.4 years (16 to 56 years) with an average follow-up of 1.5 years (0.5 to 3 years). Preoperative gapping on valgus stress radiography averaged 6.2 mm (3.5 to 14 mm), whereas postoperative gapping averaged 1.3 mm (1.0 to 2 mm). Preoperative subjective outcome scores from the International Knee Documentation Committee (IKDC) averaged 43.5 (14 to 65), and postoperative scores averaged 76.2 (54 to 88). All patients noted an improvement in side-to-side instability symptoms at final follow-up.[14]

REFERENCES

1. Tibor LM, Marchant MH, Taylor DC, et al. Management of medial-sided knee injuries, part 2: posteromedial corner. *Am J Sports Med*. 2011;39(6):1332-1340.
2. Loredo R, Hodler J, Pedowitz R, et al. Posteromedial corner of the knee, MR imaging with gross anatomic correlation. *Skeletal Radiol*. 1999;28:305-311.
3. Marchant MH, Tibor LM, Sekiya JK, et al. Management of medial-sided knee injuries, part 1: medial collateral ligament. *Am J Sports Med*. 2011;39(5):1102-1113.
4. Hughston J, Eilers A. The role of the posterior oblique ligament in repairs of the acute medial (collateral) ligament tears of the knee. *J Bone Joint Surg Am*. 1973;55:923-955.
5. Griffith CJ, LaPrade RF, Johansen S, et al. Medial knee injury: Part 1, static function of the individual components of the main medial knee structures. *Am J Sports Med*. 2009;37:1762-1770
6. LaPrade RF, Bernhardson AS, Griffith CJ, et al. Correlation of valgus stress radiographs with medial knee ligament injuries: an in vitro biomechanical study. *Am J Sports Med*. 2010;38:330-338.
7. Corten K, Hoser C, Fink C, et al. Case reports: a Stener-like lesion of the medial collateral ligament of the knee. *Clin Orthop Relat Res*. 2010;468(1):289-293.
8. Miller MD, Osborne JR, Gordon WT, et al. The natural history of bone bruises. A prospective study of magnetic resonance imaging-detected trabecular microfractures in patients with isolated medial collateral ligament injuries. *Am J Sports Med*. 1998;26:15-19.
9. LaPrade RF, Engebretsen AH, Ly TV, et al. The anatomy of the medial part of the knee. *J Bone Joint Surg Am*. 2007;89:2000-2010.
10. Coobs BR, Wijdicks CA, Armitage BM, et al. An in vitro analysis of an anatomic medial knee reconstruction. *Am J Sports Med*. 2010;38:339-347.
11. Wijdicks CA, Griffith CJ, LaPrade RF, et al. Radiographic identification of the primary medial knee structures. *J Bone Joint Surg Am*. 2009;91:521-529.
12. Griffith CJ, Wijdicks CA, LaPrade RF, et al. Force measurements on the posterior oblique ligament and superficial medial collateral ligament proximal and distal divisions to applied loads. *Am J Sports Med*. 2009;37:140-148.
13. Wijdicks CA, Brand EJ, Nuckley DJ, et al. Biomechanical evaluation of a medial knee reconstruction with comparison of bioabsorbable interference screw constructs and optimization with a cortical button. *Knee Surg Sports Traumatol Arthrosc*. 2010;18:1532-1541.
14. LaPrade RF, Wijdicks CA. Surgical technique: development of an anatomic medial knee reconstruction. *Clin Orthop Relat Res*. 2012;470:806-814.

Chapter 86

Multiligament Knee Reconstruction: The Pittsburgh Approach

Karl F. Bowman Jr, Rodrigo Salim, and Christopher D. Harner

Chapter Synopsis

- The term *multiligamentous knee injury* implies partial or complete rupture of at least two of the ligamentous stabilizers of the knee in varying combinations. The diagnosis and management of these injuries presents a clinical challenge to even the most experienced orthopedic surgeon. It is important to remember that the spectrum of injury varies widely and that every knee is different. An individualized treatment plan needs to be established for each patient after classification of the pattern of instability and identification of associated pathology. A detailed discussion of the diagnosis, treatment options and alternatives, and risks and complications of surgical intervention should be performed before one obtains surgical consent and proceeds to the operating room.

Important Points

- Dislocation should be suspected in a knee with gross instability in two or more ligament groups and warrants a high index of suspicion for associated vascular and nerve injuries.
- Acute surgical indications include the presence of vascular injury requiring intervention, open or irreducible knee dislocation, and compartment syndrome.
- Relative indications for early intervention include displaced meniscus tears and grade 3 injury to the posterolateral corner structures.
- Delayed and/or staged surgery is acceptable in many patients to decrease the risk of arthrofibrosis. We routinely wait 6 to 8 weeks to allow for resolution of acute inflammation and restoration of quadriceps strength and knee range of motion.
- The examination under anesthesia is a critical step in the final surgical plan. In most patients we consider it more important than magnetic resonance imaging (MRI) in assessing the degree of ligamentous laxity.

- Expect clinical outcomes after multiligamentous knee injuries to be less successful than after standard anterior cruciate ligament (ACL) surgery.
- Be prepared for any and all complications!

Clinical and Surgical Pearls

- Be specific with the diagnosis, including the timing of injury, grade of injury, and associated injuries.
- Carefully plan the operative management of multiligamentous injuries, and perform electively when well rested.

Surgical Sequence

- Perform cruciate reconstructions first, and pass and fix grafts on the femoral side.
- Perform collateral ligament repair or reconstruction after cruciate grafts have been passed.

Posterolateral Corner Repair and Reconstruction Pearls

- Acute repair of complete avulsions should be performed within 10 to 14 days.
- One third of acutely injured knees can be repaired.
- Stage cruciate reconstruction after posterolateral corner repair or reconstruction.
- Identify and protect the peroneal nerve.

Medial Collateral Ligament Reconstruction Pearls

- We almost always delay medial collateral ligament (MCL) surgery for 6 to 8 weeks.
- MCL reconstruction is rarely required, and almost all MCL injuries can be repaired.
- Tibial-sided injuries are less likely to heal.
- Use MRI to define level of injury before surgery, and target management to address the specific injury location.
  - Proximal—Advance ligament and tie over screw and washer at the anatomic footprint.

Continued

–   Middle—Advance posterior oblique ligament (POL) to tighten the MCL midsubstance.
–   Distal—Elevate and advance the native ligament. Secure with screw and washer at the anatomic insertion.

Graft Tensioning

- ACL—full extension
- Posterior cruciate ligament (PCL)—90 degrees of knee flexion with an anterior drawer
- Lateral collateral ligament (LCL)—30 degrees of flexion with gentle tibial internal rotation
- Popliteofibular ligament—30 degrees of flexion with gentle tibial internal rotation
- MCL—30 degrees of knee flexion
- POL—near full extension

Clinical and Surgical Pitfalls

- Check frequently for preoperative and postoperative deep vein thrombosis (DVT) and use appropriate prophylaxis. Do not hesitate to obtain a venous duplex Doppler scan if there is a clinical suspicion of DVT.
- Beware of posterior horn and root tears of the medial meniscus associated with PCL injuries.
- Always find and assess any injury to the peroneal nerve during posterolateral corner reconstructions. If encountered, be aggressive with bracing and early range of motion to prevent contractures before the return of neurologic function (if any).
- Postoperative rehabilitation and return to work or sports is slower than with primary ACL surgery.

The diagnosis and management of the multiple ligament–injured knee presents a clinical challenge to even the most experienced orthopedic surgeon. We consider *multiligamentous knee injury* to be a spectrum that can range from a cruciate plus a collateral ligament injury to a bicruciate (dislocated knee) injury with or without collateral involvement. It is important to remember that the severity of injury varies widely and that every knee is different. Certain ligaments can be partially injured and may heal with nonoperative management (medial collateral ligament [MCL]; posterior cruciate ligament [PCL]). The most commonly encountered multiligamentous injuries at our institution are combined anterior cruciate ligament (ACL)–MCL and PCL–posterolateral corner (PLC) injuries, followed by bicruciate ruptures with an associated collateral ligament tear. Treatment strategies should follow basic clinical guidelines, which may need to be adjusted on an individual basis.[1]

PREOPERATIVE CONSIDERATIONS

These injuries typically have one of three presentations: immediately after a traumatic event in the emergency room, in the clinical setting after acute evaluation and stabilization, and in the setting of chronic instability. Assessment begins with a thorough history and physical examination to establish the mechanism of injury; to characterize the functional, employment, and athletic status of the patient; and to identify concomitant injuries and prior knee pathology. Initial evaluation must be performed expeditiously to identify indications for emergent intervention and minimize potentially limb-threatening complications including compartment syndrome, popliteal artery lacerations, and peroneal nerve

injuries. Dislocation should be considered in knees with gross instability of two or more ligaments because more than 50% reduce spontaneously before evaluation.[2]

The physical examination of the knee begins with assessing for abrasions, lacerations, previous surgical scars, and the presence of significant intra-articular or lower extremity swelling. A careful neurovascular examination to detect pulse asymmetry and distal motor or sensory deficits is performed, and concern for arterial injury should prompt urgent evaluation with noninvasive vascular studies (ankle-brachial indexes [ABIs]), computed tomography (CT) angiography, or popliteal arterial angiography.[3] Characterization of the pattern of ligamentous instability is performed with an evaluation of patellar stability and Lachman, anterior and posterior drawer, and varus and valgus testing at full knee extension and 30 degrees of flexion. Additional rotatory testing including a dial test and evaluation of posteromedial and posterolateral rotatory instability is performed as indicated. It is important to evaluate clinical laxity with the tibiofemoral joint initially reduced, because abnormal positioning of the joint may lead to overestimation or underestimation of tibial translations, especially during posterior drawer or rotatory testing. Comparison with the contralateral extremity allows detection of subtle clinical laxities, although swelling, pain, and guarding may interfere with the ability to accurately identify and grade ligament injuries. We grade all injuries with the International Knee Documentation Committee (IKDC) standard clinical laxity scale (grade 1, 3 to 5 mm; grade 2, 5 to 10 mm; grade 3, more than 10 mm). By definition, a partial ligamentous injury is categorized as grade 1+ or 2+, and a complete tear as grade 3+.[4]

We obtain standard radiographs of both knees in all patients to evaluate for fracture, associated arthritis, and joint reduction. The presence of subtle findings including avulsion fracture, joint subluxation, and patellar height is also assessed. Magnetic resonance imaging (MRI) assists in the grading of ligamentous injuries and identification of pathology of the menisci, chondral surfaces, and related structures.[5] The MRI findings are reviewed with the direct input of our musculoskeletal radiology colleagues before an individualized treatment plan is established.

Acute surgical indications include vascular injuries requiring intervention, open or irreducible knee dislocation, and compartment syndrome. We previously reported on performance of ligamentous repair or reconstruction within 1 to 3 weeks of injury,[4,6] although we now prefer delaying surgery to allow for resolution of the acute inflammatory phase of injury (i.e., swelling), interval healing of previous surgical interventions (e.g., vascular repair, fasciotomy), restoration of knee range of motion (ROM), and the return of quadriceps motor control. Relative indications for acute surgical intervention (within 14 days) in our hands include grade 3 PLC avulsions and displaced longitudinal meniscal tears; anatomic repair can be performed before the onset of significant scarring or retraction. Primary cruciate ligament reconstruction can be deferred for 6 to 8 weeks with frequent clinical evaluation to assess the pattern of ligamentous instability and detection of factors including deep vein thrombosis (DVT) or wound complications. A detailed discussion of the diagnosis, the treatment options and alternatives, and the risks and complications of surgical intervention is performed before surgical consent is obtained and the procedure is begun.

SURGICAL TECHNIQUE
Anesthesia

The choice of anesthesia is determined in conjunction with the patient, anesthesiologist, and surgeon. Influential factors include the patient's age, medical comorbidities, and previous anesthetic history. A general anesthetic is routinely used, with muscular relaxation required only during the examination under anesthesia. Adjuvant regional anesthesia with indwelling femoral and sciatic catheters is allowed for pain control after an appropriate postoperative neurovascular examination has been performed.

Positioning

The patient is identified in the preoperative holding area, and the informed consent is reviewed. The operative extremity is marked with the word "yes" and the surgeon's initials within the surgical field. A small bump is placed under the ipsilateral sacroiliac joint, and a

lateral post is placed at the level of the greater trochanter. A 10-pound sandbag is secured to the operative table with tape to allow the limb to rest at 90 degrees of knee flexion without manual assistance. A tourniquet is not used during our surgical procedures. The contralateral extremity is padded to the level of the SI joint with surgical foam. A Foley catheter is routinely placed to manage intraoperative fluid balance during the procedure. Intravenous antibiotics are administered for routine prophylaxis within 60 minutes of the skin incision.

Surgical Landmarks, Incisions, and Portals

The surface anatomy is identified and the planned surgical incisions are marked. Important landmarks include the inferior patellar pole, tibial tubercle, Gerdy tubercle, fibular head, and medial and lateral joint lines. The soft spot at the fibular neck is palpated and marked to correspond to the expected location of the peroneal nerve. The anterolateral portal is placed 2 to 3 mm lateral to the edge of the patellar tendon at the level of the inferior pole of the patella, and the anteromedial portal is placed 1 cm medial to the patellar tendon at the same level. A careful assessment of the presence of patella alta or baja is performed to allow consistent placement of the arthroscopic portals with respect to the joint line. A superolateral outflow portal is placed 1 cm proximal to the superior pole of the patella between the vastus lateralis and the iliotibial (IT) band. If a posteromedial portal is required, the site is determined during arthroscopy with a spinal needle (Fig. 86-1).

The surgical incisions are injected with 0.25% bupivacaine and 1:100,000 epinephrine for hemostasis. Our standard anterior surgical incision for tibial tunnel placement and hamstring autograft harvest is longitudinally centered between the anterior and posterior borders of the anteromedial tibial cortex approximately 3 cm distal to the joint line. An anterior longitudinal incision from the midpatella to the distal aspect of the tibial tubercle, overlying the medial border of the patellar tendon, is used for patellar ligament autograft harvest, and a 6-cm longitudinal incision centered over the proximal patella and quadriceps tendon is used for quadriceps tendon autograft harvest. Lateral procedures are performed through a 12-cm curved incision centered between the biceps femoris tendon and IT band proximally and the fibular head and Gerdy tubercle distally. Medial ligament injuries are addressed through a proximal extension of the anteromedial tibial incision that is centered over the junction of the middle and posterior third of the medial femoral condyle and extends toward the distal edge of the vastus medialis obliquus (VMO). We attempt to preserve the largest skin bridge possible (minimum 7 cm) between incisions

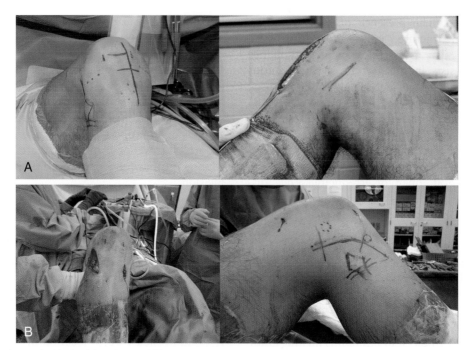

Figure 86-1. Balanced skin incision for multiligamentous knee reconstructions. **A,** Anterior cruciate ligament reconstruction, lateral meniscus repair, and medial collateral ligament repair with use of a bone–patellar tendon–bone autograft. **B,** Posterior cruciate ligament and posterolateral corner reconstruction. The fibular head and expected location of the peroneal nerve are identified.

to minimize wound healing complications. Midline incisions are avoided.[7]

Examination Under Anesthesia

The examination under anesthesia is the most important step in determining the final surgical plan. In most patients we consider it more important than the MRI findings for assessing the degree of ligamentous injury. We use fluoroscopy to directly compare the amount of pathologic laxity with the contralateral extremity. Our standard examination includes anterior and posterior drawer, Lachman, varus and valgus, and medial and lateral rotational tests. These tests are performed with the tibiofemoral joint initially reduced to prevent underestimation or overestimation of pathologic motion (Fig. 86-2).

Specific Steps

Box 86-1 outlines the specific steps of the procedure.

Cruciate Ligament Reconstruction[8]

The majority of cruciate ligament injuries encountered in adults are complete intrasubstance tears that are not amenable to primary repair and require reconstruction. We perform an anteromedial portal technique for ACL reconstruction and an all-arthroscopic single-bundle

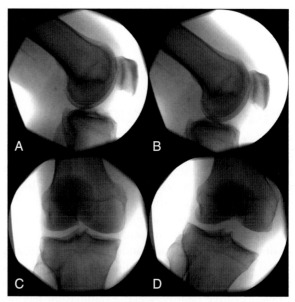

Figure 86-2. The examination under anesthesia of a patient with a grade 3 anterior cruciate ligament (ACL) injury, grade 2 posterior cruciate ligament (PCL), and grade 3 medial collateral ligament (MCL) is shown. An ACL reconstruction and proximal MCL repair were performed, and the PCL was treated nonoperatively. Fluoroscopy is used to evaluate the amount of pathologic laxity encountered. It is important to begin with the joint in a reduced position to avoid underestimation or overestimation of laxity.

BOX 86-1 Surgical Steps

- Cruciate ligament reconstruction
- Posterolateral corner and lateral collateral ligament injury repair
- Isolated lateral collateral ligament reconstruction
- Popliteofibular ligament reconstruction
- Repair of medial collateral ligament (MCL) and posterior oblique ligament
- Repair of proximal (femoral side) MCL injuries
- Repair of distal (tibial side) MCL injuries
- Repair of midsubstance MCL injuries
- Wound closure

---

transtibial technique for PCL reconstruction. The senior author (C.D.H.) routinely delays cruciate reconstruction for 6 to 8 weeks to allow for resolution of swelling, return of full knee ROM, and quadriceps control. This approach also allows autograft tissues to be used while decreasing the risk of arthrofibrosis from the graft harvest. Use of fresh-frozen allograft tissue has the advantages of avoidance of donor site morbidity, decreased surgical time, and potentially decreased pain and stiffness postoperatively. Disadvantages include slower graft incorporation and risk of disease transmission.[9] We prefer the use of an autograft for ACL reconstruction and will frequently use allograft tissue for PCL reconstructions. Bicruciate ligament reconstructions are performed in a specific sequence to ensure appropriate tunnel placement and minimize the risk of convergence (Fig. 86-3). We begin with establishing the most technically demanding tunnel (PCL tibial tunnel), followed by the ACL femoral tunnel and the PCL femoral tunnel, and finish with the ACL tibial tunnel. The ACL tibial tunnel is placed on the anteromedial tibial cortex, and the PCL tibial tunnel is placed on the anterolateral cortex (Fig. 86-4). Fluoroscopy is used intraoperatively to confirm that the ACL reconstruction is placed in the anatomic tibial and femoral footprints, and the PCL reconstruction is placed in the center of the AL bundle on the femoral side and in the center of the native insertion on the tibial side.[10] The tunnels are drilled and sequentially dilated to the appropriate diameter. The grafts are then passed from tibia to femur and secured on the femoral side with suspensory fixation (e.g., screw and washer, EndoButton [Smith & Nephew, Andover, MA]). Appropriate deployment of the femoral fixation device is confirmed on fluoroscopy. The senior author does not use interference screws. The PCL is initially tensioned at 90 degrees of knee flexion with an anterior drawer applied to the tibia, followed by ACL graft tensioning in full extension.[8] Final cruciate graft tensioning and tibial fixation are delayed until completion of collateral ligament repair or reconstruction.

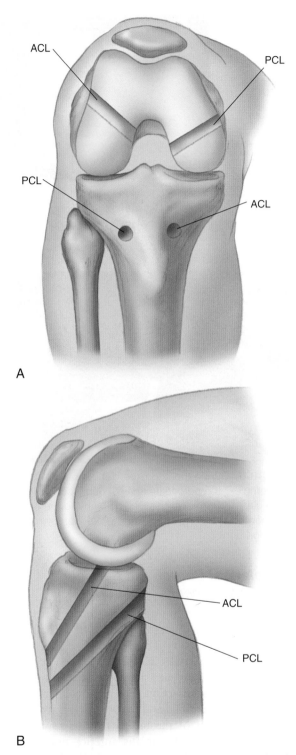

Figure 86-3. Careful planning of bone tunnel position during multiligamentous knee reconstruction is important to prevent convergence. We place our PCL tunnel distal to the ACL tunnel and set the drill guide to a larger angle to ensure that our tunnels are appropriately spaced. *ACL,* Anterior cruciate ligament; *PCL,* posterior cruciate ligament.

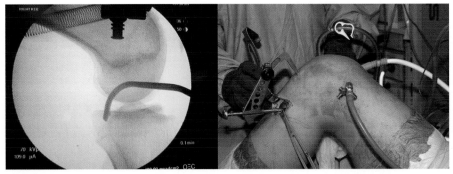

Figure 86-4. The anatomic tibial insertion of the posterior cruciate ligament (PCL) is visualized via a posteromedial portal. A commercially available PCL guide set to 55 degrees is advanced through the anteromedial portal and placed immediately distal and lateral to the PCL tibial insertion. Fluoroscopic imaging confirms appropriate guide location before drilling of the tibial tunnel.

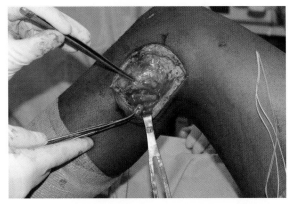

Figure 86-5. During the exposure of the posterolateral corner complex, the peroneal nerve is identified and carefully cleared from scar tissue. Any injury to the nerve is documented and correlated with the preoperative examination findings.

Posterolateral Corner and Lateral Collateral Ligament

PLC complex injuries are addressed through a lateral exposure through the interval between the IT band and biceps femoris complex. The IT band at the Gerdy tubercle may be partially elevated subperiosteally to facilitate exposure of the lateral collateral ligament (LCL) and popliteal insertion. The peroneal nerve must also be carefully identified and released as it travels from the posterior aspect of the biceps femoris toward the fibular neck and into the tibialis anterior muscle (Fig. 86-5). Any evidence of injury is recorded and correlated to the preoperative examination findings.

In certain patients, the PLC complex will have a distal soft tissue or bony avulsion injury that can successfully be repaired in the acute setting (<14 days) (Fig. 86-6). These injuries are repaired with No. 2 braided nonabsorbable sutures or the use of a screw and soft tissue washer to secure the biceps femoris and LCL complex to the proximal fibula (Figs. 86-7 and 86-8). After 14 days, significant scarring and retraction may

be encountered, making primary repair much more difficult and increasing the risk of iatrogenic peroneal nerve injury during the surgical exposure. Reconstruction is usually necessary if the injury is chronic or if midsubstance attenuation exists.

Isolated Lateral Collateral Ligament Reconstruction

If the examination under anesthesia demonstrates increased varus opening at full knee extension with no evidence of rotational instability then an isolated reconstruction of the LCL may be performed (Fig. 86-9). Our current method for reconstruction uses a 7- to 8-mm Achilles tendon allograft with a bone plug placed into the intramedullary space of the proximal fibula, tensioned proximally through a femoral bone tunnel. During the surgical exposure, palpation of the deficient LCL can usually be facilitated by placing the knee in the figure-four position. The fibular insertion is identified and dissected free from its attachment. A guidewire is carefully advanced longitudinally into the proximal fibula (Fig. 86-10). After fluoroscopic confirmation of the guidewire placement, a reamer is used to open the intramedullary canal and sequentially dilated to fit the bone plug (Fig. 86-11). The allograft bone plug is placed into the bone tunnel and secured with a metal interference screw (Fig. 86-12). The native LCL is then reflected proximally and the inferior portion of the native attachment near the lateral femoral epicondyle is identified. A guidewire is placed and inspected under fluoroscopy. A blind-end tunnel is then reamed to a depth of 30 mm. The femoral tunnel is angled proximally and anteriorly to prevent penetration of the articular surface. Nonabsorbable sutures are used to whipstitch the proximal graft end, and it is advanced through the bone tunnel to the medial femoral cortex. The LCL graft is tensioned at 30 degrees of knee flexion with a valgus force applied and secured over an AO post placed on the medial femoral cortex. The native LCL is then oversewn onto the graft for reinforcement.

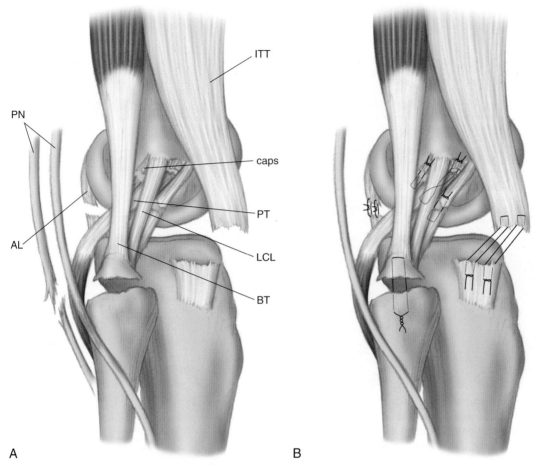

Figure 86-6. Acute avulsions of the posterolateral corner (PLC) complex are best managed in the first 7 to 14 days after injury before the onset of retraction and scarring. Structures that may be involved include the IT band *(ITT)*, lateral collateral ligament *(LCL)*, biceps tendon *(BT)*, popliteus tendon and popliteofibular ligament *(PT)*, arcuate ligament *(AL)*, and posterolateral capsule *(caps)*. Associated injury to the peroneal nerve *(PN)* should be suspected in the setting of acute PLC injuries.

Popliteofibular Ligament Reconstruction

If a significant amount of external rotational instability exists compared with the contralateral side, then a reconstruction of the popliteofibular ligament complex is performed (Fig. 86-13). These injuries will frequently occur in the setting of varus laxity and may require concomitant LCL reconstruction. Graft requirements for this reconstruction are a single-strand soft tissue autograft or allograft.

Through the previously described lateral approach, the popliteus tendon is identified inferior and anterior to the LCL insertion, elevated subperiosteally off its insertion, and tagged with a No. 2 nonabsorbable suture. A 7-mm femoral tunnel is then drilled in the anatomic insertion of the popliteus tendon to a depth of 30 mm. A second tunnel is created in the proximal fibula, distal and medial to the intramedullary tunnel

created for the LCL reconstruction. A guidewire is passed from anterior, distal, and medial to posterior, proximal, and lateral and evaluated under fluoroscopy. If the location is appropriate, a 6-mm drill is used to open the tunnel, followed by dilatation to 7 mm. Great care must be taken to avoid fibular fracture or tunnel convergence during fibular tunnel preparation. The proximal graft end and tagged native popliteus tendon are combined and advanced into the femoral tunnel to a depth of 25 mm, and the distal graft end is brought underneath the LCL (native or reconstruction) and passed through the fibular tunnel from posterior to anterior with the assistance of a Hewson suture passer. The femoral graft is secured over an post and washer on the anteromedial femoral cortex. The PF reconstruction is then tensioned at 30 degrees of knee flexion with gentle tibial internal rotation and secured with a bioabsorbable interference screw in the fibular tunnel.

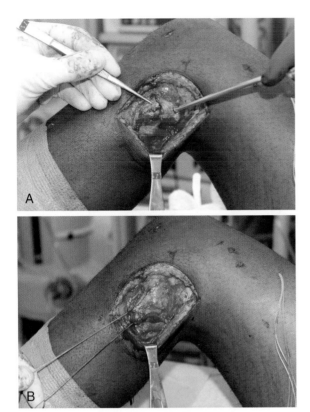

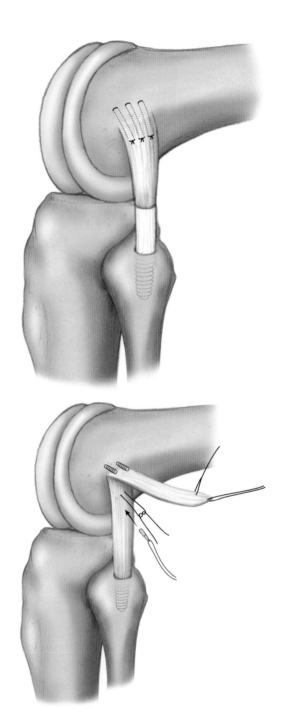

Figure 86-7. This is a combined anterior cruciate ligament tear with a distal avulsion of the lateral collateral ligament (LCL) and conjoint tendon (long and short heads of the biceps femoris). The injured tendon and LCL sleeve have been elevated off the proximal fibula and mobilized. The avulsed LCL and conjoint tendon is secured with a nonabsorbable No. 2 suture whipstitched to the edge of the ligamentous complex. Traction is applied distally to restore the native ligament tension.

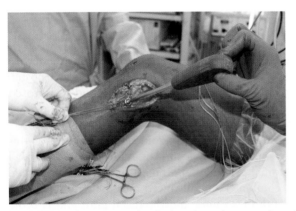

Figure 86-8. A screw and soft tissue washer are placed into the proximal fibula to reattach the avulsed PLC at its anatomic insertion site and tightened with the knee at 30 degrees of flexion.

Figure 86-9. A schematic representation of the single-bundle anatomic lateral collateral ligament reconstruction. This reconstruction can be performed as an isolated lateral procedure or combined with an anatomic reconstruction of the popliteus and popliteofibular ligament. *(Modified from Cole BJ, Harner CD. The multiple ligament injured knee. Clin Sports Med. 1999;18:241-262.)*

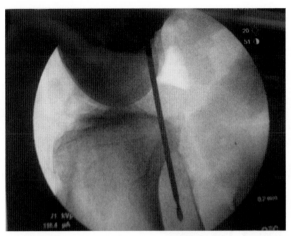

Figure 86-10. A guidewire is carefully advanced into the intramedullary canal of the proximal fibula and checked under fluoroscopy. Orthogonal images are obtained to confirm central placement within the intramedullary canal. The peroneal nerve is protected at all times.

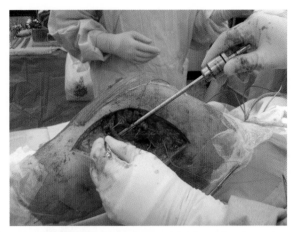

Figure 86-11. The fibular tunnel for lateral collateral ligament reconstruction is carefully reamed by hand over a guidewire with care taken not to fracture the cortex or injure the peroneal nerve. The tunnel is then carefully dilated to the appropriate size to avoid fracture.

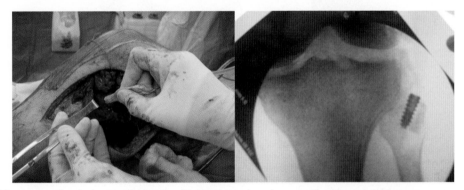

Figure 86-12. The bone plug is inserted into the fibular tunnel and secured with an interference screw. Fluoroscopic imaging is used to confirm the placement of the interference screw within the proximal fibula.

Medial Collateral and Posterior Oblique Ligament

Our current management of concomitant MCL patholaxity in the setting of a multiligament reconstruction depends on the location and grade of injury. In most patients we delay surgery for 6 to 8 weeks to allow swelling to subside and knee ROM and quadriceps control to return. On occasion we will perform an acute MCL repair in the setting of a severe combined injury, but this is the exception and not the rule.

The location of injury is noted on the MRI scan and correlated with the findings of the valgus stress examination under anesthesia. If grade 3 laxity is present with the knee in full extension, the surgical procedure is tailored to the location of MCL pathology identified via MRI. A standard medial longitudinal incision based over the posterior third of the medial femoral condyle is opened to the underlying fascial layer, with care taken to identify and protect the saphenous nerve and its branches (Fig. 86-14). The plane between the posterior edge of the MCL and the leading edge of the POL is identified and incised longitudinally, and the flaps are elevated (Fig. 86-15). Care must be taken to avoid injuring the medial meniscus, which lies directly beneath this layer. The location of MCL injury then dictates the repair performed.

Proximal (Femoral Side) Medial Collateral Ligament Injuries

If the examination and imaging findings are consistent with a proximal MCL tear, the ligament is elevated from its attachment on the medial femoral condyle, then the anterior and posterior margins are whipstitched with No. 2 nonabsorbable sutures. The ligament is then tensioned proximally with the knee placed at 30 degrees of flexion. A 6.5-mm cancellous AO screw and spiked soft tissue washer are drilled and advanced into the native MCL footprint on the medial femoral condyle and secured. This allows for restoration of the MCL tension with an anatomic repair. The POL is then reapproximated to the posterior edge of the MCL with No. 2

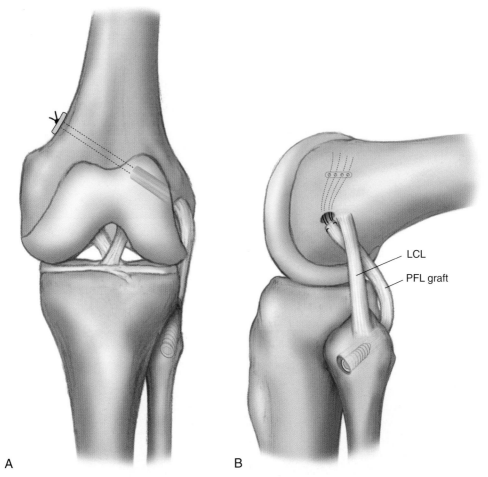

A   B

Figure 86-13. A schematic representation of the anatomic popliteofibular ligament reconstruction performed with a soft tissue graft. This construct anatomically restores the popliteus complex while incorporating the native popliteus tendon. *LCL,* Lateral collateral ligament; *PFL,* popliteofibular ligament. *(Modified from Cole BJ, Harner CD. The multiple ligament injured knee.* Clin Sports Med. *1999;18:241-262.)*

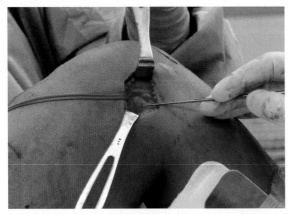

Figure 86-14. A standard medial longitudinal incision based over the posterior third of the medial femoral condyle is sharply incised to the underlying fascial layer, with care taken to identify and protect the saphenous nerve and its branches.

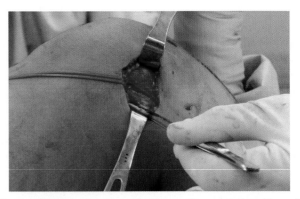

Figure 86-15. The plane between the posterior edge of the medial collateral ligament and the leading edge of the posterior oblique ligament is identified and incised longitudinally and the flaps elevated. The medial meniscus lies directly below this interval, and careful dissection is performed to avoid iatrogenic meniscal injury.

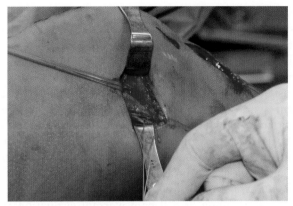

Figure 86-16. Significant grade 2 to 3 midsubstance injuries to the MCL are treated with an imbrication of the posterior oblique ligament (POL) into the MCL.

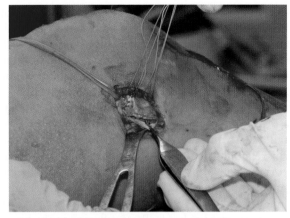

Figure 86-17. The anterior edge of the POL is tagged with interrupted No. 2 nonabsorbable sutures placed in a horizontal mattress configuration.

nonabsorbable sutures placed in a horizontal mattress fashion and tied with the knee near full extension.

Distal (Tibial Side) Medial Collateral Ligament Injuries

Distal (tibial side) MCL injuries are managed in a similar fashion to proximal (femoral side) injuries. The distal ligament is elevated subperiosteally with a curved osteotome. The anterior and posterior edges are whipstitched with No. 2 nonabsorbable sutures and tensioned distally. An 18-gauge spinal needle is used to localize the native tibial insertion 2 to 3 cm distal to the joint line. This is checked fluoroscopically to prevent articular penetration and avoid any previously placed cruciate ligament tunnels. A 6.5-mm cancellous AO screw and spiked soft tissue washer are placed through the substance of the MCL and tightened at 30 degrees of knee flexion. The POL is then reapproximated as previously described.

Midsubstance Medial Collateral Ligament Injuries

Significant midsubstance injuries to the MCL are treated with imbrication of the POL to reinforce and tension the attenuated midsubstance fibers. After the MCL and POL interval has been opened and any meniscal repair performed, the anterior edge of the POL is tagged with No. 2 nonabsorbable sutures placed in an interrupted horizontal mattress pattern (Figs. 86-16 and 86-17). The sutures are advanced in a pants-over-vest pattern into the midsubstance of the MCL and tied at 30 degrees of knee flexion, imbricating the ligament and restoring tension (Fig. 86-18).[11] If persistent laxity exists, this repair may be reinforced with a soft tissue allograft inserted directly into bone at the native femoral and tibial MCL attachments with bone tunnels or suture anchors and repaired to the native MCL in a side-to-side fashion. We have not had to perform an MCL reconstruction for MCL laxity in over 5 years.

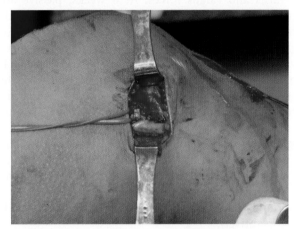

Figure 86-18. The sutures are passed into the midsubstance of the medial collateral ligament (MCL) in a pants-over-vest fashion, passed with the knee at 20 to 30 degrees of flexion, and tied at full knee extension. This restores the tension within the MCL by imbricating the posterior oblique ligament.

Wound Closure

After graft tensioning and confirmation of knee stability, the surgical wounds are thoroughly irrigated with an antibiotic solution. A standard layered closure of the wound is performed and sterile dressings applied. A postoperative brace locked in extension is applied before the conclusion of anesthesia. The calf is palpated to ensure that an iatrogenic increase of the intracompartmental pressures has not occurred as a result of bleeding or arthroscopic fluid extravasation.

POSTOPERATIVE CONSIDERATIONS AND REHABILITATION

General guidelines for rehabilitation of the multiligamentously injured knee include promoting tissue healing, decreasing pain and swelling, restoring full motion, increasing muscular strength and endurance, improving proprioception, enhancing dynamic stability of the knee, and reducing functional limitations and disability. Patients are initially immobilized in a hinged knee brace locked in full extension. For PCL reconstructions, a pillow is placed underneath the calf to provide an anterior tibial force while the patient rests. DVT prophylaxis is tailored to the individual preoperative risk factors. Early rehabilitation focuses on protecting the repair, restoring quadriceps strength and tone, and achieving terminal knee extension. Initial exercises include isometric quadriceps contractions, straight-leg raises, and calf pumps performed at home. Passive flexion to 90 degrees is initiated at 3 to 4 weeks after surgery under the guidance of a physical therapist to avoid posterior tibial sag or varus and valgus forces. At 6 weeks, passive and active-assisted ROM activities are initiated and the brace is discontinued if quadriceps control is restored, with full knee flexion expected by 12 weeks postoperatively. Crutch weight bearing is progressed from touchdown weight bearing to full weight bearing over this period unless a lateral repair or reconstruction has been performed, necessitating partial weight bearing in an extension brace for a total of 8 weeks. Strengthening exercises are increased progressively, and running is permitted at 6 months if 80% quadriceps strength is achieved. Return to sedentary work is allowed as early as 2 weeks, return to heavy labor at 6 to 9 months, and sports participation at 9 to 12 months postoperatively.[12]

RESULTS

Because of the variable injury patterns, surgical techniques, and outcome measures, the results of multiligamentous knee reconstructions are difficult to report and compare. Our results have been consistent with other reports of surgical outcomes after knee dislocation with allograft cruciate ligament reconstruction.[4]

Our treatment protocol for the management of multiligamentous knee injuries offers acceptable functional outcomes, ROM, and stability, particularly in those treated in the acute setting. The majority of patients are able to perform their activities of daily living without difficulty, but return to competitive sports is less predictable. Patients treated for chronic knee instability appear to be more likely to report functional limitations than patients treated within 3 weeks of their injury.

Complications

Complications are rare but may have significant consequences if not identified and treated promptly. Vascular injury and compartment syndrome may result from the initial trauma, and any evidence of acute knee dislocation or pulse asymmetry should be evaluated with ABIs. If the ABI scores are less than 0.9 for the affected extremity or a sufficient concern for arterial injury exists, imaging with either a CT angiogram or formal angiography is indicated, with vascular surgery consultation. Increasing pain or evidence of compartment syndrome should also be managed aggressively with fasciotomy, if indicated. Because of the amount of soft tissue injury and subsequent inflammation after acute multiligamentous injuries, the treating orthopedist should have a high index of suspicion for DVT in the preoperative and postoperative settings. Complaints of increased swelling or calf pain warrant evaluation and venous duplex ultrasound to detect DVT and initiate an appropriate course of anticoagulation. Additional postoperative complications include surgical site infection and stiffness. Patients are seen within 3 days after surgery for a wound check and dressing change. Wound drainage or superficial dehiscence is monitored closely with frequent dressing changes, clinical follow-up, and surgical debridement if necessary. Postoperative knee ROM is assessed at each clinical visit, and a protocol is provided to the patient and physical therapist with expected progression of knee flexion. If flexion or extension deficits are identified, the frequency of supervised physical therapy and postoperative clinical checks is increased. If persistent extension or flexion deficits are not improved by 3 to 4 months after surgery, a manipulation under anesthesia, arthroscopic lysis of adhesions, and application of extension drop-out casting are performed.

REFERENCES

1. Cole BJ, Harner CD. The multiple ligament injured knee. *Clin Sports Med.* 1999;18(1):241-262.
2. Wascher DC, Dvirnak PC, DeCoster TA. Knee dislocation: initial assessment and implications for treatment. *J Orthop Trauma.* 1997;11(7):525-529.
3. Klineberg EO, Crites BM, Flinn WR, et al. The role of arteriography in assessing popliteal artery injury in knee dislocations. *J Trauma.* 2004;56(4):786-790.
4. Harner CD, Waltrip RL, Bennett CH, et al. Surgical management of knee dislocations. *J Bone Joint Surg Am.* 2004;86(2):262-273.
5. Casagranda BU, Maxwell NJ, Kavanagh EC, et al. Normal appearance and complications of double-bundle and selective-bundle anterior cruciate ligament reconstructions using optimal MRI techniques. *AJR Am J Roentgenol.* 2009;192(5):1407-1415.
6. Rihn JA Groff YJ, Harner CD, et al. The acutely dislocated knee: evaluation and management. *J Am Acad Orthop Surg.* 2004;12(5):334-346.
7. Müller W. *The knee: form, function, and ligament reconstruction.* Berlin; New York: Springer-Verlag; 1983, xviii, 314 p.
8. Forsythe B, Harner C, Martins CA, et al. Topography of the femoral attachment of the posterior cruciate ligament.

Surgical technique. *J Bone Joint Surg Am.* 2009;91(suppl 2 Pt 1):89-100.

9. Olson EJ, Harner CD, Fu FH, et al. Clinical use of fresh, frozen soft tissue allografts. *Orthopedics.* 1992;15(10): 1225-1232.

10. Amis AA, Jakob RP. Anterior cruciate ligament graft positioning, tensioning and twisting. *Knee Surg Sports Traumatol Arthrosc.* 1998;6(suppl 1):S2-S12.

11. Hughston JC, Eilers AF. The role of the posterior oblique ligament in repairs of acute medial (collateral) ligament tears of the knee. *J Bone Joint Surg Am.* 1973;55(5): 923-940.

12. Irrgang JJ, Fitzgerald GK. Rehabilitation of the multiple-ligament-injured knee. *Clin Sports Med.* 2000;19(3): 545-571.

Chapter 87

Arthroscopic Lateral Retinacular Release and Lateral Retinacular Lengthening

Jack Farr II, Christian Lattermann, and D. Jeff Covell

Chapter Synopsis

- Lateral release and lateral lengthening are effective procedures to improve symptoms of anterior knee pain attributable to isolated lateral compression syndrome. Although both are contraindicated as isolated procedures in patients with patellofemoral instability, these procedures may be indicated in combination with patella realignment procedures.

Important Points

- Lateral release has a specific role in treatment of patients with symptoms of lateral compression syndrome.
- Indications include tight lateral retinaculum and patellar tilt.
- History and physical examination are fundamental to patient selection.
- Isolated lateral release is of limited efficacy and often contraindicated in patients with patellar instability.
- Care must be taken to avoid an "over-release," which can lead to iatrogenic medial instability.
- Lateral retinacular release or lengthening may be indicated in combination with other patellofemoral alignment procedures in patients with patellofemoral instability.

Clinical and Surgical Pearls

- Isolated lateral release is a rather rare surgical procedure if the indications are observed correctly.

- When the procedure is done arthroscopically, hemostasis is important. The progressive technique involves control of any bleeding first with increased inflow pressure, followed by release of the tourniquet (if used); then with minimal intra-articular water pressure, final hemostasis is ensured.
- The use of a hooked electrocautery device allows cutting and hemostasis simultaneously. The device should be inserted through the lateral arthroscopic portal with the arthroscope in the medial portal, with a direct view of at the lateral retinaculum.
- As an alternative to open lateral retinacular release, lateral lengthening has the advantage of maintaining the overall integrity of the lateral retinacular restraint to the patellofemoral joint.

Clinical and Surgical Pitfalls

- Inappropriate patient selection—for example, patients with a history of instability—can lead to poor outcomes if the underlying patellofemoral pathology is not corrected.
- Excessive release can lead to iatrogenic medial patellar instability.

Lateral retinacular release, when performed for the wrong indication or with poor attention to technical details, leads to poor clinical results and a high complication rate.[1] The isolated use of retinacular release is best limited specifically to patients with lateral patellar hypercompression syndrome. Used for that indication, there are more consistently good results, although the exact diagnostic criteria for a "tight lateral retinaculum" remain elusive.

With regard to patellofemoral instability, lateral release must be used very carefully because it can easily lead to increased lateral patellofemoral instability as well as medial patellar dislocation. Contrary to intuition, the lateral retinaculum is not a ligamentous structure pulling the patella laterally but a checkrein preventing the patella from subluxing medially and/or laterally depending on the degree of flexion of the knee joint.[2]

Stringent patient selection with appropriate indications must be paramount, because failure to select patients appropriately may lead to devastating outcomes for them. The goal of this chapter is to describe the role of lateral retinacular release and lateral retinacular lengthening in treating patients with patellofemoral symptoms and illustrate the surgical approach for both of those procedures.

PREOPERATIVE CONSIDERATIONS

History

- Anterior knee pain focused in the lateral retinaculum, common in knee flexion with repetitive motions (climbing or descending stairs) or positional (prolonged immobilization of flexed knee). Often the anterior knee pain is multifactorial, and the lateral retinacular pain may be only a small component.
- Trauma (patient may recall a specific injury)—more often repetitive microtrauma of sports or work overuse.
- Extensive and correctly performed conservative measures without success (taping, bracing, stretching, and core proximal as well as local knee exercise programs).

Patients may also report primarily instability (history of recurrent subluxation or dislocation) with or without associated pain. It is important to note this distinction and to probe regarding the true cause of pain and discern the nature and role of the instability versus giving way because of transient pain or weakness.

Physical Examination

Factors affecting surgical indication are as follows:

- Range of motion (should be normal)
- Patellar tracking (may be laterally displaced)
- Patellar tilt with tight lateral retinaculum
- J-sign does not correlate with tilt, more with tracking
- Lateral patellar pain with compression

Factors affecting surgical exclusion are as follows:

- Muscular imbalance of the extremity (vastus medialis obliquus [VMO])

- Patellofemoral osteoarthritis (OA) (advanced degenerative changes)
- Patellar subluxation or dislocation
- Alignment of the lower extremity (valgus or rotational deformity)
- Excessive J-sign (lateral patellar translation as the knee moves into extension)
- Normal patellar mobility (medial or lateral patellar glide with manual pressure)
- Generalized hyperlaxity

It is essential to consider the complex nature of patellofemoral joint pain and critically assess signs of instability, taking into account the entirety of the core and lower extremity. Patients with underlying instability or malalignment issues may require additional corrective proximal and distal realignment procedures in conjunction with lateral release. Lateral hypercompression syndrome needs to be identified clinically, because this is the most common pathology that benefits from isolated lateral release. If patellofemoral instability is present, lateral retinacular release and lengthening are among several procedures that may need to be done in combination. The evaluation for patellofemoral instability includes the evaluation of femoral axial alignment, rotational alignment, patellar height, tibial tuberosity–trochlear groove (TT-TG) measurements, and trochlear dysplasia.

Imaging

Plain Radiographs

- Standard anteroposterior and lateral views
- Axial view at 30 degrees of knee flexion (Merchant view)
- Long-leg alignment view for tibiofemoral alignment
- True lateral view in 30 degrees of flexion (patellar height, patellar tilt, and trochlear morphology)[3]

Computed Tomography

- Scans at varying degrees of flexion are useful to evaluate patellar tracking.
- Calculate TT-TG distance.
- Assess patellar tilt referenced from posterior condyles.

Magnetic Resonance Imaging

- Assess soft tissue (thick lateral retinaculum, inadequate medial restraint structures).
- Evaluate cartilaginous injury.
- Calculate TT-TG.
- Assess patellar tilt and cartilaginous Caton-Deschamps ratio.

Indications and Contraindications

The indications for lateral release have become increasingly rigorous since it was first described. Ideally, this procedure is performed for patients with isolated anterior knee pain from lateral patellar compression syndrome in the presence of a tight lateral retinaculum and patellar tilt, in whom extensive conservative therapy has failed. Alternatively, lateral release may be used as an adjunct to proximal or distal realignment procedures. In these patients lateral retinacular lengthening may be preferable.

Contraindications for isolated lateral retinacular release are patellar instability, an elevated TT-TG distance, trochlear dysplasia, and lower extremity malalignment or torsion. Additional contraindications are the same as those associated with arthroscopy, including acute or chronic infections or gross anatomic abnormalities of the knee.

ARTHROSCOPIC LATERAL RELEASE

Surgical Technique

Anesthesia and Positioning

The patient is positioned and prepared for a standard arthroscopic procedure of the knee in the supine position. A tourniquet is not necessary, but if used it needs to be positioned as proximal as possible on the operative extremity. The leg is securely placed in an arthroscopic leg holder and allowed to hang over the edge of the table with the foot of the table dropped. The nonoperative leg is supported and placed out of the way in a well-padded leg holder. The type of anesthesia selected may include a general endotracheal, spinal, regional block or local anesthetic with sedation.

Surgical Landmarks, Incisions, and Portals

Landmarks
- Inferior pole of the patella
- Patella tendon
- Tibial tubercle
- Joint line
- Medial and lateral parapatellar soft spot

Incisions and Portals
- High anteromedial
- High anterolateral

Examination Under Anesthesia and Diagnostic Arthroscopy

With the patient under anesthesia, a thorough examination should be performed and includes knee range of motion, ligamentous testing, assessment of patellar tracking and patellar tilt, and manual medial-lateral patellar glide testing. This may provide key information with regard to patellar stability. Standard diagnostic arthroscopy should be performed in all compartments of the knee to address concomitant intra-articular pathology including loose bodies, ligamentous deficiencies, and articular surface defects. With flexion the normal lateral retinaculum becomes tighter and the medial soft tissues more lax. Therefore in a normal knee the patella will most typically track laterally and tilt during arthroscopy. This is *not* an indication for lateral release. The decision for a lateral release is made preoperatively as described earlier. Once again, operative notes that state a lateral release was performed because of tilt found at arthroscopy should be discouraged.

Specific Steps

Box 87-1 outlines the specific steps of this procedure.

Portal Placement

Standard high anteromedial and anterolateral portals are placed, and diagnostic arthroscopy is performed. The lateral patellar tilt should be verified by physical examination and can be visualized arthroscopically (Fig. 87-1).

Division of the Lateral Retinaculum for Release of the Patella

An electrocautery device (hooked bovie) is inserted into the joint through the anterolateral portal, and selective

> **BOX 87-1** Surgical Steps
> - Portal placement and diagnostic arthroscopy
> - Division of the lateral retinaculum for release of the patella
> - Closure

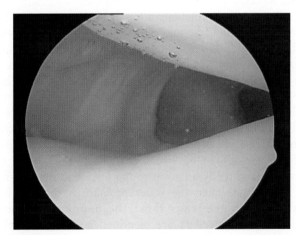

Figure 87-1. Arthroscopic view of a laterally tilted patella. Note that arthroscopic tilt is not an indication for lateral release.

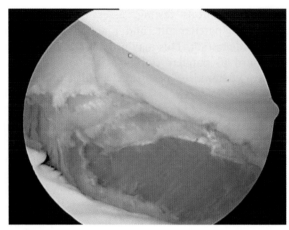

Figure 87-2. Arthroscopic release of the lateral retinaculum (typical view after complete release). Care is taken to stop immediately at subcutaneous fat to avoid skin necrosis.

division of the lateral retinacular fibers is performed under direct visualization in a layered fashion about 1 cm lateral to the lateral border of the patella. The water pressure should be kept relatively low (40 to 60 mm Hg). The release should extend proximally from the superior pole of the patella with care taken not to transect the fibers of the vastus lateralis (VL). The extent of lateral release is determined intraoperatively by manually everting the patella and assessing lateral tilt. Sufficient release is achieved when the patellar tilt has been revered to neutral—*not* the historic "turn-up sign" of eversion to 90 degrees. The fibers are divided until the fatty subcutaneous tissues are encountered. It is essential to avoid excessive release of the lateral retinaculum because this may lead to increased medial instability and subluxation, a potentially devastating complication (Fig. 87-2).

The superior geniculate artery is likely to be encountered; care should be taken to avoid cutting the artery, which would lead to significant postoperative hematoma. To avoid this complication a stepwise approach as described by Sherman and colleagues should be applied.[4] Whereas Sherman described this technique with a tourniquet, if use of the tourniquet is avoided altogether, hemostasis is achieved from start to finish. The arthroscope is positioned such that the entire length of the release can be visualized. The cautery hook is positioned directly adjacent to the release in plain sight of the scope. Then the water pressure is reduced by switching off the water flow. The tourniquet is then released; any bleeders are identified and immediately cauterized. As a final step the water is carefully drained from the knee joint under continuous observation of the retinacular edges.

Closure

Portals are closed in a standard fashion and covered with a sterile compressive dressing to minimize hemarthrosis. Postoperatively it is common to have significant swelling along the lateral retinaculum; the intra-articular water escapes into the subcutaneous tissue at the end of the surgical procedure. It is therefore important to reduce the water pressure before completion of the lateral release.

Postoperative Considerations

Rehabilitation

- Range of motion as tolerated.
- Weight bearing as tolerated.
- Rehabilitative exercises for core proximal as well as quadriceps strengthening (particularly VMO).
- Medial superior and inferior patella mobilization. Avoid lateral mobilization of the patella.

Complications

- Hemarthrosis
- Excessive release resulting in medial patellar instability
- Complications associated with knee arthroscopy

Results

In the appropriate patient, lateral release is an effective procedure to alleviate symptoms of anterior knee pain caused by lateral compression syndrome.[1,5] Only a small subset of patients with anterior knee pain will have indications for lateral release, accounting for only 2% of surgical procedures annually.[1,6] Advantages of the arthroscopic approach include minimal invasiveness, direct visualization of the release, improved hemostasis, and ability to address concomitant intra-articular pathology, particularly degenerative changes of the patellofemoral joint. When the procedure is performed in isolation with the appropriate indications, patient satisfaction can achieve high levels of success (Table 87-1).[1,7,10] Poor patient selection, failure to address issues of concomitant patellofemoral instability, or overaggressive retinacular release can lead to devastating outcomes including iatrogenic medial instability.

LATERAL RETINACULAR LENGTHENING

Surgical Technique

Anesthesia and Positioning

Anesthesia is dictated by the concomitant procedures. The patient can be positioned in an arthroscopic leg holder or supine so that the knee can be positioned in full extension and can easily be flexed.

TABLE 87-1 Clinical Results of Arthroscopic Lateral Release

Author	Follow-up	Outcomes
Gerbino et al[7] (2008)	8.5 years	140 knees 92% of patients satisfied or very satisfied 15-year survivorship of 78% on Kaplan-Meier curve for no reoperation
Ricchetti et al[8] (2007)	2 years	Systematic review of patellar instability treated with LR 77.3% success (no redislocation) 93.6% success in conjunction with soft tissue realignment LR alone inferior treatment of patellar instability compared with combined realignment procedures
Woods et al[9] (2006)	2.25 years	22 patients 85% good to excellent results IKDC score: 76 points SF-36 score: 50 (physical) and 86 (functional)
Panni et al[10] (2005)	5 years	100 patients LR (for pain): 70% satisfied LR (for instability): 50% satisfied

IKDC, International Knee Documentation Committee; *LR,* lateral release; *SF-36,* Short Form 36.

Specific Surgical Approach

The surgical approach is based on simplifying the true complex anatomy described by Merican and Amis into two layers.[11] The superficial oblique layer arises from the anterior aspect of the iliotibial band and courses to the lateral patella. This portion of the lateral retinaculum does not attach to the femur. The deep tissues are the transverse fibers and course from the femur to the patella in the same region and may also be labeled the lateral patellofemoral ligament (analogous to the medial patellofemoral ligament on the medial side). The lateral lengthening begins with exposure of the proximal lateral aspect of the soft tissues attaching to the patella. In most patients the superficial oblique fibers from the iliotibial band are discrete from the VL and vastus lateralis obliquus and are palpable. This tissue is then incised adjacent to the patella, followed by sharp elevation of this tissue plane from the deep transverse fibers (Fig. 87-3).

Most often, it is possible to separate these two tissue planes for a distance of approximately 1 to 2 cm from the patella. At this point the deep transverse fibers may be incised longitudinally.

In most patients this deep layer will be confluent with the capsule. At this point the cut edge of the deep transverse fibers, which remain attached to the femur, is then sutured directly to the superficial oblique fibers

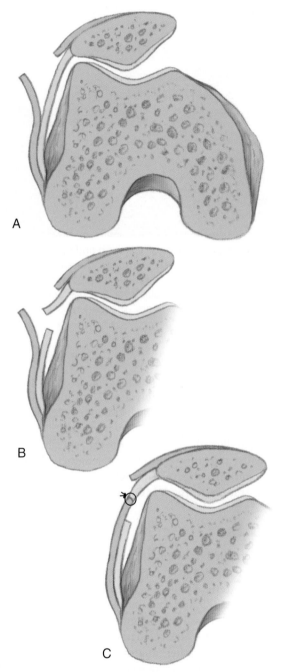

Figure 87-3. Steps for lengthening of the lateral retinaculum (axial views, right knee). **A,** Cut and reflect the superficial layer from the deep layer. **B,** Cut the deep layer approximately 1.5 cm posterior to the patella attachment. **C,** Attach the superficial layer, which is now posteriorly based to the deep fibers that are attached to the patella. *(Modified from Biedert RM. Case 3: Lateral patellar hypercompression, tilt, and mild lateral subluxation. In: Biedert RM, ed:* Patellofemoral Disorders: Diagnosis and Treatment. *Chichester, UK: Wiley; 2004.)*

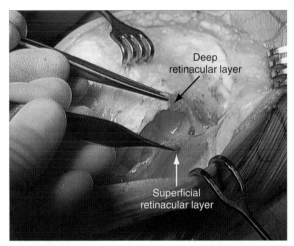

Figure 87-4. Separation of the deep and superficial layers. The anterior forceps are grasping the cut edge of the deep retinacular layer, and the more posterior forceps hold the superficial retinacular layer that has been dissected from the deep fibers. This patient is the same as in Figure 87-3B.

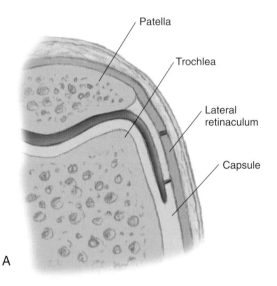

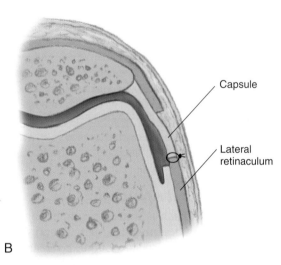

Figure 87-5. O'Neill illustration of the lateral retinacular Z-plasty that uses different terminology from that described by Fulkerson and later by Merican (see Figs. 87-6 and 87-7, respectively). It appears the O'Neill "lateral retinaculum" is equivalent to the Fulkerson "superficial oblique retinacular layer" and the O'Neill "capsule" is equivalent to the Fulkerson "deep transverse retinacular layer." *(Modified from O'Neill DB. Open lateral retinacular lengthening compared with arthroscopic release. A prospective, randomized outcome study. J Bone Joint Surg Am. 1997;79: 1759-1769.)*

that are attached to the patella (Fig. 87-4). This seals the joint with approximately 1 to 2 cm more length in the lateral retinaculum, which thus increases its laxity. This can be adjusted as necessary to optimize the medial lateral patellar displacement of the specific patient. Optionally, this approach may be lengthened to allow patellofemoral surgery through a lateral approach without trauma to the VMO.

Results

Lateral lengthening is an alternative to lateral release. It was first described as a Z-plasty type of lengthening of the lateral retinaculum by Larson in 1978 followed by Ceder in 1979 and then more recently by O'Neill in 1997 with a prospective randomized comparison of lateral release with lateral lengthening.[12-14] These reports were based on earlier anatomic descriptions of the lateral retinaculum as depicted in (Fig. 87-5). The labeling of the tissues is different from current terminology; the more superficial fibers were called the "lateral retinaculum," and the deeper fibers were called the "capsule".

Subsequently, in 1980 Fulkerson described the anatomy of the lateral retinaculum based on the dissection of 23 cadavers and one fresh specimen. He identified a superficial oblique layer and a deeper transverse layer.[15] This concept was further supported in the text *The Patellofemoral Joint* by Fox and Del Pizzo in 1993 and is depicted in Figure 87-6.[16]

Using this superficial and deep layer description of the lateral retinaculum, Biedert demonstrated an alternative lateral lengthening to the Z-plasty lengthening of

previous authors during the International Patellofemoral Study Group proceedings in Garmisch-Partenkirchen, Germany in 2000; his findings were subsequently published in 2004.[17] More recently, Merican and Amis even more precisely defined the lateral retinaculum of the knee based on 35 specimens.[11] Their descriptions added additional detail to the concepts described by Fulkerson. This article is an excellent anatomic overview to be used before one learns the procedure in the laboratory in preparation for performing the surgery. Figure 87-7

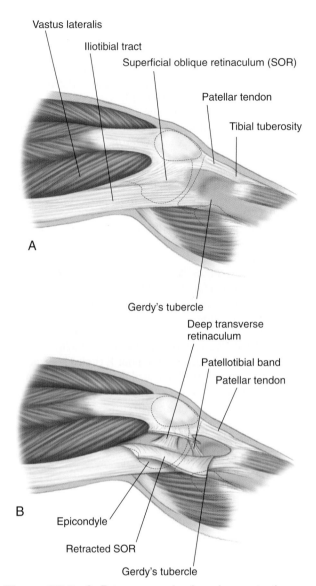

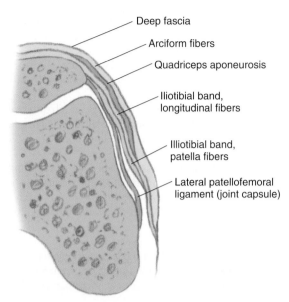

Figure 87-7. A cross-sectional diagram illustrating the components of the lateral retinaculum of the knee at the level of the lateral femoral condyle. *(Modified from Merican AM, Amis AA. Anatomy of the lateral retinaculum of the knee.* J Bone Joint Surg Br. *2008;90:527-534.)*

Figure 87-6. A, Extensor mechanism demonstrating the superior oblique retinaculum interdigitating with the longitudinal fibers from the vastus lateralis and patellar tendon. **B,** Deep transverse retinaculum with the epicondylopatellar band and patellotibial band. Note that the superior oblique retinaculum has been retracted to demonstrate the deep structures. *(Modified from Fox JM, Del Pizzo W.* The Patellofemoral Joint. *New York: McGraw-Hill; 1993.)*

illustrates the multiple complex layers of the lateral knee soft tissues. Merican and colleagues in 2009 then further defined the functional characteristics of the lateral retinaculum in a laboratory study demonstrating the different biomechanical properties of the iliotibial band–related superficial fibers and the deeper lateral patellofemoral ligament fibers.[18]

The problems with an inappropriate or overly aggressive lateral release have been described. It is obvious that with cutting of the retinaculum there is a loss of any restraints (to medial or lateral displacement) that the retinaculum offered. When used appropriately for

excessive lateral patellofemoral compression (or said another way, excessive tension in lateral structures that are functionally too short), an arthroscopically performed lateral retinacular release may be the most appropriate procedure. However, because the lateral retinaculum actually prevents excessive lateral patellar displacement after disruption of the medial restraints, lengthening rather than release of the lateral retinaculum may be useful in situations in which the medial restraints are compromised so as not to completely destabilize the patella proximally. This medial patellar instability with subluxation or dislocation is in fact a more common sequela after lateral release. Maintaining control of the lateral retinaculum while still decreasing the excessive tension in the lateral fibers would be advantageous in this setting. Finally, a subset of patients will develop postoperative extensive effusions, which will be subcutaneous by definition after lateral release. With lateral lengthening, the joint is sealed and thus this scenario can be avoided.

REFERENCES

1. Lattermann C, Toth J, Bach BR. The role of lateral retinacular release in the treatment of patellar instability. *Sports Med Arthrosc.* 2007;15:57-60.
2. Desio SM, Burks RT, Bachus KN. Soft tissue restraints to lateral patellar translation in the human knee. *Am J Sports Med.* 1998;26:59-65.
3. Maldague B, Malghem J. The true lateral view of the patellar facets. A new radiological approach of the femoro-patellar joint (author's transl). *Ann Radiol (Paris).* 1976;19:573-581.

4. Sherman OH, Fox JM, Sperling H, et al. Patellar instability: treatment by arthroscopic electrosurgical lateral release. *Arthroscopy*. 1987;3:152-160.

5. Clifton R, Ng CY, Nutton RW. What is the role of lateral retinacular release? *J Bone Joint Surg Br*. 2010;92: 1-6.

6. Fithian DC, Paxton EW, Post WR, et al. International Patellofemoral Study Group: Lateral retinacular release: a survey of the International Patellofemoral Study Group. *Arthroscopy*. 2004;20:463-468.

7. Gerbino PG, Zurakowski D, Soto R, et al. Long-term functional outcome after lateral patellar retinacular release in adolescents: an observational cohort study with minimum 5-year follow-up. *J Pediatr Orthop*. 2008;28: 118-123.

8. Ricchetti ET, Mehta S, Sennett BJ, et al. Comparison of lateral release versus lateral release with medial soft-tissue realignment for the treatment of recurrent patellar instability: a systematic review. *Arthroscopy*. 2007;23: 463-468.

9. Woods GW, Elkousy HA, O'Connor DP. Arthroscopic release of the vastus lateralis tendon for recurrent patellar dislocation. *Am J Sports Med*. 2006;34:824-831.

10. Panni AS, Tartarone M, Patricola A, et al. Long-term results of lateral retinacular release. *Arthroscopy*. 2005;21: 526-531.

11. Merican AM, Amis AA. Anatomy of the lateral retinaculum of the knee. *J Bone Joint Surg Br*. 2008;90: 527-534.

12. Ceder LC, Larson RL. Z-plasty lateral retinacular release for the treatment of patellar compression syndrome. *Clin Orthop Relat Res*. 1979;110-113.

13. Larson RL, Cabaud HE, Slocum DB, et al. The patellar compression syndrome: surgical treatment by lateral retinacular release. *Clin Orthop Relat Res*. 1978; 158-167.

14. O'Neill DB. Open lateral retinacular lengthening compared with arthroscopic release. A prospective, randomized outcome study. *J Bone Joint Surg Am*. 1997;79: 1759-1769.

15. Fulkerson JP, Gossling HR. Anatomy of the knee joint lateral retinaculum. *Clin Orthop Relat Res*. 1980; 183-188.

16. Fox JM, Del Pizzo W. *The Patellofemoral Joint*. New York: McGraw-Hill; 1993:399.

17. Biedert RM. Lateral patellar compression, tilt, and mild lateral subluxation. In Biedert RM, ed: *Patellofemoral Disorders: Diagnosis and Treatement*. Chichester, UK: Wiley, 2004:*Clin Orthop Relat Res*. 1980;376.

18. Merican AM, Sanghavi S, Iranpour F, et al. The structural properties of the lateral retinaculum and capsular complex of the knee. *J Biomech*. 2009;42:2323-2329.

Chapter 88

Medial Patellofemoral Ligament Reconstruction and Repair for Patellar Instability

Emmanuel N. Menga and Andrew J. Cosgarea

Chapter Synopsis

- Patellar instability results in substantial morbidity in active individuals. Rehabilitation remains the mainstay of treatment. Surgery is indicated in the setting of recurrent instability and failure of nonoperative measures. Multiple surgical techniques, including osteotomy and soft tissue procedures, have been described for the management of patellar instability. In the absence of malalignment as the primary abnormality, soft tissue procedures have been shown to be successful. This chapter describes techniques for the repair and reconstruction of the medial patellofemoral ligament.

Important Points

Indications

- Symptomatic lateral instability without bony malalignment
- Acute patellar dislocation and associated intra-articular abnormality (e.g., osteochondral fracture, loose body, or meniscus injury)

Contraindications

- Isolated patellofemoral pain or arthrosis
- Medial instability

Clinical and Surgical Pearls

- Patellar instability should be differentiated from patellofemoral pain.
- The position of the incisions should be modified according to the location of the tear as indicated by physical examination and preoperative magnetic resonance imaging studies.
- Femoral tunnel position requires a thorough understanding of normal anatomy.
- Before final fixation, the clinician should identify the graft length that reproduces normal lateral translation as compared with the contralateral knee (two to three quadrants of lateral translation).
- Medial patellofemoral ligament reconstruction can be combined with a distal realignment procedure if neither procedure alone provides adequate stability.
- Lateral release in the presence of excessive lateral retinacular pressure should be considered.

Clinical and Surgical Pitfalls

- When drilling the patellar tunnel, the clinician should avoid violating the anterior cortex or posterior articular surface.
- Multiple or large drill holes through the patella create stress risers and increase the risk of patellar fracture.
- Malposition of the femoral tunnel results in abnormal graft forces that can lead to excessive cartilage pressure or graft failure.
- Loss of motion is the most common complication and can be secondary to inadequate postoperative rehabilitation, tunnel malposition, or overtensioning of the graft.

Numerous surgical procedures have been described for the treatment of patellar instability, most with generally favorable success rates. The medial patellofemoral ligament (MPFL), the primary soft tissue passive restraint to pathologic lateral patellar displacement,[1] is torn when the patella dislocates.[2,3] There has been a great deal of interest recently in soft tissue procedures that address the MPFL. Techniques have been described to repair[2-5] or reconstruct[6-9] the MPFL in an attempt to restore its function as a checkrein. Regardless of which approach is taken, successful surgical treatment requires that the surgeon have a thorough understanding of the relevant anatomy and a working knowledge of patellofemoral biomechanics.

PREOPERATIVE CONSIDERATIONS

History

Patellofemoral complaints are among the most common problems encountered by physicians treating knee disorders, and instability is a distinct subset that is usually amenable to surgical treatment. Instability represents a continuum ranging from minor incidental subluxation episodes to traumatic dislocation events. Patients with frequent subluxation episodes and patients with dislocation usually experience substantial knee pain, swelling, and stiffness, resulting in interruption of their normal occupational and recreational activities.

Patellar dislocations can occur from an indirect twisting mechanism as the upper body rotates while the foot remains planted on the ground or, less commonly, from a direct blow to the medial aspect of the patella during contact sports or motor vehicle accidents when the patella is driven laterally. The patella may be spontaneously reduced as the knee is extended, or it may require a formal reduction maneuver. With initial dislocation episodes, the pain and swelling are caused by soft tissue and articular surface damage. The resulting hemarthrosis and quadriceps weakness may take several weeks to resolve. The degree of morbidity tends to decrease in patients who sustain multiple recurrent episodes.

Subluxation episodes are usually less dramatic and manifest as a feeling of instability and pain. Patients often describe the sense that the knee may "give out." These episodes usually occur with trunk rotation during physical activity and result in a variable degree of pain and swelling. The pain is usually anterior and may be bilateral, especially in patients with malalignment or diffuse ligamentous laxity. The most important clinical determination to be made is whether the pain described by the patient is associated with patellar instability, because the common clinical entity of isolated anterior knee pain (patellofemoral pain syndrome) is nearly universally treated nonoperatively.

Physical Examination

Tibiofemoral alignment is evaluated with the patient standing. The knee is then observed for intra-articular and extra-articular swelling, and the knee's range of motion is formally measured and compared with that of the contralateral leg. The soft tissues are palpated for areas of tenderness. The examiner should try to identify the area of greatest tenderness along the course of the MPFL, a procedure that usually identifies the location of the tear.

A thorough ligamentous examination is necessary to rule out concomitant cruciate or collateral ligament tears. It is not uncommon to confuse the symptoms of a torn anterior cruciate ligament with patellar instability. Medial collateral ligament injuries commonly occur at the time of patellar dislocation. Measurement of the quadriceps angle can be used as a gross assessment of the lateral force vector. During active knee extension, patellar tracking is observed, and in particular the patella is watched for a tendency to slip laterally as the knee approaches the last 20 degrees of extension when the patella is no longer constrained by the lateral trochlear ridge. Patellar translation is estimated by applying a laterally directed force to the medial side of the patella with the knee in extension. The examiner attempts to quantify the amount of translation (in quadrants) and the consistency of the end point. An indistinct or "soft" end point suggests MPFL incompetence. A sense of apprehension with this maneuver (apprehension sign) supports the diagnosis of instability. Conversely, apprehension with medial translation may suggest medial instability. Lateral retinacular tightness is assessed by attempting to lift the lateral edge of the patella (tilt test). The retinaculum is considered tight if the patella will not correct to a neutral or horizontal position.

Imaging

Radiographs

The standard radiographic series includes anteroposterior, lateral (30 degrees of flexion), tunnel, and sunrise (30 to 45 degrees of flexion) views. The tunnel view is useful for showing osteochondral lesions or loose bodies in the notch. The lateral view gives information about patellar height and trochlear morphologic features. The sunrise view shows the degree of subluxation and tilt as well as any osteochondral lesions.

Other Imaging Modalities

Computed tomography scans in the axial plane are used to evaluate patella tilt, subluxation, and trochlear morphology. Superimposed axial images through the trochlear groove and tuberosity are used to measure the tibial tuberosity–trochlear groove distance (Fig. 88-1). Patella height index calculation can be made from the sagittal images. Although computed tomography scans are ideal for showing the bony anatomy, magnetic resonance imaging shows the soft tissue injuries, including MPFL tears, meniscus tears, and chondral lesions.

Indications and Contraindications

MPFL reconstruction is indicated for patients with symptomatic recurrent lateral subluxation or dislocation episodes for whom nonoperative treatment

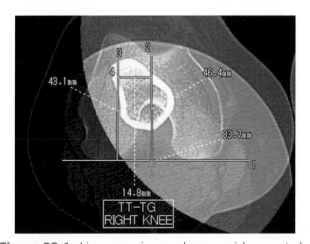

Figure 88-1. Lines superimposed on an axial computed tomography image of the right knee through the trochlear groove and tuberosity are used to measure the tibial tuberosity–trochlear groove *(line 4, TT-TG)* distance. *1,* Line drawn tangential to the posterior femoral condyles; *2,* line drawn through the deepest point of the trochlea perpendicular to the posterior epicondyle tangent; and *3,* line drawn parallel to the trochlear line through the patellar tendon center.

(including activity modification, physical therapy, and bracing) has failed. Tibial tuberosity osteotomy procedures such as the Elmslie-Trillat, which directly decrease the quadriceps angle by medializing the tibial tuberosity, have a theoretical advantage in patients with greater degrees of malalignment. The Fulkerson anteromedialization osteotomy is preferred for patients with malalignment and degenerative changes.[10] MPFL reconstruction or repair can be combined with distal osteotomy if neither alone can provide adequate stability. Lateral retinacular release is reserved for patients with excessive lateral patellofemoral pressure; it is ineffective as an isolated procedure for patients with instability.

Some authors recommend MPFL repair after first-time patellar dislocation.[3] We usually treat an initial subluxation or dislocation episode nonoperatively but may repair an acute MPFL tear when surgery is indicated for concomitant intra-articular disease (such as an osteochondral fracture, large loose body, or meniscus tear). MPFL repair may also be used to treat recurrent instability. With repeated instability episodes, the MPFL becomes attenuated and functionally incompetent. To reestablish the normal checkrein effect, the MPFL is tightened by cutting, shortening, and reattaching it at the patellar or femoral insertion or by midsubstance imbrication.

MPFL repair or reconstruction is contraindicated in patients with medial instability or isolated anterior knee pain. In patients with substantial medial patellofemoral degenerative changes, great care should be taken not to overtighten the MPFL because doing so will result in

excessive medial joint pressure and is likely to exacerbate patellofemoral pain.

SURGICAL TECHNIQUE

Anesthesia and Positioning

The procedure is performed on an outpatient basis with use of general or regional anesthesia techniques. The patient is positioned supine on a standard operating room table. A vertical thigh post is used to facilitate arthroscopic evaluation and is removed before the reconstruction is started. A tourniquet is placed around the proximal thigh on the operative side, and a compressive thigh-high stocking is placed on the contralateral leg. Prophylactic intravenous antibiotics are administered before incision.

Examination

Examination Under Anesthesia

Once adequate anesthesia has been established, a comprehensive examination is performed. It is usually easier to characterize patellar stability, translation, and tilt when the patient is anesthetized. With the knee in extension, the position of the patella is determined at rest and with a lateral translation force applied (Fig. 88-2A). Even an unstable patella will not stay dislocated unless the knee is maintained in a flexed position. It is important to compare the amount of translation on the symptomatic side with the normal lateral patellar translation in the contralateral knee. The examiner should use his or her thumb to push the patella laterally and assess the amount of translation as well as the consistency of the end point. It is also important to measure medial translation (Fig. 88-2B). Rarely, medial instability may be confused with lateral instability, especially if the patient has had an overaggressive previous lateral retinacular release. It is also important to assess the patient for lateral retinacular tightness. If the examiner is unable to evert the lateral edge of the patella to the neutral or horizontal position, and if the patient's symptoms and preoperative radiographs are consistent with excessive lateral pressure, consideration should be given to a concomitant arthroscopic lateral retinacular release.

Arthroscopic Examination

Diagnostic arthroscopy is performed via standard superolateral, inferomedial, and inferolateral portals. The suprapatellar pouch, the medial and lateral parapatellar gutters, and the posteromedial and posterolateral compartments are carefully assessed for loose bodies. The articular surfaces of the patella and trochlea are thoroughly visualized for chondral lesions. Most often, the medial facet of the patella and the proximal portion of the lateral femoral condyle are injured after traumatic

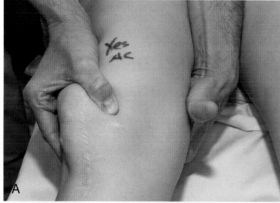

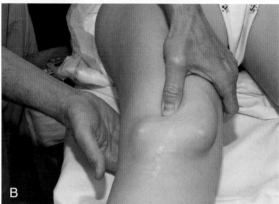

Figure 88-2. A, With the knee in extension, the position of the patella is determined with a lateral translation force applied (glide test). **B,** It is also important to measure medial translation because medial instability may occasionally be identified.

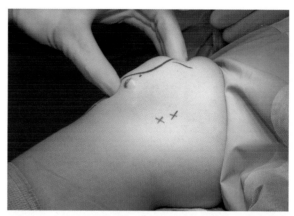

Figure 88-3. Marks are made on the skin over the adductor tubercle and the medial femoral epicondyle.

BOX 88-1 Surgical Steps

1. Medial patellofemoral ligament (MPFL) exposure and repair
2. Graft harvest and preparation for MPFL reconstruction
3. Patellar tunnel preparation and graft fixation
4. Femoral tunnel preparation
5. Graft tensioning and fixation
6. Closure

---

patellar dislocation. Hemorrhage in the soft tissue and a capsular defect along the medial edge of the patella suggest a recent traumatic avulsion of the MPFL insertion. Patellar tracking in the trochlear groove is visualized while the knee is flexed and extended. The menisci and cruciate ligaments are assessed for concomitant pathologic changes. Any substantial chondral lesions are addressed surgically with debridement, marrow stimulation, or repair techniques as indicated. Careful consideration should be given to whether large defects should be unloaded by tibial tuberosity osteotomy techniques, such as anteromedialization. If there is excessive tightness of the lateral retinaculum, an arthroscopic release may be performed, although we have not found it to be routinely necessary.

Surgical Landmarks and Incisions

A marking pen is used to identify the location of the patella and tibial tuberosity. Marks are also made over the adductor tubercle and just distally over the medial femoral epicondyle (Fig. 88-3). If an MPFL repair is to be performed, the location of the incision is marked based on the location of the MPFL tear as ascertained by preoperative clinical examination and imaging.

Specific Steps

Box 88-1 outlines the specific steps of this procedure.

1. Medial Patellofemoral Ligament Exposure and Repair

The leg is exsanguinated with an Esmarch bandage, and the tourniquet is raised while the knee is in an extended position. With a recent dislocation, it may be possible to identify the site of failure at the medial border of the patella, at the medial femoral epicondyle, or (less commonly) in midsubstance. Some authors believe that the most common site of failure is off of the femur.[3] In this location, the torn MPFL can be repaired to a stump of remaining tissue with No. 2 nonabsorbable sutures or reattached directly to a freshened bone surface with two or three suture anchors. If the MPFL is avulsed at the medial edge of the patella, the bone is freshened with a rongeur, and suture anchors are placed at the avulsion site. Repair of a midsubstance rupture is more challenging. It is not always possible to identify the location of tissue failure, and especially in chronic injury it can be difficult to determine how much to shorten the attenuated ligament. Overtightening the ligament will result in subsequent repair failure or overconstraint of the patella. We generally reserve MPFL repair techniques for patients who have experienced recent instability episodes when acute surgical intervention is indicated for concomitant intra-articular disease.

2. Graft Harvest and Preparation for Medial Patellofemoral Ligament Reconstruction

Various autologous or allogeneic graft sources are available for MPFL reconstruction. We prefer to use the gracilis tendon, which is immediately adjacent to the reconstruction site and relatively easy to harvest. An incision is made directly over the pes anserine insertion, and blunt dissection is used to expose the sartorial fascia. The superior edge of the sartorial fascia is identified anterior to the superficial medial collateral ligament. The sartorial fascia is then incised and everted to expose the underlying gracilis and semitendinosus tendons. A combination of blunt and sharp dissection is used to separate the gracilis tendon from the sartorial fascia. The free end of the tendon is tagged, and a tendon stripper is then used to harvest the gracilis tendon. Although the gracilis is smaller and shorter than the semitendinosus tendon, it is still substantially stronger than the native MPFL[11] and is almost always long enough for an adequate graft to be constructed. After the gracilis tendon has been harvested, the sartorial fascia is sutured back to its insertion on the proximal medial tibia. Allograft is used preferentially in revision procedures and may also be beneficial in patients with hyperlaxity syndromes.

The graft material is then prepared for implantation by removal of muscle and other debris from the surface. A No. 2 fiber loop (Arthrex, Naples, FL) is woven through the end of the tendon, and the tendon diameter is measured by passage of the graft through a graft sizer (Fig. 88-4).

3. Patellar Tunnel Preparation and Graft Fixation

A 2-cm incision is made along the medial border of the patella. The proximal and distal poles of the patella are palpated, and the equator of the patellar is localized. A short 2.5-mm Kirschner wire (K-wire) is drilled from medial to lateral, proximal to the equator of the patella. The surgeon must carefully advance the K-wire so that it exits the lateral edge of the patella without violating the posterior articular surface or the anterior cortex (Fig. 88-5). This position is confirmed with lateral fluoroscopy. A second 2.5-mm K-wire is drilled approximately 3 mm proximal to the first K-wire (Fig. 88-6). Both tunnels are then overdrilled with a 4.5-mm cannulated drill bit to a depth of approximately 15 mm (Fig. 88-7). The K-wires are removed, and a pituitary rongeur is used to create a 15-mm deep slot. Two short K-wires are then passed from medial to lateral through the blind tunnel to create diverging tunnels exiting the skin on the lateral side of the patella. One of the two suture ends from the graft is passed through the eyelet of one of the K-wires; the process is repeated with the second suture end and second K-wire. Both K-wires are advanced from medial to lateral across the patella, and the end of the graft is docked in the blind patellar tunnel (Fig. 88-8A). Both sutures are then retrieved through the superolateral arthroscopy portal. With the graft appropriately docked 15 mm into the blind tunnel, the

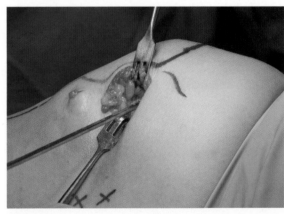

Figure 88-5. The medial border of the patella is exposed, and the K-wire is advanced so that it exits the lateral edge of the patella without violating the posterior articular surface or the anterior cortex.

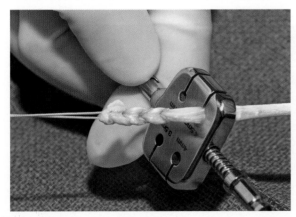

Figure 88-4. A No. 2 fiber loop is woven through the end of the tendon, and the diameter is measured.

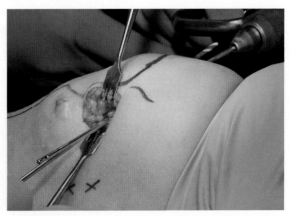

Figure 88-6. A second 2.5-mm K-wire is drilled approximately 3 mm distal to the first K-wire.

sutures are tied directly onto the surface of the lateral border of the patella through the superolateral portal over a substantial bone bridge. Aggressive manual traction on the graft confirms excellent fixation.

4. Femoral Tunnel Preparation

An incision is made over the interval between the adductor tubercle and medial femoral epicondyle (Fig. 88-8B). A crucial technical error during MPFL reconstruction surgery is to place the femoral tunnel too far proximal. Anatomic studies have reported that the femoral attachment site of the MPFL is at the medial epicondyle, which is approximately 1 cm distal to the adductor tubercle.[12,13] Others have reported the femoral attachment to be just anterior to the medial epicondyle.[14,15] One biomechanical study has suggested that malpositioning of the femoral tunnel even 5 mm too far proximal can result in substantially increased graft force and pressure applied to the medial patellofemoral joint.[16]

Once the bony landmarks are surgically exposed, a short 2.5-mm K-wire is placed just anterior to the medial femoral epicondyle (Fig. 88-9A). This position can be confirmed fluoroscopically (Fig. 88-9B). The graft is then passed through a soft tissue tunnel underneath the

medial retinaculum and the remnant of the MPFL (Fig. 88-10). The graft is then wrapped around the base of the K-wire, allowing assessment of graft isometry as the knee is flexed and extended. Minor changes in the position of the K-wire will allow fine-tuning of tunnel positioning. Once the optimal position for the femoral tunnel has been determined, the short K-wire is

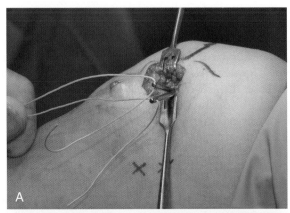

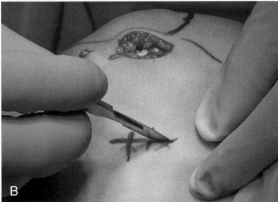

Figure 88-8. One of the two suture ends from the graft is passed through the eyelet of one of the K-wires; the process is repeated with the second suture end and second K-wire. The K-wires are advanced from medial to lateral across the patella so that the end of the graft is docked in the blind patellar tunnel (**A**). An incision is made over the adductor tubercle and medial epicondyle (**B**).

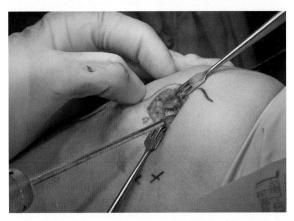

Figure 88-7. The K-wires are overdrilled with a 4.5-mm drill bit.

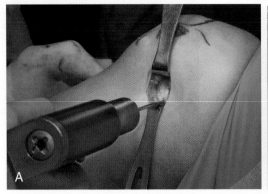
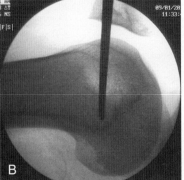

Figure 88-9. A, Once the bony landmarks have been exposed, a 2.5-mm K-wire is placed just anterior to the medial femoral epicondyle. **B,** Appropriate position of the K-wire can be confirmed fluoroscopically.

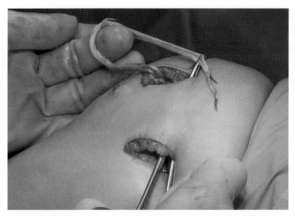

Figure 88-10. The graft is then passed through a soft tissue tunnel underneath the medial retinaculum and the remnant of the medial patellofemoral ligament.

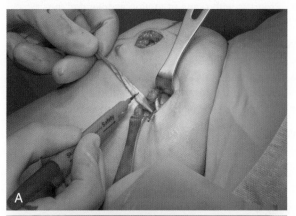

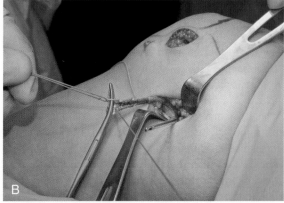

Figure 88-11. A, To allow for interference screw fixation, the graft is marked and cut 2 cm longer than the distance to the femoral tunnel. **B,** A No. 5 Ticron suture is passed through a loop woven through the femoral end of the graft with a No. 2 Ticron suture. The No. 5 Ticron suture will be used to pull the graft into the femoral tunnel, then removed after graft fixation.

exchanged for a long 2.5-mm eyelet K-wire that is then passed laterally with a slight anterior and proximal angulation. To allow for interference screw fixation, the graft is marked and cut 2 cm longer than the distance to the femoral tunnel (Fig. 88-11A). The eyelet K-wire

is then overdrilled with a 5.0- to 6.0-mm cannulated drill bit to a depth of approximately 25 mm. A No. 2 Ticron suture is then sewn through the end of the graft approximately 20 mm longer than the length of the graft to the opening of the tunnel. A No. 5 Ticron suture is passed through the loop woven through the femoral end of the graft with the No. 2 Ticron suture (Fig. 88-11B). The No. 5 Ticron suture will be used to pull the graft into the femoral tunnel, then removed after graft fixation. The suture ends are then passed through the eyelet of the K-wire, and the graft is pulled into the blind femoral tunnel as the K-wire is pulled out the lateral side of the knee.

5. Graft Tensioning and Fixation

Tension is placed on the free suture ends on the lateral aspect of the knee as the surgeon moves the knee several times through a full range of motion. As the knee flexes and extends, the amount of tension in the graft can be ascertained by the amount of traction felt on the free suture ends. In addition, the graft tension is directly palpated and visualized through the medial incision. It is extremely important not to overconstrain the graft. The knee is placed in full extension, and the patella graft length that reproduces the same amount of normal lateral translation is noted on the contralateral side (Fig. 88-12A). The knee is flexed to confirm that the graft is not too tight and that the patellofemoral joint is not overconstrained (Fig. 88-12B). Once the appropriate graft length is identified, graft fixation is achieved with a 7.0-mm bioabsorbable cannulated interference screw (Fig. 88-13). The screw is countersunk below the surface of the bone. Fixation can be augmented by sewing the graft to adjacent soft tissue at the tunnel opening. It should then be confirmed that the knee has full range of motion, the patella is no longer dislocatable, and the graft provides a firm checkrein, preventing pathologic lateral translation.

6. Closure

Subcuticular wound closure offers excellent cosmesis. Cryotherapy devices are routinely used to help control pain and swelling. Local anesthetic is injected into the soft tissue around the portals and incisions. A compressive dressing is then applied, followed by a thigh-high compression stocking and a postoperative brace locked in full extension.

POSTOPERATIVE CONSIDERATIONS

Rehabilitation

Immediately after surgery, patients are instructed in quadriceps sets, straight-leg raises, and crutch ambulation and are allowed touch-down weight bearing. The

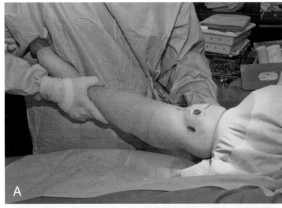

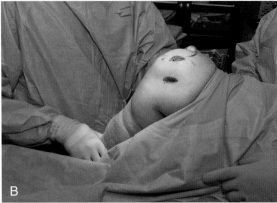

Figure 88-12. A, The knee is placed in full extension, and the patella graft length that reproduces the same amount of normal lateral translation is noted on the contralateral side. **B,** Before the graft is fixed in place, the knee is flexed and extended to confirm appropriate isometry and to confirm that the patella is not overconstrained.

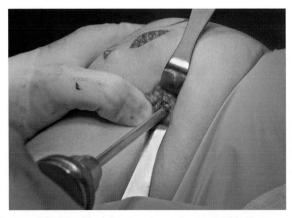

Figure 88-13. Final fixation is performed with the interference screw once isometry has been confirmed.

brace remains locked in full extension for 1 week, at which point patients are encouraged to begin knee range-of-motion exercises and to progress with weight bearing as tolerated. Patients are encouraged to attend formal physical therapy three times per week, where

BOX 88-2 Postoperative Rehabilitation Protocol

Discharge
- Ambulate with touch-down weight bearing (5 pounds maximum) in brace locked in full extension.
- Quadriceps sets, ankle pumps every hour.
- Continue intermittent ice (cooler) and elevation.

Week 1
- Clinic visit, remove portal sutures.
- Advance to 25% weight bearing in brace (brace must be locked in full extension during walking).
- Physical therapy referral three times per week for 12 weeks.
- Flexion exercises: heel slide, seated flexion, prone flexion.
- Continue knee brace until at least 6 weeks after surgery.
- Progress with range of motion as tolerated, no restriction.

Week 2
- Clinic visit, removal of incision sutures.
- Advance to full weight bearing in brace (brace must be locked in full extension during walking).
- Advance to straight leg raises with 1 pound of weight.

Week 3
- Begin stationary bike for range of motion.
- Reemphasize extension exercises.
- Advance with weights.

Week 4
- Straight-leg raises (100 repetitions daily).
- Should have at least 120 degrees of flexion.

Week 6
- Discontinue brace.

knee range of motion and quadriceps-strengthening exercises are emphasized.

The brace is unlocked for ambulation as soon as quadriceps strength is sufficient. Patients are given the goal of achieving 120 degrees of knee flexion by 4 weeks postoperatively, and the brace is generally discontinued by 6 weeks. Patients are encouraged to achieve full knee range of motion by 8 weeks and allowed to progress to jogging and sports-specific drills by 12 weeks. Most patients are able to return to sports by 4 to 5 months (Box 88-2).

Complications

As with many knee reconstruction procedures, the most common postoperative complication is loss of motion. Flexion and extension deficits may be secondary to inadequate postoperative rehabilitation. Early weight

TABLE 88-1 Published Studies Reporting Outcome after Medial Patellofemoral Ligament (MPFL) Repair or Reconstruction

Type of Procedure	Study	No. of Patients	Follow-up (years)	Results
MPFL repair	Christiansen et al[4] (2008)	42	2.0	Kujala score: 85 Redislocation: 16.7%
	Garth et al[2] (2000)	20	2.7	95% good to excellent
	Nomura et al[5] (2005)	5	5.9	Kujala score: 97.6 80% good to excellent
	Sallay et al[3] (1996)	12	3.0	Dislocation: 0 58% good to excellent
MPFL reconstruction	Deie et al[6] (2003)	4	7.4	Dislocation: 0 Kujala score: 96.3
	Drez et al[7] (2001)	15	2.6	Dislocation: 0 Kujala score: 88
	Servien et al[8] (2011)	29	2.0	69% optimal femoral tunnel position; 2 patients with apprehension
	Steiner et al[9] (2006)	34	5.5	85.3% good Kujala score: 90.7

bearing and motion exercises can minimize this risk. Flexion deficits may also be secondary to intraoperative technical errors (graft malpositioning or overtensioning). These errors could also overload the medial patellofemoral joint, resulting in pain and arthrosis, especially in the setting of a traumatic medial patellar chondral lesion. Other complications include recurrent instability, painful hardware, and patellar fracture.[8,16,17]

RESULTS

Published studies reporting outcome after MPFL repair or reconstruction have been limited by small numbers of patients, retrospective design, and lack of control groups but have been generally favorable[2,3,5-7,9] (Table 88-1). Most authors report satisfactory outcomes (good and excellent) in the range of 83% to 96%.[2,5,7,9,11] Studies reporting isolated repair of the MPFL without concomitant vastus medialis obliquus repair or isolated primary repair without a distal osteotomy or extensor mechanism realignment are associated with higher failure rates with no reduction in risk of redislocation or improvement in subjective functional score based on the Kujala knee score compared with patients undergoing nonoperative management.[4,18] Because a variety of different outcome parameters have been used, it is difficult to compare results, indicating the need for larger, multicenter controlled studies.

REFERENCES

1. Desio SM, Burks RT, Bachus KN. Soft tissue restraints to lateral patellar translation in the human knee. *Am J Sports Med.* 1998;26:59-65.
2. Garth Jr WP, DiChristina DG, Holt G. Delayed proximal repair and distal realignment after patellar dislocation. *Clin Orthop Relat Res.* 2000;377:132-144.
3. Sallay PI, Poggi J, Speer KP, et al. Acute dislocation of the patella. A correlative pathoanatomic study. *Am J Sports Med.* 1996;24:52-60.
4. Christiansen SE, Jakobsen BW, Lund B, et al. Isolated repair of the medial patellofemoral ligament in primary dislocation of the patella: a prospective randomized study. *Arthroscopy.* 2008;24:881-887.
5. Nomura E, Inoue M, Osada N. Augmented repair of avulsion-tear type medial patellofemoral ligament injury in acute patellar dislocation. *Knee Surg Sports Traumatol Arthrosc.* 2005;13:346-351.
6. Deie M, Ochi M, Sumen Y, et al. Reconstruction of the medial patellofemoral ligament for the treatment of habitual or recurrent dislocation of the patella in children. *J Bone Joint Surg Br.* 2003;85:887-890.
7. Drez Jr D, Edwards TB, Williams CS. Results of medial patellofemoral ligament reconstruction in the treatment of patellar dislocation. *Arthroscopy.* 2001;17:298-306.
8. Servien E, Fritsch B, Lustig S, et al. In vivo positioning analysis of medial patellofemoral ligament reconstruction. *Am J Sports Med.* 2011;39:134-139.
9. Steiner TM, Torga-Spak R, Teitge RA. Medial patellofemoral ligament reconstruction in patients with lateral patellar instability and trochlear dysplasia. *Am J Sports Med.* 2006;34:1254-1261.
10. Fulkerson JP, Becker GJ, Meaney JA, et al. Anteromedial tibial tubercle transfer without bone graft. *Am J Sports Med.* 1990;18:490-496; disc 496-497.
11. Amis AA, Firer P, Mountney J, et al. Anatomy and biomechanics of the medial patellofemoral ligament. *Knee.* 2003;10:215-220.
12. Smirk C, Morris H. The anatomy and reconstruction of the medial patellofemoral ligament. *Knee.* 2003;10:221-227.

13. Steensen RN, Dopirak RM, McDonald III WG. The anatomy and isometry of the medial patellofemoral ligament: implications for reconstruction. *Am J Sports Med.* 2004;32:1509-1513.

14. Feller JA, Feagin Jr JA, Garrett Jr WE. The medial patellofemoral ligament revisited: an anatomical study. *Knee Surg Sports Traumatol Arthrosc.* 1993;1:184-186.

15. Nomura E, Inoue M. Surgical technique and rationale for medial patellofemoral ligament reconstruction for recurrent patellar dislocation. *Arthroscopy.* 2003;19:E47.

16. Elias JJ, Cosgarea AJ. Technical errors during medial patellofemoral ligament reconstruction could overload medial patellofemoral cartilage. A computational analysis. *Am J Sports Med.* 2006;34:1478-1485.

17. Bollier M, Fulkerson J, Cosgarea A, et al. Technical failure of medial patellofemoral ligament reconstruction. *Arthroscopy.* 2011;27:1153-1159.

18. Camp CL, Krych AJ, Dahm DL, et al. Medial patellofemoral ligament repair for recurrent patellar dislocation. *Am J Sports Med.* 2010;38:2248-2254.

Chapter 89

Sulcus Deepening Trochleoplasty

Paulo R.F. Saggin, Paolo Ferrua, and David Dejour

Chapter Synopsis

- Deepening trochleoplasty is a procedure designed to correct high-grade trochlear dysplasia, which is one of the most important factors involved in the genesis of patellar instability. Trochlear correction improves patellar tracking, reduces the patellofemoral joint reaction force, and decreases the tibial tubercle–trochlear groove (TT-TG) value. It must be considered in patients undergoing surgery for patellar instability.

Important Points

- Indications
  - Severe trochlear dysplasia (types B and D) with patellar dislocations
- Contraindications
  - Mild trochlear dysplasia
  - Open growth plates
  - Early arthritis
- Trochlear dysplasia classification
  - Type A: Presence of crossing sign. The trochlea is still symmetric and concave.
  - Type B: Crossing sign and trochlear spur. The trochlea is flat or convex.
  - Type C: Crossing sign in addition to the double-contour sign. There is no spur; the lateral facet is convex and the medial facet is hypoplastic.
  - Type D: Combines all the mentioned signs: crossing sign, supratrochlear spur, and double-contour sign. Cliff pattern.

- Types B and D have prominence of the trochlea and increased patellofemoral reaction forces.

Clinical and Surgical Pearls

- Positioning must allow full range of motion during procedure.
- Midline incision with adapted midvastus approach.
- Adequate exposure and access to the undersurface of the trochlea.
- Intraoperative new trochlea planning.
- Adequate bone removal and achievement of a malleable osteochondral flap.
- Correction of associated abnormalities.
- Early rehabilitation.

Clinical and Surgical Pitfalls

- Avoid cartilage damage during the osteochondral flap confection—keep a safe distance from the cartilage.
- Achieve a well-molded bone bed; otherwise the new trochlea will not be adequately refashioned.
- Avoid prolonged immobilization (sometimes required for the associated procedures).
- Be alert for the indication; pain is not an indication.

Trochlear dysplasia is one of the major factors causing patellar dislocations (together with patella alta, excessive tibial tubercle–trochlear groove distance, and excessive patellar tilt). This anatomic abnormality is present in 96% of patients with patellar dislocations.[1] Trochlear osteotomy or trochleoplasty is the procedure designed to correct the abnormal shape of the trochlea, improving patellar tracking and preventing instability. It is a logical procedure from the biomechanical point of view. Despite being technically demanding, it yields good results, and therefore it should be known to surgeons dealing with the patellar dislocation population.

Trochleoplasty should be combined with other procedures to treat the other major causes of instability and is rarely performed alone.

PREOPERATIVE CONSIDERATIONS

Trochleoplasty is indicated in patients with high grade trochlear dysplasia and patellar instability, and particularly when abnormal tracking of the patella is observed during active and passive motion of the knee. As with any surgery performed in this group of patients, it is indicated after the second or third documented dislocation. The dislocation is usually confirmed if the patient has had the patella reduced by a physician, if radiographs obtained on the occasion of the trauma evidence a medial patellar bone avulsion, or if magnetic resonance imaging (MRI) confirms the medial soft tissue rupture and the associated medial patellar and lateral femoral condyle bruises. At times the history is not so clear, but the patient usually recalls the sensation of instability followed by pain, edema, and ecchymosis.

Imaging is essential to understand trochlear dysplasia and to allow its classification. Whereas normal trochleae have sulci of adequate depth, dysplastic trochleae are shallow, flat, or even convex. On lateral x-ray projections, this is represented by the crossing sign—the groove line reaches (or crosses) the line representing the superior edge of the facets. Two other features are typical of dysplastic trochleae on lateral views: the supratrochlear spur and the double contour sign. The supratrochlear spur is the same sometimes visualized in the surgical exposure, located in the superolateral aspect of the trochlea. It corresponds to an attempt to contain the lateral displacement of the patella. The double contour represents the medial hypoplastic facet, seen posterior to the lateral one in the lateral view. Based on these signs, and sometimes aided by computed tomography (CT) axial views, trochlear dysplasia may be classified into four types[2]:

- Type A: Presence of crossing sign in the lateral true view. The trochlea is shallower than normal ones, but still symmetric and concave.
- Type B: Crossing sign and trochlear spur. The trochlea is flat or convex in axial images.
- Type C: Presence of crossing sign, and in addition the double-contour sign can be found on the lateral view, representing the medial hypoplastic facet. There is no spur. In axial views, the lateral facet is convex and the medial hypoplastic.
- Type D: Combines all the mentioned signs: crossing sign, supratrochlear spur, and double-contour sign. In the axial view, there is clear asymmetry of the facets' height, also referred to as a *cliff pattern* (Fig. 89-1).

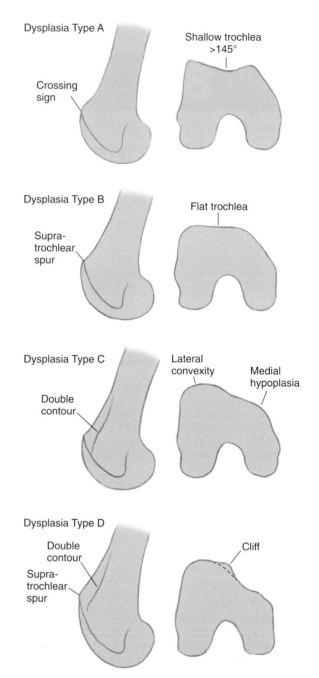

Figure 89-1. Trochlear dysplasia classification according to Dejour.

Trochleoplasty is indicated in dysplasia types B and D, when there is prominence of the trochlea. Type A is low-grade trochlear dysplasia and should not be responsible for instability, if present. Type C represents a subtype of trochlear dysplasia not suited for sulcus-deepening trochleoplasty because the trochlea is already hypoplastic and should not benefit from bone removal.

Open growth plates are a contraindication to trochleoplasty. Pain is not specifically addressed by this procedure and should not be the only element taken into account when the procedure is indicated. It should be

TABLE 89-1. Computed Tomography (CT) with Lyon Protocol

Measure	How to Measure (CT Scan)	Patients with at Least One Episode of Patellar Dislocation (Mean ± SD)	Controls (Mean ± SD)	Comments
Femoral anteversion	Angle between center of femoral head or neck and posterior condyles	15.6 ± 9.0 degrees	10.8 ± 8.7 degrees	
TT-TG	Distance between trochlear groove and tibial tuberosity in two overlapped cuts	19.8 ± 1.6 degrees	12.7 ± 3.4 degrees	Pathologic threshold is 20 mm
External patellar tilt	Angle formed by the transverse axis of the patella and posterior femoral condyles	28.8 ± 10.5 degrees Average increase of 6 degrees with quadriceps contraction	10 ± 5.8 degrees Average increase of 1.5 degrees with quadriceps contraction	Pathologic threshold without quadriceps contraction is 20 degrees
External tibial torsion	Angle formed by the tangent to the posterior aspect of the plateau and the bimalleolar axis	33 degrees	35 degrees	Too much variation, no particular significance found

SD, standard deviation; TT-TG, tibial tubercle–trochlear groove distance.

remembered that this procedure is indicated for instability. Early (or established) arthritis is another contraindication because trochleoplasty can worsen the cartilage status.

To achieve successful outcomes, associated abnormalities should be addressed in the same procedure. The TT-TG value is addressed when trochleoplasty is carried out, because the proximal part of it (the trochlear groove) is moved laterally from its native location. The other major factors involved in patellar instability should also be evaluated and treated, so plain radiographs (anteroposterior view, true lateral view, and axial view at 30 degrees of knee flexion) and CT scan with the Lyon protocol must be routine in the preoperative evaluation[1] (Table 89-1).

SURGICAL TECHNIQUE

Anesthesia and Positioning

After regional anesthesia and sedation, the patient is positioned lying supine. A lateral pad is applied to the proximal thigh, and a distal support under the foot allows the knee to be kept flexed by approximately 80 degrees. Full range of motion is possible during the procedure. A tourniquet is applied to the proximal thigh.

Specific Steps

Box 89-1 outlines the specific steps of this procedure.

1. Exposure

The incision is performed with the extremity flexed. A straight midline incision is performed from the superior

BOX 89-1 Surgical Steps

1. Exposure
2. Bone exposure
3. Trochlear planing
4. Cortical bone removal
5. Cancellous bone removal
6. Flap modeling
7. Fixation
8. Synovium reattachment
9. Associated procedures and patellar tracking checkup
10. Closure

patellar limit to the tibiofemoral articulation. A full-thickness skin flap is raised medially, and the arthrotomy is performed through the medial capsule. Proximally, the vastus medialis obliquus (VMO) is split in line with its fibers, from the superior-medial patellar edge to 4 cm proximally in the muscle belly (Fig. 89-2). The patella is briefly everted for inspection, cartilage damage rating, and adequate cartilage treatment if needed, and subsequently retracted laterally, providing adequate trochlear exposure (Figs. 89-3 and 89-4).

2. Bone Exposure

Before the osseous procedure is started, synovium must be removed from the edge of the trochlea. It is incised with a scalpel on the cartilage edge (Fig. 89-5), and a periosteal elevator is used to retract it away from the trochlear edge (Fig. 89-6). It is important to handle it carefully to keep a tissue of good quality that will allow adequate coverage by the end of the procedure.

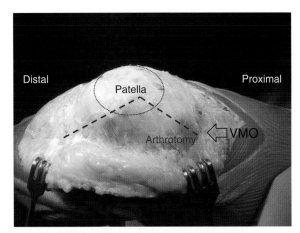

Figure 89-2. After the skin flap is raised, the arthrotomy is performed. *VMO,* Vastus medialis obliquus.

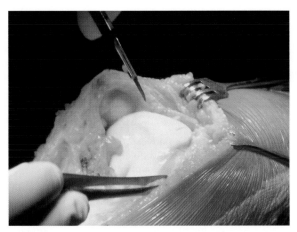

Figure 89-5. Incision of the synovium attached to the osteochondral edge.

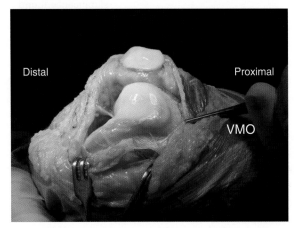

Figure 89-3. Complete exposure. The patella is everted for inspection. *VMO,* Vastus medialis obliquus.

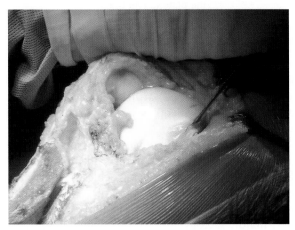

Figure 89-6. Retraction of the synovium attached to the osteochondral edge.

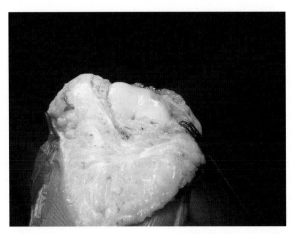

Figure 89-4. Distal view of the trochlea with the patella laterally retracted.

3. Trochlear Planing

The new trochlear groove is planed and drawn over the native one. From the intercondylar notch, a line deviating 3 to 6 degrees laterally is drawn proximally, representing the new groove. The proximal part of the new

groove is positioned according to the TT-TG value to correct a possible malalignment. The lateral margins are also drawn from the intercondylar notch through the sulcus terminalis of each condyle (Fig. 89-7).

4. Cortical Bone Removal

A strip of cortical bone corresponding to the amount of the bump must be removed. That means that the cortical bone that is present from the anterior femoral cortex to the cartilage edge must be osteotomized with a thin osteotome and removed. This creates the access to the undersurface of the trochlea and constitutes the first step to bringing the new trochlea to a normal position (not prominent) and eliminates the bump (Fig. 89-8).

5. Cancellous Bone Removal

The cancellous bone that lies under the trochlear cartilage must also be removed to reshape and reposition the new trochlea. Osteotomes and curettes are helpful in the procedure, but a drill with a specific depth guide is used for this purpose (Fig. 89-9). This depth guide is set to allow bone removal from the cartilage undersurface,

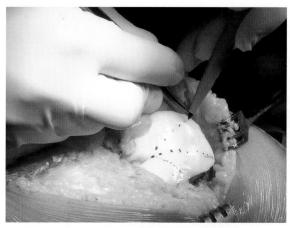

Figure 89-7. The new trochlear limits are drawn. The bottom of the sulcus is the median line drawn from the intercondylar notch deviating laterally 3 to 6 degrees. The lateral limits are drawn through the sulcus terminalis.

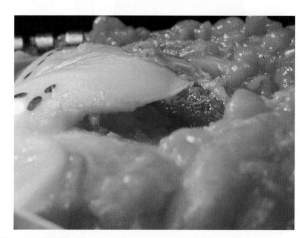

Figure 89-8. Cortical bone removed from the osteochondral edge of the proximal trochlea.

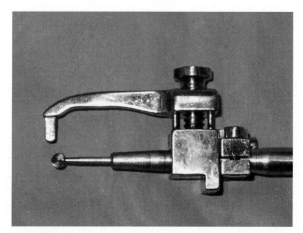

Figure 89-9. Drill with special depth guide.

producing a uniform cartilage-bone shell of 5 mm. It avoids cartilage damage and thermal necrosis, which could result from excessive bone removal. The shell produced must be sufficiently compliant to allow modeling. Without the guide, bone must be removed,

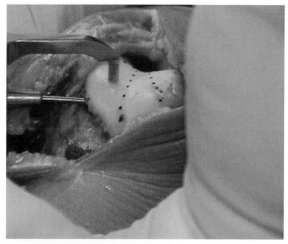

Figure 89-10. The drill with depth guide removing cancellous bone from the undersurface of the trochlea.

especially from where the new planned sulcus will lie. All bone that projects beyond the anterior femoral cortex should be removed (Fig. 89-10).

6. Flap Modeling

The cartilage-bone flap should sit flush on the underlying bone bed. The bone bed should be deepened in its central portion to re-create an adequate groove. Once the flap is adequately modeled over the bone bed and the trochlear conformation is satisfactory, fixation is performed.

7. Fixation

Absorbable sutures are used to fix the cartilage-bone flap to the underlying bone bed. One suture is passed from each facet and tied over the corresponding medial and lateral gutters; this allows pulling down of the new groove with homogenous pressure of both facets on the cancellous bone, promoting perfect healing (Fig. 89-11).

8. Synovium Reattachment

The synovium that was formerly dissected away from the osteochondral margin is sutured back to it. This protects the patellar cartilage from the femoral bone and minimizes blood loss through the exposed cancellous bone.

9. Associated Procedures and Patellar Tracking Checkup

After the procedure has been carried out and satisfactory trochlear shape has been achieved, the associated needed procedures are performed. We routinely perform an associated medial patellofemoral ligament reconstruction with or without a lateral release, depending on the tracking obtained. After the complete procedure is done, patellar tracking and stability are checked (Fig. 89-12).

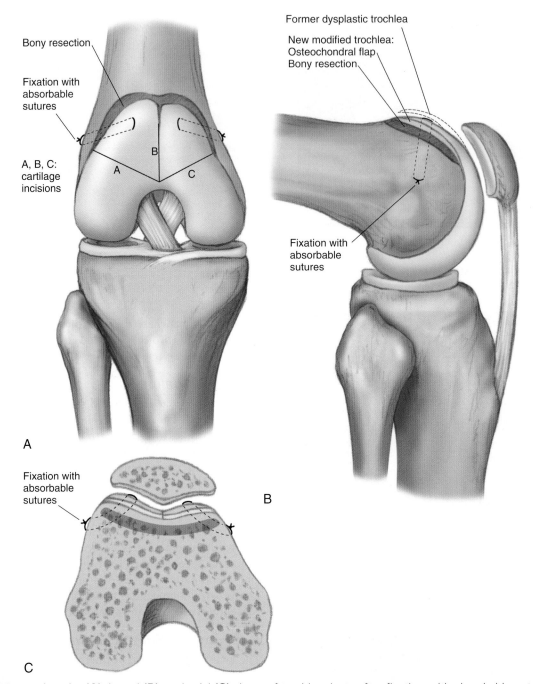

Bony resection

Fixation with
absorbable
sutures

A, B, C:
cartilage
incisions

A

Former dysplastic trochlea

New modified trochlea:
Osteochondral flap
Bony resection

Fixation with
absorbable
sutures

B

Fixation with
absorbable
sutures

C

Figure 89-11. Anterior **(A)**, lateral **(B)**, and axial **(C)** views of trochleoplasty after fixation with absorbable sutures.

10. Closure

Closure of the medial retinaculum is the final step. No drains are installed.

POSTOPERATIVE CONSIDERATIONS

Rehabilitation

Trochleoplasty does not necessitate immobilization or weight restriction, but the associated procedures must be considered. Immediate rehabilitation goals are pain and edema reduction and range-of-motion recovery. Immediate weight bearing is allowed with an extension brace, and flexion must be regained without forced or painful postures. The brace is removed when quadriceps strength allows the patient to walk. Quadriceps strengthening with weights on the foot or on the tibial tubercle is prohibited in the initial phase. Early mobilization on a continuous passive motion device improves cartilage nutrition and helps further trochlear modeling by the patella. After 45 days, cycling with weak resistance and weight-bearing proprioceptive exercises may be initiated. From the fourth to the sixth month, running can

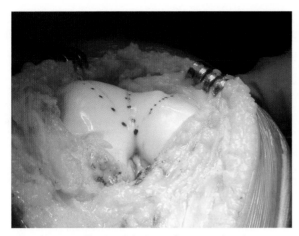

Figure 89-12. Final axial view after trochleoplasty.

be reinitiated and quadriceps reinforcement with open kinetic chain exercises from 0 to 60 degrees and minor loads are allowed. Sports return is allowed after the sixth month.

Follow-up

Control radiographs are obtained immediately postoperatively and at 6 weeks. Six months after the procedure, a CT scan is performed to document the achieved correction.

Complications

Specific complications related to trochlear surgery may include trochlear necrosis, cartilage damage, incongruence with the patella, and hypocorrection or hypercorrection. Trochlear necrosis is an issue of particular concern but it does not seem to occur, because the cartilage nutrition is not dependent on the underlying bone. Schottle[3] performed biopsies in three patients after trochleoplasty, showing cartilage cell viability and flap healing. He concluded that the risk of cartilage damage is low. Incongruence with the patella is another possible complication, especially because patellar dysplasia is common in this population. The long-term outcome is not known. Hypocorrection or hypercorrection may cause the failure of the procedure, but missed associated abnormalities must also be ruled out.

Infection, deep venous thrombosis, and sympathetic reflex dystrophy (complex regional pain syndrome) may arise after trochleoplasty just as they may arise after any surgery, requiring adequate treatment and delaying rehabilitation.

RESULTS

Trochleoplasty is effective in improving trochlear anatomy and tracking. Amis and colleagues[4] studied the patellar tracking in normal knees after simulating dysplasia and again after performing a trochleoplasty, and concluded that trochleoplasty increased stability and provided small but significant changes in patellar tracking. Fucentese and colleagues,[5] using CT scans preoperatively and postoperatively, demonstrated that trochleoplasty lateralized the trochlear groove and medialized the patella, increased the trochlear depth, decreased the lateral patellar inclination angle, decreased the sulcus angle, and increased the lateral trochlear slope, thus re-creating a more normal anatomy.

Trochleoplasty results are generally good in terms of stability and function, whereas the results for pain are less clear.

Two series reviewing deepening trochleoplasty were published in the *10èmes Journées Lyonnaises de Chirurgie du Genou* in 2002. The first group included 18 patients in whom patellar surgery for instability had failed, with a mean age of 24 years at surgery. The mean follow-up was 6 years (2 to 8 years, no patients lost to follow-up). The new surgery was indicated six times for pain and 12 times for recurrence of instability. The average number of surgeries before the trochleoplasty was two. The deepening trochleoplasty was associated with a tibial tubercle medialization in eight patients, in six with a tibial tubercle distalization, and in 18 with a VMO-plasty. All patients were reviewed clinically with the International Knee Documentation Committee (IKDC) form and radiographically; 65% were satisfied or very satisfied. The knee stability was rated A 13 times, and B five times. Twenty-eight percent of the patients had residual pain, and this was correlated to the cartilage status at surgery. Two patients developed patellofemoral arthritis. The mean patellar tilt was 35 degrees (18 to 48 degrees) in the preoperative setting, and improved to 21 degrees (11 to 28 degrees) with the quadriceps relaxed and 24 degrees (16 to 32 degrees) with the quadriceps contracted after the surgery.

In the second group there were 44 patients. They had no antecedents of patellofemoral surgery. The mean follow-up was 7 years (2 to 9 years). At the time of surgery, 22 tibial tubercle medializations, 26 distalizations, and 32 VMO-plasties were associated. These patients were also reviewed clinically with the IKDC form and radiographically. Eighty-five percent were satisfied or very satisfied. Knee stability was rated A 31 times, and B 13 times. Five percent had residual pain, but this was not correlated to the cartilage status at surgery. No patellofemoral arthritis was noted. The mean patellar tilt preoperatively was 33 degrees (24 to 52 degrees) and improved postoperatively to 18 degrees (9 to 30 degrees) with the quadriceps relaxed and 22 degrees (14 to 34 degrees) with the quadriceps contracted.

Table 89-2 summarizes the other published series.

There is considerable heterogeneity in the published series regarding the patients treated and the severity of

TABLE 89-2. Results of Published Series about Trochleoplasty

Author	Procedure	No. of Knees	Follow-up (Average)	Results	Conclusion
Verdonk et al[6] (2005)	Deepening trochleoplasty	13	18 months	Larsen-Lauridsen score: 7 poor, 3 fair, 3 well Subjective: 6 very good, 4 good, 1 satisfactory, 2 inadequate	77% satisfied with the procedure—good subjective outcome despite poor objective outcomes
Donell et al[7] (2006)	Deepening trochleoplasty	17	3 years	Kujala score improved from 48 to 75 7 patients very satisfied, 6 satisfied, 2 disappointed Boss height reduced from 7.5 mm to 0.7 mm	Good improvement in the Kujala score and high satisfaction rate
Von Knoch et al[8] (2006)	Bereiter trochleoplasty	45	8.3 years	No recurrence of dislocation 93.9% correction of trochlear dysplasia Degenerative changes in 30% 35 knees had pain preoperatively Postoperatively, pain became worse in 15 (33.4%), remained unchanged in 4 (8.8%) and improved in 22 (49%) 4 knees that had no pain preoperatively (8.8%) continued to have no pain	Good results in stability Inconsistent results for pain
Schottle et al[9] (2005)	Bereiter trochleoplasty	19	3 years	No redislocations Kujala score improved from 56 to 80 16 improved subjectively Pain improved in 12 patients and became worse in 2	Good results for instability and pain
Utting et al[10] (2008)	Bereiter trochleoplasty	42	24 months	IKDC score improved from 54 to 72 Kujala score improved from 62 to 76	Good results with function improvement
Fucentese et al[11] (2011)	Bereiter trochleoplasty	44	4 years	Kujala score increased from 68 to 90 Pain remained unchanged in 27, decreased in 14, and increased in 3 knees 27 knees ranked excellent, 10 good, 2 fair, and 5 poor	Good results Pain in most patients remained unchanged

IKDC, International Knee Documentation Committee.

their disease, the number of associated procedures, the preoperative status of the patients, and the type of procedure being undertaken. The published series also differ in follow-up and outcomes measurements. As a result, no clear conclusions can be drawn about the final and long-term outcomes. Further prospective and controlled data with rigorous statistical method are lacking and would allow better understanding of indications, long-term results, and complications of this procedure.

REFERENCES

1. Dejour H, Walch G, Nove-Josserand L, et al. Factors of patellar instability: an anatomic radiographic study. *Knee Surg Sports Traumatol Arthrosc.* 1994;2:19-26.
2. Dejour D, Le Coultre B. Osteotomies in patello-femoral instabilities. *Sports Med Arthrosc.* 2007;15:39-46.
3. Schottle PB, Schell H, Duda G, et al. Cartilage viability after trochleoplasty. *Knee Surg Sports Traumatol Arthrosc.* 2007;15:161-167.
4. Amis AA, Oguz C, Bull AM, et al. The effect of trochleoplasty on patellar stability and kinematics: a biomechanical study in vitro. *J Bone Joint Surg Br.* 2008;90:864-869.
5. Fucentese SF, Schottle PB, Pfirrmann CW, et al. CT changes after trochleoplasty for symptomatic trochlear dysplasia. *Knee Surg Sports Traumatol Arthrosc.* 2007;15:168-174.
6. Verdonk R, Jansegers E, Stuyts B. Trochleoplasty in dysplastic knee trochlea. *Knee Surg Sports Traumatol Arthrosc.* 2005;13:529-533.
7. Donell ST, Joseph G, Hing CB, et al. Modified Dejour trochleoplasty for severe dysplasia: operative technique and early clinical results. *Knee.* 2006;13:266-273.
8. von Knoch F, Bohm T, Burgi ML, et al. Trochleoplasty for recurrent patellar dislocation in association with trochlear dysplasia. A 4- to 14-year follow-up study. *J Bone Joint Surg Br.* 2006;88:1331-1335.
9. Schottle PB, Fucentese SF, Pfirrmann C, et al. Trochleoplasty for patellar instability due to trochlear dysplasia: A minimum 2-year clinical and radiological follow-up of 19 knees. *Acta Orthop.* 2005;76:693-698.
10. Utting MR, Mulford JS, Eldridge JD. A prospective evaluation of trochleoplasty for the treatment of patellofemoral dislocation and instability. *J Bone Joint Surg Br.* 2008;90:180-185.
11. Fucentese SF, Zingg PO, Schmitt J, et al. Classification of trochlear dysplasia as predictor of clinical outcome after trochleoplasty. *Knee Surg Sports Traumatol Arthrosc.* 2011;19(10):1655-1661.

Chapter 90

Management of Arthrofibrosis of the Knee

K. Donald Shelbourne and Heather Freeman

Chapter Synopsis

- Arthrofibrosis of the knee is a preventable complication that presents many challenges to the treating physician. Effective treatment involves working closely with rehabilitation staff with the overall objective being to regain symmetrical knee extension, knee flexion, and strength. A classification system for arthrofibrosis, step-by-step treatment methods, and results of this treatment approach are presented in this chapter.

Important Points

- Prevention is the best treatment for arthrofibrosis.

- Preoperative and postoperative rehabilitation is a critical aspect of treatment.

- Do not attempt to work on knee extension and flexion range of motion (ROM) at the same time. Restore symmetrical knee extension first, then work on knee flexion second.

- Patients with contracture of the patellar tendon may demonstrate some improvement of knee flexion but will not regain full symmetry.

Clinical and Surgical Pearls

- Surgical intervention depends on the classification and should focus on the following:

    1. Eliminating impingement of the anterior cruciate ligament (ACL) or ACL graft in the intercondylar notch

2. Removal of extrasynovial scar tissue anterior to the tibia and within the infrapatellar fat pad (if present)

3. Medial and lateral retinacular release to restore patellar mobility (if needed)

4. Knee manipulation to regain knee flexion (if needed)

- The use of a passive knee extension device is more effective than casting in conjunction with surgical treatment.

- Early postoperative care should focus on prevention of hemarthrosis to avoid a quadriceps muscle shutdown.

Clinical and Surgical Pitfalls

- Good quadriceps muscle control is needed so that the hamstring muscles do not go unopposed and pull the knee into flexion, making extension difficult to maintain. Also, contraction of the quadriceps stretches the patellar tendon to full length and prevents shortening of the patellar tendon.

- There is no specific timeframe for surgical intervention or how long patients should take to complete preoperative rehabilitation. Rehabilitation can be a lengthy process, but it is imperative that patients fully maximize knee extension and flexion before surgery.

- It is counterproductive to work on knee extension and flexion ROM at the same time. Similarly, it is counterproductive to work on strengthening and ROM at the same time.

Arthrofibrosis is the proliferation of fibrotic tissue within and surrounding a joint. It results in decreased range of motion (ROM), pain, decreased function, and subsequent strength loss secondary to disuse. In the knee joint, arthrofibrosis is a potential complication after fracture treatment or intra-articular surgery, including arthroscopy, anterior cruciate ligament (ACL) reconstruction, and total knee arthroplasty. Arthrofibrosis is a difficult condition to treat, and precautionary measures should be taken to prevent this potential postoperative complication.

Arthrofibrosis of the knee results in the loss of extension, and in some patients loss of knee flexion also occurs. Loss of knee extension is usually more symptomatic compared with loss of flexion.[1]

Arthrofibrosis is most effectively treated via a multidisciplinary approach, with the physician, rehabilitation staff, and patient working closely together. The treatment should be viewed as a process that includes intensive rehabilitation, followed by arthroscopic scar resection when needed and postoperative rehabilitation. In addition, patients often require a lot of emotional support and encouragement throughout this process and must be well informed and actively involved in their own care.

PREOPERATIVE CONSIDERATIONS

Physical Examination

Normal ROM of the knee may include some degree of hyperextension and varies from person to person. Therefore ROM of the uninvolved knee must be assessed first to gain a comparison point, and any difference between the uninvolved and involved knee ROM is noted as a deficit. Hyperextension of the knee is often overlooked, but is a normal finding in most knees. DeCarlo and Sell[2] found that 95% of males and 96% of females have some degree of knee hyperextension; the mean for males was 5 degrees, and the mean for females was 6 degrees. Knee extension must be assessed with the patient supine and both heels propped on a bolster, allowing the knees to fall into hyperextension (Fig. 90-1). Unless extension is measured this way and compared with that of the opposite, normal knee, a slight loss of knee extension could easily be overlooked. The amount of knee extension and flexion loss is noted and can be used to classify the severity of arthrofibrosis to assist with treatment planning (Table 90-1).[3]

Physical examination should also include an assessment of patellar mobility, quadriceps muscle control, observed muscle atrophy, and patella height. Decreased patellar mobility is observed in patients with type 3 or 4 arthrofibrosis, and patients with type 4 arthrofibrosis will have a shortened patellar tendon.

Imaging

Bilateral standing posteroanterior, lateral, and Merchant view radiographs should be obtained. It is important to measure patellar height and compare it between the involved and uninvolved knees to detect any side-to-side difference. The length of the patellar tendon can be measured on the lateral radiograph from the inferior pole of the patella to the tibial tubercle. The normal values for this measurement can vary considerably, making a side-to-side comparison necessary for detection of tendon contraction. Patients with type 4 arthrofibrosis will demonstrate patella infera from a contracted patellar tendon.

A Merchant view radiograph,[4] in which both patellae are viewed, can be used to detect disuse osteopenia in the involved patella. This is a sign that the patient has been significantly favoring the involved leg by standing with the weight shifted onto the uninvolved leg and avoiding use during other activities of daily living.

Magnetic resonance imaging (MRI) is useful in determining the extent of scar formation and proliferation within the knee and surrounding tissues.

Surgical Planning

The optimal timing for surgical intervention will vary considerably among patients with arthrofibrosis. It is important for patients and clinicians to understand that treatment of arthrofibrosis is a process that is not isolated to surgical intervention alone. Appropriate and directed preoperative and postoperative rehabilitation is a crucial aspect of caring for patients with this condition.

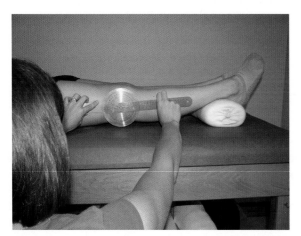

Figure 90-1. Measurement of knee extension with the heels propped on a bolster to allow the knees to fall into hyperextension. This also allows for a visual side-to-side comparison.

TABLE 90-1. Classification of Arthrofibrosis[3]

	Knee Extension	Knee Flexion	Other Features
Type 1	≤10-degree deficit*	Normal	Passively straightens with overpressure
Type 2	>10-degree deficit*	Normal	Unable to fully extend with overpressure
Type 3	>10-degree deficit*	≥25-degree deficit*	Decreased medial and lateral movement of patella
Type 4	>10-degree deficit*	≥30-degree deficit*	Patella infera on radiographs

*All range-of-motion deficits are based on comparison with the range of motion of the normal, uninvolved knee.

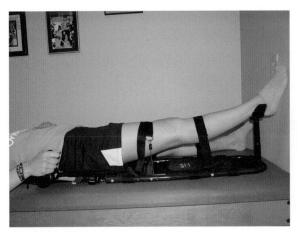

Figure 90-2. A passive knee extension device is used to provide a patient-controlled, prolonged stretch to the knee.

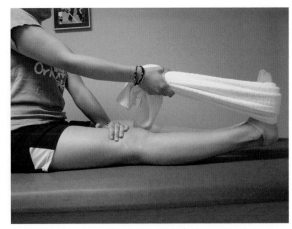

Figure 90-3. Towel stretch exercise to regain symmetrical passive knee extension.

The decision of when to proceed with surgery is based not on timeframes, but rather on the progress made with rehabilitation. Patients with type 1 arthrofibrosis may be able to regain symmetrical knee extension with rehabilitation alone, and surgical intervention may not be necessary. When needed, surgical intervention for arthrofibrosis is most successful when performed after the patient has worked diligently to improve knee ROM but has reached a plateau and can no longer make improvements with rehabilitation alone. In addition, the patient must be mentally prepared for surgery and have a full understanding of the plan of care, the postoperative rehabilitation required, and the prognosis of this condition.

Rehabilitation

Preoperative rehabilitation is divided into two distinct phases: the primary focus of the first phase is to maximize knee extension, and the goal of the second phase is to maximize knee flexion without any loss of knee extension. In our experience, working on knee extension and flexion at the same time is counterproductive, and patients become frustrated with the lack of progress. Similarly, working on lower extremity strength is also delayed until maximal or full ROM has been achieved.

Owing to the difficulty in regaining knee extension in patients with arthrofibrosis, we routinely prescribe the use of a passive knee extension device (Kneebourne Therapeutic, Noblesville, IN) in this patient population (Fig. 90-2). This device provides a patient-controlled, sustained stretch to the knee to help patients regain symmetrical knee extension, including hyperextension. The patient can use this device independently at home three to five times per day for 10 to 15 minutes per session. Patients also perform towel stretch (Fig. 90-3), prone hang, and heel prop exercises to improve knee

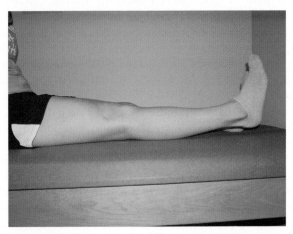

Figure 90-4. The active heel-lift exercise is important to ensure that good quadriceps muscle control is achieved. Without good quadriceps muscle control, the hamstring muscles are unopposed and pull the knee into a flexed position.

extension. In addition, patients work to improve quadriceps muscle control with the goal of regaining the ability to perform an active heel lift (Fig. 90-4) and achieve active hyperextension.

Whenever a patient loses knee extension and cannot fully extend the knee, it becomes difficult to stand with weight shifted onto that leg because the joint cannot "lock out." Consequently, patients develop the habit of favoring the involved leg, and this perpetuates further strength and ROM loss. Therefore it is also important to encourage the patient to begin standing with the weight shifted onto the involved leg and attempting to lock the knee out straight to combat the deconditioning associated with habitual disuse.

While working to improve extension, it is important to note the location of any pain or discomfort during the extension exercises because this is an indication of the underlying cause of knee extension loss. If a patient

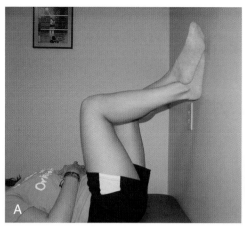
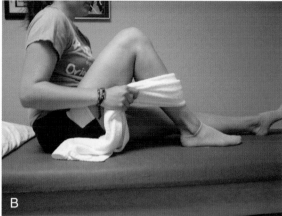

Figure 90-5. The wall slide **(A)** and heel slide **(B)** are exercises to improve knee flexion. These exercises are started once extension has been maximized.

feels pain or discomfort posteriorly during extension exercises, it is likely a result of shortened posterior soft tissue structures, whereas anterior knee pain is a result of the proliferation of abnormal tissue blocking the intercondylar notch. Early in the rehabilitation process, most patients feel soreness or discomfort in both locations; however, patients who have maximized knee extension with rehabilitation but still have a mechanical block to full extension will report only anterior soreness or discomfort with stretching.

Once knee extension has been maximized, the patient may begin the second phase of rehabilitation to work on knee flexion. It is important to monitor ROM closely during this phase to make sure that knee extension does not begin to decrease. If any loss of knee extension occurs as flexion exercises are introduced, the knee flexion exercises are discontinued until knee extension is restored. The heel slide and/or wall slide exercise can be used to improve knee flexion (Fig. 90-5).

Indications and Contraindications for Surgery

Surgical intervention for arthrofibrosis is indicated for patients who continue to have ROM deficits in the affected knee compared with the opposite, uninvolved knee despite rehabilitation. Contraindications include an acute inflammatory process of the knee from recent injury or surgery, or lack of mental preparedness to undergo the surgery and participate in the postoperative rehabilitation.

SURGICAL TECHNIQUE

The goal of surgical intervention for arthrofibrosis is to remove any mechanical block to full ROM. Shelbourne and colleagues[3] have described the arthroscopic technique and rehabilitation program based on the type of arthrofibrosis that is present.

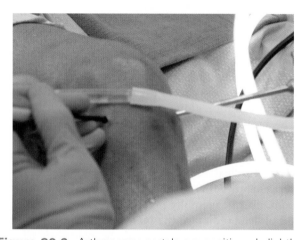

Figure 90-6. Arthroscopy portals are positioned slightly more widely than standard to allow for better visualization of the anterior aspect of the knee joint.

Anesthesia and Positioning

All patients are given general anesthesia and positioned supine on the operating table. Patellar mobility and knee ROM are evaluated under anesthesia. Throughout the surgical procedure, patellar mobility and knee ROM are reevaluated to determine if additional surgical steps are needed to remove mechanical blockages to knee extension and flexion.

The knee is injected with 20 mL of 0.25% bupivacaine and epinephrine, then prepared and draped in a sterile fashion. A tourniquet is placed on the thigh and inflated to 300 mm of pressure.

Position of Surgical Portals

Arthroscopy is performed through standard medial and lateral portals with a 30-degree scope, although the position of the medial and lateral portals is shifted slightly proximal and farther medial and lateral, respectively, to allow for better visualization of the anterior aspect of the joint (Fig. 90-6).

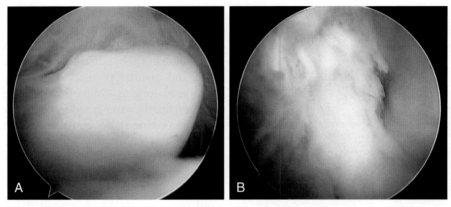

Figure 90-7. A, Cyclops lesion at the base of the anterior cruciate ligament. **B,** Anterior cruciate ligament graft after resection of Cyclops lesion.

BOX 90-1 Surgical Steps

1. Examine the area anterior to the proximal tibia for the presence of extrasynovial scar tissue formation.
2. Eliminate impingement in the intercondylar notch.
3. Remove the scar tissue distally to the level of the upper tibia and anteriorly to the horns of the menisci.
4. Excise the fibrotic capsule up to the insertion of the vastus medialis oblique and vastus lateralis muscles.
5. Perform knee manipulation after the scar resection to achieve as much knee flexion as possible.

Specific Steps

Box 90-1 outlines the specific steps of this procedure.

1. Examine the area anterior to the proximal tibia for the presence of extrasynovial scar tissue formation. The blunt trochar is used to loosen scar between the posterior patellar tendon and anterior tibia. Patients with type 2, 3, or 4 arthrofibrosis often require excision of scar tissue in this area with use of a basket forceps and menisci shaver. The surgeon must identify the anterior horn of the medial meniscus and lateral meniscus and remove any scar tissue that has formed in this area extending down to the upper tibia.
2. Eliminate impingement in the intercondylar notch. Examine the intercondylar notch and base of the ACL for the presence of a hypertrophied cyclops scar around the base of the ACL (Fig. 90-7). Place the knee into full extension and examine for impingement. Debride through excision and/or ablation until the ACL fits in the intercondylar notch without any impingement with the knee in full extension. This is typically all that is required to treat patients with type 1 arthrofibrosis. If continued graft impingement

occurs, a notchplasty or further debridement of the ACL graft may be necessary to achieve appropriate fit between the ACL and the intercondylar notch.
3. Patients with type 3 or 4 arthrofibrosis also have extrasynovial scar formation in the fibrotic infrapatellar fat pad located between the patella tendon and the tibia. Use a blunt probe to establish a plane between the patella tendon and the scar tissue. Remove the scar tissue distally to the level of the upper tibia and anteriorly to the horns of the menisci.
4. In patients with type 3 or 4 arthrofibrosis, excise the fibrotic capsule up to the insertion of the vastus medialis oblique and vastus lateralis muscles to free the patella and patellar tendon completely and help restore mobility of the patella.
5. In patients with type 3 or 4 arthrofibrosis, perform knee manipulation after the scar resection to achieve as much knee flexion as possible. Keep in mind that patients with type 4 arthrofibrosis are likely to have a remaining flexion ROM deficit owing to the shortening of the patellar tendon.

POSTOPERATIVE CONSIDERATIONS

Prevention of postoperative hemarthrosis is imperative for a good result. If a quadriceps muscles shutdown occurs, the hamstrings are unopposed and will continually pull the knee into a flexed position, making it difficult or even impossible to maintain knee extension symmetry. Furthermore, a quadriceps muscle shutdown can potentially lead to contracture of the patella tendon and patella infera. When good quadriceps muscle control is maintained, the patella tendon is engaged and stretched to its full length through active contraction of the quadriceps muscle.

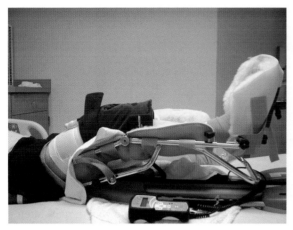

Figure 90-8. For prevention of hemarthrosis, a continuous passive motion machine is used to elevate the knee above the level of the heart, and a cold-compression device is applied to the knee immediately after surgery.

Antiembolism stockings and a cold compression device (Cryo/Cuff, DJO, Vista, CA) are applied to the knee immediately after surgery. Patients remain in the hospital for 23 hours after surgery and are given a continuous ketorolac drip for pain control and swelling prevention. We believe that there are significant physical and mental benefits to having these patients remain in the hospital overnight to ensure that they obtain full extension the day of surgery and to use the measures mentioned earlier to prevent postoperative pain and swelling.

The knee is placed in a continuous passive motion (CPM) machine set from 0 to 30 degrees to elevate the knee above the level of the heart (Fig. 90-8). Knee extension exercises are performed three or four times per day, including use of the passive knee extension device (Kneebourne Therapeutics; see Fig. 90-2), towel stretch (see Fig. 90-3), heel prop, and straight-leg raises. We have found that the use of the knee extension device several times per day is more effective and better tolerated by the patient than extension casts.[5]

Patients are discharged home with the CPM machine and instructed to remain on bed rest for the first 5 postoperative days with the knee in the CPM machine except for bathroom privileges and when completing the earlier-described exercise sessions three or four times per day. Full weight bearing is encouraged, and patients are instructed to stand with the weight shifted onto the involved knee, locking the knee out straight. This is done to reeducate the patient to use the involved leg normally and to stop the habit of favoring it by holding the knee bent and shifting the weight off the involved leg. This also serves to help promote full knee extension and good quadriceps muscle control. Patients may ambulate without an assistive device but may use one if needed for balance. Additional details about the postoperative rehabilitation progression and

results of this treatment method have been published previously.[5]

Similar to the preoperative rehabilitation program, postoperative rehabilitation focuses first on knee extension and quadriceps muscle control, then targets knee flexion as long as symmetrical knee extension is maintained; finally, strengthening is begun once ROM has been maximized. We consider symmetrical strength to be within 10% of that of the uninvolved limb when tested isokinetically. Care must be taken to ensure that ROM does not decrease when the strengthening phase is begun. If this occurs, discontinue the strengthening and focus on ROM only until it is regained. Patients must also be reeducated and encouraged to shift weight onto the involved leg and use it normally during activities of daily living; otherwise, relative strength loss compared with the uninvolved knee will be perpetuated.

This can be a long, arduous process for patients with arthrofibrosis, and care must be taken to monitor for loss of ROM during each phase and adjust the rehabilitation accordingly. The goal is to regain symmetrical knee ROM and strength compared with the opposite, uninvolved knee. Patients with type 4 arthrofibrosis are not expected to regain full knee flexion symmetry owing to the contracture of the patellar tendon, but some improvement in flexion is usually achieved.

RESULTS

Arthrofibrosis is an extremely difficult condition to treat, and therefore prevention is the best form of treatment. Acute surgery performed on a swollen knee,[6-8] concomitant medial collateral ligament repair with ACL reconstruction,[6,8,9] and poorly designed or supervised perioperative rehabilitation programs[8,10] have all been associated with increased risk of arthrofibrosis. In recent years there has been a shift from immobilization to immediate ROM after ACL reconstruction as part of an effort to decrease the risk of development of arthrofibrosis.

When arthrofibrosis does occur, it is important for the physician and rehabilitation staff to work closely together to establish a plan of care working toward the goals outlined earlier. The results of 33 patients treated with the protocol described in this chapter have been previously published.[5] Mean ROM of the involved knee improved from 0-8-117 degrees (degrees of hyperextension–degrees of extension short of 0 degrees–degrees of flexion) preoperatively to 3-0-134 degrees postoperatively, compared with 5-0-147 degrees in the uninvolved knee. All patients demonstrated improved ROM, and 29 of 33 achieved higher subjective survey scores.

Overall, greater ROM was associated with better subjective knee scores. Patients who achieved normal ROM according to International Knee Documentation

TABLE 90-2. International Knee Documentation Committee (IKDC) Criteria for Grading Knee Range of Motion*

	Normal	Nearly Normal	Abnormal	Severely Abnormal
Extension difference (degrees)	≤2	3-5	6-10	>10
Flexion difference (degrees)	≤5	6-15	16-25	>25

*Range of motion is compared with that of the opposite knee, including hyperextension.

Committee (IKDC) criteria (Table 90-2) had a mean IKDC subjective survey score of 72.6, which was significantly higher than that of patients who did not achieve normal ROM ($P = .04$). The mean IKDC subjective survey score was 68.8 for patients who achieved nearly normal ROM, 63.0 for patients with abnormal ROM, and 45.8 for patients with severely abnormal ROM.

Harner and colleagues[6] reported similar findings in their study of patients with ROM loss after ACL reconstruction. In their study, seven patients subjectively rated their knee as "fair" or "poor" on a modified version of the Cincinnati Knee Rating Scale; all of these subjects had at least 5 degrees of extension loss. Cosgarea and colleagues[11] also found that subjects with less extensive arthrofibrosis involvement and better ROM outcomes had better functional outcomes.

CONCLUSIONS

The best treatment for arthrofibrosis is prevention; however, a combined approach of directed rehabilitation and arthroscopic scar resection when needed has shown encouraging results. The use of a patient-controlled knee extension device is now preferred over the use of extension casting. Patients, physicians, and rehabilitation staff must be committed to the entire process, including extensive preoperative and postoperative rehabilitation.

REFERENCES

1. Paulos LE, Rosenberg TD, Drawbert J, et al. Infrapatellar contracture syndrome. An unrecognized cause of knee stiffness with patella entrapment and patella infera. *Am J Sports Med*. 1987;15:331-341.
2. DeCarlo MR, Sell K. Normative data for range of motion and single-leg hop in high school athletes. *J Sport Rehab*. 1997;6:246-255.
3. Shelbourne KD, Patel DV, Martini DJ. Classification and management of arthrofibrosis of the knee after anterior cruciate ligament reconstruction. *Am J Sports Med*. 1996;24:857-862.
4. Merchant A. Classification of patellofemoral disorders. *Arthroscopy*. 1988;4:235-240.
5. Biggs-Kinzer A, Murphy B, Shelbourne KD, et al. Perioperative rehabilitation using a knee extension device and arthroscopic debridement in the treatment of arthrofibrosis. *Sports Health*. 2010;2:417-423.
6. Harner CD, Irrgang JJ, Paul J, et al. Loss of motion after anterior cruciate ligament reconstruction. *Am J Sports Med*. 1992;20:499-506.
7. Mayr HO, Weig TG, Plitz W. Arthrofibrosis following ACL reconstruction: reasons and outcome. *Arch Orthop Trauma Surg*. 2004;124:518-522.
8. Shelbourne KD, Wilckens JH, Mollabashy A, et al. Arthrofibrosis in acute anterior cruciate ligament reconstruction. The effect of timing of reconstruction and rehabilitation. *Am J Sports Med*. 1991;19:332-336.
9. Noyes FR, Mangine RE, Barber SD. The early treatment of motion complications after reconstruction of the anterior cruciate ligament. *Clin Orthop Relat Res*. 1992;277:217-228.
10. Noyes FR, Berrios-Torres S, Barber-Westin SD, et al. Prevention of permanent arthrofibrosis after anterior cruciate ligament reconstruction alone or combined with associated procedures: a prospective study in 443 knees. *Knee Surg Sports Traumatol Arthroscopy*. 2000;8:196-206.
11. Cosgarea AJ, DeHaven KE, Lovelock JE. The surgical treatment of arthrofibrosis of the knee. *Am J Sports Med*. 1994;22(2):184-191.

Distal Realignment for Patellofemoral Disease

Jack Farr II, Christian Lattermann, and D. Jeff Covell

Chapter Synopsis

- Tibial tubercle transfer (TTT), often performed in conjunction with other proximal realignment procedures, is an effective procedure to alter patellofemoral forces and optimize load bearing to articular cartilage in patients with patellofemoral disease. A comprehensive understanding of patellofemoral pathology and its multifactorial nature is critical before TTT and necessitates evaluation of the entirety of the extremity.

Important Points

- Medialization of the tibial tubercle is indicated for an objective increased tibial tuberosity–trochlear groove (TT-TG) distance with or without patellar instability. Tuberosity surgery is most commonly performed as a component of a comprehensive approach to patellofemoral compartment pathology.

- Anteromedialization (AMZ) of the tibial tubercle is indicated as for tibial tuberosity medialization (TTM) in patients with patellofemoral chondrosis or in combination with cartilage restoration procedures.

- TTT is contraindicated in patients with a normal TT-TG distance, axial malrotation, or areas of chondrosis, which have increased loads after TTT, as well as those with standard contraindications to osteotomy.

- Patients have patellofemoral pain and may have a history of patellar instability or dislocation. Additional findings may include intermittent effusion, crepitation, and loose body sensation. Often, previous nonsurgical and surgical interventions have failed.

Clinical and Surgical Pearls

- The goal for all tuberosity surgeries is "normalization" of the tuberosity position—that is, the surgery is not just to medialize or to anteriorize.

- Although computed tomographic scans are not obtained routinely, most patients have undergone a magnetic resonance imaging evaluation, which is useful for defining the regions of any chondrosis. This will aid in the planning of tubercle surgery (e.g., AMZ to unload a distal lateral area of chondrosis).

- The magnetic resonance imaging evaluation may have been performed at another facility, but it is still possible for the radiologist to go back to the images and to measure the TT-TG distance and the Caton-Deschamps ratio.

- The mean TT-TG distance of asymptomatic patients is 13 mm.

- The TT-TG distance is abnormal above 20 mm.

- The steepest AMZ angle is 60 degrees. For the typical 15 mm of elevation, this results in medialization of approximately 8 mm, which would normalize the elevated TT-TG distances in the majority of patients.

- An elevated Caton-Deschamps ratio (patella alta) would suggest that a component of distalization be added to normalize the position of the tibial tuberosity.

- Always measure hip internal and external rotation in the prone position. If there is excessive internal hip rotation, this implicates an increase in femoral anteversion, which should then be evaluated with computed tomography (hip, knee, and ankle), which will also detect excessive tibial external rotation.

- Preoperative rehabilitation prepares the limb and patient for recovery.

- Rehabilitation must emphasize proximal and core musculature and not just local muscles.

- The combination of cartilage restoration with AMZ (when specific chondral lesions are noted) may allow improved outcomes compared with either procedure alone.

- Be alert for pain that is disproportionate to the surgery. Early intervention (including sympathetic blocks) may avoid progression to classic complex regional pain syndrome.

Continued

Clinical and Surgical Pitfalls

- Tibial tuberosity overmedialization increases medial patellofemoral forces and may lead to patellofemoral chondrosis and arthrosis.

- Medial tibiofemoral forces also increase with tuberosity medialization, so be very careful in considering the procedure in a varus knee to avoid acceleration of medial compartment wear.

- Warn patients of hardware pain and the potential need for removal.

- AMZ significantly weakens the tibia until healing. Early weight bearing will lead to an increased tibial fracture rate.

- Whereas a "little" medialization may be beneficial, more is not better. The goal is to normalize the TT-TG distance.

- Tibial tuberosity surgery cannot substitute for correction of patholaxity of the medial patellofemoral ligament (MPFL) causing patellar dislocations.

- The lateral release with tibial tuberosity surgery is only to balance the soft tissue. Overzealous lateral release may cause both medial iatrogenic dislocations and paradoxically an increase in lateral patholaxity.

- Tibial tuberosity surgery is contraindicated when the apparent lateral position is from a combination of excessive femoral anteversion and tibial external rotation.

- In patients with extreme trochlear dysplasia, the "bump" at the entrance to the trochlea will continue to interfere with tracking unless it is directly addressed.

- Too much anteriorization can cause problems with skin healing and may significantly rotate the patella, causing abnormal contact areas.

- AMZ outcomes are poor with proximal pole, panpatellar chondrosis or if there is trochlear chondrosis.

- Patella infera is a complicated problem and should be treated with a continuum of care; tuberosity surgery must have a thorough, scientifically based role if it is contemplated in that situation.

Although the emphasis of this chapter is on tibial tuberosity surgery for patellofemoral disease, the multifactorial nature of patellofemoral dysfunction requires an acknowledgment that a patellofemoral problem is rarely addressed by a single surgical treatment. Tibial tuberosity repositioning must be examined with a full appreciation of proximal soft tissue balance, limb rotation, and articular cartilage disease (grade, site, and extent). Although positive outcomes were initially reported for many distal realignment patellofemoral surgeries, early positive results often deteriorated markedly over time. With the Hauser[1] posterior medial tuberosity transfer, although stability was maintained, patellofemoral cartilage degeneration predictably occurred over time. Thus, in general, patellofemoral surgery not only must address the acute problem but do so without causing intermediate and long-term problems such as chondrosis and arthrosis. Application of a more scientific approach to patellofemoral dysfunction has led to the identification of the importance of the medial patellofemoral ligament (MPFL) in restraint to lateral patellar instability, and it has refined and focused the limited role of lateral release to isolated, documented patellar tilt rather than global patellofemoral pain or instability. Likewise, the role of tibial tuberosity surgery for patellofemoral dysfunction continues to evolve both as an isolated procedure and in conjunction with proximal patellofemoral surgery.

Indications espoused for tuberosity surgery (often in combination with proximal soft tissue surgery) at one point included patellofemoral pain, instability, chondrosis, and arthrosis. Straight tibial tuberosity medialization (TTM) was initially associated with the names of specific surgeons, including Roux,[2] Elmslie, and Trillat[3]; anteriorization with Maquet[4]; and anteromedialization (AMZ) with Fulkerson.[5] These tuberosity surgeries have, at times, been used to treat static patellar subluxation, recurrent lateral patellar instability, patellar pain, and patellofemoral chondrosis. Tuberosity surgery for treatment of recurrent or chronic patellofemoral dislocation or subluxation was based on the assumption that the primary pathologic process was in an increased Q (quadriceps) angle; for pain and chondrosis, elevation was promoted as the preferred procedure to dramatically decrease patellofemoral stress. Whereas it is obvious that repositioning of the distal point of the Q angle (tibial tuberosity) surgically does modify the Q angle, today the MPFL is accepted as the main restraint to lateral patellar instability. In fact, the Q angle, which formed the rational basis for planning of a TTM, is being questioned as a benchmark in light of the poor intraobserver reproducibility of the measurement as reviewed by Post.[6] In addition, Fithian has questioned the role of TTM for lateral patellar instability. At the annual meeting of the American Orthopaedic Society for Sports Medicine in 2005, he presented a case series of recurrent lateral patellar instability treated by MPFL reconstruction with or without TTM. The results were the same in both groups. On the other hand, it must be acknowledged that Carney et al[1] has reported excellent long-term results in prevention of recurrent patellar instability with TTM, although critics note that his report is a clinical outcomes series without radiographs that might have demonstrated arthrosis (as predicted to occur with excessive medialization of the tuberosity in biomechanical studies by Kuroda et al[7]). Furthermore, because the extent of medialization with TTM has been variably defined, critics could imply that (1) some of the patients with instability successfully treated by TTM experienced spontaneous healing of the MPFL, (2) the MPFL lesion was marginally injured, or (3) the TTM "overmedialized" the tuberosity and constrained the patella into stability.

From a basic science approach, the initial tuberosity surgery focused on the action of the various force vectors on patellar position and motion and on the effect of tuberosity position on those vectors. However, the equation is more complicated; Teitge and colleagues,[8] Powers and colleagues,[9] Heino and colleagues,[10] and others have emphasized the importance of the "other half" of the joint in motion—the trochlea and associated tibiofemoral torsion. Furthermore, Dejour and colleagues[11] have drawn attention to the importance of trochlear morphologic features (dysplasia) in patients with lateral patellar instability. In a comparative study, Paulos and colleagues[12] reviewed the efficacy of derotational high tibial osteotomy in the setting of significant tibial torsion, reporting that patients receiving derotational procedures had improved outcomes and had more symmetrical gait patterns than patients who underwent proximal-distal realignment. This finding was echoed by Fouilleron and colleagues,[13] who reported very high satisfaction rates after derotational osteotomy for patients with femorotibial malrotation. Continued investigation is needed to better define the role of derotational osteotomies. In an attempt to objectify tuberosity surgery, we must define normal and abnormal positions of the tuberosity. We must in addition consider the extent of femoral internal torsion and tibial external torsion as per Teitge[8] and Heino and colleagues.[10]

This objective approach to limb coronal and axial alignment from hip to ankle also measures (at the knee) an objective alternative to the Q angle, that is, the tibial tuberosity–trochlear groove (TT-TG) distance (Fig. 91-1). The TT-TG distance, as popularized by Dejour,[14] quantitates the concept of tibial tuberosity malalignment locally at the knee. Studies suggest that a TT-TG distance of more than 15 to 20 mm is abnormal; most asymptomatic patients have distances that are less than 15 mm. Likewise, anteriorization was first shown mathematically to reduce patellofemoral stress, but direct measurement with pressure-sensitive film, real-time pressure transducer arrays, and finite element analysis modeling such as by Cohen and Ateshian show that although stresses are typically reduced with anteriorization, there is a unique response for each knee, and a global 50% force reduction cannot be assumed. More recently, measures of trochlear contact pressures by Rue

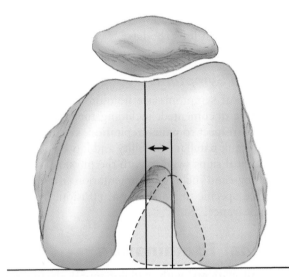

Figure 91-1. Tibial tuberosity to trochlear (femoral) groove distance is measured between perpendicular lines drawn from posterior condyles through the deepest aspect of the trochlea and the midpoint of the patellar tendon attachment of the proximal tibial tuberosity.

and colleagues[15] confirmed the utility of straight anteriorization in reducing patellofemoral contact pressure. Thus load transfer should play an important role in surgical planning, as opposed to the assumption that there will be an absolute decrease in stress. With use of these and other objective parameters, further studies may objectively quantify the preoperative pathologic process to aid in planning of tuberosity surgery.

PREOPERATIVE CONSIDERATIONS

History

Subgroups considered for tuberosity surgery include patients with static subluxation of the patella, those with patellofemoral chondrosis that requires load optimization, and those with recurrent lateral instability with or without static subluxation. The history will be highly variable for each subgroup, from insidious onset of patellofemoral pain to pain that began after a patellar instability episode. The standard patellofemoral history as outlined by Post[6] should be elicited. Function aspects need to be documented, including the amount of energy needed to cause instability and the degree of stress necessary to cause pain. Prior surgical operative notes are useful, as are the intraoperative images.

Typical History
- Failure of prolonged appropriate physical therapy and bracing
- Patellofemoral area pain with prolonged flexed knee position, stairs, or squats
- Giving way with either pain or patellar inability

- Patellofemoral crepitation and intermittent effusion and occasional loose bodies
- Often prior chondroplasty and lateral release

Signs and Symptoms

Patellofemoral symptoms are ubiquitous but nonetheless must be documented, including functional impairments with respect to pain, crepitation, swelling, giving way, and frank patellar instability and loose body sensations. Clinical signs overlap with the physical examination findings and include documentation of crepitation during the specific arc of motion, effusion, and loose body appearance.

Physical Examination

As for all patients with patellofemoral dysfunction, a standard examination of the knee and the entire functional kinetic chain from the pelvis to the foot is performed. A standard patellofemoral examination as detailed by Post pays particular attention to the following:

- Focal site or sites of maximal pain (especially at prior scars) or diffuse pain with any touch (to suggest chronic regional pain syndrome; see the discussion of contraindications)
- Patellar displacement (measured in trochlea quadrants)
- Patellar height (normal, infera, alta)
- Tuberosity position relative to the center of the trochlea (Q angle less reliable)
- Limb rotation (femoral and tibial internal and external rotation)
- Muscle bulk and strength, with attention to the vastus medialis obliquus
- Patellar tracking through active and passive range of motion
- Individual variations of adequacy of the MPFL
- Patellar tilt or extent of eversion, especially with prior lateral release
- Patellar crepitation (document angle of flexion at which this occurs)
- Apprehension: classic lateral versus global versus medial
- Fulkerson medial instability test

Imaging

Radiography

- Standard weight-bearing anteroposterior and true lateral views
- Shallow flexion angle axial view (i.e., Merchant view)
- Long-limb alignment to evaluate coronal limb malalignment

- Rosenberg (skier's) weight-bearing posteroanterior view

Other Modalities

Magnetic resonance imaging with or without contrast enhancement will add information about the extent and position of articular cartilage disease. Magnetic resonance imaging or computed tomography delineates patellofemoral morphologic features (extent of dysplasia), evaluates congruity of the patella in the trochlea, and provides objective measurement of the TT-TG distance and patellar height, with the understanding that cartilage contour does not always match bone contour.

Technetium bone scan may indicate areas of overload and arthrosis or suggest complex regional pain syndrome (sympathetically mediated pain).

Indications and Contraindications

Indications for Tibial Tuberosity Medialization

- Objective measurement of an increased TT-TG distance and symptoms, which can be directly related to abnormal stress secondary to resultant force vectors. The joint has normal or nearly normal articular surfaces of the patellofemoral compartment.
- Objective measurement of a markedly increased TT-TG distance in patients undergoing MPFL reconstruction or repair in an effort to decrease abnormal stress to the MPFL.
- Potentially, patients with the diagnosis of static chronic patellar subluxation, in addition to recurrent patellofemoral instability, who are undergoing MPFL surgery. In this situation TTM is performed in an effort to improve patellofemoral joint congruity, thus improving contact area, which may decrease stress.
- Objective measurement of an increased TT-TG distance in a patient who has undergone patellofemoral arthroplasty and in whom chronic patellar subluxation is demonstrated after correct implantation and adequate lateral release and MPFL repair or reconstruction.

Indications for Anteromedialization

- As for TTM, but with chondrosis in the distal lateral region of the patella with an intact trochlea or minimal trochlear chondrosis. (Restated, this includes excessive lateral compression with tilt, chronic static patellar subluxation, and a combination as described originally by Fulkerson.)
- As in the preceding, but with more extensive chondrosis (grade, distribution, and trochlear chondrosis). AMZ may be combined with cartilage restoration procedures when AMZ can decrease stress to the restored region.

Contraindications to Tibial Tuberosity Medialization

- Normal TT-TG distance
- Abnormal femoral anteversion or tibial torsion as per Teitge
- Problem not explained by an increased TT-TG distance
- Medial patellofemoral chondrosis that would be subjected to increased loading after TTM
- Grade III or higher (Outerbridge or International Cartilage Repair Society) chondrosis of the patella or trochlea
- Standard contraindication to knee osteotomy, such as nicotine use, nonspecific pain, infection, inflammatory arthropathy, marked osteoporosis (which would compromise fixation), complex regional pain syndrome, patella infera, and arthrofibrosis
- Relative contraindication in the markedly varus knee that could result in increased stress to the medial tibiofemoral compartment after TTM as per Andrish

Contraindications to Anteromedialization (without Cartilage Restoration)

- As for contraindications to TTM and when AMZ would be expected to increase the stress in areas of damaged cartilage (e.g., proximal patellar pole after impact chondrosis, diffuse midwaist patellar chondrosis, or medial facet chondrosis
- Trochlear chondrosis of grade II or higher

SURGICAL PLANNING

The goal of medialization is normalization of the tuberosity position rather than overmedialization, so preoperative radiographic or clinical assessment of TT-TG distance is useful in planning.

Concomitant Procedures

If lateral release and MPFL repair (or reconstruction) are performed in conjunction with TTM or AMZ, the procedure order is lateral release, then tuberosity surgery, and finally MPFL surgery. If cartilage restoration is planned in addition to the TTM or AMZ, these procedures can be performed concomitantly to reduce total knee exposure to surgery and to ease the patient's rehabilitation.

SURGICAL TECHNIQUES

Anesthesia and Positioning

The less invasive TTM can be performed with the patient under local anesthetic with sedation. TTM as well as AMZ may be performed by use of regional blocks (femoral and sciatic), with a postoperative femoral nerve block for prolonged pain control. Alternatively, epidural, spinal, or general anesthetics may be used according to the surgeon's preference. Both AMZ and TTM are performed with the patient in the supine position, often with a roll under the ipsilateral pelvis to decrease external rotation. They are often performed with the foot of the operating table elevated and a side post used for the arthroscopic portion of the procedure rather than with the foot in the dependent position.

Surgical Landmarks, Incisions, and Portals

Figure 91-2 details the surgical landmarks, incisions, and portals for this procedure.

Landmarks

- Patella
- Trochlear margins
- Patellar tendon attachment to tibial tuberosity
- Gerdy tuberosity
- Crest of tibia

Portals and Approaches

- The arthroscopic portion of the procedure is performed through standard anteromedial and anterolateral portals with the option of an additional proximal portion to view patellar tracking in the trochlea.
- For the isolated TTM, a longitudinal 5-cm incision is made lateral to the tibial tuberosity.
- AMZ is performed either through an oblique 12-cm incision from the anterolateral portal to the midline distally or directly in the midline beginning 2 cm proximal to the patellar tendon attachment to the tibial tuberosity and continuing distally.

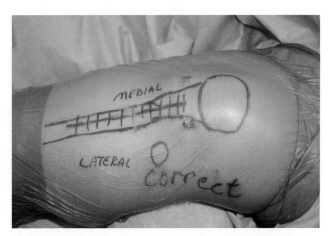

Figure 91-2. Skin landmarks for anteromedialization incision include patella, patellar tendon, tibial crest, and Gerdy tuberosity.

Structures at Risk

- Anterior tibial artery
- Deep peroneal nerve
- Patellar tendon
- Sites of long-term overload (leading to chondrosis)

Examination Under Anesthesia and Diagnostic Arthroscopy

Under anesthesia, the range of motion (comparison of passive patellar tracking to known preoperative active range of motion) and the full extent of patellar displacement and tilt are documented. Diagnostic arthroscopy allows mapping and grading of all areas of chondrosis. These findings enter into final planning and in some instances suggest cancellation of the tuberosity surgery in light of discovery of a contraindication.

The arthroscopic examination documents the associated tibiofemoral and patellofemoral chondral (grade and region lesions) and morphologic features of the pathologic process. This information allows fine-tuning of the tuberosity surgery for the indications listed previously. Arthroscopic chondral treatment may be performed as indicated, followed by titration of the lateral release, if necessary. For patients with reversible patellar tilt and significant medial patellar displacement (two trochlear quadrants), a lateral release will not be performed; for patients with patellar tilt and medial patellar displacement (one trochlear quadrant or less), a limited lateral release or step-cut lateral lengthening will be titrated to allow reversal of tilt and to achieve two quadrants of medial patellar displacement.

Specific Steps

Box 91-1 outlines the specific steps of this procedure.

Tibial Tuberosity Medialization

Figure 91-3 demonstrates tibial tuberosity medialization.

BOX 91-1 Surgical Steps

1. Exposure
2. Planning of the osteotomy
3. Performance of the osteotomy
4. Tubercle fixation

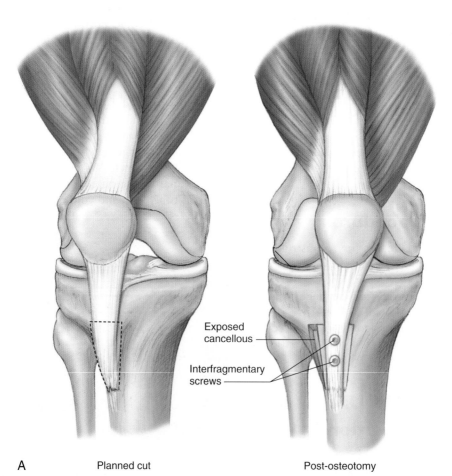

A   Planned cut   Post-osteotomy

Exposed cancellous —

Interfragmentary screws —

Figure 91-3. A, Overview of tibial tuberosity medialization.

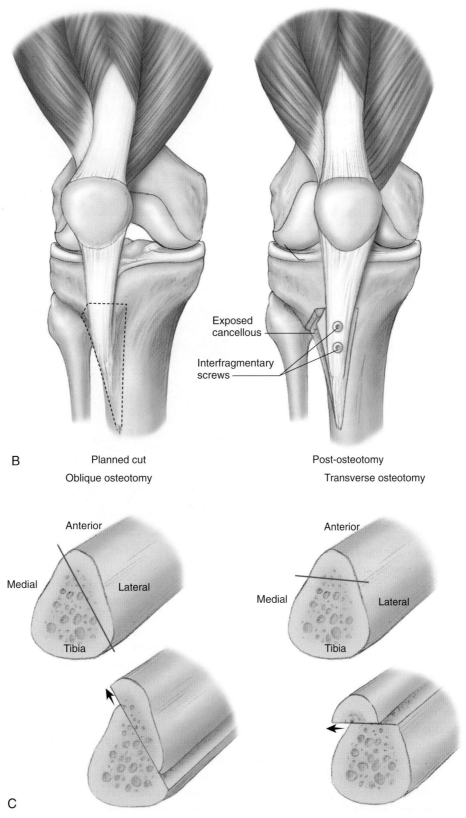

B   Planned cut   Post-osteotomy

Oblique osteotomy   Transverse osteotomy

Exposed cancellous

Interfragmentary screws

Anterior

Medial   Lateral

Tibia

Anterior

Medial   Lateral

Tibia

C

Figure 91-3. cont'd. B, Overview of anteromedialization. **C,** Orientation of the oblique anteromedialization osteotomy *(left)* and of the flat osteotomy of tibial tuberosity medialization *(right).*

1. Exposure

The skin incision is based on whether the TTM is an isolated or combined surgery. The standard longitudinal incision is made lateral to the tibial tuberosity, with approximately 2 cm of the incision above the tuberosity and 3 cm of the incision below the tuberosity. It may be modified to a more universal direct anterior longitudinal approach as dictated by concomitant surgery. The patellar tendon is identified, and the lateral release (if it is performed) is extended along the lateral border of the patellar tendon with emphasis on hemostasis. A 1.5-cm subperiosteal exposure of the lateral aspect of the tibial tuberosity is performed.

2. Planning of the Osteotomy

The coronal plane cut is referenced from the anterior joint lines to be flat in the coronal plane. If there is a desire to unload the distal lateral patella, the cut is made with a mildly anteriorly directed slope (Fig. 91-3C).

3. Performance of the Osteotomy

A 1.5-cm deep cut in the axial plane is performed just proximal to the protected patellar tendon proximal attachment to the tibial tuberosity. A second bone cut begins at the posterior aspect of this cut and extends distally for approximately 5 cm while remaining 1.5 cm posterior to the crest of the tibial tuberosity. With the distal anterior tibial crest kept intact, the tuberosity is rotated medially, making a greenstick fracture at the distal portion of the osteotomy. The tuberosity is medialized to the extent that that TT-TG distance is normalized, but not overmedialized.

4. Tuberosity Fixation

The tuberosity is temporarily fixed with a Kirschner wire. Patellar tracking is viewed, and if it is acceptable, the tuberosity is fixed with interfragmentary screws (the screws are aimed medially, with care taken to avoid vascular injury).

Anteromedialization

1. Exposure

If the AMZ is an isolated procedure, begin the midline longitudinal incision midway between the patella and tuberosity and extend it distally 10 to 15 cm. Alternatively, the incision can course from the anterolateral portal to the same point on the tibial crest distally. Proximal extension may be performed to allow concomitant patellofemoral cartilage restoration. The patellar tendon is exposed subcutaneously. The lateral aspect of the patellar tendon is released, isolated, and protected. This lateral peripatellar tendon incision is extended proximally to the lateral release (noting the specific lateral release indications discussed earlier) and then distally along the anterior tibial crest to begin

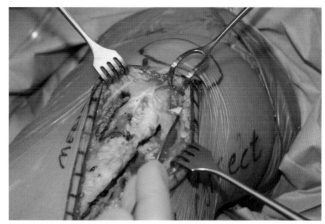

Figure 91-4. The pointer is at the distal extent of the arthroscopically performed lateral release. The peripatellar tendon and lateral tibial crest incision sites are marked. Note that a tourniquet was not used during this procedure.

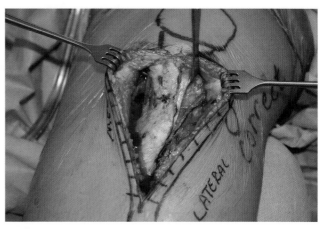

Figure 91-5. An Army-Navy retractor demonstrates that both margins of the patellar tendon have been released.

elevation of the anterior compartment musculature (Fig. 91-4). To allow anteriorization, a release is also performed immediately adjacent to the patellar tendon medially. The freed patellar tendon is protected with a retractor (Fig. 91-5). The anterior compartment musculature is subperiosteally dissected, and a retractor is positioned at the posterior extent of the lateral tibial wall to protect the posterior neurovascular structures (Fig. 91-6).

2. Planning of the Osteotomy

With use of a commercially available AMZ osteotomy system (Tracker, Mitek, Raynham, MA), the osteotomy starting entrance position is planned by placing the cutting block jig medial to the patellar tendon attachment to the tibial tuberosity (Fig. 91-7). The planned osteotomy begins adjacent to the medial patellar tendon and courses laterally as it runs distally to allow the osteotomy to exit distally and laterally (a triangle shape). A drill guide–like arm is inserted into the cutting block.

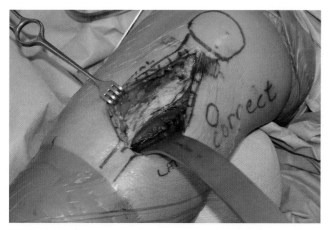

Figure 91-6. The anterior compartment musculature has been subperiosteally elevated from the lateral wall of the tibia and held with a custom retractor.

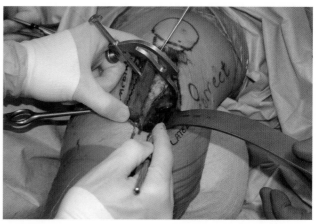

Figure 91-8. The tip of the slope selector guide (highlighted by the probe) shows where the osteotomy will exit. In moving the cutting block more medial and the tip of the slope selector more anterior up the wall of the tibia, the angle of the slope is decreased. With the osteotomy exiting just anterior to the posterior wall, the steepest slope (approximately 60 degrees) is obtained.

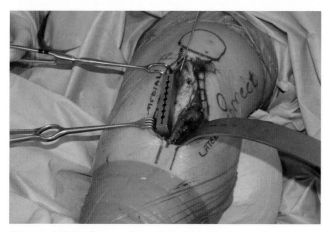

Figure 91-7. The cutting block is angled laterally as it extends distally from the medial aspect of the patellar tendon attachment to the tuberosity, which makes a thin shingle of bone distally to allow the necessary repositioning of the tuberosity. The nerve hook is retracting the medial edge of the patellar tendon.

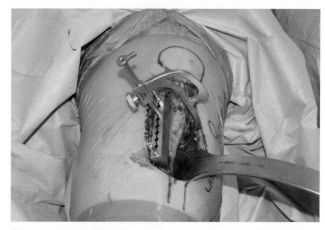

Figure 91-9. After the desired slope and cutting block position have been selected, the cutting block is temporarily fixed to the tibia with pins through drill holes. Note that the cutting block is positioned more laterally at the distal aspect.

The tip of the slope selector arm predicts the lateral wall exit of the oblique osteotomy (Fig. 91-8). The top (osteotomy exit) should be on the lateral wall of the tibia, always anterior to the posterior wall. With the cutting block immediately adjacent to the patellar tendon attachment medially and the slope selector tip just anterior to the posterior wall, the slope is approximately 60 degrees (see Fig. 91-3C). By moving the cutting block medially and the slope selector anteriorly, the slope can be decreased, for example to 45 degrees. A smaller angle provides increased medialization relative to anteriorization—that is, the suggested anteriorization of 1.2 to 1.5 cm is "constant," and thus with a steep slope (60 degrees) the medial displacement would be 0.6 to 0.75 cm; for a 45-degree slope, the same elevation would allow 1.2 to 1.5 cm of medialization.

3. Performance of the Osteotomy

With the desired slope selected, the cutting block is temporarily fixed to the tibia with pins through drill holes (Fig. 91-9). The oblique cut is made with an oscillating saw cooled with saline. The saw is directly observed as it exits on the lateral wall of the tibia anterior to the retractor (Fig. 91-10). The cutting block is removed. The oblique cut is finished proximally and distally with use of the original bone cut as a capture saw guide (Fig. 91-11). For finishing of the proximal osteotomy, an osteotome connects the posterolateral wall saw exit site to the lateral aspect of the patellar tendon attachment to the tibial tuberosity (Fig. 91-12).

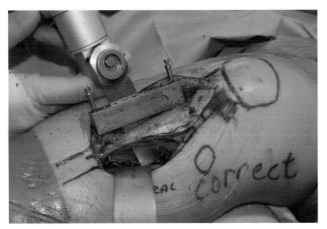

Figure 91-10. The saw is observed at all times as it exits the posterior aspect of the lateral wall. The retractor helps protect underlying tissues.

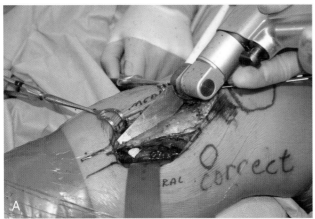

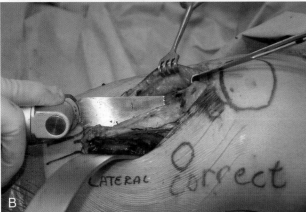

Figure 91-11. After the main portion of the oblique cut has been made through the jig, the cutting block is removed and the osteotomy is used as a capture guide to finish the distal (**A**) and proximal (**B**) aspects of the oblique cut.

With a change in the angle of the osteotome, the last bone cut connects the previous cuts that have extended just proximal to the patellar tendon attachment to the tibial tuberosity medially and laterally. At this point, the tuberosity pedicle is free to rotate up the inclined slope.

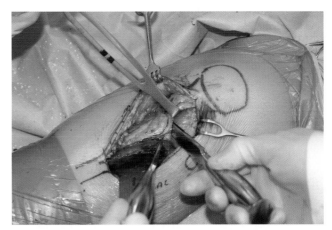

Figure 91-12. The two osteotomes represent the final proximal cuts. The more posterior osteotome courses from the proximal extent of the posterior oblique cut to the lateral attachment of the patellar tendon to the tuberosity. The second osteotome connects the lateral cut just made to the cut already present on the medial aspect of the patellar tendon attachment to the tuberosity. Note the retractor protecting the patellar tendon. Also note that the angles of the cuts are quite different.

4. Tuberosity Fixation

The completed oblique cut allows movement of the tuberosity pedicle up the included plane, affecting the desired anteromedialization. The tuberosity is temporarily fixed with Kirschner wire, and the anteriorization and medialization are measured (Fig. 91-13). The tuberosity is fixed with an interfragmentary technique, with avoidance of vascular structures as discussed by Miller (Fig. 91-14).

POSTOPERATIVE CONSIDERATIONS

Follow-up

- Standard knee management includes a protective brace locked at or near extension initially, compression, cryotherapy, elevation, and possible continuation of the femoral nerve block (Fig. 91-15). The limb is observed for compartment syndrome and any problems with skin healing.
- Sutures and staples are removed at 7 to 10 days.
- Radiographs are typically obtained perioperatively and then at 6 weeks postoperatively. For comparison of preoperative and postoperative radiographs, see Figure 91-16.

Rehabilitation

- The less extensive osteotomy of the TTM allows the patient to begin bearing weight with crutches as tolerated. AMZ requires limited weight bearing with

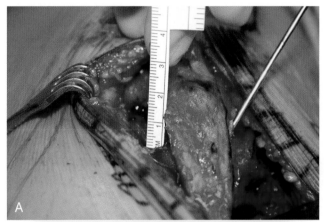

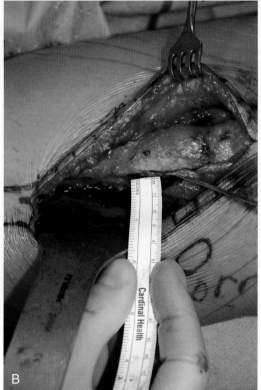

Figure 91-13. After the tuberosity has been repositioned up the slope of the osteotomy, it is fixed temporarily with a K-wire, and the anteriorization (**A**) and medialization (**B**) are checked.

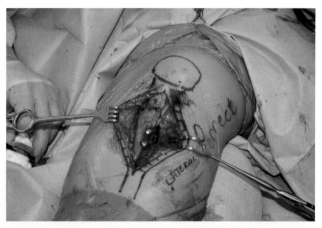

Figure 91-14. The tibial tuberosity is fixed with two 4.5-mm interfragmentary screws in the new position.

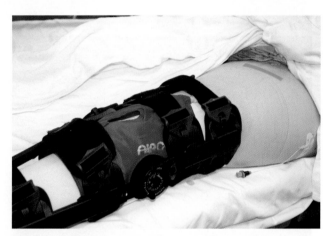

Figure 91-15. Postoperative management with antithrombotic hose, a cryotherapy device, and a hinged brace locked in extension or 0 to 30 degrees. Note the two catheters proximally for the femoral and sciatic regional nerve blocks. The sciatic catheter is removed immediately after surgery; the femoral catheter may be used for added pain control.

two crutches for 6 weeks to minimize fracture. The initial protective brace may be discontinued when the patient is safe and has excellent quadriceps control.

- Early postoperative exercises serve to improve venous flow, to maintain quadriceps function, and to maintain patellar mobility. The patient is rapidly progressed to a comprehensive core proximal muscle strengthening program and range-of-motion exercises. Depth, grade, and region of chondral lesion and restoration will dictate the type and flexion angle of patellofemoral loading exercises.

- The AMZ is protected with a brace locked in full extension or 0 to 30 degrees for ambulation; the brace is removed for supine heel slides. The stationary bike is started for early range of motion.

Complications

Complications are similar to those of any open bone procedure of the knee. These include fracture, malunion, loss of fixation, nonunion, infection, thromboembolic phenomenon, compartment syndrome, sympathetically mediated pain, arthrofibrosis, patellar infera, and long-term progression of patellofemoral chondrosis. In addition, failure to address preoperative surgical indications may lead to postoperative complications.

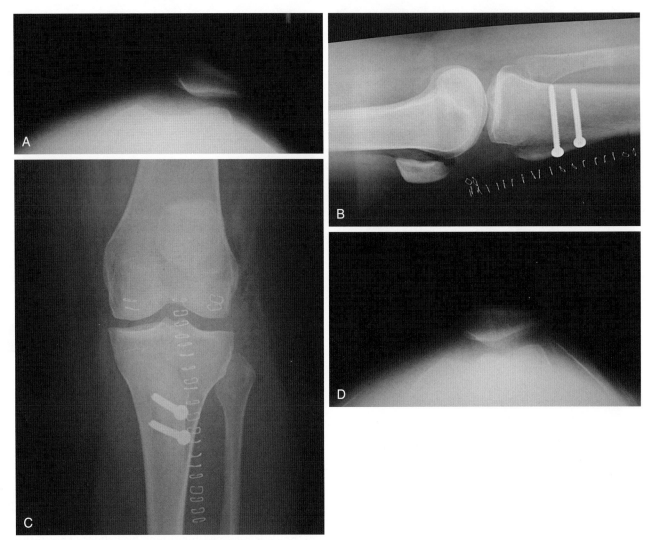

Figure 91-16. Radiographs of the procedure described here. **A,** Preoperative Merchant view with chronic static subluxation (no instability). **B,** Lateral view showing tuberosity elevation and fixation. **C,** Anteroposterior view showing medialization. **D,** Postoperative Merchant view with improved centralization of the patella.

TABLE 91-1. Results of Short- and Long-Term Case Series for Tibial Tuberosity Medialization (TTM) and Anteromedialization (AMZ)

Investigator	Surgery Type	Follow-Up (Average)	Outcomes
Akgun et al[17] (2010)	AMZ	2.6 years	12/17 good to excellent
Barber et al[18] (2008)	TTM	98 months	91.4% prevention of redislocation, all patients with functional improvement
Bellemans et al[19] (1997)	AMZ	32 months	Lysholm scores: preoperative, 62; postoperative, 92
Buuck and Fulkerson[20] (2000)	AMZ	8.2 years	86% good and excellent
Cameron et al[21] (1986)	AMZ	2 years	82% good and excellent
Caton et al[22] (2010)	TTM plus proximalization or distalization	2 years	76.8% stability when combined with distalization; 83% good to excellent when combined with proximalization
Carney et al[23] (2005)	TTM	26 years	54% good and excellent
Carofino et al[24] (2008)	AMZ	2 years	12/17 good to excellent
Endres et al[25] (2011)	TTM	10 years	16.18 good to excellent results; majority returned to same level of sporting activity
Fulkerson[26] (1983)	AMZ		All patients experienced substantial relief of pain
Fulkerson et al[27] (1990)	AMZ	35 months	89% good and excellent
Karamehmetoglu[28] (2007)	AMZ	28 months	85.7% excellent, very good, or satisfied
Karataglis et al[29] (2006)	TTM	40 months	73% very satisfactory and satisfactory
Koeter et al[30] (2007)	AMZ	28 months	All patients had improved pain and function scores
Naranja et al[31] (1996)	TTM plus anteriorization	74.2 months	53% good and excellent
Pidoriano et al[32] (1997)	AMZ	46.8 months	72% improvement
Pritsch et al[33] (2007)	TTM with or without proximalization or distalization	6.2 years	72.5% good to excellent
Sakai et al[34] (1996)	AMZ	5 years	20/21 satisfactory
Shen et al[35] (2007)	AMZ	67.3 months	Kujula score: preoperative, 43.9; postoperative, 88.9
Tecklenburg et al[36] (2010)	TTM	38 months	Postoperative scores: IKDC, 80.4; Kujala, 88
Tjoumakaris et al[37] (2010)	AMZ	46 months	97% returned to preinjury sports

IKDC, International Knee Documentation Committee.

RESULTS

Both short- and long-term case series for TTM and AMZ demonstrate high percentages of good and excellent results (Table 91-1). However, these are case series and need interpretation within the ranking of evidence-based medicine. Indeed, Mani and colleagues[16] showed that medialization of the tibial tubercle led to a subsequent external rotation of the tibia in cadaveric studies, thereby partially offsetting the intended surgical correction. Alterations of tibiofemoral kinematics may influence contact pressure on cartilage and could affect long-term results. In addition, these results need to be reviewed with biomechanical studies (i.e., Cohen and Kuroda) in mind.

REFERENCES

1. Hauser EDW. Total tendon transplant for slipping patella: a new operation for recurrent dislocation of the patella. 1938. *Clin Orthop Relat Res.* 2006;452:7-16.
2. Roux C. Luxation habituelle de la rotule: traitement operatoire. *Rev Chir Orthop Reparatrice Appar Mot.* 1888;8: 682-682.
3. Trillat A, Dejour H, Couette A. Diagnostic et traitement des subluxations recidivantes de la rotule. *Rev Chir Orthop Reparatrice Appar Mot.* 1964;50:813-824.
4. Maquet P. Advancement of the tibial tuberosity. *Clin Orthop Relat Res.* 1976;115:225-230.
5. Fulkerson JP. Anteromedialization of the tibial tuberosity for patellofemoral malalignment. *Clin Orthop Relat Res.* 1983;177:176-181.

6. Post WR. Clinical evaluation of patients with patellofemoral disorders. *Arthroscopy.* 1999;15:841-851.

7. Kuroda R, Kambic H, Valdevit A, et al. Articular cartilage contact pressure after tibial tuberosity transfer. A cadaveric study. *Am J Sports Med.* 2001;29:403-409.

8. Teitge RA, Faerber WW, Des Madryl P, et al. Stress radiographs of the patellofemoral joint. *J Bone Joint Surg Am.* 1996;78:193-203.

9. Powers CM, Ward SR, Fredericson M, et al. Patellofemoral kinematics during weight-bearing and non–weight-bearing knee extension in persons with lateral subluxation of the patella: a preliminary study. *J Orthop Sports Phys Ther.* 2003;33:677-685.

10. Heino Brechter J, Powers C, et al. Quantification of patellofemoral joint contact area using magnetic resonance imaging. *Magn Reson Imaging.* 2003;21:955.

11. Dejour H, Walch G, Neyret P, et al. [Dysplasia of the femoral trochlea]. *Rev Chir Orthop Reparatrice Appar Mot.* 1990;76:45-54.

12. Paulos L, Swanson SC, Stoddard GJ, et al. Surgical correction of limb malalignment for instability of the patella: a comparison of 2 techniques. *Am J Sports Med.* 2009; 37:1288-1300.

13. Fouilleron N, Marchetti E, Autissier G, et al. Proximal tibial derotation osteotomy for torsional tibial deformities generating patello-femoral disorders. *Orthop Traumatol Surg Res.* 2010;96:785-792.

14. Dejour H, Walch G, Nove-Josserand L, et al. Factors of patellar instability: an anatomic radiographic study. *Knee Surg Sports Traumatol Arthrosc.* 1994;2:19-26.

15. Rue JPH, Colton A, Zare SM, et al. Trochlear contact pressures after straight anteriorization of the tibial tuberosity. *Am J Sports Med.* 2008;36:1953-1959.

16. Mani S, Kirkpatrick MS, Saranathan A, et al. Tibial tuberosity osteotomy for patellofemoral realignment alters tibiofemoral kinematics. *Am J Sports Med.* 2011;39: 1024-1031.

17. Akgün U, Nuran R, Karahan M. Modified Fulkerson osteotomy in recurrent patellofemoral dislocations. *Acta Orthop Traumatol Turc.* 2010;44:27-35.

18. Barber FA, McGarry JE. Elmslie-Trillat procedure for the treatment of recurrent patellar instability. *Arthroscopy.* 2008;24:77-81.

19. Bellemans J, Cauwenberghs F, Witvrouw E, et al. Anteromedial tibial tubercle transfer in patients with chronic anterior knee pain and a subluxation-type patellar malalignment. *Am J Sports Med.* 1997;25:375-381.

20. Buuck D, Fulkerson J. Anteromedialization of the tibial tubercle: A 4- to 12-year follow-up. *Oper Tech Sports Med.* 2000;8:131-137.

21. Cameron HU, Huffer B, Cameron GM. Anteromedial displacement of the tibial tubercle for patellofemoral arthralgia. *Can J Surg.* 1986;29:456-458.

22. Caton JH, Dejour D. Tibial tubercle osteotomy in patellofemoral instability and in patellar height abnormality. *Int Orthop.* 2010;34:305-309.

23. Carney JR, Mologne TS, Muldoon M, et al. Long-term evaluation of the Roux-Elmslie-Trillat procedure for patellar instability: a 26-year follow-up. *Am J Sports Med.* 2005;33:1220-1223.

24. Bicos J, Carofino B, Andersen M, et al. Patellofemoral forces after medial patellofemoral ligament reconstruction. *J Knee Surg.* 2006;19:317-326.

25. Endres S, Wilke A. A 10 year follow-up study after Roux-Elmslie-Trillat treatment for cases of patellar instability. *BMC Musculoskelet Disord.* 2011;12:48.

26. Fulkerson JP. Anteromedialization of the tibial tuberosity for patellofemoral malalignment. *Clin Orthop Relat Res.* 1983:176-181.

27. Fulkerson JP, Becker GJ, Meaney JA, et al. Anteromedial tibial tubercle transfer without bone graft. *Am J Sports Med.* 1990;18:490-496.

28. Karamehmetoğlu M, Oztürkmen Y, Azboy I, et al. [Fulkerson osteotomy for the treatment of chronic patellofemoral malalignment]. *Acta Orthop Traumatol Turc.* 2007;41: 21-30.

29. Karataglis D, Green MA, Learmonth DJA. Autologous osteochondral transplantation for the treatment of chondral defects of the knee. *Knee.* 2006;13:32-35.

30. Koëter S, Diks MJF, Anderson PG, et al. A modified tibial tubercle osteotomy for patellar maltracking: results at two years. *J Bone Joint Surg Br.* 2007;89:180-185.

31. Naranja RJ, Reilly PJ, Kuhlman JR, et al. Long-term evaluation of the Elmslie-Trillat-Maquet procedure for patellofemoral dysfunction. *Am J Sports Med.* 1996;24: 779-784.

32. Pidoriano AJ, Weinstein RN, Buuck DA, et al. Correlation of patellar articular lesions with results from anteromedial tibial tubercle transfer. *Am J Sports Med.* 1997;25: 533-537.

33. Pritsch T, Haim A, Arbel R, et al. Tailored tibial tubercle transfer for patellofemoral malalignment: analysis of clinical outcomes. *Knee Surg Sports Traumatol Arthrosc.* 2007;15:994-1002.

34. Sakai N, Koshino T, Okamoto R. Pain reduction after anteromedial displacement of the tibial tuberosity: 5-year follow-up in 21 knees with patellofomoral arthrosis. *Acta Orthop Scand.* 1996;67:13-15.

35. Shen HC, Chao KH, Huang GS, et al. Combined proximal and distal realignment procedures to treat the habitual dislocation of the patella in adults. *Am J Sports Med.* 2007;35:2101-2108.

36. Tecklenburg K, Feller JA, Whitehead TS, et al. Outcome of surgery for recurrent patellar dislocation based on the distance of the tibial tuberosity to the trochlear groove. *J Bone Joint Surg Br.* 2010;92:1376-1380.

37. Tjoumakaris FP, Forsythe B, Bradley JP. Patellofemoral instability in athletes: treatment via modified Fulkerson osteotomy and lateral release. *Am J Sports Med.* 2010;38: 992-999.

Chapter 92

Management of Proximal Tibiofibular Instability

Nate Kopydlowski and Jon K. Sekiya

Chapter Synopsis

- Dislocation of the proximal tibiofibular joint is a very uncommon condition that is easily misdiagnosed without clinical suspicion of the injury. Injuries to the joint are more commonly atraumatic and should be treated with surgery only after all other therapies have been exhausted. Reconstructive procedures are recommended for patients whose source of pain is instability in the joint as opposed to arthritis.

Important Points

- Atraumatic instability is more common and often misdiagnosed.
- All nonsurgical therapies should be attempted before surgical intervention.
- Protection of the peroneal nerve during surgery helps to prevent injury and relieves symptoms common to this injury.
- The reconstructive procedure is recommended for patients whose pain is a result of joint instability.
- The arthrodesis procedure is recommended for patients in whom the correction of joint instability would not relieve pain, such as patients with proximal tibiofibular joint arthritis.

Clinical and Surgical Pearls

- History and physical examination are very important for diagnosis.
- Proximal tibiofibular joint instability is a very unusual and uncommon condition.
- All other clinical possibilities should be ruled out before a diagnosis is made.
- Injection of steroid and anesthetic into the joint can relieve pain and confirm a positive diagnosis.
- Reconstruction is recommended to maintain correct anatomic function and rotation of the joint.

Clinical and Surgical Pitfalls

- Resecting and protecting the peroneal nerve during surgery can prevent peroneal nerve palsy.
- Fibular resection during an arthrodesis procedure can decrease ankle pain and instability after surgery.
- Limit patients to passive flexion until 6 weeks to reduce the stress that is applied to the reconstructed ligaments (prevent biceps femoris from pulling on the fibular head).

Instability of the proximal tibiofibular joint is a very rare condition that is often misdiagnosed when there is no suspicion of the injury. The proximal tibiofibular joint ligaments both strengthen the joint and allow it to rotate and translate during ankle and knee motion. Instability of the joint can be a result of an injury to these ligaments. The clinical presentation of joint injury can range from common idiopathic subluxation with no history of trauma, to less common high-energy traumatic dislocations that may be associated with long bone fracture. Successful diagnosis of the injury can be improved by a better understanding of the biomechanics of the joint and a clinical suspicion of the injury when symptoms are present.

Treatment for proximal tibiofibular joint stability requires that nonsurgical management be attempted first for patients with atraumatic subluxation of the proximal tibiofibular joint. Initial management of traumatic joint dislocation should involve closed reduction under local anesthesia, followed by surgical intervention if reduction fails. We recommend joint reconstruction to repair the proximal tibiofibular joint, which will retain the functional anatomy and rotation of the joint, over arthrodesis, especially in children and athletes.

PREOPERATIVE CONSIDERATIONS

Patient History

History of Atraumatic Injury

Atraumatic proximal tibiofibular joint subluxation is the more common presentation of proximal tibiofibular joint instability. Atraumatic subluxation is thought to result from injury to the anterior ligament and to the anterior capsule of the joint, and it can be associated with Ehlers-Danlos syndrome, muscular dystrophy, and generalized laxity.[1] Subluxation typically occurs in patients who have no history of inciting trauma but may have generalized ligamentous laxity; the condition is not commonly bilateral. Joint subluxation is common in adolescents, typically girls, and results from hypermobility of the joint, in which symptoms can decrease with skeletal maturity.[2] Some studies have shown that congenital dislocation of the knee can also be associated with atraumatic superior dislocation of the proximal tibiofibular joint.[1]

History of Traumatic Injury

Traumatic dislocations of the proximal tibiofibular joint are uncommon and are normally caused by high-energy injury or a fall on a twisted knee. The most common traumatic dislocations are in an anterolateral direction, followed by posteromedial and superior dislocations. Anterolateral dislocation commonly stems from injury to the anterior and posterior capsular ligaments, and commonly the lateral collateral ligament.[1,2] The common cause of traumatic anterolateral dislocation is a fall on a flexed knee, or a violent twisting motion during an athletic activity.[3] The hyperflexed knee results in relaxation of the biceps femoris tendon and the lateral collateral ligament, and the violent twisting of the body creates a torque that pushes the fibular head laterally to the edge of the lateral tibial metaphysis.[1,2] The forced plantar flexion and ankle inversion forces the laterally displaced fibular head anteriorly.[1]

Clinical Presentation

The early recognition of instability in the proximal tibiofibular joint is necessary to optimize management of the injury and to avoid potential misdiagnosis. Early diagnosis of this injury can prevent further injuries to the joint that are harder to treat, such as chronic or fixed subluxation. Many common injuries can cause the same symptoms as proximal tibiofibular dislocation; therefore the integrity of the surrounding ligamentous

structures should be investigated before a diagnosis is made. Proximal tibiofibular dislocation is commonly missed initially when high-energy trauma results in other traumatic fractures as well, such as injury to the tibial plateau or shaft, injury to the ipsilateral femoral head or shaft, ankle fracture, or knee dislocation.[1,2]

Atraumatic dislocation of the proximal tibiofibular joint is easily misdiagnosed when there is no clinical suspicion of the injury, owing to its association with a wide range of symptoms that mirror many common knee injuries. Patients with subluxation of the proximal tibiofibular joint commonly report pain over the joint that is aggravated by direct pressure over the fibular head. Flexing the knee to 90 degrees to relax the lateral collateral ligament and biceps femoris tendon, then moving the fibular head anteriorly and posteriorly, can test instability of the joint. Although many patients do not note symptoms during daily activities, symptoms may develop during activities that require sudden changes in direction. Patients often report symptoms such as knee instability and giving way during these activities, as well as clicking and popping during daily activities.[3]

Traumatic dislocations commonly cause pain along the lateral knee that radiates into the region of the iliotibial band and the patellofemoral joint and is increased with palpation of the prominent fibular head and ankle motion.[4] The patient's pain commonly limits the range of motion, especially knee extension, and motion of the ankle; the patient's ability to bear weight on the affected leg is also limited by pain. It is common for patients to also have transient peroneal nerve injuries, especially with posteromedial dislocation.[1,2]

Physical Examination Techniques

Suspicion of atraumatic injury to the proximal tibiofibular joint warrants extensive inspection during the physical examination of the knee. Most patient histories do not reveal any mechanism of injury to the proximal tibiofibular joint, and symptoms of lateral knee pain can be very misleading. The examination of patients with atraumatic subluxation or chronic instability should be performed with the knee flexed to 90 degrees. The proximal tibiofibular joint should be palpated for tenderness, and laxity should be evaluated by translating the fibular head anteriorly and posteriorly with the thumb and index finger and asking the patient if the symptoms are reproduced or if there is any apprehension.[4] The stability of the proximal tibiofibular joint is typically increased by full extension of the knee; if it is not, the lateral collateral ligament and posterolateral structures may also be injured.

During significant trauma, traumatic dislocations of the tibiofibular joint are commonly missed, so the physical examination of this joint is a significant part of the comprehensive knee examination. The integrity of the ankle and functional status of the peroneal nerve should also be assessed during the physical examination, because of the association of nerve, syndesmotic ligament, and interosseous membrane damage with this injury. The relative avascularity of the area of the proximal tibiofibular joint prevents the presentation of knee effusion with an isolated injury, but there may be a prominent lateral mass.[1] Anterolateral dislocations often manifest with severe pain near the proximal tibiofibular joint and along the stretched biceps femoris tendon, which may appear to be a tense, curved cord.[1] Dorsiflexing and everting the foot, as well as extending the knee, emphasize pain at the proximal tibiofibular joint. The diagnosis of joint instability can be confirmed by steroid and local anesthetic injection into the joint under fluoroscopic guidance, if pain is relieved.

Imaging Techniques

The integrity of the proximal tibiofibular joint is best visualized through plain radiographs. Plain radiographs should be taken from anteroposterior, lateral, and oblique (45 to 60 degrees internal rotation of the knee) views, with comparison views from the contralateral knee, or from the preinjury knee if possible.[5] When a diagnosis is suspected but not clearly established by plain radiographs, axial computed tomography has been found to be the most accurate imaging modality for detection of injury of the proximal tibiofibular joint.[6] Magnetic resonance imaging (MRI) can also confirm a diagnosis of recent dislocation, based on the presence of pericapsular edema of the joint and edema of the soleus at its fibular origin of the popliteus muscle, but this finding is often absent in chronic and atraumatic cases.[7]

Indication and Contraindications

In many patients with proximal tibiofibular instability, the ability to perform daily tasks is reduced, especially sports activities that require quick changes in direction. The goal of instability correction is to restore patients to normal function through nonsurgical methods, such as closed reduction or physical therapy. Symptomatic atraumatic subluxation of the proximal tibiofibular joint can commonly be treated with nonsurgical treatment. Pediatric patients with atraumatic subluxation can have generalized ligamentous laxity and self-limiting symptoms that normally resolve with skeletal maturity. Traumatic joint dislocation should be treated by closed reduction. When surgical intervention is necessary for patients without arthritis, joint and ligament reconstruction should be performed to preserve the

anatomy and rotation of the joint. Patients with arthritis pain in the proximal tibiofibular joint should undergo an arthrodesis procedure to alleviate the joint pain that a ligament stabilization procedure will not correct.

Before undergoing surgery, patients with atraumatic proximal tibiofibular instability should be cautioned regarding the risk of recurrence. Patients who have sustained a traumatic dislocation of the proximal tibiofibular joint and who have not undergone nonsurgical physical therapy or closed reduction procedures to attempt to correct the instability and reduce pain should not participate in surgical intervention. Also, patients who are unwilling or unable to comply with the postoperative rehabilitation regimen should not undergo surgical management.

NONSURGICAL TREATMENT

Symptomatic atraumatic subluxation of the proximal tibiofibular joint can often be treated successfully through nonsurgical management. Patients with substantial pain should be immobilized in a cylinder cast for 2 to 3 weeks to help to reduce symptoms.[1,2] If instability symptoms continue, lower hamstring and gastrocnemius muscle strengthening can be combined with a supportive 1-cm strap to lessen symptoms. The strap should be placed below the fibular head and worn only as needed during activities that produce symptoms, to prevent peroneal palsy. It is also important to modify activities to avoid knee hyperflexion during the nonsurgical management of instability. Joint pain can also be relieved by a fluoroscopically guided injection of local anesthetic and steroid into the joint capsule.

Traumatic proximal tibiofibular dislocation should first be treated through a closed reduction procedure under local anesthesia or intravenous sedation.[3] Closed reduction should be performed with the knee in 80 to 110 degrees of flexion, and by applying pressure to the fibular head in the posteromedial direction. Reduction may fail if the fibular head is wedged on the lateral tibial ridge by the lateral collateral ligament. After reduction, an audible pop may be heard; the lateral collateral ligament and poster lateral structures should be examined for stability. Reductions are normally stable if there were no concomitant ligamentous injuries. Many other authors recommend soft dressing without immobilization, and crutch-assisted weight bearing progressing to full weight bearing over 6 weeks.[8] Ogden's study showed that 57% of patients who were immobilized after closed reduction later required surgical intervention for continuing symptoms.[2]

SURGICAL TECHNIQUE

Box 92-1 outlines the specific steps of this procedure.

Reconstruction
Dissection and protection of peroneal nerve
Creation of allograft tunnel
Allograft preparation
Allograft insertion and fixation
Incision closure

Arthrodesis
Dissection and protection of peroneal nerve
Joint preparation
Tibial autograft harvest
Fibular resection
Autograft preparation and insertion
Incision closure

Anesthesia and Examination

The procedure can be performed with the patient under general endotracheal anesthesia. The patient is placed in a supine position on the operating table, and all of the bony prominences are well padded. A tourniquet is placed thigh high on the operative leg, and the lower extremity is prepared and draped in usual sterile fashion. The instability of the joint should be assessed and compared with the stability of the contralateral joint, with the patient under anesthesia, by flexion of the knee to 90 degrees and manipulation of the fibular head posteriorly and anteriorly.

Landmarks and Incision

The anatomic landmarks, including the Gerdy tubercle, the fibular head, and the border of the biceps femoris, are demarcated with a marking pen. After preparation, the incision is demarcated in a curvy linear configuration along the border of the biceps femoris and around the joint line, as well as the fibular head (Fig. 92-1A). The planned incision site is injected with a mixture of 0.25% bupivacaine (Marcaine) and epinephrine. The incision is made with a No. 10 blade along the planned incision demarcation, and the skin and subcutaneous tissue are divided down to the fascia level through a combination of sharp dissection and electrocautery (Fig. 92-1B).

Peroneal Nerve Dissection (Fig. 92-1C)

Dissection and protection of the peroneal nerve should be performed in all patients to protect the nerve, as well as to relieve symptoms that are present in many patients. Identify the peroneal nerve as it courses around the posterior aspect of the fibular head, and perform a neurolysis out around the fibular neck. The nerve should be freed proximally and distally until the nerve dangles free posteriorly away from the intended area of work and marked with a small vessel loop. Dissect the knee between the biceps femoris tendon and the peroneal nerve, identifying the posterior portion of the fibula, and dissect the lateral head of the gastrocnemius off the tibia to expose the posterior portion of the tibia.

Reconstruction

Allograft Tunnel Creation (Fig. 92-1D)

- A Henning retractor should be placed in the interval between the lateral head of the gastrocnemius, the biceps femoris tendon, the peroneal nerve, and the posterior capsule of the knee to protect the posterior structures of the knee.
- A guide pin is drilled in an anterior-to-posterior direction through the fibular head in the anatomic insertion sites over the anterior and posterior tibiofibular ligaments.
- The guide pin should be overdrilled with a 6-cm reamer, and a Hewson suture passer is used to place a passing suture through the tunnel.
- With use of an anterior cruciate ligament (ACL) guide, the second guide pin is drilled from anterior to posterior through the tibia directly inferior to the Gerdy tubercle, with the posterior structures protected.

Allograft Preparation (Fig. 92-1E)

- The tibialis anterior allograft or autograft (usually semitendinosus) is thawed in antibiotic solution, the ends are whipstitched with a No. 2 nonabsorbable braided suture, and the graft is trimmed to fit a 6-mm passer tunnel.

Allograft Insertion and Fixation (Fig. 92-1F)

- The graft is pulled from anterior to posterior through the fibula and then in a posterior-to-anterior direction through the tibia.
- Right-angle forceps are used to create a tunnel underneath the anterior compartment musculature, and the graft is passed medially to laterally underneath muscle compartment.
- The appropriate length of the graft that creates the desired tension to form an anterior and posterior tibiofibular ligament is then determined.
- The whipstitched fiber wires are then tied together with multiple square knots under the anterior compartment with the fibula reduced.
- An additional No. 2 nonabsorbable braided suture is placed in a figure-of-eight through the anterior portion of the fibula, to pin the fibular head to the graft and stabilize it in the reduced position.
- The C-arm is then used to confirm that the positioning of the fibular head is anatomically correct.

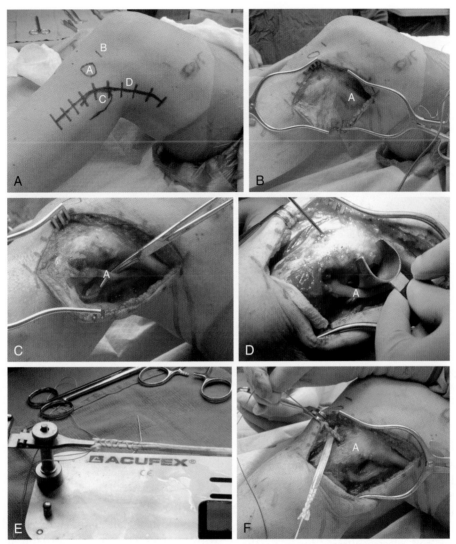

Figure 92-1. Proximal tibiofibular reconstruction (left knee). **A,** Demarcation of Gerdy tubercle *(A)*, the joint line *(B)*, the fibular head *(C)*, and the incision *(D)* in a curvy linear pattern. **B,** Dissection down to level of fascia of the biceps femoris *(A)* by sharp dissection and electrocautery. **C,** Dissection and protection of the peroneal nerve *(A)*. **D,** Drilling of fibular head guide pin with protection of posterior knee vessel and peroneal nerve *(A)* by Henning retractor. **E,** Preparation of tibialis anterior allograft with No. 2 nonabsorbable braided whipstitch. **F,** Insertion and fixation of allograft through tibia and fibula head *(A)*.

Fusion

Arthrodesis correction of proximal tibiofibular instability should be performed only when patients have arthritis pain in the joint. This procedure predisposes the ankle joint to increased pain and instability by preventing rotation of the fibula, transferring rotational forces to the ankle. Resecting part of the fibula during the procedure can reduce this pain and instability.[9]

Joint Preparation (Fig. 92-2A)

- The peroneal nerve should be dissected and protected throughout the procedure with the technique described earlier.

- The joint is exposed, and osteotomes and curettes are used to denude the bone joint surfaces to bleeding subchondral bone.
- Use a rongeur and make sure no cartilage is left in the joint, and confirm with the C-arm that the fibular head is in the correct anatomic position within the joint.

Autograft Harvest

- The cancellous autograft is harvested from the Gerdy tubercle by drilling a 5-mm hole in the tubercle, and autograft bone grafts are procured.
- The wound is then copiously irrigated and covered with a wet sponge.

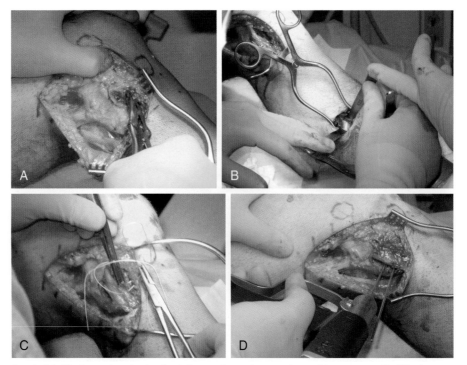

Figure 92-2. Proximal tibiofibular arthrodesis. **A,** Joint surface destruction with rongeur. **B,** Fibular resection at the junction of the proximal and middle third of the fibula. **C,** Periosteum closure over bone allografts. **D,** Drilling of guide pins for partially threaded cancellous screws.

Fibular Resection (Fig. 92-2B)

- The fibular resection is performed through a 4- to 5-cm longitudinal incision at the junction of the proximal and middle third of the fibula.[9]
- The subcutaneous tissue is then bluntly dissected down to the muscle fascia; the fascia is then split via blunt dissection and electrocautery down to the fibula that is isolated with Hohman retractors.
- To prevent reunion of the bone, 1 cm of the fibula is excised with a small oscillating saw and an osteotome, and the wound is copiously irrigated and covered with a wet sponge.

Autograft Preparation and Insertion

- The cancellous autograft obtained from the Gerdy tubercle is pulverized into little pieces with the fibulectomy piece so that it can be packed into the tibiofibular joint.
- The proximal tibiofibular joint is then filled with the pieces from the autografts, and the periosteum is closed over the joint to hold the grafts in place (Fig. 92-2C).
- The joint is stabilized with two cannulated 4.5-mm partially threaded cancellous screws that are placed, under direct C-arm visualization, through the fibular head into the tibia (Fig. 92-2D).
- The position of the proximal tibia in relation to the distal fibula is checked to verify that the distal fibula

has not been displaced and an acceptable position has been maintained.

Incision Closure

The periosteal soft tissues are closed over the screw, with interrupted No. 0 absorbable braided sutures, so that it will not come in contact with the peroneal nerve. A drain is placed in the incision, which is closed with interrupted No. 0 absorbable braided sutures, followed by 3-0 absorbable monofilament sutures in interrupted buried fashion and a running No. 4-0 absorbable monofilament suture. The wounds are sterilely dressed, and the knee is placed in a range-of-motion knee brace locked at full extension.

POSTOPERATIVE CONSIDERATIONS
Follow-up

- The patient may be kept overnight for pain management.
- The sutures are removed 6 to 8 days later.

Rehabilitation

- Knee should be kept in range-of-motion brace at all times for 6 weeks.

TABLE 92-1. Clinical Case Studies of Proximal Tibiofibular Instability Repair

Author	Procedure Performed	Follow-up	Outcome
Ogden[1] (1974)	Arthrodesis without fibular resection	2-17 years	100% complained of ankle pain and instability (N = 3)
Ogden[1] (1974)	Arthrodesis with fibular resection	1-7 years	100% free of symptoms (N = 4)
Ogden[2] (1974)	Fibular head resection	17 months	Patient was asymptomatic (N = 1)
Giachino[11] (1986)	Reconstruction with biceps femoris tendon	17-22 months	Both patients had no recurrent symptoms (N = 2)
van den Bekerom et al[12] (2004)	Fixation with a cancellous screw	3-6 months	Pain alleviated in 88%
Levy et al[13] (2006)	Temporary fixation with cannulated screw	8 months	Patient was pain free and returned to sports (N = 1)
Robinson et al[8] (2007)	Temporary tricortical screw fixation	1 year	Patient had full range of motion and no pain (N = 1)
MacGiobain et al[14] (2008)	Temporary Kirschner wire fixation	12 weeks	Patient returned to sports after 12 weeks (N = 1)
Horst and LaPrade[15] (2010)	Anatomic reconstruction with hamstring autograft	2 years	Both patients had improved IKDC and Cincinnati knee survey scores (N = 2)

IKDC, International Knee Documentation Committee.

- Patients need to be able to achieve full hyperextension symmetrical with contralateral knee by 4 weeks.
- The knee should only be flexed passively for the first 6 weeks.
- After 6 weeks, weight bearing can begin as tolerated with crutches.
- Full range of motion must be achieved by 3 months.
- Gait and range of motion should be normal by 5 months.
- Slow jogging and advanced strength training with weights can begin after 5 months.
- Patient can return to sports activities after 7 months when strength has returned, when patient can sprint and change direction without a limp, and when clinical examination findings are satisfactory.

Complications

- Damage to neurovascular structures resulting in peroneal nerve palsy
- Risk of reoperation
- Failure to resolve instability; recurrent or worsening instability
- Stiffness and loss of motion
- Need for hardware removal

RESULTS

Clinical studies of the proximal tibiofibular joint confirm that reconstruction or temporary fixation has better outcomes than arthrodesis procedures. Patients who undergo arthrodesis, or fibular head resection, may have symptoms because of damage to the epiphyseal plate of the proximal fibula, which can lead to unequal growth of the tibia and fibula in children.[10] Patients who have undergone an arthrodesis procedure may also experience chronic ankle joint pain and instability owing to the prevention of fibular rotation.[1,2] There are few long-term clinical studies of proximal tibiofibular joint instability because instability is uncommon and many diagnoses are missed. The details of clinical studies of proximal tibiofibular instability repair are presented in Table 92-1.

REFERENCES

1. Ogden, JA. Subluxation and dislocation of the proximal tibiofibular joint. *J Bone Joint Surg Am.* 1974;56(1): 145-154.
2. Ogden JA. Subluxation of the proximal tibiofibular joint. *Clin Orthop Relat Res.* 1974;(101):192-197.
3. Sekiya JK, Kuhn JE. Instability of the proximal tibiofibular joint. *J Am Acad Orthop Surg.* 2003;11(2): 120-128.
4. Sijbrandij S. Instability of the proximal tibio-fibular joint. *Acta Orthop Scand.* 1978;49(6):621-626.
5. Resnick D, Newell JD, Guerra Jr J, et al. Proximal tibiofibular joint: anatomic-pathologic-radiographic correlation. *AJR Am J Roentgenol.* 1978;131(1):133-138.
6. Keogh P, Masterson E, Murphy B, et al. The role of radiography and computed tomography in the diagnosis of acute dislocation of the proximal tibiofibular joint. *Br J Radiol.* 1993;66(782):108-111.

7. Axe MJ, Snyder-Mackler L. Proximal tibiofibular dislocation/sublaxation. *J Orthop Sports Phys Ther.* 2008;38(2):87.

8. Robinson Y, Reinke M, Heyde CE, et al. Traumatic proximal tibiofibular joint dislocation treated by open reduction and temporary fixation: a case report. *Knee Surg Sports Traumatol Arthrosc.* 2007;15(2):199-201.

9. Ebraheim NA, Elgafy H, Xu R. Bone-graft harvesting from iliac and fibular donor sites: techniques and complications. *J Am Acad Orthop Surg.* 2001;9(3):210-218.

10. Van Seymortier P, Ryckaert A, Verdonk P, et al. Traumatic proximal tibiofibular dislocation. *Am J Sports Med.* 2008;36(4):793-798.

11. Giachino AA. Recurrent dislocations of the proximal tibiofibular joint. Report of two cases. *J Bone Joint Surg Am.* 1986;68(7):1104-1106.

12. van den Bekerom MP, Weir A, van der Flier RE. Surgical stabilisation of the proximal tibiofibular joint using temporary fixation: a technical note. *Acta Orthop Belg.* 2004;70(6):604-608.

13. Levy BA, Vogt KJ, Herrera DA, et al. Maisonneuve fracture equivalent with proximal tibiofibular dislocation. A case report and literature review. *J Bone Joint Surg Am.* 2006;88(5):1111-1116.

14. MacGiobain S, Quinlan JF, O'Malley N, et al. Isolated proximal tibiofibular joint dislocation in an elite rugby union player. *Br J Sports Med.* 2008;42(4):306-307.

15. Horst PK, LaPrade RF. Anatomic reconstruction of chronic symptomatic anterolateral proximal tibiofibular joint instability. *Knee Surg Sports Traumatol Arthrosc.* 2010;18(11):1452-1455.

Index

Note: Pages numbers followed by letters *b* refer to boxed material, those followed by *f* refer to figures, and those followed by *t* refer to tables.